CHEMORADIATION: AN INTEGRATED APPROACH TO CANCER TREATMENT

CHEMORADIATION: AN INTEGRATED APPROACH TO CANCER TREATMENT

CHIEF EDITOR

Madhu J. John, M.D.
Clinical Associate Professor
University of California, San Francisco
Director, Radiation Oncology Services
Kaweah Delta Cancer Care Center
Visalia, California
The Cancer Center at St. Agnes
Fresno, California

ASSOCIATE EDITORS

Marshall S. Flam, M.D., F.A.C.P.
Clinical Associate Professor
Department of Medicine
University of California, San Francisco
The Cancer Center at St. Agnes
Fresno, California

Sewa S. Legha, M.D., F.A.C.P.
Professor, Department of Medicine
Department of Medical Oncology
University of Texas, M.D. Anderson Cancer Center
Houston, Texas

Theodore L. Phillips, M.D., F.A.C.R.
Professor and Chairman
Department of Radiation Oncology
University of California, San Francisco
San Francisco, California

Foreword by Vincent T. DeVita, Jr., M.D.

Lea & Febiger

PHILADELPHIA · BALTIMORE · HONG KONG
LONDON · MUNICH · SYDNEY · TOKYO

A WAVERLY COMPANY
1993

Lea & Febiger
Box 3024
200 Chester Field Parkway
Malvern, Pennsylvania 19355-9725
U.S.A.
(215) 251-2230

Executive Editor—Michael Brown
Manuscript Editor—Denise Wilson
Production Manager—Samuel A. Rondinelli

Publication Rights

R. Tagore

MacMillan and Co. Ltd.
St. Martin's Street, London, 1945

Library of Congress Cataloging-in-Publication Data

Chemoradiation : an integrated approach to cancer treatment / Madhu J.
John . . . [et al.].
p. cm.
Includes bibliographical references and index.
ISBN 0-8121-1482-5
1. Cancer—Adjuvant treatment. 2. Cancer—Chemotherapy.
3. Cancer—Radiotherapy. I. John, Madhu J.
[DNLM: 1. Combined Modality Therapy. 2. Neoplasms—radiotherapy.
QZ 269 C517]
RC271.A35C44 1993
616.99′406—dc20
DNLM/DLC
for Library of Congress 92-48953
CIP

NOTE: Although the author(s) and the publisher have taken reasonable steps to ensure the accuracy of the drug information included in this text before publication, drug information may change without notice and readers are advised to consult the manufacturer's packaging inserts before prescribing medications.

Reprints of chapters may be purchased from Lea & Febiger in quantities of 100 of more. Contact Sally Grande in the Sales Department.

PRINTED IN THE UNITED STATES OF AMERICA

Print number: 5 4 3 2 1

For Mummie and Babu
with much love—MJJ

and

For Shama, Laura, Kuldip, and Joan
with gratitude for their forbearance—MJJ, MSF, SSL, and TLP

In the meanwhile, the air is filling with the perfume of promise.

From: The "Gitanjali" (song offerings)
Rabindranath Tagore

FOREWORD

Is it appropriate today to have an entire text that focuses on the subject of using radiation therapy and chemotherapy together? Yes. First, there is increasing evidence that the combination works, often in common and difficult-to-treat tumors, such as lung, rectal, and head and neck cancers, and sometimes even in the real tough cancers like those that originate in the pancreas. While the clinical advantage in these tumors is sometimes marginal, the biologic observation that something is there to be gained is important and, unfortunately, has not been properly exploited. This text reviews the trials, tribulations, and recent results of some of these studies in the appropriate disease-oriented chapters.

Part of our problem in applying chemoradiation therapy, it must be admitted, is the way we grew up as specialists, each often seeing his part of the disease with little appreciation for the opposite number. Cancer, of course, has always been smarter than we are: it flourishes on piecemeal approaches to its attack. Thus, the old approach of surgery first, then radiation, then chemotherapy—each after the other has failed—was born on tradition, in the order of the birth of the specialties, not science. So were the schedules we use: five treatments a week for radiotherapy; chemotherapy on days one and eight, both conveniently falling during clinic times during the work week—but cancer also grows on weekends. These idiosyncrasies are the constraints imposed on clinical trials by the exigencies of practice, and the economics of medicine, that unfortunately take precedence over the design of scientifically-based clinical trials. So we find ourselves, almost 100 years after the introduction of radiotherapy, and 46 years after the introduction of chemotherapy, in the position of knowing we can do better using both modalities together but with a woeful lack of good information on how to do it. A good place to start is to collect all the best information in one place so it can serve as a nidus for future growth. By definition, that may be called a book and for that reason alone this text is a valuable addition to the field.

There is another, perhaps more important reason for a book focusing on this subject. We are beginning to understand the biology of cancer in ways we only dreamed of in the past. The unraveling of the signaling systems used by cells to communicate with each other, and the homology of the gene products of those systems, in many cases, with products of oncogenes and suppressor genes, has finally put the subject of the control of cell growth on a higher plane. Evidence is emerging that cancer, as we know it in the clinic, results from the accumulation of a series of damaging events to the genes that control these signaling systems. It seems highly plausible that in any given cancer population there is a heterogeneity of cells with different degrees of ability to respond to signals. The paradox of chemotherapy that cures the least differentiated tumors is probably best explained by the vulnerability created in these cells by their "inability to hear" and their resultant repeated entry into the cell cycle. Those that are better differentiated retain some capacity to behave in a normal fashion, but their presence may be the reason for drug failures, which may require radiotherapy or other means of attack. It is also likely that all malignant cells still have to be destroyed; this requires that we be able to describe the degree of this type of heterogeneity in tumor populations with newer molecular techniques. If we can, this will allow us to anticipate the need for the rational use of combined modality therapies, including the innovative use of chemotherapy with radiotherapy and biologicals.

As one who has often espoused the conviction that cancer is a systemic disease from the start, and thus systemic therapy needs to be initiated earlier, even as the initial therapy (primary or neoadjuvant chemotherapy), and more often, to control micrometastases, I also have to allow for the fact that new data suggest that events that control the propensity to metastasize may not occur simultaneously with events that determine malignancy, and thus there may be a therapeutic window during which efforts to control the primary will take precedence over concern for systemic disease. While this may be accomplished with greater ease with newer, more sophisticated radiotherapy techniques alone, it also may involve the use of chemotherapy with a slightly different intent. We are also beginning to see therapeutic attempts to attack the metastatic process itself which may allow us to freeze-frame metastatic deposits and approach them with methods of treatment that do not resemble those we have developed by habit and convention.

Finally, as one peruses the studies collected in this text one is often struck by the fact that, in the past, we have rarely combined therapies without making significant compromises. It does no good to control distant metastases if you can't control the primary, but in many cases, less attention has been given to improving the radiation part of the study design, and the longterm results suggest little progress, or reveal a weakness in the study and requires a new trial and another five years of work. This has recently been the case in studies of nonsmall-cell lung cancer, in which it was evident that systemic therapy can be effective in controlling distant metastases and even in prolonging survival if the study design allows the use of a workable model (i.e., Stage IIIA and B disease), but the practicality of the approach was compromised by the lack of control of the primary disease with radiotherapy. In drug-curable tumors, the addition of radiotherapy always looks good if the chemotherapy that is given is compromised, and it often is by the use of less effective drug combinations and arbitrary dose reductions, or omissions of drugs altogether, without testing the effect. This is true in many studies of Hodgkin's disease, and it has left us in the dark as to whether we should be using these therapies together routinely—many years after we have been certain that both modalities can cure Hodgkin's disease. In short, we need to do better at designing these kinds of trials.

In fairness, we have made considerable progress, when one considers that not too many years ago it was difficult to do these studies at all. Still, we can do better by facing the cancer cell on equal terms. The cancer cell doesn't specialize and we have to overcome the pressures of our specialization in order to take advantage of all the new biologic information and the many intriguing intimations of benefit from more intelligent use of chemotherapy and radiotherapy together. This text is a good place to start.

Vincent T. DeVita, Jr., M.D.
Benno C. Schmidt Chair in Clinical Oncology
Attending Physician and Member
Program of Molecular Pharmacology and Therapeutics
Memorial Sloan-Kettering Cancer Center
New York, New York

PREFACE

The last two decades have been notable for the gradual yet perceptible change in our thinking, our research, and the manner in which we approach the treatment of cancer. We have realized that a number of cancers, hitherto considered local diseases (breast cancer, for example), require a combination of local and systemic treatments for a successful outcome. Improvements in surgical techniques, refinements in megavoltage radiotherapy delivery, and the introduction of less toxic chemotherapeutic drug analogs, while certainly impacting treatment acceptability and morbidity, have not had a marked effect on the survival of cancer patients, particularly when modalities are viewed and used in isolation. Inasmuch as "multidisciplinary" and "multimodality" approaches to cancer management were the oncologic buzzwords of the 1970s and 1980s, oncologists of various disciplines continue to view each other with a certain suspicion and intransigence. This is a result of lack of knowledge of "other" modalities as much as it is due to a commitment to a particular discipline.

This book is an attempt to enjoin the local discipline of radiotherapy with the systemic modality of chemotherapy into the increasingly accepted science of chemoradiation. Although pediatric malignancies were the first to benefit from this liaison, several adult solid tumors and leukemias are now being treated successfully by combining the two disciplines. The combination of radiation with systemic agents in the treatment of cancer began almost simultaneously with the discovery of the x-ray. Part I of this book surveys the relatively brief and often erratic history of this combination. The term "chemoradiation" refers to the myriad ways in which all types of systemic agents are combined with radiotherapy. It therefore encompasses the use of protectors, antagonists, modifiers, and cytokines, in addition to the conventional chemotherapeutic agents, with various types and techniques of radiotherapy. It is not restricted to any particular manner of drug delivery and includes the oral, intramuscular, intravenous, and infusional administration of drugs with radiotherapy. It also includes the sequential, alternating, and concurrent use of radiotherapy and drugs. The theoretic rationale for these three ways of delivering chemoradiation are discussed separately in Part II. The specific interactions and interferences of various drugs with radiotherapy are also included. Part III details the clinical data available in the treatment of cancers of various sites. Part IV summarizes available data on the adverse effects related to the use of chemoradiation in various anatomical sites. Acute and longterm toxicity grading systems and some possible means of decreasing these toxicities are also included in Part IV. Part V includes a sampling of investigatory protocols being conducted by various research groups and one oncologist's insight into what chemoradiation might offer in the future.

This book offers a comprehensive outlook on the subject of chemoradiation: it reviews the clinical and toxicity data available to date, details the biologic and theoretic rationale for its use, and suggests some promising means of investigation for the future. We believe that the medical student and the oncologist, the general surgeon and the family practitioner, the radiobiologist and the theoretical scientist will all find something of use and/or interest to them. We hope that our excitement and passion about the subject is contagious so that more medical personnel will venture into it. Oncologically speaking, it can only make things better.

Fresno, California — Madhu J. John

ACKNOWLEDGMENTS

My interest in the subject of combining drugs and radiotherapy was initially provoked and then fostered through the years by Giulio D'Angio. I am sure there are several generations of oncologists who have benefited from his sense of history, his heartfelt passion in his work, and his ability to impart his enthusiasm and intelligence (in small portions at least). On their behalf, my thanks.

I am indebted to Carrie Randazzo, who transcribed every part of this book into the computer format, proofread every chapter several times, and displayed remarkable poise and fortitude in dealing with 64 busy authors and one occasionally difficult editor.

Gratitude is due to several staff members of Kaweah Delta District Hospital and the Kaweah Delta Cancer Care Center, in Visalia, California, who helped in various ways but mostly with their time. I would especially like to mention Jeannine Hinkel, our librarian, who helped on many occasions with computer searches and references with little notice.

Chapter 46, a compendium of current research protocols using chemoradiation, was gleaned from material provided by Michael Friedman at the National Cancer Institute, Harry Bartelink of the Netherlands Cancer Institute, and my co-editor Theodore Phillips from the University of California, San Francisco. Nick Nair Inc. designed the graphic presentations of select protocols. The quietly elegant hard cover and the vivid contemporary imagery of the book jacket are the creations of Nanda Nair, M. Arch., Los Angeles.

This book was conceived five years ago. I am grateful to Lea & Febiger for their continued faith in the project through all this time. Special thanks are due to Kenneth Bussy, Michael Brown, Tanya Lazar, Denise Wilson, and Sam Rondinelli for their kindness in guiding this novice through the various phases of planning and production.

The authors involved in writing this book deserve our congratulations and thanks for their generosity in the considerable time spent on their difficult and often uncharted projects and for the quality and expertise that is evident in their work.

Above all, I wish to thank my co-editors Marshall Flam, Sewa Legha, and Theodore Phillips. Unquestionably, this book would not be here today without them. In addition to critically reviewing every chapter in this book, they have written several on subjects in which they have national and international reknown. Their reputations persuaded Lea & Febiger to embark on this project, and their considerable influence enabled us to assemble such a distinguished and literate group of authors.

M.J.J.

CONTRIBUTORS

Jaffer A. Ajani, M.D.
Assistant Professor
Department of Gastrointestinal Oncology
The University of Texas M.D. Anderson Cancer Center
Houston, Texas

Mohamed K. Ali, M.D., Ph.D.
Professor of Medicine
Chief, Cardiopulmonary Section
The University of Texas M.D. Anderson Cancer Center
Houston, Texas

David Bardenstein, M.D.
Assistant Professor of Ophthalmology and Pathology
Case Western Reverse University, School of Medicine
Director, Ocular Oncology Service
Director, Ocular Pathology Service
University Hospitals of Cleveland
Cleveland, Ohio

Kevin P. Barton, M.D.
Fellow, The University of Chicago
Pritzer School of Medicine
Chicago, Illinois

Jacob D. Bitran, M.D.
Clinical Professor of Medicine
University of Chicago
Lutheran General Hospital
Parkridge, Illinois

Karl G. Blume, M.D., F.A.C.P.
Professor of Medicine
Stanford University Medical Center
Department of Medicine
Bone Marrow Transplantation Program
Stanford, California

Nancy J. Bunin, M.D.
Assistant Professor of Pediatrics
University of Pennsylvania
School of Medicine
Staff Physician, Division of Oncology
The Children's Hospital of Philadelphia
Philadelphia, Pennsylvania

Stephen K. Carter, M.D.
President
Pharmaceutical Research and Development Division
Briston-Myers Squibb Company
Wallingford, Connecticut

Nelson J. Chao, M.D.
Assistant Professor of Medicine
Stanford University Medical Center
Department of Medicine
Assistant Director
Bone Marrow Transplantation Program
Stanford, California

Devron H. Char, M.D.
Director of Ocular Oncology
Professor of Ophthalmology, Radiation Oncology and the Francis I. Proctor Foundation
University of California, San Francisco
Department of Ophthalmology
San Francisco, California

C. Norman Coleman, M.D.
Professor and Chairman
Joint Center for Radiation Therapy
Harvard Medical School
Boston, Massachusetts

Robert L. Comis, M.D.
Vice President of Medical Science
Fox Chase Cancer Center
Philadelphia, Pennsylvania

Louis S. Constine III, M.D.
Associate Professor of Radiation Oncology and Pediatrics
University of Rochester Medical Center
Rochester, New York

John A. Cook, M.D.
Radiation Oncology Branch
National Cancer Institute
National Institutes of Health
Bethesda, Maryland

James D. Cox, M.D.
Professor of Radiotherapy
Vice President for Patient Care and Physician-in-Chief
University of Texas, M.D. Anderson Cancer Center
Houston, Texas

Giulio J. D'Angio, M.D.
Vice Chairman and Clinical Director
Department of Radiation Oncology
School of Medicine
Hospital of the University of Pennsylvania
Philadelphia, Pennsylvania

Marshall S. Flam, M.D., F.A.C.P.
Clinical Associate Professor
Department of Medicine
University of California, San Francisco
The Cancer Center at St. Agnes
Fresno, California

Stephen J. Forman, M.D.
Director, Department of Hematology and Bone Marrow Transplantation
Department of Medical Oncology/Hematology
City of Hope National Medical Center
Duarte, California

Michael A. Friedman, M.D.
Associate Director
Cancer Therapy Evaluation Program
Division of Cancer Treatment
National Cancer Institute
Bethesda, Maryland

Karen K. Fu, M.D., F.A.C.R.
Professor
Department of Radiation Oncology
University of California, San Francisco
San Francisco, California

James H. Goldie, M.D., F.R.C.P.C.
Head, Division of Medical Oncology
Cancer Control Agency of B.C.
Vancouver, British Columbia, Canada

Leonard L. Gunderson, M.D., M.S.
Chairman
Division of Radiation Oncology
Mayo Clinic
Rochester, Minnesota

J. Michael Hamilton, M.D.
Chief, Clinical Investigation Section
NCI—Navy Medical—Oncology Branch
Bethesda, Maryland

Terence S. Herman, M.D.
Chief of Radiation Oncology
Dana-Farber Cancer Institute
Associate Professor in Radiation Oncology
Harvard Medical School
Boston, Massachusetts

Harold A. Hopkins, Ph.D.
Associate Professor
Division of Radiobiology & Biophysics
University of Virginia Health Sciences Center
Charlottesville, Virginia

Richard T. Hoppe, M.D., F.A.C.R.
Professor
Department of Radiation Oncology
Stanford University Medical Center
Stanford, California

Sandra J. Horning, M.D.
Associate Professor of Medicine
Stanford University Medical Center
Division of Oncology
Stanford, California

Madhu J. John, M.D.
Clinical Associate Professor
University of California, San Francisco, CA
Director, Radiation Oncology Services
Kaweah Delta Cancer Care Center
Visalia, California
The Cancer Center at St. Agnes
Fresno, California

David H. Johnson, M.D.
Associate Professor of Medicine
Division of Oncology
Department of Medicine
Vanderbilt University
Nashville, Tennessee

A. Robert Kagan, M.D.
Chief
Department of Radiation Oncology
Kaiser Permanente Medical Center
Los Angeles, California

Robert F. Kallman, Ph.D.
Professor
Division of Radiobiology Research
Department of Radiation Oncology
Stanford University Medical Center
Stanford, California

Timothy J. Kinsella, M.S., M.D.
Professor and Chairman
Department of Human Oncology
University of Wisconsin Clinical Cancer Center
Madison, Wisconsin

Ritsuko Komaki, M.D.
Associate Professor of Radiotherapy
Department of Radiotherapy
The University of Texas M.D. Anderson Cancer Center
Houston, Texas

Sewa S. Legha, M.D.
Professor, Department of Medicine
Department of Medical Oncology
University of Texas, M.D. Anderson Cancer Center
Houston, Texas

Victor A. Levin, M.D.
Professor,
Bernard W. Biedenharn Chair in Cancer Research,
Department of Neuro-Oncology
The University of Texas M.D. Anderson Cancer Center
Houston, Texas

William B. Looney, M.D., Ph.D., D.Sc.
Professor & Director
Division of Radiobiology & Biophysics
University of Virginia Health Sciences Center
Charlottesville, Virginia

Robert A. Lustig, M.D.
Attending Radiation Therapist
Cooper Hospital
University Medical Center
Clinical Associate Professor
Robert Wood Johnson Medical School
Camden, New Jersey

Moshe H. Maor, M.D.
Professor
Department of Radiotherapy
The University of Texas M.D. Anderson Cancer Center
Houston, Texas

James A. Martenson, Jr., M.D.
Consultant
Division of Radiation Oncology
Mayo Clinic
Rochester, Minnesota

Marsha D. McNeese, M.D.
Associate Professor of Radiotherapy
Department of Radiotherapy
M.D. Anderson Cancer Center
Houston, Texas

Robert S. Miller, M.D.
Associate Professor
Department of Medical Oncology
University of California, Davis
Sacramento Center for Hematology and Medical Oncology
Sacramento, California

James B. Mitchell, Ph.D.
Deputy Chief
Radiation Oncology Branch
National Cancer Institute
National Institutes of Health
Bethesda, Maryland

David Murray, Ph.D.
Associate Professor
Department of Experimental Radiotherapy
The University of Texas M.D. Anderson Cancer Center
Houston, Texas

Anantha K. Murthy, M.D.
Associate Professor of Radiology
Department of Therapeutic Radiology
Rush Medical College
Rush-Presbyterian-St. Luke's Medical Center
Chicago, Illinois

Stacy R. Nerenstone, M.D.
Helen & Harry Gray Cancer Center
Hartford Hospital
Hartford, Connecticut

Theodore L. Phillips, M.D., F.A.C.P.
Professor and Chairman
Department of Radiation Oncology
University of California, San Francisco
San Francisco, California

Miljenko V. Pilepich, M.D.
Director
Department of Radiation Oncology
C. McAuley Health Center
Ann Arbor, Michigan

Tyvin A. Rich, M.D.
Associate Professor
Department of Clinical Radiotherapy
The University of Texas M.D. Anderson Cancer Center
Houston, Texas

Mack Roach III, M.D.
Assistant Professor
University of California, San Francisco
Department of Radiation Oncology
San Francisco, California

Regina Rochford, R.N., B.S.N., ONC.
Radiation Oncology Services
Kaweah Delta Cancer Care Center
Visalia, California

Rey Rodriguez, M.D.
PG-4 Resident in Radiation Oncology
Department of Human Oncology
University of Wisconsin-Madison
Madison, Wisconsin

Philip Rubin, M.D., F.A.C.R.
Professor
University of Rochester School of Medicine
Chairman, Department of Radiation Oncology
University of Rochester Medical Center
Rochester, New York

Anthony H. Russell, M.D.
Clinical Assistant Professor
Department of Gynecologic Oncology
University of California, Davis
Radiation Oncology Center
Sutter Memorial Hospital
Sacramento, California

Richard L. Schilsky, M.D.
Associate Professor of Medicine
The University of Chicago
Cancer Research Center
Chicago, Illinois

Sidney A. Scudder
Assistant Professor of Medicine
Division of Hematology/Oncology
University of California, Davis Medical Center
Sacramento, California

William U. Shipley, M.D.
Professor, Department of Radiation Medicine
Massachusetts General Hospital Cancer Center
Harvard Medical School
Boston, Massachusetts

Sol Silverman, M.D.
Chairman
Department of Oral Medicine
University of California, San Francisco
San Francisco, California

Stephen R. Smalley, M.D.
Associate Professor
Department of Radiation Oncology
University of Kansas Medical Center
Kansas City, Kansas

Philip J. Stella, M.D.
C. McAuley Health Center
Ypsilanti, Michigan

Samuel G. Taylor, M.D.
Associate Professor of Medicine
Section of Medical Oncology
Department of Internal Medicine
Rush Medical College
Rush-Presbyterian-St. Luke's Medical Center
Chicago, Illinois

Beverly A. Teicher, Ph.D.
Associate Professor of Pathology and Radiation Therapy
Dana-Farber Cancer Institute
Harvard Medical School
Boston, Massachusetts

Frank M. Torti, M.D.
Associate Professor of Medicine
Stanford University and Veterans Affairs Medical Center
Palo Alto, California

Andrew T. Turrisi, III, M.D.
Associate Professor
Department of Michigan Medical School
Ann Arbor, Michigan

Srinivasan Vijayakumar, M.D., DMRT
Assistant Professor of Radiation and Cellular Oncology
University of Chicago Medical Center
Chicago, Illinois

Everett E. Vokes, M.D.
Associate Professor of Medicine and Radiation and Cellular Oncology
University of Chicago Medical Center
Section of Hematology/Oncology
Chicago, Illinois

CONTENTS

Color Figures Appear Following Page 172.

Section C. MECHANISMS OF RESISTANCE TO CHEMORADIATION

Part III CLINICAL APPLICATIONS

Part IV TOXICITY

Section A. ORGAN-SPECIFIC TOXICITY

Section B. TOXICITY GRADING CRITERIA

Section C. POTENTIAL METHODS OF DECREASING CHEMORADIATION TOXICITY

Part V FUTURE TRENDS

Part I

INTRODUCTION

Chapter 1

HISTORICAL PERSPECTIVE

GIULIO J. D'ANGIO

Holmes and Schultz, in their review of the early years of x-ray treatment of cancer, recorded that x-radiation was first used by Grubbe to treat a woman with cancer of the breast. This occurred in Chicago on January 29, 1896, only one month after Roentgen's epochal report in a relatively obscure German publication on December 28, 1895 (1,2). The news of the innovation had spread so swiftly and so widely that the human mind rapidly grasped the implications and applications of the x-ray.

The following chapters of this history are not all happy ones, as the side effects of ionizing radiations soon became evident, but the ingenuity and perspicacity of the early workers continued. By March 1896, radiation dermatitis had been clearly established by E. Thomson, who performed experiments on his own skin (2). Deleterious effects on deeper tissues were documented in 1903 by Perthes, who conducted perhaps the first laboratory radiobiologic experiments. He showed that the growth of irradiated limbs of young chicks was stunted compared to their untreated counterparts (3). Almost from the beginning, the benefits of ionizing radiations were explored with an expanding awareness of the damage they caused in normal tissues, especially the immature or rapidly growing.

Burchenal has reviewed the much longer history of anticancer medication (4), which stretches back millennia and has progressed slowly until recent years. Many of the compounds used hundreds of years ago, albeit with limited if any efficacy, were based on metals. Burchenal points out the fact that platinum-containing preparations are now among the most active of those used for cancer therapy (5). In fact, colloidal lead was employed with irradiation in the 1920s and was believed to increase local radiotherapy (RT) effects (6,7). Many compounds have been enlisted in attempts to enhance radiation effects. In 1905, Billings started what is probably the first such trial. He reasoned that benzene could be combined with irradiation in treating leukemia because both are myelotoxins (8). Other substances used in the early years were detailed by Kligerman; they range in complexity from distilled water to halogenated pyrimidines (9–11).

Rationales for the use of chemicals with radiation varied. Stathmokinetic drugs such as colchicine were first believed to have anticancer activity; subsequent studies of the vinca alkaloids, also stathmokinetic, established vinblastine and vincristine as effective drugs. Attempts were made to exploit the ability of these drugs to "freeze" mitosis for radiotherapeutic purposes. There was hope that cells escaping from mitotic delay would be synchronized and, thus, more vulnerable to carefully timed RT. Experiments along these lines were abortive, however, because the cell cycles soon became asynchronous (12).

Professor J.S. Mitchell and colleagues pursued another rationale. They noted that synthetic vitamin K (menadiol sodium diphosphate, Synkayvite) blocked nucleic acid synthesis (13,14). Laboratory and clinical studies combining RT and Synkayvite followed, with some encouraging results. Benefits seemed highly dependent on precise timing of the two agents; perhaps for that reason, Synkayvite is no longer under active investigation. Purine and pyrimidine antagonist antimetabolites are not used as radiation enhancers but are often part of combined modality programs, especially in pediatrics. Halogenated pyrimidine analogs, however, are the objects of continued research. In the 1950s, Heidelberger and colleagues synthesized 5-fluorouracil (5-FU), the first antimitotic conceived and prepared specifically as a counterfeit molecule designed to confound normal nucleic acid synthesis (11). 5-FU was quickly used in clinical trials and in combination with radiation therapy for a variety of human cancers (9). It was found that local radiation reactions are enhanced, but cancer control rates were generally disappointing despite the promise and brilliance of the concept (15). However, 5-FU, combined with other agents, still has a role in treatment of selected cancer patients (16).

Following an analogous and elegant rationale, halogenated pyrimidines were synthesized by Djordjevic and Szybalski and studied by them and by Kaplan et al as radiation sensitizers (17,18). Despite supportive laboratory evidence, these compounds, iododeoxyuridine (IUdR), bromodeoxyuridine (BUdR), and their congeners, have not yet fulfilled their promise, although clinical trials are still under way (19,20).

Combination chemoradiation using antimetabolites was in vogue several years ago. One of the first formal trials was mounted by the Radiation Therapy Oncology Group (RTOG) for patients with head and neck cancers. Patients receiving combined therapy with methotrexate and RT developed more pronounced reactions, thus demonstrating an interaction, but no survival benefit could be demonstrated (21,22).

The antibiotic Actinomycin D (AMD) is widely used in pediatrics. During early clinical trials, AMD was found through serendipitous observations to interact with radiation therapy, as had been suggested by Schulte (23). These interactions are clinically significant for both normal tissues and certain childhood cancers. AMD given with radiation therapy enhances RT effects, as do some of the compounds previously discussed (24,25). AMD has an additional predictable effect that is seen in many patients: it can reactivate latent RT effects in previously irradiated normal tissues, the so-called "recall" or "flare" reaction, a phenomenon first reported in 1959 (24). These properties are shared by two other antibiotics with carcinolytic properties, the anthracyclines doxorubicin (Adriamycin/ADR) and daunomycin. AMD and ADR are used individually and together with RT in many pediatric protocols. The ability of these drugs to augment RT effects early during the RT course and to recall previous radiation related injury is well documented.

Enhanced early reactions and flares, separately or together, can increase the potential for normal tissue injury, which can occur even though the radiation dose per se might be well within tolerance limits (26). Understanding of these combined therapy adversities has had a profound influence on the RT employed in multimodal oncology regimens when radiation enhancing and reactivating drugs are used. Radiation oncologists have accepted the elimination of RT, or RT dose reductions in order to avoid injuries, while being secure in the demonstration that effective chemotherapeutic agents contribute to local control as well as to the ablation of distal micrometastases (26–29). The three national Wilms' tumor studies have succeeded in identifying prognostic subsets in this pediatric population, progressively fine-tuned components of multimodal therapies, and have offered a prototype for a systematic approach to oncologic research (27,28).

Other classes of active anticancer compounds, needed for both local and systemic control, are known to combine with RT to produce unexpected toxicities, albeit in less overt fashion. Examples include leukoencephalopathy after brain irradiation plus the antimetabolite methotrexate given systemically to leukemic children, more likely when RT precedes the drug, and the increased eighth-nerve damage after cranial-base RT plus cisplatinum used for brain tumors and certain parameningeal sarcomas (30,31).

This overview has been limited to RT combined with active anticancer agents. Mention must be made of combinations of RT and substances that are not carcinolytic. The list includes attempts to exploit the photosensitizing porphyrins, and the oxygen effect (e.g., hyperbaric oxygen) and efforts to widen the therapeutic ratio through radiosensitizers like misonidazole and radioprotectors such as WR-2721 (32–38). The lessons learned from combined chemoradiation effects, both good and bad, have been duplicated in chemotherapy experience. Multiple drugs are known to be better than single agents in controlling many diverse diseases while at the same time multiplying the toxic manifestations. An appreciation of these competing effects led Li et al (1956) and Ross et al (1965) to devise the first multiple-drug regimens for solid tumors employing agents with differing toxicities (39,40). Their reports of success in women with choriocarcinoma treated with regimens based on methotrexate and AMD were seminal and led to many effective multi-agent regimens, including mechlorethamine, Oncovin (vincristine), procarbazine, and prednisone (MOPP) in Hodgkin's disease (41). However, combinations of drugs that are toxic for specific organs, although by different mechanisms, can have devastating effects. For instance, the tubular nephrotoxicity of ifosfamide given to patients previously exposed to cisplatinum, with its predominantly glomerular injury, can lead to profound kidney damage (42).

This discussion has not mentioned any of the countless meritorious and relevant laboratory studies that will be covered in later chapters. The omission here was not to deny their importance but to emphasize that many of the signal observations have been those made in the clinic. Trial therapies certainly must be built on sound radiobiologic, pharmacologic, and pharmacokinetic bases. Nonetheless, it remains for the alert clinician to detect unexpected combined therapy responses, not only to protect patients from iatrogenic morbidities but to exploit combined treatment effects for possible clinical benefit.

REFERENCES

1. Roentgen WC. Ueber eine neue Art von Strahlen: Sitzungsberichte der Physikal-Medicine. Gesselschaft, Wuerzburg. 137:132, 1895.
2. Holmes GW, Schultz MD. Therapeutic Radiology. Philadelphia, Lea and Febiger, 1950.
3. Perthes G. Ueber den Einfluss der Roentgenstrahlen auf epithelial Gewebe insbensondere auf das Carcinom. Archiv Fuer Klinische Chirurgie 71:955, 1903.
4. Burchenal JH. The historical development of cancer chemotherapy. *In:* Clinical Chemotherapy. Kuemmerle HP, Berkarda B, Karrer K, Mathe G (Eds). New York, Thieme-Stratton, Inc., 1984, p. 3.
5. Rosenberg G, VanCamp L, Trosko JE, Mansour VH. Platinum compounds: A new class of potent antitumor agents. Nature 222:385, 1969.
6. Ullmann HJ. Combination of colloidal lead and irradiation in cancer therapy. JAMA 89:1218, 1927.
7. Wood FC. Effects of combined radiation and lead therapy. JAMA 89:1216, 1927.
8. Billings F. Discussion of paper by Dr. Francis Wood, Irradiation treatment of leukemia. Proceedings of the Association of American Physicians, 1922. JAMA 79:67, 1922.
9. Kligerman MM. The role of combination radiation and chemotherapy. Proceedings of the Conference on research on the radiotherapy of cancer. American Cancer Society, 1961, p. 147.
10. Sugiura K. Effect of injections of distilled water on growth of irradiated mouse sarcoma 180. Am J Roentgenol 43:533, 1940.
11. Heidelberger C, Chaudhari NK, Dannenberg P, et al. Fluorinated pyrimidines, new class of tumor-inhibitory compounds. Nature 179:663, 1957.
12. Cardinale A. Personal communication, February 1992.
13. Mitchell JS. Clinical assessment of tetrasodium 2-methyl-1:4-naphthohydroquinone diphosphate as radiosensitiser. *In:* British Empire Cancer Campaign; Thirty-First Annual Report Covering the Year 1953. London, England, British Empire Cancer Campaign, 1954, p. 245.
14. Mitchell JS. Laboratory studies and clinical radiotherapeutic trials of some chemical radiosensitizers. Acta Radiol Suppl 116:431, 1954.
15. Vermund H, Gollin FF, Ansfield FJ. Clinical studies of 5-fluorouracil as adjuvant of radiotherapy. Front Radiat Ther Oncol 4:132, 1969.
16. Moertel CG, Fleming TR, Macdonald JS, et al. Levamisole and fluorouracil for adjuvant therapy of resected colon carcinoma. N Engl J Med 322:352, 1990.
17. Djordjevic B, Szybalski W. Genetics of human cell lines, III. Incorporation of 5-bromodeoxyuridine and 5-iododeoxyuridine into the deoxyribonucleic acid of human cells and its effect upon radiation sensitivity. J Exp Med 112:509, 1960.
18. Kaplan HS, Smith KC, Tomlin PA. Effect of halogenated pyrimidines on radiosensitivity of E. coli. Radiat Res 16:98, 1962.
19. Berry JR. Radiotherapy plus chemotherapy: Have we gained anything by combining them in the treatment of human cancer? Front Radiat Ther Oncol 4:1, 1969.
20. Speth PA. Iododeoxyuridine (IUdR) incorporation into DNA of human hematopoietic cells, normal liver and hepatic metastases in man: As a radiosensitizer and as a marker for cell kinetic studies. Int J Radiat Oncol Biol Phys 16:1247, 1989.

21. Kramer S. Use of methotrexate and radiation therapy for advanced cancer of the head and neck. Front Radiat Ther Oncol 4:116, 1969.
22. Kramer S. Methotrexate and radiation therapy in the treatment of advanced squamous cell carcinoma of the oral cavity, oropharynx, supraglottic larynx and hypophyarnx (Preliminary report of a controlled clinical trial of the Radiation Therapy Oncology Group). Can J Otolaryng 4(2):213, 1975.
23. Schulte G. Erfahrungen mit neunen cytostatischen Mittein bei Haemoblastosen und Carcinomen und die Abgrenzung ihrer Wirkungen gegen Roentgentherapie. Z Krebsforsch 58:400, 1952.
24. D'Angio GJ, Farber S, Maddock CL. Potentiation of x-ray effects by actinomycin-D. Radiology 73:175, 1959.
25. D'Angio GJ. Clinical and biologic studies of actinomycin-D and roentgen irradiation. Am J Roentgenol 87:106, 1962.
26. Tefft M, Lattin PB, Jereb B, et al. Acute and late effects on normal tissues following combined chemo-radiotherapy for childhood rhabdomyosarcoma and Ewing's sarcoma. Cancer 137(Suppl):1201, 1976.
27. D'Angio GJ, Evans A, Breslow N, et al. The treatment of Wilms' tumor: Results of the Second National Wilms' Tumor Study. Cancer 47:2302, 1981.
28. D'Angio GJ, Breslow N, Beckwith JB, et al. Treatment of Wilms' Tumor Results of the Third National Wilms' Tumor Study. Cancer 64:349, 1989.
29. Maurer HM. The Intergroup Rhabdomyosarcoma Study: Update–November 1978. NCI Monogr 56:61, 1981.
30. Price RA, Jamieson PA. The central nervous system in childhood leukemia. II. Subacute leukoencephalopathy. Cancer 35:306, 1975.
31. Packer RJ, Meadows AT, Rorke B, et al. Long-term sequelae of cancer treatment on the central nervous system in childhood. Med Pediatr Oncol 15(5):241, 1987.
32. Loken MK. Porphyrins as modifiers of effects of roentgen rays. Radiology 69:201, 1957.
33. Thomlinson RH, Gray LH. The histological structure of some human lung cancers and the possible implications for radiotherapy. Br J Cancer 9:539, 1955.
34. Churchill-Davidson I. The oxygen effect in radiotherapy–historical review. *In:* Frontiers of Radiation Therapy and Oncology. Meyer J and Vaeth SM (Eds). San Francisco, Karger, 1968.
35. Urtasun RC, Chapman JD, Brand P. Phase I study of high-dose metronidazole: A specific in vivo and in vitro radiosensitizer of hypoxic cells. Radiology 117:129, 1975.
36. Urtasun RC, Coleman CN, Wasserman TH. Keynote address: Clinical trials with hypoxic cell sensitizers: Time to retrench or time to push forward? Int J Radiat Oncol Biol Phys 10:1691, 1984.
37. Yuhas JM, Storer JB. Differential chemoprotection of normal and malignant tissues. J Natl Cancer Inst 42:331, 1969.
38. Kligerman MM, Turrisi AT, Urtasan RC, et al. Final report on Phase I trial WR-2721 before protracted fractionated radiation therapy. Int J Radiat Oncol Biol Phys 14:1119, 1988.
39. Li MC, Hertz R, Spencer DB. Effect of methotrexate therapy upon choriocarcinoma and chorioadenoma. Proc Soc Exp Biol Med 93:361, 1956.
40. Ross GT, Goldstein DP, Hertz R, et al. Sequential use of methotrexate and actinomycin D in the treatment of metastatic choriocarcinoma and related trophoblastic disease in women. Am J Obstet Gynecol 93:223, 1965.
41. DeVita VT Jr, Simon RM, Hubbard SM, et al. Curability of advanced Hodgkin's disease with chemotherapy: Long-term follow-up of MOPP-treated patients at the National Cancer Institute. Ann Int Med 92:587, 1980.
42. Goren MP, Pratt CB, Meyer WH, et al. Mesna excretion and ifosfamide nephrotoxicity in children. Cancer Res 49:7153, 1989.

Part II

BIOLOGY OF CHEMORADIATION

Section A

THEORETICAL CONSIDERATIONS

Chapter 2

TERMINOLOGY FOR CHEMORADIATION EFFECTS

THEODORE L. PHILLIPS

INTRODUCTION

Combinations of chemotherapy and radiotherapy have been used in cancer management for over 25 years. Early in the development of the combined modalities, empirical regimens were employed, but more recently two principal objectives have emerged. The first objective is to increase local–regional control through the interaction of the two cytotoxic modalities. The second is to improve survival through the reduction of failure due to distant metastases by means of the action of the drugs on sites that are not irradiated. The intended denouement is, of course, to improve survival through reduction of both local failure and distant metastasis.

Possible reasons for combining radiation therapy and chemotherapy can be based on a number of effects. When chemotherapy is used in conjunction with radiation therapy, it may sterilize micrometastases outside the radiation field or it may increase the response of tumor cells to radiation through various mechanisms. These mechanisms include inhibiting repair of sublethal or potentially lethal radiation damage and conferring some degree of additivity of cytotoxicity in the radiation target volume (1).

Since hypoxic tumor cells are generally resistant to radiation, reduction of the tumor mass by chemotherapy may improve the blood supply and lead to reoxygenation, thereby increasing radiation tumor-cell kill. Cell kinetics may be perturbed by chemotherapy, which would be beneficial if radiation is delivered during a more sensitive cycle phase or detrimental if increased proliferation follows an approach such as neoadjuvant chemotherapy. Reduction of proliferation during radiotherapy by a chemotherapeutic agent would be beneficial.

Radiation therapy could improve the response to chemotherapy by decreasing the tumor mass, which would lead to improved blood supply and drug delivery. Radiation may also induce increased cell proliferation and enhanced sensitivity for cell cycle active agents. However, when administered during the time of drug damage repair, radiation therapy may inhibit the repair of drug-damaged cells.

Because of the complexity of the interaction between the two modalities, which can be seen from the brief discussion above, a clear definition of terminology is essential. In the past, such loose terms as "sensitization" or "synergism" have been used to describe situations in which an apparent improvement in response occurred. Such oversimplification should be avoided, and more specific terminology appropriate to the actual type of drug–radiation interaction should be employed.

The remainder of this chapter will discuss the techniques for comparing tumor and normal tissue response and the proper terminology for describing such comparisons. It will cover the types of interactions that may occur between drugs and radiation, citing specific terminology for these reactions, and will then discuss specific terminology for effects that occur within the target volume for radiotherapy. Finally, a presentation of the analysis of interaction isobolograms will be provided.

PARAMETERS OF TUMOR RESPONSE

In considering the interaction of radiation and chemotherapy in a chemoradiation approach to tumor treatment, one must individually analyze the concepts of tumor response and tumor control as well as the concepts of toxicity and maximum tolerated tissue injury before determining whether the result is an improved therapeutic effect. It is important to keep in mind the types of responses that occur within tumor and normal tissue and the possible alterations in these responses by the interaction of radiation and chemotherapy (2).

It is common to measure tumor response by the percent of reduction in tumor area or volume that may occur after treatment. This approach is used particularly in the chemotherapy literature. It must be realized that this approach is very inaccurate in terms of comparing one regimen to another and particularly in comparing single versus combined modality treatments. **Tumor size reduction** is a complex interaction between inhibition of proliferation, tumor cell death and loss, and tumor proliferation. It is possible that an increase in clonogenic cells has occurred although, for instance, an apparent partial response (greater than 50% reduction in volume) is manifest. Thus, comparison of tumor response data for two different modalities, for example comparing a combined modality approach to a single modality, can lead to inaccurate conclusions.

More accurate measurements are those of **tumor regrowth delay** and tumor control or complete clinical eradication of tumor for a defined time period. Regrowth delay, the time it takes a tumor to shrink and regrow to either the original volume or a volume 2 to 4 times greater than the original, correlates well with cell kill. Thus, in animal systems, regrowth delay is applicable where direct cell survival measurements are not possible (3). **Tumor cure,** often expressed as a 50% tumor control probability in animal systems, correlates well with eradication of all clonogenic tumor cells in 50% of the population. Therefore, in assessing tumor response, it is preferable to use the endpoints of regrowth delay or a fixed level of tumor control probability (4).

PARAMETERS OF TOXICITY

The term **toxicity** may be used to cover all forms of detrimental reactions experienced by the patient or by an experimental animal. Because this may occur in many organ systems, the overall term "toxicity" is difficult to quantify. Tissue-specific toxicities, on the other hand, may be clearly quantifiable and traced to an injury to a single or a limited number of cell populations within the target organ (5). Thus, the term toxicity should always be defined in terms of response of a specific organ system (6). Ideally, this response should be described by a dose-response relationship, which can be quantified, or by endpoints that are suited for analysis by calculations of the probability of a 50% response (7). In clinical practice, this is often not possible. Grading systems, which are as linear as possible, can be utilized to compare toxicities for specific organs.

In most clinical situations, there is a maximum tolerable level of toxicity in each organ, which is compatible with a worthwhile quality of life following a specific treatment course. These interactions are expressed graphically in Figure 2–1. It can be seen that tumor control probability increases with increasing dose, as does toxicity. When a maximum tolerated level of toxicity is reached, the dose cannot be clinically exceeded, and this limits tumor control probability.

QUANTIFICATION OF TUMOR AND NORMAL TISSUE EFFECTS

Since the nature of the interaction between radiation and chemotherapy in terms of less than or greater than additive effects is generally unknown (see below), it is necessary to derive a term that will be usable for all observed reactions. The term **dose-effect factor** (DEF) has been coined to define the observed effects of combined radiation and chemotherapy. The dose-effect factor is defined as follows: $DEF = RDE/RDE_D$, where RDE = the radiation dose required to achieve an effect without the presence of the drug and RDE_D = the radiation dose required to achieve the same effect in the presence of the chemotherapy treatment. If the dose-effect factor can be determined for

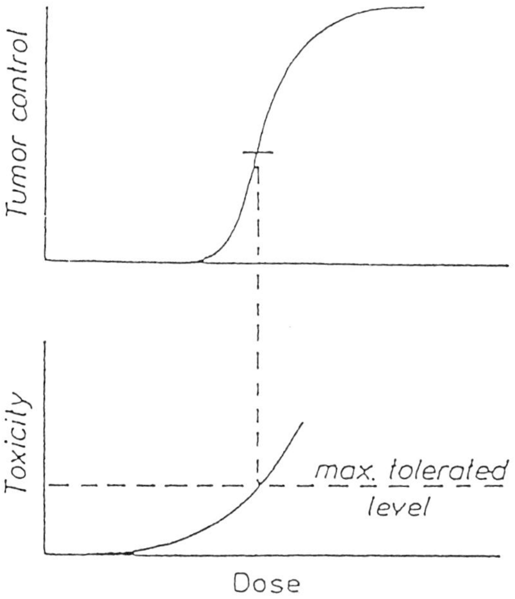

Fig. 2–1. The maximum level of tumor control that can be achieved with a given form of therapy depends on the dose level that produces a maximum tolerable level of toxicity and upon the shape of the dose-response curve for tumor control. (From Steel GG, Peckham MJ. Int J Radiat Oncol Biol Phys 5:85, 1979. Copyright 1979, Pergamon Press Ltd.)

both the tumor and the normal tissue, then a second value, the **therapeutic ratio,** can be derived (1).

Various terms have been used to describe improvements in treatment. Nonquantitative phrases such as "improved therapeutic result," "clinical benefit," or "synergistic response" have been used. However, these terms may not truly represent an improvement in the therapeutic ratio, which requires that the increased effect seen in the tumor is greater than that seen in the relevant and critical normal tissue included in the radiation target column. It is possible to use dose-effect factors derived for pertinent tumor and normal tissue to calculate the therapeutic ratio. The therapeutic ratio (TR) is defined as follows: $TR = DEF_T/DEF_{NT}$, where DEF_T and DEF_{NT} are the dose-effect factors for tumor and normal tissues, respectively. When the therapeutic ratio calculated in this manner is greater than 1, then benefit has generally occurred.

GENERAL TYPES OF INTERACTION BETWEEN RADIATION AND CHEMOTHERAPY

Spatial Cooperation

The term **spatial cooperation,** which was originally described by Steel and Peckham (8), describes the situation in which the targets for radiation and for chemotherapy lie in different sites within the body. An example is that of the acute lymphocytic leukemia of childhood, in which combination chemotherapy is used to treat the generalized disease and particularly the bone marrow, intrathecal methotrexate is used to treat subclinical disease in the spinal axis, and radiation is used to treat deep-lying tumor cells within the brain. This is the most specific example of spatial cooperation. In most other situations, the drug has access to the organ and tumor being irradiated and may cause additional reactions within that target volume. It is reasonable to use this term to describe situations in which control of disease outside the radiation volume is achieved by chemotherapy.

As described by Steel and Peckham, when the strategy of spatial cooperation is employed, one should independently use the most effective chemotherapy and the most effective radiotherapy for the two different areas of disease in question. Often, the two modalities may be temporally separated in their administration. Constraints are imposed by the need for at least some degree of toxicity independence. If the use of the combination in an attempt to achieve spatial cooperation requires significant dose reduction of either agent, it may lead to less than the response achieved with a single agent. Although toxicity independence is ideal, it is not generally possible in combined chemotherapy and radiotherapy, with few exceptions; thus, one must deal with relative toxicity in normal tissue and tumor when determining whether a combined modality regimen is beneficial.

Enhancement

In any situation in which increased response occurs within the radiation target volume in the presence of a chemotherapeutic regimen, the term **enhancement** should be used. It is not possible to determine whether such enhancement is additive, supra-additive, or subadditive, as described below. Enhancement should be used to describe any increase in effect greater than that observed with either chemotherapy or radiotherapy alone. Enhancement of tumor response is highly desirable, but often enhancement of normal tissue response will also occur. To determine whether an advantageous situation exists, the dose-effect factors and therapeutic ratio calculations should be performed as described above.

Diminution

The term **diminution** can be used to describe a decrease in effectiveness when chemotherapy is combined with radiotherapy. The response observed is less than that observed with either modality alone and may include inhibition, antagonism, and protection. **Inhibition** can be defined as the situation in which the combined effect is less than that seen with the more active of the two agents alone. **Antagonism** occurs when the combined effect is less than that of the less active agent. The term **protection** is reserved for situations in which the effect of one agent is decreased by another agent which itself is inactive in causing the effect observed. This occurs with sulfhydryl radioprotectors, which themselves have no antitumor or normal tissue effects.

SPECIFIC TERMINOLOGY FOR EFFECTS WITHIN THE TARGET VOLUME

As discussed above, it is often difficult to define the exact type of interaction that occurs when looking in vivo in animal systems and particularly when looking at clinical data. Spatial cooperation does not come into play here. The following presents a number of other interactions pertinent to the primary tumor volume that should be emphasized.

Enhancement Effects

The enhancement effects that can be observed include additivity, supra-additivity, and subadditivity. **Additivity** occurs when the total response at the target volume is equal to the sum of responses expected from each of the two agents alone. Additivity can be quantitated easily if complete cell survival curves are available for the two modalities and if these cell survival curves are linear. The situation becomes much more complex, as discussed below under isobolograms, if the response curves are not linear and if such quantitative information is not available. The term **supra-additivity** is used to describe responses that exceed the possible range of additive responses, including corrections for nonlinearity of survival curves. This is a situation in which the response observed is greater than that which would be seen if two independent agents with linear dose-response curves were given and the cell kill from each added. Again, the complex definition of additivity must be employed and truly defined as supra-additivity. It is possible to apply the term "synergism" to situations of true supra-additivity, but supra-additivity is the preferred term. **Subadditivity** occurs when the response observed is less than that expected when the cell kill for each agent is combined, again using corrections for nonlinear survival curves to define such additivity.

Diminution Effects

Inhibition occurs when the combined effect of two agents, i.e., radiation and chemotherapy, is less than that seen with the more active agent alone in the specific tumor or normal tissue target. **Antagonism** occurs when the combined effect is less than the less active agent alone. The term protection should be reserved for situations in which the effect of one agent is decreased by another agent that is inactive for the effect under consideration. Examples of this are the use of WR-2721 to reduce the bone marrow toxicity of cyclophosphamide and renal toxicity of cisplatinum, as well as to reduce bone marrow and small intestinal toxicities by radiation.

ANALYSIS OF CHEMORADIATION INTERACTIONS BY ISOBOLOGRAM

Determination of additivity and other degrees of interaction is simple when the dose-response curves for radiation and chemotherapy are linear. This is, however, not generally the case, as can be seen in Figures 2–2

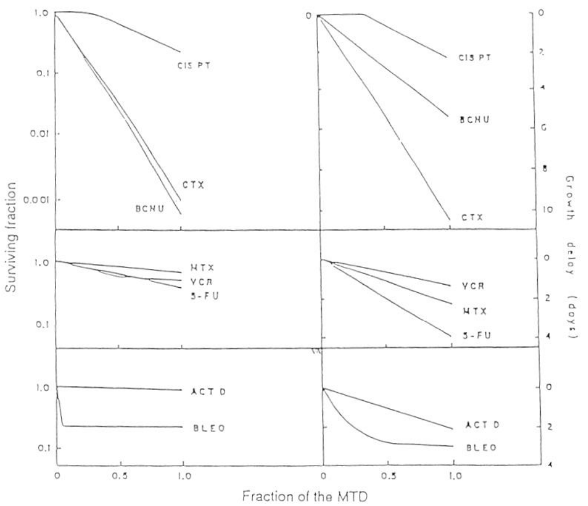

Fig. 2–2. Comparison of dose-response curves obtained in two assays. Left: in vivo/in vitro assay (log-linear plot). Right: growth delay assay (linear-linear plot) with delay increasing from top to bottom for comparison with survival data. Drugs are grouped approximately according to class, with alkylating agents at the top, antimetabolites in the middle, and others at the bottom. CIS PT: cisplatin; BCNU: carmustine; CTX: cyclophosphamide; MTX: methotrexate; VCR: vincristine; 5-FU: fluorouracil; ACT D: dactinomycin; BLEO: bleomycin; MTD: maximum tolerated dose. (From Begg AC, et al. Cancer Res 40(1):145, 1980.)

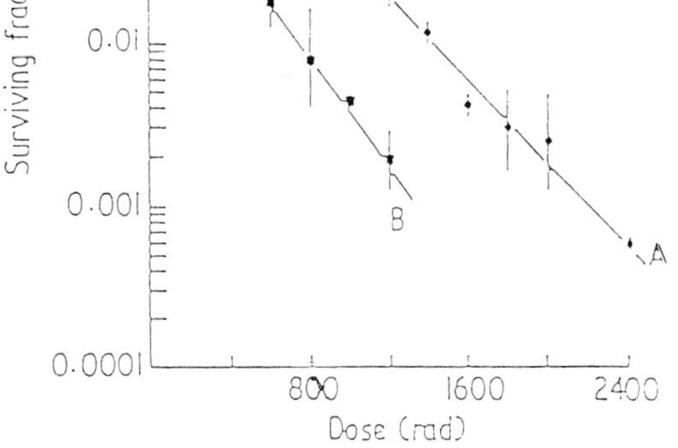

Fig. 2–3. In vivo dose-response curves of EMT6 tumors grown and irradiated as flank tumors (●) or lung nodules (■). Bars represent + *1* SE. (From Begg AC, et al. Cancer Res 40(1):145, 1980.)

and 2–3. Figure 2–2 demonstrates that the response to a variety of chemotherapy agents is extremely variable. In a few instances, such as with cyclophosphamide and carmustine (BCNU), it is linear, but for other drugs there is either a very shallow response, a biphasic response, or in some cases, little or no response. As shown in Figure 2–3, radiation dose-response curves for tumors in vivo are complex with initial shoulders, linear portions, and secondary resistant populations due to hypoxia and other factors. Thus, it is necessary to apply more complex analysis to determine whether greater than additive effects are observed (9).

If the dose-response curves are linear, as shown in curve A in the upper portion of Figure 2–4, the effects are truly additive. If the dose of agent A is plotted versus the dose of agent B to yield the same level of survival, it will result in a straight line that intersects the axes at the point of maximum doses of agent A or agent B.

Most dose-response curves are nonlinear and cannot be made so by any simple math-

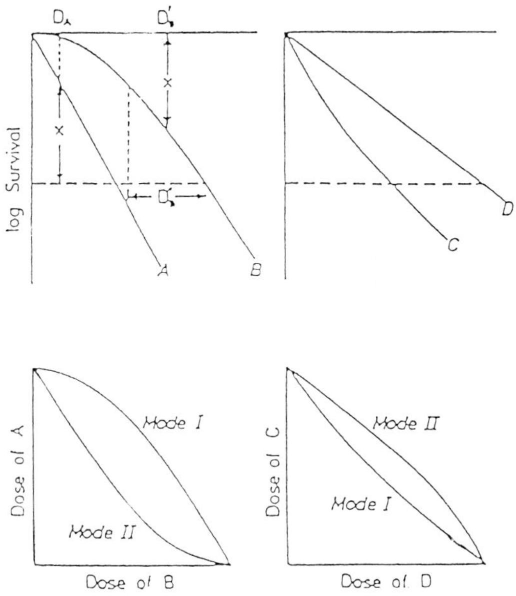

Fig. 2–4. Method of calculating envelope of additivity for two pairs of cytotoxic agents (A + B and C + D), where one of each pair has a nonlinear dose-response curve. (From Fu KK, et al. *In:* Cell Survival after Low Doses of Radiation. London Institute of Physics, 1975, p. 251, IOP Publishing Limited.)

ematical transformation. Thus, the question is, if the dose-response curves are not extremely far from linear, can we rule out an apparently large interactive effect as more or less additive? The various panels of Figure 2–4 illustrate the methods of calculating what Steel and Peckham have defined as the **envelope of additivity.** This is best understood by using the examples shown in Figure 2–4. If the dose of each agent that gives log survival values adds up to the level shown by the dotted line in the upper left panel, i.e., measuring from 100% survival down for each agent, one obtains the plots in the lower left panel labeled Mode I. Note that this addition has been performed by taking the dose increments starting from zero that give the log survivals adding up to level S, which is defined by the horizontal dotted line.

A second mode of calculation is possible, however. In this mode, one takes the dose increment that gives the required contribution to the total effect in any region of the dose-response curve, up to the limit S. The most extreme case will occur when this is measured in the steepest part of the survival curve. Note that for curves A and B, the Mode I line lies above the Mode II line in the isobologram in the lower left panel, and the intervening space is known as the envelope of additivity. Any responses within this volume can be considered as additive. In the upper right set of curves, the analysis for Mode I and Mode II injury leads to the opposite effect, with Mode II lying above Mode I because of the decreasing slope of curve C as compared to the increasing slope of curve B.

The reason for using Modes I and II is the fact that survival can be considered either to have been unaffected by the other treatment (i.e. Mode I) or that the other treatment has acted like an initial dose of the second treatment, yielding the Mode II type of analysis. A simple consideration of radiation survival curves with a shoulder reveals the validity of this approach. In the Mode I analysis, the shoulder would occur in both curves; in the Mode II analysis, the linear portion of both curves would be used and would be simply additive, creating a linear isobologram. Mode I calculation is inaccurate in this case, because it suggests that radiation is supra-additive with itself. Since it is unknown in many situations whether treatments are truly additive to themselves or are supra- or sub-additive, the only possible response is to calculate an envelope of additivity using both the Mode I and Mode II analysis.

TIMING OF ADMINISTRATION OF RADIATION AND CHEMOTHERAPY

Disparate timing schedules may be used to combine radiation and chemotherapy in the treatment of cancer. The time of administration has a major effect on cell killing in both normal tissues and tumors (see Table 2–1). Maximum drug kill relative to the time of radiation varies by as much as −18 to +48 hours in terms of the time of drug delivery. Thus, it is extremely important to define the sequence of administration and clearly evaluate the various sequences available to determine the most effective combination. Generally, timing of radiation and chemotherapy delivery may be divided into remote, sequential, simultaneous, and alternating.

Remote

Remote administration refers to the situation in which the drug and radiation are given at times separated sufficiently to eliminate interaction of cell kill by one agent on the cell kill by the other agent. This is an endpoint that is difficult to define: although the cellular interactions may disappear within 48 hours in terms of inhibition of repair and other molecular interactions, the interaction in terms of depopulation may last

Table 2–1. Times of Maximum and Minimum Cell Killing in Intestinal Crypt Cells

Drug	Maximum (h)	Minimum (h)
Bleomycin	−6	+48
Carmustine	−2	+24
Cisplatin	0	+2
Cyclophosphamide	−18	+18
Dactinomycin	−6	+48
Doxorubicin	+12	0
Fluorouracil	+24	+48
Mechlorethamine	−12	−48
Methotrexate	−12	+24
Vincristine	+48	−48

Note: Drug administration time is relative to radiation time.

for weeks or months. Clearly, the administration cannot be so remote that tumor regrowth will have achieved original or greater levels; however, it may be so remote as to allow normal tissue repair if this is more rapid than tumor repopulation. Remote administrations have been termed clinically as **adjuvant,** i.e., delivery of chemotherapy after the irradiation, and **neoadjuvant,** i.e., delivery of the chemotherapy regimen before the course of radiotherapy. Both of these remote approaches have been taken in order to minimize radiation toxicity. It should be noted, however, that both remote approaches minimize the chance for positive interaction within the tumor target volume.

Sequential

Sequential administration, defined as the close approximation of radiation and chemotherapy, is the next step above remote administration. A course of chemotherapy may be given and radiation begun one or a few days later or vice versa.

Simultaneous

Simultaneous schedules include delivery of chemotherapy during a course of radiation so that the drug is present during a significant number of radiation treatment fractions. Although this approach may maximize toxicity in normal tissues, it may also maximize tumor response as described above. If the enhancement of tumor response is greater than that of normal tissue, a beneficial reaction still occurs.

Alternating

A number of schedules have been derived that apply the alternating approach in which a chemotherapy regimen, either single or multi-agent, is alternated on a weekly or monthly basis or even more frequently with a shortened course of radiation. These regimens attempt to reduce toxicity to normal tissues and enhance tumor response by delivery of each agent when enhanced sensitivity to the other has been induced by the first agent. At least two cycles of each agent must be delivered for this to qualify as an alternating regimen, rather than a sequential or even a remote regimen.

SUMMARY

It can been seen from this discussion that the interaction of radiation and chemotherapy is quite complex. It is important to avoid such vague and general terms such as "synergism" and "sensitization" and to attempt to define the specific interactions that occur as additive, supra-additive, or subadditive. Determination of the dose-effect factor and the therapeutic ratio is useful in evaluating combined modality regimens. Finally, one must always keep in mind whether the goal is to achieve spatial cooperation or enhanced response in the local–regional irradiated volume.

REFERENCES

1. Fu KK, Phillips TL. Biological rationale of combined radiotherapy and chemotherapy. *In:* Hematology-Oncology Clinics of North America. Vokes EE (Ed). Philadelphia, WB Saunders, 1991, p. 737.
2. Phillips TL, Fu KK. The interaction of drug and radiation effects on normal tissues. Int J Radiat Oncol Biol Phys 4:59, 1978.
3. Begg AC, Fu KK, Kane LJ, Phillips TL. Single-agent chemotherapy of a solid murine tumor assayed by growth delay and cell survival. Cancer Res 40(1):145, 1980.
4. Fu KK, Phillips TL, Wharam MD, Kane LJ. The influence of growth and irradiation conditions on the radiation response of the EMT6 tumor. *In:* Cell Survival After Low Doses of Radiation. Alper T (Ed). London Institute of Physics, 1975, p. 251.
5. Luk KH, Ross GY, Phillips TL, Goldstein LS. The interaction of radiation and cis-diaminedichloroplatinum (II) in intestinal crypt cells. Int J Radiat Oncol Biol Phys 5(8):1417, 1979.
6. Phillips TL, Fu KK. Quantification of combined radiation therapy and chemotherapy effects on critical normal tissues. Cancer 37:1186, 1976.
7. Phillips TL, Ross GY, Goldstein LS, Begg AC. The interaction of radiation and bleomycin in intestinal crypt cells. Int J Radiat Oncol Biol Phys 5(9):1509, 1979.
8. Steel GG, Peckham MJ. Exploitable mechanisms in combined radiotherapy-chemotherapy: The concept of additivity. Int J Radiat Oncol Biol Phys 5:85, 1979.
9. Wharam MD, Phillips TL, Kane L, Utley JF. Response of a murine solid tumor to in vivo combined chemotherapy and irradiation. Radiology 109(2):451, 1973.

Chapter 3

NEOADJUVANT COMBINED MODALITY THERAPY

JAMES H. GOLDIE

INTRODUCTION

The term **adjuvant chemotherapy** was developed to encompass the use of systemic drug treatment as part of the management of localized malignancies known to be at high risk for systemic relapse. The term was initially used for circumstances in which surgery was the form of local–regional therapy; early use of adjuvant treatment was based on the hypothesis that surgical removal of a tumor was associated with increased risk of dissemination of metastatic disease. The induction of surgically induced metastases is not a major problem from the standpoint of systemic relapse; the problem is that micrometastases may have occurred long before definitive local–regional therapy. Under these circumstances, the role of adjuvant chemotherapy is to eliminate micrometastatic disease before it has reached the stage of overt clinical recurrence.

A variety of experimental animal models and early clinical trials support the concept that systemic chemotherapy may be more likely to affect cure if utilized when the overall tumor burden in the patient is low.

While most adjuvant chemotherapy programs are used in conjunction with surgery as the primary treatment modality, nothing precludes the use of chemotherapy in conjunction with radiation, if radiation is being employed as the means of local control. The following chapter reviews some of the biological processes that may be involved in determining the utility of adjuvant chemotherapy. Also presented is the specific role that chemotherapy may be able to play in conjunction with radiation.

MODELS OF CHEMOTHERAPEUTIC ACTION AND DRUG RESISTANCE

The studies of Skipper and colleagues convincingly demonstrated that virtually all of the so-called cytotoxic anticancer drugs produced similar quantitative effects on target neoplastic cells (1). These workers were able to show that a given dose of a specific antitumor drug always killed about the same proportion or fraction of tumor cells, irrespective of the absolute number of tumor cells that were present in the host animal. This is the **fractional cell kill** or **log kill effect,** which produces cell survival curves for antitumor agents that are similar to those seen with ionizing radiation.

Typically, antitumor agents produce two types of cell survival curves (2). The first type, which is seen with the alkylating-agent type of DNA-binding drugs, is basically a log linear dose-response relationship such that increasing doses progressively produce a greater fractional cell kill. The second type consists of an initial log linear dose response followed by a plateau of the cell killing curve so that further increases in dose do not result in further reductions in cell viability. This is seen with a variety of agents, such as vinca alkaloids, epidiphylotoxins, cytosine arabinoside, and methotrexate. These are all agents that are believed to exert their main cell-killing effects at a specific point in the cell cycle. Therefore, there is a significant time dependency with respect to their quantitative cell killing action. If the duration of exposure to these agents is significantly increased, to a duration equal to one to two cell cycle lengths, then the plateau shape in the survival curve tends to be lost, as a high proportion of the target cells passes through the vulnerable point in the cell cycle.

Deviations from the simple repetitive log kill effect are seen, however, if treatment is started in an experimental animal with a high tumor burden. The first one or two cycles may be associated with a significant log kill but, as further applications of treatment are administered, it is noted that the overall cell kill progressively diminishes. It is soon evident that one is dealing with a recurring tumor cell population that is unresponsive to the treatment that was initially effective (3).

Harvesting the recurrent tumor cells in these circumstances and transplanting them into a suitable host confirm that an alteration has occurred in the properties of the neoplastic cells, rendering them resistant to a specific antitumor agent. This process of selection for drug resistance has many similarities to the circumstances that are commonly encountered in the clinic. Treatment in a clinical setting may initially produce regression followed by relentless regrowth of the tumor. A large body of experimental work in both laboratory and clinical systems has confirmed that this type of treatment failure appears to be associated with selection for drug-resistant variant cells that arise within the initial tumor cell population (4,5).

If one assumes that drug-resistant tumor cells arise through a process of spontaneous mutation and are selected by the antitumor drug, then it is possible to develop a mathematically based theory describing the process and draw a number of inferences relating to treatment optimization (6). Regarding adjuvant chemotherapy, two of these inferences are of particular importance. The first concerns the relationship between overall tumor burden and the likelihood that drug-resistant cells are present within the neoplastic population. For any given value of the mutation rate to resistance, it can be demonstrated that the probability of the presence of resistant mutants will be directly linked to the total number of tumor cells present when treatment is commenced. Secondly, early in the growth of the tumor, there is a significant probability that no resistant mutants will appear and, therefore, therapy directed at smaller tumor burdens has a greater likelihood of success.

The association between tumor burden and curability has been clearly demonstrated in a number of experimental systems and seems to be true for many clinical situations (7,8). This relationship strongly supports the use of chemotherapy in an adjuvant mode whenever it is a feasible. Clearly, there are a number of types and classes of malignancy that present at an advanced stage at first diagnosis, so the opportunity for adjuvant chemotherapy is not amenable. But for many of the slower growing epithelial-derived malignancies that are seen in middle and later life, the primary neoplasm may present months or years before distant metastases become apparent. Adjuvant chemotherapy has its greatest potential in this situation, which is the focus of current clinical research.

EVOLUTION OF DRUG RESISTANCE IN TUMORS

A large amount of experimental and clinical data are available that support the hypothesis that phenotypic variability with respect to drug sensitivity commonly occurs within tumor cell populations (9,10). Drug-resistant variants to all of the clinically useful antineoplastic agents can be readily produced in experimental systems and appear to have their counterparts in the clinic as well. Moreover, tumor cells display a capacity to demonstrate resistance to many drugs concurrently, either through the sequential accumulation of phenotypic changes that render them resistant to a series of individual drugs or through broader phenotypic changes that have the capacity to demonstrate resistance to a large variety of agents through one single phenotypic alteration. An example of this latter mode of resistance is the recently described multidrug-resistant phenotype (11), in which mutant cells that express significant levels of a membrane glycoprotein are capable of demonstrating high orders of resistance to a large variety of toxic heterocyclic compounds. These compounds tend to be substances drawn from the natural product environment and include many of the most useful antineoplastic agents.

The biologic basis of this evolution of drug resistance in tumors has been the subject of considerable study and debate. It has been proposed that neoplastic cells are fundamentally genetically unstable and, as part of this pattern of genetic instability, they will generate a large number of genotypic and phenotypic variants, some of which will express high orders of drug resistance. The molecular basis for this genetic instability is still unclear, but the consequences seem unambiguous. Unlike normal cells, which show little or no tendency to alter their inherent drug sensitivity over time, tumor cells will typically evolve variants that display significant degrees of drug resistance. This process appears to be dramatically enhanced under the conditions of selection imposed by the therapeutic application of cancer chemotherapeutic agents.

We have proposed a model for this process (6) that involves somatic mutations occurring within the tumor cell population. These mutations result in the steady production of new variant cells that differ from their parents by their degrees of drug sensitivity to a variety of antineoplastic agents. The probability of these mutants arising is directly related to the actual size of the tumor burden being considered (or more technically, to the total number of cell divisions that the neoplastic burden has undergone). Therefore, large or biologically older tumors will be expected to contain significant numbers of drug-resistant cells. Conversely, small tumors that are young in a biological sense may not have yet evolved significant levels of drug resistance and will therefore be more susceptible to drug-induced cure.

MODELS OF RADIATION EFFECT

The effect of radiation on cell viability is a subject of enormous complexity. In the following section, we will not attempt to deal with this issue in any more than a superficial manner. Our focus is to devise a simple model of radiation effect that may have heuristic value predicting optimal drug and radiation combinations.

A single dose of ionizing radiation will produce an initial shoulder in the cell survival curve followed by a log linear reduction in cell viability (12). The extent of the reduction of cell viability will be dictated both by the dose of radiation and by the inherent radiation sensitivity of the target cell population. A number of factors are known to contribute to the magnitude of the cell-killing effect, including factors such as degree of hypoxia of the target cells and the general microenvironment in which the affected cells are located at the time of treatment.

Clinical radiotherapeutic schedules involve repeated applications of dosage fractions over an extended period of time so that the overall net cell kill is related not only to the cumulative killing effect of each dose but also to the amount of cell regrowth that occurs between applications of therapy. However, in a simple first approximation, we can say that a particular dose of radiation can be expected to produce a specific fractional cell kill on a population of proliferating neoplastic cells. The overall biologic effect will not be too dissimilar from the application of a single dose of an alkylating agent type of chemotherapy drug when this is given on a single occasion.

The question of whether tumor cell populations are heterogeneous with respect to inherent radiation sensitivity is an issue that is still subject to debate and has not yet been definitively resolved. However, for purposes of developing a simple model of treatment effects, we will assume that no heterogeneity in terms of radiation sensitivity exists within the hypothetical tumor and that the magnitude of the cell killing will be dictated primarily by the magnitude of the dose (to within the limits of normal tissue tolerance).

The total amount of radiation that can be delivered to a local regional site is primarily limited by the normal tissue tolerance adjacent to the tumor. This puts an upper limit on the total dose that can be given. Therefore, it is not realistic to discuss models of radiation effect in which essentially unlimited doses or fractions of radiation can be applied to a single anatomical location. We will, therefore, in the subsequent discussion, assume that the delivered radiation dose is fixed and cannot be exceeded above this level and that the amount of radiation given will be insufficient on its own to totally eradicate the tumor (otherwise, there would be no necessity to involve other forms of treatment).

MODELS OF CHEMORADIATION EFFECT

The theoretical model of drug resistance described above lends itself to both a mathematical and computer-based approach to simulate treatment effects on tumor populations of differing burden and degrees of resistance and to identify treatment strategies that will be optimal in terms of eradicating a tumor population with the highest degree of probability.

As mentioned previously, commencing treatment as early as possible in the evolution of the tumor is an optimal strategy. Another involves the use of multiple drugs given more or less concurrently to reduce the probability that there will be cells present in the tumor that are resistant to all of the drugs available in the treatment protocol. In other words, it would be maximally effective to give drugs A, B, C, and D concurrently, as opposed to giving the same agents in a sequential fashion, because the latter strategy would permit the tumor time to evolve resistance to the last drugs employed in the protocol.

There are definite limits to the feasibility of giving several antitumor agents simultaneously, even if one is able to minimize the degree of nonoverlapping toxicity. Most of the useful neoplastic agents have significant toxic effects on the rapidly proliferating cells of the bone marrow and upper aerodigestive tract; combinations of these agents given in full dose will produce at least additive toxicity on the vulnerable normal cell systems, with the risk of producing serious or fatal side effects before the tumor population is eradicated.

One role of mathematical modeling is to identify strategies that will come closest to achieving the therapeutic effect of simultaneous multiagent therapy without at the same time producing the inevitable toxicity that such strategies may yield.

Provided certain biologic and mathematic conditions can be satisfied, a rational and potent strategy utilizes effective noncross-resistant chemotherapeutic agents in an alternating as opposed to a sequential fashion (13). That is, if we assume that we have drugs A and B, which are similar in every respect except that drug A will effect cells resistant to drug B and vice versa and that the simultaneous use of A and B is precluded because of toxicity, then the most effective strategy is to utilize these agents in an alternating fashion, e.g., AB AB AB, etc. This makes intuitive sense and can be readily demonstrated on a theoretical, mathematical basis as well. If we assume that cells that are resistant to one drug will, if given time, evolve to a double level of resistance, then those strategies that will most rapidly deplete a single level of resistant mutants will prove to be most effective, with the highest probability of generating drug-induced cure.

Attempts to apply this theoretical approach at the clinical level have been fraught with some difficulty. While the agents ideally should be noncross-resistant, the most important criterion that must be met is that each agent (or combination of agents in a particular protocol) should be quantitatively equivalent to the other. Relatively small deviations in this quantitative symmetry will result in scenarios in which strict one-to-one alternation no longer emerges as the optimal strategy. Instead, we are faced with much more complex interwoven strategies that might involve three courses of drug A and then one of drug, B followed by three courses of A, etc. The theoretical basis for these more complex strategies has been analyzed by Day (14). We are left with a somewhat pessimistic conclusion that while alternating chemotherapy may be attractive on theoretical grounds, it may be difficult to put into actual clinical practice.

Despite this, several types of alternating chemotherapeutic strategies have been evaluated; a reasonable proportion appears to show some advantage over sequential chemotherapy. In many studies, the difference was not great but in none did it appear that the alternating approach was inferior to sequential treatment. As mentioned above, the alternating strategy appeared to yield definite advantages in at least some circumstances (15).

TREATMENT STRATEGIES

Since theoretical studies and certain clinical trials suggest that the sequencing of therapeutic agents can be an important determinant of therapeutic result, then this permits us to examine the question of sequencing of radiation and chemotherapy.

As discussed above, there is some uncertainty as to whether true heterogeneity with respect to intrinsic radiation sensitivity does occur within tumors. Even if it does not, studies suggest that radiation and drug resistance in cells may not be closely linked, so it is reasonable to assume that cells that are resistant to a particular drug or drug combination need not display altered sensitivity to radiation.

Under these conditions, one can look at sequencing strategies of radiation and chemotherapy in which the effect of radiation is modeled as a chemotherapeutic agent that is noncross-resistant with the drug component of the treatment protocol. The major differences from the standpoint of treatment modeling are that the radiation effect is confined to a discrete anatomical location and, unlike drugs, it can be given only for a limited and fixed dose to a certain predetermined effect. Given these assumptions, we can then examine in more detail the effect of radiation and chemotherapeutic sequencing.

COMBINED MODALITY TREATMENTS

In the following sections, we will describe two models of combined modality treatment that are based on the above principles and assumptions and that can be put into a form that can be tested at the clinical level.

Early Versus Late Application of Radiation

There are two specific scenarios that can be examined in the instance of combined modality treatment that lend themselves to testing at the clinical level. This is basically to determine whether it is more effective to apply radiation early in the treatment program, i.e., prior to the initiation of chemotherapy, or to apply it late after induction chemotherapy, with radiation then being used in a "consolidating" mode.

There are theoretical advantages to both approaches, and it may even appear to make better intuitive sense to use chemotherapy to shrink the tumor down to a size that can then be eradicated by follow-up radiation. Since we would not expect the chemotherapy to select for radiation-resistant cells, then progressively shrinking the localized tumor mass may yield a residual tumor population that is small enough to be cured by an appropriate program of radiotherapy.

The theoretical advantages of employing radiation first and then following up with the chemotherapy include the fact that even if the local tumor mass cannot be eradicated by radiation, unless the proportion of chemotherapy-resistant cells in the tumor was extremely high, the effect of the radiation would be to "dilute out" the drug-resistant subpopulation as the tumor shrinks under the impact of the radiation. We would then be left with a small residual population of tumor cells that should be basically drug sensitive and can be eliminated by an appropriate program of chemotherapy (Fig. 3–1).

There are disadvantages to both treatment approaches, concerning the hypothetical behavior of drug-resistant cells that may arise within the tumor. In the first approach, in which chemotherapy is employed first, we know that by definition this will not eliminate any drug-resistant cells that are already present in the tumor, a likely scenario with most solid tumors of clinical dimensions.

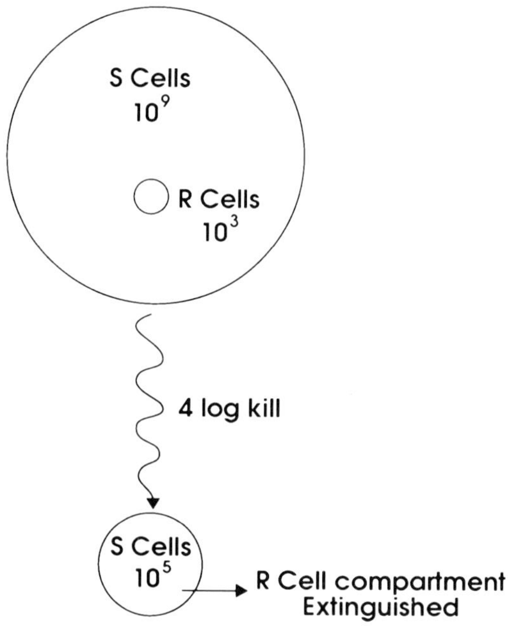

Fig. 3–1. Schematic diagram indicating theoretical effect of radiation being applied to a tumor mass that contains a small but non-negligible proportion of drug-resistant cells. If it is assumed that the radiation functions in a nondiscriminant mode (that is, equally toxic to the drug-sensitive and drug-resistant cells), then a dose of radiation that will reduce the total tumor population by four logs will be expected on average to extinguish the entire drug-resistant population. In a real tumor, it is assumed that the drug-resistant cells are distributed more or less uniformly throughout the tumor and that there are no privileged sanctuaries for them.

During the program of chemotherapy, such drug-resistant phenotypes will have an opportunity to metastasize outside the radiation treatment field and cause eventual relapse and death. Conversely, if we examine the behavior of drug-resistant cells in the situation in which radiation is used first, then this subpopulation will be reduced in tandem with the drug-sensitive population during the period of treatment. Metastasis may still occur and at the same rate as in the previous situation. But now, because we are reducing both drug-sensitive and drug-resistant populations with radiation, the probability of a resistant metastasis becoming disseminated will be reduced.

The relative superiority of one strategy over another is heavily dependent on the rate at which metastases are generated within the tumor mass. If the proportion of drug-resistant to drug-sensitive cells is relatively high, then the probability of a proportion of the metastases being drug resistant at the time of distant seeding will be correspondingly high. Thus, the late use of radiation is less effective than those programs in which radiation is used early. This supports the use of some type of alternating radiation chemotherapy approach, as described above, or a program of combined modality therapy in which radiation and chemotherapy are commenced simultaneously.

Alternating Chemoradiation

As a variation of the strategies described above, it can also be demonstrated both clinically and experimentally that alternating chemotherapy and radiotherapy may offer advantages over the sequential application of these modalities. The fundamental rationale for this derives from similar arguments to those that were developed for the use of alternating noncross-resistant chemotherapy. This approach is described in greater detail in Chapter 4. Provided that certain assumptions are made about the behavior of the individual tumor cells and their states of drug and radiation resistance, alternating therapy emerges as a practical strategy that is supported by a consistent body of experimental data.

The concept of alternating chemotherapy and radiotherapy is illustrated in Figures 3–2 to 3–4, which are based on actual experimental data comparing observed outcomes to a computer simulation. To complete the computer simulation studies, a number of tumor and treatment modality parameter values were be measured or estimated. These parameters included the total number of tumor cells, the proportion of tumor cells that had clonogenic capacity, the fraction of drug-sensitive cells that exhibited radiation resistance, and the fraction of drug-resistant cells that exhibited radioresistance. Also, estimates were made of the mutation rate to drug resistance and the log kills of the doses of radiation and chemotherapy.

In Figure 3–2, we see the effect of administering radiation alone, which resulted in some minor reductions in tumor size followed by regrowth of the whole tumor, including the clonogenic or stem cell compart-

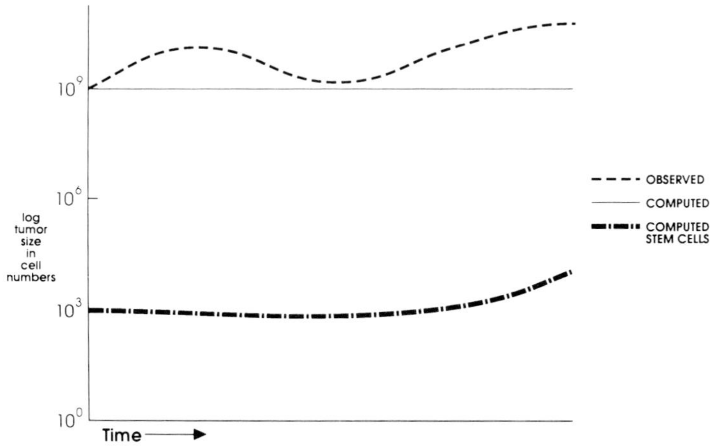

Fig. 3–2. Experimental radiotherapy of rat hepatoma 3942A. The actual observed gross tumor volume is indicated on the graph and the computer-estimated results for total cell number and stem cell compartment are added.

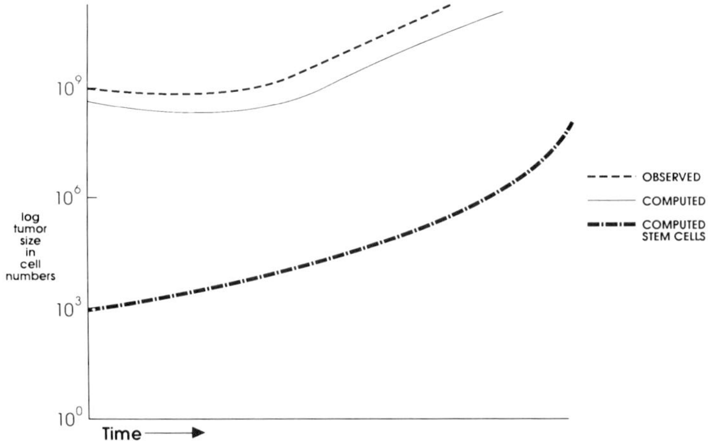

Fig. 3–3. Same system as in Figure 3–2; the results of chemotherapy treatment are displayed.

ment. The computer simulation predicted that the therapy would not be curative, as confirmed by observation.

Figure 3–3 shows the observed and the predicted outcomes when chemotherapy alone was applied. The use of chemotherapy on its own was even less effective than radiation, resulting in only a minimal perturbation in tumor growth followed by sustained regrowth during therapy. This demonstrated a close concordance between the simulated and observed results.

Thus, we can see that neither chemotherapy nor radiotherapy independently was capable of producing significant therapeutic effects in this particular experimental tumor. In Figure 3–4, radiation was alternated with chemotherapy at the same doses that were used in the previous two experiments. There is a close correlation between the observed and predicted behavior of the gross tumor mass, which showed a progressive decline during the course of therapy. However, it is interesting to note the behavior of the stem cell compartment, which the computer simulation indicated had been extinguished early in the treatment program, suggesting that these tumor-bearing animals should have been cured. When longer observation was carried out, the residual tumor mass progressively involuted, resulting in indefinite survival of the treated animals.

For this approach to be successful, it is necessary for chemotherapy and radiotherapy each to be effective in producing therapeutic action against cells that are resistant to the other therapeutic modality. Although the effects are only additive in a quantitative

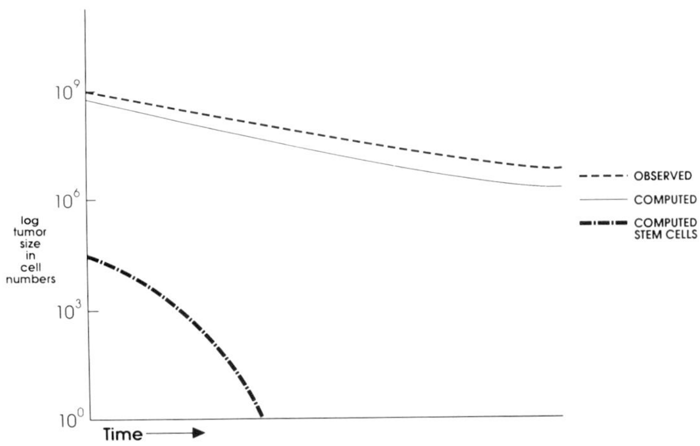

Fig. 3–4. Same system as in Figures 3–2 and 3–3; the graph shows results with alternating radiotherapy and chemotherapy. Note that both measured and computed graphs for the total cell number show progressive decline over time, and the computer simulation indicates early extinction of the tumor stem cell compartment predicting cure. With longer follow-up than is indicated on the graph, it was noted that the residual tumor mass contracted progressively until impalpable and that the animals survived indefinitely.

sense, they qualitatively result in a profound synergistic effect because the two treatment modalities combined can result in cure of the tumor, which is not possible by using either modality alone. For a detailed description concerning how the simulation studies were carried out technically, the reader is referred to our work in Arriagada (16).

CONCLUSIONS

This simple modeling approach suggests that the combined use of chemotherapy and radiotherapy cannot simply be carried out in an arbitrary fashion but depends on the predominating treatment failure, i.e., either local failure to eradicate the tumor or distant failure. In clinical situations in which distant failure is common, the modeling approach strongly supports the use of radiation therapy early in the treatment program rather than in a late consolidating mode.

There will be circumstances in which drug-resistant metastases will evolve early in the growth of the tumor, before diagnosis and before primary local regional therapy is commenced. These situations may be palliated by single modality or combined modality therapy but are incurable with existing therapeutic tools. The sequencing or simultaneous modality approach may be effective in neoplasms in which the evolution of high levels of drug-resistant distant metastases occurs as a relatively late event and in which prompt elimination of the local–regional mass will greatly diminish the likelihood of this unfavorable event. The cure of the tumor under these circumstances depends on sufficient courses of effective systemic chemotherapy to deal with any metastatic burden, which should be drug sensitive.

It is not possible by currently available means to measure the key biologic states of the tumor that would dictate the most effective strategy. However, because the different treatment strategies are sufficiently distinct and are technically feasible to apply at the clinical level, one can examine appropriate clinical trials to determine which sequencing approach yields the best results. Clinical studies examining different aspects of this sequencing approach have already been completed in some centers and are under way in others. While no unambiguous conclusions can be reached at this time, the clinical work performed to date appears to allay one important and serious concern. With appropriate dosage adjustments and modern methods of supportive care, it is possible to put patients through fairly rigorous combined modality treatment programs without unacceptable morbidity. Thus, ethical concerns that might otherwise have impeded the clinical testing of these theoretical concepts appear to be satisfied. Ongoing and recently completed clinical trials should provide more clear-cut answers to the question of whether appropriate sequencing and early concurrent use of chemotherapy and radiation have the potential to significantly improve treatment results.

REFERENCES

1. Skipper HE, Schabel FM Jr, Wilcox WS. Experimental evaluation of potential anticancer agents XII: On the criteria and kinetics associated with curability of experimental leukemia. Cancer Chemother Rep 35:1, 1964.
2. Bruce WR, Valeriote FA. Normal and malignant stem cells in chemotherapy. *In:* Proliferation and Spread of Neoplastic Cells. 21st Annual Symposium on Fundamental Cancer Research at MD Anderson Hospital and Tumor Institute. Baltimore, Williams & Wilkins, 1968, p. 409.
3. Skipper HE. Cancer Chemotherapy I: Reasons for success and failure of treatment of murine leukemias with the drugs now employed treating human leukemias. Ann Arbor, University Microfilms International, 1978, p. 1.
4. Brockman RW. Mechanisms of resistance. *In:* Antineoplastic and Immunosuppressive Agents. Sartorelli AC, Johns DG (Eds). Berlin, Springer-Verlag, 1974, p. 352.
5. Goldie JH, Coldman AJ. The genetic origin of drug resistance and neoplasms: Implications for systemic therapy. Cancer Res 44:3643, 1984.
6. Goldie JH, Coldman AJ. A mathematic model for relating the drug sensitivity of tumours to their spontaneous mutation rate. Cancer Treat Rep 63:1727, 1979.
7. Salmon SE. Kinetic rationale for adjuvant chemotherapy for cancer. *In:* Adjuvant Therapy of Cancer. Salmon SE, Jones SE (Eds). Amsterdam, Elsevier, 1977, p. 15.
8. DeVita VT Jr. The relationship between tumour mass and resistance to chemotherapy. Cancer 51:1209, 1983.

9. Claes Trope. Different susceptibilities of tumor cell subpopulations to cytotoxic agents and therapeutic consequences. *In:* Tumor Cell Heterogeneity, Origins and Implications. Owens AH, Coffey DS, Baylin SB (Eds). New York, Academic Press, 1982, p. 147.
10. Young RC. Drug resistance: The clinical problem. *In:* Drug Resistance in Cancer Therapy. Ozols RF (Ed). Norwell, Massachusetts, Kluwer Academic Publishers, 1989, p. 1.
11. Gerloch JH, Kartner N, Bell DR, et al. Multidrug resistance. Cancer Surv 5:25, 1986.
12. Wheldon TE. Radiotherapy treatment strategies. *In:* Mathematical Models in Cancer Research. Wheldon TE (Ed). Philadelphia, Adam Hilger, 1989, p. 134.
13. Goldie JH, Coldman AJ, Gudauskas GA. Rationale for the use of non-cross-resistant chemotherapy. Cancer Treat Rep 66:439, 1982.
14. Day R. Treatment sequencing, uncertainty and asymmetry: Protocol strategies for combination chemotherapy. Cancer Res 46:3876, 1986.
15. Goldie JH, Coldman AJ. Application of theoretical models to chemotherapy protocol design. Cancer Treat Rep 70:127, 1986.
16. Goldie JH, Coldman AJ, Ng V, et al. A mathematical and computer based model of alternating chemotherapy and radiation therapy in experimental neoplasms. *In:* Treatment Modalities in Lung Cancer. Antibiotics and Chemotherapy. Arriagada R (Ed). Basel, Karger, 1988, p. 11.

Chapter 4

EXPERIMENTAL AND CLINICAL RATIONALE FOR ALTERNATING CHEMOTHERAPY AND RADIOTHERAPY IN HUMAN CANCER MANAGEMENT

WILLIAM B. LOONEY AND HAROLD A. HOPKINS

INTRODUCTION

"Clinical schedules for delivery of radiotherapy and chemotherapy have evolved independently. The underlying therapeutic strategy for the clinical utilization of chemotherapy has evolved from the necessity of using large doses separated by long time periods of 3–4 weeks, to allow primarily for gastrointestinal tract and bone marrow recovery. The underlying therapeutic strategy for the clinical utilization of radiotherapy has evolved from the necessity of using small daily radiation doses to avoid major damage to the normal tissue surrounding the tumor. However, there is no reason to believe that these methods of delivery represent optimal therapies. There are >100 different cancers. Clinical success to date is primarily the result of specific clinical protocols utilizing one or more treatment modalities to obtain an effective therapeutic ratio between the eradication of the specific tumor and the toxic effects on the host" (1).

Knowledge of the most effective strategies for the integration of chemotherapy and radiotherapy is a prerequisite for integrating these established modalities with new treatment modalities such as biologic response modifiers. Well-defined clinical protocols to determine how to interact more effectively between chemotherapy and radiotherapy offer the greatest potential for more rapid improvement in treatment.

Substantial changes have occurred in the management of cancers of the head and neck (2–12), breast (13–15), bladder (16,17), lung (18–30), esophagus (31,32), rectum (33), anal canal (34), and of sarcomas (35,36). These have resulted from the greater use of chemotherapy and radiotherapy and the decreased use of radical surgery. In spite of these changes in therapeutic strategy, no definitive answer has been obtained to the question of the most effective strategy for integration of chemotherapy and radiotherapy in cancers with demonstrated clinical responsiveness to both treatment modalities. Furthermore, no general consensus exists concerning the optional treatment of either chemotherapy or radiotherapy alone for a large number of cancers.

THERAPEUTIC STRATEGIES

The various means by which chemotherapy and radiotherapy can be combined (see Chapter 2 for terminology) may be categorized and briefly described as follows.

1. **Concomitant:** Utilizing chemotherapy and radiotherapy together.
   a. Continuous: Radiotherapy is administered continuously on consecutive days until the total course of radiotherapy is given. Chemotherapy may be given every 3 to 4 weeks as in conventional chemotherapy alone or by continuous or daily infusion. The use of chemotherapy and radiotherapy at the beginning of induction therapy permits both modalities to be administered with the greatest intensity over the shortest period of

time. This strategy also provides the means of minimizing the buildup of cross-resistant tumor cells, because there is a "zero time" interval between delivery of the two modalities. It also provides initial treatment of micrometastases. The greatest disadvantage is increased toxicity, as demonstrated in the management of Hodgkin's disease.

   b. Intermittent: Radiotherapy is given at the same time as conventional chemotherapy, intermittently every 3 to 4 weeks.

2. **Sequential:** A full course of chemotherapy and a full course of radiotherapy are administered separately in time. The full course of chemotherapy may be given first, followed by a full course of radiotherapy, or vice versa. One of the major advantages of this strategy is that host toxicity is reduced by avoiding the excessive toxicities when the two modalities are given concomitantly. One of the primary disadvantages is that the intensity of treatment is reduced, thereby increasing the possibility of repopulation of the tumor during treatment. Also, if a full course of chemotherapy is given before radiotherapy, then the possibility of a buildup of chemoresistant tumor cells is increased.
3. **Alternating:** This strategy evolved in attempts to maximize the advantages of concomitant and sequential treatment and minimize the disadvantages of these extensively used strategies for utilizing chemotherapy and radiotherapy. Chemotherapy is given intermittently every 3 to 4 weeks as in conventional (single modality) chemotherapy. Radiotherapy is given between successive courses of chemotherapy. The objective is to provide temporal separation of delivery of both modalities so that both chemotherapy and radiotherapy can be given at the initiation of induction therapy without compromise of the intensity or full therapeutic dose of either modality. This approach is designed to reduce toxicity by temporal separation of delivery of chemotherapy and radiotherapy, to minimize the buildup of the resistance of the tumor cells to either modality, and to provide early chemotherapy for treatment of micrometastasis.

The alternating strategy has evolved from clinical studies at the Institute Gustave Roussy (IGR), Paris, and from experimental studies at the University of Virginia (UVA), in attempts to maximize the advantages of concomitant and sequential treatments and to minimize the disadvantages of these extensively used strategies for utilizing chemotherapy and radiotherapy.

Using the experimental solid tumor 3924A, a cure rate of 50% or greater was obtained with an alternating cyclophosphamide (CP) and radiotherapy protocol, with acceptable toxicity to the host, as opposed to no cures from three or more courses of either modality alone at total doses that exceeded the permissible levels of damage to the host. The most effective cancer chemotherapeutic dose and schedule for induction therapy were first determined for CP given alone. The flexibility of radiotherapy permitted total radiation dose escalation within the fixed chemotherapy schedule for three courses, until a tumor cure rate of 50% or greater was realized. Escalating the radiation dose while holding the chemotherapy dose and schedule constant permits scientific analysis of the results of interacting chemotherapy and radiotherapy with only one major variable, i.e., total radiation dose. Thus, an untreatable situation with one modality has been transformed into a treatable situation by simply alternating two modalities. The alternate use of chemotherapy and radiotherapy allowed twice the recovery time from each modality and resulted in reductions in toxicity to within clinically acceptable limits for both modalities without loss of tumor control and cure rates.

The Goldie-Coldman Model on Therapeutic Resistance*

It was possible to correlate the predictions of the Goldie-Coldman model and the UVA experimental results (37). Under the condi-

*This section gives results from a collaborative effort with JH Goldie, AJ Coleman, and V Ng, Division of Medical Oncology and Division of Epidemiology and Biometry, Cancer Control Agency of British Columbia, Vancouver, British Columbia, Canada.

tions used in the UVA study, the alternating of courses of chemotherapy and radiotherapy emerges as a powerful strategy capable of producing cures. The basis for this enhanced therapeutic effect is not completely understood, but the mathematical analysis suggests that an important component is the ability of each modality to extinguish subpopulations of tumor cells that are resistant to the other mode of therapy.

The Goldie-Coldman model was used to analyze the UVA experimental results of giving four courses of CP (150 mg/kg) every 11 days, four courses of radiation (1500 cGy) every 11 days, and four courses of CP alternating with radiation every 11 days. No cures were obtained with either radiation or CP alone; however, a cure rate greater than 50% was obtained when the two modalities were alternated.

These findings are consistent with the somatic mutation model of increasing proportions of tumor cells in 3924A becoming resistant to increasing numbers of courses of radiation alone (T_R) or cyclophosphamide alone (T_C). The findings were also consistent with the Goldie-Coldman model, showing that a one-course alternation of radiation and cyclophosphamide for three cycles (T_R–T_C–T_R–T_C–T_R–T_C) is better than a three-course alternating regimen (T_R–T_R–T_R–T_C–T_C–T_C). The somatic mutation model indicates a tumor cure probability of 0.37 for the three-course regimen, contrasted with a tumor cure probability of 0.57 for a one-course alternation.

The modeling approach used for chemotherapeutic effects assumes that cells are either sensitive or resistant to the drug in question. The log of the probability that a sensitive cell will survive the drug is linearly related to the dose, i.e., log-kill law. Resistant cells survive administration of the same drug at the therapeutic dose with probability (1). The behavior of tumor cells upon irradiation is assumed to be analogous for radiosensitive cells and to act with diminished effect on radioresistant cells. These assumptions may be viewed as approximations that reduce the number of parameters to be used in the model while preserving many essential properties of the effects involved. Cells are assumed to spontaneously mutate to drug resistance at a rate α per cell division. The parameter is referred to as the mutation rate. As a first approximation, it will be considered that a fixed proportion of the dividing cells are in the radioresistant state. A further parameter, F, was introduced to measure overlap in each type of resistance due to the same cause, i.e., the possible location of cells in regions of the tumor that are both hypoxic and inaccessible to the drug. Thus, this parameter, has some ability to estimate the magnitude of such joint resistance to the two modalities. Unfortunately, this formulation does not contain a model of the host in order to assess the toxic effect of various treatment combinations and schedules. Therefore, it is not possible to assess the effect of combinations on overall survival but only the effect on the tumor. The relationship of the effects of treatment on the host and tumor is discussed below in the following sections.

We would like to reemphasize that in this model, it was assumed that chemotherapy resistance arose through the mechanism of spontaneous mutation. The question of the mechanism of radioresistance was deliberately left open, except to specify that the absolute number of radioresistant cells would increase with increasing tumor size and that radiation- and chemotherapy-resistant states did not completely overlap. The process of radioresistance could be related to local microenvironmental effects, intrinsic genetic changes, or some combination of the two. It suffices for a simple simulation of the data for the process to behave as described in the model.

The Hryniuk Dose Intensity Concept

The optimum dose intensity is not known for any disease. However, considerable evidence has recently accumulated indicating that treatment outcome correlates well with dose intensity.

Hryniuk defines dose intensity as the amount of drug delivered per unit time, expressed as mg/m^2/week (regardless of schedule) (38,39). **Relative dose intensity** is the amount of drug delivered per unit time compared to an arbitrarily chosen standard single-drug regimen, expressed as a decimal fraction. Dose intensity given after dose reduction and time delays due to toxicity is called **received dose intensity.** To calculate dose intensity, it is necessary to assume that scheduling does not directly determine antitumor effect, drugs in a combination are equivalent in activity, different administration routes produce equivalent effects, and no significant interactions occur between drugs given simultaneously.

Hryniuk makes the following points.

1. Scheduling determines toxicity and thereby limits the dose intensity that can be tolerated.
2. Scheduling may also govern antitumor effect directly; however, normal host tissue makes the determination of the direct effects on the tumor difficult in clinical studies.
3. More sophisticated research techniques such as the response surface methodology of Carter, Wampler, and Stablein (40) may eventually ascertain whether scheduling directly determines antitumor effect.
4. The concept of dose intensity complements the Goldie-Coldman hypothesis. Well-defined experimental solid tumor systems provide the means for determining the relationship between toxicity and antitumor effects and the complex relationships between tumor burden, total therapeutic dose, dose intensity, and scheduling. The concepts of the Goldie-Coldman model and the concept of dose intensity elucidated by Hryniuk were derived for chemotherapy; however, both concepts can also be adapted readily for radiotherapy and for radiotherapy used with chemotherapy.

EXPERIMENTAL CHEMORADIATION

Solid Tumor Models

From six different tumors with different morphological, cell kinetic, biochemical, biologic, and growth (doubling times, 1 to 24 days) characteristics, two were selected for the experimental program. **3924A** is responsive to radiation and to the representatives of three major classes of chemotherapeutic agents we have evaluated, i.e., 5-FU, doxorubicin, and CP. The other tumor, **H-4-II-E,** is resistant to radiation and to these three chemotherapeutic agents. The experimental work to be presented relates to studies with 3924A. This experimental solid tumor fulfills the primary criterion that we wished to address with regard to the clinical relevance of the experimental studies. This criterion was that the tumor was responsive to both chemotherapy and radiotherapy, but cures could not be obtained by either chemotherapy or radiotherapy alone when the limitations of tumor response and host toxicity were taken into consideration.

The kinetics of cell proliferation and tumor growth are as follows: the actual doubling time for 3924A is 104 hours (hr), the potential volume doubling time is 42 hr, and the cell cycle time is 27.4 hr. The different phases of the cycle are: T_{G1}, 14 hr; T_S, 9.3 hr; T_{G2}, 3.7 hr; and T_M, 0.4 hr. The 1-hr thymidine labeling index is 17.6, the growth fraction is 0.65, and the cell loss factor is 0.60 (41).

The use of the concepts derived from experimental animal tumor models in the design of clinical protocols offers several advantages. In experimental systems, endpoints are available (cure rate, tumor growth delay, and animal survival) that are similar to endpoints used in a cancer clinical trial (complete and partial response rates, time to progression, and patient survival). In experimental animal systems, however, the opportunity exists for more precise measurements and a wider range for varying the independent variables. Treatment strategies may be explored that later may be adapted for use in clinical protocols. Although the findings from experimental animal models may not be directly applicable to cancer treatment in man, the concepts may be adapted and used in specific clinical situations.

Multiple Radiation Fractions Per Day with Chemotherapy

The rationale for multiple fractions per day (MFD) radiation is that normal tissue recovers more rapidly than tumor tissue and it allows a shorter total time to deliver the radiation dose. A 50% cure rate could be achieved with 6,000 cGy administered as MFD and alternated with CP, whereas it was necessary to administer a total of 11,250 cGy with single daily fractions alternated with CP to achieve a 50% cure rate.

The increased effectiveness of MFD radiation compared to daily fractions indicates a therapeutic advantage for this schedule since normal tissues are expected to show a dose-sparing effect. Addition of CP to the intermittent MFD schedule appears to further enhance effectiveness of MFD radiation by eliminating daily dose sparing of tumor, in addition to its own cell-killing effect (44).

The schedules for treatments with radiation alone or alternated with CP are shown in Table 4–1. The MFD radiation was given as 250 cGy per fraction on days 1, 2, 12, 13, 23, and 24. For the alternating schedule, CP was given on the day following each short course of MFD radiation in each cycle, on days 3, 14, and 25. The length of each treatment cycle, 11 days, allows recovery of bone marrow from the effects of the chemotherapy (43). Taylor et al have used intermittent combined chemotherapy and radiotherapy in the management of head and neck cancers (7).

Tumor Growth Delay

It is important to know the extent of tumor cell kill for a particular regimen and whether different agents or modalities interact to increase the proportion of cells killed. In addition to tumor cell kill, cure rates also depend upon the size of the tumor at initial treatment and the extent of regrowth during the treatment period. Growth delay, on the other hand, is relatively insensitive to small differences in tumor size at treatment and to repopulation during treatment, provided an appropriate volume is chosen for the endpoint.

Recently, we have utilized the simple relationship between tumor growth delay (GD) and surviving fraction (SF)

$$SF = \tfrac{1}{2}^{GD/Td}$$

to transform tumor regrowth data into the surviving fraction form (44). Survival curves can then be constructed for treatment

Table 4–1. Alternating Chemotherapy and Multiple Fractions Per Day Radiotherapy; Cyclophosphamide Given 1 Day After Each of 3 Courses of Radiation

A. *Schedule of Treatments*

	Day in Cycle										
	1	2	3	4	5	6	7	8	9	10	11
1st Cycle (Days 1–11)	R[a]	R	C[b]								
2nd Cycle (Days 12–22)	R	R	C								
3rd Cycle (Days 23–33)	R	R	C								

B. *Results*

Total No. Fractions	Total Dose (cGy)	Partial Response[c,d]	Tumor Cures[c,e]	Median Growth Delay	Median Survival (Days)	Lung Metastases[c]
12	3000	7	0	91	101	7
18	4500	7	3	117	>130[f]	0
24	6000	5	5	—	>130[f]	1
30	7500	3	6	—	>130[f]	0

[a]Radiation given as 250 cGy per fraction on days 1, 2, 12, 13, 23, 24.
[b]Cyclophosphamide 150 mg/kg or 0.9 g/m^2, given on days 3, 14, and 25.
[c]Ten animals were in each group.
[d]>50% reduction in tumor volume, compared to volume at first treatment.
[e]No tumor found at time of sacrifice.
[f]Day of sacrifice.

schedules that employ radiotherapy and chemotherapy alone or in combination, with treatment durations extending over several weeks. By using a constant for the doubling time (Td), relative data can be obtained that preserve the variation between treatments and between experiments.

Figure 4–1 shows SF as calculated from GD for radiotherapy alone and in combination with CP, with the radiotherapy given as one fraction per day. The Td is assumed to be constant between all treatments at 5.2 days. Treatments were initiated with radiotherapy for 10 days, then CP was given on day 11, and radiotherapy was resumed on day 12, for three courses of CP and 30 days radiotherapy. Using parameters derived from single dose data of D_0 = 406 cGy and n = 1.63, with f representing the number of fractions, the multifraction, multitarget, single-hit model

$$\text{Model I: } SF = [1 - (1 - e^{-D/D_0})^n]^f$$

closely fits our data for 30 daily fractions given at 100 to 375 cGy/day (Fig. 4–1) (44). In Figure 4–1, the solid symbols are the actual data points and the line is the response predicted by the model. The curve is concave downward because the total dose was increased by increasing the dose per fraction. This agreement between prediction and observation indicates that repair of sublethal radiation damage is completed between fractions and that the radiosensitivity of the tumor is unchanged as treatment continues. These data for the 3924A tumor are not consistent with the linear-quadratic model since a plot of ln SF/fD vs. D does not yield a straight line. Survival data obtained for tumors treated with daily radiation alternated with three courses of CP (open symbols) are in agreement with a simple additive effect of the two individual modalities in the combination.

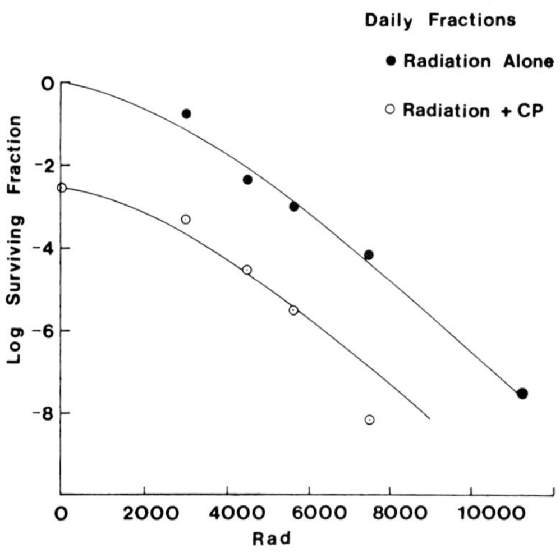

Fig. 4–1. Surviving fraction as calculated from growth delay data for 3924A after 30 daily radiation fractions, alone and alternated with CP. Solid lines were calculated from the multitarget model: $SF = [1 - (1 - e^{-D/D_0})^n]^f$ with D_0 = 406 cGy and n = 1.63. (Reprinted with permission from Hopkins HA, Looney WB. *In:* Interactions Between Antitumour Drugs and Radiation. Hill BT, Bellamy AS (Eds). Boca Raton, FL, CRC Press, Inc., 1990, p. 69.)

An MFD schedule was devised by increasing the number of 250-cGy fractions given over 2-day periods. These courses were given on days 1 to 2, 12 to 13, and 23 to 24. When both CP and radiation were given, the CP was given 1 day after each radiation course on days 3, 14, and 25 (Table 4–1). Model I gives a straight line (Fig. 4–2, dashed lines) because D, the dose per fraction, was constant while f, the number of fractions, was varied. The experimental data are not well represented by the model (44). MFD radiation is more effective than predicted by the model at the higher radiation doses. However, the steeper-than-expected slope for the experimental data could be accounted for by modifying the term D in the multifraction, multitarget, single-hit model by substituting Dx − a for D, where D = dose per fraction, x = number of fractions per day, and a = the recovered dose per day. The assumption is that the effective dose for MFD schedules is related to the dose per day, not the dose per fraction. The model then becomes:

$$\text{Model II: } SF = (1 - [1 - e^{-\{Dx-a\}/D_0}]^n)f'$$

where f′ is the number of days during which radiation is given. Reasonable representations of the experimental data were obtained for radiation alone when a = 200 cGy, and for radiation and CP when a = 0 (Fig. 4–2, solid lines).

Apart from the steeper-than-expected slope for our MFD radiation schedule when used alone, further advantage for this sched-

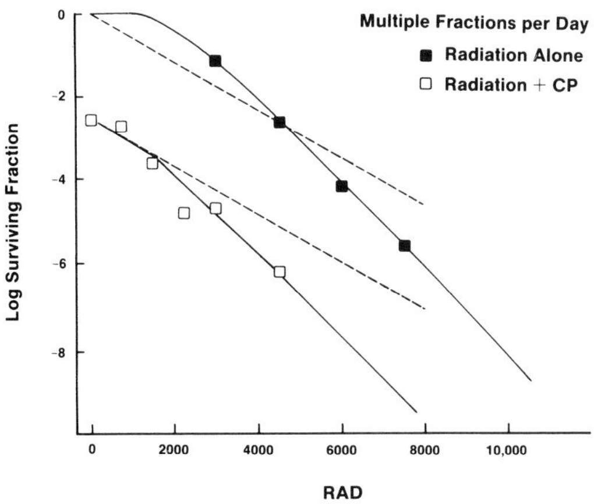

Fig. 4–2. Surviving fraction for hepatoma 3924A after MFD radiation, alone and alternated with CP. Dashed lines were calculated from Model I: $SF = [1 - (1 - e^{-D/D_0})^n]f$ with $D_0 = 460$ cGy, $n = 1.63$, and $D = 250$ cGy per fraction. Solid lines were calculated from Model II: $SF = (1 - [1 - e^{-\{Dx-a\}/D_0}]^n)^{f'}$ with x = number of fractions per day, $f' = 6$, $a = 0$ cGy for radiation + CP and $a = 200$ cGy for radiation alone. (Reprinted with permission from Hopkins HA, Looney WB. *In:* Interactions Between Antitumor Drugs and Radiation. Hill BT, Bellamy AS (Eds). Boca Raton, FL, CRC Press, Inc., 1990, p. 69.)

ule was obtained when used with CP. CP appeared to give an additive response with daily radiation fractions (Fig. 4–1) but a greater than additive response with MFD radiation (Fig. 4–2).

Since local tumor control was obtained at the higher radiation doses with daily fractions when given with CP, the surviving fraction necessary to achieve the tumoricidal dose (TCD_{37}) was calculated for the model and compared with the observed local control data. This is the calculated log SF at which one tumor cell survives and for which a 37% cure rate would be expected (45). The following was assumed: (a) at the TCD_{37} only one clonogenic cell survives, (b) all tumor cells are clonogenic at the initial treatment, (c) the initial tumor cell number for 250-mm^3 tumors is 0.7×10^8 cells, and (d) the doubling time of 5.2 days corresponds to a relative growth rate of 1.1426 per day. For daily fractions, the calculated log SF at the TCD_{37} was found to be −9.7, which for the model combined with CP (Fig. 4–1), would be attained at a total radiation dose of 10,900 cGy + CP. This is close to the actual value because 50% cures were obtained at 11,250 cGy + CP.

For MFD radiation, the calculated log SF at the TCD_{37} was −9.2, which for Model II with CP (Fig. 4–2), would be attained at a dose of 7400 cGy + CP. This estimate exceeds the actual TCD_{37} by more than 1400 cGy, since 50% cures were obtained at 6000 cGy. The observed cure rates were 30% at 4500 cGy, 50% at 6000 cGy, and 60% at 7500 cGy (Table 4–1).

In experiments in which radiation was given as daily fractions and the dose per fraction was varied, a plot of log surviving fraction/total radiation dose versus dose per fraction did not yield a straight line, indicating that the data for 3924A would not fit with the linear-quadratic model. Withers, Taylor, and Maciejewski (46) have indicated that simple isoeffects formulae for changes in fractionation patterns in clinical radiotherapy cannot ever be valid because normal tissues and tumors vary, not only in their sensitivity to changes in fraction size, but also in their repopulation kinetics. Furthermore, repopulation kinetics change during treatment. Withers et al also indicated that there may be a spectrum of α/β ratios for different tumors or within similar tumors of different kinetic characteristics. Wide individual variations in tumor regrowth characteristics are likely, not only among tumors of different sites but also within tumors of the same site in different patients. Thus, the linear-quadratic model has many limitations regarding its utilization in the design of clinical protocols for radiotherapy alone. The introduction of chemotherapy further complicates the use of the linear-quadratic model in clinical protocols designed to determine the most effective strategy for utilizing chemotherapy and radiotherapy. This assessment of the linear-quadratic model based on clinical radiotherapeutic studies is similar to the assessment made in UVA experimental studies utilizing chemotherapy and radiotherapy. The UVA experimental data could be fit into a multifraction, multitarget, single-hit model, but not a linear-quadratic model.

Tumor Cell Survival

Three independent methods have been utilized to assess the changes in rates of tumor cell depopulation and repopulation before, during, and after treatment. They are as follows: 1) the change in number of tumor cells in the "S" phase of the cell cycle determined by autoradiographic methods, 2) the incorporation of [^{3}H]thymidine into tumor DNA determined by biochemical methods and used as an index for changes in cellular proliferation rates, and 3) the instantaneous rate of change of the tumor growth rates determined by biomathematical methods from changes in tumor volume. Repeated measurements of the tumor volume has provided a noninvasive way of assessing relative changes in the total cell number of tumors before, during, and after treatment (Fig. 4–3) (1).

The DNA-specific activity in the CP-treated (150 mg/kg) tumors was depressed below control value for 4 to 5 days before recovery began; then it increased to a maximum at day 9 (Fig. 4–4). Changes in tumor growth rate following four 150-mg/kg doses of CP given every 11 days were determined biomathematically and are shown in Figure 4–3. The time of maximum tumor growth rate was well defined at 13 to 15 days after treatment, even with an escalation of the chemotherapy dose by a factor of 5 (50 to 250 mg/kg) (Table 4–2). This was also true after large single doses of radiation. Similar results were also obtained from studies of the chemoresistant and radioresistant tumor H-4-II-E after chemotherapy and radiotherapy (41).

The accelerated rate after treatment provides information relative to tumor cell re-

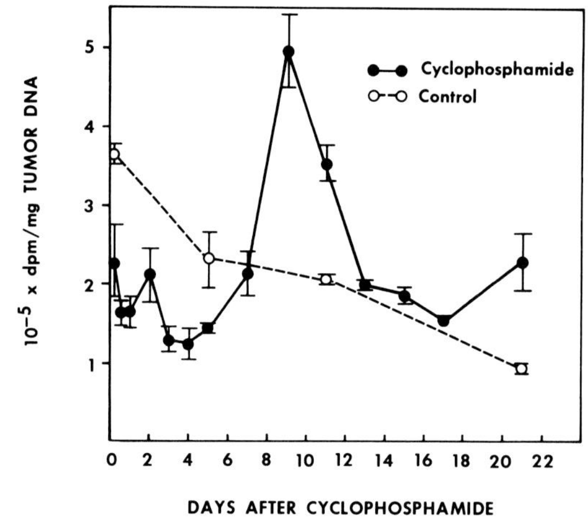

Fig. 4–4. Effect of cyclophosphamide (150 mg/kg) on [^{3}H] thymidine incorporation into DNA of hepatoma 3924A. Bars = SE; dpm = disintegrations/min. (From Looney N. NCI Monogr 6:85, 1988, IOP Publishing Ltd.)

population following treatment. The volume doubling times in the two experimental solid tumors in the rat used in our studies were 4 days and 2 days, respectively, for 3924A and H-4-II-E. Even though the volume doubling time varied by a factor of 2, T_{min} was similar in both tumors following chemotherapy and radiotherapy. Over a wide dose range for both radiation and chemotherapy (5-FU, Adriamycin, and CP), T_{min} was 5 to 11 days after treatment. Previous biochemical and histologic studies in both 3924A and H-4-II-E have shown that this time course for tumor volume reduction is related to tumor cell

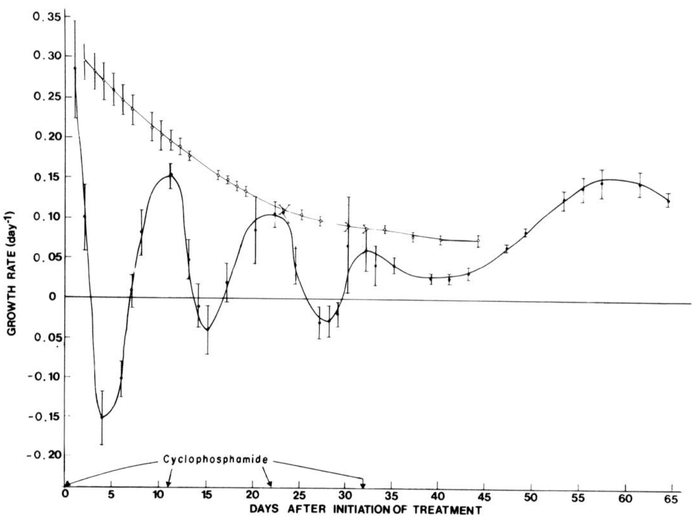

Fig. 4–3. Changes in tumor growth rate following four doses of cyclophosphamide (150 mg/kg). Upper curve = control; lower curve = cyclophosphamide treatment. Points = mean of instantaneous growth rates for ten 3924A tumors on indicated day after treatment. Bars = SE. The T_{max} occurred 10, 11, and 15 days after administration of the fourth and final dose on day 33. (From Looney WB. Special lecture: Alternating chemotherapy and radiotherapy. NCI Monogr 6:85, 1988, IOP Publishing Ltd.)

Table 4–2. Changes in Tumor Volume and Tumor Growth Rates Following Increasing Doses of Cyclophosphamide (3924A)

Treatment	Tumor Growth Delay (Days)	T_{min}(Days)	T_{max} (Days)	Tumor Growth Rate** Day^{-1} at T_{max}
250 mg/kg	17.5 ± 1.39*	9.86 ± 0.40*	15.75 ± 0.16*	0.383 ± 0.023
200 mg/kg	16.3 ± 0.92	8.40 ± 0.43	13.40 ± 0.37	0.254 ± 0.021
150 mg/kg	12.8 ± 0.49	8.50 ± 0.22	14.33 ± 0.16	0.349 ± 0.030
100 mg/kg	10.7 ± 0.41	8.10 ± 0.88	14.00 ± 0.49	0.350 ± 0.024
50 mg/kg	5.8 ± 0.54	5.00 ± 0.33	13.10 ± 0.96	0.289 ± 0.019

*Standard error of the mean.
**Growth rates for untreated tumors at these times were 0.171 ± 0.012, 0.161 ± 0.011, 0.156 ± 0.011, 0.167 ± 0.011 and 0.128 ± 0.014 at T_{max} for 50, 100, 200, and 250 mg/kg cyclophosphamide, respectively.
Tumor Growth Delay: Increase in time (days) required for treatment tumors to reach a volume of 1000 mm^3. Tumors of control group reach 1000 mm^3 in 4.1 ± 0.69 days.
T_{min}: Time of minimum tumor volume.
T_{max}: Time of maximum tumor growth.

destruction and removal following chemotherapy and radiotherapy.

The effects of treatment on the tumor result in cell loss, with a reduction in tumor size. Our studies and many others on solid tumors have shown that the growth rate at T_{max} 14 days after 150 mg/kg CP, was greater (0.35 day^{-1}) than the control tumor growth rate at the initiation of the experiment (0.30 day^{-1}) and over twice that of the control tumor (0.15 day^{-1}) at the time of T_{max} on day 14 (Table 4–2).

It has been demonstrated that the growth rate of solid tumors is inversely related to size. If there is a marked reduction in tumor volume as a result of treatment, then the smaller tumor will grow at a faster rate. In this case, they are growing at rates comparable to tumors 14 days younger. The fact that the growth rate of treated tumors at T_{max} is greater than the growth rate of control tumors at V_o (volume at treatment) raises a less likely but intriguing question: are the growth rates of the tumors accelerated following therapeutic insult in a manner similar to the accelerated proliferation of host organs such as bone marrow and gut to therapeutic insult? If this is the case, then it would suggest that the tumors are reacting similarly as normal tissue does to therapeutic insults. It would also suggest that the tumor is more responsive to host control mechanisms than previously realized.

Tumor Volume

Tumors may become less responsive to chemotherapy with advancing size as a consequence of a decreasing growth fraction. We found that 3924A exhibits little difference in the time required to grow to a specified volume (8 or 40 times initial volume) after treatment with CP at the LD_{10}, for initial tumor volumes ranging from 250 mm^3 to 10,000 mm^3 (Table 4–3). However, if growth delays are derived in the usual way as the difference between treated and control groups at a common tumor volume, they will appear to decrease with increasing tumor size at the time of treatment. This apparent contradiction is a consequence of a change in the slope for untreated control tumors from an initial doubling time of ~2 days to a terminal doubling time of ~4.2 days at volumes larger than 3000 mm^3, while tumors regrowing after treatment exhibit only the terminal growth rate (44). This difference is kept relatively constant between treatments and between experiments by always starting treatment when tumors are approximately the same size (250 mm^3). The additional observations (Table 4–2) that regrowth began at similar times after treatment and that median survivals from the time the tumor was injected were similar for all groups (except for the one treated at largest size) provide further evidence that the effect of CP is independent of tumor size at the time of treatment over a wide range of tumor volumes.

The log SF (log surviving fraction) at the TCD_{37} was estimated to be −9.7 for daily radiation combined with CP. The log SF at the TCD_{37} with MFD radiation combined with CP was estimated to be −9.2. It should be noted (Table 4–3) that a tumor with a

Table 4–3. Effect of 150 mg/kg Cyclophosphamide (CP) on 3924A When Administered to Tumors of Various Sizes

V_o[a]	Tumor Cell Number	Time to $8V_o$[b]		Time to $40V_o$[c]		Onset of Visible Regrowth[d]	Relative Lifespan[e]
		CP	Control	CP	Control		
~250	0.7×10^8	24	3.3	33	8.5	14	1.56
~500	1.4×10^8	23	4.1	34	11	13	1.42
~1000	2.8×10^8	22	5.7	33	14	13	1.37
~2000	5.6×10^8	22	7.2	35	16	12	1.42
~5000	1.4×19^9	25	9.8	—	—	11	1.37
~10,000	2.8×10^9	24	10	—	—	12	1.00[f]

[a]Tumor volume (mm^3) at treatment.
[b]Time in days required for tumor to reach 8 times the volume at treatment.
[c]Time in days required for tumor to reach 40 times the volume at treatment.
[d]Days after treatment.
[e]Median lifespan from inoculation with tumor for treated rats ÷ similar data for untreated rats.
[f]Death occurs before full effect of CP can be expressed.

volume of 250 mm^3 would have 0.07×10^9 cells. This provides the information for further studies to assess the quantitative interrelationship between tumor burden, host toxicity, and the dose intensity for the most effective scheduling of chemotherapy and radiotherapy.

Distant Metastases

Experimental animal tumor models can also provide data on the appropriateness of particular regimens in preventing or treating metastases. Solid tumor model 3924A metastasizes to the lungs, but this is not apparent unless the lifespan of the animal is increased by subcurative treatment of the tumor to prolong the life of the rat. Pulmonary metastases were prevalent among animals given radiation daily or as MFD over periods of 3 to 4 weeks at total doses ranging from 3000 to 11,250 cGy. Multiple doses of CP, each at the level that was lethal to 10% of the animals, did not cure the primary tumor but appeared to delay the appearance of metastases. Treatment schedules that alternated the delivery of multiple 250-cGy fractions of radiation during 2-day periods with CP at a dose of 150 mg/kg for a total of three courses were effective in curing the primary tumor and eliminating pulmonary metastases (see Tables 4–1 and 4–5) (47). The clinical implication of these experimental results is that initiation of intense chemotherapy and radiotherapy at the onset of treatment should increase the possibility of eliminating the primary and metastatic dissemination.

Chemoradiation Scheduling Assessment*

In 1958, Box (42) suggested the potential usefulness of the statistical design and analytical procedures that have been developed for the explanation of response surfaces. Cox (48) developed an approach utilizing the hazard function or instantaneous failure rate to relate failure-time to treatment variables. This statistical model has been studied extensively and is widely used by statisticians analyzing failure data. Carter et al (49) demonstrated that the multivariant logistic function quadratic is an acceptable model to relate the probability of a favorable treatment outcome to treatment levels. Once the dose-response surface is estimated in this manner, it can be explored to determine the significance of single or multiple drug combinations alone or with radiotherapy and to estimate optimal treatment levels.

Survival times and times to 40 V_o (40 × volume at the time of initiation of treatment) for the combination chemotherapy–radiotherapy studies were analyzed using Cox's hazards model (48) with time-varying covariants, as described by Carter et al (40). In this approach, the relationship between the

*This section was completed as a collaborative effort with W.H. Carter, Jr. and E.D. Campbell, Department of Biostatistics, Medical College of Virginia, Virginia Commonwealth University, Richmond, Virginia.

instantaneous risk of death or of V = 40 V_0 at time t, \(t), and the treatment variable is given by

$$(1)\ \backslash(t) = >\lambda_0(t)\ \exp$$
$$(\beta_1 x_1 + \beta_2 x_2 + \beta_{12} x_1 x_2 + \tau_1 x_1 t + \tau_2 x_2 t + \tau_{12} x_1 x_2 t)$$

where $\lambda_0(t)$ is the instantaneous risk of death or of V = 40 V_o at time t for animals in the control group,

β_1 is an unknown constant associated with the effect of radiation,

β_2 is an unknown constant associated with the effect of CP,

β_{12} is an unknown constant associated with the interaction between radiation and CP,

τ_1 is an unknown constant that allows for the possibility of the effect of radiation to change over time,

τ_2 is an unknown constant that allows for the possibility of the effect of CP to change over time,

τ_{12} is an unknown constant that allows for the possibility of the effect of the interaction between radiation and CP to change over time,

x_1 and x_2 are doses of radiation and CP, respectively, and t is any value of time (in days) > 0.

The model parameters, β_1, β_2, β_{12}, τ_1, τ_2, and τ_{12}, were estimated by the method of maximum likelihood.

The hazard analysis was performed using the T40 V_o data (Fig. 4–5). The τ's in Equation (1) were significant ($p < 0.05$), indicating time by treatment interactions. These indicate that the effect of radiation, the effect of CP, and the effect of the interaction between the two is not constant but varies with time. A high probability of longterm tumor control is not achieved by radiation alone at doses to 9000 cGy; CP is also required.

Tumor cell survival as well as animal survival or lifespan after noncurative treatment can be estimated from the T40 V_o data. In previous experiments, data were obtained on animal survival after treatment and were reported as median survival. By combining the acute toxicity data with the calculated day of death (LS), derived from the relationship between T40 V_o and animal survival, the relative advantage for particular courses of treatment may be assessed using the most relevant endpoint from the clinical perspective, survival.

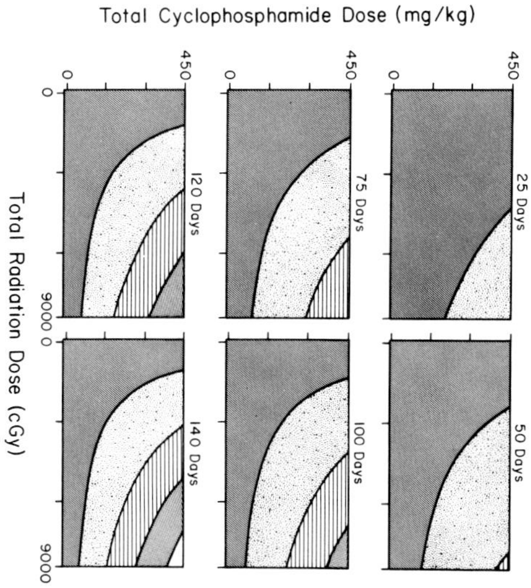

Fig. 4–5. Contour plots of cyclophosphamide versus total radiation dose from hazard analysis showing dose regions having similar log relative risks of tumor volume reaching 40 V_o on the specified day. Log relative risk levels represented by the various shadings are (from lower left to upper right): +11.04 to −177; −177 to −554; −554 to −931; −931 to −1308; −1308 to −1496.

The hazard analysis was performed using the animal survival data (Fig. 4–6). The τ's in Equation (1) were significant ($p < 0.0001$), indicating time by treatment interactions. The most immediate consequence of these terms is that for survival greater than 100 days, Figure 4–6 suggests that high doses of radiation in addition to moderate doses of CP are required to lower the risk of death; for survival less than 100 days, it appears that radiation alone is associated with a decrease in the risk of death.

Conclusions

Extensive UVA experimental studies have demonstrated that multiple fractions per day (MFD) radiotherapy given intermittently in short courses and alternated with chemotherapy is more effective than alternating single daily radiation fractions with chemotherapy (1,47,51–55). Therefore, the effect

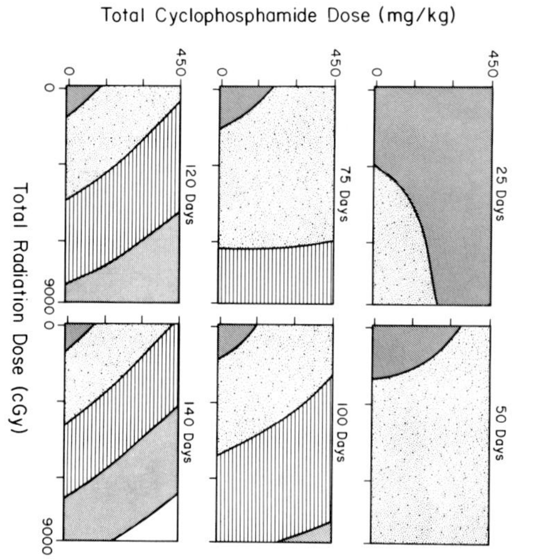

Fig. 4–6. Contour plots of cyclophosphamide versus total radiation dose from hazard analysis showing dose regions having similar log relative risks of death on the specified day. Log relative risk levels represented by the various shadings are (from lower left to upper right): +1.509 to −2.73; −2.73 to −11.2; −11.2 to −19.76; −19.76 to −28.2; −28.2 to −32.4.

Table 4–4. Tumor Growth Delay for Varying Intervals Between MFD Radiation and Cyclophosphamide (CP)

Treatment	Median Growth Delay* (Days)
MFD Radiation Alone (2500 cGy)**	33
CP Alone (150 mg/kg)	20
Additive Effect Radiation Alone + CP Alone	53
Radiation–11–CP***	48
Radiation–7–CP	51
Radiation–4–CP	53
Radiation–1–CP	51
CP–0–Radiation	49
CP–1–Radiation	48
CP–4–Radiation	64
CP–7–Radiation	57
CP–11–Radiation	60

*Growth Delay: The increase in number of days required to reach 40 times the initial tumor volume, compared with untreated controls. Ten rats/group.

**Radiation given as 10 250-cGy fractions over 2-day period.

***MFD Radiation followed 11 days later by cyclophosphamide.

of temporal separation of modalities was examined using the newer MFD radiation schedules. The results of this study, summarized in Table 4–4, show only an additive effect for growth delay when radiation was given 11, 7, 4, or 1 day(s) before CP, and the same additive effect when the two modalities were given concomitantly. Growth delays for schedules in which radiation was given 4, 7, or 11 days after CP were significantly greater than the concomitant group ($p \leq 0.005$). Therefore, these results with the newer radiation schedule confirm the earlier conclusion that administration of the two modalities concomitantly gives no therapeutic advantage when compared with longer intervals between modalities (51,55). Furthermore, the results indicate that increased therapeutic effectiveness can be realized even after temporal separation of delivery of each of the modalities. This offers the clinical potential for an increased therapeutic ratio by one modality increasing the therapeutic effectiveness of the other.

A schedule that alternates delivery of MFD radiotherapy and CP at intervals of 7 days is shown in Table 4–5. This schedule provides for recovery of bone marrow during the 14-day interval between successive doses of chemotherapy and for recovery of mucosa adjacent to the tumor during the 7-day interval between radiotherapy and chemotherapy. The 7-day interval may also benefit from treatments being given at the onset of the accelerated proliferation after previous treatment as discussed above (Fig. 4–5). The tumor cure rate was 10% in the group given 6000 cGy, 70% in the group given 7500 cGy, and 60% in the group given 9000 cGy (Table 4–5).

These results demonstrate the superiority of alternating CP with intermittent MFD radiation schedules over alternating CP with daily radiation schedules. It should be noted that the protocol of three courses of daily radiation (total radiation dose, 7500 cGy) alternated with CP was given over a 32-day period with no cures (Fig. 4–7), while the protocol of three courses of intermittent MFD (total dose, 7500 cGy) alternated with CP was given over a 35-day period with a 70% tumor cure rate (Fig. 4–8). One of the most significant clinical ramifications of

Table 4–5. Alternating Chemotherapy and Multiple Fractions Per Day Radiotherapy With Cyclophosphamide Given 7 Days After Each of 3 Courses of Radiation

A. *Schedule of Treatments*

	Day in Cycle													
	1	2	3	4	5	6	7	8	9	10	11	12	13	14
1st Cycle (Days 1–14)	R[a]	R						C[b]						
2nd Cycle (Days 15–28)	R	R						C						
3rd Cycle (Days 29–42)	R	R						C						

B. *Results*

Total No. Fractions	Total Dose (cGy)	Partial Response[c,d]	Tumor Cures[c,e]	Median Growth Delay	Median Survival (Days)	Lung Metastases[c]
18	4500	9	0	136	161	5
24	6000	9	1	—	>171[f]	2
30	7500	3	7	—	>172[f]	0
36	9000	4	6	—	>172[f]	1

[a]Radiation given as 250 cGy per fraction on days 1, 2, 15, 16, 29, 30.
[b]Cyclophosphamide 150 mg/kg or 0.9 g/m^2, given on days 8, 22, and 36.
[c]Ten animals were in each group.
[d]>50% reduction in tumor volume, compared to volume at first treatment.
[e]No tumor found at time of sacrifice.
[f]Day of sacrifice.

these findings is that relatively long periods of time (±7 days) can elapse between modalities without loss of therapeutic effectiveness. These results demonstrate that small daily radiation doses given continuously with CP are less effective than MFD radiation doses given intermittently with CP.

CLINICAL APPLICATIONS

These experimental findings are consistent with conclusions drawn from the clinical management of Stage IIIB Hodgkin's disease at Stanford University. Hoppe, Horning, and Rosenberg concluded in 1985 (56) that excessive toxicity occurred when the two modalities were given concomitantly. They had previously concluded that temporal separation of delivery of the two modalities by alternating chemotherapy and radiotherapy was the most effective way to manage Stage IIIB Hodgkin's disease.

Clinical studies by Amdur et al (57) have demonstrated that split courses of daily radiation are less effective in the treatment of head and neck cancer than continuous daily radiation. The UVA experimental studies demonstrate that successful treatment (i.e., tumor cure rate of 50% or greater) can be realized if MFD radiation is given intermittently. Both clinical and experimental studies demonstrate that intermittent ("split-course") daily radiation schedules are less effective than continuous daily radiation schedules. This indicates the MFD should be employed clinically if "split courses" are used.

However, in cancers such as small cell carcinoma of the lung, which are very chemosensitive and radiosensitive, daily radiation dose schedules can be effectively used in combination with chemotherapy. The clinical data of Tubiana, Arriagada, Le-Chevalier, and their associates at the IGR (18,22–24) have demonstrated an interval of 7 days between chemotherapy and radiotherapy and an additional 7-day interval between courses without any treatment resulted in complete response rate of 79% and a 5-year relapse-free survival rate of 16%. This was

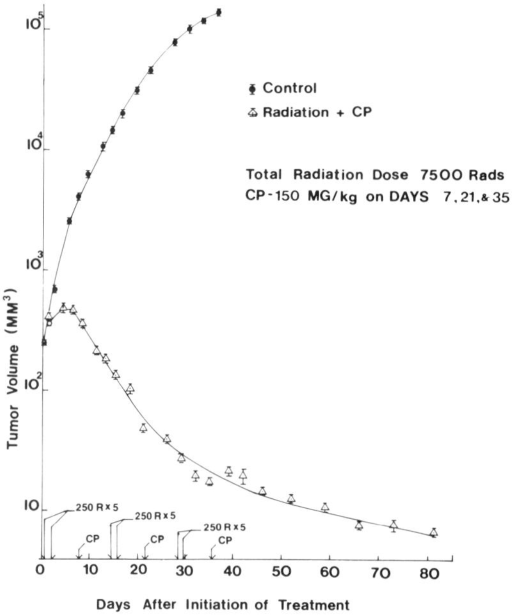

Fig. 4–7. Changes in mean tumor volume ± S.E.M. following daily radiation treatment alone and in combination with cyclophosphamide. Total radiation dose: 7500 cGy. Daily fractions of 250 cGy were given over three 10-day periods for a total of 30 fractions. Cyclophosphamide (150 mg/kg) was given on days 10, 21, and 32 for only the combined group. (From Looney WB, et al. Semin Oncol 16:176, 1989.)

accomplished in 109 patients who had minimal early or late effects from treatment.

ALTERNATING CHEMORADIATION IN CANCER MANAGEMENT

Theoretical Aspects

Demonstration of the therapeutic responsiveness of the tumor to each modality is a primary prerequisite for future clinical investigations into more effectively combining chemotherapy and radiotherapy. For example, if a 50% complete response rate can be achieved by one modality, then giving the other modality to which the tumor is also responsive offers the possibility of increasing the response rate up to 100%. Since complete response is necessary for tumor cure, the more effective integration of chemotherapy and radiotherapy offers the possibility of substantially increasing therapeutic response.

Tubiana (23,52) has illustrated, by way of calculations based on cell number, the respective roles of radiotherapy and chemotherapy in control of a clinical tumor. For a 100-g tumor (10^{11} cells) in which 1% of the tumor cells are clonogenic (10^9 cells), the tumor control dose (TCD) is approximately 6000 cGy in 30 fractions, if average radiosensitivity is assumed (D_{50} = 200 cGy). If 50% of the cells are killed by the chemotherapy (equivalent to partial remission), leaving 5 × 10^8 cells, the TCD is 5800 cGy. If 90% of the cells are killed by the chemotherapy, leaving 10^8 cells, the TCD is still 5400 cGy. Since the limit of tumor detection by current imaging methods is a tumor 4 to 6 mm in diameter, a complete response by current techniques could still have in the order of 10^7 to 10^8 tumor cells (perhaps 10^5 to 10^6 clonogenic cells). These calculations, which neglect the additional dose needed to compensate for tumor repopulation during the treatment period, serve to emphasize the necessity of

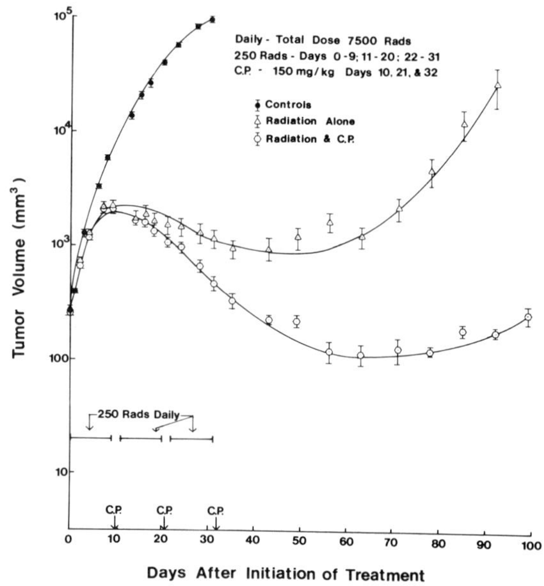

Fig. 4–8. Changes in mean tumor volume following MFD irradiation in which cyclophosphamide was given 7 days after each of three courses of radiation (R) on days 0 and 1, 14 and 15, and 28 and 29. Total radiation dose was 7500 cGy. (From Looney WB, et al. Semin Oncol 16:176, 1989.)

maintaining the full dose of radiotherapy in schedules that combine chemotherapy and radiotherapy. Administering both modalities with the greatest intensity possible during induction therapy is of paramount importance to minimize the chance of recurrence of the tumor at the primary site and to eradicate micrometastases that have already been seeded.

Goldie and co-workers (58,59) proposed that drug resistance results from somatic mutations in tumor cell populations and that a "front-loaded," first-line treatment strategy with the most effective agents possible in the highest dosages possible represents the clinician's best approach. Hryniuk (39) has emphasized the importance of drug dose in determining results of chemotherapy. In theory, the optimum dose intensity should simply be a mathematic expression derived from two known constants: optimum total dose and optimal duration of treatment. In clinical practice, neither of these is known.

The concept of dose intensity proposed by Hryniuk complements the Goldie-Coldman hypothesis. Well-defined experimental solid tumor systems provide the means for determining the relationship between host toxicity, antitumor effects in relationship to tumor burden, total therapeutic dose, as well as its relationship to dose intensity and scheduling.

Scheduling determines toxicity and thereby limits the dose intensity that can be tolerated. Scheduling may also govern antitumor effect directly; however, normal host tissue makes the determination of the direct effects on the tumor difficult in clinical studies. More sophisticated research techniques such as those using response surface methodology developed by Carter and associates are now being employed in collaborative studies with the objective of determining the significance of different drug combinations with different radiation-dose combinations to estimate optimum treatment levels. This provides a powerful tool in current and future studies to assess the relationship between the scheduling of chemotherapy and radiotherapy and dose intensity, antitumor effects, tumor burden, and host toxicity (animal survival). Results of these collaborative studies in our experimental solid tumor systems should provide valuable insights on how this may be utilized to determine the optimum total doses of chemotherapy and radiotherapy and the optimum duration of treatment for different cancers.

No clinical evidence is available that conclusively demonstrates that giving the two modalities concurrently results in synergism. If the two modalities are only additive when given concurrently, no therapeutic gain is realized by giving the two modalities together compared with the temporal separation of the delivery of the two modalities. In addition, a reduction in the therapeutic ratio can occur, as in Hodgkin's disease, as a result of increased toxicity if given concomitantly. Clinical studies have demonstrated that large intermittent doses of chemotherapy given every 3 to 4 weeks can be effective in successfully managing chemosensitive and radiosensitive cancers, such as Hodgkin's lymphoma. It would seem logical to assume that large amounts of radiation given intermittently can similarly be successfully used in radiosensitive tumors.

The effectiveness of alternating chemotherapy and radiotherapy, in both clinical and experimental studies, could be attributed in part to preventing the buildup of subpopulations of resistant tumor cells as postulated by the Goldie-Coldman hypothesis. In 1984, Goldie and Coldman discussed resistance in the context of their model as follows.

> "Overcoming a heterogenous population of cells would dictate that ideally all of the active agents should be used concurrently. Because of their considerable toxicity to normal cells, there are definite limits to the number of antineoplastic agents that can be given simultaneously without major reductions in drug dosage. Because lowering the dose will not only reduce the fractional cell kill for that particular agent but will also in effect raise the mutation rate and resistance to it, it is clear that significant dose reductions to accommodate more drugs will at some point become a self-defeating strategy. We are then confronted with the problem as to how to use most effectively a larger number of cytotoxic agents than can be safely administered concurrently. Analysis of this problem leads to the conclusion that one solution is to alternate at each cycle between 2 roughly equivalent treatment programs. These could represent single agents but in practice would

more often constitute complex drug combinations themselves. Alternating chemotherapy can therefore be seen as a mechanism to allow one to introduce therapeutic diversity early into the treatment program" (60).

It has been demonstrated that the growth rate of solid tumors is related to size. If there is a marked reduction in tumor volume as a result of treatment, then the smaller tumor will grow at a faster rate. Extensive clinical studies have been carried out on primary and metastatic tumor volume changes in the lung because of the ability to measure changes in tumor volume from serial chest radiographs (61–65). Other studies have evaluated changes in tumor size at different organ sites. Welin (66) evaluated the rates and patterns of growth of 375 tumors of the large intestine and rectum by using serial double-contrast media. Order (67) employed computerized axial tomography (CAT) scanning techniques to evaluate tumor volume changes in liver. Newer methods of quantitatively determining tumor volume changes following cancer treatment should provide the means for more accurate assessment of tumor response to therapy.

van Peperzeel (65) made a detailed evaluation of changes in lung tumor volumes before, during, and after radiotherapy. She found that the nadir for tumor volume reduction (T_{min}) for 11 patients with primary and metastatic lung tumors following radiation was 5.7 ± 0.45 days (range, 3 to 7 days). This close range for T_{min} occurred in a variety of tumors with volume doubling times that varied by a factor of 13 (17 to 228) days. In addition to primary squamous cell and anaplastic carcinoma of the bronchus, metastatic tumors of the testicles, as well as liposarcomas and fibrosarcomas were included in the study. The T_{min} in dogs with pulmonary metastases was 5 days; volume doubling time was 27 days. The volume doubling times in the two experimental solid tumors in the rat used in our studies were 4 days and 2 days, respectively, for 3924A and H-4-II-E. Even though the volume doubling time varied by a factor of 2, T_{min} was similar in both tumors following chemotherapy and radiotherapy (Table 4–6). Over a wide dose range for both radiation and chemotherapy (5-FU, Adriamycin, and CP), T_{min} was 5 to 11 days after treatment.

Therefore, the temporal events leading to T_{min} in man, dogs, and rats are similar for a wide variation of tumors with markedly different growth rates. Accelerated tumor growth rates were found in 10 of 11 patients treated with radiation by van Peperzeel (Table 4–6). Tumor volume changes were determined by Malaise et al (63) in 27 patients with lung metastases from a variety of primary tumors before and after 1000 cGy radiation as a single dose of two doses of 500 cGy given 3 hours apart. The growth rate of lung metastases following radiation was 3 to 5 times faster than the rate before radiation. The close temporal relationship of accelerated growth following treatment in the three species suggests that host response may play a more important role in this phenomenon than had previously been realized.

Experimental Aspects

The times from initiation of treatment until the beginning of complete response in six different solid tumors in man (small cell and nonsmall cell carcinomas of the lung, testicular cancer, malignant melanoma, metastatic breast cancer, and metastatic sarcoma) are shown in Table 4–7. Median time to complete response in the six different tumor types varied from 30 to 73 days. The human tumors were arranged in ascending order of tumor growth rates based on the determinations of Frei (68). The volume doubling times for these tumors varied from 25 to 100 days. Comparable times for complete response were present in both clinical and experimental induction therapy. The mean time to complete response varied from 23 to 65 days for 3924A, in which varying radiation dose-per-fraction schedules were combined with chemotherapy.

This section relates to the complete response of experimental and human cancer after induction therapy. Therefore, objectives of the section relate to therapeutic strategies that will permit the most effective use of both chemotherapy and radiotherapy during induction therapy. Because complete tumor response is a prerequisite for cure, it is of primary importance in clinical studies designed to achieve this objective.

Considerable interest has been directed toward the question of tumor repopulation during and after treatment. This occurs in

Table 4–6. The Time for Minimum Tumor Volume (T_{min}) and Maximum Tumor Growth Rate (T_{max}) in Man and Experimental Animals After Radiotherapy and Chemotherapy

I. Primary Solid Tumors

Treatment	3924A		H-4-II-E	
	T_{min}(days)[1]	T_{max}(days)[2]	T_{min}(days)[1]	T_{max}(days)[2]
A. Rats				
5-FU (50–200 mg/kg)	6–9	9–14	~8	~15
Adriamycin (5–10 mg/kg)	6–11	14–16	5–9	12–17
Cyclophosphamide (50–250 mg/kg)	5–10	14–16	7–8	11–14
Single dose radiation (750–4000 cGy)	7–11	13–23	5–9	9–16

II. Primary and Metastatic Lung Tumors[3]

Treatment	T_{min}(days)	T_{acc}(days)[4]
B. Man Single dose radiation (300–700 cGy)	5–10	8–40
C. Dogs Single dose radiation (150–300 cGy)	5–6	5–15
D. Mice Single dose radiation (210 cGy)	~2	~3

[1]T_{min}: Time of tumor volume minimum post treatment (days).
[2]T_{max}: Time of tumor growth rate maximum immediately following T_{min}.
[3]H.A. van Peperzeel, European Journal of Cancer 8:665–675, 1972.
[4]T_{acc}: Time interval of accelerated growth following T_{min}.

cancers that have been unsuccessfully depopulated. Trott and Kummermehr (69) have indicated that an independent estimate of the repopulation potential of human tumors can be gained from the latency time to local recurrence after potentially curative radiotherapy. The method is based on the assumption that postirradiation subclinical growth is not much different from proliferation during radiotherapy.

It has been proposed that **potential tumor volume doubling time** (T_{pot}) might be better than actual tumor volume doubling in the clinical assessment of tumor regrowth (69–71). Potential doubling time is derived from the labeling index and the duration of S-phase (T_S). The difference between the actual doubling time derived from serial determinations of tumor volume changes and the potential doubling time is the cell loss factor. The high cell loss fractions of 90 to 99% that have been reported for many human cancers suggest that minor errors in the determination of the labeling index may have resulted in major errors in estimating the potential doubling times (71). In addition, the large variation in the labeling indices found within and between tumors introduces another major source of error in the accurate and reproducible estimates of potential volume doubling times before, during, and after treatment in clinical studies. Repeated determinations of tumor labeling indices in the same patient are not feasible at present for large-scale clinical studies. Most human tumors are not readily accessible for repeated sampling. Begg et al (72) described a method for determining T_S from a single biopsy using in vivo labeling with bromodeoxyuridine (BrdUrd) and flow cytometry. Wilson et al (73) recently demonstrated the potential advantage of this single biopsy technique in a report on three human tumors. The usefulness of this technique in selecting a particular radiotherapy schedule for a particular patient will await the data currently being gathered on a range of tumor types so that correlations can be made with

Table 4–7. Time From Beginning of Induction Therapy to Beginning of Complete Response (Days)

SECSG[1] Protocol Number Treatment[4]	Solid Tumor Type	Tumor Volume Doubling Times[2] (Days)	Number of Complete Resonders[3]	Median Time to Complete Response[3] (Days)
78 GU 240 ABV	Testicular Cancer	25	203	66
78 LUN 328 CAV + RT	Limited Extent Small Cell Lung Cancer	40	38	47
79 LUN 252 CAV	Extensive Small Cell Lung Cancer	40	26	40
77 MEL 312 A, ACT, AMP C and M	Malignant Melanoma	42	7	30
78 SAR 327	Metastatic Sarcoma	45	Only 2 CRs	44 and 77
77 BRE 324 CAF	Metastatic Breast Cancer	90	Only 2 CRs	35 and 66
78 LUN CAMF	Nonsmall Cell Lung Cancer	100	5	73

[1]Southeastern Cancer Study Group
[2]Emil Frei III, Design of Models for Testing Cancer Therapeutic Agents, Van Nostrand Reinhold Co., New York, 1981.
[3]Data courtesy of Dr. A.A. Bartolucci, Director, SECSG Statistical Center.
[4]Treatment abbreviations as follows: A—Adriamycin; ACT—Actinomycin; AMP—Amphotericin, B—Bleomycin; C—Cyclophosphamide; F—Folinic Acid; M—Methotrexate; V—Vincristine; RT—Radiotherapy.

other characteristics of the tumors and response to treatment.

Efforts are currently under way in cancer centers to test the relationship between the inherent radiosensitivity of human tumor cells measured in primary or early passage cultures and the response of the individual patient's tumor to radiation therapy (74). The intrinsic radiosensitivity of human tumor cell cultures correlates with the clinical radiosensitivity of several different tumor histologies, as evidenced by analyses of low-dose parameters of radiation survival curves generated from a large number of cell lines (75). Such radiosensitivity has therefore served as a basis for attempts to develop predictive assays of tumor radiocurability. Peters (76) has pointed out that the majority of prognostic factors are empiric rather than mechanistic and have been determined by retrospective analysis of factors influencing the outcome of treatment. Such prognostic indicators can be powerful and accurate predictors of radiation response, but because they are empiric, they simply predict a favorable or unfavorable treatment outcome while offering no prima facie basis for selecting possible superior alternative treatments. Peters further states that the prognostic factors determining the probability of tumor control in any given patient are multifactorial. It is not unreasonable, however, to expect that cellular radiosensitivity and other radiobiologically based predictive assays will refine the discrimination of existing prognostic factors and, more importantly, offer a means of selecting patients on a rational basis for appropriate trials of new treatment strategies. At present, this method is not ready for generalized clinical utilization.

The potential for noninvasive methods for repeated assessment of tumor volume changes is discussed below, in view of the current limitations of these methodologies for clinical studies in general. The rate of growth in solid tumors is inversely proportional to tumor volume. It has been demonstrated in the UVA experimental studies that large doses of either radiation or CP will result in a latent period followed by well-defined periods of accelerated tumor growth. These experimental results suggest potentially exploitable clinical possibilities. Changes in growth rates for some human tumors may be calculated from repeated noninvasive determinations of tumor volume using tumor-imaging techniques. This could provide quantitative assessment of therapeutic response as well as a sensitive method of continuous monitoring during the course of treatment. If well-defined periods of maximum tumor growth rate occur clinically as in the UVA experimental results, there is the potential for increasing the therapeutic effectiveness by giving the second modality at the time of maximum tumor cell proliferation induced by the previous modality.

Clinical Aspects

The successful treatment of Stage IIIB Hodgkin's disease represents a major clinical advance in the effective utilization of chemotherapy and radiotherapy in cancer management. At Stanford University in 1979, Hoppe et al (77) obtained a complete response rate of 87% from alternating chemotherapy and radiotherapy in patients with extensive Hodgkin's disease. In 1984, Halberg (78) presented a follow-up of the Stanford study and concluded that alternating chemotherapy and radiotherapy was superior to either chemotherapy alone, radiotherapy alone, or split-course chemotherapy and radiotherapy. Our experimental studies are consistent with the basic clinical tenets that have evolved from these clinical studies.

The results of the clinical protocols at Stanford University with MOPP and radiation in the clinical management of patients with Stage IIIB Hodgkin's disease were updated by Hoppe, Horning, and Rosenberg in 1985. Patients treated with total lymph node irradiation (TLI) alone had a very poor outcome—only 15% longterm disease-free survivors (56). Giving both modalities together resulted in excessive toxicity —over 50% of the patients treated with TLI followed by MOPP were longterm disease-free survivors. This result, however, is little better than could be expected after treatment with MOPP alone. In contrast, the alternating program of chemotherapy and radiotherapy has proven superior to these other approaches, with 76% of these patients having longterm disease-free survival. The UVA experimental results have demonstrated the critical importance of the intensity of the delivery of the first two courses of treatment. Clinical results have confirmed that the first two courses are the most important. For example, Henkelman, Hagemeister, and Fuller, at the M.D. Anderson Hospital and Tumor Institute, have demonstrated that only two cycles of MOPP and radiotherapy for Stage IIIB Hodgkin's disease are as effective as more extensive treatment.

The clinical data of Tubiana, Arriagada, LeChevalier, and their associates at the IGR (19,23–24) were developed simultaneously but independently from the experimental studies at UVA. Their clinical use of alternating radiotherapy and chemotherapy was based on two clinical observations. For lung cancer and other solid tumors, longterm results obtained with concomitant or sequential regimens have been disappointing, and high toxicity has resulted from concomitant administration of the two modalities. The

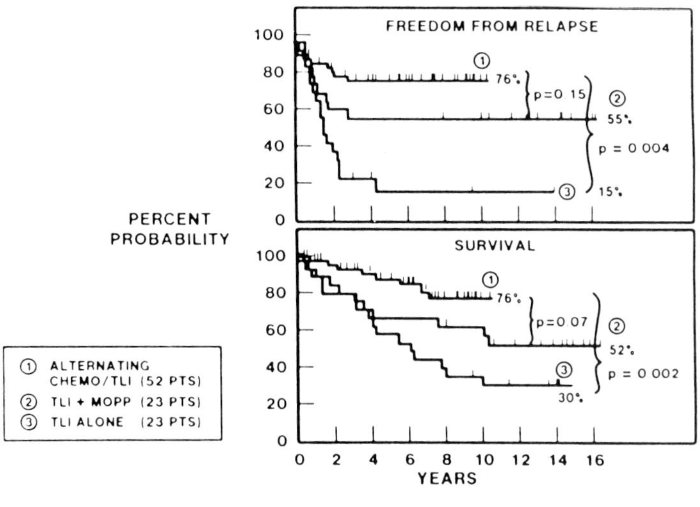

Fig. 4–9. Longterm relapse-free and actuarial survival for patients with Stage IIIB Hodgkin's disease treated with total lymphatic irradiation (TLI), TLI with MOPP given sequentially, and alternating chemotherapy and TLI. (From Halberg FE, et al. Int J Radiat Oncol Biol Phys 10(suppl 2):105, 1984, Pergamon Press Ltd.)

poor results suggested a low efficacy, probably related to a high tumor repopulation or to early development of chemoresistance. The basic concept of this new alternating chemotherapy/radiotherapy regimen was to maintain the chemotherapy schedule, so that any reduction in its effectiveness would be avoided, and to add other agents without cross-resistance to it as early as possible. After a few unsuccessful attempts, a schedule was used in which courses of radiotherapy were delivered in the middle of the traditionally long rest period of 3 to 4 weeks between successive courses of chemotherapy. A relatively large amount of radiotherapy could be given between courses of chemotherapy without changing the chemotherapy schedule. This also allowed a recovery period between modalities of nearly a week in which no therapy was delivered. The clinical data from IGR show that the alternating regimen produces an excellent complete response rate of 79% and a five-year relapse-free survival rate of 16% in limited small cell lung cancer. Therefore, current clinical and experimental results indicate that the alternating chemotherapy/radiotherapy approach offers considerable potential for substantial improvement in cancers responsive to both treatment modalities.

FUTURE PROSPECTS FOR ALTERNATING CHEMORADIATION

The results of both clinical and experimental studies bring into much sharper focus the need to concentrate on giving treatment with both modalities with the greatest intensity possible during the first two courses of induction therapy. This underscores the possibility for substantial improvement in cancer management by utilizing new approaches such as alternating chemotherapy with newer delivery methods of radiotherapy (hyperfractionated or accelerated fractions), which has the potential for greater destruction of tumor within acceptable limits of host toxicity.

Two pilot studies initiated in the United States address the question of how to more effectively use chemotherapy and radiotherapy for small cell carcinoma of the lung. Johnson et al of the Eastern Cooperative Oncology Group (ECOG) have initiated a pilot study (18) of alternating chemotherapy and hyperfractionated radiotherapy for the treatment of limited-stage small cell lung cancer. Turrisi, at the University of Pennsylvania, entered 23 patients with limited SCLC in a trial from July 1984 through March 1987. Concurrent platinum (DDP) and etoposide (VP-16) chemotherapy was used with 150 cGy radiotherapy two times daily to a total dose of 4,500 cGy in 3 weeks (see Chapter 26).

The primary clinical question is whether larger amounts of chemotherapy and radiotherapy can be delivered by alternating chemotherapy with multiple fractions of radiotherapy per day than with concomitant delivery. If temporal separation of delivery (7 days) of the two modalities can achieve comparable therapeutic response with reduced toxicity, then it may be possible to increase one modality or the other until a substantial cure rate is achieved. If administering both modalities concurrently achieves a substantially better therapeutic response, even though toxicity is increased but manageable, this would be the most effective approach. A prospective randomized trial comparing these two new approaches with a conventional sequential treatment regimen is necessary to answer this question. A phase II single-arm pilot study is in progress by Mandell, Ghavimi, and LaQuagla, at the Memorial Sloan-Kettering Cancer Research Institute in children having rhabdomyosarcoma with gross residual or metastatic disease. This study provides an illustration of intensive induction therapy employing alternating intensive multi-agent chemotherapy and hyperfractionated radiotherapy. The preliminary results indicate that the mode of alternating chemotherapy and radiotherapy, as employed in this pilot study, is well tolerated. Dr. Mandell and associates conclude that the alternating regimen offers a significant improvement in protocol compliance over previous protocols using concomitant chemotherapy and radiotherapy, without any apparent compromise in local primary control or survival rates with a median follow-up suggestive of adequate elapsed time for the appearance of most relapses and deaths in advanced rhabdomyosarcoma.

Head and neck cancers fulfill the basic criteria for further studies, because extensive clinical studies have demonstrated that head and neck cancers are responsive to both treatment modalities. The following clinical protocol design is based on concepts derived from the UVA experimental results and clinical studies. The chemotherapy dose schedule was held constant and the total radiation dose was escalated until a 50% or greater cure rate was realized in the experimental studies.

Merlano et al, at the Italian National Institute for Cancer Research in Genoa, Italy, recently reported on a cooperative randomized study comparing the effectiveness of induction therapy giving radiotherapy sequentially in one arm with an alternation of chemotherapy and radiotherapy in a second arm (5,81). The complete response rate in the alternating arm was significantly better than the complete response on the sequential arm.

Saunders et al (6) and Dische and Saunders (82) have demonstrated that 5040 cGy can be delivered in 12 consecutive days (150 cGy three times daily) by giving continuously hyperfractionated, accelerated radiotherapy for the treatment of nonsmall cell carcinoma of the lung and head and neck cancers. The results of Al-Sarraf et al (2) and Martin et al (83) showed that three courses of cisplatin and 5-FU given on days 1, 22, and 43 resulted in a 46 to 48% complete response rate. The clinical protocol design shown in Table 4–8 proposes the use of these three cycles of 5-FU and cisplatin and that the chemotherapy dose and schedule be held constant in view of the high complete response rate. The three fractions (150 cGy) per day used in the Saunders et al protocol were reduced to two fractions per day in this protocol to reduce toxicity because chemotherapy is also given. It is proposed that 2100 cGy be given in each of three courses over 7-day periods, as 150 cGy/fraction twice daily (total dosage, 6300 cGy) (Table 4–8). This approach would permit total radiation dose escalation by increasing the frequency of daily fractions. All other parameters would be held constant so that a systematic assessment of increased therapeutic effectiveness with increasing total radiation doses could be obtained. For example, the total dose could be increased to 9450 cGy by simply increasing the number of fractions from two to three per day at intervals of approximately 6 hours or decreased to 3150 cGy by reducing the number of fractions from two to one per day. It should be noted that the proposed protocol permits the delivery of both radiation and chemotherapy in 7 to 9 weeks, a fraction of the 24 weeks of a conventional six-course induction regimen for chemotherapy alone. More courses of chemotherapy can be given if control of the primary tumor and metastases is not accomplished by alternating three courses of chemotherapy and radiotherapy.

The three primary therapeutic strategies for giving radiotherapy while holding the

Table 4–8. Summary of Therapeutic Strategies for Utilizing Chemotherapy and Radiotherapy in Cancer Management (Head and Neck Cancer)

(A) *Concomitant*						
1) *Continuous*						
Treatment	*First Cycle*		*Second Cycle*		*Third Cycle*	
5-FU & Cisplatin	Days 1–5		Days 22–27		Days 43–47	
Radiation	Days 1–20 ←6300→ cGy					
2) *Intermittent*						
5-FU & Cisplatin	Days 1–5		Days 22–27		Days 43–47	
Radiation	Days 1–7 ←2100 cGy→		Days 22–29 ←2100 cGy→		Days 43–50 ←2100 cGy→	
(B) *Sequential*						
5-FU & Cisplatin	Days 1–5		Days 22–27		Days 43–47	
Radiation						Days 48–68 ←6300 cGy→
(C) *Alternating*						
5-FU + Cisplatin	Days 1–5		Days 22–27		Days 43–47	
Radiation		Days 10–16 ←2100 cGy→		Days 31–37 ←2100 cGy→		Days 52–58 ←2100 cGy→

dose and time of delivery of three courses of chemotherapy constant is shown in Table 4–8. This diagrammatic representation is not intended for use in specific clinical protocols. It is shown to illustrate how future clinical protocols may be developed to answer key questions and systematically evaluate the different ways to utilize the two modalities by obtaining scientifically valid answers to these key questions.

Concomitant radiotherapy can be given either continuously in 47 days or intermittently in 50 days. If radiotherapy is given concomitantly at the beginning of chemotherapy, this would have the advantage of treatment with the greatest intensity over the shortest time period. In addition, this would minimize the buildup of cross-resistant tumor cells. The administration of chemotherapy at the beginning of treatment would also address the problem of micrometastases. The major disadvantage would be toxicity from giving both modalities together.

The intermittent administration of chemotherapy and radiotherapy given concomitantly can be given in essentially the same time as concomitant administration (50 vs. 47 days). This has the advantage of maintaining the overall intensity of treatment with periods for host recovery between courses. This has been the approach that Taylor et al have used (7,80). However, toxicity is encountered in the management of head and neck cancer, which results from giving the two modalities together on an intermittent basis.

Sequential administration of chemotherapy and radiotherapy would have the least toxicity. However, the time for delivery of both modalities is increased to 68 days, compared to 47 days when given together (Table 4–8). The reduction in the overall intensity of treatment would reduce the effectiveness of therapy. In addition, giving all of the chemotherapy first would increase the possibility of the buildup of chemoresistant tumor cells.

Alternating chemotherapy and radiotherapy could be given with a small reduction in the intensity of delivery of the two modalities. The treatment could be given in 58 days, as opposed to 47 and 50 days for the concomitant administration of chemotherapy and radiotherapy given either continuously or intermittently. It would have similar advantages as concomitant administration with regard to minimizing the buildup of cross-resistant tumor cells and the management of micrometastases. It would also have the advantage of reduced toxicity by not giving chemotherapy and radiotherapy together as well as periods of no treatment with either modality to reduce host toxicity. A more conservative plan, recently proposed to reduce toxicity, increased the chemotherapy cycle from 21 to 28 days (53). If the patients can tolerate this regimen, then it would be possible to increase the intensity of delivery of treatment by reducing the cycle to 21 days as proposed here (see Table 4–8).

Clinical studies employing new concepts such as the concept of alternating chemotherapy and radiotherapy, which evolved from clinical studies at the Institute Gustave Roussy and experimental studies at UVA, can benefit from the Goldie-Coldman hypothesis, the concept of dose intensity proposed by Hryniuk, and the ability to assess the interrelationship of treatment on the host and tumor by the response surface methodologies devised by Carter.

Tumor depopulation and repopulation before, during, and after treatment have been assessed by multiple independent methods in well-defined experimental solid tumor systems. Information gained from the assessment of changes in tumor growth rates by biochemical, autoradiographic, and biomathematical methods and changes in total tumor cell number by biochemical and biomathematical methods has provided data for the development of experimental protocols to assess the use of chemotherapy and radiotherapy. These results have provided the necessary information to design protocols to transform an untreatable solid tumor with either modality alone to a successfully treatable solid tumor (cure rates of 50% or greater) by the more effective use of both modalities in induction therapy. Multiple methods of assessing depopulation and repopulation should provide a more comprehensive picture of the changes that occur in humans before, during, and following treatment.

Future clinical investigations designed to determine the most effective way of utilizing chemotherapy and radiotherapy should first establish that the cancer is clinically responsive to each modality. Then, it will be necessary to determine by clinical studies the greatest therapeutic index that can be attained by determining the maximum therapeutic effectiveness within acceptable limits of host toxicity.

REFERENCES

1. Looney WB. Special lecture: Alternating chemotherapy and radiotherapy. NCI Monogr 6:85, 1988.
2. Al-Sarraf M, Kish J, Ensley J, Tapazoglou E. Combined modality therapy in patients with locally advanced squamous cell carcinoma of the head and neck: Wayne State University (WSU) experience. *In:* Neo-Adjuvant Chemotherapy. Jacquillat C, Weil M, Khayat D (Eds). Paris, John Libbey Eurotext Ltd, 1988, p. 67.
3. Leyvraz S, Bernasconi S, Capasso P, et al. Accelerated treatment with alternating hyperfractionated radiotherapy and chemotherapy of advanced, inoperable squamous cell carcinoma of the head and neck. *In:* Neo-Adjuvant Chemotherapy. Jacquillat C, Weil M, Khayat D (Eds). Paris, John Libbey Eurotext Ltd, 1988, p. 71.
4. Looney WB, Hopkins HA. The experimental basis of new strategies in combining chemotherapy and radiotherapy. *In:* Combined Radiotherapy And Chemotherapy In Clinical Oncology. Horwich A (Ed). London, Edward Arnold, 1992, p. 23.
5. Merlano M, Grimaldi A, Benasso M, et al. Neoadjuvant chemotherapy versus alternating chemo-radiotherapy in head and neck cancer. *In:* Neo-Adjuvant Chemotherapy. Jacquillat C, Weil M, Khayat D (Eds). Paris, John Libbey Eurotext Ltd, 1988, p. 333.
6. Saunders MI, Dische S, Fowler JF, et al. Radiotherapy employing three fractions on each of twelve consecutive days. Acta Oncol 27:163, 1988.
7. Taylor SG, Murthy A, Caldarelli DD, et al. Use of concurrent chemotherapy and radiation in head and neck cancer. *In:* Neo-Adjuvant Chemotherapy. Jacquillat C, Weil M, Khayat D (Eds). Paris, John Libbey Eurotext Ltd, 1988, p. 79.
8. Nissenbaum M, Browde S, Bezwoda WR, et al. Treatment of advanced head and neck cancer: Multiple daily dose fractionated radiation therapy and sequential multimodal treatment approach. Med Pediatr Oncol 12:204, 1984.
9. Fu K. Concurrent radiotherapy and chemotherapy for advanced head and neck cancer. *In:* Head and Neck Cancer. Wittes RE (Ed). New York, Wiley, 1985.
10. Wang CC, Blitzer PH, Suit HD. Twice-a-day radiation therapy for cancer of the head and neck. Cancer 55:2100, 1985.
11. Byfield JE, Sharp TR, Frankel SS, et al. Phase I and II trial of five day infused 5-fluorouracil and radiation in advanced cancer of the head and neck. J Clin Oncol 2:406, 1984.
12. Taylor SG IV, Murthy AK, Showel JL, et al. Improved control in advanced head and neck cancer with simultaneous radiation and cisplatin/5-FU chemotherapy. Cancer Treat Rep 69:933, 1985.
13. Door A, Bader J, Friedman MA. Locally advanced breast cancer: Current status and future directions. Int J Radiat Oncol Biol Phys 16:775, 1989.
14. Jacquillat Cl, Weil M, Auclerc G, et al. Results of a conservative treatment combining neoadjuvant chemotherapy and radiotherapy in 252 patients with breast cancer. *In:* Neo-Adjuvant Chemotherapy. Jacquillat C, Weil M, Khayat D (Eds). Paris, John Libbey Eurotext Ltd, 1988, p. 129.
15. Lippman ME, Swain SM, Egan EF, et al. Neoadjuvant chemotherapy in the combined modality approach of locally advanced nonmetastatic breast cancer. *In:* Neo-Adjuvant Chemotherapy. Jacquillat C, Weil M, Khayat D (Eds). Paris, John Libbey Eurotext Ltd, 1988, p. 143.
16. Rosso R, Venturini M, Michelottii A. Alternating chemotherapy and radiotherapy treatment in patients with infiltrating bladder cancer. *In:* Neo-Adjuvant Chemotherapy. Jacquillat C, Weil M, Khayat D (Eds). Paris, John Libbey Eurotext Ltd, 1988, p. 459.
17. Scher H. Neo-adjuvant therapy of invasive bladder tumors. *In:* Advances in Urologic Oncology. Williams R, Carroll P (Eds). New York, Macmillan Publishing Co., 1989.
18. Johnson D, Chairman, Lung Cancer Committee, and his associates of the Eastern Cooperative Oncology Group (ECOG). Personal communication, 1988.
19. Arriagada R, LeChevalier T, Baldeyrou P, et al. Alternating radiotherapy and chemotherapy schedules in small cell lung cancer, limited disease. Int J Radiat Oncol Biol Phys 11:1461, 1985.
20. Johnson B, Grayson J, Woods E, et al. Limited stage small cell lung cancer treated with concurrent etoposide/cisplatin plus bid chest radiotherapy. Proceedings of the American Society of Clinical Oncology, 25th Annual Meeting, 8:228, 1989.
21. Le Chevalier T, Arriagada R, Baldeyrou P, et al. Carcinomes bronchiques a petites cellules

limites. Resultats d'un protocole d'alternance de chimiotherapie et de radiotherapie chez 165 malades. *In:* Neo-Adjuvant Chemotherapy. Jacquillat C, Weil M, Khayat D (Eds). Paris, John Libbey Eurotext Ltd, 1988, p. 89.
22. Tubiana M. The 1987 Franz Buschke Lecture: The role of radiotherapy in the treatment of chemosensitive tumors. Int J Radiat Oncol Biol Phys 16:763, 1989.
23. Tubiana M, Arriagada R, Cosset JM. Sequencing of drugs and radiations: The integrated alternating regimen. Cancer 55(Suppl):2131, 1985.
24. Tubiana M. The combination of radiotherapy and chemotherapy. *In:* Treatment Modalities in Lung Cancer (Antibiotics and Chemotherapy Series). Arriagada R, Le Chevalier T (Eds). Farmington, CT, S Karger, 1988, p. 1.
25. Turrisi AT, Glover DJ, Mason BA. A preliminary report: Concurrent twice-daily radiotherapy plus platinum-etoposide chemotherapy for limited small cell lung cancer. Int J Radiat Oncol Biol Phys 15:183, 1988.
26. Feld R, Evans WK, DeBoer G, et al. Combined modality induction therapy without maintenance chemotherapy for small cell carcinoma of the lung. J Clin Oncol 2:294, 1984.
27. Arcangeli G, Righini R, Nervi C, et al. Pilot study of multiple-fraction daily radiotherapy alternating with chemotherapy in patients with stage IV non-oat cell lung cancer. Cancer Treat Rep 69:25, 1985.
28. Choi CH, Suit HD. Evaluation of rapid radiation treatment schedules utilizing two treatment sessions per day. Radiology 116:703, 1975.
29. Bleehan NM, Cox JD. Radiotherapy for lung cancer. Int J Radiat Oncol Biol Phys 11:1001, 1985.
30. Lokich J, Chaffey J, Neptune W. Concomitant 5-fluorouracil infusion and high-dose radiation for stage III non-small cell lung cancer. Cancer 64:1021, 1989.
31. John MJ, Flam MS, Mowry PA, et al. Radiotherapy alone and chemoradiation for nonmetastatic esophageal carcinoma. Cancer 63:2397, 1989.
32. Seydel HG, Leichman L, Byhardt R, et al. The Radiation Therapy Oncology Group, Preoperative radiation and chemotherapy for localized squamous cell carcinoma of the esophagus: A RTOG study. Int J Radiat Oncol Biol Phys 14:33, 1988.
33. Gastrointestinal Tumor Study Group. Prolongation of the disease-free interval in surgically treated rectal carcinoma. N Engl J Med 312:1465, 1985.
34. Papillon J. Concomitant radiochemotherapy in the management of epidermoid carcinoma of the anal canal. *In:* Neo-Adjuvant Chemotherapy. Jacquillat C, Weil M, Khayat D (Eds). Paris, John Libbey Eurotext Ltd, 1988, p. 51.
35. Mandell LR, Ghavimi F, Exelby P, Fuks Z. Preliminary results of alternating combination chemotherapy (CT) and hyperfractionated radiotherapy (Hart) in advanced rhabdomyosarcoma (RMS). Int J Radiat Oncol Biol Phys 15:197, 1988.
36. Rosen G, Marcove R, Cacavio A, et al. Osteogenic sarcoma in adults: The value of neoadjuvant chemotherapy. *In:* Neo-Adjuvant Chemotherapy. Jacquillat C, Weil M, Khayat D (Eds). Paris, John Libbey Eurotext Ltd, 1988, p. 499.
37. Goldie JH, Coldman AJ, Hopkins HA, Looney WB. A mathematical and computer based model of alternating chemotherapy and radiation therapy in experimental neoplasms. *In:* Treatment Modalities in Lung Cancer. Arriagada R, Le Chevalier T. (Eds). Antibiot Chemother 41:11, 1988.
38. Hryniuk W, Levine MN. Analysis of dose intensity for adjuvant chemotherapy trials in stage II breast cancer. J Clin Oncol 4:1162, 1986.
39. Hryniuk WM. The importance of dose intensity in the outcome of chemotherapy. *In:* Advances in Oncology. Hellman S, DeVita V, Rosenberg S (Eds). Philadelphia, JB Lippincott Co, 1988, p. 121.
40. Carter WH Jr, Wampler GL, Stablein DM. Regression Analysis of Survival Data in Cancer Chemotherapy. New York, Marcel Dekker, Inc., 1983, p. 79.
41. Looney WB, Hopkins HA, Kovacs CJ, et al. Single and combined (radiation-cyclophosphamide) modality therapy in experimental solid tumors. Adv Radiat Biol 10:305, 1983.
42. Box GEP. In discussion of: An Experimental Design in Combination Chemotherapy by N. Mantel. Ann N Y Acad Sci 909(76):931, 1958.
43. Hopkins HA, Looney WB. Interactions between cyclophosphamide and radiation. *In:* Interactions Between Antitumour Drugs and Radiation. Hill BT, Bellamy AS (Eds). Boca Raton, FL, CRC Press, 1990, p. 69.
44. Hopkins HA, Looney WB. Solid tumor models for the assessment of different treatment modalities: XXVI. Estimates of cell survival from tumor growth delay after alternating radiotherapy and chemotherapy. Int J Radiat Oncol Biol Phys 13:217, 1987.
45. Wheldon TE. Can dose-survival parameters be deduced from in situ assays? Br J Cancer 41(Suppl IV):79, 1980.
46. Withers HR, Taylor JMG, Maciejewski B. The hazard of accelerated tumor clonogen repop-

ulation during radiotherapy. Acta Oncol 27:131, 1988.
47. Looney WB, Hopkins HA. Administration of radiation or cyclophosphamide versus alternated radiation and cyclophosphamide treatment of primary tumor and pulmonary metastases. NCI Monogr 6:145, 1988.
48. Cox DR. Regression models and life tables. J R Stat Soc B 34:187, 1972.
49. Carter WH, Wampler GL, Crews SL, Howells R. On determining the levels of treatment to optimize the probability of a favorable response. Cancer Treat Rep 61:849, 1977.
50. Looney WB, Hopkins HA. Solid tumors as a model for the development of antineoplastic therapy, Methods Cancer Res 19:304, 1982.
51. Looney WB, Trefil JS, Hopkins HA, et al. Solid tumor models for the assessment of different treatment modalities: V: Therapeutic strategy for sequential chemotherapy with radiotherapy. Proceedings National Academy of Science, USA, 74:1983, 1977.
52. Looney WB, Hopkins HA, Tubiana M. Experimental and clinical studies alternating chemotherapy and radiotherapy. Cancer Metastasis Rep 8:53, 1989.
53. Looney WB, Hopkins HA. Modification of radiotherapy by radiosensitizers and cancer chemotherapeutic agents, Part II. Semin Oncol 16:176, 1989.
54. Looney WB, Hopkins HA. The relationship of experimental, theoretical and clinical studies of alternating chemotherapy and radiotherapy in the management of lung cancer. *In:* Treatment Modalities in Lung Cancer (Antibiotics and Chemotherapy Series). Farmington, CT, 5 Karger, 1988, p. 35.
55. Hopkins HA, Ritenour ER, MacLeod MS, Looney WB. The effect of varying the time between irradiation and cyclophosphamide on growth response of hepatoma 3924A. Int J Radiat Oncol Biol Phys 5:1455, 1979.
56. Hoppe RT, Horning SJ, Rosenberg SA. The concept, evolution and preliminary results of the current Stanford clinical trials for Hodgkin's disease. Cancer Surv 4:459, 1985.
57. Amdur MD, Parsons JT, Mendenhall WM, et al. Split-course versus continuous-course irradiation in the postoperative setting for squamous cell carcinoma of the head and neck. Int J Radiat Oncol Biol Phys 17:279, 1989.
58. Goldie JH, Coldman AJ, Gudauskas GA. Rationale for the use of alternating non-cross-resistant chemotherapy. Cancer Treat Rep 66:439, 1982.
59. Goldie JH. New thoughts on resistance to chemotherapy. Hosp Pract 18:165, 1983.
60. Goldie JH, Coldman AJ. The genetic origin of drug resistance in neoplasms: Implications for systemic therapy. Cancer Res 44:3643, 1984.
61. Breur K. Growth rate and radiosensitivity of human tumours. I. Growth rate of human tumours. Eur J Cancer Clin Oncol 2:157, 1966.
62. Dutreix J, Tubiana M, Wambersie A, Malaise EP. The influence of cell proliferation in tumours and normal tissues during fractionated radiotherapy, Eur J Cancer 7:205, 1971.
63. Malaise EP, Charbit A, Chavaudra N, et al. Change in volume of irradiated human metastases. Investigation of repair of sublethal damage and tumour repopulation. Br J Cancer 26:43, 1972.
64. Tubiana M, Malaise EP. Combination of radiotherapy and chemotherapy: Implications derived from cell kinetics. *In:* Lung Cancer: Progress in Therapeutic Research. Muggia F, Rozenweig M (Eds). New York, Raven Press, 1979, p. 51.
65. van Peperzeel HA. Effects of single doses of radiation on lung metastases in man and experimental animals. Eur J Cancer Clin Oncol 8:665, 1972.
66. Welin S, Youker J, Spratt JS Jr. Rates and patterns of growth of 375 tumors of the large intestine and rectum observed serially by double contrast enema study (Malmo technique). Am J Roentgenol Radium Ther Nucl Med 90:673, 1963.
67. Order SE, Klein JL, Ettinger D, et al. Phase I–II study of radiolabeled antibody integrated in the treatment of primary hepatic malignancies. Int J Radiat Oncol Biol Phys 6:703, 1980.
68. Frei E III. Models and the Clinical Dilemma. *In:* Design of Models for Testing Cancer Therapeutic Agents. Fidler IJ, White RJ (Eds). New York, Van Nostrand Reinhold Co., 1981, p. 248.
69. Trott KR, Kummermehr J. What is known about tumour proliferation rates to choose between accelerated fractionation or hyperfractionation? Radiother Oncol 3:1, 1985.
70. Parsons J, Bova FJ, Million RR. A re-evaluation of technique for squamous cell carcinoma of the head and neck. Int J Radiat Oncol Biol Phys 6:1645, 1980.
71. Fowler JF. Potential for increasing the differential response between tumours and normal tissues: Can proliferation rate be used? Int J Radiat Oncol Biol Phys 12:641, 1985.
72. Begg AC, McNally NJ, Shrieve DC, Karcher H. A method to measure the duration of DNA synthesis and the potential doubling time from a single sample. Cytometry 6:620, 1985.
73. Wilson GD, McNally NJ, Dische S, Bennett MH. Cell proliferation in human tumours

measured by in-vivo labelling with bromodeoxyuridine. Br J Radiol 61:419, 1988.

74. Brock WA, Baker FL, Peters LJ. Radiosensitivity of human head and neck squamous cell carcinomas in primary culture and its potential as a predictive assay of tumor radiocurability. Int J Radiat Oncol Biol Phys 56(5):751, 1989.
75. Fetil B, Deschavanne PJ, Debieu D, et al. Correlation between PLD repair capacity and the survival curve of human fibroblasts in experimental growth phase: Analysis in terms of several parameters. Radiat Res 116(1):74, 1988.
76. Peters LJ. The Regaud Lecture: Inherent radiosensitivity of tumor and normal tissue cells as a predictor of human tumor response. Radiother Oncol 17(3):177, 1990.
77. Hoppe RT, Portlock CS, Glatstein E, et al. Alternating chemotherapy and irradiation in the treatment of advanced Hodgkin's disease. Cancer 43:472, 1979.
78. Halberg FE, Hoppe RT, Rosenberg SA, et al. Alternating chemotherapy and irradiation in advanced Hodgkin's disease. J Radiat Oncol Biol Phys 10(Suppl. 2):105, 1984.
79. Henkelmann GC, Hagemeister FB, Fuller LM. Two cycles of MOPP and radiotherapy for stage III A and stage III B Hodgkin's disease. J Clin Oncol 6:1293, 1988.
80. Taylor SG IV, Murthy AK, Showel JL, et al. Improved control in advanced head and neck cancer with simultaneous radiation and cisplatin/5-FU chemotherapy. Cancer Treat Rep 69:933, 1985.
81. Merlano M, Vitale V, Rosso R, et al. Treatment of advanced squamous-cell carcinoma of the head and neck with alternating chemotherapy and radiotherapy. N Engl J Med 327:1115, 1992.
82. Dische S, Saunders MI. Continuous, hyperfractionated, accelerated radiotherapy (CHART). Proceedings of the 17th International Congress of Radiology. Br J Cancer 59(3):325, 1989.
83. Martin M, Hazan A, Vergnes L, et al. Randomized study of fluorouracil and cisplatinum as neoadjuvant therapy in head and neck cancer: A preliminary report. Proceedings of 17th International Congress of Radiology, 1989, p. 329.

Chapter 5

A MODEL FOR CONCURRENT CHEMORADIATION IN CLINICAL TRIALS

MADHU J. JOHN

Opinions are divided regarding the biological justification for using radiotherapy and chemotherapy simultaneously against human tumors. There is considerable experimental data from in vitro and in vivo systems suggesting that normal tissue effects are enhanced without the temporal separation of these two modalities. On the other hand, there is a growing body of empirical clinical data suggesting that concurrent chemotherapy and radiotherapy increases tumor cure rates as measured by survival with acceptable increases in adverse effects on normal tissues. In this chapter, a conceptual model of concurrent chemoradiation is presented. According to this construct, it should be the preferred method of combination of the two modalities in treating human cancers and should be subjected to verification by appropriately designed clinical trials, especially in therapy-resistant locally advanced tumors. The biological and clinical rationale for simultaneous chemoradiation will be addressed, followed by an evaluation of empirical clinical data that show increased survival with this approach.

MODEL FOR CONCURRENT CHEMORADIATION

A model for concurrent chemoradiation is described in Figure 5–1. Its origins are diverse: Steel and Peckham's treatise on the conceptual and biologic basis of chemotherapy–radiotherapy interaction (1); the Goldie-Coldman mathematical model of spontaneous mutation and their strategy of scheduling treatments (2,3); the Norton-Simon hypothesis and Day's "worst drug rule" (4,5); and the design and results of empirical clinical trials in cancers of the esophagus, cervix, and anal canal (6). For descriptive purposes, the model is divided into two sequential phases: Phase A, or induction–consolidation, and Phase B, or consolidation–maintenance. Phase B may not be required in some tumors, may be separated from Phase A by a time interval, or may be continuous with Phase A.

PHASE A: INDUCTION—CONSOLIDATION

Phase A constitutes the entire treatment course or the bulk of radiation and chemotherapy doses. Its aim is to achieve maximal broad-spectrum tumor cell kill in a heterogenous primary tumor site and eradicate subclinical micrometastases at other sites. It generally lasts over a 4- to 5-week period unless the intensity of radiotherapy and/or chemotherapy and its resultant toxicity necessitate a split in the treatment course.

Radiotherapy

Daily doses greater than 180 cGy are generally not tolerated in concurrent chemoradiation. Total doses of 3600 to 4500 cGy over a 4- to 5-week period are usually well tolerated without interruption at most tumor sites. In others, total doses of > 6000 cGy are possible. If necessary, reduced fields may be used at the 3000 or 3600 cGy level for some and at higher doses for others. Hyperfractionation (120 to 150 cGy twice daily) may be attempted over part or all of this phase of treatment to achieve a larger nominal dose. As a strategical means of achieving late intensification (explained

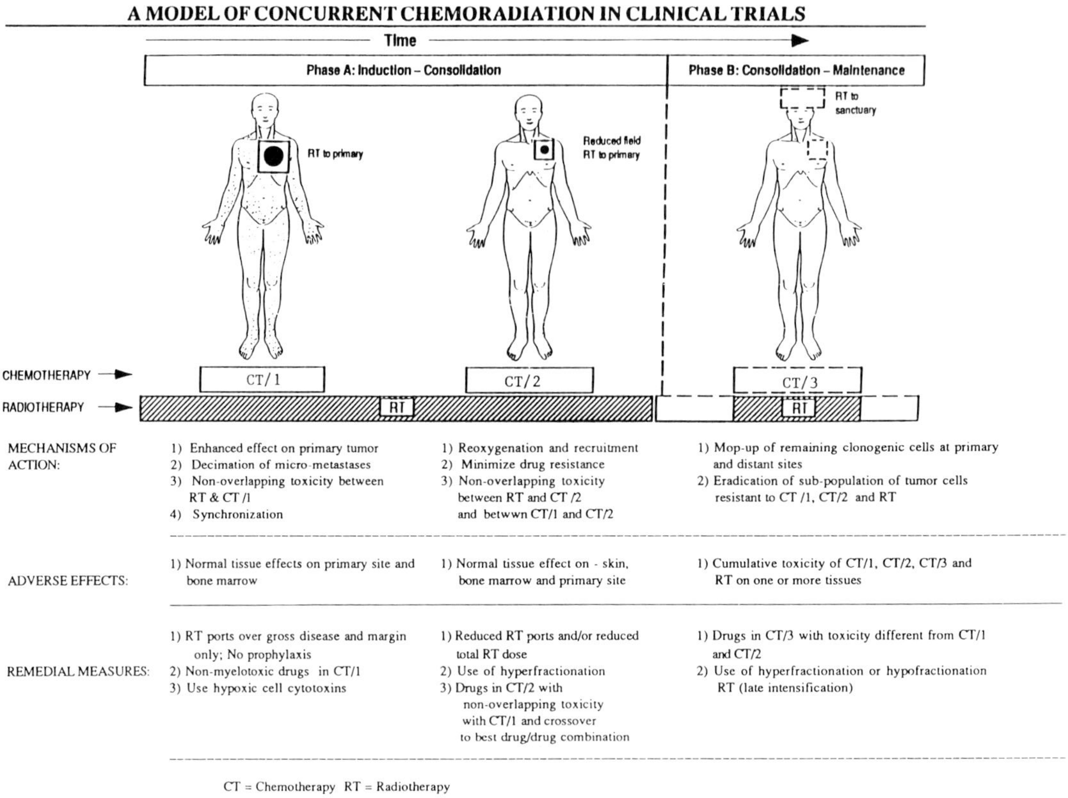

Fig. 5–1.

later in this chapter), hyperfractionation is preferably given over the last week or weeks of Phase A. Accelerated fractionation (180 cGy to 200 cGy twice daily) or hypofractionation (600 to 250 cGy in one to four fractions, respectively, per week) has not been attempted previously with concurrent chemotherapy (with the exception of malignant gliomas) and is likely to decrease the therapeutic ratio.

The radiotherapy (RT) field covers only aggregates of tumor, such as the primary tumor site and enlarged lymph nodes, with minimal margins. No attempt is made to cover subclinical potential disease sites unless no active chemotherapeutic agent is available for use in this phase of treatment. For example, the supraclavicular nodal area is not to be covered by the radiotherapy field in primaries of the middle and lower third of the esophagus unless palpable nodes are present in that region. This reduces the volume of pulmonary tissue that is prone to radiotherapy–chemotherapy interaction and toxicity. Whenever possible, RT fields should be reduced to conform to the reducing primary tumor.

Chemotherapy

In general, as many drugs as can be used without compromising (due to acute toxicity) the total RT dose to be given during this phase of treatment should be administered. In practical terms, two or three cycles of combination chemotherapy are delivered during this induction–consolidation phase of therapy (CT/1 and CT/2). Depending on the number of drugs in each combination, the dose of each drug should be reduced to one-third to two-thirds of the normal dose when the drug is administered with concurrent radiotherapy.

Choice of Drugs

In terms of function, two general types of drugs are available for use against most human tumors; both should be exploited if possible.

The first category includes those with proven clinical activity against the tumor in question. Their mechanism of action in relation to radiotherapy may be by enhancement, including additive, subadditive, or supra-additive effects. (See Chapter 2 for definitions of these terms.) An example of this group of drugs would be 5-fluorouracil (5-FU) + mitomycin C in cervical cancer. Both drugs exhibit moderate activity against cervical cancers; while 5-FU enhances radiotherapy effect with supra-additivity, mitomycin C interacts by simple additivity. However, this category of drugs may not interact with radiotherapy at all (or very little) at the RT target site. In this case, their mechanism of interaction may be by spatial cooperation or independent action, including toxicity independence (7,8). As part of the late intensification process, these drugs are usually reserved for use in the latter part of Phase A (or in Phase B).

The second category of drugs that are used in Phase A include those that enhance or increase radiation effect by sensitization without significant activity against the specific tumor. An example of this type of drug would be 5-FU in lung cancer.

A third category of drugs that may be used in Phase A of the model would interact by enabling larger overall doses of radiotherapy or chemotherapy to be used, e.g., the radioprotector WR-2721 (see Chapter 45). In addition, others may allow for a continuous (rather than a split) course of chemoradiation. For example, granulocyte-macrophage colony-stimulating factor (GM-CSF) may negate the need for a treatment split required by myelotoxicity. In general terms, this category of drugs should not be used if their toxicity overlaps with the drugs from either of the first two categories. Also, they are preferably delivered early in Phase A, to allow for uninterrupted radiotherapy and unmodified doses of planned chemotherapy and/or to minimize the time interval in a split course of therapy.

A fourth category of drugs that must be included in Phase A is hypoxic cell cytotoxins or bioreductive agents, such as SR-4233 and mitomycin C. Brown and Koong have shown that such cytotoxins are superior to hypoxic cell radiosensitizers when combined with fractionated radiotherapy on a tumor model with varying components of hypoxic cells (9). These agents are best given early in the first drug combination cycle (CT/1) for two reasons: metastatic phenotypes or chemoradiation-resistant variants develop from hypoxic tumor cells and their development is related to time (10); and there is some evidence that the process of reoxygenation, which is to be expected with fractionated radiotherapy, confers an increased metastatic efficiency on these previously hypoxic cells (11).

Time Sequence of Administration

The time interval between chemotherapy administration and a radiation dose or fraction may not appear important because drugs and radiotherapy are being given concomitantly in this model. However, the phenomenon of supra-additivity should be exploited whenever possible; otherwise only simple additivity would be obtained. For example, two to five fractions of radiotherapy may be given before starting a 4- to 5-day 5-FU infusion in cervical cancer, because maximal enhancement of radiotherapy takes place within the first 48 hours of 5-FU infusion following radiotherapy (12).

Mode of Administration

There is considerable in vitro and in vivo experimental data showing that infusion (rather than bolus injection) of 5-FU is required for enhancing the cytotoxicity of radiotherapy for human tumor cells because this enhanced effect is strongly dependent on drug concentration and duration of exposure with relation to radiotherapy (12,13). There are also clinical data in esophageal, anal canal, and cervical cancers showing that the combination of infusional 5-FU and radiotherapy is extremely well tolerated, particularly with regard to myelotoxicity seen following bolus injections of the drug (14–16). This comparative reversal of toxicity is particularly fortuitous, because bone-marrow depression is the single most common problem that impedes the timeliness and quantitative delivery of most chemoradiation regimens.

The need for prolonged infusion of cisplatinum in order to achieve a supra-additive effect in combination with continuous low-dose-rate radiotherapy has been noted (17). This has implications that could be utilized in combining cisplatinum and intracavitary cesium/radium applications for advanced cancers of the cervix (16).

Variation of Drug Combinations

It is recommended that as many different drug combinations as possible be used in Phase A of the chemoradiation model, i.e., CT/1 should differ from CT/2. There are three possible advantages in undertaking this measure.

1. There will be a greater chance of increasing the therapeutic ratio if the sites of primary toxicity of the drugs in CT/1 are different from those of drugs in CT/2.
2. If drugs of different types or categories are utilized in two or more cycles during Phase A, it is more likely that subpopulations in a heterogenous tumor that are resistant to one drug would succumb to another. Several drugs, such as hydroxyurea, vincristine, and 5-FU, are cell cycle dependent, with maximal cell kill in different phases of the cell cycle. Thus, if two phase-specific drugs are used during two different periods within Phase A, a variable synchronization could result, which would enhance cell kill in three different phases specific to the two drugs and radiotherapy.
3. Finally, a well-documented phenomenon of pleomorphic drug resistance exists, whereby certain cells within a tumor mutate and become resistant to several groups of drugs (cross-resistance) (3). This mutation may not be caused by the initial drug used to challenge the tumor. However, resistance is far less likely to develop if drugs from different categories or with different modes of action, are used.

Mechanics of Interaction in Phase A

The various mechanisms of chemoradiation interaction include the following.

1. An increased effect on primary tumor burden by enhancement, whether by supra-additivity, subadditivity, or simple additivity.
2. Elimination of micrometastases by independent action.
3. Nonoverlapping toxicity between various drugs and between the drugs and radiotherapy.
4. Variable synchronization by phase-specific drugs and fractionated radiotherapy.
5. Minimizing development of drug resistance.

Other possible mechanisms include:

1. Reoxygenation and recruitment: due to combining the effect of radiotherapy and drugs, reoxygenation of hypoxic and resistant subpopulations of tumor cells are likely to take place sooner than with either chemotherapy or radiotherapy alone. Cells in the resting phase (Go) are more likely to be recruited into the proliferative phases that are more radiosensitive and chemosensitive.
2. Relevant experimental work by Hill et al suggests that tumor cells mutate spontaneously to become metastatic cells when tumors reach a critical size (18). Another possibility of progressive increase in metastatic phenotypes with increasing size of tumor does exist. In either case, the delivery of multiple cytotoxic agents (drugs and radiotherapy) within a short period of time increases the likelihood that these phenotypes will not develop.

PHASE B: CONSOLIDATION—MAINTENANCE

Phase B treatment may or may not be required, depending on the tumor type. For example, delivery of 4140 to 4500 cGy of continuous radiotherapy with two cycles of concomitant 5-FU and mitomycin C chemotherapy yields over 86 to 100% disease-free cure rates in cancers of the anal canal (27). On the other hand, in advanced cancers of the head and neck region, radiotherapy and concurrent cisplatinum chemotherapy could proceed uninterrupted to a total of

7000 cGy. In early cancers of the esophagus, Coia et al report the tolerance and effectiveness of 6000 cGy of uninterrupted radiotherapy and three cycles of concomitant combination chemotherapy consisting of 5-FU and mitomycin C (28). In more advanced cancers of the esophagus, John et al require a 3-week split after 3800 to 4140 cGy of radiotherapy and two cycles of combination chemotherapy before proceeding with additional chemoradiation (29).

In general terms, however, it is preferable in the framework of this model to continue chemoradiation into Phase B without interruption but without sacrificing the preferred intensity of chemoradiation (particularly chemotherapy) during Phase A.

Radiotherapy

An additional 900 cGy to 2500 cGy may be delivered through reduced external RT ports if conventional daily fractions of 180 cGy are used. This dose is dependent on the primary tumor site and the intensity of the concurrent chemotherapy that is being given. For example, head and neck cancers require and tolerate 7000 cGy with concurrent cisplatinum only; anal canal cancers may not require this additional dose when 4100 cGy to 4500 cGy is given with concurrent 5-FU + mitomycin C (in Phase A).

In Phase B, accelerated fractionation or hyperfractionation is preferred to conventional fractionation. In some tumor types, this additional radiotherapy may be delivered in the form of intracavitary, interstitial, or intraluminal therapy, as in cervical and esophageal cancers.

It is during this phase that radiotherapy to sanctuary sites, such as cranial radiotherapy in small cell cancers of the lung, is to be delivered.

Chemotherapy

Additional chemotherapy (with or without concurrent radiotherapy) is of greater importance in this consolidation–maintenance phase of treatment. The tumor burdens at the primary and potential distant sites have presumably been largely eliminated. A fresh set of chemotherapeutic agents would eliminate most remaining tumor cells, clonogenic or otherwise, at the reoxygenated primary tumor site and subclinical metastatic sites.

By using yet another combination of drugs in this phase of treatment, there is a greater opportunity to eliminate any subpopulation of tumor cells that may have become resistant to CT/1 and CT/2. The drug that has the greatest single-agent activity against the primary tumor must always be included in this combination. In addition, the particular combination of drugs in CT/3 must be formulated with an eye on nonoverlapping of toxicity with the drugs in CT/1 and CT/2. If such a combination of drugs does not exist for a particular tumor type, the combination of drugs in CT/1 could be substituted. The potential for cumulative toxicity of this set of drugs is reduced by the time interval between delivery of CT/1 in Phase A and CT/3 (same as CT/1) in Phase B.

Mechanism of Interaction in Phase B

Virtually all of the mechanisms elaborated in Phase A may be interplayed in Phase B as well. The mechanisms of critical importance in this consolidation–maintenance phase would be those with activity against subpopulations of tumor cells resistant to treatment in Phase A, as well as spontaneously mutant subpopulations that may have formed during the life cycle of the tumor cells.

The mechanism of reoxygenation of hypoxic and resistant tumor cells into sensitive and proliferative phase cells would also be important but less critical in this consolidation–maintenance phase of the model.

RATIONALE

Theoretical Advantages

It is generally agreed that, except for its potentially unacceptable cumulative toxicity, the use of concurrent radiotherapy and chemotherapy would be advantageous in the treatment of locally advanced cancers that are not amenable to treatment by either modality alone. The advantages for such an approach would be the potential to achieve *maximal tumor-cell kill in the shortest period of time.*

The desire to minimize tumor burden is paramount because of the well-documented relationship between tumor mass and curability of human malignancies (19,20). The reasons that this goal of minimal tumor burden must be achieved within the shortest period of time are varied: the natural history of experimental tumors as a function of time is characterized by increases in tumor burden, the development of drug-resistant or radioresistant subpopulations within a tumor, and an increased rate of metastatic phenotypes (based on the hypotheses of either the mutational or nonmutational origin of metastases) (3,20–22).

Based on the somatic mutation theory, Goldie et al proposed a strategy of combining noncross-resistant drugs in alternating treatment schedules (3). The work of Hill et al suggested that tumors reach a critical size or volume before "explosively" generating metastatic phenotypes (18). Goldie considered the development of such phenotypes analogous to that of drug-resistant, (and therefore radiation-resistant) mutants from a tumor that had reached the critical or threshold size (23). In a nonmutational scenario, the metastatic variant would gradually increase in number as the tumor grew larger. In either case, it can be seen that, according to the Goldie-Coldman hypothesis, the critical need is for maximal tumor kill within the least amount of time (maximum kill, least time) so that metastatic phenotypes or chemoradiation-resistant phenotypes do not develop. The concurrent use of chemotherapy and radiation fulfills the dual aspects of this necessity.

The Norton-Simon hypothesis stated that the rate of tumor regression was directly related to the chemotherapy/radiation dose and the growth rate of the tumor prior to any treatment (4). Hence, in a heterogenous tumor, the slower-growing clones of cells would be smaller in number and more resistant than faster-growing clones. According to Day's "worst drug rule," the worse or less effective drug (A) should be used initially for a relatively prolonged period to decrease or eliminate the faster-growing, relatively sensitive clones. The more "effective" drug (B) would then be effective in eliminating the slow-growing resistant clones (5). Norton and Day have provided a mathematical prediction of cure rates for various permutations of drugs A and B (Table 5–1) (5). It can be seen that the increased use of the worse drug (A) provides the maximal tumor

Table 5–1. Cure rates for selected treatment schedules, where A is "Worst Drug"—An illustration of Day's "Worst Drug Rule"

Drug Cumulative Dose		Schedule		Cure Rate When	
A	B			A and B Are Symmetric	A Is Worse
12	0	12A	(AAAAAAAAAAAA)	0.0003	0.0003
9	3	9A3B	(AAAAAAAAABBB)	0.15	0.15
9	3	[3AB]	(AAABAAABAAAB)	0.23	0.23
9	3	[B3A]	(BAAABAAABAAA)	0.40	0.39
9	3	3B9A	(BBBAAAAAAAAA)	0.41	0.39
6	6	6A6B	(AAAAAABBBBBB)	0.32	0.22
6	6	[3A3B]	(AAABBBAAABBB)	0.44	0.20
6	6	[AB]	(ABABABABABAB)	0.52	0.15
6	6	Comb.*	(A/2 + B/2 × 12)	0.62	0.12
6	6	[BA]	(BABABABABABA)	0.52	0.10
6	6	[3B3A]	(BBBAAABBBAAA)	0.44	0.09
6	6	6B6A	(BBBBBBAAAAAA)	0.32	0.08
3	9	3A9B	(AAABBBBBBBBB)	0.41	0.01
3	9	[A3B]	(ABBBABBBABBB)	0.40	0.005
3	9	[3BA]	(BBBABBBABBBA)	0.23	0.002
3	9	9B3A	(BBBBBBBBBAAA)	0.15	0.001
0	12	12B	(BBBBBBBBBBBB)	0.0003	0.0003

*Combination chemotherapy: half the dose of A and B together in each course.

(Reprinted with permission from Norton L, et al. *In:* Important Advances in Oncology 1991. Devita VT, Hellman S, Rosenberg SA (Eds). Philadelphia, JB Lippincott, 1991, p. 57.)

cell kill. When the two drugs A and B are more or less equal in effectiveness, the simultaneous schedule of A + B at reduced doses provides the best results—at least 10% over the alternating schedule and 20% over the sequential schedule.

In addition, concurrent chemoradiation would be an alternative strategy to avoid cosmetic or functional deficits of surgery in certain anatomical areas (head and neck, lower gastrointestinal tract) or to avoid surgery at sites where considerable operative mortality is expected (esophagus).

The Extrapolation of Experimental Models to Clinical Practice

The theoretical advantages of concurrent chemoradiation notwithstanding, several investigators, such as Tubiana, Fu, and Looney, have advocated the temporal separation of the two modalities in clinical studies (24,25,26). Their position was primarily based on experimental studies on normal tissue responses. Moreover, most of these experimental data on normal tissue responses were based on single doses of radiotherapy and chemotherapy, in contradistinction to clinical practice, in which both modalities are administered in fractionated doses—specifically to ameliorate the normal tissue response.

There is also considerable skepticism regarding the validity of the actual model systems used in experimental studies of combining radiotherapy and chemotherapy. The major discrepancies between these systems and human tumors include vast differences in blood supply and cell heterogeneity. Even in the realm of late normal tissue effects, no satisfactory animal model systems exists that may be extrapolated readily to humans (27,28).

There are several (at least six) ways in which chemotherapy could interact with radiotherapy on the cellular level. There are an equal number of factors that influence their combined effect on the clinical level, including drug and radiation dose, fractionation sequence, and dose rate (8,23,25). The lack of compatible tumor and animal model systems to study the various permutations and combinations of these factors and models of interaction makes suspect the extrapolation of data from these experimental models to clinical practice.

Yet, several investigators have recommended, as clinical strategies, the neoadjuvant use of chemotherapy with radiotherapy or surgery or the alternating use of radiotherapy and chemotherapy (see Chapters 3 and 4). Their recommendations may have been modulated on the veritable certainty of increased normal tissue effects when the two modalities are given simultaneously. In doing that, they may have overlooked several strategies that could be employed to circumvent or minimize the toxicities of simultaneous chemotherapy and radiotherapy. More importantly, they may have bypassed the virtually assured probability of greater tumor cell kill with concurrent chemoradiation.

On the other hand, there may be several clinical situations in which the parameters of tumor growth and/or doubling time are such that treatment time is not critical, as may be the case in Hodgkin's disease. There may be situations in which tumor regression is highly dose-dependent. In such cases, simultaneous chemoradiation would be clearly inappropriate, because adequate doses of chemotherapy and/or RT cannot be administered without prohibitive toxicity. The use of alternating or sequential chemoradiation is then preferred. Both of these strategies are, in a way, temporally exaggerated (in accordion fashion) forms of concurrent chemoradiation.

Empirical Clinical Experience with Concurrent Chemoradiation

In 1980, several previous chemoradiation trials covering various tumor sites and carried out in a randomized, controlled fashion in the previous decade were summarized by Phillips (8). These included several pediatric tumors, such as Wilms' tumor, rhabdomyosarcoma, and Ewing's sarcoma, in which chemotherapy was used concurrently with radiotherapy as well as following it. The positive results of these trials were in the form of increased local control, decreased distant metastases, or both. In adults, controlled studies showed that various anticancer drugs given during and after radiotherapy significantly improved survival in colorectal and pancreatic cancers, as well as in malignant gliomas, advanced head and neck cancers, and small cell carcinoma of the lung.

In the 1990s, this strategy of combining chemotherapy and radiotherapy in concurrent fashion has been successively used in cancers of the anal canal, esophagus, cervix, vagina, head and neck region, bladder, and nonsmall cell cancer of the lung (refer to respective chapters). Several of these clinical trials have been pilot or uncontrolled studies. However, the sheer volume and the consistency of positive results of these studies have been convincing enough that the oncologic community is unlikely to go back to the standard and unsatisfactory use of radiotherapy or surgery alone in the treatment of some of these cancers, even in the absence of prospective randomized trials. Our experience with chemoradiation in cancers of the anal canal, cervix, and esophagus were partly instrumental in the genesis of this model; they will be elaborated later in this chapter.

The acute adverse effects of concurrent chemoradiation have certainly been increased (without increased mortality), but longterm follow-up that is available in several primary sites, such as the anal canal and esophagus, has failed to show any unusual or even expected late effects. (See Chapters 21 and 25.)

On the other hand, the strategy of neoadjuvant chemotherapy prior to radiotherapy or surgery while showing improved local control has yet to show improved survival in studies involving head and neck cancers and anal canal tumors (29,30). In cancers of the esophagus, this approach has yielded improved survival in a few instances but has had no impact on the considerable morbidity and mortality attributable to surgery (31,32).

The strategy of alternating chemotherapy and radiotherapy has yielded short-term positive results in Hodgkin's disease, non-Hodgkin's lymphoma, and small cell cancer of the lung (24). The results of this approach in cervical cancers and inflammatory breast cancer are awaited (24).

THERAPEUTIC IMPLICATIONS

Reduction of Radiotherapy and Chemotherapy Dose

A profound difficulty for several investigators in accepting a concurrent chemoradiation approach to clinical tumors appears to be the reduced radiotherapy dose used in empirical clinical trials. In 1961, Kligerman felt that in the treatment of solid tumors, "doses of radiation close to tolerance are probably necessary when used in combination with chemotherapeutic agents" (33). Tubiana, while advocating an alternating drug and radiotherapy approach, commented that the two modalities "should be given up to full doses in order to be effective" (24). Such full-dose chemoradiation combinations would result in prohibitive toxicity and have been clearly shown not to be necessary in pediatric malignancies such as Wilms' tumor, neuroblastomas, some brain tumors, and in CNS prophylaxis for acute leukemias (see Chapters 17 and 38).

In point of fact, several clinical trials in cancers of the anal canal, cervix, and esophagus, in adults in whom concurrent chemotherapy and radiotherapy in reduced doses have been utilized, have shown greater efficacy in terms of increased local control, decreased distant metastases, and overall survival using reduced doses of radiotherapy and chemotherapy compared to reports using radiotherapy alone (Table 5–2). At least for anal canal and esophageal cancers, the apparent superiority of chemoradiation can-

Table 5–2. Reduced Doses of RT in Concurrent Chemoradiation Clinical Trials of Various Tumor Sites

Site	RT Dose (cGy)	5-Yr. Survival (%)	5-Yr. Survival (%) With RT Alone
Anal Canal (15,34)	3000 to 4500	70–96	58–79
Esophagus (14,39)	4500 to 5000	50*	18*
Cervix (16)	3600 external	90	28

*2-year survival
RT = Radiotherapy

not be attributed to mere compensation by chemotherapy for inadequate RT.

It is true that one might have to gradually increase radiotherapy and chemotherapy doses in a chemoradiation regimen to further boost survival rates, such as in esophageal cancer (31). In such cases, two alternative methods are feasible.

1. The alternating chemotherapy–radiotherapy approach (i.e., CT→RT→CT→RT . . .).
2. Concurrent chemotherapy and radiotherapy tempered by split course of the combination (i.e., RT+CT→Rest→RT+CT→Rest→RT+CT.

The latter alternative would be wholly consistent with the concurrent chemoradiation model. Theoretically, it should be preferred to the alternating model unless the rest period (in the concurrent model) is in excess of the doubling time of the tumor in question.

In practical terms, the duration of the rest period in the concurrent model depends on the site and intensity of combined toxicity and may vary from 0 to 21 days. For example, a complete course of adequate concurrent radiotherapy and chemotherapy can be given without a rest period in anal canal and cervical cancers. On the other hand, our experience with concurrent chemoradiation in esophageal cancers requires a 21-day split after an induction–consolidation phase of treatment (Phase A) (14).

A third variable of physician and/or patient acceptability probably exists. To take the anal canal experience again, while most patients in the series at Fresno–UCSF have not required a split or rest period due to often severe perineal dermatitis (15), the RTOG experience has been contrary. Most centers participating in a prospective chemoradiation protocol for anal cancer (#87-04) required a split before completing two cycles of 5-FU ± mitomycin C and 4500 cGy of pelvic RT*.

Therapeutic Ratio

The radiobiologic concept of therapeutic ratio (TR) has been frequently cited as the central issue in the evaluation of chemoradiation at the clinical level. It refers to acute and intermediate (not late) toxicity. The problems regarding the extrapolation of experimental data to one clinical situation has been described above. The fairly severe normal tissue reactions seen in experimental studies are generally avoidable in modern oncologic practice. Finally, since the therapeutic ratio refers to both tumor and normal cells, the probability of obtaining improved survival without altering the therapeutic ratio exists, and clinical examples of this phenomenon are available.

$$\text{Thus, if } TR_{RT} = \frac{\text{Effect on tumor}}{\text{Effect on normal tissue}} = \frac{X}{Y}$$

$$\text{and } TR_{CT+RT} = \frac{X+1}{Y+1}$$

$$\text{Then } TR_{RT} = TR_{CT+RT}$$

Anal Canal Cancer

Evaluation of several clinical trials of chemoradiation in anal canal cancer shows that acute normal tissue effects on the bone marrow and perineal skin are markedly increased compared to trials using radiotherapy alone (34,35). These effects, however, are transient and clinically manageable. The consistently superior disease-free survival rates with chemoradiation suggest, therefore, that both tumor and normal tissue effects are increased and, as a consequence, the therapeutic ratio is unlikely to have increased. Furthermore, longterm follow-up available in several reports does not confirm our fears of late effects with chemoradiation (see Chapter 25).

Esophageal Cancer

The Fox Chase experience with early esophageal cancers is an example of a chemoradiation trial showing an increased or unchanged therapeutic ratio (36). While the cure rates were superior, there was no evidence of increased esophagitis or fistula formation. The myelotoxicity, though increased, was apparently tolerable. The Leichman experience with chemoradiation is an

*John M. Personal review of RTOG records, July 1991.

example of an apparent decrease in therapeutic ratio, whereby treatment–morbidity was considered excessive and prohibitive even though no treatment-related mortality ensued (37).

Cervical Cancer

The NCOG-RTOG pilot study for advanced cervical cancer suggested that the chemoradiation used in their regimen was within acceptable limits, with a Grade 3 and 4 toxicity level of 10% (38). The external radiotherapy actual pelvic dose, however, was approximately 20% less than conventional treatment. For a true comparison of therapeutic ratios, the central dose would have to be increased by 20%, a decision that would have to be made on the basis of effectiveness of that protocol regimen. In other words, increasing therapeutic ratio need not be the central impetus in determining the specifics of a chemoradiation regimen.

Combining Chemotherapy and Surgery

The concept of combining surgery and chemotherapy (which for purposes of brevity we will term "chemosurgery") offers the ideal theoretical scenario for the management of human tumors generally resistant to conventional treatment approaches, be it radiotherapy or surgery alone or a combination of radiotherapy and surgery. This is because the substitution of surgery for radiotherapy in our model offers the certainty of decreasing tumor burden in the shortest possible time period.

On the practical side, however, a model for chemosurgery has to contend with the **operative mortality** of some surgical procedures, such as esophagectomy, the **functional morbidity** of others, such as laryngectomy, "commando" operations for head and neck neoplasms, anterior-posterior resections for lower gastrointestinal malignancies, and the inherent **inadequacy** of still others, such as pelvic node dissections in gynecological and genitourinary malignancies.

There is also the matter of locally advanced tumors that, by their anatomical extent, make adequate surgery impossible. A classic example of such disease is Stage III lung cancers, in which nodal involvement and attachment of tumors to vital structures would make surgery untenable.

SUMMARY

The advantage of using radiotherapy and chemotherapy concurrently in sensitive systems is that enhanced tumor cell kill is a virtual certainty in experimental and human tumors. The primary disadvantage of concurrent chemoradiation regimens is the possibility of increased normal tissue damage. The tactic of temporally separating these two modalities in a sequential or alternating manner is meant to increase the therapeutic ratio by decreasing normal tissue effects while not retarding the enhanced effect on tumor cells when combining the two modalities. These two alternate means of chemoradiation delivery are largely based on unsatisfactory experimental in vitro and in vivo models. Extrapolation from these data to clinical trials is therefore suspect.

A large number of empirical clinical studies with concurrent chemoradiation in locally advanced cancers of various tumor sites has been reported, showing increased survival compared to radiotherapy or surgery alone. These trials have generally showed increased but transient and acceptable acute toxicities and no outward longterm toxicities. A model for concurrent chemoradiation, based on several mathematical and biological models and these empirical studies, is presented for possible use in clinical trials for locally advanced tumors (with a high probability of subclinical micrometastases) in general and specifically for those that do not respond to local modalities of surgery and radiotherapy.

The means by which the two modalities can be combined concurrently with impunity and the advantages therein can be deduced from known mechanisms of interaction. This model offers potential methods of increasing the acceptability of normal tissue effects without relinquishing the enhanced activity of concurrent chemoradiation on tumor cells.

REFERENCES

1. Steel GG, Peckham MJ. Exploitable mechanisms in combined radiotherapy–chemo-

therapy: The concept of additivity. Int J Radiat Oncol Biol Phys 5:85, 1979.
2. Goldie JH, Coldman AJ. A mathematical model for relating drug sensitivity of tumors to their spontaneous mutation rate. Cancer Treat Rep 63:1727, 1979.
3. Goldie JH, Coldman AJ, Gudauskas G. Rationale for the use of alternating non-cross-resistant chemotherapy. Cancer Treat Rep 66:439, 1982.
4. Norton L, Simon R. Tumor size, sensitivity to therapy, and the design of treatment schedules. Cancer Treat Rep 61:1307, 1977.
5. Norton L, Day R. Potential innovations in scheduling of cancer chemotherapy. *In:* Important Advances in Oncology 1991. DeVita VT, Hellman S, Rosenberg SA (Eds). Philadelphia, JB Lippincott, 1991, p. 57.
6. John MJ, Flam MS, Mowry PA. Clinical potential of synchronous radiotherapy and chemotherapy for advanced squamous cell carcinoma. NCI Monogr 6:375, 1988.
7. Steel GG. Terminology in the description of drug-radiation interactions. Int J Radiat Oncol Biol Phys 5:1145, 1979.
8. Phillips TL. Clinical and experimental alterations in the radiation therapeutic ratio caused by cytotoxic chemotherapy. *In:* Radiation Biology in Cancer Research. Meyn RE, Withers HR (Eds). New York, Raven Press, 1980, p. 567.
9. Brown JM, Koong A. Therapeutic advances of hypoxic cells in tumors: A theoretical study. J Natl Cancer Inst 83(3):178, 1991.
10. Rice GC, Ling V, Schimke RT. Frequencies of independent and simultaneous selection of Chinese hamster cells for methotrexate and doxorubicin (Adriamycin) resistance. Proc Natl Acad Sci USA 84:9261, 1987.
11. Young SD, Hill RP. Effects of reoxygenation on cells from hypoxic regions of solid tumors: Anticancer drug sensitivity and metastatic potential. J Natl Cancer Inst 82(5):371, 1990.
12. Looney WB, Hopkins HA, MacLeod MS, Ritenour R. Solid tumor models for the assessment of different treatment modalities. XII. Combined chemotherapy–radiotherapy: Variation of time interval between time of administration of 5-fluorouracil and radiation and its effect on the control of tumor growth. Cancer 44:437, 1979.
13. Byfield JE, Calabro-Jones P, Klisak I, Kulhanian F. Pharmacologic requirements for obtaining sensitization of human tumor cells in vitro to combined 5-fluorouracil or ftorafur and x-rays. Int J Radiat Oncol Biol Phys 11:791, 1985.
14. John MJ, Flam MS, Mowry PA, et al. Radiotherapy alone and chemoradiation for non-metastatic esophageal carcinoma. A critical review of chemoradiation. Cancer 63:2397, 1989.
15. John MJ, Flam MS, Lovalvo L, et al. Feasibility of nonsurgical definitive management of anal canal carcinoma. Int J Radiat Oncol Biol Phys 13:299, 1987.
16. John M, Cooke JK, Flam M, et al. Preliminary results of concomitant radiotherapy and chemotherapy in advanced cervical carcinoma. Gynecol Oncol 28:101, 1987.
17. Fu KK, Lam KN, Rayner PA. The influence of time sequence of cisplatin administration and continuous low dose rate irradiation (CLDRI) on their combined effects on a murine squamous cell carcinoma. Int J Radiat Oncol Biol Phys 11(12):2119, 1985.
18. Hill RP, Chambers AF, Liug V, et al. Dynamic heterogeneity: Rapid generation of metastatic variance in mouse B-16 melanoma cells. Science 224:998, 1984.
19. DeVita VT Jr. The relationship between tumor mass and resistance to chemotherapy. Cancer 51:1209, 1983.
20. Tannock IF. Tumor growth and cell kinetics. *In:* The Basic Science of Oncology. Tannock IF, Hill RP (Eds). New York, Pergamon Press 1987, p. 14.
21. Schiffer LM. Cellular proliferation in tumor and in normal tissues. *In:* Principles and Practices of Radiation Oncology. Perez CA, Brady LW (Eds). Philadelphia, JB Lippincott Co., 1987, p. 56.
22. Goldie JH, Coldman, AJ. The genetic origin of drug resistance in neoplasms: Implications for systemic therapy. Cancer Res 44:3643, 1984.
23. Goldie JH. Scientific basis for adjuvant and primary (neoadjuvant) chemotherapy. Semin Oncol 14(1):1, 1987.
24. Tubiana M, Arriagada R, Cossett JM. Sequencing of drugs and radiation, the integrated alternating regimen. Cancer 55:2131, 1985.
25. Fu KK. Biological basis for the interaction of chemotherapeutic agents and radiation therapy. Cancer 55:2123, 1985.
26. Looney WB. Special lecture: Alternating chemotherapy and radiotherapy. NCI Monogr 6:85, 1988.
27. Perez CA, Brady LW. Introduction: Relevance of radiobiologic concepts in clinical radiation therapy. *In:* Principles and Practice of Radiation Oncology. Perez CA, Brady LW (Eds). Philadelphia, JB Lippincott Co., 1987, p. 1.
28. Howes AE, Coleman NC, Phillips TL, Sutherland R. Combined modality therapy using cytotoxic agents and radiation therapy. Am J Clin Oncol 11(3):304, 1988.
29. Tannock IF, Browman G. Lack of evidence for a role of chemotherapy in the routine man-

agement of locally advanced head and neck cancer. J Clin Oncol 4:1121, 1986.
30. Michaelson RA, Magill GB, Quan SH, et al. Preoperative chemotherapy and radiation therapy in the management of anal epidermoid cancer. Cancer 51:390, 1983.
31. Roth JA, Pass HI, Flanagan M, et al. Randomized clinical trial of preoperative and postoperative adjuvant chemotherapy with cisplatinum, vindesine and bleomycin for carcinoma of the esophagus. J Thorac Cardiovasc Surg 96:242, 1988.
32. Kelsen DP. Chemotherapy for loco-regional and advanced esophageal cancer. Cancer Updates 2(10):1, 1988.
33. Kligerman MM. The role of combination radiation and chemotherapy. Conference on Research on the Radiotherapy of Cancer. American Cancer Society, 1961, p. 147.
34. Hughes LL, Rich TA, Delclos L, et al. Radiotherapy for anal cancer: Experience from 1979–1987. Int J Radiat Oncol Biol Phys 17(6):1153, 1989.
35. Cummings BJ, Keane TJ, Thomas GM, et al. Results and toxicity of the treatment of anal canal carcinoma by radiation therapy or radiation therapy and chemotherapy. Cancer 54:2062, 1984.
36. Coia LR, Engstrom PF, Paul A. Non-surgical management of esophageal cancer. Report of a study of combined radiotherapy and chemotherapy. J Clin Oncol 5:1783, 1987.
37. Leichman L, Herskovic A, Leichman CG, et al. Nonoperative therapy for squamous-cell cancer of the esophagus. J Clin Oncol 5(3):365, 1987.
38. John MJ, Flam MS, Sikic B, et al. Preliminary results of concurrent radiotherapy and chemotherapy in advanced cervical carcinoma. A Phase II prospective intergroup NCOG-RTOG study. Gynec Oncol 37:1, 1990.
39. John MJ. Esophageal carcinoma. *In:* Medical Radiology. Concomitant Continuous Infusion Chemotherapy and Radiation. Rotman M, Rosenthal CJ (Eds). Berlin, Springer-Verlag, 1991, p. 247.

Section B

MECHANISMS OF INTERACTION OF SPECIFIC CHEMOTHERAPEUTIC AGENTS WITH RADIATION

Chapter 6

BASIC MECHANISMS OF RADIATION CELL INJURY

THEODORE L. PHILLIPS AND KAREN K. FU

INTRODUCTION

The effects of ionizing radiation on cells and tissues were appreciated quite soon after the discovery of x-rays in 1895 by Roentgen and the subsequent discovery and isolation of radium and its daughter products by the Curies. It was noted very early that radiation would cause reactions of the skin and complete regression of skin malignancies.

Important milestones in the application of radiation to cancer therapy include the development of higher energy x-ray tubes, artificially produced radioactive isotopes, and more recently, high-energy x-ray sources with particular emphasis on linear accelerators. The use of radiotherapy came of age with the discovery that fractionated irradiation over several days or weeks was more efficacious than single exposures and resulted in less normal tissue damage (1,2). Great strides have been made with the availability of remote loading systems for the use of artificial isotopes and the use of high-energy accelerators.

The biologic effects of radiation were not only observed in the treatment of cancer but, in the early years, through the employment of x-rays in physics experiments, in diagnostic radiology, and in industry. Chronic skin injuries, hair loss, and other effects were noted in radiation workers. It soon became evident that radiation could have marked deleterious effects on cells and tissues and that chronic exposure could lead to the subsequent induction of malignancy (3). These observations led to research by the early radiobiologists in the 1920s and 1930s using animals and plants. Discoveries included the effects of radiation on genetic makeup, the effect of oxygen on radiation sensitivity, and the pathologic effects of radiation on various organs. The development of atomic energy and atomic weapons led to a great increase in radiobiologic research during World War II and after. This work has made great strides through the introduction of cell culture techniques, cytogenetics, and molecular biology, which have allowed an increase in our understanding of the mechanisms of cell killing by radiation and the kinetics of killing and repair.

RADIATION PHYSICS

Understanding the biologic effects of radiation requires a knowledge of the way in which radiations interact with cells and tissues to produce the events that lead to cell injury (4). All radiations used in radiotherapy produce damage in cells, tissues, or tumors through their ability to cause ionization and free radical formation in the target volume. **Ionization** occurs when either charged particles, uncharged particles, or electromagnetic photons interact with cell components, including both the water and the organic molecules. Obviously, a charged particle will cause ionization on its own and subsequent free radical formation. Uncharged particles loosen charged particles from the nucleus and cause ionization. Photons interact with electrons in the atomic shell. As a result of this interaction, the electrons are ejected from their orbits and then cause ionization and free radical formation. For ionization to occur, the charged particle must have an energy of at least 10 KeV. Charged particles may be emitted by natural radioactive decay or may be produced in high-energy accelerators. Likewise, uncharged particles (i.e., neutrons) can be created in decay reactions, in atomic reactors, and in accelerators. Photons are created by bombarding a target with electrons and creating x-rays or through the natural decay of radioactive elements. Some radioactive decay releases gamma-rays rather than photons, but in terms of biologic interactions, they are similar.

Microdosimetric Distributions

The distribution of energy along the track of a particle or photon is not diffuse or uniform but is variable and focal. The track of any charged particle is composed of spurs, short tracks, and blobs of ionization. These short tracks and blobs, also called **delta rays,** and occur at the end of the electron penetration range. Thus, even with photon irradiation, absorption results in a range of energy densities from low to quite high. This mixture of ionization density is part of the reason that one apparently sees two components of injury, i.e., a repairable and a nonrepairable type. At least part of the explanation for that phenomenon will be described in depth below (5).

Initial Chemical Products

The cell may be viewed by the radiation chemist as an array of diffusing macromolecules surrounded by an aqueous solution of rapidly diffusing salt molecules of low molecular weight. Within this array, two types of effects are caused by the interaction of the ionizing particles and the aqueous/molecular system. **Direct effects** are defined as radiation-induced changes that result from ionizations causing free radical formation directly within the target molecules, i.e., the DNA macromolecules. **Indirect effects** are defined as radiation-induced changes in the critical target molecules that result from ionizations and free radicals formed in the intracellular water, which then reacts secondarily with the critical target molecules.

The initial radiochemical events in mammalian cells occur over a short time scale of approximately 10^{-11} to 10^{-10} seconds. In terms of direct effect, when the target molecule is ionized, a positively charged molecule and an electron are formed. This then decays into a target molecule containing a free radical, defined as a molecule with neutral charge containing an unpaired outer electron. Such free radicals are very reactive, have excess energy, and a lifetime of 10^{-5} seconds or less (6).

Because water molecules comprise a great proportion of the total cell mass, interactions in water play a major role in indirect lethal radiation damage. It is generally estimated that at least about 70% of injury is due to indirect action secondary to primary ionizations in water. The initial reaction includes the formation of H_2O^+ and e^-. H_2O^+ then reacts with H_2O to form H_3O^+ and the OH radical. The electron (e^-) reacts with H_2O to form H_2O^-, which then dissociates into a hydrogen radical and a hydroxyl ion. The free electron may also react with H^+ to form a hydrogen radical or with H_2O to form a hydrated electron (e^-aq). These reactions take place within small volumes over the time scale of 10^{-14} to 10^{-10} seconds. Recombination processes can produce H_2 and H_2O_2. The bottom line is that the reactions involving the interaction of water and photons yield the hydrogen free radical, the hydroxyl free radical, an aqueous electron, hydrogen, hydrogen peroxide, and the hydroxyl ion. Of these, the hydroxyl and hydrogen radicals are the most strongly oxidizing and the aqueous electron is the most strongly reducing species. In terms of producing cell inactivation, the hydroxyl radical is the most important.

It is important to understand the time scale of these basic radiochemical interactions. The initial excitations and ionizations occur over 10^{-12} to 10^{-18} seconds, and the indirect effect through water radicals occurs over 10^{-6} to 10^{-12} seconds. In contrast, removal of products such as H_2O_2 by enzymatic methods is much slower and cell death itself occurs on a longer time scale. Because of the short life of free radicals, their diffusion distance is limited and the area over which they will act is a small fraction of the total cell volume.

RADIATION BIOLOGY

Critical Targets and Initial Lesions

All eukaryotic cells retain certain common features of internal organization, in addition to specialized functions and chromosomal organizations that occur in different species, tissues, and organs. These features include a functional nucleus, a nuclear membrane, mitochondria for energy production, ribosomes for the synthesis of protein, Golgi apparatus, and secretory organelles, as well as endoplasmic reticulum and lysosomes. The cell is surrounded by an envelope consisting of a lipoprotein membrane; the integrity of this membrane is vital to the cell, and the membrane wall has complex receptor structures. The exact site of important radiation injury in the cell has been debated for many years. For a time, it was thought that enzyme damage or membrane damage was the key event. However, the multiplicity of these structures and the small dose of radiation necessary to kill a cell made it difficult to understand how damage to these structures could lead to cell death. Extremely high doses (i.e., 50,000 cGy or more) can cause instantaneous cell death through damage to cell organelles and to the ribosomes. A better understanding of the nature and function of the nucleus, the complete elucidation of the structure of DNA, and the structure and function of chromosomes have led to the understanding of the function of the nucleus and its radiation sensitivity (7).

Various probes have been used to demonstrate that the nucleus is the primary target of radiation-induced cell death. Some studies have demonstrated with short-range, heavy charged particle beams that the cross section for inactivation of the cell is similar to the size of the cell nucleus. These experiments concluded that the passage of a single heavy ion through the nucleus was sufficient to inhibit the colony-forming ability of the cell. These results have been substantiated by experiments using a particle irradiation from a polonium source. In these experiments, it was shown that up to 25,000 cGy delivered to the cytoplasm had no effect on cell proliferation, whereas small doses to the nucleus resulted in cell inactivation.

Additional experiments in which radioactive isotopes are incorporated into the DNA have given further support to the theory that *the nucleus and the DNA are the primary sites of inactivation.* Such studies indicate that the contribution of cytoplasmic damage to radiation-induced reproductive cell death is minimal. Additional recent experiments using 125-Iodine incorporated into the DNA indicate that the DNA itself is the most sensitive target in the cell if reproductive or mitotic cell death is the endpoint.

Radiation injury to the cell is generally detected by two different experimental techniques. At the microscopic level, damage to chromosomes may be detected through the study of chromosome and chromatid aberrations. At the chemical level, damage to the DNA may be detected through a variety of techniques, including ultracentrifugation, pulsed field gel electrophoresis, and neutral elution, all of which can measure the size of the resultant DNA fragments.

If one studies the structure of chromosomes, which is visible at the time of metaphase, various abnormalities can be detected that differ according to the time of irradiation relative to the DNA synthetic cycle. Damage prior to the synthesis or S-phase yields chromosome aberrations, i.e., damage to both sister chromatids. Damage that occurs after S-phase yields chromatid aberrations. Both chromosome and chromatid aberrations are thought to be due to direct or indirect radiation injury mediated through ionization first and then through free radical formation. These radiochemical lesions result in the breakage of the chromosomes and either dissociation of the broken fragments, which leads to deletions, or to misrepair. Misrepair may lead to aberrations such as translocation, dicentrics, and ring formation. Chromosomes may, of course, be rejoined in some situations and restored to a completely normal structure. Examples of chromosome and chromatid aberrations are shown in Figure 6–1. Such misrepaired chromosomes, as well as the loss of DNA caused by deletions, will not yield normal segregation of chromosomal material into daughter cells and will lead to daughter cells deficient in components necessary for the synthesis of vital proteins required for subsequent divisions. Certain aberrations, such as anaphase bridges, can actually freeze the cell in mitosis, preventing cell division.

There is a close relationship between cell lethality, as measured by colony-forming ability, and the incidence of either chromosome aberrations or translocations, which can be measured by recently developed chromosome-staining techniques (Fig. 6–2). The incidence of aberrations or translocations is related to the dose of radiation,

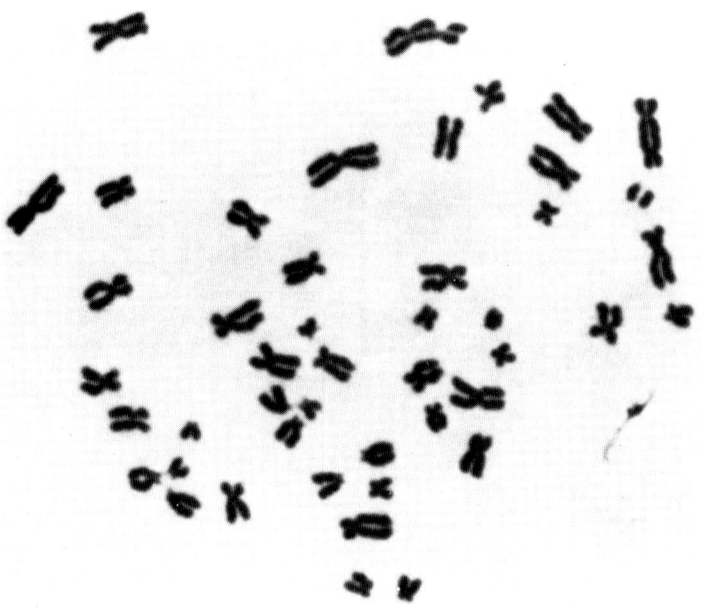

Fig. 6–1. Chromosome preparation from irradiated human leukocytes. At the top of the figure, a chromatid deletion is seen, and in the upper right hand corner, a dicentric chromosomal aberration appears. (Photomicrograph courtesy of Sheldon Wolff.)

and the exact number that will occur is also related to the nature of the radiation. Different responses occur with low-linear energy transfer (LET) photon-type irradiation, as used in conventional x-ray therapy, and with high-LET sources such as neutrons or alpha particles. The number of chromosome lesions relates closely to cell survival and is also modified in a similar way by radiation energy, oxygen concentration, linear energy transfer, and dose rate (8).

Cellular radiosensitivity also correlates with the total chromosome volume and the total DNA content. In plants, the larger the mean chromosome volume, the greater the radiosensitivity. There is a close correlation between the presence of an aberrant chromosome at the first postradiation division and the subsequent inability of the damaged cells to form a colony of more than 50 cells. The ability to form a colony of more than 50 cells is generally the definition of cell survival in a cell culture experiment. Evidence suggests that cell lethality following irradiation is secondary to chromosomal damage. The lethal event is probably an unrepaired or misrepaired double-stranded DNA break that yields a chromosome break, aberration, or translocation.

In the past 20 years, there have been major advances in the knowledge of DNA chemistry and in the nature of DNA synthesis repair processes following damage to DNA by chemicals, ultraviolet light, and ionizing radiation. DNA injury is generally classed as double-strand breaks, single-strand breaks, base damage, and cross linking. All four of these lesions can be stable and are the result of free radical formation in the DNA.

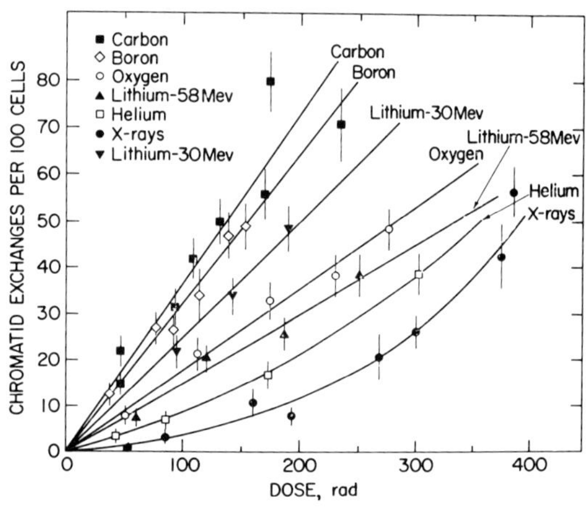

Fig. 6–2. Incidence of chromosome exchanges per 100 cells as a function of radiation dose for x-rays and various high-LET-charged particles. (From Elkind MM, Whitmore FG, Alescio T. Science 143:145, 1964; Copyright 1964 by the AAAS.)

Many studies using various endpoints have shown that ionizing radiation induces large numbers of single-strand DNA breaks that are very efficiently repaired by mammalian cells. Evidence suggests that single-strand breaks are rejoined efficiently at 37°C with first-order kinetics in less than one cell cycle, except for those that constitute a portion of a double-strand break. It can be calculated that after exposure to approximately 200 cGy, up to 50,000 single-strand breaks and approximately 40 double-strand breaks will occur. Since this dose is usually only lethal to 50% of the cells on average, it is clear that a significant number of double-strand breaks must be repaired. It is possible that 40 breaks is an overestimate and that a proportion of the double-strand breaks are repaired back to a normal state rather than misrepaired or left unrepaired. New techniques such as chromosome painting and staining, with cell analysis and flow cytometry, as well as the use of pulsed-field gel electrophoresis may allow the resolution of this question.

There are obvious interactions between the chromatin, DNA, and other components of the chromosome, including the structural proteins and the enzymes that control the coiling and uncoiling of the DNA. Additional information concerning this and the number and nature of the genes involved in repair is being accumulated each year. It is clear, however, that the lethal lesion represents an unrepaired or misrepaired double-strand break associated with or yielding a misrepaired chromosome. Such lesions are not compatible with unlimited subsequent cell divisions.

Figure 6–2 indicates the relationship between the number of chromatid exchanges observed for low- and high-LET radiations as a function of radiation doses. The shape of these curves, although inverted, compares well with the shape of cell-survival curves as determined by clonogenic assays.

Types of Cell Death

Cell death following irradiation has generally been divided into two types on a phenomenologic basis. The first is known as **interphase** or **intermitotic** death. With this type of lesion, cells become pyknotic and die before entering mitosis. This type of cell death is particularly common among some subpopulations of lymphocytes but may be seen in a number of other cell types, such as salivary gland cells.

The second type of cell death is **mitotic, proliferative,** or **clonogenic.** In this type, cells are unable to maintain continuous division, often defined as the inability to form a colony of at least 50 cells. Often, one or two mitoses undergo transversion with subsequent giant cell formation and failure of colony development. Other cells may mature, enlarge, and die without entering mitosis, but the delay indicates that this is a mitotic rather than an interphase death. This type of cell death is most important in controlling tumor cell growth; it appears that the clonogenic cells of most tumors undergo mitotic death.

The measurement of mitotic death was markedly expedited by the development of mammalian cell culture techniques in the 1950s and the subsequent development techniques for cloning tumor cells in vitro directly after radiation exposure in vivo. Mitotic death is important not only in tumors but in the regeneration of most epithelial structures, such as skin, mucosa, and intestinal lining, as well as bone marrow.

With the ability to measure cell survival using clonogenic assays (initially with bacteria and more recently with mammalian cells in appropriate medium), established cell lines, or even primary explants, it is possible to generate survival curves with various types of radiation. Figure 6–3 shows a survival curve generated for Chinese hamster cells irradiated in suspension and assayed by monolayer culture. This figure also shows the effect of oxygen concentration on cellular radiosensitivity. It can be seen that the curves have an apparent initial shoulder and do not extrapolate directly to a surviving fraction of 1.0. This shallow initial slope and the greater slope at higher doses, which occurs with low-LET radiations, has been explained by two popular theories.

The first and the longest in use is the **single-hit, multitarget theory,** which is expressed by the following equation:

$$\frac{S}{S_o} = 1 - (1 - e^{-D/DO})^n$$

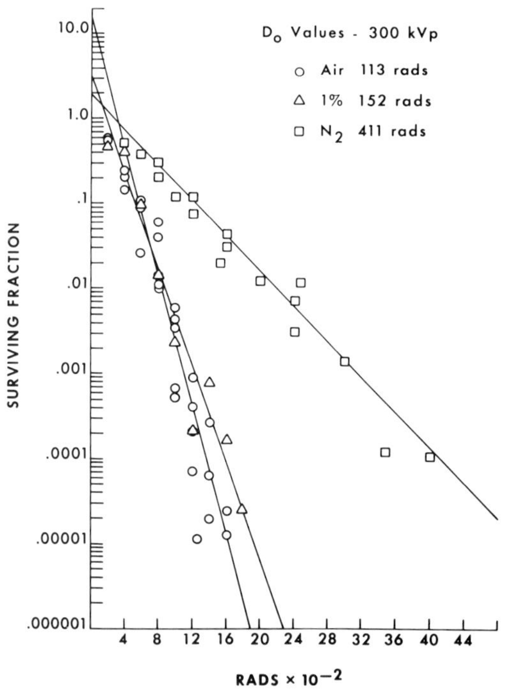

Fig. 6–3. Survival of B14FAF Chinese hamster cells irradiated in suspension and assayed by monolayer culture as a function of graded radiation doses and oxygen concentration. (From Steel GG, et al. Radiother Oncol 9:299, 1987.)

where S/S_0 is the fraction of cells surviving after a dose (D), and D_0 is the reciprocal of the slope of the terminal exponential portion of the cell survival curve. This model postulates that a finite number of targets exist within the cell (i.e., "n" targets), each of which must be hit before cell lethality occurs. Such a relationship makes the assumption that no cell kill will occur at small radiation doses. This seems unlikely, based on recent experiments that can measure survival after small radiation exposures. While this formula fits well for bacterial cells, which may have two nuclei that must be inactivated, it does not fit the preponderance of available mammalian cell data. This formula tends to underestimate cell kill at small doses (i.e., at 200 cGy per exposure as used in radiotherapy) and is driven basically by survival after large doses.

A more reasonable fit appears to occur using the **linear-quadratic theory.** This theory assumes that there are two components of damage by radiation, i.e., one that is repaired and one that is not. Irreparable damage, called **alpha damage,** is linearly related to dose and is similar to that seen with chromosome aberrations using high-LET radiations. The second component, the **beta component,** is related to the square of the dose and assumes repair. The linear-quadratic equation is written as follows:

$$\frac{S}{S_o} = e^{-(\alpha D + \beta D^2)}$$

where S/S_0 is the fraction of cells surviving after a dose D.

This equation is widely used in describing the radiobiology of cellular systems and has been applied not only to cell culture data but to in vivo normal tissue injury studies.

Cell Survival In Vivo and In Vitro

The survival of mammalian cells has been shown to be qualitatively similar, whether the cells are irradiated as established cell lines in vitro and cultured in liquid medium or agar or whether they are irradiated in situ and subsequently assayed by explantation or in vivo colony counting. It was previously thought that all mammalian cells had rather similar sensitivities, with particular reference to the single-hit multitarget theory. All cells appear to have D_0 in the range of 100 to 200 cGy and extrapolation numbers between 1.5 and 4.

As more accurate cell culture methods and particularly the ability to follow single cells are developed, it becomes clear that there is a great variation in survival at doses below 300 cGy among different cell lines. At these low doses, the alpha component in the linear-quadratic theory is dominant; thus, the initial slope of the curve will be determined by the alpha component. Cells appear to have differing degrees of ability to repair double-strand breaks; thus, their alpha values can vary widely, yielding great differences in survival after 200- or 300-cGy exposures. It is true that survival after a single dose of 1000 cGy is relatively similar among all mammalian cell lines, with the exception of ultrasensitive bone marrow stem cells, lymphocytes, spermatogonia, and oocytes. When responsive tumors are irradiated under different conditions, one can see that great variations in sensitivity are seen due to factors other than inherent cellular radiosensitivity. Figure 6–4 illustrates three survival curves for the EMT6/SF tumor. In the curve showing the greatest sensitivity, the cells were irradiated in vitro after passage in vitro. It can be seen that the initial slope and the terminal slope are steeper than the other two curves, which were obtained either with cells removed from tumors grown in vivo and irradiated in vitro or were irradiated in vivo and then assayed in vitro.

Clearly, the environment of the cell and its growth conditions at the time of radiation markedly influence its sensitivity (9). One could postulate that the EMT6 cell in vitro is in maximum growth phase—few cells are noncycling and they exhibit the greatest degree of sensitivity. Cells taken from the in vivo situation will be, in many cases, noncycling, deprived of nutrients, and in other ways rendered more radioresistant. Cells treated in vivo have the same characteristics but are also hypoxic and therefore more resistant.

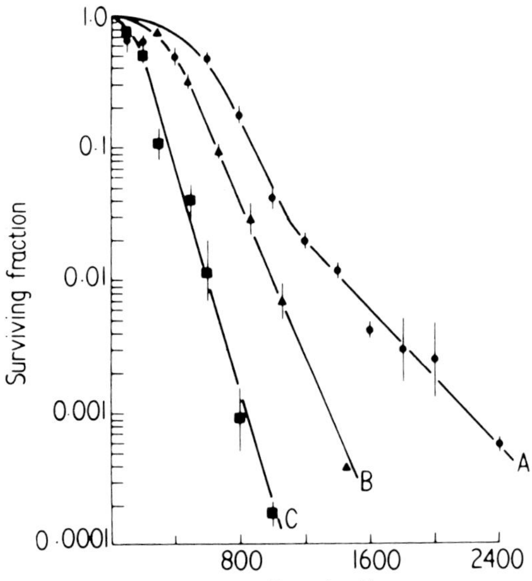

Fig. 6–4. Survival of EMT6/SF tumor cells irradiated either in vivo as flank tumors (closed circles), in vitro immediately following suspension from flank tumors (closed triangles), or in vitro after passage in vitro (closed squares). (From Fu KK, Phillips TL, Wharam MD, Jr., Kane LJ. The influence of growth and irradiation conditions on the radiation response of the EMT6 tumor. Proc 6th L. H. Gray Conf, 1974, Cell Survival after Low Doses of Radiation. Institute of Physics, Bristol Publishing Office, England, 1975, IOP Publishing Ltd.)

An important concept has been introduced recently: cell survival at low doses, particularly after 200 cGy (10,11). There is a wide variation of survival after 200 cGy among human cell lines studied. Important recent observations have been made of cells freshly explanted from human tumors. It has been shown that survival after 200 cGy varies widely among individual tumors of the same histology and among different tumor types such as the small cell carcinoma, which is relatively radiosensitive, and the melanoma, which is relatively radioresistant.

MODIFIERS OF CELL KILLING

Many physiologic and chemical modifiers have been shown to significantly change the shape of the survival curve in terms of alpha as well as beta injury. One of the most potent modifying agents is **oxygen.** The survival of Chinese hamster cells irradiated in vitro in air, in 1% oxygen, and in nitrogen has been shown in Figure 6–3. A marked change in the slope of these survival curves occurs when cells are irradiated in nitrogen, and only a slight change occurs when they are irradiated in 1% oxygen as compared to irradiation in air. This relationship is known as **the oxygen effect;** it is clear that only small quantities of oxygen are required for maximum sensitization of cells. The effect of oxygen is measured by the **oxygen enhancement ratio** (OER), which is calculated by dividing the dose required to cause a given level of survival in nitrogen by the dose required for the same level of survival in air. OERs range from about 2.1 to 3.2 in mammalian cells for low-LET radiations.

The mechanism by which oxygen sensitizes cells is of interest and may also relate to interaction of radiation and chemotherapy at the chemical level. The best accepted theory was proposed by Chapman et al and is shown in Figure 6–5. It can be seen that direct and indirect effects cause DNA free radicals, which can then be repaired by reduction or fixed by oxidation through reaction with electron affinic compounds of which oxygen is the prime example. Other chemical species have this property as well and have been explored as hypoxic cell sensitizers in clinical trials of radiotherapy.

Another major modifier of cellular radiosensitivity is **dose rate.** As discussed previ-

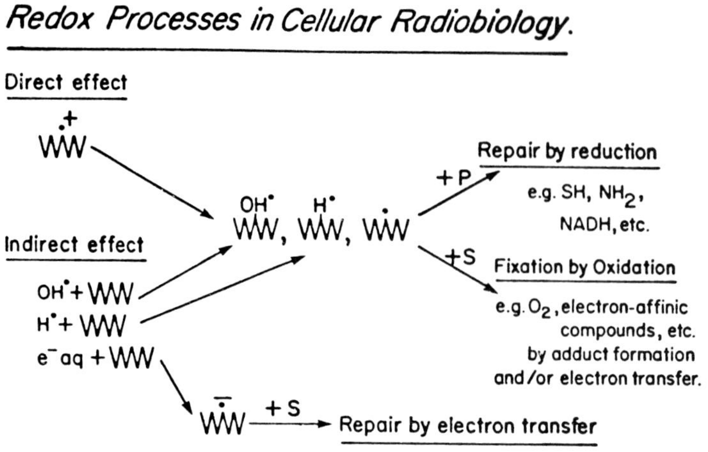

Fig. 6–5. Redox processes in cellular radiobiology. WW = cellular target molecule, P = radical reducing species, S = radical oxidizing species. (From Chapman JD, et al: Chemical radiosensitization studies with mammalian cells growing in vitro. In: Radiation Research: Biomedical, Chemical, and Physical Perspectives (OF Nygaard, HI Adler, WK Sinclair, eds). Orlando, Academic Press, 1981, p. 757.)

ously, cells are capable of repairing radiation injury by repairing single-strand breaks and, to some extent, by properly rejoining double-strand breaks. Figure 6–6 is an example of the survival of intestinal crypt cells irradiated in vivo at dose rates between 0.5 and 280 cGy per minute. Survival curves become less steep at decreasing dose rates until they

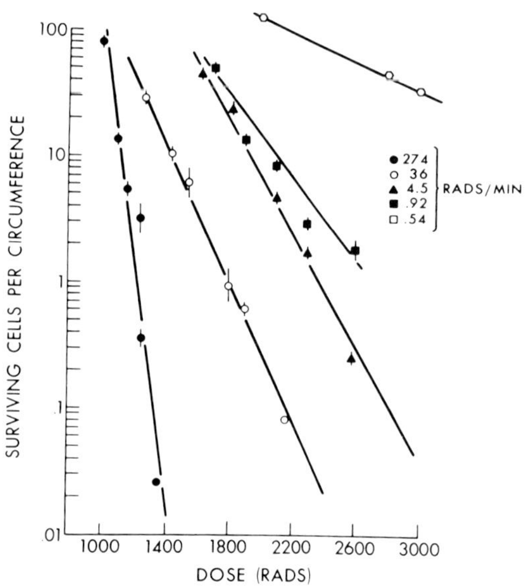

Fig. 6–6. Response of mouse jejunal crypt cells to [137]Cesium irradiation with decreasing dose rates as shown. Corrected surviving crypt cells per circumference plotted versus radiation dose in rads (cGy). (From Fu KK, Phillips TL, Kane LJ, Smith V. Radiology 114:709, 1975.)

approach the initial slope of the survival curve, as defined by the alpha term in the linear-quadratic theory.

Radiation quality can also markedly influence cell survival, as previously discussed relative to chromosome and chromatid aberrations. High-LET radiations generally yield only alpha type damage and therefore result in a linear survival curve (Fig. 6–7) for 15 MeV neutrons as compared to tumor cells irradiated in situ and assayed in vitro following [137]Cesium irradiation.

As will be discussed elsewhere in this volume, other **chemical modifiers** of radiation response exist in addition to the hypoxic cell sensitizers mentioned above. Halogenated pyrimidines incorporated into the DNA make it up to three times more radiosensitive, and when high percentages of the thymidine are replaced, the survival curves are composed primarily of alpha components. Cytotoxic chemicals may modify the sensitivity of cells by either selective killing or modification of repair and will be discussed at length in other chapters (12).

BIOLOGIC RESPONSES AT THE CELLULAR LEVEL

The cell undergoes many changes following radiation exposure. Recently, Wolff demonstrated that small doses of radiation can induce repair enzymes and make cells more resistant to subsequent irradiation. Others, beginning with Elkind et al, have shown that

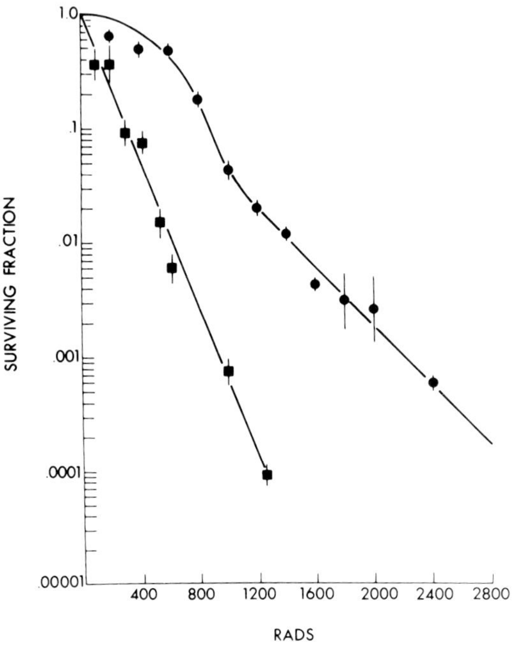

Fig. 6–7. Response of EMT6/SF tumor cells irradiated in situ and assayed in culture with ^{137}Cesium or 15-MeV neutrons in air-breathing mice. ● = ^{137}Cesium, ■ = 15-MeV neutron. (From Fu KK, Phillips TL, Rowe JR. Cancer 34:48, 1974.)

if radiation doses are divided into two exposures, a significant decrease in killing will occur as compared to a single dose of the same sum total. This can be seen at dose rates of greater than 3 cGy/min. This type of repair, termed **sublethal damage repair,** is associated with increasing survival as a function of time between doses up to a maximum time, which is generally between 3 and 6 hours. A subsequent decrease in survival may be observed in split-dose experiments due to cellular progression through the cycle and at least partial synchronization. These phenomenon are illustrated by Figure 6–8 from original work published by Elkind. Sublethal damage repair is exhibited by almost all mammalian cells, either exposed in culture or tested in vivo. A few types, such as oocytes and spermatogonia and certain lymphocytes, do not appear to show sublethal damage repair. Such repair occurs less after high-LET radiation, appears to occur efficiently during low-dose-rate irradiation, and may be blocked by certain cytotoxic chemicals and other agents.

A second type of repair is known as **potentially lethal damage repair.** This is demonstrable in cell cultures that are held under plateau phase growth conditions and denied fresh medium for a period before subculturing. Potentially lethal damage repair may be very important in tumor therapy, because it could be modified by various fractionation schemes or by chemotherapy.

Both sublethal damage and potentially lethal damage may be modified by a number of

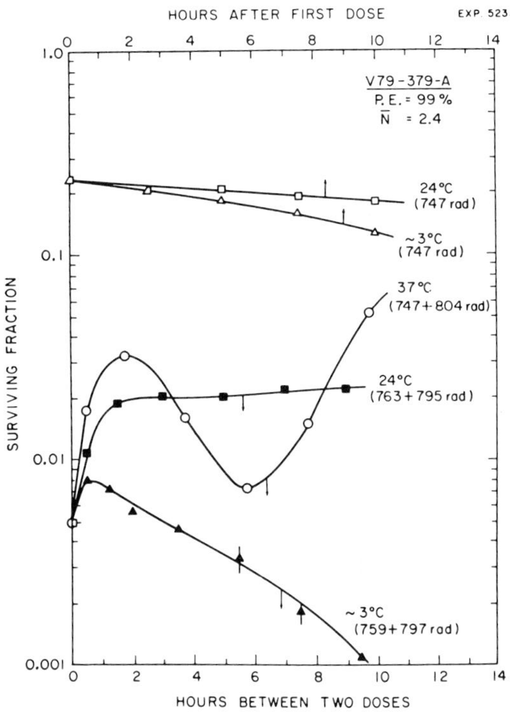

Fig. 6–8. Survival of Chinese hamster cells exposed to 2.5-MeV x-rays in single (upper curves) or split-fraction irradiations with the doses shown. Cells exposed and incubated between exposures at the temperatures shown or after the first dose only. Note that the repair of sublethal damage increases survival but that secondary decrease in survival occurs with longer intervals for the cells irradiated with two fractions at 96.8° F (37° C) because of progression through the cell cycle. Cells held at 75.2° F (24° C) do not progress and show a plateau in survival. Cell sensitivity increases with exposure to 37.4° F (3° C). (From Elkind MM, et al. Radiat Res 25:359, 1965.)

classical modifiers of radiation. Under severe hypoxia, sublethal damage repair is reduced or eliminated. With high-LET radiations, both sublethal and potentially lethal damage repair are absent.

CELL CYCLE EFFECTS

Viable cells, which are evaluated by the clonogenic assay and are subject to mitotic death, will at some time enter the cell cycle, progress from the resting or G_0 stage through the presynthetic period or G_1, through DNA synthesis or S-phase, through a postsynthetic period known as G_2, and then through mitosis. Study of cell cycle effects was initially made possible by the use of thymidine labeled with tritium. Recently, this is done more readily using halogenated pyrimidines, iododeoxyuridine (IUdR), or 5-bromodeoxyuridine (BUdR) with antibodies against DNA that have incorporated these agents, which then can be stained and evaluated using automated cell analysis or flow cytometry techniques. It is now easy, in disaggregated cell populations, to characterize the DNA as pre- and postsynthetic by labeling with halogenated pyrimidines to accurately calculate the labeling index and the potential doubling time.

Position in the cell cycle influences inherent radiosensitivity (Fig. 6–9). In general, cells that are in S-phase are most resistant and those that are in mitosis, at the G_1–S interphase, are most sensitive. Cells in mid-G_1 and in late S are most resistant. The variation in sensitivity by a factor of at least 2.5 appears to occur if one compares the sensitivity during mitosis to sensitivity in late S-phase. Both the potential doubling time and the variation in sensitivity through the cycle can be important in human cancer therapy if it is possible to irradiate the cells during the more sensitive phase of the cycle.

As intimated above, the relative potential for cells to repopulate is based on both the fraction of the population that is in cell cycle and the length of the cell cycle. It can be expressed by the term **potential doubling time** or T_{pot}.

The potential doubling time will not necessarily describe the actual observed growth of the tumor, because a second major influence on observed tumor volume is the cell

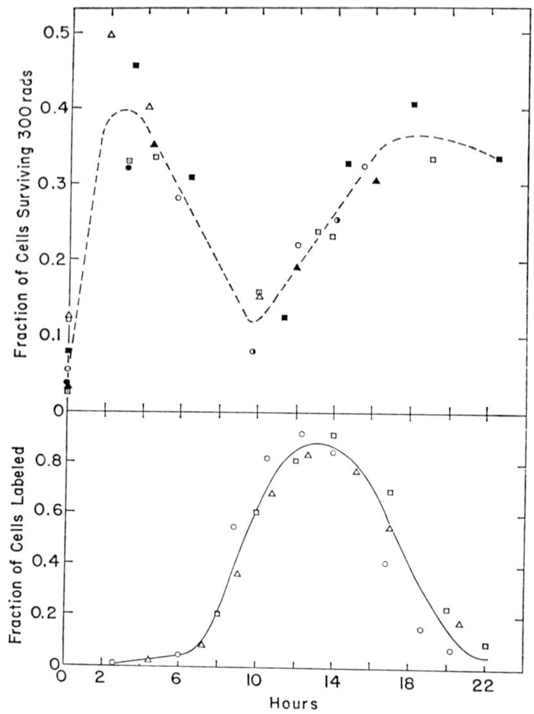

Fig. 6–9. The relationship between the fraction of cells surviving a single x-ray dose and the time interval following synchronization by selection of mitotic cells. The lower curve shows the pattern of DNA synthesis for cells similarly synchronized. From this it can be deduced that the first peak in the upper curve takes place during the G_1 period and that the second peak in the upper curve occurs in conjunction with the end of the synthetic period or late S. (From Terasima T, Tolmach LJ. Biophys J 3:11, 1963 by copyright permission of the Biophysical Society.)

loss factor, which can be as high as 90% in some squamous cancers. Thus, it is highly possible that a tumor could appear to be growing, yet if this were due to the accumulation of dead cells, the clonogenic number could actually be decreasing. The opposite occurs when tumors appear to shrink yet can be shown to have increases in the number of clonogenic cells.

There is wide variation in the proportion of cells that are in cycle or in the growth fraction of tumors between at least 10 and 80%. The total tumor volume doubling time will vary according to the growth fraction, the cell cycle time, and the cell loss factor "ϕ." The definition of ϕ is as follows:

$$\phi = 1 - T_p/T_d$$

in which T_p is the potential doubling time and T_d is the actual doubling time observed from direct measurements of tumor volume.

It has been recognized recently that the two most important values that could be measured in human tumors to predict their radiation response are the previously discussed surviving fraction after 200-cGy exposure and the T_{pot}. The former would determine whether sufficient cell kill could occur at standard 200-Gy fractions and the latter whether significantly shorter overall treatment times would be beneficial because rapid repopulation induces cells with a short potential doubling time (13).

FRACTIONATION EFFECTS IN CHEMORADIATION

As discussed previously, both cell repopulation and cell repair of sublethal and potentially lethal damage are extremely important factors in the outcome of fractionated radiation therapy, in terms of both normal tissue damage and tumor control. The major factors that influence this have been dubbed "the four Rs of radiotherapy" by Withers and include **repair** of sublethal damage, **reoxygenation, repopulation,** and **reassortment** into different and sometimes more sensitive or more resistant phases of the cell cycle. With more recent knowledge, a fifth factor may be added, namely the inherent cellular **radiosensitivity** as described by the surviving fraction at 200 cGy.

It is evident from experimental data that all five of these major factors influencing radiotherapy can be modified by cytotoxic chemotherapy. Repair of sublethal damage can clearly be inhibited by agents such as Actinomycin D. There is evidence that platinum compounds given at the time of irradiation will also suppress or delay sublethal damage repair. In addition, radiation may inhibit drug repair, as has been seen in intestinal crypt cells with bleomycin and carmustine (BCNU).

Repopulation can be inhibited by cytotoxic chemotherapy. This may be extremely important when chemotherapy is used in simultaneous combination with radiotherapy. Radiotherapy clearly induces repopulation, and drugs that are cell cycle specific could be quite effective in reducing or eliminating this problem. Other agents that are cytostatic rather than cytotoxic have been discovered recently.

Reoxygenation may be enhanced through drug killing of subpopulations of cells and shrinkage of the tumor. Reassortment, likewise, may be induced by drugs that would kill cells in the mitotic phase, cause synchronization, and then potentially allow irradiation to be more effective at selected subsequent time intervals.

SUMMARY

Radiation primarily kills cells through eliminating their ability to proliferate. This effect is secondary to damage to the DNA and resultant chromosome aberrations or translocations that prevent unlimited mitosis.

Such killing is influenced by many factors, including the nature of the radiation, the dose rate, the inherent sensitivity of the cells, and chemical and physical modifiers.

Extensive repair systems exist for the elimination of most radiation-induced lesions, and the remaining lesions are all important in determining cell survival.

Repair of sublethal radiation injury, repopulation, reoxygenation, reassortment of the cell cycle, and inherent cellular radiosensitivity are all important in determining tumor and normal tissue injury in clinical radiotherapy. All five are potentially modified by chemotherapy. This leads to the conclusion that the combination of chemotherapy and radiotherapy can be extremely powerful in the improvement of tumor response, as long as the parallel injury in normal tissue is understood and controlled.

REFERENCES

1. Thames HD, Hendry JS. Fractionation in Radiotherapy. London, Taylor and Francis, 1987.
2. Withers HR, Thames HD. Dose fractionation and volume effects in normal tissues and tumors. Am J Clin Oncol 11:313, 1988.
3. Hall EJ. Radiobiology for the Radiologist. 3rd ed. Philadelphia, JB Lippincott, 1988.
4. Johns HE, Cunningham JR. The Physics of Radiology. 4th ed. Springfield, IL, CC Thomas, 1983.
5. Fowler JF. The linear-quadratic formula and

progress in fractionated radiotherapy. Br J Radiol 62:679, 1989.
6. Ward JF. DNA damage produced by ionizing radiation in mammalian cells: Identities, mechanisms of formation, and reparability. Prog Nucleic Acid Res Mol Biol 35:95, 1988.
7. Meyn RE, Withers HR. Radiation Biology in Cancer Research. New York, Raven Press, 1980.
8. Steel GG, Deacon JM, Duchesne GM, et al. The dose-rate-effect in human tumour cells. Radiother Oncol 9:299, 1987.
9. Steel GG, Peacock JH. Why are some human tumours more radiosensitive than others? Radiother Oncol 15:63, 1989.
10. Peters LJ. Inherent radiosensitivity of tumor and normal tissue cells as a predictor of human tumor response. Radiother Oncol 17:177, 1990.
11. Chapman JD, Peters LJ, Withers HR (Eds). Prediction of Tumor Treatment Response. New York, Pergamon Press, 1989.
12. Fu KK, Phillips TL. Biologic rationale of combined radiotherapy and chemotherapy. Vokes EE (Ed). Hematol Oncol Clin North Am 5:737, 1991.
13. Withers HR, Taylor JMG, Maciejewski B. The hazard of accelerated tumor clonogenic repopulation during radiotherapy. Acta Oncol 27:131, 1988.

Chapter 7

ANTIMETABOLITES

TYVIN A. RICH AND DAVID MURRAY

INTRODUCTION

The combined use of antineoplastic drugs and radiation for the treatment of malignant disease is increasing because of widespread agreement that such combinations can improve the therapeutic ratio. Better survival and quality of life have been achieved with chemoradiation for patients with nonmetastatic squamous cell cancers of the esophagus (1) or the anus (2) and for patients with adenocarcinomas of the pancreas and rectum (3). Antimetabolites constitute one type of antineoplastic agent used in chemoradiation. Some chemoradiation treatment schedules employ a single antimetabolite, usually the halogenated pyrimidine 5-fluorouracil (5-FU); others combine 5-FU with additional chemotherapeutic agents, such as cisplatinum or mitomycin, and most recently leucovorin (folinic acid-SF) or levamisole to exploit the phenomena known as biochemical (4) or immunologic (5) modulation. The term **modulation** here refers either to increased cytotoxicity as measured in cell culture studies or to increased chemotherapeutic effectiveness as gauged by improved therapeutic effect in the clinic.

This chapter reviews the results of clinical investigations of combined antimetabolites and radiotherapy (RT), from which some insight into the mechanisms of interaction between these modalities can be inferred. Some antimetabolites have also been combined with RT in laboratory studies in an effort to understand how the fundamental processes of x-ray-induced DNA damage and its repair can be manipulated to therapeutic advantage. Such studies hold the promise that better treatments will eventually be developed on the basis of rational mechanistic considerations.

MECHANISMS OF ACTION

Antimetabolites are chemotherapeutic agents that act by fraudulent incorporation into or interaction with cellular biochemical machinery, thus altering normal pathways of intermediary and primary DNA or RNA metabolism. These agents are primarily the nucleoside analogs that become incorporated into DNA, such as 6-mercaptopurine, 6-thioguanine, cytosine arabinoside (Ara-C), and 5-azacitidine. Other antimetabolites, such as hydroxyurea (HU), methotrexate (MTX), and 5-FU, can also inhibit the intermediary synthesis of endogenous nucleotides required for DNA synthesis (Fig. 7–1).

5-FU is unique in that it can incorporate directly into RNA (as a uracil analog), while both 5-FU and its deoxyribonucleoside derivative, 5-fluorodeoxyuridine (5-FUdR), can be converted to 5-fluorodeoxyuridylate (5-FdUMP) and thus inhibit thymidylate synthase, DNA synthesis, and, potentially, DNA-repair processes. Other halogenated pyrimidines, such as 5-iododeoxyuridine (5-IUdR) and 5-bromodeoxyuridine (5-BUdR), and to some extent 5-FUdR, are incorporated directly into the DNA of S-phase cells in place of thymidine. These halogenated nucleosides also have cytotoxic properties, but only 5-FUdR has achieved widespread use as a chemotherapeutic agent.

Nucleoside analogs, such as 5-BUdR, are used to sensitize the tumor cells to the effects of radiation by replacing up to 25% of the thymidine in the DNA. Such preirradiation treatments with both 5-BUdR and 5-IUdR increase the initial yield of radiation-induced DNA single-strand and double-strand breaks while having little or no effect

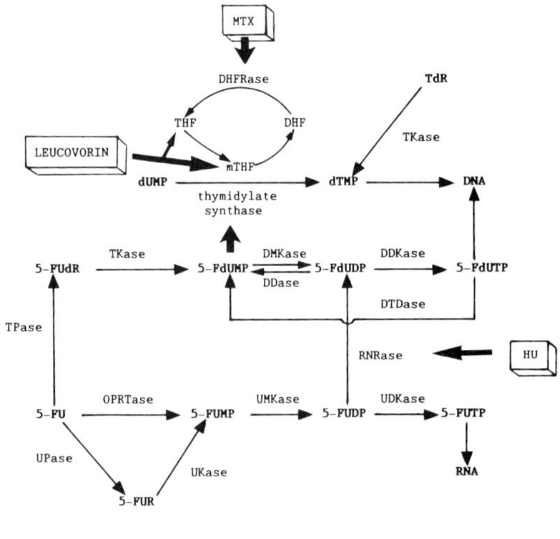

Fig. 7–1. Metabolic pathways important to the interaction between modulated 5-FU and RT.

KEY:

UPase:	uridine phosphorylase
UKase:	uridine kinase
UMKase:	uridine monophosphate kinase
UDKase:	uridine diphosphate kinase
OPRTase:	orotate phosphoribosyltransferase
TPase:	thymidine phosphorylase
TKase:	thymidine kinase
DMKase:	deoxynucleoside monophosphate kinase
DDKase:	deoxynucleoside diphosphate kinase
DDase:	deoxyuridine diphosphatase
DTDase:	deoxyuridine triphosphate diphosphohydrolase
RNRase:	ribonucleotide reductase
DHF:	dihydrofolate
DHFRase:	DHF reductase
THF:	tetrahydrofolate
mTHF:	5,10-methylene THF

on their repair (6,7). These data are consistent with a mechanism of radiosensitization in which the incorporated halogen atoms react with radiation-induced hydrated electrons, resulting in additional DNA chain scission reactions. Without such reactions, these electrons would contribute little to DNA strand breakage (8). For 5-FU, the situation is different; although it may also be incorporated into DNA (9), the importance of this pathway in both cytotoxicity and radiosensitization has not been fully established. Indeed, it is sometimes difficult to detect 5-FU residues in DNA because UTP hydrolase can eliminate 5-FUTP before it can be incorporated and because uracil DNA glycosylase can remove 5-FU residues that do become incorporated (9,10). The halogenated pyrimidines (BUdR and IUdR) and fluoropyrimidines (5-FU and FUdR) are also discussed in Chapter 11.

INTERACTION WITH RADIATION

Cellular Kinetics

Cytotoxic antimetabolites that have been combined with RT in the clinic include 5-FU, MTX (11), and HU (12). Ara-C, although a mainstay in the treatment of myeloproliferative and lymphoproliferative diseases, has been studied with RT mainly in the laboratory setting (13). A valid starting point for understanding the interaction between these drugs and x-rays is to consider the influence of cellular kinetics on the sensitivity of cells to these treatments. The cytotoxic mechanisms of the separate treatment components are fairly well understood. The inhibition of intermediary DNA synthesis by an antimetabolite results in a cytotoxic effect that is observed in cycling cells but not in resting (G_0) cells (9). Antimetabolite cytotoxicity is thus proliferation-dependent, i.e., antimetabolites are **cycle-specific agents.** The cellular kinetics, or the rate of turnover of the cell populations in both tumor and normal tissues, correlate strongly with early treatment effects (14). For example, cell killing by either MTX or HU in high doses is preferential for cycling cells in vitro and reaches a plateau after about 24 hours. Cell killing by 5-FU is also considered to be cycle specific and is exponential (15), although some reports indicate it to be phase specific (9). Cell killing by x-rays alone is phase specific; mitotic cells are generally the most sensitive and late S-phase cells are the most resistant, while G_1 and G_2 cells are intermediate (14).

The combination of drugs and RT, however, has many possible modes of action. One reason for combining two cytotoxic agents is to improve selectively the therapeutic effect on the tumor. From a clinical perspective, this need not necessarily involve a direct interaction between the two agents. Such effects can be considered generally within a framework delineated by Steel and Peckham (16), who described four modes through which the coadministration of two cytotoxic agents may result in an increased therapeutic ratio.

(I) Enhancement of the tumor response compared to that of normal tissue.
(II) Normal-tissue toxicity independence.
(III) Spatial cooperation (where disease at one anatomical site that is insensitive to one agent is controlled by the second agent).
(IV) Normal tissue protection without concomitant protection of tumor cells.

Modes I, II, and III are the most likely to occur in the clinical application of antimetabolites and RT, since both agents are individually cytotoxic.

Modes II and III may be important clinically, but they are not dependent upon any form of interaction between the two agents. Mode I effects, on the other hand, require that the two agents interact either at the biochemical or cellular levels. Indeed, the numerous demonstrations that 5-FU enhances the radiosensitivity of cells in vitro strongly suggests such an interaction. These interactive effects can be of several types. For example, the magnitude of the effect on DNA of both drugs and RT can vary according to the cell's position in the cycle (14). In a heterogenous population of tumor cells, the response to treatment will vary depending on the percentage of cycling cells present as well as on the rate of cell proliferation. Both RT and antimetabolites can cause cell-cycle delay (14). Some of the effects of combination therapy may therefore be related to the first agent, causing a parasynchronization (via cell-cycle delay and/or phase-specific cytotoxicity) that results in an increased sensitivity of the remaining cells to the second agent. Redistribution of the cells into more radioresistant phases of the cell cycle could also result in some degree of radioprotection.

Another explanation for the enhanced effects of concurrent treatment is the possible enhancement by the antimetabolite of the damaging effects of RT or vice versa. For example, a consequence of the deranged DNA metabolism induced in a proliferating cell by an antimetabolite is that the cell may become more susceptible to the cytotoxic effects of a second anticancer agent, including other antimetabolites and RT. Other possibilities, such as the modification of radiation-induced DNA damage by 5-FU or inhibition by 5-FU of the repair of such DNA damage, will be discussed below.

With respect to Mode I effects, evidence suggesting a supra-additive or synergistic interaction between 5-FU and RT came from early laboratory studies by Heidelberger and colleagues (17) that showed that combining individual doses of 5-FU and RT, which themselves were not curative, could result in tumor cures. Although full dose-response relationships were not established for the two agents, the dose levels used for each agent had acceptable normal-tissue toxicity in rodents; thus, clinical trials were warranted and were pursued enthusiastically, beginning over 30 years ago (18). Randomized clinical trials showed a greater-than-expected local control rate for 5-FU plus RT, compared to RT alone, for squamous cell carcinomas and adenocarcinomas and some increase in early effects in normal tissues. With the publication of these laboratory data and subsequent clinical studies of 5-FU and RT, thc phrase "radiosensitizer" was coined to describe the interaction between these cytotoxic modalities.

The increased hematological and gastrointestinal (GI) toxicity observed following the administration of single (bolus) injections of 5-FU during RT (19) indicated that radiosensitization was, unfortunately, not restricted to the tumor. Reactions of normal tissues in the irradiation volume were also increased compared to RT alone, but they were deemed acceptable, possibly because the RT doses used were relatively low. Larger studies confirmed that there was a relatively steep 5-FU dose-response relationship for severe systemic side-effects; administration of more than 15 mg/kg per day for 3 days at the beginning of RT led to unacceptably severe acute hematological and GI toxicity and some fatality (20). These studies suggested that in antimetabolite–RT combinations, there is an optimal drug dose above which the therapeutic ratio may decrease because normal tissue reactions are too severe. The magnitude of radioenhancement is thus limited by the acceptability of early normal-tissue reactions. However, there is no a priori reason to expect there to be greater cytoxic effects in tumors than in normal tissues. Nonetheless, the use of concurrently administered antimetabolites and RT remains popular, because an improvement in tumor control has been achieved without prohibitive toxic effects in normal tissue.

With the knowledge that normal-tissue reactions are heightened by the combined treatment, an important aspect of future treatment techniques will be to avoid unnecessary involvement of normal tissue. Multiple-field RT treatment, using high-energy beams, can produce a high-dose envelope of radiation around the target with a rapid decline in x-ray dose in the surrounding normal tissues. Thus, by tailoring the RT portal around the target, even a small enhancement of RT effects to both tumor and normal tissues may appear as preferential tumor enhancement.

Recent studies by Weinberg and Rauth (21) of squamous cell carcinoma (SCC VII) in animals demonstrated that 5-FU and RT are additive when analyzed by the isobologram method. These results differ from the observations of supra-additivity in the studies of Heidelberger et al (17).

Clinical and laboratory studies indicate that cytotoxic doses of antimetabolites are necessary for radioenhancement; thus, the third of Steel and Peckham's modes, spatial cooperation, may play some role, particularly in those clinical situations in which the systemic therapy administered with RT has proven value in the control of micrometastatic disease (3). There is little evidence that antimetabolites act through the fourth mode of interaction.

Since antimetabolite cytotoxicity is predominantly proliferation dependent, the limiting normal-tissue reactions (which have occurred largely in the bone marrow, skin, and GI mucosa) may overlap with the early normal-tissue responses to RT alone. The chemoradiation effects observed in normal tissues, particularly those seen with antimetabolites plus RT, are similar to those seen with accelerated RT (22). This analogy may be useful from several perspectives. The basis of enhancement lies in the kinetic model, and the mechanism for improved results with combined modality therapy rests on the recruited stem-cell population or the accelerating repopulating clonogen (23,24). Repopulation during RT may be an important phenomenon underlying treatment failure from RT alone, based on the analysis of the clinical data on time to recurrence, split-course RT, and prolongation of overall treatment time (23,24). Chemoradiation may theoretically improve local tumor control beyond that provided by RT alone, since the tumor cells accounting for radiotherapeutic failure may be more susceptible to cycle-specific agents. This radiobiologic explanation for interaction does not require the effect to be supra-additive but suggests a greater relevance of the timing of the administration of the drug, which targets its cytotoxic effects toward the repopulating cells during RT. In this regard, the assessment of tumor-cell kinetics during treatment could potentially aid in selecting those patients whose tumors show marked repopulation and in whom the timely use of cycle-specific agents could target susceptible tumor cells.

Timing of Modalities

Ideally, a knowledge of individual tumor cell kinetics could be used to optimize administration schedules of cycle-specific agents. The use of tumor or normal-tissue cell kinetic data from individual patients is presently not practical for scheduling treatments of antimetabolites and RT because of the lack of widely available methods for accurately assessing such parameters. However, some of the newer methods for estimating the labeling index (LI), S-phase duration, and tumor potential doubling time (T_{pot}), by 5-BUdR incorporation and monoclonal antibody techniques, may be useful for assessing kinetic parameters in the future (25). For example, it may be reasonable to treat patients whose tumors have a relatively high pretreatment LI and short T_{pot} values with antimetabolites and RT early in the treatment course, which may be when the highest proportion of cells are in cycle. Alternatively, the proportion of cycling cells may increase in the latter part of a course of fractionated RT. Based on recent evidence from clinical radiobiologic analysis of the time factor in head and neck squamous cell cancers, stem-cell recruitment or repopulation may become relevant in the fourth week of conventional RT (900 to 1000 cGy/week in five fractions) (23,24). In this case, a better timing for antimetabolite therapy may be when the rate of repopulation in the tumor stem cell compartment is increasing. Another approach would be to give antimetabolites with each fraction of RT, especially in those cases where the tumor kinetics are not known, so that any cells recruited into the cycle during a course of RT will be exposed to the drug.

In the United States, RT is usually administered according to fractionation schemes in which at least five daily fractions are given per week in doses of 180 to 200 cGy. For convenience, the initial clinical trials of chemoradiation administered maximum permitted doses of intravenous chemotherapy with several of the initial RT treatments. Increased early toxicity in the bone marrow, mucous membranes, and GI tract was an expected consequence of the cycle-specific agents used. In general, there have been few reports that late toxicity from chemoradiation is greater than expected from RT alone (26). The lack of increased late effects may be partly a result of the use of a lower total radiation dose in the combined protocols. Most clinical trials of single antimetabolites, such as 5-FU or HU, with RT have generally started with lower (by 10% to 15%) total RT doses because of the conviction that the combined treatment should be more effective than RT alone. In a study in which high doses of RT were administered concurrently with 5-FU, greater late effects than those seen with RT alone were reported (27); however, this has not been found universally. The current state of the art of chemoradiation using antimetabolites with RT has thus been empirically derived, with a major emphasis on the reactions in normal tissue. New directions for research will require a more detailed understanding of tumor and normal-tissue cell kinetics, as well as further comparisons of drug administration methods and scheduling.

Pharmacology of Antimetabolites

Bimolecular investigations into the mechanisms of cytotoxicity for combinations of these agents, and their respective roles in potentiation, could serve as a useful guide in the design of new clinical studies. One of the most extensively studied antimetabolites combined with radiation, 5-FU, and its deoxyribonucleoside derivative, 5-FUdR, may serve as a paradigm for understanding the mechanisms of drug-radiation interaction. 5-FU is a pyrimidine base in which the hydrogen in the 5 position of uracil has been replaced by flourine. The related nucleoside compound, 5-FUdR, has an added deoxyribose, thus creating an analogue of d-uridine and d-thymidine. Once inside the cell, these free bases and nucleoside must be phosphorylated to stimulate cytotoxic activity.

5-FU can be converted to 5-FUdR by thymidine phosphorylase and can then be phosphorylated by thymidine kinase to form 5-FdUMP (Fig. 7–1). Along with the cofactor 5,10-methylene tetrahydrofolate, 5-FdUMP forms a stable ternary complex with thymidylate synthase, resulting in the inhibition of thymidylate synthesis and causing cell death by thymidine starvation (28). 5-FdUMP may also undergo further phosphorylation to 5-FdUTP, which can be fraudulently incorporated into DNA, a process that has been associated with DNA fragmentation and inhibition of DNA chain elongation (29,30). Fluoropyrimidine incorporation occurs during semiconservative DNA synthesis, with resulting nick and gap formation caused by uracil-DNA glycosylases that excise incorporated 5-FU residues.

Another cytotoxic mechanism may be caused by 5-FUdR, inhibiting DNA-repair processes through alteration of precursor nucleotide pools so that "housekeeping" replacement of pyrimidine bases following physiologic turnover cannot be effectively maintained (31). The use of preirradiation 5-FU or protracted 5-FU during fractionated RT could also alter pool sizes at a magnitude sufficient to affect DNA-repair mechanisms (see below).

5-FU can also be converted to 5-fluorouridine monophosphate (5-FUMP). This can occur by two different pathways: (1) direct conversion by orotate phosphoribosyltransferase (OPRT) in the presence of phosphoribosyl pyrophosphate (PRPP); or (2) intermediate conversion to the ribonucleoside 5-fluorouracil riboside (5-FUR) by uridine phosphorylase followed by formation of 5-FUMP by uridine kinase (Fig. 7–1). This analogue can then be further phosphorylated to 5-fluorouridine triphosphate (5-FUTP), which can be incorporated into RNA, potentially affecting the processing of RNA (32–36); ribosomal RNA may be particularly sensitive in this regard. There is a great deal of heterogeneity in the metabolism of 5-FU, as illustrated by the studies of Houghton and

Houghton (37), who showed that human colorectal carcinoma xenografts may differ in their predominant metabolic pathways of 5-FU metabolism. One group of tumors used predominantly OPRT to metabolize 5-FU into ribonucleotides, whereas another group used the uridine phosphorylase/uridine kinase pathway (37). Such heterogeneity in the metabolism of 5-FU by human tumor cells may be an important consideration in fluoropyrimidine radioenhancement. Thus, 5-FU and 5-FUdR, while structurally similar, are actually quite different drugs that do not necessarily share patterns of mechanism of action, sensitivity, or cross-resistance. The mechanisms for the cytotoxic (and possibly the radiosensitizing) effects of 5-FU and 5-FUdR are potentially related to any of three pathways: inhibition of thymidylate synthase, effects resulting from incorporation of 5-FU into DNA, and, for 5-FU in particular, through additional effects on RNA metabolism.

Studies of 5-FU cytotoxicity have shown that there is considerable biochemical variability in 5-FU metabolism and that this relatively disadvantageous factor may be overcome by administering the drug over prolonged time intervals (38). Some of the differences in 5-FU metabolism seen in human tumors (caused by the differential rates of 5-FU conversion into ribonucleotides over short time intervals) may be diminished during these extended time periods. A second reason that longer drug exposure intervals could improve the therapeutic index is related to increased incorporation into DNA or RNA, or both, which could lead to an increased disruption of cellular function.

Optimal administration schedules have not been established for most antineoplastic agents, and because antimetabolites have been among the longest available and most studied agents, they were among the first to be tested extensively by infusion schedules. In pilot studies of GI cancer, the maximum tolerated dose of 5-FU was 15 mg/kg per day for three consecutive days when combined with conventionally fractionated RT (20). More intensive intravenous/bolus drug treatment resulted in unacceptable acute toxic effects, including bone marrow suppression, stomatitis, and fatal complications.

Since the administration schedule that achieves maximal dose intensity may not be the same for all drugs, especially when given with RT, there is a sound rationale for investigations into the pharmacodynamic response to any drug as a function of concentration and duration of exposure. The simplest of these functions is the concentration-time product [C × T]. Antimetabolite cytotoxicity demonstrates a marked time dependency; the cytotoxicity is greater when the duration of exposure is increased by prolonged infusion. In other words, for the same value of [C × T], longer exposure times will result in greater cell killing (39). For example, when HT-29 cells were exposed to 5-FU in vitro for 1 hour at 240 ng/ml, the surviving fraction was 0.07, whereas 1 ng/ml of 5-FU for 240 hours resulted in a surviving fraction of 0.002 (38). These data support the argument that exposure time may be more important than peak drug levels, especially for chemotherapeutic agents like 5-FU, which have a very short serum half-life (about 10 minutes). 5-FU in the prodrug form, ftorafur, is available in an oral preparation, and frequent daily dosing could be considered as an alternative treatment to continuous intravenous infusion.

Infusional schedules of 5-FU, on which there are some clinical data, include the 5-day schedule of 25 to 30 mg/kg (1000 mg/m^2) per 24 hours. Important aspects of the pharmacology of 5-FU infused by this schedule are evident from the work by Byfield and colleagues (40), who showed that the infusion schedule and dose of 5-FU may be critical in obtaining clinical radiosensitization. At constant drug infusion levels of about 20 mg/kg per 24 hours, they found reproducible serum concentrations that were linearly related to the administered dose. At lower dose levels, little or no 5-FU could be detected in the serum, possibly because the 5-FU did not saturate the metabolic pathways into which it is actively incorporated. The data also suggest that there may be a minimum effective duration of exposure to 5-FU (at least exceeding the cell-cycle time) and that the cytotoxic effect is inversely related to the administered dose as the exposure time is increased (39).

Mechanisms of Antimetabolite-Radiation Interaction

Early in vitro studies of the cellular basis for the interaction between 5-FU and radiation centered on cell recovery processes, mainly because the fact that postirradiation 5-FUdR decreased the survival of irradiated cells in the classic study by Phillips and Tolmach (41) was taken to signify that the drug enhanced the lethal expression of potentially lethal damage (PLD). Thus, 5-FU and 5-FUdR must somehow inhibit the ability of cells to recover from PLD. We attempted to see whether 5-FU altered the ability of log-phase human colon cancer cells to recover from that form of PLD that is expressed by incubating the cells with hypertonic (0.5 M) saline (42). However, irradiated cells treated with 5-FU were so sensitive to hypertonic conditions that no cells survived the treatment, precluding any estimate of PLD-recovery kinetics. Studies by Berry (43), Byfield et al (44), and Nakajima et al (45) all showed that 5-FU had no effect on recovery from sublethal damage (SLD) in HeLa cells, HT-29 human colon adenocarcinoma, and mouse L cells, respectively. Similarly, Kim et al (46) found that 5-FUdR had no effect on SLD recovery in HeLa cells.

There have been relatively few direct studies of the molecular mechanism(s) underlying the radioenhancing effects of 5-FU. Because 5-FU is active when given after irradiation (44,47,48) it is often presumed that postirradiation 5-FU radiosensitizes cells by inhibiting the repair of some type of radiation-induced DNA damage. However, the repair of single-strand breaks was unchanged in cervical cancer cells treated with up to 2.5 mg/ml 5-FU (49) and in CHO cells treated with 100 ug/ml 5-FU (50). Similarly, postirradiation 5-FU (100 ug/ml) had no effect on double-strand break repair in human colon cancer cells (42). Thus, radioenhancement by postirradiation 5-FU does not appear to be accompanied by any effect on the overall rate of ligation of DNA strand breaks. Inhibition of double-strand break repair was observed in human adenocarcinoma cells following protracted preirradiation treatment with 5-FUdR (51), in which prolonged inhibition of thymidylate synthase and perturbation of nucleotide pools were in evidence, supporting the notion that using different treatment protocols will produce very different effects and that 5-FU and 5-FUdR probably have different mechanisms of action.

Another possible mechanism for postirradiation enhancement involves the misrepair of radiation damage. Physical methods of measuring DNA strand break repair give no information about the fidelity of such repair, and one could envisage that the combined damage from radiation and 5-FU could be misrepaired and converted to a lethal lesion, perhaps because of the simultaneous action of repair systems on both types of damage, an increased level of 5-FU misincorporation into the DNA of irradiated cells, or a combined effect of 5-FU and radiation on nucleotide metabolism (see above). Rather than considering DNA damage per se, perhaps we should remember that both 5-FU and radiation alter DNA metabolism; for example, they both suppress DNA synthesis. Their combined effects on such processes may therefore be very important. For example, treatment of HeLa cells for up to 6 hours with 1 uM 5-FUdR delays the expression of radiation-induced suppression of DNA synthesis (52).

In the above discussion, we have presumed that 5-FU somehow enhances radiation-induced cell killing, i.e., that the effectiveness of the combination is the result of a radioenhancement phenomenon. However, it is not improbable that it is the cytotoxicity of 5-FU that is enhanced by prior irradiation, i.e., that the effectiveness is the result of a chemoenhancement effect and that radiation may alter the subsequent pathways of 5-FU metabolism. Because one of the requisites for 5-FU radioenhancement is that the 5-FU treatment alone is cytotoxic (40), the influence of cellular metabolism on 5-FU conversion into 5-FdUMP, 5-FdUTP, and 5-FUMP (and thus on thymidylate synthase inhibition and DNA/RNA incorporation) may be very important. For example, the supra-additive effect of 5-FU and RT could involve increased incorporation of the 5-FU into RNA, potentially magnifying the disruption of RNA processing and function observed in unirradiated cells (see above). In this regard, RT may be "modulating" the effect of 5-FU, a concept that is plausible within the framework of our current understanding of mechanisms by which 5-FU cytotoxicity can be increased.

Modulation of 5-FU by biochemical means rather than by RT is being used currently, based on the laboratory findings that alterations in the metabolism of 5-FU can increase cytotoxicity and clinical usefulness.

In the postoperative adjuvant treatment of rectal cancer, future trials will integrate RT with newer, modulated, 5-FU regimens such as 5-FU-levamisole and 5-FU-leucovorin (53); however, the optimization of these newer chemoradiation regimens is greatly hampered by the fact that the cellular and molecular mechanisms underlying their therapeutic advantage are poorly understood. A fuller understanding of these interactions could greatly clarify future directions for new treatment schedules and may result in optimized treatment. For example, an increased inhibition of DNA synthesis by 5-FU-leucovorin and likewise by RT, could shunt 5-FU metabolism into RNA. Further studies of the effects of radiation on the incorporation of 5-FU into cellular RNA and its effect on RNA processing are clearly warranted on the basis of the marked effect of 5-FU on RNA metabolism in unirradiated cells (32–36). Levamisole or leucovorin could modulate these processes, as discussed above; in this regard, biochemical modulation of the inhibitory effect of 5-FU on thymidylate synthase, for example by leucovorin, could have possible therapeutic advantages when combined with RT. New trials of RT and 5-FU modulated with leucovorin will be needed to determine whether the therapeutic ratio will be improved, because information about the early and late toxic effects of this combination on normal tissues is sparse.

Many of the clinical trials of 5-FU chemoradiation in the 1970s and 1980s used bolus 5-FU with the first 3 days of RT and, in some studies, during the last week of RT after the recovery of blood counts (3,54,55). Longer radioenhancement schedules for 5-FU have employed infusions of 5 to 7 mg/kg (300 mg/m^2) per 24 hours for 5 to 7 days per week, given over 25 to 35 days (56). In a prospective, randomized comparison, this schedule was as well tolerated as bolus 5-FU administration, whereas the continuous infusion method was shown to have a higher therapeutic index; thus, there may be an equally sound rationale for its use as a radiosensitizer as compared with the schedule using higher doses (1000 mg/m^2 per 24 hours) for a shorter time (5 days). The optimal duration of treatment or the best drug dosage will be dictated by host toxic reactions.

OTHER ANTIMETABOLITES

MTX is historically one of the most extensively used antimetabolites; its activity is related to its structural analogy to folic acid. MTX has frequently been used with RT (57), although little or no data exist on the use of its structural analogs. The major mechanism of action of MTX is a cycle-specific inhibition of the enzyme dihydrofolate reductase (DHFR); a secondary target of action is the enzyme thymidylate synthase. For a variety of biochemical reasons, DHFR appears to be the principle target for cytotoxicity, but there are no data that clearly implicate this mechanism as the basis for the interaction between MTX and RT.

When MTX has been combined with RT, the dosages recommended have been up to 200 mg/m^2 by bolus administration one to two times per week with RT (57). At higher dosages, the frequency must be decreased and the treatment cycles lengthened to every 2 to 4 weeks. Folinic acid has to be administered after high doses of MTX to reduce bone marrow toxicity.

HU interferes with DNA synthesis by inhibiting ribonucleotide reductase, and it has been used extensively in the combined modality treatment of women with squamous cell carcinomas of the uterine cervix (58). It has been given orally at a dose of 80 mg/kg every third day, starting on the first day of RT and continuing for 12 weeks.

SUMMARY

Optimal chemoradiation treatments have probably not been realized because the complexity of interaction between two or more antineoplastic agents is great and because the best combination of therapies depends not only on the response of the tumor but also on the response of the normal tissues. Combinations of RT and an antimetabolite are currently being studied in a variety of clinical protocols; 5-FU chemoradiation is probably the most popular.

At the present time, clinicians do not have to dwell on the notion of additivity versus supra-additivity; instead, they must understand the empirical relationships of combined modality therapy in order not to exceed normal tissue tolerance. To do otherwise may undermine the basic goal of combined modality therapy. In other words, the therapeutic index is currently a more clinically relevant concept than the actual mechanism of any underlying interaction. Clearly, whether antimetabolites and RT interact in an additive or supra-additive manner is dependent on the system being studied, whereas the therapeutic index will be influenced by the therapeutic conditions, the tumor system, the specific endpoints examined, and by definitions of local control and normal tissue toxicity in the experimental setting. The modeling of in vitro and in vivo laboratory data may be intellectually attractive, but for practical reasons, the results of clinical trials usually guide the conceptualization of the interaction between cytotoxic agents.

The key to success in the clinic has thus been based on the selection of the chemotherapy agents, the dosages, the timing of administration with respect to RT, and the methods of administration employed. There are currently no universally accepted protocols for chemoradiation nor has any specific chemoradiation protocol using antimetabolites demonstrated a clear superiority. Prospective testing with rigorous criteria for tumor and normal tissue responses will be necessary to determine optimal therapeutic combinations, with the expectation that toxicity (early or late) will be the limiting factor.

In the last decade, an important aspect of this research has been the wide acceptance of the need to administer 5-FU as a prolonged infusion during a course of RT. The relative importance of drug treatment schedules, routes and methods of drug administration, and the radiation dose and fractionation scheme will require further study before improved results can be anticipated. From a better understanding of the bimolecular mechanisms of interaction, it is reasonable to predict that improved clinical results will ultimately be achieved.

Acknowledgment

This work was supported in part by grants CA06294 and CA16672 from the National Cancer Institute.

REFERENCES

1. Rich T, Ajani J. Radiotherapy for esophageal cancer. *In:* Gastrointestinal Cancer: Current Approaches to Diagnosis and Treatment. Levin B (Ed). Austin, TX, University of Texas Press, 1988, p. 261.
2. Cummings BJ. Anal cancer. Int J Radiat Oncol Biol Phys 19:1309, 1990.
3. Douglass HO, Stablein DM, Thomas PRM. An organized multi-institutional interdisciplinary evaluation of the role of radiation therapy alone or combined with chemotherapy in treatment of adenocarcinoma of the gastrointentinal tract. NCI Monogr 6:253, 1988.
4. Rustum YM, Trave F, Zakrzewski SF, et al. Biochemical and pharmacologic basis for potentiation of 5-fluorouracil action by leucovorin. NCI Mongr 5:165, 1987.
5. Moertel CG, Fleming TR, Macdonald JS, et al. Levamisole and fluorouracil for adjuvant therapy of resected colon cancer. N Engl J Med 322:352, 1990.
6. Kinsella TJ, Dobson PP, Mitchell JB, Fornace AJ. Enhancement of x-ray induced DNA damage by pre-treatment with halogenated pyrimidine analogs. Int J Radiat Oncol Biol Phys 13:733, 1987.
7. Ling LL, Ward JF. Radiosensitization of Chinese hamster V79 cells by bromodeoxyuridine substitution of thymidine: Enhancement of radiation-induced toxicity and DNA strand break production by monofilar and bifilar substitution. Radiat Res 121:76, 1990.
8. Zimbrick JD, Ward JF, Myers LS. Studies on the chemical basis of cellular radiosensitization by 5-bromouracil substitution in DNA. II. Pulse and steady-state radiolysis of bromouracil-substituted and unsubstituted DNA. Int J Radiat Biol 16:525, 1969.
9. Valeriote F, Santelli G. 5-fluorouracil (FU). *In:* Cell Cycle Effects of Drugs. Dethlefsen LA (Ed). Oxford, Pergamon Press, 1986, p. 85.
10. Schuetz JD, Wallace HJ, Diasio RB. DNA repair following incorporation of 5-fluorouracil into DNA of mouse bone marrow cells. Cancer Chemother Pharmacol 21:208, 1988.
11. Jackson RC. Biological effects of folic acid antagonists with antineoplastic activity. *In:* Cell Cycle Effects of Drugs. Dethlefsen LA (Ed). Oxford, Pergamon Press, 1986, p. 112.
12. Sinclair WK. The combined effect of hydroxyurea and x-rays in Chinese hamster cells in vitro. Cancer Res 28:190, 1988.
13. Iliakis G. Radiation-induced potentially lethal damage: DNA lesions susceptible to fixation. Int J Radiat Oncol Biol Phys 53:541, 1988.
14. Denekamp J. Cell Kinetics and Cancer Therapy. Springfield, IL, CC Thomas, 1982.

15. Bruce WR, Meeker BE, Valeriote FA. Comparison of the sensitivity of normal haematopoietic and transplanted lymphoma colony-forming cells to chemotherapeutic agents administered in vivo. J Natl Cancer Inst 37:233, 1966.
16. Steel GG, Peckham MJ. Exploitable mechanisms in combined radiotherapy-chemotherapy: The concept of additivity. Int J Radiat Oncol Biol Phys 5:85, 1979.
17. Heidelberger C, Chaudhari HC, Daunenberg P, et al. Studies on fluorinated pyrimidines. II. Effects of trans-planted tumors. Cancer Res 18:305, 1958.
18. Schein PS, Gore ME, Buckman RA. Radiation therapy and 5-fluorouracil. Drugs Exp Clin Res 8:587, 1982.
19. Moertel CG, Childs DS, Retemeier RJ. Combined 5-fluorouracil and supervoltage radiation therapy of locally unresectable gastrointestinal cancer. Lancet 2:865, 1969.
20. Moertel CG, et al. Advanced gastrointestinal cancer. Mayo Clin Proc 39:767, 1964.
21. Weinberg MJ, Rauth AM. 5-Fluorouracil infusions and fractionated doses of radiation: Studies with a murine squamous cell carcinoma. Int J Radiat Oncol Biol Phys 13:1691, 1987.
22. Peters LJ, Ang KK, Thames HD. Accelerated fractionation in the radiation treatment of head and neck cancer. Acta Oncol 27:185, 1988.
23. Withers JR, Maciejewski B, Taylor JMG, Hlimak A. Accelerated repopulation in head and neck cancer. Front Radiat Ther Oncol 22:105, 1988.
24. Withers HR, Taylor JMG, Maciejewski B. The hazard of accelerated tumor clonogen repopulation during radiotherapy. Acta Oncol 27:131, 1988.
25. Begg AC. Derivation of cell kinetic parameters from human tumors after labelling with bromodeoxyuridine and iododeoxyuridine. Brit Inst Radiol Rep 19:113, 1989.
26. Thomas PRM, Lindblad AS, Stablein, et al. Toxicity associated with postoperative therapy for adenocarcinoma of the rectum. Cancer 57:1130, 1986.
27. Fletcher GH, et al. Chemotherapy as an adjuvant to surgery and radiation therapy. *In:* Proceedings of the Ninth International Cancer Congress. Berlin, Springer-Verlag, 1967, p. 177.
28. Danenberg PB, Montag BJ, Heidelberger C. Studies on fluorinated pyrimidines. IV. Effects on nucleic acid metabolism in vivo. Cancer Res 18:329, 1958.
29. Scheutz JD, Collins JM, Wallace HJ, Diazio RB. Alteration of the secondary structure of newly synthesized DNA from murine marrow cells by 5-fluorouracil. Cancer Res 46:119, 1986.
30. Lonn V, Lonn S. Interaction between 5-fluorouracil and DNA of human colon adenocarcinoma. Cancer Res 44:3414, 1984.
31. Yoshioka A, Tanaka S, Hiraoka O, et al. Deoxyribonucleoside triphosphate imbalance. J Biol Chem 262:8235, 1987.
32. Spears CP, Shani J, Shahinian AH. Assay and time course of 5-fluorouracil incorporation into RNA of L1210/0 ascites cells in vivo. Mol Pharmacol 27:302, 1985.
33. Greenhalgh DA, Parish JH. Effect of 5-fluorouracil on cytotoxicity and RNA metabolism in human colonic carcinoma cells. Cancer Chemother Pharmacol 25:37, 1989.
34. Greenhalgh DA, Parish JH. Effect of 5-fluorouracil combination therapy on RNA processing in human colonic carcinoma cells. Br J Cancer 61:415, 1990.
35. Takimoto CH, Cadman EC, Armstrong RD. Precursor-dependent differences in the incorporation of fluorouracil in RNA. Mol Pharmacol 29:637, 1986.
36. Takimoto CH, Tan YY, Cadman EC, Armstrong RD. Correlation between ribosomal RNA production and RNA-directed fluoropyrimidine cytotoxicity. Biochem Pharmacol 36:3243, 1987.
37. Houghton JA, Houghton PJ. Elucidation of pathways of 5-fluorouracil metabolism in xenografts of human colorectal carcinoma. Eur J Cancer Clin Oncol 19:807, 1983.
38. Calabro-Jones PM, Byfield JE, Ward JF, Sharp TR. Time-dose relationships for 5-fluorouracil cytotoxicity against human epithelial cancer cells in vitro. Cancer Res 42:4413, 1982.
39. Ratain MJ, Vogelzang NJ. Experimental rationale for continuous infusion chemotherapy. *In:* Cancer Chemotherapy by Infusion. Lokich JJ (Ed). Chicago, Precept Press, 1987, p. 12.
40. Byfield JE. The clinical use of 5-fluorouracil and other halopyrimidines as radiosensitizers in man. *In:* Cancer Chemotherapy by Infusion. Lokich J (Ed). Chicago, Precept Press, 1987, p. 479.
41. Phillips RA, Tolmach LJ. Repair of potentially lethal damage in x-irradiated HeLa cells. Radiat Res 29:413, 1961.
42. Hughes LL, Luengas J, Rich TA, Murray D. Radiosensitization of cultured human adenocarcinoma cells by 5-fluorouracil: Effects on cell survival, DNA repair, and cell recovery. Int J Radiat Oncol Biol Phys, 1992, in press.
43. Berry RJ. Effects of some metabolic inhibitors on x-ray dose-response curves for the survival of mammalian cells in vitro, and on early re-

covery between fractional x-ray doses. Br J Radiol 39:458, 1966.
44. Byfield JE, Calabro-Jones P, Klisac I, Kulhanian F. Pharmacologic requirements for obtaining sensitization of human tumor cells in vitro to combined 5-fluorouracil or ftorafur and x-rays. Int J Radiat Oncol Biol Phys, 8:1923, 1982.
45. Nakajima Y, Miyainoto T, Tanabes M, et al. Enhancement of mammalian cell killing by 5-fluorouracil in combination with x-rays. Cancer Res 39:3763, 1979.
46. Kim JH, Eidinoff ML, Laughlin JS. Recovery from sublethal x-ray damage of mammalian cells during inhibition of synthesis of deoxyribonucleic acid. Nature 204:598, 1964.
47. Vietti T, Eggerding F, Valeriote F. Combined effect of x-radiation and 5-fluorouracil on survival of transplanted leukemic cells. J Natl Cancer Inst 47:865, 1971.
48. Byfield JE. Useful interactions between 5-fluorouracil and radiation in man: 5-fluorouracil as a radiosensitizer. *In:* Antitumor Drug-Radiation Interactions. Hill BT, Bellamy AS (Eds). Boca Raton, CRC Press, 1990, p. 87.
49. Byfield JE, Lee YC. Effect of 5-fluorouracil and actinomycin D on repair of DNA single-strand breaks in cervix cancer cells. J Natl Cancer Inst 50:573, 1973.
50. Rich TA, et al. Effects of continuous post-irradiation low dose 5-fluorouracil on log- and plateau-phase CHO cells. *In:* Proceedings of Chemical Modifiers of Cancer Treatment. Abstract no. 6–21. Clearwater, FL, 1985.
51. Bruso CE, Shewach DS, Lawrence TS. Fluorodeoxyuridine-induced radiosensitization and inhibition of DNA double strand break repair in human colon cancer cells. Int J Radiat Oncol Biol Phys 19:1411, 1990.
52. Saha BK, Tolmach LJ. Delayed expression of the x-ray-induced depression of DNA synthetic rate in HeLa S3 cells. Radiat Res 66:76, 1976.
53. Adjuvant therapy for patients with colon and rectum cancer. National Institutes of Health Consensus Statement Development Conference 8(4), 1990.
54. Moertel CG, Frytak S, Hahn RG, et al. Therapy of locally unresectable pancreatic carcinoma: A randomized comparison of high dose (6000 rads) radiation alone, moderate dose radiation (4000 rads + 5-fluorouracil), and high dose radiation + 5-fluorouracil. Cancer 48:1705, 1981.
55. Gastrointestinal Tumor Study Group: A comparison of combination chemotherapy and combined modality therapy for locally advanced gastric carcinoma. Cancer 49:1771, 1982.
56. Rich TA, Lokich JJ, Chaffey JT. Pilot study of protracted venous infusion of 5-fluorouracil and concomitant radiation therapy. J Clin Oncol 3:402, 1985.
57. Gupta MK, Pointon RCS, Wilkinson PM. A randomized clinical trial to contrast radiotherapy with radiotherapy and methotrexate given synchronously in head and neck cancer. Clin Radiol 38:575, 1987.
58. Piver MS, Khalil M, Emrich LJ. Hydroxyurea plus pelvic irradiation versus placebo plus pelvic irradiation in non-surgically staged Stage IIIB cervical cancer. J Surg Oncol 42:120, 1989.

Chapter 8

ALKYLATING AGENTS

MACK ROACH III, MADHU J. JOHN, AND ROBERT F. KALLMAN

INTRODUCTION

Alkylating agents were the first group of chemotherapeutic drugs found to have specific anticancer properties (1). Their primary site of action is the DNA molecule, and they are known to affect DNA synthesis, inhibit DNA repair, and cross-link and break DNA strands.

Several alkylating agents are currently in use against human leukemias and solid tumors in standard combination regimens and in protocols using bone marrow transplantation. They include nitrogen mustard, phenylalanine mustard (melphalan/alkeran), cyclophosphamide, nitrosoureas bischloroethylnitrosourea (BCNU; carmustine), chloroethylcyclohexylnitrosourea (CCNU; lomustine), and methyl-CCNU, busulfan, chlorambucil, and thiotriethylene phosphoramide (Thio-TEPA). In addition, cisplatinum and mitomycin-C function primarily by their alkylating action. The nitrosoureas, cisplatinum, and cyclophosphamide have important clinical relevance in chemoradiation interactions and will be discussed at some length in this chapter. Mitomycin-C, an antibiotic, is described in Chapter 9.

As a class, alkylating agents function through different mechanisms (2,3). They generate unstable ions, which attach themselves to different target sites on the DNA molecule, and tend to be mutagenic and carcinogenic. Their activity tends to be enhanced by nitroimidazoles, glutathione depletion, and hyperthermia. With the exception of nitrosoureas, alkylating agents tend not to cross the blood-brain barrier. Probably because of different sites of alkylation, both their antitumor spectrum and toxicity vary greatly. Of all chemotherapeutic agents currently available, alkylating drugs are least prone to the development of drug resistance, perhaps the single most important factor responsible for limiting chemotherapy efficacy.

Antitumor activity is present against a wide range of tumors, including several leukemias, lymphomas, gliomas, multiple myeloma, head and neck cancers, and gastrointestinal and gynecologic cancers. Although bone marrow toxicity is the usual dose-limiting toxicity of alkylating agents, a wide range of other toxicities, such as cardiotoxicity (cyclophosphamide), hepatic and central nervous system toxicity (nitrosoureas), gastrointestinal (GI) toxicity (melphalan), ototoxicity, and nephrotoxicity (cisplatinum), have been noted. Table 8–1 provides a comprehensive description of cisplatinum, nitrosoureas, and cyclophosphamide, with particular reference to their interaction with radiation.

PLATINUM COMPOUNDS

The combined use of platinum-containing compounds (PCCs) and radiation (RT) has evoked more interest than any other combination in chemoradiation. PCCs have proven to be among the most active agents in the treatment of cancer. Originally described as a salt by Peyrone in 1845, cis-diamminedichloroplatinum (II) (CDDP), or cisplatinum, did not gain widespread clinical use until the early 1980s (4). Over the last 10 years, CDDP has become the drug to which all others are compared for their effectiveness in primary tumors arising within such diverse sites as the lung, the head and neck, the testis, the ovary, the cervix, and the esophagus. Although newer PCCs have been identified, none have been proven to have greater antitumor activity than CDDP.

Table 8–1. Properties of Alkylating Agents

Drugs	Mechanism of Action	Interaction with RT	Intermediates	Cell-cycle Specificity	Metabolism	Half-life	Toxicity
Cisplatinum	Interstrand and intrastrand DNA cross-linking	1. Type "b" or biochemical by inhibition of sublethal radiation damage repair 2. Type "c" or chemical interaction mediated by free radicals	Cisplatinum-DNA adducts	Most active in G1 but generally phase nonspecific	Excreted through kidneys—90%; Bile—10%	Biphasic-initial, 30 minutes; terminal, 24–38 hours	1. Nephrotoxicity 2. Ototoxicity 3. Emesis 4. Peripheral neuropathy 5. Mild myelotoxicity
Nitrosoureas	1. DNA damage through cross-links 2. DNA repair inhibition 3. Thiol depletion	"Fixing" of radiation-induced DNA damage	1. Carbonium ions 2. Isocyanites	Late G1 and early S phase	Crosses blood-brain barrier; 80% excreted in urine	Biphasic-initial 6 minutes; terminal 68 minutes	1. Myelotoxicity 2. Emesis 3. Lung and kidney toxicity, rarely
Cyclophosphamide	1. Alkylation of DNA 2. Decreasing DNA Synthesis	1. Decrease in sublethal radiation repair 2. Increased sensitivity to radiation	1. Phosphoramide 2. Nornitrogen	Late G1, early S, and M	Metabolites, 50% protein bound; eliminated by liver and kidneys	4–6.5 hours	1. Leukopenia 2. Alopecia 3. Emesis 4. Hemorrhagic cystitis 5. Cardiotoxicity (high doses)

The failure of several prospective randomized trials to demonstrate an improvement in survival with RT and CDDP-based combined modality therapy has dampened some of the initial enthusiasm for this approach (5–10). Combined RT and CDDP-based combined modality therapy is supported by several other clinical studies as well as recent animal studies. Using clinically relevant treatment schedules, these animal studies emphasize the critical schedule dependence of CDDP/RT interactions (11–17) and provide a basis for future clinical trials as well as further animal studies. In this section, we discuss issues pertinent to understanding platinum-radiation interactions and concepts relevant to future clinical trials.

Although various PCCs have undergone extensive investigation, the similarities and differences in the interactions with radiation have yet to be fully defined. The following discussion will be limited to CDDP, although similar mechanisms of interactions are likely to occur between radiation and other PCCs. A brief review of the effects of platinum alone precedes the discussion of the combined effects.

Mechanism of Action

CDDP is a square coplanar neutral dichloro complex (see Figure 8–1). The antitumor activity of CDDP is dependent on the species bound to the central platinum atom and the relative position of the ligands (18). The two sites in the cis configuration appear to be responsible for the antitumor activity, because the trans analogs are much less active (19). Preservation of neutrality also appears to be an essential condition for activity in vivo, since penetration of the cell membrane is by diffusion, not by a carrier-mediated transport system. After entering the cell, CDDP is trapped by rapid aquation.

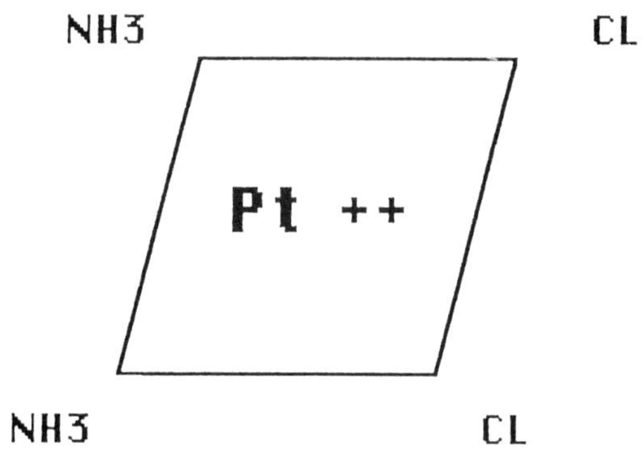

Fig. 8–1. The basic structure of cis-diamminedichloroplatinum (II) (cisplatinum).

CDDP has been shown to be a cell-cycle-specific inhibitor of DNA synthesis in a number of cell lines (20). Cells deficient in DNA repair capacity are particularly sensitive (21–23). CDDP-induced interstrand and intrastrand cross-linking of DNA resembles that seen with bifunctional alkylating agents (24). The primary binding site appears to be the N-7 guanine base, but binding also occurs to the 6-NH_2 and N-7 of adenine and to the 4-NH_2 and N-3 of cytosine. The most common adducts formed and the interaction most likely to be clinically relevant are mediated through the formation of intrastrand DNA-DNA cross-links. The formation of interstrand breaks is a much rarer and slower event, making up less than 1% of Pt-DNA adducts formed ($T_{1/2}$ = 3.5 hours). This, coupled with its failure to correlate with cytotoxicity in several studies, makes the genesis of interstrand breaks unlikely to be the mechanism through which CDDP activity can be explained (25–27).

Although most investigators have accepted DNA as the accepted target for CDDP-induced cytotoxicity, this explanation has been questioned in some recent studies. Sorenson et al (28) have suggested that the induction of cell death might be mediated through the process of apoptosis (programmed cell death), with the degradation of DNA being an early and possibly essential step.

A number of mechanisms have been proposed to explain the induction of resistance to CDDP, including amplification and expression of the mdr-1-gene (29), increased levels of glutathione (GSH) (30,31), metallothionein detoxification (32,33), increased glutathione-S-transferase levels, increased DNA repair mechanisms, amplification and/or increased expression of proto-oncogenes (29), or increased levels of XPE-binding factor (a probe for UV-damaged DNA) (34). The extent to which these or other mechanisms are responsible for what we experience clinically as progressive disease remains to be seen.

As an alternative to the conventional view of resistance, Carmichael and Hickson (35) have argued that perhaps this is a normal cellular response. They suggest that tumor responsiveness may reflect a state of hypersensitivity caused by the loss or abnormalities of certain normal cellular constituents, such as enzymes, that are involved in DNA repair.

The pharmacologic characteristics of CDDP in humans have been studied extensively and are complex (36). Within hours of intravenous administration, approximately 90% of CDDP becomes protein bound, but apparently the active cytotoxic species is contained in the ultrafiltrate or "unbound fraction." Biphasic or triphasic declines have been noted in the total and free plasma CDDP until approximately 2 hours, after which the two diverge (37,38). The biphasic decline in the plasma ultrafiltrate is characterized by an initial half-life of between 15 and 30 minutes and a prolonged terminal half-life of 24 to 38 hours (39,40).

The clinically limiting toxicities associated with CDDP are dependent upon the schedule of administration, the dose, the solutions used as vehicles during delivery of the drug, and the nature of ancillary support (e.g., the use of aggressive antiemetics). Classically, nausea and vomiting (the most common toxicities) and nephrotoxicity (the most severe toxicity) were considered to be the dose-limiting toxicities for CDDP (41,42). With the emergence of metoclopramide in the early 1970s and ondansetron and other serotonin antagonists more recently, nausea and vomiting have become more manageable (43).

Nephrotoxicity, the dose-limiting toxicity that frequently complicated the administration of CDDP in the late 1970s and early 1980s, became much less of a problem with the recognition of its critical dependence on the chloride concentration (42). A high chloride concentration apparently results in a decrease in the levels of the toxic aquatic species in the renal tubules, without compromising the antitumor activity. With the elimination of nephrotoxicity as the most critical dose-limiting toxicity, ototoxicity and a cumulative dose-related peripheral neuropathy have emerged as the major dose-limiting toxicities (24,37). Active investigation is currently under way to address these limiting toxicities.

The ability to manage dose-related toxicities due to CDDP may be more critical for some tumor types than others. Tumors demonstrating a relatively steep dose-response to CDDP might justify the use of higher doses and higher morbidity, when such doses are required for cure (e.g., salvage treatment of testicular tumors) (45). However, two recent randomized trials on poor risk germ cell and nonsmall cell lung cancer demonstrated clinical responses that were most consistent with a relatively flat dose-response curve (46,47). These studies suggest that higher doses may not be justified when CDDP is used alone. The steepness of the dose-response curve for CDDP interactions with RT remain to be defined and may determine the extent to which drug toxicities will limit the use of combined modality therapy.

Platinum-Radiation Interactions

More than 20 years ago, the first experimental model demonstrated enhanced cytotoxicity when radiation was combined with CDDP (48). Since then, much work has been done investigating its interactions with radiation. Although there are in vitro and in vivo systems that fail to demonstrate beneficial interactions between CDDP and radiation, the preponderance of evidence leaves little doubt that such interactions do exist. What remains to be defined are the mechanisms through which such interactions occur and, more importantly, the significance of such interactions. Unfortunately, it is probably much easier to identify suboptimal ways to combine these modalities than to identify the doses and schedules most likely to maximize the potential therapeutic benefits (49).

Several excellent reviews summarizing the available experimental and clinical studies related to CDDP-radiation interactions are available in the literature (50–52). We will attempt to highlight only those recurring themes found in these reviews that deserve special attention.

Interactions between radiation and CDDP could be mediated by fast free-radical-related mechanisms and/or by slow biochemical mechanisms. These two mechanisms have been called **radiation chemical** and **radiation biochemical,** respectively, by some investigators (52,53). Experimental evidence supporting both mechanisms can be found in the literature. The tendency for one or the other to dominate appears to depend on the dose of platinum, the schedule used, the experimental model, and other conditions (e.g., hypoxic vs. oxic conditions).

Radiation chemical potentiation (or a "Type C" interaction) is reported to occur only when CDDP and radiation are present simultaneously and may be modified by the addition of free radical scavengers. Neither pre-irradiation nor postirradiation results in enhancement. Richmond et al (54,55) found that in bacterial systems, this type of potentiation required that 50 μmol/1 of CDDP be free in solution during irradiation in order to enhance hypoxic radiation sensitivity, while in tissue culture only 10 μmol/1 was required. A tissue concentration equivalent of 10 μmol/1 is achievable soon after the administration of CDDP, with doses that are typically used in the clinic (range of 20 to 100 mg/m^2), but high free CDDP levels are transient and much of the tissue CDDP is thought to be bound (36,56). The extent to which this mechanism can realistically be taken advantage of in the clinic is uncertain.

In an effort to quantify the magnitude of the interactions between radiation and chemotherapy, a number of investigators have used animal models and have calculated the dose-effect factor (DEF), which is defined as follows.

$$\text{DEF} = \frac{\text{dose to achieve a specific effect without drug}}{\text{dose to achieve a specific effect with the drug present}}$$

An example of an in vivo system in which the CDDP/radiation interactions might be compatible with a Type C interaction is shown in Figure 33–2. Using this system, when CDDP and radiation were given concurrently, Tanabe and co-workers (16) observed the highest DEFs reported (peak value DEF = 2.0). The DEF pattern shown in Figure 33–1 suggests a critically time-dependent interaction, perhaps corresponding to peak free CDDP levels. Several other schedules that were studied demonstrated enhancement that could not be explained by a Type C interaction. These data suggest that more than one type of interaction may occur.

Most experimental studies have demonstrated an enhancement of radiation effects by CDDP under conditions most compatible with a radiation biochemical (or "Type B" interaction) mechanism. This mechanism is reported to require lower CDDP levels and is not as time dependent (52). Most frequently, this interaction has been attributed to CDDP "inhibition of sublethal damage repair" caused by radiation. Inhibition of potentially lethal radiation damage repair, inhibition of tumor repopulation, or perturbation of cellular kinetics, as well as other mechanisms, have been proposed as possible explanations for the observed interactions (57).

Sublethal damage is classically described by comparing split-dose radiation with single-fraction irradiation. For example, suppose that 1500 cGy causes Y_1 amount of cell kill when given as a single fraction. If, instead, two fractions of 750 cGy are given, separated by a relatively short time interval (e.g., a few minutes), Y_1 amount of cell kill will still occur. As the time interval is increased (e.g., a few hours), substantially less cell killing will be observed. This increase in cell survival suggests that some portion of the damage caused by the initial fraction of radiation has been repaired. When the same doses of radiation and the same schedule are used in the presence of CDDP, less repair (more damage) occurs.

This is summarized below as follows.

1500 cGy = Y_1 (amount of cell kill)

750 cGy + 4 hours + 750 cGy = Y_2 (amount of cell kill)

where $Y_2 \ll Y_1$

750 cGy + 4 hours + 750 cGy + CDDP = Z (amount of cell kill)

where $Z > Y_2$

This phenomenon, which is reflected by the difference between Z and Y_2, is referred to as sublethal damage repair (SLDR). In some cases, the degree of inhibition of SLDR appears to be dependent on the dose or concentration of CDDP and the intrinsic sensitivity of the tumor to CDDP.

Although the inhibition of SLDR and, consequently, the enhancement of DEF are important quantitatively, the therapeutic ratio is of more practical importance, and this is conveniently expressed by a related parameter: the therapeutic gain factor (TGF) (16).

TGF is defined as follows.

$$TGF = \frac{\text{DEF tumor}}{\text{DEF normal tissue}}$$

If a drug enhances the effects of radiation on normal tissues as much as it does on tumor tissues, so that TGF = 1, there may be no advantage of using CMT over radiation alone.

Identification of an organ-specific TGF requires knowledge of not only an appropriate quantitative endpoint (e.g., breathing rate to measure late pulmonary toxicity in the mouse, see Chapter 33) but the appropriate time when this should be measured. For example, Moulder et al (58) found the greatest enhancement of CDDP plus radiation-induced nephrotoxicity was present 3 months after irradiation. Thus, TGF calculated on the basis of comparing an early tumor response with the early response of a late-responding normal tissue might severely underestimate late toxicity.

Clinical Applications

As discussed above, full recognition of the potential benefits of CDDP and radiation-based CMT depends on optimizing the scheduling and pharmacologic variables, as well as the intrinsic sensitivity of the tumors and normal tissues that are relevant in site-specific TGFs. The failure to take into account at least these known factors is likely to result in an underestimate of the potential benefits associated with the combined use of CDDP and RT.

Among the diseases for which the combined use of platinum and radiation has shown the most promise are advanced cancers of the head and neck, esophagus, lung, cervix, and bladder. Numerous pilot studies have suggested potential benefits in using a wide range of doses and schedules, but carefully controlled randomized studies have demonstrated that indiscriminately combining these two modalities does not result in improved survival (5–9). The most promising studies have generally been those in which the radiation and CDDP have been given concurrently (12,14).

The available experimental evidence provides reaffirmation of the promise and the need for continuing investigations to define how best to combine platinum-based compounds with radiation for different diseases. The critical nature of the tumor cell line, the schedule dependence, and specific dose-effect relationships underscore the need to test new ideas using systems that have clinical relevance.

NITROSOUREAS

Mechanism of Action

The chloroethyl nitrosoureas (BCNU, CCNU and methyl-CCNU) have a wide range of antitumor activity in animal systems but clinically are of primary interest in human gliomas in conjunction with radiotherapy. Their lipophilic nature allows them to cross the blood-brain barrier.

BCNU is administered intravenously, but both CCNU and methyl-CCNU are rapidly absorbed following oral administration. Nitrosoureas disappear rapidly 6 to 22 minutes after administration. BCNU has a biphasic half-life with an initial phasc half-life of 6 minutes followed by a second phase half-life of 68 minutes (2,59).

Nitrosoureas undergo chemical decomposition to both active intermediates as well as inert products. The reactive intermediates such as carbonium ions are capable of alkylation with DNA damage through cross-links. These intermediates are therefore responsible for the antitumor and cytotoxic properties of nitrosoureas. Other important mechanisms include DNA repair inhibition and thiol depletion, which are mediated by carbamoylation by other highly reactive intermediates called isocyanates (3,59). Peak levels of all these metabolites appear within 1 to 6 hours following administration. The primary mode of excretion is through urine.

Cell cycle responses, as gauged by cell cultures and animal sarcomas studies, have consistently indicated that cells in the late G1 and early S phase are most vulnerable to nitrosoureas. In addition, these drugs appear to synchronize cells at the G2 phase (60,61). Similar synchronization by radiotherapy at the late S1, G2 phases would thus create a facile milieu for cell kill by a drug with particular lethality toward cells in S, G2 phases (for example, etoposide). Moreover, the sensitivity of M-phase cells to radiation may provide greater cell kill when combining radiotherapy and nitrosoureas.

Nitrosoureas-Radiation Interaction

Tissue culture studies of combination effects of nitrosoureas and radiation have shown increased cell killing compared to that obtained with either the drug or radiation alone (60–64). Cell survival curves have been modified by combinations of nitrosoureas and radiation. The effect appears to be that of a decrease in the shoulder and the slope of cell survival curves suggesting decreased repair of sublethal damage and increased sensitivity to radiation respectively (64).

Experimental animal tumor models such as the KHT sarcoma, the rat 9L brain tumor, and EMT-6 tumor have been used to study nitrosourea-radiation interaction (61,64,65). These studies have shown increased survival, decreased distant metastases, and increased local control with combined treatment compared to radiation alone.

Thus, both experimental tissue cultures and animal tumor models show increased cell kill with nitrosoureas-radiation administration. According to the Phillips classification (Chapter 2), the combination effect could be through spatial cooperation, additivity or supra-additivity, or a combination of any of these three mechanisms.

Also, the degree of modification of cell kill appears to be related to timing of administration of nitrosoureas in relation to radiation delivery. In quantifying normal tissue injury using mouse models, Phillips found maximal injury when BCNU was administered 2 to 12 hours before irradiation (65). Phillips also noted that the administration of BCNU 1 to 8 hours and 6 hours after irradiation of the EMT-6 mouse mammary tumor and the KHT mouse sarcoma, respectively, resulted in a favorable therapeutic ratio when intestinal crypt cells were the limiting normal tissue (65, 66). Wheeler, in a study of fractionated radiotherapy and BCNU on rats with intracerebral 9L tumors, suggested that the administration of BCNU 16 hours prior to radiation treatment resulted in superior survival spans compared to BCNU given at shorter intervals prior to irradiation (64,67).

These seemingly contrary radiobiologic studies are summarized best by Deen, whose work suggests that nitrosoureas fix radiotherapy-induced DNA damage (64,68,69). It is suggested that the BCNU administration should be within 6 to 16 hours before (or after) a radiation fraction because DNA cross-linking is produced by most intermediate products of nitrosoureas, because the process of cross-linking takes place over a period of approximately 6 hours in most in vivo studies, and because active nitrosourea intermediates have relatively short half-lives. In the treatment of human tumors, due to altered pharmacokinetics and lengthier cell cycle phases, nitrosoureas may be given 16 to 24 hours before (or after a multifractionated radiation course) the radiation fraction for maximal tumor kill in most clinical situations and particularly in the treatment of intracranial tumors.

Clinical Applications

Nitrosoureas were originally developed in order to provide antineoplastic activity against brain tumors. Their lipid solubility allowed them to penetrate the blood-brain barrier, a property uncharacteristic of several other alkylating chemotherapeutic agents. By themselves, their effectiveness against malignant gliomas appears to be limited by toxicity. A number of studies exist using nitrosoureas-radiation combinations in cerebral astrocytomas, brain stem gliomas, anaplastic ependymomas and medulloblastomas. Nitrosoureas have been used as initial therapy in combination with radiotherapy in primary brain tumors or in combination with other chemotherapeutic agents for recurrent brain tumors (see Chapters 15 and 17). Nitrosoureas are capable of palliating patients with glioblastomas and recurrent gliomas by improving their general performance status and quality of life (70). This combination may be useful in improving survival of patients with gliomas when given postoperatively in conjunction with radiotherapy (71,72).

A recently published randomized trial by the Brain Tumor Cooperative Group indicated that multidrug chemotherapy with radiotherapy conferred no particular benefit to patients with malignant glioma (80% of patients had glioblastoma multiforme) compared to BCNU and radiotherapy (73). Packer et al, in a study of 108 children with medulloblastoma or primitive neuroectodermal tumors, showed that CCNU-containing chemotherapy appeared to benefit these children, particularly those prospectively assigned to poor risk groups (74). McDonald noted responses of 6 to 18 months in patients with systemic metastases from anaplastic oligodendroglioma (75).

Nitrosoureas have significant activity against metastatic malignant melanoma. But combinations of dacarbazine and nitrosoureas have not shown significant improvement in response compared to dacarbazine alone (76). The combination of radiotherapy and nitrosoureas in malignant melanoma may be worthwhile to study. Fermand et al reported seven of eight patients were alive 9 to 17 months following nitrosoureas, melphalan, and etoposide combination chemotherapy and total body irradiation in patients with aggressive multiple myeloma (77).

Roosen et al, at Dusseldorf University, have proposed intra-arterial nimustine (ACNU) as a potentially useful tool to be used prior to postoperative radiotherapy in glioblastoma multiforme, based on results of a study on 35 patients (78).

Toxicity

As with other alkylating agents, administration of nitrosoureas is commonly associated with nausea, vomiting, hematopoietic depression, pulmonary fibrosis, and/or pneumonitis. High cumulative doses of these drugs can cause hepatic and renal toxicity and gonadal atrophy, especially in children (3). Carcinogenesis, as a specific toxicity of nitrosoureas, is complicated by the inherent natural history of secondary malignancies in patients with diseases such as leukemias, multiple myeloma, and lymphomas and in patients given a combination of nitrosoureas with other chemotherapeutic alkylating agents that are also known carcinogens (3). Depending on the site (and dose to a lesser extent) of concurrent or sequential radiotherapy, any and all of these potential toxicities may be enhanced with nitrosoureas.

Unlike other chemotherapeutic agents and even other alkylating agents, the hematopoietic depression secondary to nitrosoureas is usually manifest 3 to 6 weeks after its administration and lasts another 2 to 3 weeks (79). Thrombocytopenia and leukopenia (in that order) are the usual manifestations; consequently, cycles of nitrosoureas are given every 6 to 8 weeks. The implication is that in conjunction with radiotherapy, reduced doses of one or the other modality may be required or the modalities may have to be temporally separated.

Upper GI disturbances and pulmonary toxicity of nitrosoureas are dose related (3,80). This has grave repercussions in combined modality therapy with radiotherapy because both the GI tract and pulmonary tissues are particularly prone to irradiation. In practical terms, the use of nitrosoureas and total body irradiation (TBI) currently employed in autologous bone marrow transplantation deserves caution. BCNU with TBI has reportedly resulted in a 21% incidence of a syndrome characterized by pulmonary infiltrates and fibrosis, sometimes culminating in respiratory failure within 3 weeks of treatment (81).

Carcinogenesis, a late complication of antineoplastic therapy (both radiotherapy and chemotherapy), has long been reported in humans. Nitrosoureas, like most alkylating agents, are highly carcinogenic (2,61). However, because they are predominantly used in conjunction with radiotherapy in malignant gliomas, which are usually associated with contracted life spans, and because of the long latent period for the expression of carcinogeneity, nitrosoureas are not usually associated with secondary malignancies. In patients with colon carcinoma, adjuvant treatment with 5-FU and methyl-CCNU has been shown to have a beneficial effect on survival (Chapter 24). However, most oncologists hesitate to use methyl-CCNU in such cases and opt to use 5-FU alone or in conjunction with other drugs and/or radiotherapy.

Summary

Nitrosoureas share several features of activity, toxicity, and pharmacokinetics with other alkylating agents. However, they are uniquely different from other alkylators in other aspects. Nitrosoureas decompose rapidly after administration into active and inactive intermediates. Their antitumor and toxic activities may be attributable to different intermediates, and their lipid-soluble nature provides them with an ability to penetrate the blood-brain barrier.

Both in vitro and in vivo studies of nitrosoureas and radiotherapy suggest enhanced cell killing when combined. While there are conflicting reports of the appropriate timing of these two modalities, the consensus appears to be that nitrosoureas are best made available in tissues in the immediate period around a radiotherapy fraction.

Clinically, nitrosoureas are most commonly used with radiotherapy in the treatment of malignant gliomas and have an apparent salutary effect on the more poorly differentiated tumors such as glioblastoma multiforme. Nitrosoureas have wide antineoplastic activity; their experimental use with radiotherapy in the management of advanced malignancies that are resistant to conventional treatment is desirable.

CYCLOPHOSPHAMIDE

Mechanisms of Action

Cyclophosphamide (CP) also has a wide spectrum of antitumor activity and has been used primarily in lymphomas and lung, cervical, and ovarian cancers. CP is inactive biologically but is metabolized into active compounds by hepatic microsomal enzymes (2,3). Eighty percent of administered cyclophosphamide is oxidized into 4-keto-cyclophosphamide and carboxyphosphamides. These compounds have little cytotoxic properties and are excreted through urine. Secondary metabolism of these compounds yield metabolites such as phosphoramide mustard and nornitrogen mustard, which appear to be responsible for the cytotoxic properties of CP (3). Like most alkylating agents, these intermediates produce alkylation of DNA by attacking nucleophilic sites and decreasing DNA synthesis, thereby causing eventual cell death (2,3,59).

Cyclophosphamide is well absorbed orally and is normally administered by the oral or intravenous route. The systemic availability of the parent drug, when given orally, may be inversely dose dependent, varying between 100% for 100-mg doses and 74% for 300-mg doses (3). However, the peak plasma concentrations of both the parent compound and its active metabolites are directly dose dependent. Plasma half-life of CP varies between 3 and 10 hours. A plateau of plasma-alkylating activity is maintained for more than 6 hours. The wide variation of CP plasma half-life may be due to modulation of hepatic enzymes by previous exposure to drugs such as phenobarbital (82). CP is mostly cleared by the liver; about 15% is eliminated in the urine, and small amounts are occasionally detected in cerebrospinal fluid.

Cell-cycle responses, as gauged by cell culture and animal tumor models, have shown that similarly to nitrosoureas, cells in late G1, early S, and M phases of the cell cycle are most sensitive to CP (60). Progress in delay would therefore appear in late S and G2 phases. Both nitrosoureas and CP are thus cycle-specific agents, with proliferating cells being more sensitive than resting cells.

Cyclophosphamide-Radiation Interaction

In a series of studies on the hepatoma 3924A experimental solid tumor in rats, Looney et al demonstrated that the alternating use of CP and multiple radiation fractions achieved an enhanced effect or additive cell kill compared to either the drug or radiation given alone (83). Once again, cell survival curve modification appears to be that of a decrease in the shoulder as well as the slope, indicating a decrease in sublethal repair and increased sensitivity to irradiation. These are described in greater detail in Chapter 4 by Looney and Hopkins.

Enhanced normal-tissue response to CP in combination with radiotherapy has been shown in the central nervous system, lung, small intestine, esophagus, and skin (66,84,85). This enhancement has been noticed when the drug is given before, during, and after irradiation, often in combination with other drugs. However, in a review of experience with several mouse tumors, Phillips noted an augmented tumor response without increased normal tissue response when CP was administered 3 to 24 hours following irradiation (66).

Other toxicities related to CP, which can potentially be increased with radiotherapy, include cardiotoxicity, gonadal atrophy myelotoxicity, hemorrhagic cystitis, and carcinogenesis. Cardiac toxicity has been noted in patients receiving more than 2 mg/kg of CPM prior to bone marrow transplantation

(86). Both testicular germ cell aplasia and ovarian atrophy have been reported secondary to CP (87). Carcinogenesis secondary to alkylating agents is well established, and CP is not an exception. The combined use of radiotherapy with CP-containing chemotherapy regimens in Hodgkin's and non-Hodgkin's lymphoma should be of particular concern. Relative sparing of platelets is characteristic of CP myelotoxicity (88), but this may be offset by concurrent irradiation of bone-marrow reserve.

Hemorrhagic cystitis is a unique toxicity of the alkylating agents CP and ifosfamide. Since cystitis of varying degrees can result from pelvic irradiation, the additional use of CP in sequential or concurrent form could potentially enhance this toxicity. The incidence of such cystitis may be lowered (and the condition treated) by adequate hydration, frequent bladder emptying, bladder irrigation with N-acetylcysteine, and the use of sodium 2-mercaptoethanesulfonate (MESNA) and conjugated estrogen (3,89).

Clinical Applications

Cyclophosphamide has a wide antineoplastic spectrum. It has been used alone or in combination with other drugs against a variety of human tumors in conjunction with radiotherapy.

In small cell lung cancer, CP combined with Adriamycin and VP-16 yielded a 35% survival at 5 years. When consolidation thoracic radiotherapy was added sequentially to those patients not achieving a complete response, an additional 4% were alive at 5 years (90). CP combined with five other drugs given over 16 weeks produced 67% and 38% complete response rates, respectively, in patients with limited and extensive small cell carcinoma of the lung (91).

A CP-containing chemotherapy combination (CHOP-Bleo) and involved field irradiation for early diffuse large cell lymphomas resulted in 10-year survival rates of 74% for Stage I and 51% for Stage II patients (92). A similar combination for advanced and high-grade non-Hodgkin's lymphoma achieved a median survival of 43 months in 60 patients (93).

Combinations of CP and fractionated total body irradiation is often used in the treatment of acute leukemias (94). Combinations of CP-containing chemotherapy and radiotherapy are used in several pediatric tumors, including rhabdomyosarcoma, neuroblastoma, and Ewing's sarcoma, adult cancers of the breast and ovary, and soft-tissue sarcomas such as leiomyosarcomas (2).

SUMMARY

Cyclophosphamide is a cyclic ester of nitrogen mustard mechlorethamine, the original alkylating chemotherapeutic agent. It is absorbed easily through the oral route and has a variable plasma half-life of ranging from 3 to 10 hours. The parent drug is inactive; its cytotoxic metabolites are phosphoramide mustard and nornitrogen mustard. It is primarily cleared in the liver.

CP targets various components of DNA, resulting in major disruption of DNA replication and transcription. Cells in the G1 and early S phase of the cell cycle, compared to other phases, are particularly prone to CP.

Alkylating agents, including CP, have a wide spectrum of activity against human tumors. They also have a range of normal tissue toxicities, including effects on the bone marrow, heart, GI tract, and lung. All alkylating agents are teratogenic and carcinogenic. Their mode of interaction with radiation is probably additive. Finally, compared to other classes of drugs, alkylating agents are least susceptible to the phenomenon of multidrug resistance. For these reasons, most alkylators are best utilized in combination with other drugs when exploiting the drug-radiation interaction.

REFERENCES

1. Rhoads CP. Nitrogen mustards in treatment of neoplastic disease. JAMA 131:656, 1946.
2. Wittes RE, Leland-Jones B, Fortner C, Hubbard SM. Chemotherapy: The properties and uses of single agents. *In:* Manual of Oncologic Therapeutics 1989/1990. Wittes RE (Ed). Philadelphia, JB Lippincott, 1989, p. 91.
3. Colvin M, Chabner BA. Alkylating agents. *In:* Cancer Chemotherapy. Principles and Practice. Chabner BA, Collins JM (Eds). Philadelphia, JB Lippincott, 1990, p. 276.
4. Basolo F, Pearson, RG. The trans effect in metal complexes. Prog Inorg Chem 4:381, 1962.
5. Taylor SG, Applebaum E, Showel JL, et al. A randomized trial of adjuvant chemotherapy in

head and neck cancer. J Clin Oncol 3:672, 1985.
6. Toohill RJ, Anderson T, Byhardt RW, et al. Cisplatin and fluorouracil as neoadjuvant therapy in head and neck cancer. Arch Otolaryngol Head Neck Surg 113:758, 1987.
7. Final Report of the HNCP. Adjuvant chemotherapy for advanced head and neck squamous carcinoma. Cancer 60:301, 1987.
8. Schuller DE, Metch B, Stein DW, et al. Preoperative chemotherapy in advanced resectable head and neck cancer: Final report of the Southwest Oncology Group. Laryngoscope 98:1205, 1988.
9. Martin M, Hazan A, Vergnes L, et al. Randomized study of 5-fluorouracil and cisplatin as neoadjuvant therapy in head and neck cancer: A preliminary report. Int J Radiat Oncol Biol Phys 19:973, 1990.
10. Toohill RJ, Duncavage JA, Malin TC, et al. The effects of delay in standard treatment due to induction chemotherapy in two randomized prospective studies. Laryngoscope 97:407, 1987.
11. Perry MC, Eaton WL, Propert KJ, et al. Chemotherapy with or without radiation therapy in limited small-cell carcinoma of the lung. N Engl J Med 316:912, 1987.
12. Herskovic A, Martz K, Al-Sarraf M, et al. Comparison of radiotherapy (RT) to radiochemotherapy combination: A Phase III Trial. Proceedings of ASCO, 1991, p. 401.
13. Jacobs C, Makuch R. Efficacy of adjuvant chemotherapy for patients with resectable head and neck cancer: A subset analysis of the head and neck contracts program. J Clin Oncol 8:838, 1990.
14. Bachaud J, David J, Boussin G, Daly N. Combined postoperative radiotherapy and weekly cisplatin infusion for locally advanced squamous cell carcinoma of the head and neck: Preliminary report of a randomized trial. Int J Radiat Oncol Biol Phys 20:243, 1991.
15. Kanazawa H, Rappacchietta D, Kallman RF. Schedule-dependent therapeutic gain from the combination of fractionated irradiation and cis-diamminedichloroplatinum (II) in C3H/Km mouse model systems. Cancer Res 48:3158, 1988.
16. Tanabe M, Godat D, Kallman RF. Effects of fractionated schedules of irradiation combined with cis-diamminedichloroplatinum II on the SCCVII/ST tumor and normal tissues of the C3H/Km mouse. Int J Radiat Oncol Biol Phys 13:1523, 1987.
17. Schwachofer JHM, Crooijmans, RPMA, Hoogenhout J, et al. Effectiveness in inhibition of recovery of cell survival by cisplatin and carboplatin: Influence of treatment sequence. Int J Radiat Oncol Biol Phys 20:1235, 1991.
18. Zwelling LA, Kohn KW. Mechanism of action of cis-dichlorodiammineplatinum (II). Cancer Treat Rev 63:1439, 1979.
19. Cleare MJ. Some aspects of platinum complex chemistry and their relation to anti-tumor activity. J Clin Hematol Oncol 7:1, 1977.
20. Fraval HNA, Roberts JJ. G1 phase Chinese hamster V79-379A cells are inherently more sensitive to platinum bound to their DNA than mid S phase or asynchronously treated cells. Biochem Pharmacol 28:1575, 1979.
21. Howle JA, Gale GR. Cis-dichlorordiammineplatinum (II). Persistent and selective inhibition of deoxyribonucleic acid synthesis in vivo. Biochem Pharmacol 19:2757, 1970.
22. Harder HC, Rosenberg B. Inhibitory effects of antitumor platinum compounds on DNA, RNS and protein synthesis in mammalian cells in vivo. Int J Cancer 6:207, 1970.
23. Howle JA, Thompson HS, Stone AE, et al. Cis-dichlorodiammineplatinum (II): Inhibition of nucleic acid synthesis in lymphocytes stimulated with phytohemagglutin. Proc Soc Exp Biol Med 137:820, 1971.
24. Calabresi P, Parks RE. Chemotherapy of neoplastic diseases. *In:* The Pharmacological Basis of Therapeutics. 6th Ed. Gilman A, Goodman L (Eds). New York, Macmillan Publishing Co., 1980, p. 1298.
25. Dewitt L. Combined treatment of radiation and cis-diamminedichloroplatinum (II): A review of experimental and clinical data. Int J Radiat Oncol Biol Phys 13:403, 1987.
26. Laurent G, Erickson LC, Sharkey NA, Kohn KW. DNA crosslinking and cytotoxicity induced by cis-diamminedichloroplatinum (II) in human normal and tumor cell lines. Cancer Res 41:3347, 1981.
27. Zwelling LA, Anderson T, Kohn KW. DNA-protein and DNA interstrand cross-linking by cis- and trans-platinum (II) diamminedichloride in L1210 mouse leukemia cells and relation to cytotoxicity. Cancer Res 39:365, 1979.
28. Sorensen CM, Barry MA, Eastman A. Analysis of events associated with cell cycle arrest at G2 phase and cell death induced by cisplatin. J Natl Cancer Inst 82:749, 1990.
29. Hamilton TC, Ozols RF, Dabrow MB. Multidrug resistance to alkylating agents and platinum compounds: State of our knowledge. Oncology 4:101, 1990.
30. Lai G-M, Hamilton TC, Fojo AT, et al. Increased DNA repair in cisplatin (CP) resistant human ovarian cancer (HOC) cell lines. Proc Am Assoc Cancer Res 29:300, 1988.

31. Lai G-M, Young RC, Hamilton TC, Ozol RF. Modulation of DNA repair by buthionine sulfoximine in a cisplatin resistant human ovarian cancer cell line. Proc Am Assoc Cancer Res 30:490, 1989.
32. Hamer DH. Metallothionein. Annu Rev Biochem 55:913, 1986.
33. Kelly SL, Basu A, Teicher BA, et al. Overexpression of metallothionein confers resistance to anticancer drugs. Science 241:1813, 1988.
34. Chu G, Chang E. Cisplatin-resistant cells express increased levels of a factor that recognizes damaged DNA. Proc Natl Acad Sci USA 87:3324, 1990.
35. Carmichael J, Hickson ID. Keynote address: Mechanisms of cellular resistance to cytotoxic drugs and x-irradiation. Int J Radiat Oncol Biol Phys 20:197, 1991.
36. Gandara DR, Wiebe VJ, Perez EA, et al. Cisplatin rescue therapy: Experience with sodium thiosulfate WR2721 and diethyldithiocarbamate. Crit Rev Oncol Hematol 10:353, 1990.
37. Patton TF, Himmelstein KJ, Belt R, et al. Plasma levels and urinary excretion of filterable platinum species following bolus injection and IV infusion of cis-dichlorodiammineplatinum (II) in man. Cancer Treat Rep 62:1359, 1978.
38. Reece PA, Stafford I, Russell J, et al. A model for ultrafiltrate plasma platinum disposition in patients treated with cisplatin. Cancer Chemother Pharmacol 20:26, 1987.
39. Reece PA, Stafford I, Russell J, et al. Creatinine clearance as a predictor of ultrafiltrate platinum disposition in cancer patients treated with cisplatin: Relationship between peak ultrafiltrate platinum plasma levels and nephrotoxicity. J Clin Oncol 5:304, 1987.
40. Corden BJ, Fine RL, Ozols RF, Collins JM. Clinical pharmacology of high-dose cisplatin. Cancer Chemother Pharmacol 14:38, 1985.
41. DeGregorio MW, Wilber JR, Crowley TJ, Cadman EC. Clinical pharmacology of high-dose cisplatin. Cancer Chemother Pharmacol 15:183, 1985.
42. Ozols RF, Corden BJ, Jacob J, et al. High-dose cisplatin in hypertonic saline. Ann Intern Med 100:19, 1984.
43. Perez EA, Hesketh PJ, Gandara DR. Serotonin antagonists in the management of cisplatin-induced emesis. Semin Oncol 18(Suppl 3):73, 1991.
44. Gandara DR, Perez EA, Wiebe V, DeGregorio MW. Cisplatin chemoprotection and rescue: Pharmacologic modulation of toxicity. Semin Oncol 18(Suppl 3):49, 1991.
45. Ozols RF. Cisplatin dose intensity. Semin Oncol 16(Suppl 6):22, 1989.
46. Gandara DR, Tanaka MT, Crowley J, Livingston RB. Comparison of standard dose cisplatin, high dose cisplatin, and high dose cisplatin plus mitomycin in metastatic non small cell lung cancer: Preliminary results of a Phase III study. Abstract 843. Proceedings of ASCO 10:246, 1991.
47. Nichols CR, Williams SD, Loehrer PJ, et al. Randomized study of cisplatin dose intensity in poor-risk germ cell tumors: A Southeastern Cancer Study Group and Southwest Oncology Group protocol. J Clin Oncol 9:1163, 1991.
48. Zak M, Drobnik J. Effect of cis-dichlorodiammineplatinum (II) on the postirradiation lethality in mice after irradiation with x-rays. Strahlentherapie 142:112, 1971.
49. Begg AC, Cisplatin and radiation: Interaction probabilities and therapeutic possibilities. Int J Radiat Oncol Biol Phys 19:1183, 1990.
50. Douple EB, Richmond RC. A review of platinum complex biochemistry suggests a rationale for combined platinum-radiotherapy. Int J Radiat Oncol Biol Phys 5:1335, 1979.
51. Dewit L. Combined treatment of radiation and cis-diamminedichloroplatinum (II): A review of experimental and clinical data. Int J Radiat Oncol Biol Phys 13:403, 1987.
52. Coughlin CT, Richmond RC. Biologic and clinical developments of cisplatin combined with radiation: Concepts, utility, projections for new trials, and the emergence of carboplatin. Semin Oncol 16(Suppl 6):31, 1989.
53. Adams GE. Molecular mechanisms of cellular radiosensitization and protection. *In:* Radiation Protection and Sensitization. Morosen HL, Quintilliano M (Eds). London, Taylor and Frances, 1970, p. 3.
54. Richmond RC. Toxic variability and radiation sensitization by dichlorodiammineplatinum (II) complexes in S typhimurium cells. Radiat Res 99:596, 1984.
55. Richmond RC, Powers EL. Radiation sensitization of bacterial spores by cis-dichlorodiammineplatinum (II). Radiat Res 68:251, 1976.
56. Mattox DE, Sternson LA, Von Hoff DD, et al. Tumor concentration of platinum in patients with head and neck cancer. Arch Otolaryngol 91:271, 1983.
57. Fu KK, Phillips TL. Biologic rationale of combined radiotherapy and chemotherapy. Hematol Oncol Clin North Am 5:737, 1991.
58. Moulder JE, Holcenberg JS, Barton KA, et al. Renal irradiation and the pharmacology and toxicity of methotrexate and cisplatinum. Int J Radiat Oncol Biol Phys 12:1415, 1986.
59. Kaufman SD, Weitzman S. The clinical pharmacology of anticancer drugs. *In:* Radiation-

drug Interaction in the Treatment of Cancer. Sokol GH, Maickel RP (Eds). New York, John Wiley and Sons, 1980, p. 63.
60. Bhuyan GK, Scheidt LG, Fraser TJ. Cell cycle phase specificity of antitumor agents. Cancer Res 32:398, 1972.
61. Hill SA, Keng PC, Siemann DW. Survival in subpopulations of cells derived from solid KHT sarcomas by centrifugal elutriation following treatment of CCNU and miso. Int J Radiat Oncol Biol Phys 10:1615, 1984.
62. Siemann DW, Hill SA. Enhanced tumor response through therapies combining CCNU, miso and radiation. Int J Radiat Oncol Biol Phys 10:1623, 1984.
63. Begg AC, Fu KK, Vannar J, Phillips TL. Combination therapy of a solid murine tumor with 1,3-bis(2-chloroethyl)-1-nitrosourea and irradiation. Int J Radiat Oncol Biol Phys 5:1559, 1979.
64. Wheeler KT, Deen DF, Wilson CB, et al. BCNU-modification of the in vitro radiation response. Int J Radiat Oncol Biol Phys 2:79, 1977.
65. Phillips TL. Clinical and experimental alterations in the radiation therapeutic ratio caused by cytotoxic chemotherapy. *In:* Radiation Biology in Cancer Research. Meyor RE, Withers HR (Eds). New York, Raven Press, 1980, p. 567.
66. Phillips TL. Tissue toxicity of radiation-drug interactions. *In:* Radiation-drug Interactions in the Treatment of Cancer. Sokol GH, Maickel RP (Eds). New York, John Wiley and Sons, 1980, p. 175.
67. Loheeler KT, Kaufman K, Feldstein M. Response of a rat brain tumor to fractionated therapy with low doses of BCNU and irradiation. Int J Radiat Oncol Biol Phys 5:1553, 1979.
68. Deen DF, Williams ME, Wheeler KT. Comparison of the CCNU and BCNU modification of the in vitro radiation response in 9L brain tumor cells of rats. Int J Radiat Oncol Biol Phys 5:1541, 1979.
69. Deen DF. Personal communication, 1991.
70. Solero CL, Mondfardini S, Broombilla C, et al. Controlled study with BCNU vs. CCNU as adjuvant chemotherapy following surgery plus radiotherapy for glioblastoma multiforme. Cancer Clin Trials 2:32, 1979.
71. Stewart DJ. The role of chemotherapy in the treatment of gliomas in adults. Cancer Treat Dev 16(3):129, 1989.
72. Shapiro WR, Green SB, Burger PC. Randomized trial of three chemotherapy regimens and two radiotherapy regimens in postoperative treatment of malignant glioma. Brain Tumor Cooperative Group Trial 8001. J Neurosurg 71(1):1, 1989.
73. EORTC Brain Tumor Group. Effect of CCNU on survival rate of objective remission and duration of disease free interval in patients with malignant brain gliomas. A final evaluation. Eur J Cancer 14:851, 1978.
74. Packer RJ, Sutton LN, Goldwein JW, et al. Improved survival with the use of adjuvant chemotherapy in the treatment of medulloblastoma. J Neurosurg 74(3):433, 1991.
75. McDonald DR, O'Brien RA, Gilbert JJ, Cairncross JE. Metastatic anaplastic oligodendroglioma. Neurology 39:1593, 1989.
76. Legha SS. Current therapy for malignant melanoma. Semin Oncol 16(Suppl):34, 1989.
77. Fermand JP, Levy Y, Gerota J, et al. Treatment of aggressive multiple myeloma by high-dose chemotherapy and total body irradiation followed by blood stem cells autologous graft. Blood 73(1):20, 1989.
78. Roosen N, Kiwit JC, Lins E, et al. Adjuvant intraarterial chemotherapy in the management of World Health Organization grade IV gliomas of the brain. Cancer 64:1984, 1989.
79. DeVita VT, Carbone PP, Owens AH, et al. Clinical trials with 1,3-bis(2-chloroethyl)-1-nitrosourea. NSC-409962. Cancer Res 25:1876, 1978.
80. Crittenden D, Tranum BL, Huot A. Pulmonary fibrosis after prolonged therapy with 1,3-bis(2-chloroethyl)-1-nitrosourea. Chest 72:372, 1977.
81. Litam JP, Dail DH, Spitzer G, et al. Early pulmonary toxicity after administration of high-dose BCNU. Cancer Treat Rep 65:39, 1981.
82. Alberts DS, van Daalen Wetters T. The effects of phenobarbital on cyclophosphamide antitumor activity. Cancer Res 36:2785, 1973.
83. Looney WB, Longerbeam MG, Hopkins HA, Carter WH. Solid tumor models for the assessment of different treatment modalities. XXI. Comparison of different radiation dose schedules alone or in combination with cyclophosphamide. Cancer 51:1012, 1983.
84. Byfield JE. Central nervous system toxicities from combined therapies. Front Radiat Ther Oncol 12:228, 1979.
85. Patel AR, Shah PC, Rhee HC, et al. Cyclophosphamide therapy and interstitial pulmonary fibrosis. Cancer 38:1542, 1976.
86. Steinherz LJ, Steinherz PG. Cyclophosphamide cardiotoxicity. Cancer Bulletin 37:231, 1985.
87. Kumar R, Biggart JD, McEvoy J, et al. Cyclophosphamide and reproduction function. Lancet 1:568, 1972.
88. Nissen-Meyer R, Host H. A comparison between the hematological side effects of cyclophosphamide and nitrogen mustard. Cancer Chemother Rep 9:51, 1960.

89. Liu YK, Harty JI, Steinbock GS, et al. Treatment of radiation or cyclophosphamide induced hemorrhagic cystitis using conjugated estrogen. J Urol 144(1):41, 1990.
90. Armstrong JG, Rosenstein MM, Scher HI, et al. Limited small-cell lung cancer: Prognostic significance of a complete response to the induction phase of chemotherapy followed by thoracic irradiation. Radiology 178(3):875, 1991.
91. Taylor CW, Crowley J, Williamson SK, et al. Treatment of small-cell lung cancer with an alternating regimen given at weekly intervals: Southwest Oncology Group pilot study. J Clin Oncol 8(11):1811, 1990.
92. Velasquez WS, Fuller LM, Jagannath S, et al. Stages I and II diffuse large cell lymphomas: Prognostic factors and long term results with CHOP-bleo and radiotherapy. Blood 77(5):942, 1991.
93. Koppler H, Pfluger KH, Eschenbach I, et al. CHOP-VP16 chemotherapy and involved field irradiation for high-grade non-Hodgkin's lymphomas. A phase II multicentre study. Br J Cancer 60(1):79, 1989.
94. Clift RA, Buckner CD, Appelbaum FR, et al. Allogeneic marrow transplantation in patients with acute myeloid leukemia in first remission: A randomized trial of two irradiation regimens. Blood 76:1867, 1990.

Chapter 9

ANTIBIOTICS

MADHU J. JOHN AND SEWA S. LEGHA

INTRODUCTION

Antibiotics have the widest spectrum of antitumor activity, next to alkylating agents. They are natural products isolated from fermentation products of the various species of Streptomyces. The antineoplastic activity of antibiotics is due to inhibition of DNA and/or RNA synthesis. Their cytotoxic properties preclude their use as an antibacterial. Since they have effects on several phases of the cell cycle, antibiotics tend to be nonphase-specific antineoplastic agents. Similar to alkylating agents, antibiotics tend to be dose-limited by myelotoxicity. However, some have unique toxicities that are of particular relevance to interaction with radiotherapy. A classic example is the cardiotoxicity of anthracyclines, particularly doxorubicin, which can be exacerbated by mediastinal irradiation. The pulmonary and mucous membrane toxicities of bleomycin are also of particular concern when combined with radiotherapy for the treatment of head, neck, and thoracic tumors.

Antibiotics have a wide range of activity against human tumors, including cancers of the breast, lung, stomach, head and neck, testes, lymphomas, and several pediatric malignancies. The most important of these, particularly regarding chemoradiation, are anthracyclines, bleomycin, Actinomycin D, and mitomycin C. Table 9–1 describes the pertinent features of these antibiotics and their interactions with radiation.

ANTHRACYCLINES

Daunorubicin (daunomycin), doxorubicin (Adriamycin), idarubicin, and epirubicin are anthracycline glycoside common antibiotics in clinical use. Adriamycin and daunomycin, which are fermentation products of Streptomyces peucetius, were first introduced for clinical use in Italy in 1967 (1) and are still the most commonly used anthracyclines. Both have a tetracyclic ring structure attached to a sugar (daunosamine). Daunorubicin is used as part of a combination of several drugs for acute leukemias. Adriamycin is used for several malignancies, including cancers of the breast, lung, stomach, testes, bladder, thyroid, and ovary, for Hodgkin's and non-Hodgkin's lymphoma, for sarcomas of soft tissue and bone, and for acute leukemias, among others. The following is a description of Adriamycin alone, due to its broad-spectrum activity and its predominant clinical use among anthracyclines today.

Mechanisms of Action

Adriamycin (ADR) is usually administered in doses of 60 to 75 mg/m^2 intravenously every 21 days. Variations of drug administration include divided doses on days 0 and 7 or three consecutive days (days 0 to 2), once weekly bolus injections, and continuous infusions over 48 to 96 hours every 3 weeks. ADR is not absorbed from the gastrointestinal (GI) tract. About one-half of the ADR dose given intravenously is excreted in bile; another 10% is excreted in urine. It is non-cell-cycle specific, having activity in all phases of the cell cycle.

ADR is widely distributed in plasma and tissues. Its plasma clearance is triphasic, with half-lives of 8 to 25 minutes (distribution in tissues), 1.5 to 10 hours (metabolism), and 24 to 48 hours (release from binding sites); the mean half-life is 16 hours. ADR is predominantly metabolized in the liver (50 to

Table 9–1. Features of Antibiotics and their Interaction with Radiation

Drug	Mechanisms of Action	Interaction with RT	Intermediates	Cell-Cycle Specificity	Metabolism	Half-Life	Toxicity
Adriamycin	Hydroxyl and other free radical formation or topoisomerase II dependent DNA damage	Decreasing "n" or extrapolation number of radiation survival curve	Semiquinone Quinone Methide	Non-cell-cycle specific	50% metabolized in liver	Triphasic, mean–16 hours	1. Myelosuppression 2. Cardiotoxicity 3. Mucositis 4. Gastrointestinal
Mitomycin C	Alkylation leading to cross-linking of DNA strands; direct action on hypoxic cells	Additive or supra-additive	Semiquinone Hydroquinone	Late G1, Early S	Biodegraded in liver, kidney, heart, and spleen	Less than 20 minutes	1. Myelosuppression 2. Interstitial pneumonitis 4. Gastrointestinal
Actinomycin D	DNA binding, inhibition of RNA, and protein synthesis	Increased sensitivity of irradiated cells, inhibition of repair of sublethal radiation damage	None identified	Non-cell-cycle specific	Excreted mainly in urine, bile and feces	36 hours	1. Myelotoxicity 2. Nausea, vomiting, diarrhea 3. Pulmonary toxicity 4. Recall phenomenon
Bleomycin	DNA scission reaction between base pairs; negligible effect on hypoxic cells	Additive; some repair of sublethal radiation damage	Activated bleomycin-Fe(II)–O_2 complex	M and G_2	50% excreted in urine in 24 hours	1 hour	1. Mucositis 2. Pulmonary fibrosis 3. Esophagitis 4. Lack of myelotoxicity

60%); liver dysfunctions can lead to higher serum levels of the drug and usually require dose reduction (2,3,4).

ADR enters the cell by free diffusion through the cell membrane and may be actively ejected in some cases by P170-glycoprotein, a membrane protein (5). Most of the drug settles on the nucleus, and part of this nuclear drug is intercalated into the DNA molecule. Here, ADR affects the enzyme topoisomerase-II, which promotes DNA strand breakage (6). It is also known that ADR can undergo one or two electron reduction to reactive compounds, such as hydrogen peroxide and the hydroxyl radical (OH°), which can cause massive damage to DNA and cell membranes (7). ADR, however, circulates predominantly as the parent drug; its only common metabolite is doxorubicinol.

Thus,

$$\text{ADR} \xrightarrow[\text{reduction}]{\text{1 electron}} \text{semiquinone free radical} \longrightarrow \begin{array}{l}\text{superoxide, hydrogen peroxide}\\ \text{and hydroxyl radicals}\end{array}$$

$$\text{ADR} \xrightarrow[\text{reduction}]{\text{2 electron}} \begin{array}{c}\text{quinone}\\ \text{methide}\end{array} \longrightarrow \text{deoxyaglycone}$$

Legha et al have shown that the cytotoxic or antineoplastic activity of ADR is related to area under the curve (AUC) or exposure time (8). However, concentration has been shown to be more important than length of exposure (9,10). The cardiotoxicity of ADR is a function of the peak serum levels of the drug (8).

Interaction with Radiation

Tumors

The interaction of Adriamycin with radiation has been studied in a variety of cell lines, including normal tissue elements such as bone marrow stem cells and animal and human tumor cells (11–15). The consistent findings from these studies include the following.

1. ADR reduced the extrapolation number ("n") of cells in culture (see Chapter 6 for explanation) (11–13). In other words, it reduced the threshold of a radiation survival curve. This effect was seen when the drug was administered 3 hours prior to or in between a fractionated radiation course. Radiation followed by ADR had a similar but far less pronounced effect.
2. Secondly, ADR did *not* affect sublethal radiation damage (SLD) or potentially lethal radiation damage (PLD)(13–15).

In practical terms, this translates to a potential for ADR to reduce radiation fraction sizes in radioresistant tumors.

Normal Tissue

The clinical augmentation of radiation reactions by anthracyclines has been reported in several normal tissues, including the skin, lung, GI tract, and heart. In almost every instance, the reaction is in the form of a "recall" phenomenon, in which patients developed toxicity in a previously irradiated site. Donaldson initially reported on the radiation recall phenomenon in the skin of children treated with ADR (16). Similar reactions on the skin and lung were reported by Cassady et al (17).

ADR given to mice 24 hours prior to irradiation resulted in increased upper GI and pulmonary toxicity (18). ADR given 2 hours or 2 days after radiotherapy resulted in marked modification of radiation survival curves for intestinal crypt cells in LAF mice (19). However, Belli summated the often contradictory results of in vitro and in vivo experience of radiotherapy and ADR interaction and concluded that cellular systems rather than animal models may be better suited to study their combination effect on normal tissues (20). Clinical manifestations of severe gastroenteritis have been reported with abdominal irradiation and ADR as part of combined modality therapy, especially in children (21,22).

Anthracyclines can cause both acute and chronic cardiac failure. Acute failure can be manifest by arrhythmias, pericarditis, and congestive heart failure. With bolus administration of ADR (every 21 to 28 days), cumulative injury to myocardium occurs, culminating in characteristic myocardial fibrosis and chronic congestive heart failure (CHF). Clinical risk of CHF is minimal at cumulative doses below 350 mg/m^2; a dose limit of 550 mg/m^2 is usually imposed by medical oncologists. However, these guidelines for ADR delivery are unreasonable in circumstances in which mediastinal radiotherapy has been previously given or is contemplated. A combination of 2000 cGy to the heart and 250 mg/m^2 of ADR is estimated to cause approximately a 10% incidence of clinically evident cardiotoxicity (7,8,23). This may be clinically relevant in the treatment of Hodgkin's disease and small cell lung and breast cancer. The interaction of radiotherapy and ADR on the heart may be mitigated by modifying radiation delivery (decreasing total dose and fraction size), decreasing the cardiac volume irradiated, or increasing the interval between radiotherapy and ADR delivery, preferentially administering radiotherapy prior to ADR when feasible and by administering ADR as prolonged continuous infusion over 48 to 96 hours. The subject of cardiac toxicity secondary to chemoradiation is elaborated in Chapter 35.

Other common side effects of ADR, which may be aggravated or prolonged by radiotherapy, include mucositis, myelotoxicity, and hair loss. The incidence and severity of these adverse effects depend on the parameters of delivery listed above. The basis for common toxicity may be related to identical action by radiotherapy and anthracycline on stem cell population (bone marrow, gastrointestinal system, and/or the endothelial cell linings of blood vessel walls).

Clinical Applications

ADR has a wide spectrum of antineoplastic activity. In combination with radiotherapy, however, its activity in Hodgkin's and non-Hodgkin's lymphoma, breast cancer, lung cancer, and sarcoma of bone and soft tissues is particularly important. In bone-marrow transplantation, the use of radiotherapy and ADR has profound implications in terms of cardiotoxicity and myelotoxicity.

In Hodgkin's disease, mediastinal radiotherapy is frequently used with ADR-containing (ABVD) chemotherapy combinations (Chapter 19). Conventional fields in mantle radiotherapy use gradient doses for different cardiac volumes; 20 to 50% of cardiac volumes receive 1800 to 3000 cGy in conventional fractions of 170 to 200 cGy daily before appropriate blocks are utilized. These doses may have to be modified when large mediastinal masses are treated initially with radiotherapy. Similar problems may be anticipated in non-Hodgkin's malignant lymphoma when Adriamycin-containing regimens such as M-BACOD and COPBLAM are used and when radiotherapy is directed to "bulky" disease sites. Infradiaphragmatic radiotherapy and ADR must be used with caution in malignant lymphomas because of the potential for enhanced GI effects (21,22).

ADR is frequently a part of multidrug regimens used with whole body radiotherapy (TBI) in bone-marrow transplant programs, malignant lymphomas, leukemias, and breast cancer (see Chapter 18). There is some clinical evidence that the skin erythema or volar erythema seen with TBI and ADR may be less pronounced with increasing temporal separation of the two modalities. Other toxicities, such as cardiotoxicity and myelotoxicity, may be reduced with fractionated (rather than single large fraction) TBI (see Chapters 18 and 35).

Rosenthal and Rotman noted an 86% response rate in 11 patients with soft-tissue sarcomas treated with 120-hour continuous infusion of ADR every 3 weeks and gradually increasing doses of concurrent radiotherapy starting at 100 cGy (24).

The use of infusional ADR with vinblastine and dexamethasone (VAD) in patients with multiple myeloma refractory to alkylating agents resulted in a 65% response rate (25). ADR-containing regimens in small-cell lung cancer may become less popular than previously, either because of the resurgence of thoracic radiotherapy as part of combined modality therapy or the superiority of the cisplatinum-etoposide combination (see Chapter 26).

Summary

ADR, the prototype anthracycline, has significant activity against a wide range of human tumors. Its optimal clinical use is subverted by a distinctive cardiotoxicity and sometimes by myelotoxicity. As a result, it is invariably used as part of multidrug regimens, particularly in lymphomas and hematological malignancies.

ADR has been shown in the laboratory and clinically to render tumors and normal tissues increasingly susceptible to radiation damage. The biologic basis of radiation-ADR interaction appears to be at the level of the stem cell or the endothelial lining of blood vessels.

In practical terms, the combination of thoracic irradiation and ADR is limited by cardiac and pulmonary toxicity, abdominal irradiation and ADR is limited by GI toxicity, and TBI and ADR are limited by myelotoxicity. Hundreds of anthracycline analogs have been studied and found to be lacking in comparable activity to ADR if they possess less cardiotoxicity or myelotoxicity. Nevertheless, imaginative combinations of various radiotherapy fractionation and dose-delivery schemes and prolonged infusions of ADR constitute possible means of exploiting anthracycline-radiation interaction.

MITOMYCIN C

Mitomycin C (MMC), an antibiotic extracted from Streptomyces caespitosus, has a broad antineoplastic spectrum and has been used generally in combination with other chemotherapeutic agents against several human tumors since 1958, when it was first introduced (26). As a single-agent, its use is tempered by dose-limiting bone-marrow toxicity, and its action against hypoxic or anaerobic cells makes MMC a fundamentally superior drug to combine with radiation, to which hypoxic cells are inherently resistant. Thus, while a large number of clinical studies combining MMC (alone or with other drugs) with radiation have shown increased survival and/or local control (27), trepidation exists concerning combination of the drug with radiation when radiation fields encompass sizable areas of bone-marrow reserve.

Mechanisms of Action

Mitomycin C is usually administered intravenously but is also used for topical treatment of bladder tumors through the intravesical route. It has also been used intraarterially in GI and gynecologic tumors. After its administration intravenously, MMC is widely distributed with high concentrations in the kidneys, heart, and tongue. The half-life is about 20 minutes. MMC is rapidly biodegraded primarily by the liver and secondarily by the spleen, kidneys, brain, and heart. The large number of biodegrading sites is probably why liver and renal functions are not critical parameters for MMC dose modification. MMC is usually administered in doses of 10 to 15 mg/m^2 by bolus intravenous injection every 4 to 6 weeks to allow for bone-marrow recovery (1,27,28).

Alkylation of DNA is the principal mechanism of action of MMC. Parent MMC, in its oxidized form, is inactive. In aqueous solutions under anaerobic conditions, MMC is reduced by enzymatic or acidic action into its active intermediate radicals semiquinone and hydroquinone. The enzyme systems that facilitate this activation include NADPH-cytochrome, P-450 reductase, xanthine oxidase, and NADPH-cytochrome c_2 reductase. Monofunctional alkylation is the most common interaction, but bifunctional alkylation (which accounts for only 10% of the interactions) is responsible for cross-linking with DNA strands and, therefore, the cytotoxicity of MMC. Under aerobic conditions, MMC is similarly reduced to semiquinone and hydroquinone radicals, which interact with oxygen to form highly cytotoxic hydroxyl radicals, hydrogen peroxide, and a sulphoxide radical anion. Other mechanisms of MMC action include inhibition of DNA and protein synthesis. Cells in late G1 and early S phases are more sensitive to MMC (1,27–31). The principal mechanism of MMC action can be summarized as follows:

Oxidized MMC (inactive) → Reduction by enzyme + acidic systems → semiquinone and hydroquinone (free radicals) → 10% Bifunctional alkylation → Cross-link with DNA → cytotoxity

Interaction with Radiation

Tumors

The interaction of MMC with radiation has been studied both in vitro and in vivo, primarily with EMT6 mouse mammary tumor cells or implanted tumors (32–34). This tumor is particularly suitable for MMC-radiation interaction studies because it has significant capability to repair both sublethal and potentially lethal radiation damage and because it contains a sizable percentage of hypoxic cells. These characteristics closely parallel those of human tumors.

Rockwell and co-authors, who have studied this subject extensively in the laboratory, have arrived at the conclusion that the combination of MMC with radiation results in additive or supra-additive tumor cell kill (31–35). The supra-additive effect may perhaps be related to the differential effect of radiation and MMC on aerobic and hypoxic cells in a heterogenous tumor population. Figure 9–1 relates the differential effect on aerobic and hypoxic cells in EMT6 tumors.

Other characteristics of MMC-radiation interaction as gauged by Rockwell and other investigators in various in vivo tumor systems can be summarized as follows.

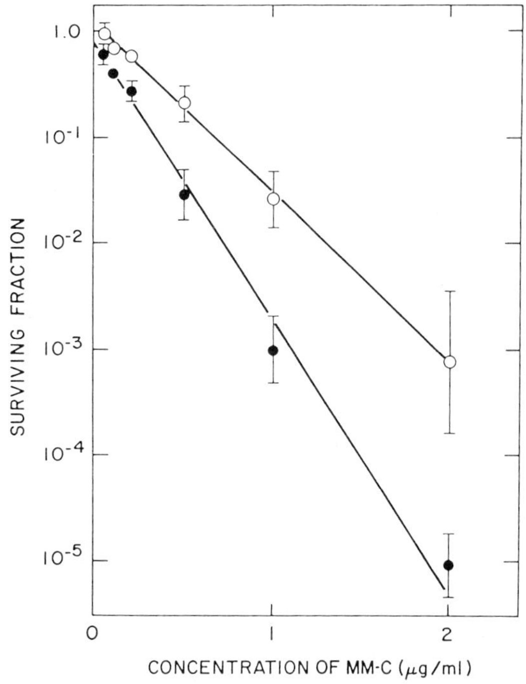

Fig. 9–1. Differential toxicity of mitomycin C for aerobic (○) and hypoxic (●) EMT6 cells. (From Rockwell S. Int J Cancer 38:229, 1986. Copyright © 1986 Wiley-Liss. Reprinted by permission of Wiley-Liss, A Division of John Wiley and Sons, Inc.)

1. MMC does not significantly change the slope of the radiation dose-response curve and vice versa. In other words, each modality does not appear to increase the sensitivity of a tumor to the other (32,35).
2. The cell-cycle responses to radiation and MMC are different and may therefore be used in complementary fashion in human experiments. While cells in G1 phase are most sensitive to MMC, they are generally radioresistant. Cells in the M and late S phase are radiosensitive but relatively resistant to MMC. Early S phase cells are sensitive to both radiation and MMC (28,35,36).
3. Studies with various tumor systems suggest that the additive or supra-additive effects of MMC and radiation are best realized when the drug is given immediately before or after radiation. The enhanced effect is less discernible when MMC is given long after radiation (32,35,37).
4. The effects of lower-dose-rate radiation on murine tumors are enhanced by MMC in either additive or supra-additive fashion, as studies by Fu et al have shown (38,39). The clinical implications of these studies cannot be overemphasized. While most clinical and laboratory chemoradiation studies have focused on conventional external (medium dose rate) radiotherapy, the results of Fu's studies open up another sizable clinical area of intracavitary, intraluminal, and interstitial therapy for potential use with chemotherapeutic agents (38,39).

Normal Tissue

The interaction of MMC and radiation on several target normal tissues has been studied in the laboratory. Results suggest that, in most cases, a therapeutic gain may be obtained but that bone-marrow, intestinal, and lung toxicities can be dose-limiting to both MMC and radiation.

Bone-marrow toxicity of radiotherapy is volume related and can be irreversible (see Chapter 31). The acute toxicity of MMC is related to stem cells in the bone marrow, such as CFU-S and CFU-GM, and results in relatively prolonged depression of white cells and platelets in peripheral blood. These two factors probably account for the fact that both medical and radiation oncologists are generally leary of combining MMC and radiation in chemoradiation protocols. On the other hand, the differential effects of radiation and MMC on aerobic and hypoxic tumor cells may be too good an advantage to pass off entirely. Moreover, antitumor activity of MMC is sizable in doses producing negligible host toxicity, and ultimate local tumor control is not necessarily predicated by total radiation dose in a chemoradiation setting (35).

An increase in intestinal crypt reactions in mice receiving MMC and radiation compared to radiation alone has been noted both with medium and low dose rates (36,38). Nausea, vomiting, and diarrhea are frequent side effects of MMC. Radiation may enhance these toxicities, depending on the area being treated. Enhanced pulmonary toxicity has been noted in mice receiving combined MMC and radiation compared to radiation alone (40,41). But there were some contradictory data regarding dose-response, in that mice treated with higher doses of radiation with MMC developed less pulmonary toxicity compared to lower doses of radiation with MMC. In humans, pulmonary toxicity secondary to MMC is characterized by dry cough, dyspnea, and diffuse interstitial infiltrates. The pattern of radiation-induced pulmonary toxicity is similar except that the distribution usually parallels the treatment volume. However, the incidence of these reactions is low enough compared to tumor reactions so that therapeutic gain is preserved.

Thus, while radiobiological data suggest increased therapeutic ratio in several animal systems with combinations of MMC and radiation, caution should be taken in transposing these data to the treatment of human cancers for several reasons.

1. In clinical settings, MMC is rarely given alone with radiotherapy; it is often combined with other drugs (such as 5-FU), which may have similar bone marrow, pulmonary, or GI adverse effects.
2. Late MMC-related toxicities such as subcutaneous necrosis have been observed in patients who had previously received radiation at the site where MMC was subsequently administered. Late nephrotoxicity and cardiotoxicity have also been reported in humans secondary to MMC (27).
3. Bone-marrow, pulmonary, and intestinal toxicity secondary to radiotherapy are all volume related. The clinician should reconsider standard radiation treatment volumes when administering MMC in the peri-irradiation period. For example, investigators at Wayne State University discontinued the use of MMC in combination with radiotherapy for cancer of the esophagus due to pulmonary toxicity. This may have been a result of the standard use of large radiation fields that encompassed large volumes of pulmonary tissues. Such toxicity can be decreased by markedly curtailing pulmonary treatment volumes without dropping MMC from the regimen for esophageal cancer (Chapter 21).

Clinical Applications

By administering MMC in bolus injections every 4 to 6 weeks, clinicians have been able to circumvent the drug's bone-marrow toxicity limitations and to use the drug to advantage in a wide variety of tumors. MMC has been used alone or in combination with other drugs and/or radiation in the treatment of lung, breast, esophageal, gastric, colorectal, cervical, pancreatic, and prostatic cancers. By itself, MMC has recorded 15 to 35% response rates against the above human tumors (27). It has an even higher response rate when administered topically against superficial bladder tumors (27).

Several retrospective studies have suggested enhanced local control and survival when combinations of 5-FU, MMC, and radiotherapy were used in treating cancers of the esophagus, anal canal, cervix, and vulva.

These are described in Chapters 21, 25, and 28, respectively. Cummings et al have shown retrospectively that relapse-free survival rates in anal cancer were greater in patients receiving the 5-FU + MMC combination compared to patients receiving 5-FU alone with radiotherapy (42). A recently concluded Radiation Therapy Oncology Group (RTOG) prospective randomized study on anal cancer shows an improvement in local control for patients receiving 5-FU + MMC + radiotherapy versus those receiving 5-FU + radiotherapy (43). In these and other studies, the addition of MMC to 5-FU + RT appears to increase acute GI and bone-marrow toxicity to an acceptable degree and does not translate to late or chronic toxicity in general.

Thomas et al conducted a series of protocols employing various combinations of 5-FU, MMC, and pelvic ± para-aortic radiotherapy for Stage IIB to IVA cervical cancer (44). Logistic regression studies indicated that the treatment variable showing a statistically significant effect in complications was the use of MMC ($p = 0.0053$). The complications reported were primarily related to the GI tract.

Weissberg et al, in a prospective randomized trial in patients with head and neck cancer, reported that patients receiving radiotherapy + MMC had a 75 ± 7% 5-year survival rate compared to 55 ± 5% survival in patients receiving radiotherapy alone (45).

Summary

The ultimate nemesis of radiation therapy in a tumor population is considered to be the hypoxic cell. The basis of fractionated radiotherapy is its theoretical capability of progressively aerating a core of hypoxic tumor cells. MMC has a distinctive property of being more lethal to hypoxic cells. Thus, the combination of MMC and radiation should, theoretically, decimate or eliminate most tumor populations if given in sufficient doses. Major obstacles are the dose-limiting marrow toxicity of MMC, along with its pulmonary toxicity and related GI disturbances. All of these may be enhanced by radiation, depending on the volume of marrow, lung parenchyma, and intestine exposed to radiotherapy.

There are several ways to optimize the enhanced effect of MMC when given with radiotherapy. For maximal effect, MMC is given immediately before or immediately after medium-dose-rate radiation fraction or low-dose-rate irradiation. To minimize toxicity, it may be necessary to reduce MMC and/or radiation dose per fraction, limit radiation treatment volumes, alternate MMC use with other alkylating drugs to reduce development of resistance to MMC, and use biologic response modifiers that are chemoprotectors and radioprotectors, particularly to reduce marrow toxicity.

All of these methods have been used singly or in unison during clinical combinations of MMC and radiotherapy. It is likely that the awareness of the therapeutic efficacy of this combination will gradually overcome the current wariness with which oncologists view MMC.

ACTINOMYCIN-D

Dactinomycin or Actinomycin-D (AMD) was the first modern antineoplastic agent noted to enhance radiation reaction in normal and tumor tissues. In 1959, D'Angio et al noted increased effects on skin and tumors in children with Wilms' tumor treated with AMD and radiotherapy (46).

AMD is one of several actinomycins derived from a soil Streptomyces. It is, however, the only one that is used clinically. The biologic effects of this drug are due to its binding to DNA, which results in inhibition of RNA and protein synthesis. It modifies radiation effects on normal and tumor cells by affecting sublethal radiation damage (SLD) and potentially lethal radiation damage (PLD). It is used in combination with other drugs, surgery, and radiotherapy in the management of several childhood tumors, such as Wilms' tumor, Ewing's sarcoma, rhabdomyosarcoma, and in a few adult tumors, such as choriocarcinoma and testicular cancer.

Mechanisms of Action

AMD is only administered intravenously because it is absorbed poorly by the oral route and causes local irritation of tissues. It is usually given as daily bolus intravenous injections for 5 days. It is widely and rapidly distributed in tissues, particularly the liver, spleen, kidneys, and salivary glands. Its beta or plasma half-life is about 36 hours. AMD is primarily excreted in the urine (up to 30%) in bile (about 10%) and in feces (about 15%) (1,2,47). No major metabolites are known to exist.

Structurally, this antibiotic consists of a central phenoxazone ring with two symmetrical polypeptide chains attached to it. AMD acts by strongly binding with DNA at multiple sites and by preventing the formation of RNA chains and protein synthesis. AMD does not appear to interact with other drugs; however, it may be part of a multidrug resistant phenotype with cross-resistance to vincristine and Adriamycin (48).

Interaction with Radiation

The nature of AMD-radiation interaction has been extensively studied by several investigators on mammalian cells (49–56). Although there are some contradictory data, a few generalizations may be derived.

1. At certain concentrations, AMD increases radiation sensitivity (decreased D_o).
2. AMD decreases the repair of sublethal radiation damage (SLD).
3. Both of the above effects are independent of the cell-cycle phase.

With work primarily conducted on Chinese hamster cells in culture, Elkind et al (54,55) first demonstrated that AMD inhibited sublethal radiation damage by showing that the survival increases present between two radiation fractions or doses were suppressed when modest concentrations of AMD were present. Also, while the D_o of this cell line (with radiation alone) was between 145 and 160 cGy, pretreatment by AMD resulted in a decrease of D_o to 91 cGy (56). Both of these effects appeared to be independent of the cell-cycle phase at the time of treatment with AMD.

Normal Tissue

AMD appears to be an enhancer of radiation injury to every type of tissue. The interaction of AMD and irradiation has been studied extensively in mammalian cells in culture, particularly with respect to enhanced effects on the skin, intestine, and pulmonary tissues.

Skin: AMD has been shown to increase early skin reactions induced by radiation (49,50). The intensity of this reaction appears to be related to the timing of drug-radiation delivery. For example, Lelieveld et al reported enhanced skin effect on normal mice when AMD was given after radiotherapy (50). Steel et al, on the other hand, barely noted any such enhancement when the drug was given 13 to 14 days prior to irradiation (51). These findings appear to correlate with the clinical observations of AMD-radiation reactions initially described by D'Angio (52). The classic "recall phenomenon" relating to the resurgence of erythema in previously irradiated skin provoked by AMD administration is described in greater detail in Chapter 36.

Gastrointestinal Tract: Phillips et al have described dose-enhancing factors (DEF) ranging from 1.3 to 1.6 for AMD given 2 hours before radiation based on studies with endpoints in intestinal crypt cell kill and esophageal lethality (53,64,65). Similar to the effect on skin, the administration of AMD 7 days before irradiation showed no enhancing effect (65).

Lungs: Several investigators have shown DEF values of 1.3 to 1.6 for AMD in combination with thoracic irradiation in animals (53,66). This enhancement of pulmonary effects was also related to the timing of AMD administration, with maximal effects recorded when the drug was given from 2 hours before to 2 hours after irradiation. Clinical manifestation of interstitial pneumonitis secondary to AMD-radiation interaction was also described first by D'Angio (46,52).

Tumors

Most laboratory studies of AMD and radiation interaction have been performed to study the nature of their interaction rather than their effect on any specific tumor. Others have been performed to refine dose schedules of the drug itself (57–63). Valeriote et al studied AMD effectiveness against murine leukemias and normal cells and suggested that daily divided doses be preferred to the single-dose schedule because the former was less toxic and equally carcinolytic (57). Bases used cultured HeLa cells to describe the enhancement of radiation effect by AMD (58). Several other in vivo or in vitro studies on tumor cell lines or clonogenic tumor assays have shown that the tumor-cell survival after AMD exposure is dependent on the product of drug concentration and time of exposure (C × T). In other words, there is no specific advantage in continuous or prolonged infusions of AMD compared to bolus injections of the drug (59–61).

Clinical Applications

Due to the wide range of tissues affected by its administration and the need for relatively high concentrations of the drug for significant antitumor activity, AMD is usually used in combination with other drugs and occasionally with radiation in several childhood tumors (27,28). Postoperatively, it is combined with vincristine (and radiation in advanced stages) in the treatment of Wilms' tumor. In Ewing's sarcoma, adjuvant therapy consists of combination chemotherapy, sometimes including AMD. In rhabdomyosarcoma, AMD is combined with vincristine (early stages) and cyclophosphamide (later stages) as standard therapy following local therapy with surgery and/or radiation.

Patients with low-risk gestational trophoblastic decrease or choriocarcinoma are treated with AMD alone (10 to 12 μg/kg daily for 5 days every 2 weeks as necessary) or with methotrexate. In high-risk patients, AMD is often combined with chlorambucil and methotrexate, although newer combinations are available. AMD is also an ingredient of the Memorial Hospital VAB-6 protocol for nonseminomatous testicular neoplasms.

Toxicity

Myelotoxicity is a dose-limiting toxicity of AMD. Thrombocytopenia and leukopenia, with nadirs from 14 to 21 days after administration, can be expected. Acute nausea, vomiting, and diarrhea often occur and, when severe, may be another dose-limiting toxicity.

Mucositis manifesting as stomatitis or proctitis is not uncommon. Erythema, dry or moist desquamation, and tanning of the skin are frequent complications. The "recall phenomenon" of erythema confined to previously irradiated skin, while traditionally ascribed to AMD, is found with other drugs as well, including Adriamycin and methotrexate. This erythema is frequently more intense than the erythema caused by radiotherapy or the drug alone. Reversible alopecia frequently manifests itself 1 week or more after AMD administration. Finally, the drug is markedly toxic when applied topically and, hence, extravasation of the drug can cause local necrosis.

Summary

AMD has a wide spectrum of activity against neoplasms. However, it is toxic to almost every tissue system in cytotoxic doses. For this reason, it is normally given in lower doses in combination with other drugs. It may be administered with radiation in lesser concentrations. Its interaction with radiation is noncycle specific. While AMD in higher-than-tolerated doses may be supra-additive with radiation, clinically acceptable doses of AMD may be additive in interaction with radiation. And because its action on cells is independent of cell-cycle phase, the possibility of activity against a subpopulation of cells inherently resistant to radiation exists and can be potentially exploited.

BLEOMYCIN

Bleomycins are several glycopeptides that are fermentation products of Streptomyces verticillus. All bleomycins contain a unique component (bleomycinic acid) with different terminal alkylamine groups. The bleomycin that is clinically used as an antineoplastic agent is actually a combination of two closely related peptides, bleomycin A2 and bleomycin B2 (67). It has important activity in head and neck cancer, testicular cancer, and malignant lymphomas. Contrary to other antineoplastic antibiotics and indeed to most commonly used antineoplastic agents, bleomycin is uniquely minimally toxic to the bone marrow. For these reasons, bleomycin alone or in combination with other drugs has been used extensively in Hodgkin's and non-Hodgkin's lymphomas and in testicular cancer. No other drug has been tested in combination with radiation as frequently as bleomycin in head and neck cancers.

Bleomycin A2, the predominant peptide in clinical bleomycin, is prepared by chemical synthesis. The original compound fermented from Streptomyces verticillus is a copper-bound complex: Cu(II)-bleomycin. It has no antitumor activity. Clinically active forms of bleomycin contain iron-bound complexes: Fe(II)-bleomycin. Three synthetic bleomycin analogs, pepleomycin, liblomycin, and tallysomycin, have been found to have markedly lesser pulmonary toxicity than bleomycin and are therefore receiving considerable attention in Phase I and II trials (68,69).

Mechanisms of Action

Bleomycin produces single- and double-strand breaks in DNA (otherwise termed "DNA scission reaction"). This action starts with the conversion of a bleomycin-Fe(II) complex to an activated bleomycin-Fe(II)–O_2 complex with the help of NADPH and NADH. The second step is a induction of DNA breaks mediated by free superoxide and hydroxyl radicals produced by the reduction of molecular oxygen (67). There is evidence that DNA strand breakage occurs in the presence of oxygen and ceases in an anaerobic environment (70).

Thus:

Bleomycin-Fe(II)	→	Oxidation NADPH, NADH	→	Activated bleomycin-Fe(II)–O_2 bleomycin-Fe(III)	→	Free radical (OH° and O_2°) generation	→	Single- and double-strand DNA breaks between base pairs

Bleomycin (BLM) can be given subcutaneously, intramuscularly, or intravenously. It is usually administered in doses of 10 to 20 units/m^2 once or twice weekly. By continuous infusion, doses of 5 to 15 units/m^2 daily are tolerated for 4 to 7 days. BLM is rapidly distributed in most tissues, where a soluble enzyme called bleomycin hydrolase inactivates it by cleaving ammonia from the drug. High concentrations of the drug remain in tissues such as the lungs and skin, which lack this enzyme; these organs are therefore particularly prone to bleomycin toxicity. The plasma half-life of the drug is 1 hour, and about 50% of unchanged bleomycin is excreted in urine within 24 hours (28).

Interaction with Radiation

Tumors

BLM was first reported in 1972 to have a potential radiosensitizing effect in experimental systems (71,72). It was suggested that the drug might inhibit SLD and/or interact synergistically with radiotherapy. Subsequent studies were more equivocal regarding the mode of BLM-radiation interaction (73,74). As methodological problems were solved, investigations were better designed and more tumor models became available. The nature of BLM-radiation interaction became less speculative. The salient points of the interaction may be described as follows.

1. BLM has little effect on hypoxic cells and probably does not enhance radiation effects in such cells (75,76).
2. Both BLM and radiation are effective in decimating well-oxygenated proliferative cells and have similar cell-cycles sensitivities (M and G2 phases) (77,78).
3. BLM-radiation interaction in tumors and normal tissues is probably additive (40,79).

Normal Tissue

BLM, by itself, is known to cause marked tissue responses in skin, mucosa, and lungs. In combination with radiation, especially when administered concurrently, there is a marked enhancement of such tissue reactions.

Skin/Mucous Membranes: BLM has been noted to cause either an additive or a supra-additive effect with fractionated radiation on skin and mucus membranes (40,79). This effect is particularly important because bleomycin has been extensively used in the treatment of head and neck cancers. The enhanced skin reactions seen with BLM-radiation interaction have been primarily acute in nature but can also manifest as late fibrosis (Fig. 9–2) (80,81).

Lungs: Radiation-induced pulmonary toxicity is known to be enhanced by BLM both in animal systems and in clinical trials (40,82,83). BLM, by itself, is known to cause pulmonary fibrosis. A cumulative dose limit of 400 units keeps the risk of this toxicity

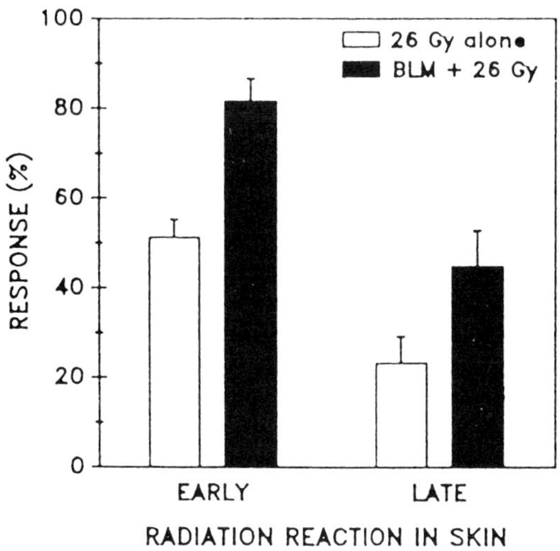

Fig. 9–2. An increased acute and late skin effect is induced when bleomycin is given simultaneously with radiation to mouse feet. (From von der Maase H. Br J Radiol 67:697, 1984.)

below 5%. Since this pathology is frequently seen with lung irradiation as well, it follows that BLM and thoracic irradiation should be combined with utmost caution, if at all. Catane et al reviewed 115 patients treated with this combination and there was a 10% incidence of fatal pulmonary toxicity (83).

Animal studies have indicated that the pulmonary toxicity of bleomycin is due to collagen synthesis following damage to pulmonary arterioles and veins. There is some indication that this damage may be prevented by the anti-inflammatory agent indomethacin and by dehydroproline (67).

Miscellaneous: Enhanced depletion of intestinal crypt cells has been noted experimentally when combining BLM with radiation (40,84). Once again, this finding has repercussions in the use of BLM with abdominal irradiation. The initial enthusiasm for combining BLM with radiation was based on the minimal myelotoxicity noted with the drug. This particular lack of toxicity of BLM use is apparently unaltered by combination with radiotherapy (85). Finally, the relationship between acute toxicity and the timing of administration of the drug in relation to irradiation appears settled. The increased normal-tissue responses that are seen with simultaneous or near-simultaneous use of BLM and radiation may be temporized or even eliminated by increasing the temporal separation of the two modalities (85).

Clinical Applications

BLM-radiation interaction has been most extensively studied clinically in head and neck cancer. Taylor has summarized these findings in Chapter 14 and in other sources (86). The following factors should be considered when combining BLM and radiation in the clinic.

1. Concurrent BLM and radiation require that the cumulative BLM dose be limited to 5 mg/kg given 2 or 3 times weekly; higher doses would require treatment interruptions or suboptimal doses of radiotherapy. Fu et al found increased disease-free and overall survival at 3 years in patients treated with a cumulative dose of 5 mg/kg bleomycin given twice weekly with radiation for oropharyngeal cancers (87).
2. Survival advantages are seen only in predominantly well-differentiated tumors such as oropharyngeal and laryngeal cancers. In fact, the 1980 study by Shanta and Krishnamurthi on oral cancers may be cited as the reason for the multiple clinical trials on head and neck cancers using BLM and radiotherapy in subsequent years (88).
3. The majority of BLM-radiotherapy trials in head and neck cancers show no benefit over radiotherapy alone and are characterized by excessive and sometimes prohibitive mucosal toxicity.

BLM, when used as a single agent, has a 15% response rate in esophageal cancer. The combination of cisplatin, vindesine, and bleomycin is one of the most effective used in this disease, with a response rate of 47% (89). Leichman et al reported a median survival of 22 months in 20 patients treated with a BLM-containing four-drug regimen and concurrent radiotherapy. This protocol, however, was abandoned due to the "prohibitive" pulmonary toxicity (90). Most such clinical trials, however, do not show benefits in combining BLM with radiation on esophageal cancer (91,92).

Saito has reported a 64% 3-year survival in patients with carcinoma of the uterine cervix treated with BLM and standard radiotherapy compared to a 42% survival in those treated with radiotherapy alone ($p < 0.05$) (93). A few studies have reported beneficial but statistically insignificant effects with BLM and radiation in the treatment of nonsmall cell lung cancer and astrocytoma (94,95). Promising retrospective studies on cancers of the penis, vulva, and skin treated with this combination have also been reported (28,96).

Toxicity

The use of BLM in combination with radiotherapy in clinical trials of various sites was motivated by the lack of bone-marrow toxicity from this drug or with the BLM-radiation combination. The results of these trials have been severely compromised by other BLM toxicities, particularly that of acute mucositis and pulmonary fibrosis. Statistically significant increased mucositis has been observed in head and neck cancer patients treated with BLM-radiation compared to radiation alone (96,97). Einhorn et al reported that five out of 13 patients (38%) treated with BLM-radiation developed pulmonary fibrosis, including three who died as a result of this toxicity (82). Vermund et al reported 75% and 56% incidences of esophagitis and mucositis in patients treated with the combination, compared to 17% and 38% treated by radiation alone (98).

Summary

Of all single drugs used in combination with chemoradiation, BLM appears to have been studied the most in clinical trials. This might have transpired due to the unbridled acceptance of earlier in vitro and in vivo studies showing synergistic BLM-radiation interaction. These studies were flawed because inappropriate tumor models and methods of evaluation were used (72,85).

Nevertheless, a wealth of information regarding BLM-radiation interaction exists. It appears that the use of BLM alone with radiation may be useful clinically, but only in well-differentiated oropharyngeal tumors and only as long as BLM is given in small doses of 5 to 15 units per week. This is because BLM is active (as is radiation) against actively proliferating cells and is cell phase specific to the M and G2 phases of the cell cycle.

In tumors that are less well-differentiated and have a sizable proportion of hypoxic cells, the BLM-radiation combination is less effective. The higher doses of BLM utilized to overcome this ineffectiveness have resulted in excessive mucositis and pulmonary fibrosis, thereby reducing the therapeutic ratio. As a result, the effects of BLM-radiation interaction on cancer are currently being investigated clinically in tumors such as malignant lymphomas, only in combination with other drugs.

REFERENCES

1. Kaufman SD, Weitzman S. The clinical pharmacology of anti-cancer drugs. *In:* Radiation-Drug Interactions in the Treatment of Cancer. Sokol GH, Maickel RP (Eds). New York, Wiley Medical, 1980, p. 63.
2. Chabner BA, Myers CE, Olivero LT. Clinical pharmacology of anti-cancer drugs. Semin Oncol 4:165, 1977.
3. Benjamin RS, Riggs, LE, Bachur NR. Pharmacokinetics and metabolism of Adriamycin. Clin Pharmacol Ther 14:592, 1973.
4. Legha SS. The anthracyclines and mitoxantrone. *In:* Cancer Chemotherapy by Infusion. Lokich JJ (Ed). Chicago, Precept, 1990, p. 197.
5. Kartner H, Riordan JR, Ling V. Cell surface P-glycoprotein associated with multi-drug resistance in mammalian cell lines. Science 221:1285, 1983.
6. Tewey KM, Chen GI, Nelson EM, et al. Intercalative anti-tumor drugs interfere with the breakage-reunion reaction of mammalian DNA topoisomerase. J Biol Chem 259:9182, 1984.
7. Myers CE, Chabner BA. Anthracyclines. *In:* Cancer Chemotherapy. Principles and Practice. Chabner BA, Collins JM (Eds). Philadelphia, JB Lippincott, 1990, p. 356.
8. Legha SS, Benjamin RS, Mackay B, et al. Reduction of doxorubicin cardiotoxicity by prolonged continuous intravenous infusion. Ann Intern Med 96:133, 1982.
9. Eichholtz-Wirth H. Dependence of the cytostatic effect of adriamycin on drug concentration and exposure time in vitro. Br J Cancer 41:886, 1986.
10. Nguyen-Ngoc T, Vrignaud P, Robert J. Cellular pharmacokinetics of doxorubicin in cultured mouse sarcoma cells originating from autochthonous tumors. Oncology 41:55, 1986.
11. Hellman S, Hannon E. Effects of adriamycin on the radiation response of murine hematopoietic stem cells. Radiat Res 67:162, 1976.

12. Belli JA, Piro AJ. The interaction between radiation and adriamycin damage in mammalian cells. Cancer Res 37:1624, 1977.
13. Byfield JE, Lynch M, Kulhanian F, Chan PYM. Cellular effects of combined adriamycin and x-irradiation on human tumor cells. Int J Cancer 19:194, 1977.
14. Bistrovic M, Nagy B, Maricic Z, Kolaric K. Interaction of adriamycin and radiation in combined treatment on mouse L-cells. Eur J Cancer 14:411, 1977.
15. Dritschilo A, Piro AJ, Belli JA. Interaction between radiation and drug damage in mammalian cells: The effect of adriamycin and actinomycin-D on the repair of potentially lethal radiation damage. Int J Radiat Oncol Biol Phys 35:549, 1979.
16. Donaldson SS, Glick JM, Wilbur JR. Adriamycin activating a recall phenomenon after radiation therapy. Ann Intern Med 81:407, 1974.
17. Cassady JR, Richter MP, Piro AJ, Jaffe N. Radiation-Adriamycin interactions: Preliminary clinical observations. Cancer 36:946, 1975.
18. Sherman DM, Carabell SC, Belli JA, Hellman S. The effect of dose rate and Adriamycin on the tolerance of thoracic radiation in mice. Int J Radiat Oncol Biol Phys 8:45, 1982.
19. Phillips TL, Wharam MD, Margolis LW. Modification of radiation injury to normal tissues by chemotherapeutic agents. Cancer 35:1678, 1975.
20. Belli JA. Radiation damage interactions with actinomycin-D and Adriamycin. *In:* Antitumor Drug-radiation Interactions. Hill BT, Bellamy AS (Eds). Boca Raton, CRC Press, 1990, p. 23.
21. Stein RS. Radiation-recall enteritis after actinomycin-D and Adriamycin therapy. South Med J 71:960, 1978.
22. Ramsom JL, Norak RW, Kumar APM, et al. Delayed gastrointestinal complications after combined modality therapy of childhood rhabdomyosarcoma. Int J Radiat Oncol Biol Phys 8:45, 1982.
23. Billingham ME, Bristow MR, Glatstein E, et al. Adriamycin cardiotoxicity: endomyocardial biopsy evidence of enhancement by irradiation. Am J Surg Pathol 1:17, 1977.
24. Rosenthal CJ, Rotman MZ. Concomitant continuous infusion Adriamycin and radiation. Evidence of synergistic effects in soft tissue sarcoma. *In:* Concomitant Continuous Infusion Chemotherapy and Radiation. Rotman MZ, Rosenthal CJ (Eds). Berlin, Springer-Verlag, 1991, p. 271.
25. Alexanian R, Barlogie B, Dixon D. High-dose glucocorticoid treatment of resistant multiple myeloma. Ann Intern Med 105:8, 1986.
26. Wakaki S, Marumo H, Tomioka K. Isolation of new fractions of antitumor mitomycins. Antibiot Chemother 8:228, 1958.
27. Verweij J, Hartigh J, Pinedo HM. Antitumor antibiotics. *In:* Cancer Chemotherapy. Principles and Practice. Chabner BA, Collins JM (Eds). Philadelphia, JB Lippincott, 1990, p. 382.
28. Wittes RE, Leyland-Jones B, Fortner C, Hubbard SM. Chemotherapy: The properties and uses of single agents. *In:* Manual of Oncologic Therapeutics 1989-1990. Wittes RE (Ed). Philadelphia, JB Lippincott, 1989, p. 99.
29. Tyer UN, Szybalski W. Mitomycin and porfiromycin chemical mechanism of activation and cross-linking of DNA. Science 145:55, 1964.
30. Lin AJ, Cosby LA, Chansky CW, et al. Potential bioreductive alkylating agents. 1. Benzoquinone derivatives. J Med Chem 15:1247, 1972.
31. Rockwell S. Cytotoxicities of mitomycin-C and x-rays to aerobic and hypoxic cells in vitro. Int J Radiat Oncol Biol Phys 8:1035, 1982.
32. Rockwell S. Effects of mitomycin-C alone and in combination with x-rays on EMT6 mouse mammary tumors in vivo. J Natl Cancer Inst 71:765, 1983.
33. Kenncdy KA, Teicher BA, Rockwell S, Sartorelli AC. The hypoxic tumor cell: A target for selective cancer chemotherapy. Biochem Pharmacol 29:1, 1980.
34. Rockwell S. Effects of some proliferative and environmental factors on the toxicity of mitomycin-C to tumor cells in vitro. Int J Cancer 38:229, 1986.
35. Rockwell S, Sartorelli AC. Mitomycin-C and radiation. *In:* Anti-tumor Drug-radiation Interactions. Hill BT, Bellamy AS (Eds). Boca Raton, CRC Press, 1990, p. 125.
36. Siemann DW, Keng PC. Responses of tumor cell subpopulations to single modality and combined modality therapies. NCI Monogr 6:101, 1988.
37. Rauth AM, Mohindra JK, Tannock IF. Activity of mitomycin-C or aerobic and hypoxic cells in vitro and in vivo. Cancer Res 43:4154, 1983.
38. Fu KK, Rayner DA, Lain KN. Modification of the effects of continuous low dose rate irradiation by concurrent chemotherapy infusion. Int J Radiat Oncol Biol Phys 10:1473, 1984.
39. Fu KK, Lain KN, Rayner PA. The combined effects of continuous low dose rate irradiation and concurrent infusion of mitomycin-C, cisplatinum and 5-fluorouracil on mice murine tumors. Endocuriether Hyperthermia Oncol 2:157, 1986.
40. von der Maase H. Experimental studies in interactions of radiation and cancer chemother-

apeutic drugs in normal tissues and solid tumors. Radiother Oncol 7:47, 1986.
41. von der Maase H, Overgaard J, Vaeth M. Effect of cancer chemotherapeutic drugs on radiation-induced lung damage in mice. Radiother Oncol 5:245, 1986.
42. Cummings BJ, Keane TJ, O'Sullivan B, et al. Epidermoid anal cancer: Treatment by radiation alone or by radiation and 5-fluorouracil with and without mitomycin-C. Int J Radiat Oncol Biol Phys 21:1115, 1991.
43. Flam M. Personal communication. January 1992.
44. Thomas G, Dembo A, Fyles A, et al. Concurrent chemoradiation in advanced cervical cancer. Gynecol Oncol 38(3):446, 1990.
45. Weissberg JB, Papac RJ, Son YH, et al. Randomized clinical trial of mitomycin-C or an adjuvant to radiotherapy in head and neck carcinoma. Int J Radiat Oncol Biol Phys 17(1):3, 1989.
46. D'Angio GJ, Farber S, Maddock CL. Potentiation of x-ray effects by actinomycin D. Radiology 73:175, 1959.
47. Tattersall MHM, Sodergren JE, Sengupta SK, et al. Pharmacokinetics of actinomycin D in patients with malignant melanoma. Clin Pharmacol Ther 17:701, 1975.
48. Pastan I, Gottesman M. Multidrug resistance in human cancer. N Engl J Med 316:1388, 1987.
49. Redpath JL, Colman M. The effect of Adriamycin and actinomycin D on radiation-induced results in mouse feet. Int J Radiat Oncol Biol Phys 5:483, 1979.
50. Lelieveld P, Scoles MA, Brown JM, Kallman RF. The effect of treatment on fractionated schedules with the combination of x-irradiation and six cytotoxic drugs on the RIF-1 tumor and normal mouse skin. Int J Radiat Oncol Biol Phys 11:111, 1985.
51. Steel GG, Adams K, Peckham MS. Lung damage in C57B1 mice following thoracic irradiation: Enhanced by chemotherapy. Br J Radiol 52:741, 1979.
52. D'Angio GJ. Clinical and biological studies of actinomycin D and roentgen irradiation. Am J Roentgenol 87:106, 1962.
53. Phillips TL, Margolis L. Radiation pathology and the clinical response of lung and esophagus. Front Radiat Ther Oncol 6:254, 1972.
54. Elkind MM, Whitmore GF, Alescio T. Actinomycin D suppression of recovery in x-irradiated mammalian cells. Science 143:145, 1964.
55. Elkind M, Sakamoto K. Combined effects of x-irradiation and chemotherapeutic drugs (nitrogen mustard and actinomycin D). Front Rad Ther Oncol 4:53, 1969.
56. Elkind MM, Kano E. Actinomycin D and radiation fractionation studies in asynchronous and synchronous Chinese hamster cells. Radiat Res 44:484, 1970.
57. Valeriote F, Vietti T, Tolen S. Kinetics of the lethal effect of actinomycin D on normal and leukemic cells. Cancer Res 33:2658, 1973.
58. Bases RE. Modification of the radiation response determined by single-cell technics: Actinomycin D. Cancer Res 19:1223, 1975.
59. Galbraith WM, Mellet LB. Disposition of (^{3}H) actinomycin D in tumor-bearing mice. Cancer Res 36:1242, 1976.
60. Wu PC, Ozols RF, Hatanake M, Boone OW. Anti-cancer drugs: Effect on the cloning of Raji lymphoma cells. J Natl Cancer Inst 68:115, 1982.
61. Ludwig R, Alberts DS, Miller TP, Salmon SE. Evaluation of anticancer drug schedule dependency using an in vitro human tumor clonogenic assay. Cancer Chemother Pharmacol 12:135, 1984.
62. Piro AJ, Taylor CC, Belli JA. Interaction between radiation and drug damage in mammalian cells. I. Delayed expressions of actinomycin-D x-ray effects in exponential and plateau phase cells. Radiat Res 63:346, 1975.
63. Piro A, Taylor CC, Belli JA. Interaction between radiation and drug damage in mammalian cells. The effect of actinomycin D on the repair of sublethal radiation damage on plateau phase cells. Cancer 37:2097, 1976.
64. Phillips TL, Wharam MD, Margolis LW. Modification of radiation injury to normal tissues by chemotherapeutic agents. Cancer 35:1078, 1975.
65. Phillips TL, Fu KK. The interaction of drug and radiation effects on normal tissues. Int J Radiat Oncol Biol Phys 4:59, 1978.
66. Colman M, Zabilansky E, Redpath JL. Modification of the radiation response of mouse lung by actinomycin D: Dependence or interval between radiation and drug treatments. Int J Radiat Oncol Biol Phys 39:157, 1981.
67. Chabner BA. Bleomycin. *In:* Cancer Chemotherapy—Principles and Practice. Chabner BA, Collins JM (Eds). Philadelphia, JB Lippincott, 1990, p. 341.
68. Sikic BI, Siddik ZH, Gram TE. Relative pulmonary toxicity and antitumor effects of two new bleomycin analogs, pepleomycin and tallysomycin A. Cancer Treat Rep 64:659, 1980.
69. Takita T, Ogino T. Pepleomycin and liblomycin, new analogs of bleomycin. Biomed Pharmacother 41:219, 1987.
70. Onishi T, Iwata H, Takagi Y. Effects of reducing or oxidizing agents on the action of bleomycin. J Biochem 77:745, 1975.

71. Matsuzawa T, Onozawa M, Morita K, Kakehi M. Radiosensitization of bleomycin on lethal effect of mouse cancer cells in vitro. Strahelentherapie 144:614, 1972.
72. Jorgensen SJ. Time-dose relationship in combined bleomycin treatment and radiotherapy. Eur J Cancer 8:531, 1972.
73. Blehen NM, Gillies NE, Twentyman PR. The effect of bleomycin and radiation in combination on bacteria and mammalian cells in culture. Br J Radiol 47:346, 1974.
74. Byfield JE, Lee YC, Tu L, Kulhanian F. Molecular interactions of the combined effects of bleomycin and x-rays on mammalian cell survival. Cancer Res 36:1135, 1978.
75. Shrieve DC, Harries JW. Effects of bleomycin irradiation on euxic and hypoxic cells. Int J Radiat Oncol Biol Phys 5:1495, 1979.
76. Roizin-Towle L, Hall EJ. Studies with bleomycin and misonidazole in aerated and hypoxic cells. Br J Cancer 37:254, 1978.
77. Grau C, Overgaard J. Effect of cancer chemotherapy on the hypoxic fraction in a solid tumor measured using a local tumor central assay. Radiother Oncol 13:301, 1988.
78. Barranco SC, Humphrey RM. The effects of bleomycin in survival and cell progression in Chinese hamster cells in vitro. Cancer Res 31:1218, 1971.
79. Molin J, Sogaard PE, Overgaard J. Experimental studies on the radiation-modifying effect of bleomycin in malignant and normal mouse tissue in vivo. Cancer Treat Rev 65:583, 1981.
80. Leith JF, Lewinsky BS, Schilling WA. Modification of the response of mouse skin to x-irradiation by bleomycin treatment. Radiat Res 61:100, 1975.
81. von der Maase H. Effect of cancer chemotherapeutic drugs on the radiation-induced skin reactions in mouse feet. Br J Radiol 57:697, 1984.
82. Einhorn L, Krause M, Hornback N, Furnas B. Enhanced pulmonary toxicity with bleomycin and radiotherapy in oat cell lung cancer. Cancer 37:2414, 1976.
83. Catane R, Schwade JG, Turris AJ, et al. Pulmonary toxicity after radiation and bleomycin—A review. Int J Radiat Oncol Biol Phys 5:1513, 1979.
84. Phillips TL, Ross GY, Goldstein LS, Begg AC. The interaction of radiation and bleomycin in intestinal crypt cells. Int J Radiat Oncol Biol Phys 5:1509, 1979.
85. Overgaard J, Grau C. Interactions between bleomycin and x-irradiation. *In:* Antitumor Drug-radiation Interactions. Hill BT, Bellamy AS (Eds). Boca Raton, CRC Press, 1990, p. 53.
86. Taylor SG. Head and neck cancer. *In:* Combined Modality Cancer Therapy. Radiation and Infusional Chemotherapy. Lokich JJ, Byfield JE (Eds). Chicago, Precept, 1991, p. 75.
87. Fu KK, Phillips TL, Silverberg IJ, et al. Combined radiotherapy and chemotherapy with bleomycin and methotrexate for advanced inoperable head and neck cancer. Update of a Northern California Oncology Group randomized trial. J Clin Oncol 5:1410, 1987.
88. Shanta V, Krishnamurthi S. Combined bleomycin and radiotherapy in oral cancer. Clin Radiol 31:617, 1980.
89. Kelsen D. Chemotherapy for loco-regional and advanced esophageal cancer. Cancer Updates 2(10):1, 1988.
90. Leichman L, Herskovic A, Leichman C, et al. Nonoperative therapy for squamous cell cancer of the esophagus. J Clin Oncol 5:365, 1987.
91. Earle JD, Gelber R, Moertel CG, Hahn RG. A controlled evaluation of combined radiation and bleomycin therapy for squamous cell carcinoma of the esophagus. Int J Radiat Oncol Biol Phys 6:821, 1980.
92. Anderson AP, Berdal P, Edsmyr F, et al. Irradiation chemotherapy and surgery in esophageal cancer: A randomized clinical study. Radiother Oncol 2:179, 1984.
93. Saito M. Chemotherapy of cancer of the uterine cervix—especially combination of bleomycin and radiation. *In:* Proceedings of the 19th General Assembly of the Japan Medical Congress. Kyoto, Japan Medical Congress, 1975, p. 251.
94. Chan PY, Byfield JE, Kagan AR, Aronstam EM. Unresectable squamous cell carcinoma of the lung and its management by combined bleomycin and radiotherapy. A clinical study of the enhanced results. Cancer 37, 2671, 1976.
95. Kristiansen K, Hagen S, Kollevold T, et al. Combined modality therapy of operated astrocytomas grade III and IV. Confirmation of the value of post operative irradiation and lack of potentiation by bleomycin in survival time. A prospective multicenter trial of the Scandanavian Glioblastoma Study Group. Cancer 47:649, 1981.
96. Abe M, Shigematsu U, Kimura S. Combined use of bleomycin with radiation in the treatment of cancer. *In:* Antitumor Antibiotics. Carter SK, Umezawata H, Douros J, Sakurai Y (Eds). Berlin, Springer-Verlag, 1978, p. 189.
97. Shah PM, Shukla SN, Patel KM, et al. Effect of bleomycin-radiotherapy combination in management of head and neck squamous cell carcinoma. Cancer 48:1106, 1981.
98. Vermund H, Kaalhus O, Winther F, et al. Bleomycin and radiation therapy in squamous cell carcinoma of the upper aerodigestive tract: A phase III clinical trial. Int J Radiat Oncol Biol Phys 11:1877, 1985.

Chapter 10

PLANT DERIVATIVES: VINCA ALKALOIDS, PODOPHYLLOTOXIN DERIVATIVES

MARSHALL S. FLAM

VINCA ALKALOIDS

Periwinkle alkaloids (vinca alkaloids) are derived from the periwinkle plant (vinca rosea). Vincristine and vinblastine (Velban) are closely related structures composed of two complex, multiringed systems linked by a carbon/carbon bridge. They differ only in methyl (vinblastine) or formyl (vincristine) side chains of the large parent molecule. This minor structural difference results in two compounds differing significantly in their spectrum of clinical activity and toxicity. Vincristine is unique among anticancer drugs in its lack of myelosuppression, which in conjunction with its broad range of clinical activity has lead to its extensive use in combination chemotherapy programs against a wide variety of neoplasms. Vinblastine, on the other hand, is significantly myelosuppressive, resulting in dose-limiting neutropenia, and demonstrates a narrower spectrum of anticancer efficacy. The dose-limiting toxicity of vincristine is neurotoxicity, primarily peripheral and autonomic neuropathies (1).

Vindesine, the third vinca alkaloid in current clinical use, is a synthetic derivative of vinblastine. Vindesine appears to have a similar spectrum of activity as vincristine and vinblastine in animal tumor systems. Its toxicity profile lies between vincristine and vinblastine, demonstrating less neurotoxicity than the former (2). Tables 10–1 and 10–2 summarize the differences in anticancer activity and toxicities of the three vinca alkaloids.

Mechanism of Action

Vinca alkaloids possess cytotoxic activity by virtue of their binding to tubulin, a basic protein subunit of the microtubular apparatus that forms the spindle along which chromosomes migrate during mitosis. Their binding to tubulin inhibits the assembly of microtubules, which leads to disruption of the mitotic spindle apparatus and arrest of cells in metaphase (3). Resistance to the vinca alkaloids may result from mutations in tubulin, which leads to decreased drug binding and a decreased ability of cells to accumulate drug due to amplification of the P-glycoprotein (4).

Table 10–1 Comparative Activities of the Vinca Alkaloids

Vincristine	Vinblastine	Vindesine
Acute lymphoblastic leukemia	Germ cell tumors	Non-Hodgkin's lymphoma
Non-Hodgkin's lymphoma	Hodgkin's disease	Hodgkin's disease
Hodgkin's disease	Nonsmall cell lung carcinoma	Small cell lung carcinoma
Multiple myeloma	Breast cancer	Nonsmall cell lung carcinoma
Small cell lung carcinoma	Histiocytosis X	Breast cancer
Wilms' tumor		Esophageal cancer
Ewing's sarcoma		
Rhabdomyosarcoma		

Table 10–2 Comparative Toxicities of the Vinca Alkaloids

Vincristine	Vinblastine	Vindesine
Peripheral neuropathy*	Myelosuppression*	Mylosuppression*
Autonomic neuropathy	Constipation, paralytic ileus	Peripheral neuropathy
Inappropriate ADH syndrome	Mucositis	Gastrointestinal symptoms
Alopecia	Alopecia	Alopecia
Vesicant effects	Vesicant effects	Vesicant effects

*dose-limiting toxicity

Pharmacokinetics

The pharmacokinetic characteristics of vincristine and vinblastine are similar and include peak plasma concentrations of approximately 0.4 μM, followed by a multiphasic plasma disappearance with half-lives of <5 minutes and 164 minutes for vincristine and <5 and 190 minutes for vinblastine (5–7). Almost 70% of a dose of vincristine is excreted in the feces, primarily as metabolites resulting from hepatic metabolism and biliary excretion (8,9). The fecal excretion of vinblastine is only 10% (10). Little of either drug is excreted in the urine. Vinca alkaloids are only administered by the intravenous (IV) route. Either drug may be administered as an IV bolus, usually at weekly intervals or as a continuous infusion over 4 to 5 days (11,12). Plasma clearance of vindesine is intermediate between vinblastine and vincristine (2).

Interaction of Vinca Alkaloids and Radiation

Radioenhancement

Microtubule inhibitors have received little attention among the drugs studied for their potential radioenhancing activity (13). The fact that cells in the mitotic (M) phase are more sensitive to ionizing radiation has been demonstrated by Sinclair and Morton employing cultured Chinese hamster cells (14). Thus, vinca alkaloids should have radioenhancing activity by potentiating radiation-induced cell kill through accumulation of cells in M phase.

Storme et al have described both in vitro and in vivo experiments demonstrating that vinblastine and other microtubule inhibitors are radiosensitizers and that microtubulin inhibitors potentiate radiation-induced cell kill through accumulation of cells in M phase (13). In vivo studies employing mouse embryo cells transformed by Kirsten murine sarcoma virus (MO4 cell line) analyzed recovery from growth inhibition (RGI) after ionizing irradiation at a dose of 1000 cGy in the presence of vinblastine. A maximum proportion of M-phase arrests in the MO4 cell cultures was found after 24 hours of treatment with vinblastine, with values returning to near normal levels 24 hours after drug removal. Treatment of MO4 spheroids with vinblastine for 24 hours or longer prior to irradiation decreased RGI from 100 to 20%. No difference in RGI was observed after pretreatment with various doses of vinblastine. A decrease in RGI was observed when spheroids were incubated with vinblastine for periods of 1 to 48 hours prior to irradiation and with increasing duration of treatment. Treatment with vinblastine for 24 hours following radiation, however, did not affect RGI. The radioenhancing effect of 24-hour pretreatment with vinblastine was completely abolished when spheroids were allowed to recover from vinblastine for 16 hours or more prior to irradiation. This radioenhancing effect was not restricted to vinblastine but also occurred with vindesine and the synthetic microtubule inhibitor, tubulozole-cis. Tubulozoletrans, which does not affect microtubules, had no effect on RGI (Fig. 10–1). The addition of a third agent, 5-fluorouracil, which blocks cells in S-phase, abolished the effects of the microtubule inhibitors on the mitotic spindle, lending further support for radiosensitization rather than the combined additive cytotoxicity of radiation plus vinblastine.

Radiation Resistance

Treatment with vincristine in irradiated mammalian tumor cell lines results in no ef-

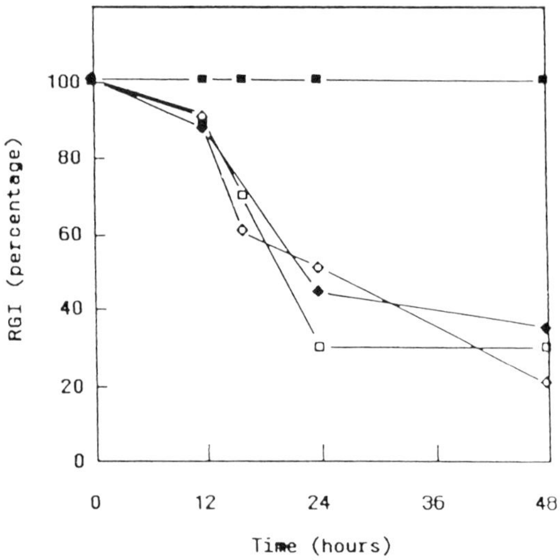

Fig. 10–1. The radioenhancing effect of microtubule inhibitors. Recovery from growth inhibition (RGI) in MO_4 spheroids treated for 12 to 48 hours prior to ionizing radiation with 0.1 μg Velban/ml (◆), 0.1 μg vindesine/ml (◇), 1 μg tubulozole-cis/ml (□), or 1 μg tubulozole-trans/ml (■). (From Storme et al. Interaction between microtubule inhibitors and ionizing radiation. *In:* Antitumor Drug Interactions. Hill BT and Bellamy AS (Eds). 1990, p. 114. Copyright CRC Press, Inc., Boca Raton, FL.)

fect on cell survival (15,16). The development of drug-resistant tumor cell lines by exposure to fractionated radiation results in resistance to vincristine that is not associated with alterations in cellular uptake of drug. In contrast, vincristine-treated L5178Y cells express resistance to vincristine and cross-resistance to doxorubicin. A comparison of the uptake of ^{3}H-vincristine into parental cells and into the resistant sublines derived following x-ray or drug exposure reveals reduced uptake and binding in vincristine-treated resistant cells compared with the parental cells. In contrast, neither ^{3}H-vincristine influx nor efflux was altered in the irradiated subline (16). Thus, the mechanisms of resistance to vincristine may differ depending upon the agent used to induce resistance.

Radioprotection

Vinca alkaloids, when appropriately administered with radiation, are capable of enhancing the recovery of normal tissues, including bone marrow and gastrointestinal epithelium, compared to treatment with radiation alone. Kovacs (17) reported increased radioresistance of intestinal epithelium when vincristine was injected 24 hours prior to radiation. Smith et al observed accelerated marrow and splenic regeneration with prolonged survival when mice were treated with colchicine, vinblastine, or vincristine before but not after radiation (18,19). A similar effect was observed by Storme et al in animals pretreated with tubulozole-cis 6 hours prior to 1750- or 2000-cGy exposure (13). This effect was not observed with 3000-cGy exposure.

Johnke et al (20) noted altered radiosensitivity of hematopoietic stem cells by vincristine pretreatment. These investigators evaluated the temporal recovery of two CFUs in marrow pretreated at various times with vincristine prior to receiving 450 cGy of radiation. The temporal recovery of the two colony forming unit (CFU) subpopulations studied was enhanced following combined vincristine and radiation with an optimal intertreatment time ranging from 12 to 24 hours. Under these optimal schedules, both CFUs studied had approached control levels by day 21; following radiation alone, the CFUs had only repopulated to 55% of control levels by day 21. When vincristine was given 1 hour prior to radiation, an insignificant radioprotective effect on either CFU population was noted. This radioprotective effect occurs at a time when CFUs are more sensitive to radiation, suggesting that vincristine may enhance recruitment of a primitive stem cell compartment that effectively repopulates the marrow following radiation. An elevation of superoxide dismutase levels localized in a bone-marrow fraction of enriched stem cells and progenitors was noted following vincristine (20). The temporal pattern of this increase, however, did not correlate with the drug-radiation schedules affording optimal radioprotection, suggesting that elevated superoxide dismutase levels are an accompanying rather than a causative factor in the mechanism responsible for vincristine-induced radioprotection.

Clinical Applications

The clinical implications of the above radiobiologic observations suggest that if vincristine and other microtubule inhibitors are to be used in conjunction with radiation, the drugs should be administered *12 to 24 hours prior to irradiation* to achieve enhanced cell kill (radiosensitization), to reduce the probability of the development of resistance to one modality prior to exposure to the second modality, and to enhance the recovery of hematopoietic tissue (radioprotective effect). Whether 24-hour continuous infusion of the vinca alkaloid prior to radiation would be more effective than bolus administration in accomplishing any of the above goals must be determined by clinical experimentation.

Pinkerton et al (21) have employed 5-day continuous infusion of vincristine (total dose, 4 mg/m^2) as part of a high-dose chemoradiotherapy regimen employing six doses of 200 cGy total body irradiation (during the 5-day vincristine infusion) followed by melphalan (180 mg/m^2) and autologous bone-marrow transplantation. The toxicities observed were mild liver function abnormalities and severe limb and jaw pain. Significant or enhanced neurotoxicity and myelosuppression were not observed.

In the clinical oncology literature, the use of vinca alkaloids as single agents in conjunction with radiation is sparse. These agents, however, have been employed in multi-agent combination chemotherapy programs in conjunction with radiation. Frequently used drug combinations employed with radiation include vincristine, cyclophosphamide, Adriamycin, and prednisone (CHOP or CVP) in the non-Hodgkin's lymphomas; velban, Adriamycin, dacarbazine, and bleomycin (ABVD) in Hodgkin's lymphoma; vincristine and/or vinblastine or vindesine with various combinations of cisplatinum, cyclophosphamide, etoposide, and mitomycin C in small cell and nonsmall cell carcinoma of the lung; and vincristine plus methyl CCNU and 5-fluorouracil in rectal and other gastrointestinal cancers. None of these clinical trials, however, are useful in separating the effects of the interaction of vinca alkaloids with radiation due to the obscuring effects of the other agents employed simultaneously in these regimens. It is doubtful that future clinical trials will allow us to do so, in view of the current trend of multi-agent chemotherapy for disease sites in which vinca alkaloids demonstrate activity.

Storme et al (13) report on a randomized Phase III trial employing 50 patients with locally advanced squamous cell carcinoma of the lung who were randomized to radiation alone (Group A) vs. radiation with vinblastine (Group B). The dose of radiation employed was 5500 cGy delivered over 6 weeks in both groups. The vinblastine group received 6-mg/m^2 weekly IV bolus injections. Response rates were 33% in Group A and 66% in Group B ($p < 0.05$). The median duration of survival was superior in the vinblastine plus radiation group (79 weeks) compared to the group that received radiation alone, whose median survival was 57 weeks ($p < 0.03$). The toxicity observed in the two groups differed in that eight out of 25 patients treated with both modalities experienced substantial dysphagia requiring hospitalization and parenteral nutritional support, whereas none of the patients in the radiation-only group experienced this toxicity ($p < 0.05$). One patient in the radiation-only group experienced radiation myelopathy. As anticipated, peripheral neuropathy was observed in some patients treated with vinblastine, but the authors did not observe any enhancement of neurotoxicity in the combined modality group.

One of the most convincing examples of a therapeutic advantage in combining radiation with chemotherapy was demonstrated for vincristine in the treatment of metastatic Wilms' tumor in the 1960s. Through studies conducted by the Southwest Cancer Chemotherapy Group, a complete remission of pulmonary metastases was demonstrated for 67% of children treated with vincristine (22). Regression proved to be temporary in most children unless therapeutic doses of radiation were also given at the sites of involvement. Vietti et al (23) treated 22 children with metastatic Wilms' tumor with combined vincristine and radiation to the metastases. Fourteen children received radiation to the lungs, four to the abdomen, and two to both sites. Radiation therapy was delayed in 20 of the 22 children from 14 to 41 days after the start of vincristine, in order to assess the effectiveness of the drug, but all patients received both vincristine and radiation therapy. The radiation dose range for the lungs was 1100 to 2013 cGy, and the abdomen received between 1500 and 4000 cGy. Sixteen children attained a complete remission, and 45% of the 22 children had no evidence of disease more than 2 years later. No pulmonary toxicity was observed. Peripheral neuropathy was observed in only three children, indicating no significant enhancement of neurotoxicity with the combination over vincristine alone. Moderate leukopenia was observed when radiation was added, probably due to the large radiation fields employed rather than to the combined effect of the two modalities.

Conclusions

The dearth of clinical trials employing vinca alkaloids and radiation without the compounding effects of other chemotherapeutic agents is unfortunate. Some suggestions for future clinical trials that might shed light on the potential interaction of vinca alkaloids and radiation are as follows.

1. Combined modality programs in lung cancer employing radiation and a vinca alkaloid as first-line treatment should be designed. Additional therapies could be added later, after the measurable effect of the initial therapy is observed. This approach, however, might be complicated by the increased potential for developing multidrug resistance due to induction of P-glycoprotein.
2. Similar regimens might be designed in the treatment of head and neck cancer or squamous cell carcinoma of the esophagus in which a vinca alkaloid is employed immediately prior to radiation therapy. Additional therapies may then be used, after a break in treatment, to allow evaluation of the initial treatment interaction. While such approaches may not offer meaningful information on survival, they may afford an opportunity to confirm some of the radiobiologic data observed in the laboratory.

PODOPHYLLOTOXIN DERIVATIVES

Etoposide (VP-16-213) is a semisynthetic derivative of podophyllotoxin, a compound extracted from the roots and rhizomes of the **podophyllum peltatum** (May apple or American Mandrake) (24). The extract, podophyllin, has been used as a treatment for warts since 1942. Clinical testing for anticancer activity of compounds derived from podophyllin was initiated in the 1950s. In the early 1970s, two synthetic glycoside derivatives, teniposide (VM-26) and etoposide (VP-16), were introduced into clinical study. The two compounds differ chemically only by the substitution of a methyl group in etoposide for a thenylidene group on the glucopyranoside sugar (24). After more than 10 years of clinical testing, no clinically significant difference between etoposide and teniposide has been identified. Etoposide has been evaluated primarily in adult tumors, whereas teniposide has been more frequently employed against pediatric malignancies.

Mechanism of Action

Etoposide differs in its mechanism of action from its parent, podophyllotoxin, and the classical spindle poisons such as colchicine, vincristine, and vinblastine in that it does not interact with tubulin or interfere with microtubular assembly (25). Rather, etoposide inhibits DNA synthesis by causing DNA strand breakage (26). Strand breakage correlates closely with cytotoxicity (27). Etoposide forms stable ternary complexes with DNA and topoisomerase-II. The enzyme then attaches covalently to DNA, forming single-strand protein-associated breaks (28). Resistance to etoposide and teniposide develops through amplification of the multidrug resistance pump (P-glycoprotein) and through alterations in formation or repair of strand breaks (29). In addition to inhibiting DNA topoisomerase-II activity, etoposide may exert its cytotoxic and antitumor action by metabolic activation in oxidation-reduction reactions to produce derivatives that can bind directly to cellular DNA (30). Thus, the cytotoxicity of etoposide may depend on a dual mechanism of DNA inactivation.

Etoposide is cell cycle dependent and phase specific; the major delay in cell progression and maximal cell killing occurs between the S and G2 phases (31).

Pharmacokinetics

Etoposide has been used in a variety of schedules and administered by both IV and oral routes. Etoposide plasma decay is biexponential, with a terminal half-life of 6 to 8 hours (32). When etoposide is administered by continuous infusion at 100 mg/m^2/day for 3 days, steady-state plasma levels in the range of 2 to 5 ug/ml are achieved in 2 to 3 hours after the start of the infusion. Upon discontinuation of the infusion, the disposition of etoposide is similar to that seen with rapid administration of the drug (33). There is no therapeutic or toxicologic advantage for continuous infusion over bolus administration. The soft gelatin capsule oral formulation has a bioavailability of 30 to 100% but averages 50% (34). Maximum tolerated IV doses are 100 mg/m^2/day for 5 consecutive days, 86 mg/m^2 /day for twice weekly doses, and 290 mg/m^2 once weekly (34). Teniposide usually is given in weekly doses of 67 mg/m^2 (34). The dose-limiting toxicity for both drugs is leukopenia.

Clinical Activity

Etoposide is most active in small cell carcinoma of the lung, particularly when used in combination with cisplatinum, with which etoposide has a potentiating effect (35). Significant activity has also been reported in Hodgkin's and non-Hodgkin's lymphomas, germ cell neoplasms, and Kaposi's sarcoma. Modest single-agent activity has been noted in nonsmall cell carcinoma of the lung, rhabdomyosarcoma, and acute leukemias.

Interaction of Etoposide and Radiation

Data regarding radiation and podophyllotoxin derivative interactions in vivo and in vitro are limited and inconclusive. Kubota et al (36) evaluated radiation sensitivity of HeLa S cells with and without etoposide (3). Exponentially growing monolayer cells were incubated with etoposide at 2.5 µg/ml for 1 hour immediately after irradiation. The combination of radiation and etoposide demonstrated a significant enhancement in cell killing, as compared with radiation alone. The difference in surviving fraction was principally due to the decrease of the shoulder of the cell-survival curve. When etoposide was combined with radiation at different time intervals in exponentially growing cells, a significant enhancement of cell killing was found immediately before and after radiation and at 6 hours after radiation. When plateau-phase cells were incubated with etoposide at 2.5 µg/ml for 1 hour immediately after radiation, no enhancement of cell killing was observed.

Hill (37) investigated the effects of pretreatment of a cell line (HN-1) derived from a squamous cell carcinoma of the tongue on drug resistance to chemotherapy when exposure to drugs occurred after fractionated irradiation of the cell cultures. In the HN-1/DXR (11) cells, resistance was expressed not only to etoposide but also to teniposide. Cross-resistance was not shown to podophyllotoxin itself. The degree of resistance to etoposide increased with increasing radiation exposure—approximately threefold after five fractions and rising to sixfold after 11 fractions as judged by the cell-survival fraction following a 24-hour exposure of cells to 1.0 µg/ml of etoposide. Resistance in this cell line was not associated with any modification in (3H)-VP-16 uptake or efflux characteristics.

Cell lines expressing resistance to etoposide resulting from prior exposure of cells in vitro to fractionated x-irradiation differ in certain essential respects from those cells in which resistance has been selected by prior exposure to the individual drugs. In these radiation-pretreated human tumor sublines, resistance to etoposide is not associated with cross-resistance to anthracyclines, alterations in drug uptake and efflux, or any detectable overexpression of the P-glycoprotein. Thus, these radiation-pretreated cells do not exhibit the classic multidrug-resistance phenotype. It is likely that other mechanisms of drug resistance are in operation. The most likely additional mechanism is reduced etoposide-induced DNA damage consistent with altered topoisomerase-II activity.

Clinical Applications

Information regarding clinical interaction of radiation and podophyllotoxin derivatives is limited. Fontana (38) described a radiation recall reaction associated with etoposide therapy. Eighteen hours following the first IV dose of etoposide and 48 hours prior to oral lomustine therapy, his patient developed a localized erythematous, urticarial eruption involving only the area of skin exposed to radiation 3 weeks previously. The skin healed completely in about 10 days; however, 3 weeks following the initial etoposide dose, the patient received an additional single dose of IV etoposide, which resulted in the development of a similar eruption with an identical distribution 8 hours following treatment.

Topical podophyllin in conjunction with visible light has been used to enhance the tumoricidal effect of ionizing radiation. Swartz et al (39) reported on a patient with locally advanced ulcerating breast carcinoma who was treated with Cobalt-60 with a total of 5000 cGy delivered to the mid-breast in 25 fractions over 48 days. A second patient was treated for a 15- × 10-cm rectal giant condyloma using a linear accelerator with a total dose of 5420 cGy. In each case, topical podophyllin (25% tincture of Benzoin) was applied once per day to the available exterior surfaces 20 minutes before treatment 4 days a week. Visible light (18.4 mW/cm^2 with 1 cm of water) was used to filter the infrared component. In both patients, bleeding ceased in days. A more rapid tumor regression with combined therapy was noted. The rectal lesion regressed to 15% of its initial area after 5 days of combined treatment. Biopsy of the chest wall demonstrated a histologic paucity of viable tumor cells in the volume treated with all modalities. Hematopoietic depression was noted.

The combination of high-dose etoposide and fractionated total body irradiation (TBI) has been employed as a preparative regimen prior to bone-marrow transplantation by Blume (40) in the United States and by Schmitz (41) in Europe. In these regimens, etoposide at a dose of 50 to 70 mg/kg was infused following 3 to 4 days of twice-daily fractions of TBI (120 to 200 cGy per fraction). Dose-limiting toxicity was mucositis and hepatotoxicity. Additional side effects included abdominal pain, diarrhea, vomiting, and a transient rash that progressed to desquamation of the palms and soles. The incidence of interstitial pneumonitis remained significant, 13 of 47 patients died of respiratory failure (40). The efficacy of this regimen in the treatment of relapsed acute leukemia was demonstrated in both series. Schmitz (41) reported 20 of 33 patients alive with 19 remaining in continuous complete remission for a median of 18 months. Blume (40) reported 16 of 33 patients alive, with 15 in continued remission (median, 12 months). The authors caution, however, against routine adoption of this regimen for its immunosuppressive potency in a clinical setting, bears an increased risk of graft rejection, because etoposide has less immunosuppresive potency than cyclophosphamide (42). Prospective randomized studies will be required to determine the role of this regimen in the treatment of leukemia. The use of high-dose etoposide in bone-marrow transplantation has been reviewed by Herzig (43).

Etoposide is currently undergoing clinical testing in combination with radiation in both small cell carcinoma and nonsmall cell carcinoma of the lung. Unfortunately, multiple other drugs are concurrently employed with etoposide. While multi-agent chemotherapy in conjunction with radiation is indeed appropriate in the treatment of lung cancer, because of the relative limited efficacy of any single agent and because of the frequent development of multiple-drug resistance, this clinical design makes it impossible to sort out the interaction between radiation and etoposide, both in terms of antitumor efficacy and toxicity. Drugs most commonly employed in conjunction with etoposide are cisplatinum, vincristine, cyclophosphamide, and Adriamycin. Radiation is delivered in a variety of schedules with conventional single fractionation and, in some studies, with twice-daily fractionation. Additionally, a variety of schedules of radiation and chemotherapy are being explored, including sequential, concurrent, and alternating programs. In the majority of randomized trials comparing a variety of combinations of drugs plus radiation, etoposide is present in all of the treatment arms, thereby making it impossible to isolate what effect etoposide has in each of the programs.

A randomized trial of cyclophosphamide, doxorubicin, and vincristine (CAV) with CAV plus etoposide (CAVE) in 231 patients with limited-stage small cell lung cancer was reported by the North Central Cancer Treatment Group (44). All patients received identical thoracic radiation consisting of 3750 cGy in 15 fractions and prophylactic cranial radiation. The addition of etoposide to the CAV regimen resulted in increased myelosuppression but not a significant improvement in survival—the median survival was 15.1 months for CAVE vs. 12.4 months for CAV ($p = 0.13$).

It is unlikely that single-agent etoposide in conjunction with radiation will be employed in the future in the treatment of lung cancer, as the trend to multiple agents in conjunction with radiation will no doubt continue to be the preferred method of clinical experimentation in the development of treatment programs for lung cancer.

Conclusions

A great deal must be learned regarding the interaction of podophyllotoxin derivatives and radiation, regarding both in vitro radiobiologic experimentation and clinical applications. There is some in vitro evidence of synergistic enhancement of cell killing when radiation and etoposide are used in proximity chronologically. However, there is documentation of reduced efficacy of etoposide if multiple fractions of radiation are administered prior to exposure to the drug. Therefore, future radiobiologic research should concentrate on identifying the optimal timing and sequence of the interaction of etoposide and radiation. While it is unlikely that future studies of lung cancer will allow single-agent etoposide interactions with radiation to be investigated, studies employing etoposide as a single agent in conjunction with radiation might be considered in the treatment of localized lymphoma, in which early stage disease could be treated with radiation alone vs. radiation plus etoposide to assess the clinical interaction. Conceivably, Phase II studies employing radiation and single-agent etoposide could be designed for resistant tumors in which other viable treatment options are limited, such as in refractory sarcomas, pancreatic carcinoma, and for postoperative recurrence of squamous cell carcinoma of the head and neck region.

REFERENCES

1. Legha S. Vincristine neurotoxicity-pathophysiology and management. Medical Toxicology 1:421, 1986.
2. Nelson RL, Dyke RW, Root MA. Comparative pharmacokinetics: Vindesine, vincristine and vinblastine in patients with cancer. Cancer Treat Rev 7(Suppl):17, 1980.
3. Owellen RJ, Hartke CA, Dickerson RM, et al. Inhibition of tubulin-microtubule polymerization by drugs of the vinca alkaloid class. Cancer Res 36:1499, 1976.
4. Kartner N, Shales M, Riordan JR, et al. Daunorubicin-resistant Chinese hamster ovary cells expressing multidrug resistance and a cell-surface P-glycoprotein. Cancer Res 43:4413, 1983.
5. Bender RA, Castle MC, Margileth DA, et al. The pharmacokinetics of ^{3}H-vincristine in man. Clin Pharmacol Ther 22:430, 1977.
6. Owellen RJ, Root MA, Haines FO. Pharmacokinetics of vindesine and vincristine in humans. Cancer Res 37:2603, 1977.
7. Lapinjoki SP, Verajankorva JM, Huhtikangas AE, et al. An enzyme-linked immunosorbent assay for the antineoplastic agent vincristine. J Immunoassay 7:113, 1986.
8. Castkem MC, Marqileth DA, Oliverio VT. Distribution and excretion of ^{3}H-vincristine in the rat and the dog. Cancer Res 36:3684, 1976.
9. Jackson DV, Castle MC, Bender RA. Biliary excretion of vincristine. Clin Pharmacol Ther 24:101, 1978.
10. Owellen RJ, Hartke CA, Haines FO. Pharmacokinetics and metabolism of vinblastine in humans. Cancer Res 37:2567, 1977.
11. Ratain M, Vogenzang NJ, Body G. Periwinkle alkaloids I: Vinblastine and vindesine. *In:* Cancer Chemotherapy by Infusion. Lokich J (Ed). Chicago, Precept Press, 1987, p. 167.
12. Jackson DV. Periwinkle alkaloids II: Vincristine. *In:* Cancer Chemotherapy by Infusion. Lokich J (Ed). Chicago, Precept Press, 1987, p. 181.
13. Storme G, Distelmans W, DeNeve W, Marcel M. Interaction between microtubule inhibitors and ionizing radiation. *In:* Antitumor Drug-Radiation Interactions. Hill BT, Bellamy AS (Eds). Boca Raton, CRC Press, 1990, p. 107.
14. Sinclair WK, Morton RA. X-ray sensitivity during the cell generation cycle of cultured Chinese hamster cells. Radiat Res 29:450, 1966.
15. Hill BT, Whelan RDH, Bellamy AS. Identification of differential drug responses and mechanism(s) of resistance in vincristine-resistant cell lines developed either by exposure to the drug or to fractionated radiation. Cancer Treat Rev 11(Suppl A):79, 1984.
16. Hill BT, Whelan RDH, Hosking LK, et al. Interactions between antitumor drugs and radiation in mammalian tumor cell lines: Differential drug responses and mechanisms of resistance following fractionated x-irradiation or continuous drug exposure in vitro. NCI Monogr 6:177, 1988.

17. Kovacs CJ. Redefining Clinical Research. *In:* Lung Cancer: Diagnostic procedures and therapeutic management with special reference to radiotherapy. Scarantino CW (Ed). New York, Springer-Verlag, 1985, p. 127.
18. Smith WW, Wilson SM. Effects of vinblastine and vincristine on survival and hemopoiesis in irradiated mice. J Natl Cancer Inst 39:1055, 1967.
19. Smith WW, Wilson SM, Fred SS. Kinetics of stem cell depletion and proliferation: Effects of vinblastine and vincristine in normal and irradiated mice. J Natl Cancer Inst 40:847, 1968.
20. Johnke RM, Kovacs CJ, Loven DP, et al. Altered radiosensitivity of hematopoietic stem cells by vincristine pretreatment: Superoxide dismutase activity as a possible mechanism. NCI Monogr 6:193, 1988.
21. Pinkerton CR, McDermott B, Phillip T, et al. Continuous vincristine infusion as part of a high dose chemoradiotherapy regimen: Drug kinetics and toxicity. Cancer Chemother Pharmacol 22:271, 1988.
22. Sutow WW, Thurman WG, Windmiller J. Vincristine sulfate in the treatment of children with metastatic Wilms' tumor. Pediatrics 32:880, 1963.
23. Vietti TJ, Sullivan MP, Haggard MF, et al. Vincristine sulfate and radiation therapy in metastatic Wilms' tumor. Cancer 25:12, 1970.
24. Isell BF, Muggia FM, Carter SK. Etoposide (VP-16): Current Status and New Developments. New York, Academic Press, Inc., 1984.
25. Loike JD, Horowitz SB. Effects of podophyllotoxin and VP-16-213 on microtubule assembly in vitro and nucleoside transport in HeLa cells. Biochemistry 15:5435, 1976.
26. Loike JD, Horowitz SB. Effect of VP-16-213 on the intracellular degradation of DNA in HeLa cells. Biochemistry 15:5443, 1976.
27. Long BH, Musial SF, Brattain MG. DNA breakage in human lung carcinoma cells and nuclei that are naturally sensitive or resistant to etoposide and teniposide. Cancer Res 46:3809, 1986.
28. Wozniak AJ, Ross WE. DNA damage as a basis for 4^1-demethylepipodophyllotoxin-9-(4,6-0-ethylidene-beta-D-glucopyranasoide) (etoposide) cytotoxicity. Cancer Res 43:120, 1983.
29. Pommier Y, Schwartz RE, Zwelling LA, et al. Reduced formation of protein-associated DNA strand breaks in Chinese hamster cells resistant to topoisomerase II inhibitors. Cancer Res 46:611, 1983.
30. Van Maanen JMS, Retel J, de Vries J, et al. Mechanism of action of antitumor drug etoposide: A review. J Natl Cancer Inst 80:1526, 1988.
31. Krishan A, Paika K, Frei E. Cytofluorometric studies on the action of podophyllotoxin and epipodophyllotoxins (VM-26, VP-16-213) on the cell cycle traverse of human lymphoblasts. J Cell Biol 66:521, 1975.
32. D'Incalci M, Farina P, Sessa C, et al. Pharmacokinetics of VP-16-213 given by different methods. Cancer Chemother Pharmacol 7:141, 1982.
33. Pfeffer M, Scalzo AJ, Nardella PA, et al. The absolute oral bioavailability and pharmacokinetics of etoposide. *In:* Etoposide (VP-16): Current Status and New Developments. Issell BF, Muggia FM, Carter SK (Eds). New York, Academic Press, 1984, p. 127.
34. Chabner BA, Myers CE. Clinical pharmacology of cancer chemotherapy. *In:* Cancer Principles and Practice of Oncology 3rd Ed. DeVita VT, Hellman S, Rosenberg SA, (Eds). Philadelphia, J.B. Lippincott, 1989, p. 384.
35. Bunn PA Jr. The role of chemotherapy in small-cell lung cancer. *In:* Etoposide (VP-16): Current Status and New Developments. Issell BF, Muggia FM, Carter SK (Eds). New York, Academic Press, 1984, p. 141.
36. Kubota N, Ikegami T, Watai K, et al. Effect of combined treatment of HeLa S_3 cells with radiation and etoposide on cell survival. Nippon Igaku Hoshasen Gakkai Zasshi 48(10):1276, 1988.
37. Hill BT. In vitro drug-radiation interactions using fractionated x-irradiation regimens. *In:* Anti-tumor Drug-radiation Interactions. Hill BT, Bellamy AS (Eds). Boca Raton, CRC Press, 1990, p. 207.
38. Fontana JA. Radiation recall associated with VP-16-213 therapy. Cancer Treat Rev 63:224, 1979.
39. Swartz MR, Rosenman J, Gunderson LL, et al. Podophyllin increases tumor radioresponsiveness. Cancer Chemother Pharmacol 7:238, 1982.
40. Blume KG, Forman SJ, O'Donnell MR, et al. Total body irradiation and high dose etoposide: A new preparatory regimen for bone marrow transplantation in patients with advanced hematological malignancies. Blood 69:1015, 1987.
41. Schmitz N, Gassman W, Rister M, et al. Fractionated total body irradiation and high dose VP-16-213 followed by allogenic bone marrow transplantation in advanced leukemias. Blood 72:1567, 1988.
42. Gassman W, Uharek L, Wottge HU, et al. Comparison of cyclophosphamide, cytarabine and

etoposide as immunosuppressive agents before allogenic bone marrow transplantation. Blood 72:1574, 1988.
43. Herzig RH. High dose etoposide and marrow transplantation. Cancer 67(Suppl 1):292, 1991.
44. Jett JR, Everson L, Teherneau TM, et al. Treatment of limited stage small-cell lung cancer with cyclophosphamide, doxorubicin and vincristine with or without etoposide: A randomized trial of the North Central Cancer Treatment Group. J Clin Oncol 8(1):33, 1990.

Chapter 11

PYRIMIDINE ANALOGS

TIMOTHY J. KINSELLA

INTRODUCTION

Halogenated pyrimidine analogs have been recognized as potential clinical radiosensitizers for almost three decades (1–6). Iododeoxyuridine (IUdR, IdUrd) and bromodeoxyuridine (BUdR, BrdUrd) are analogs of the nucleoside thymidine (dThd) and compete with dThd for incorporation into DNA (7,8), which is necessary for radiosensitization (9). Thymidine replacement is believed to result from stereochemical similarities between the van der Waal's radius of the iodine atom (2.15 Å) or bromine atom (1.95 Å) and the methyl group (2.0 Å) at the 5-position of the uridine molecule (Fig. 11–1). In recent laboratory and clinical studies, IUdR has been shown to be as effective a clinical radiosensitizer as BUdR with less systemic skin toxicity (10–12). While BUdR and IUdR share stereochemical similarities to dThd at the 5-position, the fluorinated analogs

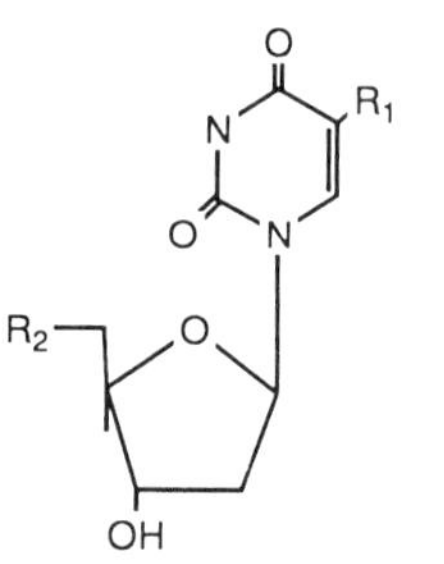

	R_1	R_2
dThd	CH_3	OH
FdUrd	F	OH
IdUrd	I	OH
5'-AdThd	CH_3	NH_2

Fig. 11–1. Structure of thymidine (dThd) and related analogs. The various analogs differ only in one substitution from dThd. Fluorodeoxyuridine (FUdR) and iododeoxyuridine (IUdR) have a halogen substitution for the methyl group at position 5, while 5′-aminodeoxythymidine (5′-AT) has an amino group instead of the hydroxyl at the 5′position.

fluorodeoxyuridine (FUdR, FdUrd) and fluorouracil (5-FU, FUra) do not and are not effectively incorporated into DNA.

HALOGENATED PYRIMIDINES

Pharmacokinetics

The halopyrimidines IUdR and BUdR, like dThd, must undergo sequential phosphorylations prior to incorporation into DNA. Figure 11–2 illustrates a schema for the endogenous (de novo) and exogenous (salvage) pathways for dThd and the halogenated pyrimidine analogs. The key enzyme in the salvage pathway is dThd kinase (TK), which is the first and rate-limiting step in the phosphorylation of both dThd and IUdR. The key enzyme in the de novo pathway of dThd is thymidylate synthase (TS). Catabolic enzymes of importance in the formation of intracellular pools of dThd and BUdR or IUdR, as well as their monophosphate forms, are cytoplasmic 5′-nucleotidase and nucleoside phosphorylase.

The salvage pathway of dThd is regulated by end-product (dTTP, IdUTP, FdUTP, BUTP) feedback inhibition of TK (13), which could limit the activation of drugs such as IUdR, BUdR, and FUdR (14) (Fig. 11–2). 5′-Aminodeoxythymidine (5′-AT) (Fig. 11–1) represents a new class of compounds capable of reducing this feedback regulatory mechanism by a direct interaction with the enzyme TK (15,16). The interaction between TK and 5′-AT is critically dependent on the presence of dTTP. In the absence of dTTP, 5′-AT competitively inhibits enzyme activity (17), whereas in the presence of dTTP, 5′-AT antagonizes the dTTP-induced inhibition of TK (15) (Fig. 11–2).

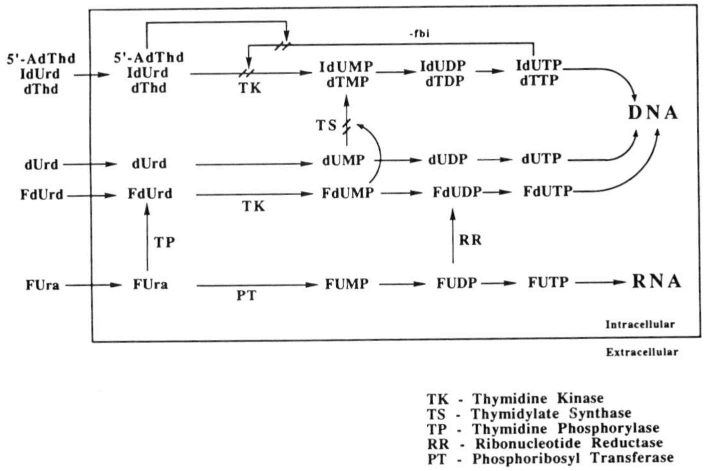

Fig. 11–2. Schema for biochemical pathways affecting the uptake and metabolism of FdUrd, 5′-AT thymidine (dThd), and its analogs (IdUrd, 5′-AT, FdUTP). dThd and IdUrd are metabolized by sequential phosphorylations to triphosphates (dTTP, IdUTP) for subsequent incorporation into DNA. The uptake of IdUrd and FdUrd (i.e., phosphorylation) is mediated by thymidine kinase (dThd kinase), which is the initial and rate-limiting enzyme in the exogenous (salvage) pathway of dThd. The endogenous (de novo) pathway of dThd is mediated by thymidylate synthase. The metabolic pathways for 5-FU are also illustrated.

5′-AT is an interesting drug for exploitation of potential clinical radiosensitization with these halopyrimidines, because it is not a substrate of the mammalian dThd kinase (18) and it is nontoxic in small animals (19). Additionally, 5′-AT has been shown to enhance the uptake of IUdR in human bladder carcinoma cell lines (647V, T24) but not in normal human urothelial cells propagated in vitro (20), suggesting a potential for differential sensitization in humans (21). Recently published data suggest that this differential response of the 647V tumor cells (compared to normal urothelial cells), to IUdR incorporation by cotreatment with 5′-AT, results from differences in regulation of TK activity, which may be pH dependent (22). Recent in vitro studies confirm enhanced radiosensitization using both 5′-AT and IUdR compared to IUdR alone (23). This biochemical modulation of IUdR is currently being tested in vivo.

The de novo pathway of dThd synthesis is also illustrated, in part, in Figure 11–2. Since IUdR and BUdR compete directly with dThd for DNA incorporation, modulation of the de novo pathway (i.e., decreased dThd synthesis) may also be important for increasing IUdR and BUdR incorporation and sensitization. The key enzyme in the de novo pathway is thymidylate synthase (TS). There are several drugs, including FUdR, 5-FU, methotrexate (MTX), N-(phosphonacetyl)-L-aspartic acid (PALA), and leucovorin, that modulate TS either directly (FUdR, 5-FU) or indirectly (PALA, MTX, and leucovorin) (24). Importantly, both leucovorin and PALA can be used as in vitro/in vivo modulators at nontoxic doses.

The pharmacology of the fluoropyrimidines is somewhat different from other halopyrimidines. Both FUdR and 5-FU inhibit TS following metabolism to FdUMP (Fig. 11–2) (25). FUdR is also a substrate of TK. Interestingly, the metabolic effects of FUdR and 5-FU differ from other nucleosides (dThd, IUdR) because their active metabolite (FdUMP) inhibits TS, resulting in the depletion of dTTP pools. This depletion of dTTP by FUdR and 5-FU is an attractive characteristic to study in vitro/in vivo mechanisms of potentiation of IUdR sensitization for two reasons: first, it can be used to evaluate the importance of regulation of TK by dTTP in the action of 5′-AT, and second, pretreatment of cells with FUdR or 5-FU can deplete dTTP pools to allow increased activation of IdUMP to the triphosphate with subsequent incorporation into DNA. Obviously, the timing of treatment with FUdR or 5-FU and IUdR requires careful study in vitro and in vivo. A recent clinical study of concomitant continuous infusions of FUdR and IUdR suggests that one can enhance IUdR incorporation into tumor cell DNA (colorectal liver metastases) by up to 2 times compared to incorporation into normal human liver (26–28).

Interaction with Radiation

Several recent in vitro investigations have focused on mechanisms of IUdR radiosensitization with potential clinical application. Incubation of exponentially growing V79 cells with IUdR and BUdR at 10^{-7} to 10^{-5} M (clinically relevant plasma steady state range) for two population doublings showed a progressive increase in percentage thymidine replacement and in radiosensitization (10). The extent of radiosensitization ($\approx 2 \times$ over control cells) appeared to be directly correlated with an increase in single-strand (SSB) and double-strand breaks (DSB) using filter elution techniques. No differences in the kinetics of SSB and DSB repair (10) were found during 3 hours of postirradiation repair. Interestingly, a higher-than-predicted ratio of SSB:DSB was found, suggesting that some excess SSB produced in IUdR- or BUdR-substituted DNA were DSB (29). The increased production of DSB in IUdR- or BUdR-treated cells immediately following x-irradiation and the persistence of more DSB after 3 hours of repair compared to irradiated controls are consistent with the hypothesis that cellular lethality is directly related to unrepaired DSB. One possible mechanism for increased DSB is the attack of a complementary DNA strand by radical intermediates (possibly uracilyl radicals) (30,31) produced in the IUdR- or BUdR-containing strand by reaction of a radiation-induced hydrated electron with IUdR or BUdR.

Phillips et al (32) have used the same in vitro cell system (exponentially growing V79 cells with a population doubling time of 7 to 8 hours) to correlate exposure time, drug concentration, and cellular incorporation of IUdR or BUdR with radiation response. At concentrations of ≥ 1 μM, the sensitizer enhancement ratio (SER) peaked after 48 to 72 hours of exposure, but required 72 to 96 hours at lower concentrations (0.1 to 1.0 μM). An important but not surprising finding by this same group was that there can be considerable variation in the concentration and exposure time ($C \times T$) for maximum radiosensitization between different cell lines. Using a human lung adenocarcinoma line (A549), they found the highest SER with 10 μM exposure for only one cell-cycle time. This finding underscores the need to investigate carefully how IUdR and BUdR are metabolized compared to dThd in different human tumor and normal cell lines. This type of biochemical study of nucleotide metabolism and possible modulation with nontoxic drugs like leucovorin and 5′-AT are undergoing laboratory testing. Such studies may have clear clinical implications, as suggested in recent publications (26,27,33).

Another potential limitation to the clinical application of IUdR or BUdR as radiosensitizers is whether any sensitization can result if IUdR or BUdR is incorporated into only one DNA strand. No previous in vitro study had compared x-radiosensitization with unifilar vs. bifilar DNA substitution in the clinically relevant range (1 to 10 μM). In a recent study (34), significant radiosensitization was found using exponentially growing V79 cells following 10 μM IUdR or BUdR for one (8% thymidine replacement) and two (16% thymidine replacement) population doublings (Fig. 11–3). By differential labeling of IUdR in DNA strands, an enhancement in x-ray-induced SSBs occurred in unsubstituted DNA in the strand basepairing with the IUdR strand and, to a lesser extent, in unsubstituted duplex DNA in the same cell. These data demonstrate that the radiolysis of IUdR-DNA produces mobile reactive intermediates that cause intermolecular damage (i.e., DNA SSB in unsubstituted DNA and resultant DSB as postulated in our previous study) (12). These intermediates (uracilyl radical) must be small and mobile in order to travel substantial distances and cause damage in adjacent unsubstituted DNA duplexes. Since IUdR incorporation into one strand can enhance radiation damage in adjacent unsubstituted DNA strands, it has greater potential as a clinical radioenhancer. This observation of significant radioenhancement with unifilar substitution in V79 cells has been confirmed in at least three different human tumor cell lines (preliminary data, unpublished). This issue has definite clinical implications because the reported doubling times of poorly radioresponsive solid tumors such as glioblastoma multiforme are 1 or more weeks (35) and unifilar substitution is a definite clinical reality.

Clinical Results

The author has conducted several pharmacologic and Phase I/II studies assessing IUdR or BUdR alone as a clinical radioenhancer (10,28,35–41). The overall results of these studies will be summarized briefly to serve as a background to support the potential clini-

	SSB[1] IdUrd[3]	SSB[1] Unsubstituted complement[4]	SSB[1] Unsubstituted duplex[5]	DSB[2]	%Trd Replacement	D_0 (Gy)	n̄
2 cycles of IdUrd	2.1	-	-	2.0	16	1.2	4.0
1 cycle of IdUrd	2.4 (A)	1.9 (B)	-	1.5	8	1.35	5.8
1 cycle of IdUrd, 1 cycle no IdUrd			1.4 (C)				
No IdUrd			1	1	0	1.7	8.5

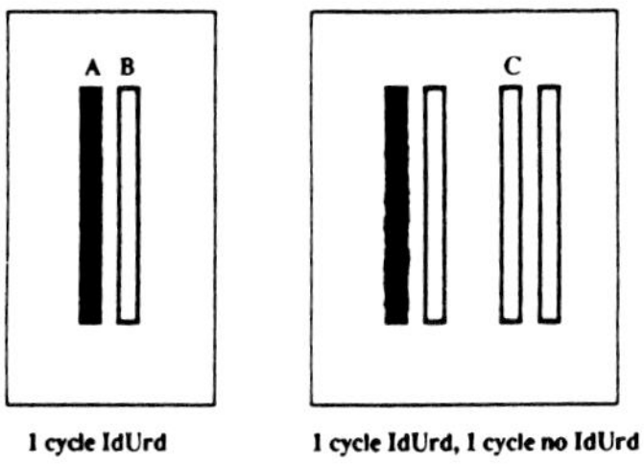

[1] DNA single strand breaks
[2] DNA double strand breaks
[3] IdUrd labeled DNA strand - ^{3}H Label
[4] Unsubstituted complementary strand DNA - ^{14}C Label
[5] Unsubstituted duplex DNA - ^{14}C Label
Note: shaded portions of figures indicate DNA single strands containing IdUrd

Fig. 11–3. Summary of the enhancement of radiation-induced strand breaks in V79 cells substituted with IdUrd.

cal significance in future studies of IUdR/BUdR.

First, IUdR or BUdR, when given as a continuous intravenous infusion, shows linear pharmacokinetics over the dose range used (250 to 1200 mg/m^2/day), with a **maximum tolerated dose (MTD) of 1000 mg/m^2/day for 14 days** (10,36). Steady-state arterial plasma ("tumor bed") levels are 4 to 6 μM at the MTD (throughout the entire 14-day infusion) (Fig. 11–4). This is a drug concentration associated with significant radioenhancement (enhancement ratios > 1.5) both in vitro (12) and in vivo, using bone marrow colony forming units (CFU-C) taken before and after the infusion (4,42). Systemic toxicity, primarily to the bone marrow, limited the period of continuous infusion to approximately 2 weeks; bone-marrow recovery was prompt, allowing for a second 2-week infusion in most patients.

Second, two different techniques were developed to measure incorporation of IUdR or BUdR into cellular DNA in normal (skin, peripheral granulocytes) and tumor cells (when available) in these clinical studies. In vitro staining of human tissue biopsy sections (skin, tumor) with an anti-IUdR/BUdR monoclonal antibody and immunohistochemistry demonstrated significantly greater tumor cell (high-grade sarcoma) incorporation (up to 50% of cells were counterstained positive) compared to normal skin (≈ 10% cells were positive by visual inspection) (10). The second technique involves more quantitative analysis of IUdR or BUdR incorporation into DNA, using high-performance liquid chromatography (HPLC) (43). In one study, up to 17% of thymidine bases in DNA of peripheral granulocytes (doubling time of 7 to 10 days) were substi-

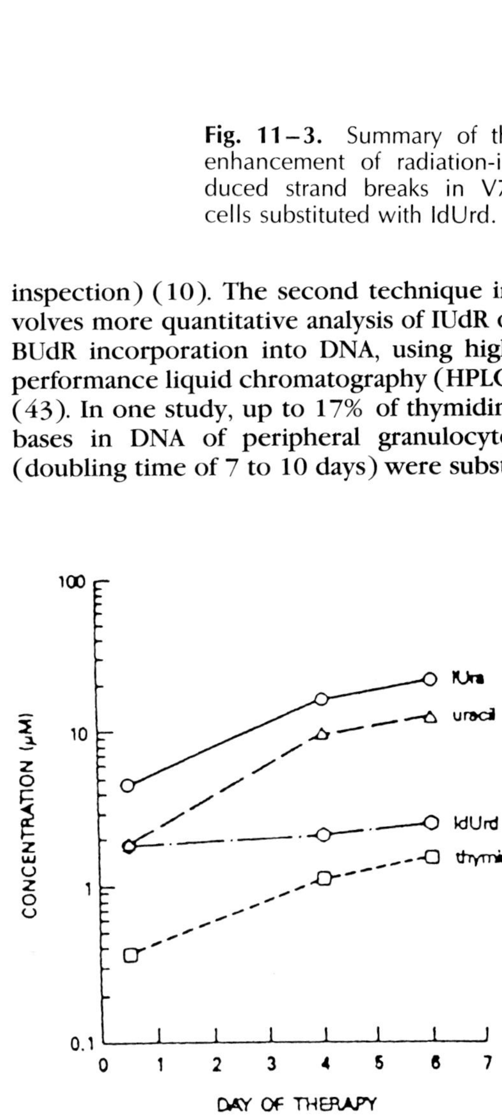

Fig. 11–4. Plasma levels of IUdR and metabolites in a typical patient receiving 1,000 mg/m^2/day of IUdR administered as a continuous IV infusion. (From Will CL, Dolwich BJ. Mol Pharmacol 29:643, 1986).

tuted, with IUdR following a 14-day continuous infusion using 1000 mg/m^2/day (37). More recently, in a clinical study of continuous infusions of IUdR for patients with liver metastases, we combined these techniques for assaying IUdR incorporation by using flow cytometry to sort monoclonal antibody positive tumor cells (employing a fluorescent conjugate) and the HPLC technique to measure thymidine substitution (26). Using duplicate pellets of single-cell suspensions of biopsies of colorectal tumor metastases and normal liver parenchyma after only a 3-day intravenous infusion of IUdR at 1000 mg/m^2/day, a median of 32% of tumor cells incorporated IUdR using flow cytometry, while the thymidine substitution in tumor DNA averaged 3% by HPLC (26). These data suggest a potential doubling time of approximately 10 days for these tumor metastases. For comparison, normal liver parenchyma showed a 5% median incorporation by monoclonal staining with < 1% thymidine substitution. Additionally, thymidylate synthase activity in tumors was twentyfold greater than in normal liver, while dThd kinase activity was twofold greater in tumors. Thus, IUdR in this trial exhibited selective incorporation into hepatic metastases compared to normal liver parenchyma (hepatocytes).

Finally, and most importantly, the clinical outcome in patients on these IUdR and BUdR studies suggests that **clinical radioenhancement** was achieved (28,38–41). These studies were designed to focus on human tumors that are poorly radioresponsive (clinically radioresistant) and are surrounded by normal tissues with low mitotic activity. Tumors selected for study included glioblastoma multiforme (labeling index of 12 to 15%) (35), high-grade (Grade 3) bone and soft tissue sarcomas (pathologically graded by extent of mitotic activity), and colorectal liver metastases (tumor doubling of ≈ 10 days as above) (28,38–41). Clinical radioenhancement was suggested by an improvement in local tumor control and survival (compared to historical controls of patients treated with radiation alone) without any associated increase in acute and late radiation effects on normal tissues (brain, bone and soft tissue, liver). For example, 17 of 28 locally advanced sarcomas treated with radiotherapy and IUdR were controlled locally (Table 11–1) with acceptable toxicity (Table 11–2). However, the design of Phase I/II studies does not involve a direct comparison of similar patients treated with standard therapy. Such Phase III studies of IUdR in high-grade gliomas and sarcomas are being performed by the Radiation Therapy Oncology Group and the National Cancer Institute. A Phase III study of BUdR and IUdR combined with conventional irradiation in anaplastic astrocytoma is being designed by the Northern California Cancer Center.

The basic strategy in these recent clinical studies was postulated by Dr. Henry Kaplan nearly 3 decades ago (44). It attempts to exploit differences in the proliferation rate of tumor compared to surrounding normal tissue. In the near future, it may be possible to better select patients for IUdR or BUdR sensitization based on high labeling indices of tumor vs. normal tissue using the monoclonal antibody technique (26,45–48). It may also be possible to reduce systemic toxicity to IUdR or BUdR by inhibiting DNA synthesis in normal self-renewal tissues (such as bone marrow) using pretreatment with hydroxyurea in "reversed-role chemotherapy" as proposed by Bagshawe (49,50).

The clinical concept of biochemical modulation of IUdR or BUdR metabolism to enhance radiosensitization is attractive and certainly challenging. One clinical challenge is optimizing the drug delivery schedule for IUdR and modulators such as the fluoropyrimidines (see basic biochemistry, Figure 11–2). Clinical studies with FUdR and 5-FU have demonstrated that the way a drug with a short half-life ($T_{1/2}$) is administered may dramatically alter its activity and toxicity. Since we documented that IUdR has a plasma $T_{1/2}$ < 5 min (36), it seems logical to use a longterm infusion (several days to weeks) for our radiosensitizing studies. One recent Phase I study attempted to enhance

Table 11–1. Local Tumor Control in 28 Patients Treated with IUdR and Radiotherapy.

Tumor Size	Bone Sarcoma	Soft-Tissue Sarcoma	Total
5–10 cm	2 of 4	4 of 5	6 of 9
10–15 cm	2 of 3	4 of 7	6 of 10
>15 cm	2 of 3	3 of 6	5 of 9
Total	6 of 10	11 of 18	17 of 28

Table 11–2. Toxicity of IUdR in 28 Patients (37,40)

Toxicity	No. of Patients	Severity	Comments
Skin rash	2	Mild	Pruritus in 1 patient
Nausea, vomiting	4	Mild	Can also be related to RT
Mucositis	8	3 Mild 5 Severe	3 patients needed hospitalization
Thrombocytopenia	23	Moderate-severe*	2 patients experienced gastrointestinal bleeding
Leukopenia	16	Mild-moderate*	1 patient experienced sepsis
Liver enzyme elevation	1	Mild	Returned to normal within 1 month

*Thrombocytopenia: moderate < 100,000 cells μl^{-1}, severe < 50,000 cells μl^{-1}. Leukopenia: mild < 2,500 cells μl^{-1}, moderate < 1,500 cells μl^{-1}. RT = Radiotherapy.

IUdR-DNA incorporation by using concomitant intravenous infusions of FUdR to block de novo thymidine synthesis (33). When IUdR and FUdR were given intravenously for 2 weeks, we noted no clinically relevant modulation of IUdR plasma levels nor enhancement of IUdR-DNA incorporation in peripheral granulocytes. Furthermore, isobologram analysis of systemic toxicity (principally bone marrow) suggested that IUdR and FUdR had additive rather than synergistic effects. Thus, we could not translate the previously published in vitro and in vivo data on IUdR and FUdR using this drug schedule. We argued that since IUdR and FUdR compete for activation by the same enzyme, thymidine kinase (see Fig. 11–2), our clinical results suggest that there may be antagonism if the enzyme is saturated. However, use of a folate analog such as methotrexate or leucovorin, which could block thymidylate synthase and de novo thymidine synthesis intracellularly without requiring activation by thymidine kinase, might be a better clinical strategy. Our preliminary in vitro results with leucovorin in a human colon cell line (HT29) demonstrates that treatment with leucovorin can significantly enhance IUdR-DNA incorporation (51). This combination of continuous intravenous infusions of IUdR and leucovorin is being studied in a proposed Phase I/II study at the University of Wisconsin.

FLUOROPYRIMIDINES

Pharmacokinetics

The metabolism of fluoropyrimidines has been studied in detail (52,53) and the major metabolic pathways are outlined in Figure 11–2. 5-FU is a structural analog of uracil with a fluorine atom in the 5-position. 5-FU was developed at the University of Wisconsin by Heidelberger over 30 years ago and remains one of the few anticancer agents whose synthesis was based on a logical rationale. Both 5-FU and FUdR have rapid transmembrane transport, and phosphorylation (similar to IUdR) is rate limiting. There are several pathways by which 5-FU may be activated (Fig. 11–2) and the dominant route of 5-FU activation can vary with different tumor cell lines. 5-FU may be converted to FUdR by dThd phosphorylase or to FdUMP by orotic acid phosphoribosyl transferase plus PRPP. FUdR, like IUdR, is then phosphorylated by TK to FdUMP, which inhibits TS. FUMP can be further phosphorylated and incorporated into RNA, or FUDP can be converted to FdUTP via ribonucleotide reductase. Incorporation of 5-FU into RNA inhibits the processing of nuclear RNA to lower molecular weight ribosomal RNA (54).

Although 5-FU is readily incorporated into RNA, it is only minimally incorporated into DNA (55–58). Two enzymatic processes are capable of excluding uracil or its analogs from DNA. dUTPase can rapidly hydrolyse FdUTP, and uracil-DNA glycosylase can remove any fluoropyrimidine that is incorporated into DNA. Thus, extensive study of fluoropyrimidine metabolism argues that any radiosensitization related to the fluoropyrimidines is probably not related to DNA incorporation. Therefore, while the metabolic pathways of the fluoropyrimidines and IUdR share similar enzymes, the biochemical mechanisms of radiosensitization are probably quite different but might be sequenced to maximize radiosensitization.

Interaction with Radiation

The mechanisms of fluoropyrimidine radiosensitization are poorly understood. To date, in vitro studies have focussed on interactions of 5-FU and radiation (59–61) with the following general conclusions: cytotoxic doses of 5-FU are necessary for radioenhancement; 5-FU is a more effective enhancer when given following irradiation and when present for extended periods; and radioenhancement does not result from inhibiting potentially lethal damage repair (PLDR). Clearly, one sees a contrast of these conclusions with those from in vitro studies of IUdR and BUdR radiosensitization where pre-incubation is necessary (1,51) and inhibiting PLDR may play an important role (9,62). Our ongoing in vitro studies of 5-FU and FUdR radiosensitization are focusing on the role of deoxyribonucleotide pool imbalances and subsequent altered DNA damage repair as a possible mechanism using two human cancer cell systems (63–65).

Clinical Results

The in vivo radiosensitizing potential of fluoropyrimidines was first described approximately 30 years ago (5,6). Two early randomized clinical trials involving bolus infusions of 5-FU and conventional fractionated radiation therapy showed improved survival compared to radiation therapy alone in gastrointestinal adenocarcinomas and head and neck squamous cell carcinomas (66,67). However, other early clinical trials were not as promising (68–70). More recently, the combination of continuous-infusion 5-FU (3 to 5 days every 3 to 4 weeks) and radiation therapy have yielded impressive tumor responses and survival benefit in various squamous cell and adenocarcinomas of the gastrointestinal tract (71–73). Weinberg and Rauth demonstrated the superiority of continuous-infusion 5-FU compared to bolus infusion 5-FU as a sensitizer to fractionated irradiation in the SCC VII in vivo tumor model (74,75). However, there are conflicting and confusing in vivo data regarding the timing and duration of the 5-FU infusion that results in greater than additive effects when combined with radiation (61). Because continuous-infusion 5-FU and radiation therapy is becoming an almost accepted clinical standard for many gastrointestinal and genitourinary (particularly bladder) tumors, further in vitro and in vivo studies of fluoropyrimidine radioenhancement are timely and most clinically relevant.

SUMMARY

In summary, there is a resurgence of interest in halogenated pyrimidines, including both the iodinated (IUdR), brominated (BUdR), and fluorinated (5-FU, FUdR) analogs as potential clinical radiosensitizers. Although these analogs share similar metabolic pathways, the mechanism(s) of radiosensitization have not been clearly defined and, indeed, are probably different. Thymidine replacement by IUdR or BUdR in DNA appears necessary for radiosensitization. To date, most clinical studies of IUdR/BUdR radioenhancement have simply attempted to select actively dividing, poorly radioresponsive tumors surrounded by relatively quiescent normal cells. It is also possible that biochemical modulation of IUdR or BUdR cellular metabolism and modulation of cell kinetics may lead to differential sensitization of tumor vs. normal cells. In contrast, DNA incorporation is unlikely to be responsible for radiosensitization using the fluoropyrimidines. Several biochemical targets for fluoropyrimidine radiosensitization are possible, including RNA effects secondary to incorporation via FUTP and alteration in DNA synthesis and/or repair mediated through inhibition of thymidylate synthase and changes in triphosphate pools. Fluoropyrimidines can also alter tumor and normal cell kinetics independently of irradiation.

REFERENCES

1. Djordjevic B, Szybalski W. Genetics of human cell lines III. Incorporation of 5-bromo- and 5-iododeoxyuridine into the deoxyribonucleic acid of human cells and its effect on radiation sensitivity. J Exp Med 112:509, 1960.
2. Erikson RL, Szybalski W. Molecular radiobiology of human cell lines V. Comparative radiosensitizing properties of 5-halodeoxycytidines and 5-halodeoxyuridines. Cancer Res 23:122, 1963.

3. Kaplan HS, Tomlin PA. Enhancement of x-ray sensitivity of E. coli by 5-bromouracil. Radiat Res 12:447, 1960.
4. Kinsella TJ, Mitchell JB, Russo A, Morstyn G, Glatstein E. The use of halogenated thymidine analogs as clinical radiosensitizers: Rationale, current status, and future prospects: Non-hypoxic cell sensitizers. Int J Radiat Oncol Biol Phys 10:1399, 1984.
5. Heidelberger C, Griesbach L, Montag BJ, et al. Studies on fluorinated pyrimidines II. Effects on transplanted tumors. Cancer Res 18:305, 1958.
6. Vermund H, Hodgett J, Ansfield FJ. Effects of combined roentgen irradiation and chemotherapy on transplanted tumors in mice. Am J Roentgenol 85:559, 1961.
7. Goz B. The effects of incorporation of 5-halogenated deoxyuridines into the DNA of eukaryotic cells. Pharmacol Rev 29:249, 1978.
8. Sirotnak FM, Barrueco JR. Membrane transport and the antineoplastic action of nucleoside analogues. Cancer Metastasis Rev 6:459, 1987.
9. Kinsella TJ, Dobson PP, Mitchell JB, Fornace AJ. Enhancement of x-ray induced DNA damage by pre-treatment with halogenated pyrimidine analogs. Int J Radiat Oncol Biol Phys 13:733, 1987.
10. Kinsella TJ, Russo A, Mitchell JB, et al. Phase I study of intravenous iododeoxyuridine as a clinical radiosensitizer. Int J Radiat Oncol Biol Phys 11:1941, 1985.
11. Kinsella TJ, Mitchell JB, Russo A, et al. Continuous intravenous infusion of bromodeoxyuridine (BUdR) as a clinical radiosensitizer. J Clin Oncol 2:1144, 1984.
12. Mitchell JB, Morstyn G, Russo A, et al. Differing sensitivity to fluorescent light in Chinese hamster cells containing equally incorporated quantities of BUdR versus IUdR. Int J Radiat Oncol Biol Phys 10:1447, 1984.
13. Breitman TR. The feedback inhibition of thymidine kinase. Biochem Biophys Acta 67:153, 1963.
14. Cohen A, Ullman B. Role of intracellular dTTP levels in fluorodeoxyuridine toxicity. Biochem Pharmacol 33:3298, 1984.
15. Fischer PH, Baxter D. Enzyme regulatory site-directed drugs. Modulation of thymidine triphosphate inhibition of thymidine kinase by 5′-amino-5′deoxythymidine. Mol Pharmacol 22:231, 1982.
16. Fischer PH, Fang TT, Lin TS, et al. Structure activity analysis of antagonism of the feedback inhibition of thymidine kinase. Biochem Pharmacol 37:1293, 1988.
17. Cheng YC, Prusoff WH. Mouse ascites sarcoma 180 deoxythymidine kinase. General properties and inhibition studies. Biochemistry 13:1179, 1974.
18. Chen MS, Shiau GT, Prusoff WH. 5′-Amino-5′-deoxythymidine: Synthesis, specific phosphorylation by herpesvirus thymidine kinase, and stability to pH of the enzymically formed diphosphate derivative. Antimicrob Agents Chemother 18:433, 1980.
19. Pavan-Langstom D, Park NH, Lass J, et al. 5′-Amino-5′-deoxythymidine: Topical therapeutic efficacy in ocular herpes and systemic teratogenic and toxicity studies (41386). Proc Soc Exp Biol Med 170:1, 1982.
20. Fischer PH, Vazquez-Padua MA, Reznikoff CA, Ratschan WJ. Preferential stimulation of iododeoxyuridine phosphorylation by 5′-aminothymidine in human bladder cancer cells in vitro. Cancer Res 46:4522, 1986.
21. Fischer PH, Vazquez-Padua MA, Reznikoff CA. Perturbation of thymidine kinase regulation: A novel chemotherapeutic approach. Adv Enzyme Regul 25:21, 1986.
22. Vazquez-Padua MA, Fischer PH, Christian BJ, Reznikoff CA. Basis for the differential modulation of IdUrd uptake by 5′AdThd among various cell types. Cancer Res 49:2415, 1989.
23. Kunugi KA, Vazquez-Padua MA, Miller EM, Kinsella TJ. Modulation of IdUrd-DNA incorporation and radiosensitization in human bladder carcinoma cells. Cancer Res 50:4962, 1990.
24. O'Dwyer PJ, King SA, Hoth DF, Leyland-Jones B. Role of thymidine in biochemical modulation: A review. Cancer Res 47:3911, 1987.
25. Spears CP, Shahinian AH, Moran RG, et al. In vivo kinetics of thymidylate synthetase inhibition in 5-fluorouracil-sensitive & -resistant murine colon adenocarcinoma. Cancer Res 42:450, 1982.
26. Speth PA, Kinsella TJ, Chang AE, et al. Selective incorporation of iododeoxyuridine into DNA of hepatic metastases versus normal human liver. Clin Pharmocol Ther 44:369, 1988.
27. Speth PA, Kinsella TJ, Chang AE, et al. Iododeoxyuridine (IdUrd) incorporation into DNA of human hematopoietic cells, normal liver and hepatic metastases in man as a radiosensitizer and as a marker for cell kinetic studies. Int J Radiat Oncol Biol Phys 16:1247, 1989.
28. Chang AE, Collins JM, Speth PA, et al. A Phase I study of intra-arterial iododeoxyuridine in patients with colorectal liver metastases. J Clin Oncol 7:662, 1989.
29. Bradley MO, Kohn KW. X-ray induced DNA double strand break production and repair in mammalian cells as measured by neutral filter elution. Nucleic Acids Res 7:793, 1979.
30. Ward JF. Molecular mechanisms of radiation-

induced damage to nucleic acid. Adv Radiat Biol 5:181, 1975.
31. Zimbrick JD, Ward JF, Myers LS. Studies on the chemical basis of cellular radiosensitization by 5-bromouracil substitution in DNA. II. Pulse and steady-state radiolysis of bromouracil-substituted and unsubstituted DNA. Int J Radiat Oncol Biol Phys 16:525, 1969.
32. Phillips TL, Bodell WJ, Uhl V, et al. Correlation of exposure time, concentration and incorporation of IdUrd in V-79 cells with radiation response. Int J Radiat Oncol Biol Phys 16:1251, 1989.
33. Speth PAJ, Kinsella TJ, Belanger K, et al. Fluorodeoxyuridine modulation of the incorporation of iododeoxyuridine into DNA of granulocytes: A Phase I and clinical pharmacological study. Cancer Res 48:2933, 1988.
34. Fornace AJ, Dobson PP, Kinsella TJ. Enhancement of radiation damage in cellular DNA following unifilar substitution with iododeoxyuridine. Int J Radiat Oncol Biol Phys 18:873, 878, 1990.
35. Hoshino T, Nagashima T, Murovic J. Cell kinetic studies of in situ human brain tumours with bromodeoxyuridine. Cytometry 6:627, 1985.
36. Klecker RW, Jenkins, JF, Kinsella TJ, et al. Clinical pharmacology of 5-iodo-2′deoxyuridine and 5-iodouracil, and endogenous pyrimidine modulation. Clin Pharmacol Ther 38:45, 1985.
37. Belanger K, Klecker R, Rowland J, et al. Incorporation of iododeoxyuridine (IdUrd) into cellular DNA in patients receiving continuous intravenous infusions. Cancer Res 46:6509, 1986.
38. Kinsella TJ, Glatstein E. Clinical experience with intravenous radiosensitizers in unresectable sarcomas. Cancer 59:908, 1987.
39. Jackson D, Kinsella TJ, Rowland J, et al. Halogenated pyrimidines as radiosensitizers in the treatment of glioblastoma multiforme. Am J Clin Oncol 10:437, 1987.
40. Kinsella TJ, Collins J, Rowland J, et al. Pharmacology and Phase I/II study of continuous intravenous infusions of iododeoxyuridine (IdUrd) and hyperfractionated radiotherapy in patients with glioblastoma multiforme. J Clin Oncol 6:871, 1988.
41. Tochner Z, Kinsella TJ, Rowland J, Glatstein E. Treatment of unresectable sarcomas of adults with hyperfractionated irradiation and iododeoxyuridine. Br J Radiol 19:101, 1989.
42. Mitchell JB, Kinsella TJ, Russo A, et al. Radiosensitization of hematopoietic precursor cells (CFU-C) in glioblastoma patients receiving intermittent intraveous infusions of bromodeoxyuridine (BUdR). Int J Radiat Oncol Biol Phys 9:457, 1983.
43. Belanger K, Collins JM. Technique for detection of DNA nucleobases by reversed-phase high-performance liquid chromatography optimized for quantitative determination of thymidine substitution by iododeoxyuridine. J Chromatogr 47:57, 1987.
44. Szybalski W. X-ray sensitization by halopyrimidines. Cancer Chemother Rep 58:539, 1974.
45. Gratzner HG. Monoclonal antibody to 5-bromo and 5-iododeoxyuridine: A new reagent for detection of DNA replication. Science 218:474, 1982.
46. Morstyn G, Hsu SM, Kinsella TJ, et al. Bromodeoxyuridine in tumors and chromosomes detected with a monoclonal antibody. J Clin Invest 72:1844, 1983.
47. Morstyn G, Kinsella TJ, Hsu SM, et al. Identification of bromodeoxyuridine in malignant and normal cells following therapy: Relationship to complications. Int J Radiat Oncol Biol Phys 10:1441, 1984.
48. Wilson GD, McNally NJ, Dunphy E, et al. The labelling index of human and mouse tumours assessed by bromodeoxyuridine staining in vitro and in vivo and flow cytometry. Cytometry 6:641, 1985.
49. Bagshawe KD. Reversed-role chemotherapy for resistant cancer. Lancet 2:778, 1986.
50. Bagshawe KD, Boden J, Boxer GM, et al. A cytotoxic DNA precursor is taken up selectively by human cancer xenografts. Br J Cancer 55:299, 1987.
51. Miller EM, Fowler JF, Kinsella TJ. Linear quadratic analysis of radiosensitivity of IUdR in human colon cancer cells. Rad Res Soc Abstract M6:64, 1990.
52. Myers CE. The pharmacology of the fluoropyrimidines. Pharmacol Rev 33:1, 1981.
53. Grem JL. Fluorinated pyrimidines. *In:* Cancer Chemotherapy. Principles and Practice. Chabner BA, Collins JM (Eds). Philadelphia, JB Lippincott Co., 1990, p. 180.
54. Will CL, Dolnick BJ. 5-fluorouracil augmentation of dihydrofolate reductase gene transcripts containing intervening sequences in methotrexate-resistant KB cells. Mol Pharmacol 29:643, 1986.
55. Lonn U, Lonn S. Progressive formation of DNA lesions during treatment with anti-metabolites without incorporation of the drugs into DNA. Mutat Res 200:243, 1988.
56. Major PD, Egan E, Herrick D, Kufe DW. 5-Fluorouracil incorporation in DNA of human breast carcinoma cells. Cancer Res 42:3005, 1982.
57. Lonn U, Lonn S. Interaction between 5-fluo-

rouracil and DNA of human colon adenocarcinoma. Cancer Res 44:3414, 1984.
58. Lonn U, Lonn S. DNA lesions in human neoplastic cells and cytotoxicity of 5-fluoropyrimidines. Cancer Res 46:3866, 1986.
59. Berry RJ. Effects of some metabolic inhibitors on x-ray dose-response curves for the survival of mammalian cells in vitro, and on early recovery between fractionated x-ray doses. Br J Radiol 39:458, 1966.
60. Nakajima V, Miyamoto Y, Tanabe M, et al. Enhancement of mammalian cell killing by 5-fluorouracil in combination with x-rays. Cancer Res 39:3763, 1979.
61. Byfield JE, Calabro-Jones P, Klisak I, Kulhanian F. Pharmacologic requirements for obtaining sensitization of human tumor cells in vitro to combined 5-fluorouracil or ftorafur and x-rays. Int J Radiat Oncol Biol Phys 8:1923, 1982.
62. Iliakis G, Kurtzman S, Pantelias G, Okavasky R. Mechanism of radiosensitization by halogenated pyrimidines: Effect of BUdR on radiation induction of DNA and chromosome damage and its correlation with cell killing. Radiat Res 119:286, 1989.
63. Meuth M. The genetic consequences of nucleotide precursor pool imbalance in mammalian cells. Mutat Res 126:107, 1984.
64. Kunz BA. Mutagenesis and deoxyribonucleotide pool imbalance. Mutat Res 200:133, 1988.
65. Snyder RD. Consequences of the depletion of cellular deoxynucleoside triphosphate pools on the excision-repair process in cultured human fibroblasts. Mutat Res 200:193, 1988.
66. Moertel CG, Childs DS, Reitemeier RJ, et al. Combined 5-fluorouracil and supervoltage radiation therapy of locally unresectable gastrointestinal cancer. Lancet 2:865, 1969.
67. Gollin FF, Ansfield FJ, Curreri AR, et al. Combined therapy in advanced head and neck cancer: A randomized study. Am J Roentgenol 114:83, 1972.
68. von Essen CF, Kligerman MM, Calabres P. Radiation and 5-fluorouracil: A controlled clinical study. Radiology 81:1018, 1963.
69. Hall BE, Good SW. Treatment of far-advanced cancer with 5-fluorouracil, used alone and in combination with irradiation. Incidence and duration of remission and survival-time data in 223 patients. Cancer Chemother Rep 16:369, 1962.
70. Stein JJ, Kaufman JJ. The treatment of carcinoma of the bladder with special reference to the use of preoperative radiation therapy combined with 5-fluorouracil. Am J Roentgenol 102:519, 1968.
71. Byfield JE, Barone RM, Sharp TR, Frankel SS. Conservative management without alkylating agents of squamous cell anal cancer using cyclical 5-FU alone and x-ray therapy. Cancer Treat Rep 67:709, 1983.
72. Keane TJ, Harwood AR, Elhakim T, et al. Radical radiation therapy with 5-fluorouracil infusion and mitomycin for esophageal squamous carcinoma. Radiother Oncol 4:205, 1985.
73. Coia LR, Paul AR, Engstrom PF. Combined radiation and chemotherapy as primary management of adenocarcinoma of the esophagus and gastroesophageal junction. Cancer 61:643, 1988.
74. Weinberg MJ, Lapointe TA, Rauth AM. Growth delay in a murine squamous cell tumor after local radiation and concurrent infusional 5-fluorouracil treatment. Int J Radiat Oncol Biol Phys 12:1449, 1986.
75. Weinberg MJ, Rauth AM. 5-Fluorouracil infusions and fractionated doses of radiation: Studies with a murine squamous cell carcinoma. Int J Radiat Oncol Biol Phys 13:1691, 1987.

Chapter 12

PERFLUOROCHEMICALS

BEVERLY A. TEICHER, TERENCE S. HERMAN, AND ROBERT A. LUSTIG

INTRODUCTION

External pressure on capillaries resulting from rapid and uncontrolled cell proliferation within malignant tumors causes blood vessels to constrict or collapse so that red blood cell passage is restricted (1–7). This effect is responsible for deficient vascular beds within solid tumors, which cause areas of severe vascular insufficiency, and often regions of frank necrosis (8–11). Thomlinson and Gray described the occurrence of small necrotic volumes in tumors at sites distant from capillaries. Based on the diffusion characteristics of oxygen, they were able to calculate that hypoxic but still viable cells would be present at distances of about 130 μm from the axis of the capillary blood vessels. This pattern of tumor growth has been observed in many animal and some human tumors.

In situ observations of growing tumors have revealed rapidly opening and closing blood vessels (7). Recently, the therapeutic significance of acute and partial hypoxia, which are consequences of vascular flux, as well as chronic hypoxia has been reviewed (12,13). As measured by radiobiologic methods (14,15) and by direct pO_2 measurements (16–18), hypoxia is present in most animal solid tumor models. Gatenby et al (19) have measured the oxygen distribution in nodal metastases of human squamous cell carcinoma and have been able to correlate the oxygen tension in these masses with the response of the tumors to radiation therapy. In 12 of 31 tumors studied, more than 26% of tumor volume contained a pO_2 less than 8 mm Hg (19). Vaupel et al (18) found that in human breast cancer xenografts growing in nude rats, the O_2 consumption rate per unit weight significantly decreased with increasing tumor mass. This decreased O_2 consumption rate of the cancer cells in vivo was the result of the increasingly deficient blood supply with increasing tumor size. Even in small tumors, however, some areas of hypoxia were commonly found (18). It now appears certain that the majority of solid tumors contain hypoxic cells, which frequently constitute 10 to 20% of the total viable tumor-cell population (20,21).

Cells grown in culture as spheroids (i.e., small balls of tightly packed cells) show central necrosis and evidence of hypoxia when grown to greater than 0.35 mm in diameter (22). It is probable, therefore, that even in occult metastases too small to be detected by standard diagnostic techniques, foci of hypoxic cells are present and have therapeutic implications.

HYPOXIC CELLS IN CANCER THERAPY

Hypoxia protects cells from the cytotoxic effects of radiation. Hypoxic cells surviving large doses of radiation are capable of either reestablishing the tumor in situ or producing tumors in other animals after transplantation (9–11). This effect is most marked after administration of large single fractions of radiation. Fractionated radiotherapy of animal tumors results in a more complex situation, because reoxygenation may occur between treatments. During reoxygenation, the tumor cells that were hypoxic at the time of irradiation become better perfused, presumably because of the death of radiosensitive euoxic cells situated between them and tumor capillaries. These previously hypoxic cells then reacquire the radiosensitivity characteristic of aerobic cells. As a consequence, the sensitivity of the tumor to subsequent irradiation is increased. Patterns of reoxygenation in tumors vary widely, however. Some tumors reoxygenate rapidly and extensively but others reoxygenate slowly (23,24).

The importance of hypoxic cells in limiting the sensitivity of human tumors to conventional, fractionated radiotherapy regimens, however, is still debated extensively. Some clinical data (25) and extrapolations from animal tumors in which reoxygenation occurs slowly suggest that hypoxic cells probably limit the curability of certain types of human cancer by fractionated radiotherapy. The relative antineoplastic selectivity of many chemotherapeutic agents in current clinical use for the treatment of cancer derives from the toxicity of the drugs to cells that are actively traversing the cell cycle. Cycle-active agents are relatively ineffective against quiescent tumor cells that are not actively cycling at the time of treatment. Cells in nutritionally deficient environments are typically noncycling. Quiescent cells are present in both animal and human tumors, and the quiescent cells of animal tumors are clonogenic (i.e., capable of proliferation).

Even for anticancer agents that are capable of readily killing noncycling cells, hypoxic cells may be resistant for the following reasons.

1. These cells may have prolonged cell-cycle times or may be blocked in their progression through the G_1 phase. Cells that remain out of mitosis for prolonged periods are better able to repair DNA damage caused by many anticancer drugs (21,23).
2. Drugs that have physicochemical properties not conducive to diffusion into tumor tissue or that are unstable or metabolized rapidly may not reach chronically hypoxic tumor cells located in regions of severe vascular insufficiency in sufficient concentrations (1,2,26).
3. Some chemotherapeutic agents require the presence of O_2 for maximal cytotoxicity (26).

PERFLUOROCHEMICAL EMULSIONS: FLUOSOL-DA

Clark and Golan (27) demonstrated in 1966 that liquid perfluorochemicals could sustain life when mice were immersed in them for long periods. Then, in 1967, Sloviter and Kamimoto (28) reported successful perfusion of rat brains with perfluorochemicals. In 1986, Geyer (29) demonstrated by total blood replacement in rats that perfluorochemicals in an emulsified form can function as well as red blood cells as oxygen carriers. However, intravenous infusions of perfluorochemical (PFC) liquids cause the death of animals because these substances are immiscible in aqueous media and thus form emboli. Therefore, these substances must be suspended as fine particles (emulsions) when they are used as artificial blood substitutes.

The size of the particles is important in relation to the retention and behavior of the particles in circulation. The half-life of a fine emulsion in rabbits (with a particle size of 0.1 μm in average diameter) was about 85 hours, whereas that of a coarse emulsion (0.25 μm in average diameter) was about 30 hours. By comparison, the average diameter for red blood cells is 5 to 10 μm. In emulsions with larger particles, the emulsion particles tend to clump and form emboli.

PFCs are metabolically inert and are transpired through the lungs. After many perfluorocarbons had been screened, perfluorodecalin was found to be the best compound with respect to the rate of excretion. It was difficult, however, to form a stable emulsion from perfluorodecalin alone; therefore, other perfluorocarbons were used in combination with perfluorodecalin (30,31). Using the mixed perfluorocarbon technique developed by Geyer, the Green Cross Corporation of Japan found that the addition of perfluorotripropylamine significantly increased the stability of the emulsion. The PFC emulsion selected for clinical testing was named Fluosol-DA.

Composition of Fluosol-DA 20%		
Perfluorodecalin	14.0	w/v%
Perfluorotripropylamine	6.0	w/v%
Pluronic-F68	2.7	w/v%
Yolk phospholipids	0.4	w/v%
Potassium olate	0.032	w/v%
Glycerol	0.8	w/v%
NaCl	0.6	w/v%
KCl	0.034	w/v%
Glucose	0.180	w/v%
$MgCl_2$	0.020	w/v%
$CaCl_2$	0.028	w/v%
$NaHCO_3$	0.210	w/v%
pH: 7.4–7.6		

The emulsion consists of 20% PFC, with seven parts of perfluorodecalin, three parts of perfluorotripropylamine, Pluronic-F68 and phospholipids as emulsifiers, and glycerol as a cytoprotecting agent. To furnish the preparation with physiologic osmolarity and oncotic pressure, Kreb's Ringers bicarbonate solution is included.

The volume of oxygen dissolved in Fluosol-DA changes linearly with oxygen partial pressure, according to Henry's law. The uptake and release of oxygen (and CO_2) are completely reversible, as with hemoglobin, and the rate is twice as fast as that of hemoglobin. The combined surface area of the particles is 1.82×10^8 cm^2 per liter available for oxygen diffusion. This is about 100 times greater than that of blood, which contains a surface area of 1.86×10^6 cm^2 oxygen-carrying particles per liter.

PFCs have limited oxygen-transport capability at ambient pressures. Oxygen content is linear with respect to oxygen tension, as opposed to blood, in which the relation is sigmoid for oxygen. Blood delivers approximately 6 vol% oxygen to tissues at ambient pressures, whereas at these same pressures, Fluosol-DA 20% can deliver only about 2 vol%. If oxygen pressure is increased to 1 atm of inspired gas ($F10_2$ 1.0), however, the amount of oxygen that can be delivered by Fluosol-DA 20% is about 6.5 vol%. Evidence suggests that a lower oxygen pressure ($F10_2$ 0.85) can be used if the concentration of perfluorochemicals is increased.

The particle size distribution of the Fluosol-DA emulsion, as determined by centrifugal sedimentation and electron microscopy, is in a narrow range, and 90% or more of the particles are smaller than 0.2 μm in diameter. The particles are coated with a layer of phospholipid and the detergent Pluronic-F68. The small size allows the emulsion particles to flow through small capillaries, leading to tissue volumes that red cells cannot reach. The corollary to this is that oxygen can at least enter areas of small capillary microcirculation. The particle size also will influence emulsion stability and viscosity. Biologically, particle size also will affect transit time, distribution, and, therefore, possibly toxicity.

COMBINING FLUOSOL-DA AND IRRADIATION

In Vivo Studies

Three times more radiation is required to kill fully anoxic cells than normally oxygenated cells. Radiosensitization, however, occurs at relatively low concentrations of oxygen—a concentration of 0.25% oxygen moves the dose-response curve halfway toward the fully aerated condition, with essentially identical dose-response curves obtained for cells in 2, 20, or 100% oxygen. Therefore, a small amount of oxygen delivered to hypoxic regions of a solid tumor would significantly increase the radiosensitivity of those tumor regions. Currently, only one perfluorochemical emulsion, Fluosol-DA 20%, has been cleared for clinical use; however, several other more concentrated perfluorochemical emulsions are currently under development. Of the new experimental emulsions, those based on perfluorocytylbromide (PFOB) and *bis*-(perfluorobutyl) ethene (F44E) appear to be most promising, primarily because of greater stability of the emulsions at room temperature and smaller volume of administration to achieve a given blood level. The potential of perfluorochemical emulsions and carbogen breathing to improve the oxygenation of hypoxic regions in the RIF-1 tumor has been investigated using oxygen microelectrodes by Song and coworkers (32,33). Measurement of intratumoral pO_2 by oxygen microelectrodes demonstrated significant increases in pO_2 when Fluosol-DA (20%) was injected into the animals and the animals breathed carbogen (95% O_2, 5% CO_2). Hiraga et al (34) found that cerebral blood flow increased approximately twofold following complete blood-PFC exchange and 1.5-fold after partial exchange. A similar 1.5-fold increase in flow was measured in intraparenchymal tumors following partial exchange. Thus, it appears that perfluorochemical emulsions are capable of improving tumor oxygenation both by serving as a carrier for oxygen and by increasing tumor blood flow.

The PFC emulsion Fluosol-DA, in combination with breathing a 100 or 95% oxygen atmosphere, has been shown to enhance the response of several solid rodent tumors to single-dose and fractionated radiation treatments (32,33,35–41).

In the application of this methodology to the clinic, questions arise regarding the lowest effective dose and the scheduling of PFC emulsion in a course of fractionated radiation therapy. We have used the Lewis lung-tumor model to address these questions in an animal tumor system (37). X-rays were delivered as 300-cGy fractions twice per day. Fluosol-DA was administered once per day at a dose of 4, 8, or 12 ml per kg of body weight (Fig. 12–1). The dose-modifying factors (DMF) observed at a tumor growth delay time of 6 days were 1.42 ± 0.16 at 4 ml/kg, 1.85 ± 0.23 at 8 ml/kg, and 2.17 ± 0.34 at 12 ml/kg. Although the dose modification seen at 12 ml/kg was greater than that seen at 8 ml/kg, this difference was not statistically significant ($p < 0.5$). Both 12 ml/kg and 8 ml/kg were significantly better than 4 ml/kg ($p < 0.0006$ and $p < 0.0024$, respectively). For all treatments, the enhancement in tumor growth delay was highly significant, as compared with results in carbogen-breathing controls ($p < 0.0001$ with 12 ml/kg and 8 ml/kg, and $p < 0.005$ with 4 ml/kg.

In clinical practice, it is unlikely that PFC emulsions would be administered daily. In an effort to mimic a clinical regimen, we administered a single dose of Fluosol-DA (12 ml/kg) on day 1 of the treatment program and delivered radiation in 200, 300, or 400 cGy fractions on days 1 to 5, one fraction per day (Fig. 12–2) (37). The DMF observed in Fluosol-DA-treated animals, when carbogen breathing was maintained for 1 hour prior to and during each radiation fraction, was 2.60 ± 0.54, which is not significantly different from the dose modification seen with Fluosol-DA/carbogen and a single dose of x-rays (37). This indicates that some effect of Fluosol-DA persists over several days or that breathing a high-oxygen-content atmosphere even after the Fluosol-DA effect is diminished can be of therapeutic benefit. In this protocol, Fluosol-DA and air breathing did not lead to dose modification. Although Fluosol-DA/air breathing, as compared with carbogen in the absence of Fluosol-DA, produced 0.5 to 1 additional days of tumor growth delay, this difference was not statistically significant.

As an approach to determining the optimal dose schedule for Fluosol-DA during a course of fractionated radiation therapy, a total dose of 16 ml/kg of Fluosol-DA was administered either as two doses of 8 ml/kg on

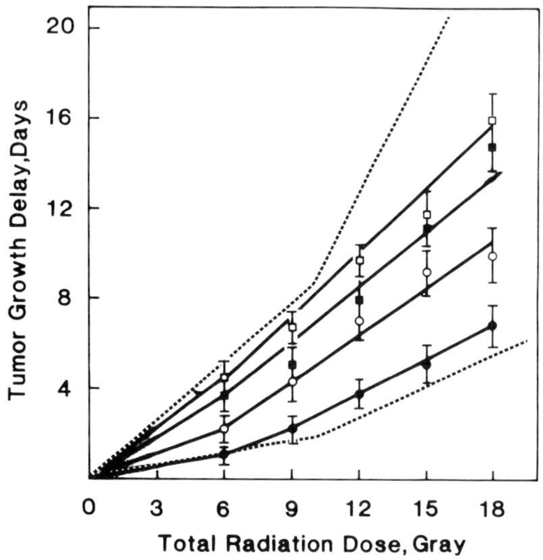

Fig. 12–1. Growth delay of the Lewis lung tumor produced by various doses of Fluosol-DA and fractionated x-ray treatment. Radiation was delivered in 300-cGy (3-Gy) fractions twice per day and Fluosol-DA administered once per day. In all groups, carbogen breathing was maintained for 1 hour prior to and during each fraction. (□) 12 ml/kg Fluosol-DA; (■) 8 ml/kg Fluosol-DA; (○) 4 ml/kg Fluosol-DA; (●) no Fluosol-DA; (---, upper) single-dose x-ray treatment and 12 ml/kg Fluosol-DA; (---, lower) single-dose x-ray treatment in the absence of Fluosol-DA. (From Teicher BA, et al. Int J Radiat Oncol Biol Phys 12:1311, 1986, Pergamon Press Ltd.)

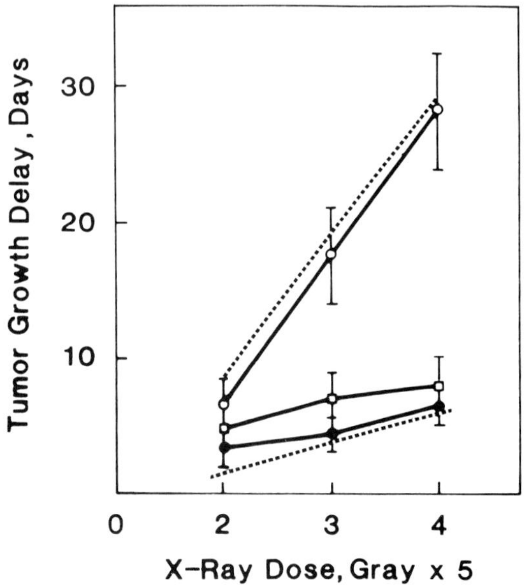

Fig. 12–2. Growth delay of the Lewis lung tumor produced by a single dose of 12 mg/kg of Fluosol-DA and five daily fractions of x-rays. (○) Fluosol-DA and 1 hour of carbogen breathing prior to and during each x-ray fraction; (□) Fluosol-DA and air breathing; (●) 1 hour of carbogen breathing prior to and during each x-ray fraction; (---, upper) Fluosol-DA and carbogen breathing with single-dose x-ray treatment; (---, lower) carbogen breathing with single x-ray treatment. (From Teicher BA, et al. Int J Radiat Oncol Biol Phys 12:1311, 1986, Pergamon Press Ltd.)

days 1 and 3 or as four doses of 4 ml/kg on days 1, 2, 3, and 4 of a 4-day protocol using the Lewis lung tumor model system (Fig. 12–3). The Lewis lung tumor was grown subcutaneously in the flanks of C578L/6J mice. Treatment was initiated when the tumors were 50 to 100 mm^3. Radiation was delivered as four daily fractions of 250, 400, or 500 cGy. Fluosol-DA was administered intravenously prior to irradiation. Carbogen breathing was maintained each day for 1 hour prior to and during each x-ray treatment. When Fluosol-DA was administered as two doses of 8 ml/kg, the DMF observed was 1.7 ± 0.3. When Fluosol-DA was given as four doses of 4 ml/kg, the DMF was 1.5 ± 0.3 compared to x-ray treatment with carbogen breathing. It appears, therefore, that administering Fluosol-DA at a therapeutic dose less frequently with carbogen breathing with every radiation fraction may produce a better treatment outcome than more frequent lower doses.

Fluosol-DA emulsion particles are taken up by the reticuloendothelial system, causing reversible hepatomegaly and splenomegaly. No enhanced radiation toxicity has been seen in sensitive normal tissues in animals treated with Fluosol-DA and oxygen breathing with radiation (42). A possibility for Fluosol-DA in radiation therapy is the use of Fluosol-DA in combination with hyperbaric oxygen, which will significantly increase the amount of oxygen carried by the PFC (43).

COMBINING FLUOSOL-DA WITH CHEMORADIATION

In Vivo Studies

With most solid tumors, however, it is unlikely that Fluosol-DA and carbogen breathing will be 100% efficient in oxygenating the entire tumor mass. It is likely that pockets of

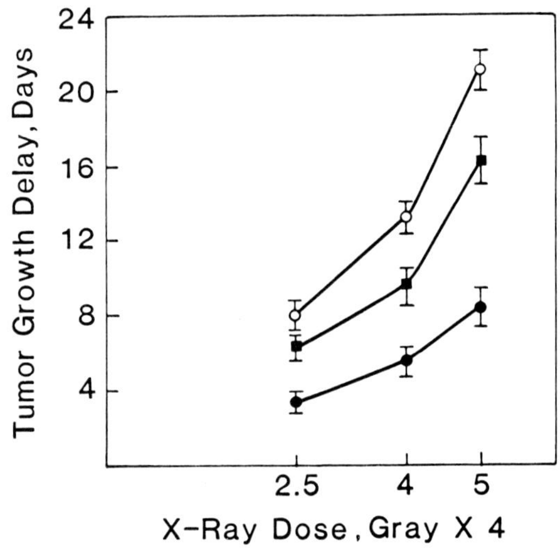

Fig. 12–3. Growth delay of the Lewis lung tumor produced by two schedules of Fluosol-DA and four daily fractions of x-rays. (●) Fractionated x-ray treatment with carbogen breathing for 1 hour prior to and during each fraction. (■) Fluosol-DA (0.1 ml; 4 ml/kg) was administered prior to each x-ray treatment with carbogen breathing 1 hour prior to and during each fraction. (○) Fluosol-DA (0.2 ml; 8 ml/kg) was administered on treatment days 1 and 3; carbogen breathing was maintained for 1 hour prior to and during each fraction (From Teicher BA. Proceedings of 35th Meeting of the Radiation Research Society; Abstract EM-1. Atlanta, GA, 1987.)

viable hypoxic cells will remain and prevent tumor cure. This residual hypoxic cell component of solid tumors must be considered in the design of curative therapeutic regimens.

Nitrosoureas

The addition of treatment with a PFC emulsion combined with breathing a high-oxygen atmosphere has been shown to improve the response of several animal tumor systems to treatment with carmustine (BCNU) as well as to other cancer chemotherapeutic agents (47,49–58). We have examined the use of Fluosol-DA and carbogen breathing with single-dose radiation treatment, BCNU, and combined drug and radiation treatment in intracranially implanted 9L gliosarcoma (59). The median enhancement in life-span produced by Fluosol-DA and carbogen breathing in addition to radiation was 2 days at 1000 cGy and 6 days at 2000 cGy, compared to radiation treatment alone (Fig. 12–4). In the group receiving 2000 cGy with Fluosol-DA and carbogen breathing, two of 20 lived 120 days. Treatment with a single intraperitoneal injection of BCNU (10 mg/kg) on day 7 post-tumor-cell implantation produced an increase in life-span of 2 days compared to untreated control animals. The combination of drug treatment with Fluosol-DA and carbogen breathing produced an increase in life-span of 26 days, which was significantly different from BCNU treatment with air breathing ($p < 0.001$) (Fig. 12–5). Finally, when BCNU, Fluosol-DA, and carbogen were combined with radiation treatment (2000 cGy), an increase in life-span of nearly 85 days compared to untreated controls was produced; 47% of patients (9 of 19) survived 120 days (Fig. 12–6) (59). These results suggest that this combination might be effective in the treatment of malignant brain tumors.

Nitroimidazoles and Hyperthermia

The antitumor efficacy of adding the nitroimidazole-radiosensitizing drugs, misonidazole and etanidazole, or hyperthermia (43°C for 30 min) to Fluosol-DA/carbogen (95% O_2/5% CO_2) and radiation was tested in the FSaIIC tumor system (60). Both the nitroimidazole drug (61–64) and hyperthermia (65–67) produced additional tumor growth delays and tumor cell cytotoxicity when given with Fluosol-DA/carbogen, either prior to or after radiation (Figs. 12–7, 12–8, and 12–9). For each of the modalities tested, the dose-modifying effect was greater when that therapy preceded rather than followed radiation (misonidazole 2.7 vs. 1.9 (63), etanidazole 2.4 vs. 1.7 (68–70), hyperthermia 4.0 vs. 1.7 (71) relative to the effect of radiation alone). Because the nitroimidazole drugs must be present prior to radiation to exert their radiosensitizing effect, the increase in tumor growth delay observed when these hypoxic cell-cytotoxic drugs

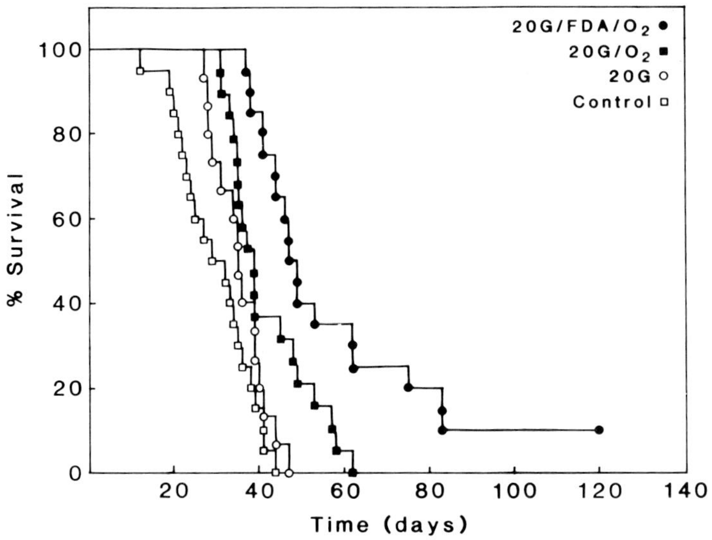

Fig. 12–4. Kaplan-Meier plot of the survival distribution for rats bearing intracranial 9L tumors. The groups shown are: untreated controls (□); 2000 cGy (20 Gy) (○); 2000 cGy (20 Gy) with carbogen breathing for 1 hour prior to and during treatment (■); and 2000 cGy (20 Gy) preceded by Fluosol-DA with carbogen breathing for 1 hour prior to and during treatment (●). (From Teicher BA, et al. Int J Radiat Oncol Biol Phys 15:1187, 1988, Pergamon Press Ltd.)

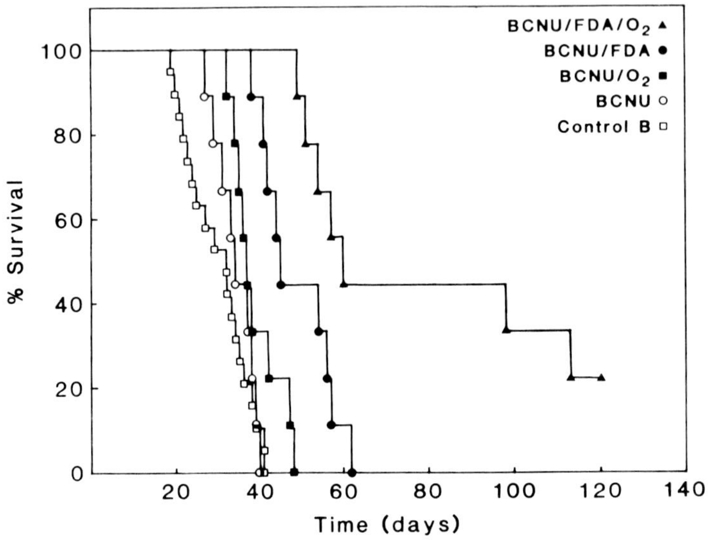

Fig. 12–5. Kaplan-Meier plot of the survival distribution for rats bearing intracranial 9L tumors. The groups shown are: untreated controls (□); BCNU (10 mg/kg) (○); BCNU (10 mg/kg) followed by 1 hour of carbogen breathing (■); BCNU (10 mg/kg) preceded by Fluosol-DA (●); and BCNU (10 mg/kg) preceded by Fluosol-DA and followed by 1 hour of carbogen breathing (▲). (From Teicher BA et al., Int J Radiat Oncol Biol Phys 15:1187, 1988, Pergamon Press Ltd.)

were administered following Fluosol-DA/carbogen and radiation suggests that Fluosol-DA and carbogen were not able to fully oxygenate the tumors and that the nitroimidazole drugs were effectively toxic to residual hypoxic cells. The treatment Fluosol-DA/carbogen → hyperthermia → radiation produced a marked increase in tumor growth delay not seen with the sequence Fluosol-DA/carbogen → radiation → hyperthermia (60). The results indicate that a treatment combination of radiation sensitizers may be more effective than radiation plus Fluosol-DA with oxygen breathing alone.

Mitomycin C and Porfiromycin

The cytotoxic effects of the addition of mitomycin C or porfiromycin on treatment with Fluosol-DA/carbogen (95% O_2/5% CO_2) breathing and radiation were also studied in the FSaIIC tumor system (72). In vitro, mitomycin C and porfiromycin are both preferentially cytotoxic to hypoxic cells (26,73–78). After in vivo exposure, however, the cytotoxicity of mitomycin C to single-cell tumor suspensions obtained from whole tumors was exponential over the dose range studied, but a plateau in cell killing was ob-

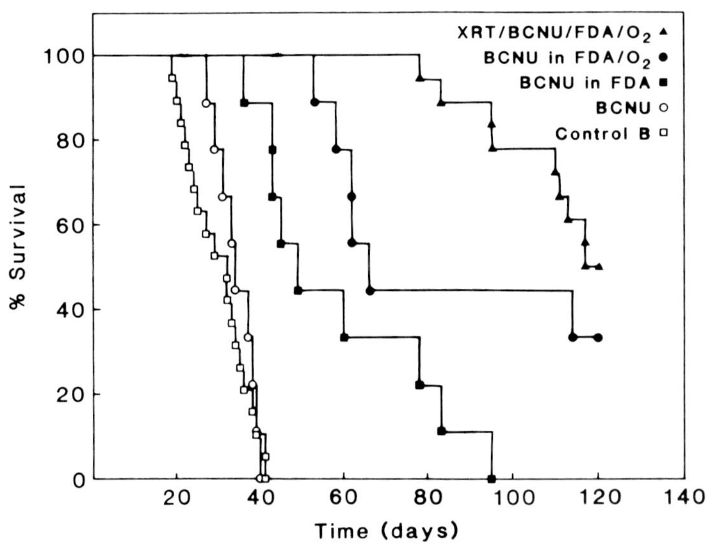

Fig. 12–6. Kaplan-Meier plot of the survival distribution for rats bearing intracranial 9L tumors. The groups shown are: untreated controls (□); BCNU (10 mg/kg) (○); BCNU (10 mg/kg) in Fluosol-DA (■); BCNU (10 mg/kg) in Fluosol-DA followed by 1 hour of carbogen breathing (●); and 2000 cGy (20 Gy) preceded by BCNU (10 mg/kg) and Fluosol-DA with 1 hour of carbogen breathing prior to and during radiation (▲). (From Teicher BA et al. Int J Radiat Oncol Biol Phys 15:1187, 1988, Pergamon Press Ltd.)

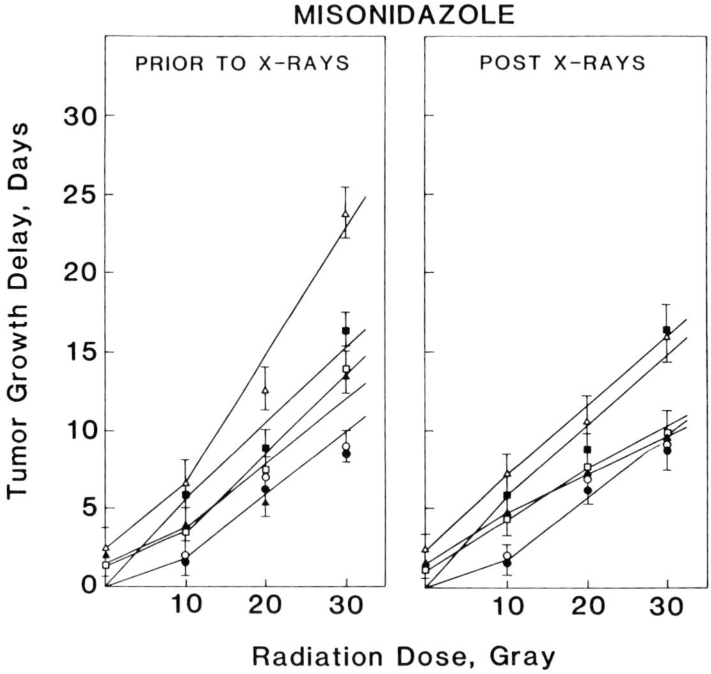

Fig. 12–7. Growth delay of the FSaIIC fibrosarcoma produced by radiation and misonidazole with Fluosol-DA with or without carbogen breathing. Misonidazole was administered either prior to or after irradiation. The treatment groups were: radiation (10, 20, or 30 Gy)/carbogen (●); Fluosol-DA (12 ml/kg) and radiation (○); Fluosol-DA/carbogen and radiation (■); misonidazole (1 g/kg) and radiation (□); misondazole-Fluosol-DA and radiation (▲); and misonidazole/Fluosol-DA/carbogen and radiation (△). (From Teicher BA et al. J Natl Cancer Inst 81:929, 1989).

served for porfiromycin (72,79,80). With Fluosol-DA/carbogen breathing and single-dose radiation, addition of either mitomycin C or porfiromycin increased the tumor cell kill achieved at 500 cGy by approximately 1.2 and 1.0 logs, respectively (Fig. 12–10). Less effect was seen with addition of the drugs at the 1000 and 1500 cGy radiation

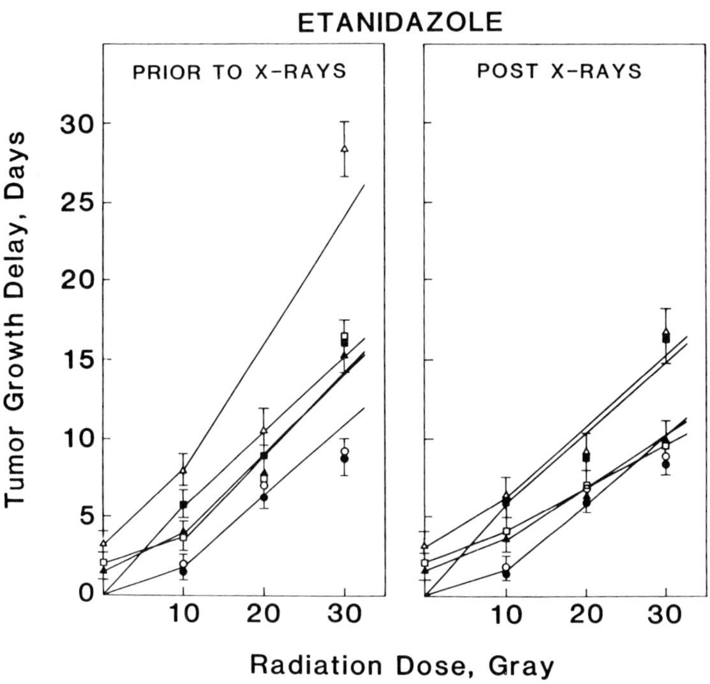

Fig. 12–8. Growth delay of the FSaIIC fibrosarcoma produced by radiation and etanidazole with Fluosol-DA with or without carbogen breathing. Etanidazole was administered either prior to or after irradiation. The treatment groups were: radiation (10, 20, 30 Gy)/carbogen (●); Fluosol-DA (12 ml/kg) and radiation (○); Fluosol-DA/carbogen and radiation (■); etanidazole (1 g/kg) and radiation (□); etanidazole/Fluosol-DA and radiation (▲); and etanidazole/Fluosol-DA/carbogen and radiation (△). (From Teicher BA et al. J Natl Cancer Inst 81:929, 1989).

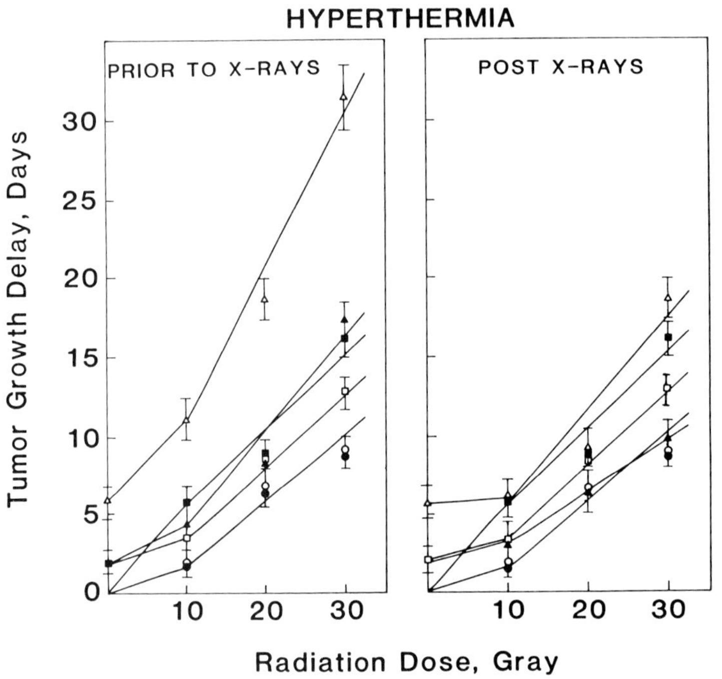

Fig. 12–9. Growth delay of the FSaIIC fibrosarcoma produced by radiation and hyperthermia with Fluosol-DA with or without carbogen breathing. Hyperthermia was administered either prior to or after irradiation. The treatment groups were: radiation (10, 20, or 30 Gy)/carbogen (●); Fluosol-DA (12 ml/kg) and radiation (○); Fluosol-DA/carbogen and radiation (■); hyperthermia (43° C, 30 min.) and radiation (□); hyperthermia/Fluosol-DA and radiation (▲); and hyperthermia/Fluosol-DA/carbogen and radiation (△). (From Teicher BA et al. J Natl Cancer Inst 81:929, 1989.)

dose levels. In tumor growth delay experiments, the addition of either mitomycin C or porfiromycin to Fluosol-DA/carbogen breathing and radiation resulted in primarily an additive increase in tumor growth delay (Table 12–1).

Administration of the fluorescent dye Hoechst 33342 to tumor-bearing mice 20 minutes prior to sacrifice followed by the preparation of a single-cell suspension from treated tumors allows separation of bright and dim cells by a fluorescently activated cell sorter. These separated populations can then be assayed for colony formation in vitro. Because the amount of dye present is a product of simple diffusion, bright cells were cells close to vessels (presumably well oxygenated) and dim cells were cells distant from vessels (presumably hypoxic) (71,81–85). Unexpectedly, the survival of Hoechst 33342 dye-selected tumor cell subpopulations (71,81–85) indicated that Fluosol-DA/carbogen breathing increased the cytotoxicity of radiation (1000 cGy) more in the bright cell subpopulation (fourfold) than in the dim cell subpopulation (twofold) resulting in an overall fourfold sparing of the dim subpopulation (Fig. 12–11). This may be because the Hoechst 33342 dye-selected bright cells contained a significant number of acutely or intermittently hypoxic cells and Fluosol-DA/carbogen may not be most successful in the population of cells that are in flux relative to vascular perfusion. Mitomycin C and porfiromycin were both more toxic to the dim cell subpopulations. Addition of mitomycin C or porfiromycin to Fluosol-DA/carbogen breathing and radiation (1000 cGy) resulted in a primarily additive effect of the drugs and radiation killing in both tumor-cell subpopulations.

Thus with mitomycin/Fluosol-DA/carbogen and radiation, there was a two-fold sparing of dim cells, and with porfiromycin in the combined treatment, there was a 1.6-fold sparing of the dim-cell population. Our results indicate that treatment strategies directed against both intermittently and chronically hypoxic tumor subpopulations can markedly increase the tumor cell-kill achieved by radiation (72).

Clinical Studies

In 1978, Makowski (86) reported on the infusion of Fluosol-DA into seven decerebrate patients who had sustained severe head injury. He infused 1000 to 1500 ml of Fluosol-DA over a period of 60 to 70 minutes via a central venous line. Changes were

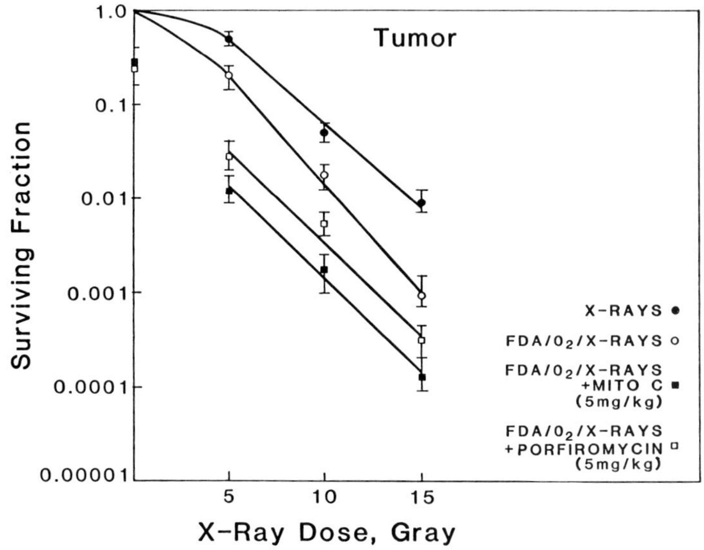

Fig. 12–10. Survival of cells from FSaIIC tumors treated with various doses of radiation alone or in combination with Fluosol-DA, carbogen or drugs. The treatment groups are: x-rays with carbogen breathing for 1 hour prior to and during treatment (●); x-rays preceded by Fluosol-DA (12 ml/kg) and carbogen breathing for 1 h prior to and during treatment (○); x-rays preceded by Fluosol-DA (12 ml/kg) and carbogen breathing for 1 h prior to and during treatment followed by mitomycin C (5 mg/kg) (■); and x-rays preceded by Fluosol-DA (12 ml/kg) and carbogen breathing for 1 hr prior to and during treatment followed by porfiromycin (5 mg/kg) (□). Points: means of three independent experiments; bars: SE. (From Holden SA, Herman TS, Teicher BA. Radiother Oncol 18:59, 1990).

noted in various hematologic parameters, all of which returned to normal within 1 hour. Ohyanagi et al (87) reported on the infusion of Fluosol-DA in normal human volunteers; 1 ml of Fluosol-DA was infused intravenously and the patient was observed for 60 minutes. Subjects were then infused at rates of 1 ml per minute for 20 to 500 ml total infusion. No changes were noted in blood pressure, pulse, or respiration. No significant changes were noted in blood count, liver enzymes, or renal function. Tremper et al (88) subse-

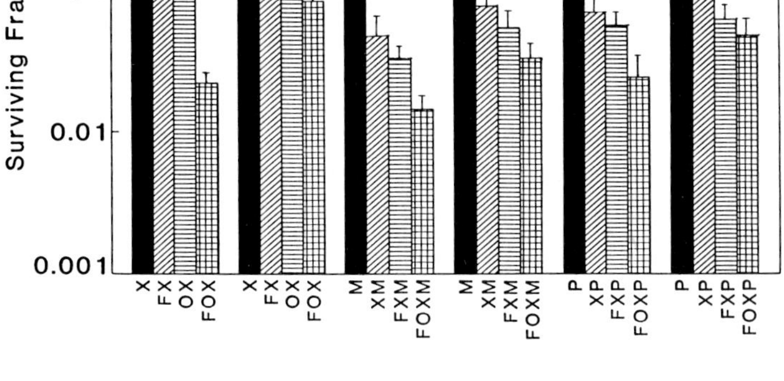

Fig. 12–11. Survival of subpopulations based on Hoechst 33342 fluorescence intensity of cells from FSaIIC tumors treated with a single dose of 10 Gray (1000 cGy) of x-rays alone or in combination. The characters beneath the bars are—X: 10 Gray (1000 cGy) of x-ray; F: Fluosol-DA (12 ml/kg); O: carbogen breathing for 1 hour prior to and during x-ray treatment; M: mitomycin C (5 mg/kg); and P: porfiromycin (5 mg/kg). Each experiment was repeated three times. Bars: SE. (From Holden SA, Herman TS, Teicher BA. Radiother Oncol 18:59, 1990.)

Table 12–1. Growth Delay of the FSaIIC Fibrosarcoma Produced by Treatment With Fluosol-DA/Carbogen Breathing and Single-Dose Radiation Combined With a Hypoxic-Cell-Selective Drug

	Hypoxic Cell Selective Drug[a]		
Treatment Group	None	Mitomycin C	Porfiromycin
Drug alone	—	5.4 ± 1.0	1.1 ± 0.5
Fluosol-DA[b] →	no effect	6.6 ± 1.2	4.8 ± 0.8
Fluosol-DA/carbogen[c] →	no effect	5.9 ± 1.0	4.5 ± 1.0
1000 cGy[d] →	1.6 ± 0.5	7.4 ± 0.8	5.5 ± 1.0
2000 cGy[d] →	6.2 ± 1.0	8.5 ± 1.5	8.6 ± 1.1
3000 cGy[d] →	8.8 ± 1.0	11.4 ± 1.7	12.3 ± 1.5
Fluosol-DA/1000 cGy[d] →	2.0 ± 0.5	6.2 ± 1.0	6.1 ± 1.3
Fluosol-DA/2000 cGy[d] →	6.9 ± 1.0	9.2 ± 1.2	11.4 ± 1.5
Fluosol-DA/3000 cGy[d] →	9.1 ± 1.0	13.3 ± 1.5	15.3 ± 1.8
Fluosol-DA/carbogen/1000 cGy[d] →	5.8 ± 1.5	9.5 ± 1.2	10.0 ± 1.5
Fluosol-DA/carbogen/2000 cGy[d] →	8.8 ± 1.5	12.7 ± 1.5	13.5 ± 1.7
Fluosol-DA/carbogen/3000 cGy[d] →	16.3 ± 2.0	18.9 ± 1.9	19.6 ± 2.1

[a]A single dose of mitomycin C (5 mg/kg) or porfiromycin (5 mg/kg) was administered by i.p. injection immediately after radiation treatment.
[b]The dose of Flusol-DA was 12 ml/kg (0.3 ml), administered intravenously.
[c]Carbogen (95% O_2/5% CO_2) breathing was initiated immediately after Fluosol-DA administration and maintained for 1 hour prior to and during radiation delivery.
[d]Radiation was delivered as a single dose to the tumor-bearing limbs.

quently reported the hemodynamic and oxygen transport effects of Fluosol-DA in an anemic patient who refused blood transfusion and required pelvic surgery. No adverse affects were noted. Subsequently, Fluosol-DA was placed in clinical trials in Japan (89) and in the United States to be used in patients who were severely anemic and refused blood products and also required surgery. Tremper (90) demonstrated that a high fraction of inspired oxygen was necessary to raise the arterial oxygen pressure significantly.

Head and Neck

A Phase I/II clinical study of adjuvant Fluosol-DA and oxygen was started in 1984; the initial results were reported by Rose et al (91). Additional patients were entered, and further results have been reported by Lustig et al (92). Advanced head and neck tumors were chosen as the initial site. These tumors are thought to contain a significant portion of hypoxic cells, which contribute to the problem of local control. In addition, evidence suggests that hyperbaric oxygen may be useful in improving local control. This study included Stage III and IV unresectable head and neck squamous cell carcinomas. Standard doses of radiation were used, with daily fractions of 180 to 200 cGy per day and total doses of 6000 to 7400 cGy. Patients were infused once a week with doses of 7 to 8 ml/kg. As the study progressed, the total volume infused over the course of treatment increased from 40 ml to 56 ml/kg. Patients breathed 100% oxygen via nasal prongs and mask for at least 30 minutes prior to and during radiation.

Eleven of 45 patients who received Fluosol-DA experienced a reaction to the test dose of 0.5 ml given intravenously prior to the start of the infusion. This generally consisted of flushing, chest pain, nausea, or low back pain. These patients were treated with Benadryl and/or steroids, and 37 were able to continue. Six of 42 patients experienced post-transfusion reactions, most often consisting of fever, chills, headache, and low back pain. The exact cause of this allergic reaction is unknown, but it is much higher in cancer patients than in patients receiving Fluosol-DA in cardiac studies. A complement activation reaction has been postulated.

Generally, these reactions are controlled with antihistamines or steroids (93). While changes in hepatic enzymes were noted in most patients, none developed symptomatic hepatomegaly or became clinically hepatotoxic. All liver function studies returned to normal in a 1- to 6-month period. No significant changes in hematologic measurements were noted.

A total of 46 patients with squamous cell carcinoma of the head and neck were entered into this study; 37 patients were evaluable for response. Nine patients were Stage III, 20 patients were Stage IV, and 8 patients had undergone previous treatment with chemotherapy and/or surgery; 28 of 37 patients (76%) received a complete response. With follow-up of 3 to 27 months, 15 patients had no evidence of disease, 6 died as a result of disease, and 6 died of other causes with local control. Of those achieving a complete response, 75% remained in remission.

At 1 year (Table 12–2), 27 patients were evaluable; 18 were alive and free of disease, 5 died of disease, and 4 died of other causes. The absolute survival at 1 year was 67% and determinant survival was 78%.

Nonsmall Cell Lung Carcinoma

In 1985, a Phase I/II study with adjuvant Fluosol-DA and oxygen was started for nonsmall cell carcinoma of the lung (94). This study included Stage II, III, or IV patients without distant metastasis and a Karnofsky of 60 or greater. Radiation therapy doses ranged from 6000 to 6600 cGy at standard fractionation. Fluosol-DA was infused once weekly at 7 to 9 ml/kg for a total dose of 42 to 49 ml/kg. The total dose in this study was lower due to concern regarding pulmonary fibrosis. Forty-five patients started therapy and 34 completed treatment. Six patients developed metastases under treatment, three died of disease-related causes, and two patients were withdrawn. A high rate of Fluosol-DA reactions was noted in this study; 36% reported a reaction to the test dose on infusion and 40% had a postinfusion reaction. However, only four patients were withdrawn due to reactions. While abnormalities were again noted in the liver enzymes, a low white count was reported in six patients, and depressed platelets under 100,000 were noted in two patients, all returned to normal within 3 to 6 months. In this study, 17 of 34 evaluable patients achieved a complete response. Thirteen subjects remained alive at 12 to 20 months.

Table 12–2 Fluosol-DA Head and Neck Study: Survival (12 Months)

Patients	Number
Evaluable	27
Alive	18
Dead from disease	5
Dead from other causes	4
Absolute survival	18/27 (67%)
Determinant survival	18/23 (78%)

Malignant Gliomas

In 1987, a Phase I/II study was opened for the treatment of high-grade malignant gliomas with adjuvant Fluosol-DA and oxygen (95). A weekly dose of 8 ml/kg of Fluosol-DA was used, given at weeks 1, 2, 3, 6, and 7 during radiation. Infusions were then increased to include one dose per week during the entire 7 weeks of therapy, for a total dose of 56 ml/kg. Following attainment of this dose level, additional doses were given of 7 ml/kg every third or fourth day for up to 3 weeks of treatment. A total of 77 ml/kg was delivered over the radiation therapy treatment course, which consisted of 6500 cGy at standard fractionation. No significant toxicities were reported. Of 18 evaluable patients at 1 year, 10 were alive, for a 1-year survival of 56%. Five patients were alive and free of disease 65 to 96 weeks from diagnosis. No long-term complications in the brain from this therapy were observed. The above studies are summarized in Table 12–3.

Works in Progress

A clinical trial involving locally advanced carcinoma of the cervix was recently started (96). This trial uses weekly Fluosol-DA infusions with oxygen breathing during external radiation therapy and during radioactive implants. This will test the usefulness of Fluosol-DA during brachytherapy treatment.

Table 12–3 Clinical Trials

Evaluable Site/Stage	Patients	RT Dose in cGy	Maximal Fluosol-DA Dose	CR	Absolute 1-Yr Survival
Head and neck	37	6600–7400	56 ml/kg	76%	67%
Lung	34	6000–6600	49 ml/kg	50%	56%
Brain/glioma	18	6500	56 ml/kg	—	56%

RT = Radiotherapy
CR = Complete Response

Chemotherapy studies with adjuvant Fluosol-DA and oxygen are currently under way. The first study uses BCNU with Fluosol-DA for recurrent gliomas of the brain in adults. The combination of Fluosol-DA and 5-fluorouracil is also under study for metastatic colon carcinoma.

FUTURE DIRECTIONS

Currently, no proven benefit of Fluosol-DA and oxygen breathing as an adjuvant to radiation therapy has been demonstrated. While improved local control has been reported in the Phase II studies, a randomized trial is yet to be concluded. While the potential to increase tumor oxygenation exists in humans, many questions remain unanswered. The pharmacokinetics of Fluosol-DA in humans are poorly understood. The intravascular half-life, as measured in the serum of patients in the head and neck study, is quite variable. Most patients had some measurable fluorocarbons at 24 hours and a few had Fluosol-DA components at 48 hours. The appropriate blood level of Fluosol-DA to achieve maximum tumor oxygenation over a course of protracted radiation therapy is unknown. Studies are in progress to further evaluate the circulating half-life of the components of Fluosol-DA. The long-range goal is to provide maximum oxygenation of the tumor during all fractions and radiation. In this regard, fractionation schemes other than standard regimens may well be the most appropriate for Fluosol-DA and oxygen. Further results and clinical trials will be necessary to completely evaluate the place of Fluosol-DA in radiation therapy.

REFERENCES

1. Thomlinson RH, Gray LH. The histological structure of some human lung cancers and the possible implications for radiotherapy. Br J Cancer 9:539, 1955.
2. Jirtle R, Clifton KH. The effect of tumor size and host anemia on tumor cell survival after irradiation. Int J Radiat Oncol Biol Phys 4:395, 1978.
3. Kjartasson I, Appelgren L, Peterson HJ. et al. Capillary blood flow, exchange and flow distribution in transplantable rat tumors. *In:* Seventh European Conference on Microcirculation. Aberdeen, Part II, Bibl. Amat., No. 12. Basel:Karger, 1978, p. 519.
4. Eddy HA. Development of the vascular system in the hamster malignant neurilemoma. Microvasc Res 6:63, 1973.
5. Endrich B, Antaglietta M, Reinhold HS, Gross JF. Hemodynamic characteristics in microcirculatory blood channels during early tumor growth. Cancer Res 39:17, 1979.
6. Tannock IF, Steel GG. Quantitative technique for the study of the anatomy and function of small blood vessels in tumors. J Natl Cancer Inst 42:771, 1969.
7. Vaupel P. Hypoxia in neoplastic tissue. Microvas Res 13:399, 1977.
8. Hirst DG. Oxygen delivery to tumors. Int J Radiat Oncol Biol Phys 12:1271, 1986.
9. Kennedy KA, Teicher BA, Rockwell SC, Sartorelli AC. The hypoxic tumor cell: A target for selective cancer chemotherapy. Biochem Pharmacol 29:1, 1980.
10. Teicher BA, Sartorelli AC. Selective attack of hypoxic tumor cells. *In:* Design of Models for Screening of Therapeutic Agents for Cancer. Fidler IJ, White RJ (Eds). New York, Van Nostrand Reinhold, 1981, p. 19.
11. Fowler JF. Chemical modifiers of radiosensitivity—theory and reality: A review. Int J Radiat Oncol Biol Phys 11:665, 1985.
12. Reynard-Bougnoux A, Lespinasse F, Malaise EP, Guichard M. Partial hypoxia as a cause of radioresistance in a human tumor xenograft: Its influence illustrated by the sensitizing effect of misonidazole and hyperbaric oxygen. Int J Radiat Oncol Biol Phys 12:1283, 1986.
13. Chaplin DJ, Durand RE, Olive PL. Acute hypoxia in tumors: Implications for modifiers of

radiation effects. Int J Radiat Oncol Biol Phys 12:1279, 1986.
14. Moulder JE, Rockwell S. Hypoxic fractions of solid tumors: Experimental techniques, methods of analysis and a survey of existing data. Int J Radiat Oncol Biol Phys 10:695, 1984.
15. Stanley JA, Shipley WV, Steel GG. Influence of tumor size on hypoxic fraction and therapeutic sensitivity of Lewis lung tumor. Br J Cancer 36:105, 1977.
16. Vaupel P, Thews G. PO_2 distribution in tumor tissue of DS-carcinosarcoma. Oncology 30:475, 1974.
17. Vaupel P, Frinak S, Bicher HI. Heterogenous oxygen partial pressure on pH distribution in C3H mouse mammary adenocarcinoma. Cancer Res 41:2008, 1981.
18. Vaupel P, Fortmeyer HP, Runkel S, Kallinowski F. Blood flow, oxygen consumption and tissue oxygenation of human breast cancer xenografts in nude rates. Cancer Res 47:3496, 1987.
19. Gatenby RA, Kessler HB, Rosenblum JS, et al. Oxygen distribution in squamous cell carcinoma metastases and its relationship to outcome of radiation therapy. Int J Radiat Oncol Biol Phys 14:831, 1988.
20. Kallman RF, Rockwell S. Effects of radiation on animal tumor models. *In:* Cancer: A Comprehensive Treatise. Vol. 6. Becker FF (Ed). New York, Plenum Press, 1977, p. 225.
21. Steel GG. Growth kinetics of tumors. Oxford, Clarendon Press, 1977, p. 147.
22. Sutherland RM, Franko AJ. On the nature of the radiobiologically hypoxic fraction in tumors. Int J Radiat Oncol Biol Phys 6:117, 1980.
23. Koch CJ, Meneses JJ, Harris JW. The effect of extreme hypoxia and glucose on the repair of potentially lethal and sublethal radiation damage by mammalian cells. Radiat Res 70:542, 1977.
24. Bedford JS, Mitchell JB. The effect of hypoxia on the growth and radiation response of mammalian cells in culture. Br J Radiol 47:687, 1974.
25. Bush RS, Jenkin RDT, Allt WEC, et al. Definitive evidence for hypoxic cells influencing cure in cancer therapy. Br J Cancer 37(Suppl III):302, 1978.
26. Teicher BA, Lazo JS, Sartorelli AC. Classification of antineoplastic agents by their selective toxicities toward oxygenated and hypoxic tumor cells. Cancer Res 41:73, 1981.
27. Clark LC, Gollan F. Survival of mammals breathing organic liquids equilibrated with oxygen at atmospheric pressure. Science 152:1755, 1966.
28. Sloviter HA, Kamimoto T. Erythrocyte substitute for perfusion of brain. Nature 216:458, 1967.
29. Geyer RP. Substitutes for blood and its components. *In:* Blood Substitutes and Plasma Expanders. Vol. 19. Jamieson GA, Greenwalt TJ (Eds). New York, A.R. Liss, 1978, p. 1021.
30. Riess JG, LeBlanc M. Solubility and transport phenomena in perfluorochemicals relevant to blood substitution and other biomedical applications. Pure Appl Chem 54:2383, 1982.
31. Riess JG. Reassessment of criteria for the selection of perfluorochemicals for second-generation blood substitutes: Analysis of structure/property relationships. Artif Organs 8:44, 1984.
32. Song CW. Increase in pO_2 and radiosensitivity of tumors by Fluosol-DA (20%) and carbogen. Cancer Res 47:442, 1987.
33. Hasegawa T, Rhee JG, Levitt SH, Song CW. Increase in tumor pO_2 by perfluorochemicals and carbogen. Int J Radiat Oncol Biol Phys 13:569, 1987.
34. Hiraga S, Klubes P, Owens ES, Cysack RL, Blasberg RG. Increases in brain tumor and cerebral blood flow by blood-perfluorochemical emulsion (Fluosol-DA) exchange. Cancer Res 47:3296, 1987.
35. Teicher BA, Rose CM. Perfluorochemical emulsion can increase tumor radiosensitivity. Science 223:934, 1984.
36. Teicher BA, Rose CM. Sensitization of solid mouse tumor to x-ray treatment by oxygen-carrying perfluorochemical emulsion. Cancer Res 44:4285, 1984.
37. Teicher BA, Rose CM. Effect of dose and scheduling on growth delay of the Lewis lung carcinoma produced by the perfluorochemical emulsion Fluosol-DA. Int J Radiat Oncol Biol Phys 12:1311, 1986.
38. Teicher BA, McIntosh NL. Optimization of Fluosol-DA administration during a fractionated radiation protocol in the Lewis lung carcinoma. Proceedings of 35th Meeting of the Radiation Research Society. Abstract EM-1. Atlanta, GA, 1987.
39. Zhang WL, Pence D, Patten M, et al. Enhancement of tumor response to radiation by Fluosol-DA. Int J Radiat Oncol Biol Phys 10:172, 1984.
40. Rockwell S. Use of perfluorochemical emulsion to improve oxygenation in a solid tumor. Int J Radiat Oncol Biol Phys 11:97, 1985.
41. Moulder JE, Fish BL. Intermittent use of a perfluorochemical emulsion (Fluosol-DA 20%) and carbogen breathing with fractionated irradiation. Int J Radiat Oncol Biol Phys 15:1193, 1988.
42. West L, McIntosh M, Gendler S, et al. Effects of intravenously infused Fluosol-DA 20% in

rats. Int J Radiat Oncol Biol Phys 12:1319, 1986.
43. Fischer JJ, Rockwell S, Martin DF. Perfluorochemicals and hyperbaric oxygen in radiation therapy. Int J Radiat Oncol Biol Phys 12:95, 1986.
44. Kokunai T, Kuwamura K. Effect of perfluorochemicals on BCNU chemotherapy: Preliminary study in a rat brain tumor model. Surg Neurol 18:258, 1982.
45. Kuwamura K, Kokunai T, Tamaki N, Matsumoto S. Synergistic effect of perfluorochemicals on BCNU chemotherapy: Experimental study in a 9L rat brain-tumor model. J Neurosurg 57:467, 1982.
46. Martin DF, Kimler BF, Evans RG, et al. Potentiation of rat brain tumor therapy by Fluosol-DA and carbogen. NCI Monogr 6:119, 1988.
47. Teicher BA, Holden SA. Survey of the effect of adding Fluosol-DA 20%/O_2 to treatment with various chemotherapeutic agents. Cancer Treat Rep 71:173, 1987.
48. Teicher BA, Holden SA, Rose CM. Effect of Fluosol-DA/O_2 on tumor cell and bone marrow cytotoxicity of nitrosoureas in mice bearing FSaII fibrosarcoma. Int J Cancer 38:285, 1986.
49. Teicher BA, Holden SA, Rose CM. Differential enhancement of melphalan cytotoxicity in tumor and normal tissue by Fluosol-DA and oxygen breathing. Int J Cancer 36:585, 1985.
50. Teicher BA, Holden SA, Rose CM. Effect of oxygen on the cytotoxicity and antitumor activity of etoposide. J Natl Cancer Inst 75:1129, 1985.
51. Teicher BA, Lazo JS, Merrill WW, et al. Effect of Fluosol-DA/O_2 on the antitumor activity and pulmonary toxicity of bleomycin. Cancer Chemother Pharmacol 18:213, 1986.
52. Teicher BA, Holden SA, Jacobs JL. Approaches to defining the mechanism of Fluosol-DA 20%/carbogen enhancement of melphalan antitumor activity. Cancer Res 47:513, 1987.
53. Teicher BA, Holden SA, Jacobs JL. Approaches to defining the mechanism of Fluosol-DA 20%/carbogen enhancement of melphalan antitumor activity. Cancer Res 47:513, 1987.
54. Teicher BA, Holden SA, Crawford JM. Effects of Fluosol-DA and oxygen breathing on adriamycin antitumor activity and cardiac toxicity in mice. Cancer 61:2196, 1988.
55. Teicher BA, Holden SA, Cathcart KNS, Herman TS. Effect of various oxygenation conditions and Fluosol-DA on the cytotoxicity and antitumor activity of bleomycin. J Natl Cancer Inst 80:599, 1988.
56. Teicher BA, Bernal SD, Holden SA, Cathcart KNS. Effect of Fluosol-DA/O_2 on etoposide/alkylating agent antitumor activity. Cancer Chemother Pharmacol 21:281, 1988.
57. Teicher BA, Herman TS, Holden SA, Cathcart KNS. The effect of Fluosol-DA and oxygenation status on the activity of cyclophosphamide in vivo. Cancer Chemother Pharmacol 21:286, 1988.
58. Teicher BA, McIntosh-Lowe NL, Rose CM. Effect of various oxygenation conditions and Fluosol-DA on cancer chemotherapeutic agents. Biomater Artif Cells Artif Organs 16:533, 1988.
59. Teicher BA, Herman TS, Rose CM. Effect of Fluosol-DA on the response of intracranial 9L tumors to x-rays and BCNU. Int J Radiat Oncol Biol Phys 15:1187, 1988.
60. Teicher BA, Herman TS, Holden SA, Jones SM. Addition of misonidazole, etanidazole or hyperthermia to treatment with Fluosol-DA/carbogen/radiation. J Natl Cancer Inst 12:929, 1990.
61. Adams GE, Ahmed I, Sheldon PW, Stratford IJ. Radiation sensitization and chemopotentiation: RSU-1069, a compound more effective than misonidazole in vitro and in vivo. Br J Cancer 49:5571, 1984.
62. Chaplin DJ, Durand RE, Stratford IJ, Jenkins TC. The radiosensitizing and toxic effects of RSU-1069 on hypoxic cells in a murine tumor. Int J Radiat Oncol Biol Phys 12:1091, 1986.
63. Frank AJ. Misonidazole and other hypoxia markers: Metabolism and applications. Int J Radiat Oncol Biol Phys 12:1195, 1986.
64. Hill RP. Sensitizers and radiation dose fractionation: Results and interpretations. Int J Radiat Oncol Biol Phys 12:1049, 1986.
65. Herman TS, Teicher BA, Jochelson M, et al. Rationale for use of local hyperthermia with radiation therapy and selected anticancer drugs in locally advanced human malignancies. Int J Hyperthermia 4:143, 1988.
66. Hofer KG. Heat potentiation of radiation damage versus radiation potentiation of heat damage. Radiat Res 110:450, 1987.
67. Dewey WC. Interaction of heat with radiation and chemotherapy. Cancer Res 44:4714S, 1984.
68. Coleman CN, Halsey J, Cox RS, et al. Relationship between the neurotoxicity of the hypoxic cell radiosensitizer SR-2508 and the pharmacokinetic profile. Cancer Res 47:319, 1987.
69. Coleman CN, Wasserman TH, Urtasun RC, et al. Phase I trial of the hypoxic cell radiosensitizer SR-2508: The results of the five to six week drug schedule. Int J Radiat Oncol Biol Phys 12:1105, 1986.
70. Dische S, Saunders MI, Dunphy EP, et al. Con-

centrations achieved in human tumors after administration of misonidazole, SR-2508 and Ro-03-8799. Int J Radiat Oncol Biol Phys 12:1109, 1981.
71. Herman TS, Teicher BA, Holden SA, Collins LC. Interaction of hyperthermia and radiation: Hypoxia and acidosis in vitro, tumor subpopulations in vivo. Cancer Res 49:3338, 1989.
72. Holden SA, Herman TS, Teicher BA. Addition of a hypoxic cell selective cytotoxic agent (mitomycin C or porfiromycin) to treatment with Fluosol-DA/carbogen/radiation. Radiother Oncol 18(1)59, 1990.
73. Kennedy KA, McGurl JD, Leonardis L, Alabaster O. pH dependence of mitomycin C-induced cross-linking activity in EMT6 tumor cells. Cancer Res 45:3541, 1985.
74. Kennedy KA, Mimnaugh EG, Trush MA, Sinha BK. Effects of glutathione and ethylxanthate on mitomycin C activation by isolated rat hepatic or EMT6 mouse mammary tumor nuclei. Cancer Res 45:4071, 1985.
75. Keyes SR, Fracasso PM, Heimbrook DC, et al. Role of NADPH: Cytochrome C reductase and DT-diaphorase in the biotransformation of mitomycin C. Cancer Res 44:5638, 1984.
76. Keyes SR, Rockwell S, Sartorelli AC. Enhancement of mitomycin C cytotoxicity to hypoxic tumor cells by dicumarol in vivo and in vitro. Cancer Res 45:213, 1985.
77. Marshall RS, Rauth AM. Modification of the cytotoxic activity of mitomycin C by oxygen and ascorbic acid in Chinese hamster ovary cells and a repair-deficient mutant. Cancer Res 46:2709, 1986.
78. Rauth AM, Mohindra JK, Tannock IF. Activity of mitomycin C for aerobic and hypoxic cells in vitro and in vivo. Cancer Res 43:4154, 1983.
79. Rockwell S. Effects of mitomycin C alone and in combination with x-rays on EMT6 mouse mammary tumors in vivo. J Natl Cancer Inst 71:765, 1983.
80. Rockwell S, Niereburg M, Irvin CG. Effects of the mode of administration of mitomycin on tumor and marrow response and on the therapeutic ratio. Cancer Treat Rep 71:927, 1987.
81. Chaplin DJ, Durand RE, Olive PL. Cell selection from a murine tumor using the fluorescent probe Hoechst 33342. Br J Cancer 51:569, 1985.
82. Chaplin DJ, Olive PL, Durand RE. Intermittent blood flow in a murine tumor: Radiobiological effects. Cancer Res 47:597, 1987.
83. Siemann DW, Keng PC. Cell cycle-specific toxicity of the Hoechst 33342 stain in untreated or irradiated murine tumor cells. Cancer Res 46:3556, 1986.
84. Siemann DW, Keng PC. Characterization of radiation resistant hypoxic cell subpopulation in KHT sarcomas. (ii) Cell Sorting. Br J Cancer 58:296, 1988.
85. Teicher BA, Herman TS, Holden SA. Combined modality therapy with bleomycin, hyperthermia and radiation. Cancer Res 48:6291, 1988.
86. Makowski H, Tentshev P, Frey P, et al. Tolerance of an oxygen-carrying colloidal plasma substitute in human beings. Proc. 4th International Symposium on Perfluorochemical Blood Substitutes. Kyoto, Japan, 1978, p. 47.
87. Ohyanagi H, Toshima K, Sekita M, et al. Clinical studies of perfluorochemical whole blood substitutes: Safety of Fluosol-DA (20%) in normal human volunteers. Clin Ther 2(4):306, 1979.
88. Tremper K, Lapin R, Levine E, et al. Hemodynamic oxygen transport effects of a perfluorochemical blood substitute, Fluosol-DA 20%. Crit Care Med 8(12):738, 1989.
89. Mitsuno T, Ohyanagi H, Naito R. Clinical studies of a perfluorochemical whole blood substitute, Fluosol-DA: A summary of 186 cases. Ann Surg 1:60, 1982.
90. Tremper K, Friedman A, Levine E, et al. The preoperative treatment of severely anemic patients with a perfluorochemical oxygen transport fluid, Fluosol-DA. New Engl J Med 307:277, 1982.
91. Rose C, Lustig R, McIntosh N, Teicher BA. A clinical trial of Fluosol-DA in advanced head and neck cancer. Int J Radiat Oncol Biol Phys 12:1325, 1986.
92. Lustig R, McIntosh-Lowe N, Rose C, et al. Phase I/II study of Fluosol-DA and 100% oxygen as an adjuvant to radiation in the treatment of advanced squamous cell carcinoma of the head and neck. Int J Radiat Oncol Biol Phys 16(6):1587, 1989.
93. Vercellottie G, Hammerschmidt D, Craddock P, Jacob H. Activation of plasma complement by perfluorocarbon artificial blood: Probable mechanism of adverse pulmonary reactions in treatment patients and rationale for corticosteroid prophylaxis. Blood 59:1299, 1982.
94. Lustig R, Lowe N, Prosnitz L, et al. Phase I/II study of Fluosol-DA and 100% oxygen breathing as an adjuvant to radiation in the treatment of unresectable non small cell carcinoma of the lung. Int J Radiat Oncol Biol Phys 19:97, 1990.
95. Evans RG, Kimler BF, Morantz RA, et al. Phase I/II study of the use of Fluosol as an adjuvant to radiation therapy in the treatment of primary high-grade brain tumors. Int J Radiat Oncol Biol Phys 19:415, 1990.
96. Bryant S. Personal Communication, May 1991.

Section C

MECHANISMS OF RESISTANCE TO CHEMORADIATION

Chapter 13

RADIATION AND CHEMOTHERAPY CYTOTOXICITY: MECHANISMS OF RESISTANCE

JOHN A. COOK AND JAMES B. MITCHELL

INTRODUCTION

At first glance, the combined use of chemotherapy and radiation therapy in cancer treatment seems to be a logical and reasonable approach. Local control of the primary tumor mass, which can often be achieved by high-dose radiation therapy combined with systemic chemotherapy to control metastatic disease, should provide an effective means of combating such a highly complex disease. If one adds to this rationale the findings that many chemotherapy drugs can enhance the effects of radiation, then the integration of both modalities becomes even more appealing.

Unfortunately, problems are encountered when the two modalities are combined. Either modality, when used in separate protocols, may cause major normal-tissue toxicity, which can be life-threatening in some instances. The onset of normal-tissue toxicity limits the dose achievable by either modality and thus compromises the administration of the drug or radiation dose delivered. The experience in most experimental models and in a number of clinical trials involving simultaneous drugs and radiation is that normal-tissue toxicity may be enhanced even further (1–3). Successful combination therapy has been achieved with various sequences of chemotherapy and radiation treatments (see Part II, section A); however, a better knowledge of the optimal timing of each modality is clearly needed.

An obstacle to effectively using combined modality approaches resides in the observation that patients frequently relapse after initial treatment and become progressively less responsive to second or third treatments (4). This is true particularly in the case of chemotherapy drugs and to a certain extent for radiotherapy. The term **resistance** has different meanings to different researchers. When a tumor fails to respond to treatment (i.e., the size of the tumor mass does not change or even enlarges during and after treatment), the tumor is often referred to as resistant. This may or may not be correct; however, to say that the tumor was **unresponsive** to treatment is a more accurate use of terminology. It is often assumed that the reason a tumor does not respond to treatment is because the cells within the tumor are inherently resistant to the treatment. This assumption may not always be true. In fact, there is considerable evidence that the physiologic environmental conditions of a tumor can render cells insensitive, while under ideal situations these cells might be inherently sensitive to a given treatment (5). In the case of chemotherapy drugs, it is conceivable that poor vascular networks in tumors limit the effective drug concentration in tumor cells and therefore compromise cell killing. Thus, there may be numerous barriers or means of interference that prevent adequate delivery of tumoricidal agents. This reality, coupled with the ever present problem of normal tissue toxicity, further complicates the effective use of combined modality treatments.

This chapter will concentrate on mechanisms of how tumors and the cells within tumors may defend against anticancer treatment modalities. A variety of factors will be considered both at the cellular and physiological levels. Most of the data discussed will highlight means by which tumors develop resistance to single modalities, with the assumption that similar mechanisms will be operative when modalities are combined.

CELLULAR SENSITIVITY

Inherent Cellular Sensitivity

It would be ideal if tumors were more sensitive to chemotherapy drugs or radiation than normal tissues, but this has never been demonstrated. Shortly following publication of the first mammalian x-ray survival curve (6), x-ray sensitivity was determined for a variety of cell types, including cell lines derived from both tumor and normal tissues (7). Most of these data until the mid-1970s was for cell lines derived from rodents. However, a distinct and consistent pattern emerged that showed hemopoietic cells to be significantly more radiosensitive than other cell types (7). This finding was also later found to be the case for human hemopoietic progenitor stem cells (8,9). Tumor-cell radiosensitivity was shown not to vary significantly among different tumor types and other normal cell types (fibroblasts, skin stem cells, intestine) (7,10,11). From the late 1970s to the 1980s, more emphasis was placed on establishing human tumor cell lines from different histological types. Recent radiosensitivity analysis of human tumor cell lines has revealed a relationship between inherent radiosensitivity, as expressed as the surviving fraction (SF_2) at 200 cGy, and the clinical responsiveness of the respective tumor type from which the cell lines were initiated (12). In general, low SF_2 values correlate with greater clinical responsiveness (see Figure 13–1). For example, small cell lung cancer (SCLC), which is initially quite responsive to radiotherapy, has in vitro x-ray SF_2 values for cell lines of 0.2. In contrast, cell lines derived from glioblastoma tumors, which are very unresponsive to radiotherapy, yield SF_2 values that range between 0.5 and 0.6 (12). Figure 13–1 shows that there is, at best, a factor of 3 difference between the most "sensitive" and "resistant" tumor cell types. While a threefold difference might seem small, when one considers a conventional course of radiation therapy consisting of 30 fractions over 5 to 6 weeks, such a variation would translate into huge differences with respect to total tumor cell kill. Surviving fractions of 0.2 vs. 0.6 can result in differences of up to 14 logs in cell kill over the course of treatment. Implicit in such an extrapolation are the assumptions that survival will remain constant for each dose delivered and that repopulation of tumor cells between doses will not be significant.

Clinically, it is known that most normal tissues are more sensitive to chemotherapy than tumors, with the possible exception of some lymphomas, leukemias, and testicular cancer. An example of such differences in the inherent cellular sensitivity among cell

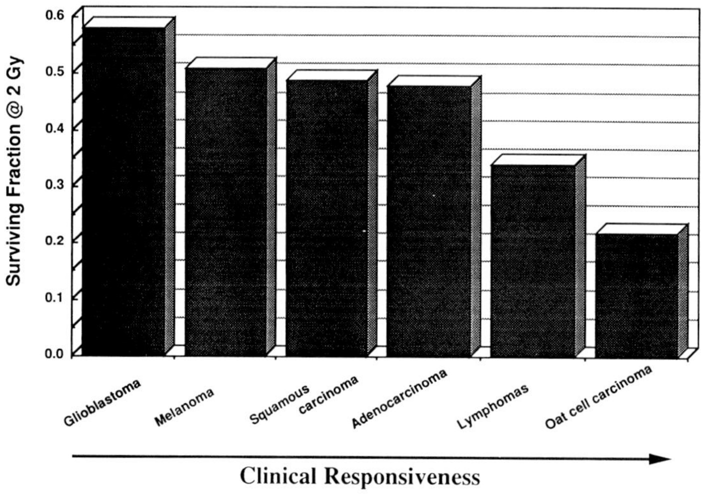

Fig. 13–1. Surviving fraction following a 200-cGy (SF_2) radiation dose compiled from 101 human tumor cell lines derived from tumors with varying responsiveness to radiation therapy. A good correlation was observed between the SF_2 of the particular tumor cell type and the clinical radioresponsiveness of the associated tumor. Low SF_2 values correlated with greater clinical responsiveness. Note that from the most to the least clinically responsive tumor, the difference is only approximately a factor of 3. (From Fertil B, et al. Int J Radiat Oncol Biol Phys 11: 1699, 1985, Pergamon Press Ltd.)

types to chemotherapy drugs is demonstrated in Figure 13–2A. Between the two human cells types (tumor and normal fibroblast), the tumor cell line is clearly more resistant (by a factor of 3) to two out of three drugs evaluated. Very little difference in sensitivity was seen for cisplatinum between the two cell types. Use of fibroblasts as representative of a normal tissue warrants reservation; however, there are few alternatives available for in vitro studies. Figure 13–2B shows that the radiosensitivity differs much less (a factor of 1.4) between these two cell types. The chemosensitivity data shown in Figure 13–2A are by no means universal, but they do serve to demonstrate that even at the in vitro level, substantial differences can exist between tumor and normal cells, with the tumor cells usually (but not always) being more resistant than normal cells.

Recent reports indicate that the introduction of various oncogenes into the cellular genome can alter the cellular response to radiation (13,14) and cisplatinum (15,16). In two reports (13,15), the introduction and expression of mutated ras oncogenes made cells more resistant to x-rays and cisplatinum. There has been some question regarding the interpretation of such experiments, particularly in the case of increased radiation resistance by oncogenes (17). Activation of oncogenes has been implicated in a variety of human malignancies. Activated oncogenes and oncogene-encoded proteins can have dramatic effects at the cellular level on multiple systems. It is not clear presently how oncogenes affect the inherent sensitivity to radiation and cisplatinum. Possibilities include alterations in repair systems, drug influx/efflux, intracellular detoxification systems, or chromatin structure.

Inherent cellular resistance to cancer treatment modalities could (and perhaps does) pose a formidable obstacle to effective therapy. What cellular attributes constitute inherent cellular resistance or different sensitivities to a cancer treatment modality? This is not an easy question and has been the focus of extensive research for many years now. The answer to the question most likely resides in the genetic makeup of the cell. Modern DNA technology will hopefully add to our understanding in the near future as to which genes are instrumental in governing the sensitivity of cells to cancer treatments. While a knowledge of the gene allows the identification of specific proteins, the manipulation of their specific functions still requires a considerable amount of understanding of cellular biochemistry and tumor physiology for beneficial approaches to cancer treatment.

Repair Systems

The ability to repair damage is a vital and necessary cellular function. Repair in this context is the "fixing" or "undoing" of damage to a structure of molecule necessary for viability and function. There are several ways in which cells could accomplish this objective. First, molecules that can "chemically" restore damaged molecules may be present in cells. An example might be a reducing species (such as glutathione, which is discussed

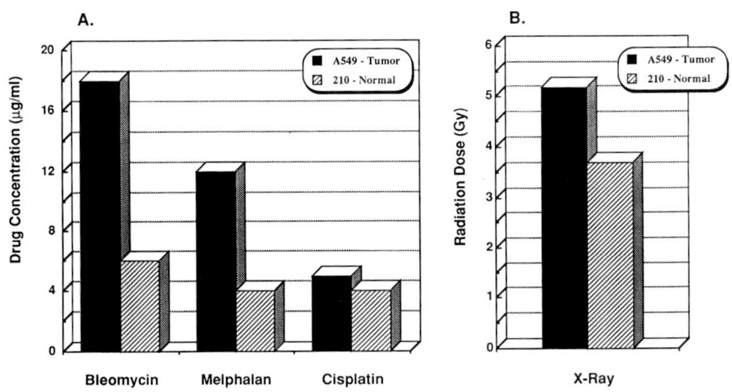

Fig. 13–2. A. Drug concentration required to reduce cell survival to 10% for human A549 human lung adenocarcinoma and normal lung fibroblast 210 cells. Exposure to all drugs listed was for 1 hour, and survival was assessed by the clonogenic assay. (Data adapted from Reed DJ, et al. Pharmacol Rev 36:25S, 1984.) B. Radiation dose required to reduce cell survival to 10% for human A549 lung adenocarcinoma and normal lung fibroblast 210 cells.

later in this chapter) that could donate electrons to oxidized (damaged) substrates. Secondly, there might be a variety of enzymatic systems that can recognize and repair damaged substrates through a set of complex and ordered reactions. Lastly, there may be cellular systems that prevent damage before it occurs. Such systems would involve detoxification of toxic species by either chemical or enzymatic means.

The exact identification of critical cellular structures or molecules and the specific type of damage rendered by anticancer modalities is by no means complete. In the case of radiation, there is considerable evidence pointing to DNA as the critical target for radiation damage (18,19), with double-strand DNA breaks as the lethal lesion (20). It is also known that radiation-induced cellular effects are due to the production of free radical species and/or direct ionization of target molecules. In contrast, there may be multiple means of imposing cellular damage by chemotherapy drugs. A case in point is the drug Adriamycin, which has several means of inducing cytotoxicity, including DNA intercalation, inhibition of topoisomerase II, and the production of toxic oxygen-related species (21). Less is known about critical cellular damage sites for other chemotherapy drugs; however, DNA by virtue of its importance and size is an obvious target. Rational use of combined chemotherapy and radiation would be greatly enhanced if we understood the mechanism(s) of how each modality works, both alone and in combination. Without this information, there will always be a certain level of risk-taking involved.

The fact that tissues can repair radiation damage was known for many years prior to its quantification at the cellular level (22). The repair of sublethal radiation damage is measured by following the clonogenic survival of cells when irradiated in a split-dose regimen and allowing various recovery times between the two doses (22). These studies, in addition to various temperature and energy inhibition studies, have identified an enzymatic process as being responsible for repair (23,24). The specific enzymes responsible for this repair have not been identified. Split-dose repair studies are difficult to conduct and interpret using chemotherapy drugs, because "acute" doses of drugs administered over a few minutes cannot usually be achieved. Even when the drug is rinsed free of the cells after a brief exposure, there is still the possibility that some amount of the drug will remain associated with the cells, thereby complicating the response to a second exposure.

One example of an enzymatic repair process for a specific class of chemotherapy agents resides with the nitrosoureas. Nitrosoureas are thought to kill cells through the formation of DNA/DNA interstrand cross-links, supposedly by chloroethylation of the O^6 position of guanine (25). Many human cells, referred to as the Mer^+ phenotype, have a repair system that effectively removes this adduct, prevents DNA/DNA intrastrand cross-links, and therefore makes them resistant to nitrosoureas (26,27). Repair deficient (Mer^-) cells are sensitive to nitrosoureas. The Mer^+ phenotype most likely contributes to the resistance of human tumors treated in the clinic with nitrosoureas.

Repair enzymes studied over recent years with regard to DNA damage include DNA polymerase alpha and beta and the topoisomerases (I and II) (28,29). Chemotoxic agents have been shown to inhibit the function of these enzymes (i.e., aphidicolin and Adriamycin) (30,31). Perhaps because of the number of enzymes involved in repair and the possibility of overlap in function, results obtained by the use of these inhibitors to study repair has been ambiguous. Other chemotherapy drugs have been shown to inhibit the repair of radiation damage by less direct means. This is usually observed by virtue of the elimination of the shoulder of the acute-dose radiation survival curve and depends on the specific sequencing of the drug and radiation exposure.

Tumor-cell enzymatic repair systems can interfere with anticancer treatment modalities. Identifying repair genes and their products, with the idea of ultimately devising effective treatment strategies to selectively modulate tumor vs. normal cell responses, is currently a major goal among oncology researchers. This will be a difficult order to fill, given that repair systems probably do not differ markedly between tumor and normal tissues. The traditional approach has been to study repair systems in genetically simpler organisms, such as bacteria or yeast, and to look for homologous features in mammalian cells. An example of this is the discovery in

Escherichia coli uvr of the ABC excision nuclease complex used to excise pyrimidine dimers induced by UVA light (32,33). Although the excision repair process has been worked out in some detail in E. coli, the enzymes responsible for excision repair in mammalian cells have not been isolated (33).

The advent of more sophisticated molecular biology techniques has also provided opportunities to isolate repair genes. One example of the molecular biology approach is the attempt to isolate the gene(s) responsible for the remarkable radiation resistance seen in Deinococcus radiodurans (34,35). This involved making a cDNA library from D. radiodurans DNA, which was used to transform E. coli. Preliminary results include the isolation of transformants with increased radiation resistance (34,35).

Another approach in identifying repair genes is the use of mutants that have been selected for extreme sensitivity to a given modality. Sensitive mutants for both radiation and some chemotherapy drugs have been isolated (36–38). Transfection of such mutant cell lines with normal DNA and selection of subsequent clones with restored normal sensitivity is the first step toward identifying repair genes. There has been some success toward this end for ultraviolet light-sensitive mutants (39,40); however, the identification and characterization of specific mammalian repair genes for x-rays and chemotherapy drugs has remained elusive.

Cellular Detoxification Systems

Recently, much attention has been directed toward cellular biochemical systems capable of detoxifying drugs (xenobiotics) and/or toxic free radical species produced by drugs or radiation. Prominent in the cell's defense armamentarium are the cytochrome p-450 system, superoxide dismutase (SOD), catalase (CAT), and glutathione (GSH) and GSH-dependent enzymes. The cytochrome p-450 system is involved in the biotransformation of drugs, which often leads to drug inactivation (41). A stimulated cytochrome p-450 system in tumor cells could pose a barrier for effective cytotoxicity for certain drugs, and this has been reported in some instances (42). SOD converts superoxide to hydrogen peroxide, and CAT can detoxify hydrogen peroxide to water. These two enzymes should be important in the detoxification of toxic oxygen-related species that can be produced by both radiation and certain radiomimetic chemotherapy drugs.

GSH, a small tripeptide molecule, assumes a pivotal role in numerous bioreductive reactions, transport, enzyme activity, protection from harmful oxidative species, and detoxification of xenobiotics (43–45), as shown in Figure 13–3. GSH S-transferase and GSH peroxidase are two enzymes that act in concert with GSH and provide the cell with a powerful means to detoxify both drugs and toxic oxygen-related species produced by drugs or radiation. Modulation of GSH levels in cells prior to treatment with several different anticancer modalities can markedly affect the cellular response (46–49). Examples of how GSH modulation can modify the cellular response to some anticancer modalities are shown in Figure 13–4. Modulation studies have been made by the introduction of agents that specifically inhibit (buthionine sulfoximine, BSO) or stimulate (oxathiozolidine, OTZ) GSH synthesis or directly introduce GSH (GSH esters) intracellularly (50–52). Figure 13–4 shows that modulation of GSH has little influence on the radiation response (49,53). However, depletion of GSH can significantly sensitize cells to bleomycin and melphalan, while elevation affords protection to both drugs (46,54). Elevated GSH or GSH-related enzymes have been correlated with in vitro resistance of human tumor cells to several chemotherapy drugs (55,56). In these cells, depletion of GSH markedly sensitizes the cells to the drugs for which they were resistant. These in vitro observations have led to the prospect of GSH

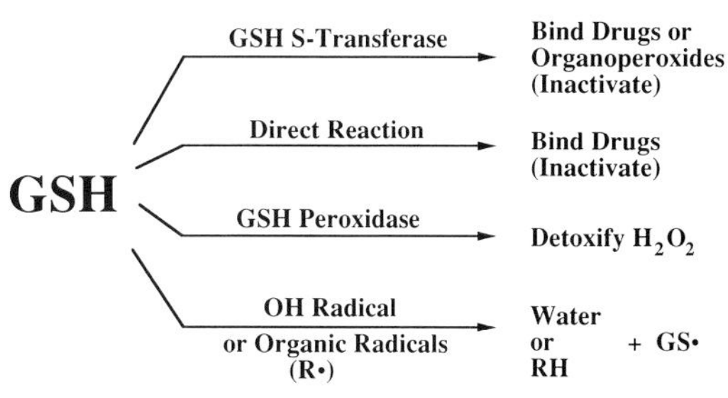

Fig. 13–3. Diagram demonstrating how GSH could protect cells from drugs or toxic oxygen-related free radical species.

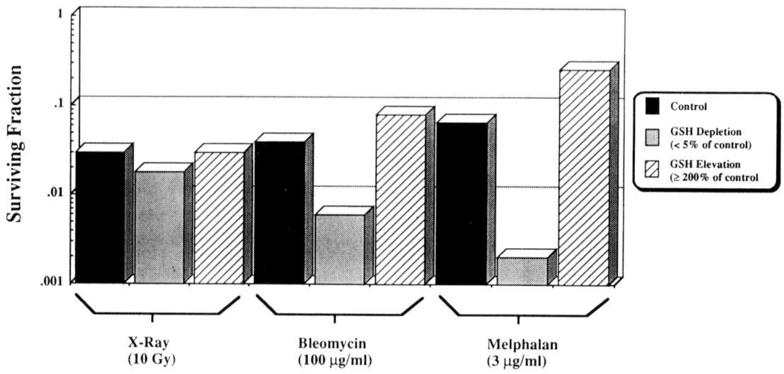

Fig. 13–4. The effects of GSH modulation on the survival of Chinese hamster V79 cells exposed to x-rays (1000 cGy) or for a 1-hour exposure to bleomycin or melphalan. BSO pretreatment yielded GSH levels <5% of control prior to drug exposure. GSH levels were elevated prior to x-ray, bleomycin, and melphalan treatment by OTZ to 200% of control levels. For bleomycin and melphalan, GSH depletion was sensitized and GSH elevation was protected. In contrast, GSH depletion or elevation had little influence on the radiation response.

depletion via BSO administration for drug-refractory tumors in the clinic.

Many human tumor cells grown in culture have been shown to have high levels of GSH (57–59). Elevated GSH levels in human lung cancer cells have also been shown to decrease the effectiveness of hypoxic-cell radiosensitizers such as SR-2508, as shown in Figure 13–5 (57,58). Notice that SR-2508 alone sensitized hypoxic cells very little; however, when cells were depleted of GSH by BSO prior to treatment, significant SR-2508 sensitization was observed. If tumor cells in vivo have corresponding high levels of GSH, the success of radiosensitizers could possibly be diminished. These findings have prompted research into the intracellular GSH levels in human tumors cells in vivo and whether high GSH levels might be predictive with regard to patient response to treatment (60,61). Attempts to deplete GSH levels in tumors prior to chemotherapy, with agents such as BSO, are currently under consideration in the clinic.

DRUG RESISTANCE

Tumor-cell drug resistance is not a new problem. The observation of drug resistance and the potential problems it posed clinically was already a topic of discussion in the 1950s (62). Using experience gained from the treatment of microbial organisms, Goldie and Coldman first proposed that the possibil-

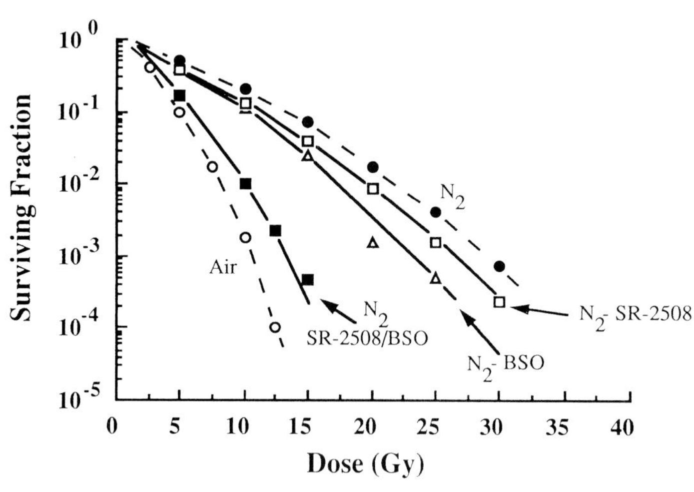

Fig. 13–5. X-ray survival curves for human lung adenocarcinoma cells under aerobic and hypoxic conditions. The nitroimidazole hypoxic cell radiosensitizer SR-2508 (1 mM) or GSH depletion (<5% of control levels) by BSO did not significantly sensitize hypoxic cells to radiation; however, the combination of GSH depletion and SR-2508 markedly sensitized hypoxic cells. (Data adapted from Phillips TL, et al. Int J Radiat Oncol Biol Phys 12:1627, 1986 and Mitchell JB, et al. Int J Radiat Oncol Biol Phys 12:1143, 1986, Pergamon Press Ltd.)

ity of two or more mutations arising and conferring resistance to tumors was probable (63). Therefore, the possibility of achieving a cure would be theoretically enhanced by using drugs that had different targets in an alternating scheme of delivery (63). However, clinical studies have demonstrated that even in the setting of multiple-agent chemotherapy, certain tumors that respond initially eventually relapse and are refractory to further treatment (4).

Genetic alterations that could lead ultimately to tumor-cell resistance might be of several classes: point mutations, gene amplification, or gross chromosomal rearrangements. In addition, mutations do not have to be within the resistant gene itself but may occur in various promoter regions, and thus may act to increase the overall expression of the protecting protein. How cells become resistant to a variety of drugs with different modes of cytotoxicity (**multidrug resistance or MDR**) is difficult to explain in that the cell population arose from a single-point mutation. One possible explanation for such resistance might be that the cell membrane was altered in order not to allow different drugs to have access to critical targets of cytotoxicity within the cell. Ling and coworkers have produced strong evidence that this is the case in an experimental in vitro model (64,65). Multidrug-resistant Chinese hamster cells have altered cell membranes that include increased amounts of a 170-kD/p-glycoprotein (p-170), which serves to pump drugs out of cells, thereby preventing toxicity. The exact mechanism by which p-170 works is not completely known; however, it is thought that drugs bind either directly to p-170 or to a carrier protein and are then extruded through the p-170 transmembrane pore and out of the cell (65). Interestingly, this p-170 protein is also present in some normal tissues, including the liver, kidney, and gastrointestinal tract, and may serve to protect the host from toxic materials. Whether pleiotropic drug resistance at the cellular level develops during therapy has not been firmly established in patients. Monoclonal antibodies that recognize p-170 receptors have been developed and are currently being used to determine whether tumor cells from patients that fail chemotherapy are positive for the presence of p-170. Preliminary findings suggest that some but not all patients who relapse after chemotherapy are positive for p-170 (66–69).

Whether the MDR phenotype is responsible for drug resistance in a cell line is determined by the reduced cytotoxicity to several different types of drugs (Adriamycin, vinca alkaloids, 5-fluorouracil). Furthermore, the reversal of drug resistance by verapamil, which has been shown to competively inhibit the p-170 efflux of several drugs (70), is also used as an indicator of the MDR phenotype (68). Although the use of verapamil in vitro to reverse drug resistance has been successful, the clinical trials of verapamil in conjunction with Adriamycin chemotherapy has been less positive (71).

The association of drug resistance due to gene amplification has also been reported, especially for drugs such as methotrexate (72). Longterm exposure to methotrexate in increasing concentrations or other environmental conditions (73) can induce gene amplification for the enzyme dihydrofolate reductase (DHFR) (72). This gene amplification leads to an overproduction of DHFR, which is the target enzyme for methotrexate-induced cytotoxicity.

Chromosomal rearrangements are common occurrences in many types of cancer (74). No mechanism regarding this type of gene rearrangement has been identified to cause drug resistance, but it may prove to be an important mechanism.

If initial drug treatments induce mutations and lead to the selection of drug-resistant populations in tumors, it could be questioned why drug resistance is not also induced in normal tissues that are dividing at a rate similar to many tumors. This is generally not seen clinically, although other factors to be discussed (environmental and cell-cycle related) may be responsible for this difference.

In the context of combined modality therapy, the question arises regarding whether cells that are resistant to cytotoxic drugs might also be resistant to radiation. There are clinical situations in which a proportion of patients who fail chemotherapy also fail radiation therapy. Likewise, there are patients who may fail chemotherapy but respond to radiation therapy. One potential mechanism, as discussed above regarding chemotherapy drug resistance, can be readily excluded for radiation resistance: the plasma cell membrane does not pose a barrier to high-energy photons. Radiation dose is delivered in an uniform manner to all parts of the cell or tissue being exposed. One approach to answering the question regarding possible radioresistance of chemoresistant cells is simply conducting x-ray survival curve experiments for cell lines that demonstrate chemoresistance. One of the first studies reported regarding this issue used Chinese hamster V79 cells and a V79 variant cell line resistant to Adriamycin (75). Figures 13–6A and 13–6B show cell-survival curves for both the parental and Adriamycin-resistant cell lines exposed to Adriamycin and x-rays. The 77A-51S cells were approximately fivefold more resistant to Adriamycin than the parental cell line at the 1% survival level. Interestingly, these cells are slightly more sensitive to x-rays than the parental cells with respect to the terminal slope of the survival curve; however, for a dose of 200

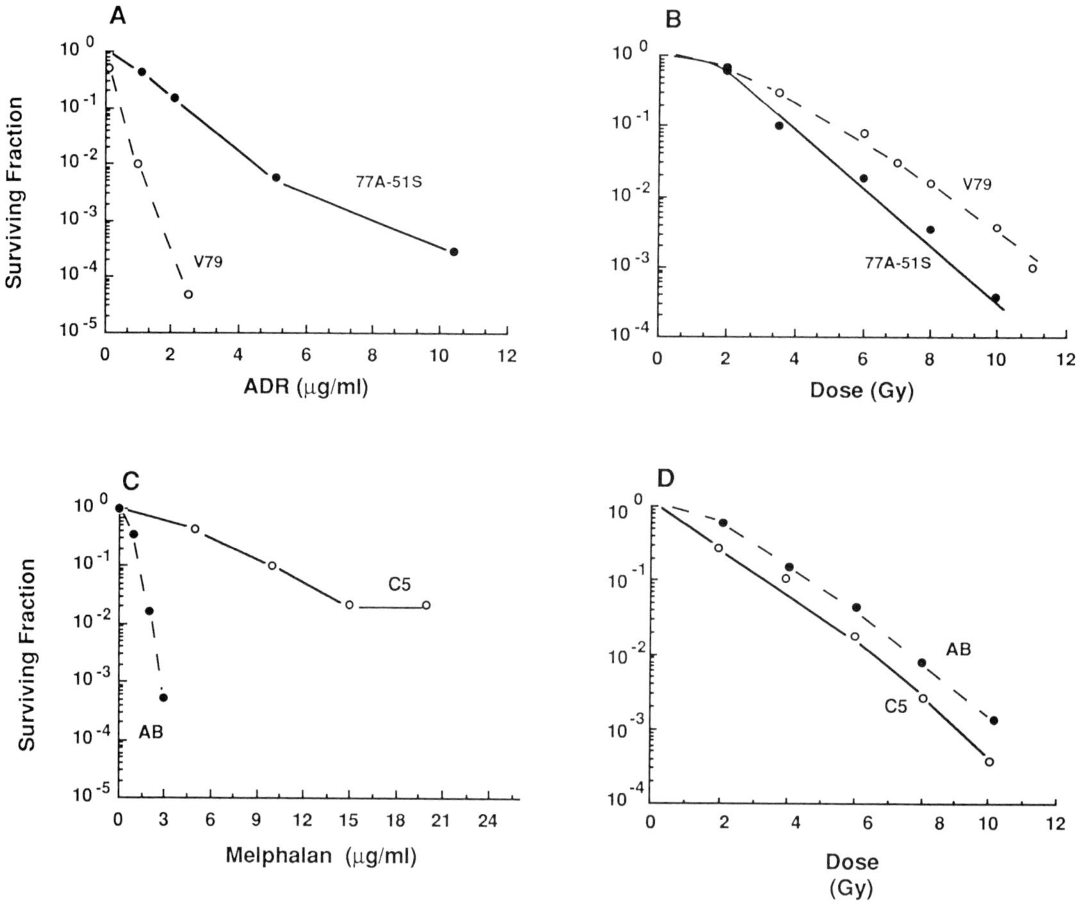

Fig. 13–6. A. Adriamycin cell-survival curves for Chinese hamster V79 and 77A-51S cells. 77A-51S cells were derived from V79 cells after prolonged exposure to increasing concentrations of Adriamycin. These cells exhibit an approximate 5-fold resistance at 1% survival to a 1-hour exposure of Adriamycin compared to the parental V79 cell line. B. X-ray survival curves of the two cell lines shown in A. The n and D_o values for the V79 cells were 740 and 130 cGy and for 77A-51S were 890 and 90 cGy, respectively. SF_2 values were similar for both cell lines. (Figures 13–6A and 13–6B: Data adapted from Belli JA, et al. Int J Radiat Oncol Biol Phys 5:1231, 1979.) C. Melphalan survival curve for parental Chinese hamster AB cells and multi-drug resistant mutant C5 cells. C5 cells were derived from AB cells following mutation induction and longterm incubation in increasing concentrations of colchicine (Ling V, et al. Cancer Treat Rep 67:869, 1983). C5 cells exhibit resistance to many different chemotherapy drugs. D. X-ray survival curves of the two cell lines shown in C. No cross-resistance to radiation was observed for the C5 cells. (Figures 13–6C and 13–6D: Data adapted from Mitchell JB, et al. NCI Monogr 6:187, 1988.)

cGy, their survival is approximately the same as the parental cell line. With this particular cell model, there is no suggestion that resistance to Adriamycin confers cross-resistance to radiation. In support of this observation are survival-curve data for two additional hamster cell lines made resistant to Adriamycin and cisplatinum (76,77). Neither of these drug-resistant variants exhibited any difference in their radiation sensitivity compared to that of the parental cell line. No difference in the radiation sensitivity was observed between a parental Chinese hamster cell line when compared to a pleiotropic multidrug-resistant variant cell line as shown in Figures 13–6C and 13–6D (78). The C5 cell line had GSH, catalase, and GSH transferase levels of 2.0-, 1.9-, and 1.9-fold higher, respectively, than the parental cell line (78). Thus, a presumed link between elevated levels of GSH and related detoxification enzymes, with a resulting increased radiation resistance, was not observed.

Increased radiation resistance in some but not all drug-resistant human tumor cell lines has recently been reported (79,80). There have been conflicting findings regarding the radiosensitivity of Adriamycin-resistant cell lines compared to the parental cell line of origin; one study showed no difference at SF_2 (79) and the other showed an approximate twofold resistance (80). Human ovarian cell lines resistant to melphalan and cisplatin were found to be resistant to x-rays (1.5-fold) when compared to the parental cell line at the SF_2 (79). The 1.5-fold difference in survival at SF_2 between the parental and drug-resistant cell line represents a potentially significant alteration in the radiation response for the drug-resistant cells. The melphalan-resistant cell line had approximately 2.4-fold higher GSH levels than the parental cell line. GSH depletion by BSO restored the normal radiosensitivity of the melphalan-resistant cell line. It was therefore inferred that increased GSH levels were responsible for the increased radiation resistance (79). This interpretation differs from others that found a minimal role for GSH in the radiation response (49,81) (see Figures 13–6C and 13–6D). GSH levels, when modulated within the same cell line over a range of 5 to 250% of control levels, were not found to modify significantly radiation sensitivity (49,53,81,82).

A related consideration is whether radiation treatment might result in altered sensitivity to chemotherapy. There are a few in vitro reports in which prior radiation exposure significantly increased the incidence of methotrexate-resistant clones (83–85), cisplatinum (85), and carmustine (BCNU) (86). The mechanism of these observations is unclear but could involve radiation-induced genomic alterations leading the methotrexate transport alterations or DHFR gene amplification in surviving cells (84). In the case of the BCNU resistance, radiation induced an increase in the O^6-methylguanine-DNA-methyltransferase (86). In the clinic, this could conceivably happen. In the case of prior exposure to x-rays inducing resistance to cisplatinum, this resistance was transient, with normal sensitivity to cisplatinum returning in 60 days following irradiation.

Hill et al reported that multiple fractions of radiation were able to induce the MDR phenotype in CHO cells (87). After the radiation treatments, these cells showed increased resistance to the vinca alkaloids, VP-16, Adriamycin, and cisplatinum; this resistance was reversed by the use of verapamil. Interestingly, these cells did not show amplification of the p-170 gene or of the p-170 mRNA; however, the cells did show an increased expression of the p-170 protein. The drug resistance induced using radiation treatments was not as high as that produced by continuous low-dose exposure to colchicine.

It should be noted that while radiation could lead to changes in inherent cellular sensitivities (as a result of genomic alterations) to subsequent chemotherapy, other possibilities exist. Radiation treatment could alter the tumor vascular supply, tumor bed, and other physiological determinants that could compromise the delivery of the drug to the clonogenic tumor cells.

CELL CYCLE/PROLIFERATION

Because events vital for cellular regeneration occur in a sequential and orderly fashion and because drugs and radiation have specific mechanisms of killing, the resistance of tumors to cancer therapies may be heavily dependent on both the time of treatment and the position of cells in the cell cycle. Therefore, the distribution of cells throughout the cell cycle, as well as the rate at which the cells move through the cell cycle, could be crucial factors in any cancer treatment protocol.

Howard and Pelc were the first to separate the interdivision time (time from one mitosis to another) and three stages: G1, S, and G2 phases (88). Later work demonstrated the presence of G_0 cells within mouse tumors; these cells did not incorporate ^{3}H-thymidine after long perfusion time and thus were considered nonproliferative but potentially clonogenic (89,90). Research has demonstrated that both qualitative and quantitative differences exist for cells in each of the five identified stages (G_0, G1, S, G2, and M); these include differences in enzyme activities, enzyme quantities, DNA replication, and DNA repair capabilities. This heterogenous nature dictates that agents that are highly toxic to some cells in a population may be without effect on others within the same population. Because exponentially growing populations have cells distributed throughout the cell cycle, it is difficult to unambiguously identify toxic mechanisms for any one agent. Identification requires the isolation of pure populations of highly synchronized cells in unique positions of the cell cycle. Fortunately, through the development of cell-synchrony techniques, purified populations of synchronized cells have been obtained; both toxicity information and an increased understanding of cytotoxic mechanisms have been the result of these techniques (91,92).

Terishma and Tolmach were the first to apply synchrony techniques to measure the sensitivity of HeLa cells to radiation throughout the cell cycle (called an age-response curve) (91). As Figure 13–7 demonstrates, there was at least a threefold variation in survival; late S-phase/early G1 cells showed the maximal resistance and mitotic cells showed the maximal sensitivity. The exact reasons for the increased and decreased sensitivity to x-rays throughout the cell cycle are still not known.

Sinclair first published an age-response curve for the drug hydroxyurea (92). As Figure 13–7 shows, hydroxyurea is toxic to S-phase cells but much less so for cells in other parts of the cell cycle. The mechanism responsible for hydroxyurea cytotoxicity is believed to involve the inhibition of ribonucleotide reductase, an enzyme important in the production of deoxyribonucleotides from ribonucleotide precursors (93). In addition to its cytotoxicity, hydroxyurea also induces cell-cycle blocks at the G1/S phase border. If applied for short periods, hydroxyurea is not toxic to non-S-phase cells, and

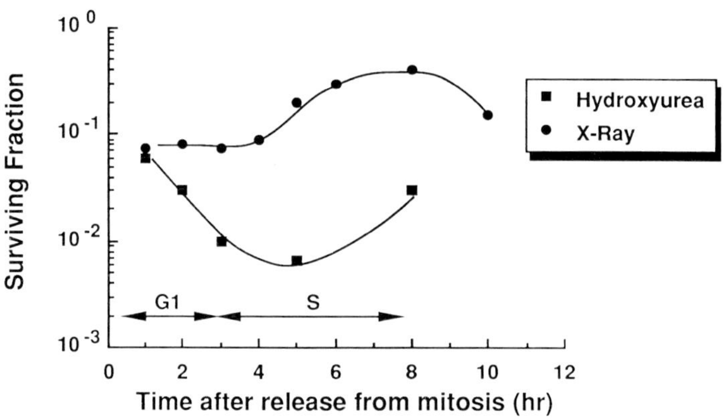

Fig. 13–7. Survival of synchronized V79 Chinese hamster lung fibroblasts to either x-rays or 1 μM hydroxyurea as a function of time after mitosis. Mitotic V79 cells were isolated by the mitotic shake-off technique of Terishma and Tolmach and plated back into petri dishes for survival studies. Various times after plating, the cells were exposed to 710 Gy of x-rays and incubated for clonogenic survival. Other mitotically synchronized populations were exposed to 1 μM hydroxyurea for various times after plating and then washed several times to remove the hydroxyurea and finally allowed time to grow for clonogenic survival. (From Sinclair WK. Cancer Res 28:198, 1968.)

once washed off, the cells will move through the cell cycle in a highly synchronous manner (92).

The importance of understanding the age response of any cytotoxic agent is twofold. First, when a combination of agents is utilized either concurrently or in alternating schedules, the most efficient agents will be those that have opposite cell-cycle specificities. An example of this principle is found in Figure 13–7, where the cell-cycle survival variations for both radiation and hydroxyurea are plotted on the same graph (94). By applying both agents simultaneously, cells resistant to radiation would be killed more efficiently by hydroxyurea (S-phase cells), while cells more resistant to hydroxyurea could be controlled by the radiation (G1 cells). Secondly, agents that nonrandomly kill off cells in one portion of the cell cycle temporarily may produce a semisynchronous population of cells (95). By prudently timing the second dose of either drug or radiation (to catch the remaining cells that move into the sensitive portion of the cell cycle), a greater degree of killing could possibly be accomplished when compared to an agent's effect on a purely asynchronous population (95). This effect has been demonstrated for in vitro systems (95) and various in vivo systems (96,97); however, it has never been clearly demonstrated to occur in the clinical situation.

Because many tumors may have a substantial fraction of G_0 cells, the continual stimulation of these cells into the cell cycle may lead to treatment failure. Primarily because many chemotherapy drugs are selectively toxic to actively cycling cells, the G_0 cells may represent an important unaffected reservoir of clonogenic cells (98). In addition, because hypoxia and poor nutrient conditions tend to be associated with cells in the G_0 stage, radiation sensitivity may also be adversely affected. Therefore, a detailed knowledge of the percentage of cells in the active portion of the cell cycle (G1, S, G2, and M), as well as information on the rate of cell turnover and loss from the tumor population, may allow tailoring of therapies to individual patients.

Durand and Vanderbyl have published data demonstrating the importance of cell-growth kinetics in the development of drug resistance (99). They treated V79 spheroids with two concentrations of cisplatinum daily over a 2- to 3-week period and followed the spheroid regrowth pattern under these cytotoxic conditions. The lower cisplatinum concentration used (0.75 μg/ml) initially reduced the number of viable cells, but subsequently the spheroids developed resistance and continued to grow. The higher concentration of cisplatinum used (0.1 μg/ml) also reduced the number of viable cells in the first week of treatment, but with further treatments, the number of viable cells remained constant and the spheroids remained at a constant size (no growth). However, they were also able to analyze the drug sensitivity of single cells from the spheroids after each drug treatment. Significantly, no increase in drug resistance was seen as a function of drug incubation time. Because there was an increase in the S-phase fraction of the spheroids as the drug-incubation time increased, Devan and Vanderbyl concluded that the spheroid drug resistance was due to an increase in the growth fraction of the cells that overcame the cytotoxicity of the cisplatinum.

Much of the cell-cycle information has been derived utilizing ^{3}H-thymidine as a radioactive marker for proliferating populations (89,100,101). Although this was adequate for in vitro work and has been applied to humans (102), this technique has not found general clinical use because of the radiation involved and the long processing times. However, new technology has been developed during the last 10 to 15 years that will hopefully provide useful cell-cycle information to the practicing oncologist in time to be of clinical use. The first of these advancements was the development of monoclonal antibodies to the halogenated pyrimidine bromodeoxyuridine (BUdR) (103). BUdR is a nonradioactive thymidine analog that, at low concentrations, is nontoxic to cells and, thus, can readily be used to identify cells that are actively moving through the cell cycle (104,105). Figure 13–8 shows a human prostatic mouse xenograft labeled in vivo with a single 4-mg/kg intraperitoneal injection of BUdR. It can be seen that a small percentage of labeled cells are found throughout the tumor, indicating a low proliferative index. Clearly, the ability to iden-

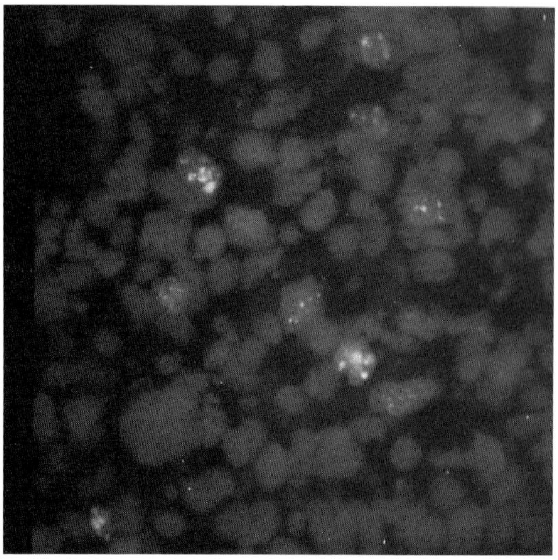

Fig. 13–8. Fluorescence photomicrograph of BUdR labeled DU-145 human prostatic tumor xenograft. Human tumor prostate cells (10^7) were injected into nude mice and allowed 3 to 4 weeks growth to develop 3- to 4-mm-size tumors. A single intraperitoneal 4-mg/kg dose of BUdR was injected, and after a 2-hour period of time, the animals were sacrificed and the tumors removed and frozen for sectioning. Frozen sections (8 to 10 μm) were labeled with propidium iodide, which labels the nucleus of all cells red, and with an anti-BUdR antibody technique, which labels all proliferating cells in S-phase with a green-yellow color. Notice that only a few cells in this field are positively labeled for BUdR, indicating significant heterogeneity with respect to cell proliferation and the proportion of cells in S-phase. (Figure 13–8 also appears in color in the color section.)

tify and quantitate the proliferating S-phase fraction within tumors is now possible and can be rapidly accomplished. Other monoclonals now available, such as Ki-67 and DNA alpha polymerase, differentiate cells that are in cycle from those that are out of cycle (106,107). These antibodies should provide information related to the growth fraction of tumors. Finally, to quantitate these labeling techniques, instruments such as flow cytometers (108) and microscope-based image analysis systems (109) have been developed and should provide rapid and accurate information on the status of tumor growth. The possibility of both studying and manipulating the cell cycle for maximum treatment response seems within reach but will require much interaction between the practicing physician and the laboratory researcher.

PHYSIOLOGIC/ENVIRONMENTAL FACTORS IN TUMOR

Hypoxia

A possible limitation of the use of ionizing radiation and possibly for chemotherapy drugs in cancer therapy is the presence of hypoxic cells within tumors. While their presence in human tumors has never been directly proven, histologic findings and experimental rodent tumor studies suggest that they are present and possibly afford a considerable obstacle to successful treatment (110,111). During rapid tumor growth, cells at some distance from capillaries can become oxygen deprived and yet remain viable for extended times. Because there is less oxygen present, fewer toxic oxygen-related radicals are formed by radiation exposure of these cells, thereby rendering them approximately three times more resistant to radiation than cells in fully aerobic conditions. One approach to reverse such radiation resistance has been the development of nitroimidazole hypoxic-cell radiosensitizers (112). Although efficient in the laboratory, there are a number of shortcomings in using these sensitizers in the clinic, including drug toxicity and achieving adequate drug concentrations in hypoxic cells during radiation.

The cytotoxicity of certain chemotherapy drugs can also be influenced by oxygen (113–115). Similar to the effects observed for radiation, cells treated with bleomycin, streptonigrin, and vincristine under hypoxic conditions are more resistant than those treated under fully aerobic conditions (113,114). In contrast, however, cells were found to be more sensitive to mitomycin C and Adriamycin under hypoxic conditions (113). Methotrexate, 5-fluorouracil, cisplatinum, and BCNU cytotoxicity was found to be the same under either aerobic or hypoxic conditions (113). Thus, similar problems regarding hypoxic-cell resistance could be encountered with certain chemotherapy drugs. Identification of tumors with significant hypoxic fractions prior to treatment would greatly aid the oncologist in selecting appropriate drugs that would target hypoxic cells.

Hypoxic cell markers are currently under evaluation with this goal in mind (116,117).

pH

The importance of pH and the various homeostasis mechanisms used by biologic systems to maintain pH in a narrow range is well documented (118). Warburg first proposed in 1930 that tumors cells had impaired respiration and thus were heavily dependent on glycolysis for energy production (119). It was subsequently shown that this generality does not hold universally and therefore is not a unique parameter for all tumors (120,121). On the other hand, measurements made on many tumors have indicated a trend toward higher rates of both anaerobic and aerobic glycolysis (121). This increased dependence can lead to an excess production of protons and, combined with poor blood flow, can induce large reductions in the extracellular pH (121). Studies have shown that many tumors have extracellular pH levels anywhere from 0.2 to 0.5 pH units lower than most normal organ systems (122,123). Although most research to date has concentrated on the advantages of low pH for increased tumor cell kill, the possibility that low pH could reduce the effectiveness of various treatment strategies has not been adequately investigated. Low pH could induce drug resistance in one of several ways: by effecting a tumor's growth status, by reducing tumor blood flow and thereby reducing extracellular drug gradients, by changing the permeability properties of a drug, by altering enzyme transport properties, and/or by selecting for cells with increased tolerance to environmental stresses.

Cells grown in culture are acutely sensitive to their incubation pH and respond to either high or low pH by reducing their growth rate (124). Because many chemotherapy drugs are more toxic to actively proliferating cells, a reduction in overall growth rate is expected to decrease the overall effectiveness of these agents. Most studies demonstrate that combined hypoxia and low pH are highly toxic conditions for cells (123,125). However, the effect of low pH on moderately hypoxic cells is unknown but would be expected to increase the rate of transition from a proliferating G1 state to a nonproliferating G_0 state. There can be cell-cycle redistributions with prolonged low pH incubation (increases in G1, decreases in S) (126). This problem has not been adequately addressed in the literature, primarily because most drug/radiation studies are done on cells given an acute exposure of low pH, whereas within a tumor, cells have likely been growing under low pH for many generations.

Studies have shown that, as the tumor mass increases, the overall pH and oxygenation status decrease (127). It has also been demonstrated that the induction of low pH conditions in tumors leads to drastic reductions in blood flow (121). Because of an increased dependence on glucose metabolism, it is possible to reduce the blood flow selectively to certain tumors without any concomitant reduction in normal tissue blood flow by injections of large doses of glucose (121). While this procedure can and does lead to increased cell killing it may lead to reductions in drug delivery and to the induction of severe hypoxia. Thus, the pH status of a patient at the time of therapy may strongly influence the pharmacokinetics of drug delivery as well as the tumor radiosensitivity.

On a molecular level, drugs can have proton-dissociable groups, which have dissociation constants in the range of biologic systems (6.6 to 7.8). In addition, depending on the environment they are evolved in, proteins operate most efficiently at specific pH values. These two events operating simultaneously (protein function and drug physical state) can act to severely reduce uptake efficiency of cells (123). Thus, pharmacokinetics as measured in the blood plasma may not adequately describe the pharmacokinetics within tumors.

Finally, it has become increasingly apparent that cells that develop tolerance to one type of environmental stress may be resistant to other types of stresses (128). An example of this is the increased resistance to Adriamycin cytotoxicity that cells exhibit when made tolerant to ethanol or heat treatments (128). Mutant cells, which are more resistant to low pH effects, have been isolated; however, whether these cells will be more resistant to various toxic drugs is unknown (129).

TUMOR CELL HETEROGENEITY

A factor that most likely generates resistance of tumor cells to cancer treatments is heterogeneity. Heterogeneity can be expressed through either environmental, genetic, or cellular differences; tumors often express all three. Environmental factors already discussed include the oxygen status, nutrient status, and pH status. Genetic factors include the ploidy status, gene amplification, and variations in gene expression. Cellular differences arise from the interplay of environmental and genetic factors and are found in the growth status, cell-cycle times, and the cellular turnover rate. Another factor that is rarely emphasized is the number of cellular types found within tumor biopsies. Figure 13–9A shows several volume distributions of various tumor and normal tissue biopsies. It is clear that several populations are present in both the tumor and normal samples. This appears to be a trivial factor; however, when analysis is attempted to define the presence of tumor-specific markers (such as enhanced growth factor expression or proteins involved in drug resistance) or levels of drug detoxification systems, problems can occur. An example of this difficulty is seen in Figure 13–9B, in which the quantitation of GSH was attempted using a GSH-specific fluorescent probe, monochlorobimane (130). In many of the tumor biopsies that we have analyzed for average GSH content, normal-tissue GSH levels are either the same or higher. However, these bulk measurement techniques may severely underestimate the GSH content of tumor cells, as in Figure 13–9B, which shows the results obtained from the analysis of variations of GSH content within tumor and normal-tissue biopsies. The fluorescence profiles demonstrate a number of points. First, there are a number of distinct populations of cells with varying GSH contents. Secondly, differences in GSH content can vary by amounts greater than three- to fivefold. Finally, a portion of tumor cells within a biopsy can have a significantly greater GSH content than the normal tissue from which the tumor arose. The dilution of tumor biopsies by normal tissue can be substantial, in that some tumor specimens may contain from 40 to 60% lymphocytes. Until tumor-specific markers can be identified and techniques can be developed to sort or separate tumor cells from biopsies, the information derived by these bulk techniques could be misleading.

A final and often overlooked aspect of heterogeneity is the problem of dose or drug delivery to tumors. Drug doses are often quantitated by measurements of the peak plasma concentrations or the concentration and duration of exposure ($C \times T$) parameter and tumor levels are expected (or anticipated) to reflect these levels. There are few studies that actually measure drug levels in tumors in human cancer treatment protocols (21). Studies done with Adriamycin have indicated a pronounced lack of penetration of the drug into human tumors (21). This must lead one to ask whether drug resistance occurs not because resistant phenotypes are selected for, but rather because inadequate drug concentrations are achieved for good cell kill.

A result of our lack of knowledge of drug levels within tumors is exemplified by the clinical experiences with hydroxyurea. As discussed above, hydroxyurea has a number of important cytostatic and cytotoxic properties (92). However, clinical experience with hydroxyurea has been disappointing. Thus, with the exception of cervical cancer trials, where it is combined with radiotherapy, hydroxyurea has been dropped from clinical protocols (131). It should be stressed that none of the clinical trials assessed whether enough drug got to the treated tumors or whether any cytostatic or synchrony effects were induced (131). This is not a trivial factor, as hydroxyurea is not effective either as a cytotoxic or as a cytostatic drug below a 1000-μM level (131). While it is a valid point that cell-cycle technology in the past was not sufficiently advanced to measure these events adequately, this is currently not the case.

CONCLUSIONS

In this brief review, we have discussed potential ways by which genetic, biochemical, or physiologic factors can reduce the effectiveness of radiation and chemotherapy drugs. Perhaps this survey has imposed many more questions than answers, for this is indeed a complex area. The current tendency is to classify all failures of cancer treatment, by chemotherapy or radiation therapy, as

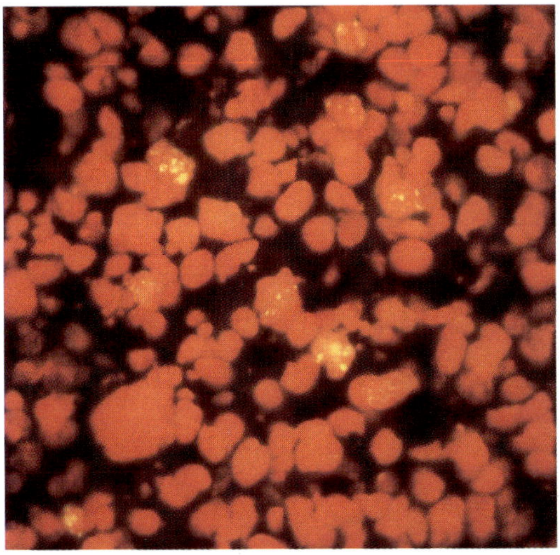

Fig. 13–8. Fluorescence photomicrograph of BUdR labeled DU-145 human prostatic tumor xenograft. Human tumor prostate cells (10^7) were injected into nude mice and allowed 3 to 4 weeks growth to develop 3- to 4-mm-size tumors. A single intraperitoneal 4-mg/kg dose of BUdR was injected, and after a 2-hour period of time, the animals were sacrificed and the tumors removed and frozen for sectioning. Frozen sections (8 to 10 μm) were labeled with propidium iodide, which labels the nucleus of all cells red, and with an anti-BUdR antibody technique, which labels all proliferating cells in S-phase with a green-yellow color. Notice that only a few cells in this field are positively labeled for BUdR, indicating significant heterogeneity with respect to cell proliferation and the proportion of cells in S-phase.

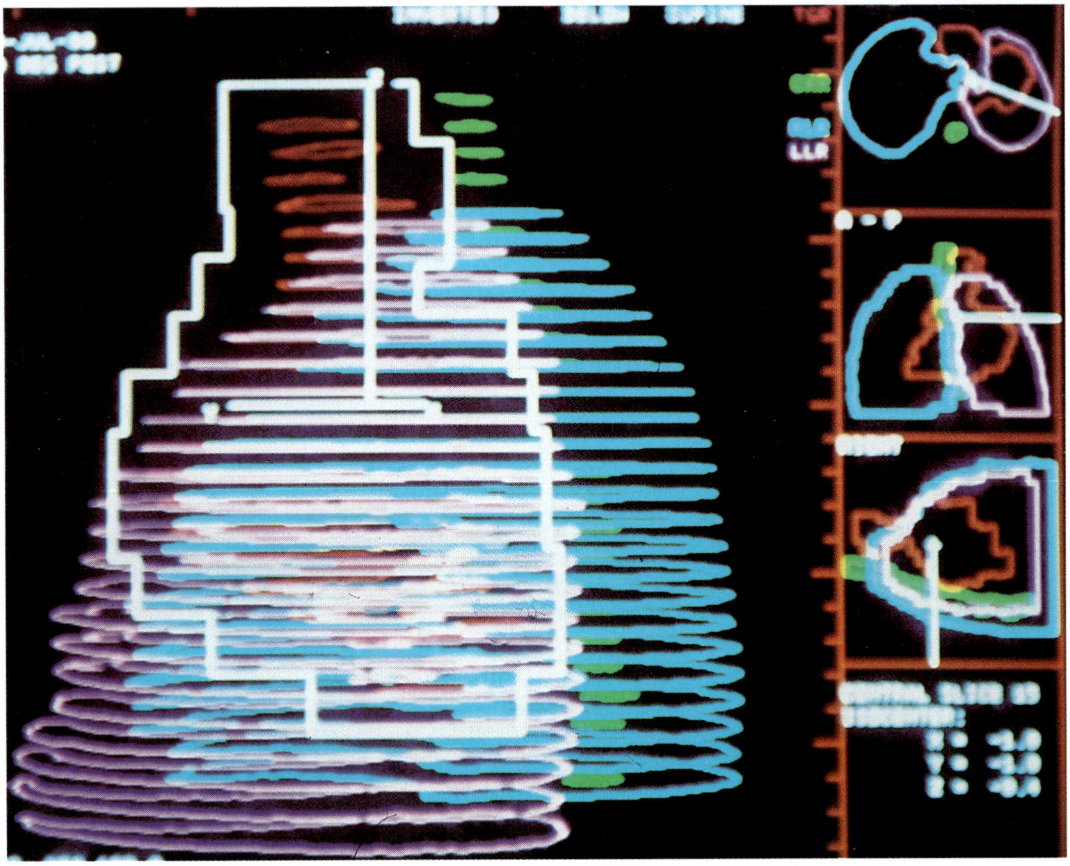

Fig. 27–1. Beam's eye view, from a 20-degree left posterior oblique perspective, of a patient's lungs (blue and purple contours), spinal cord (green contours), and composite target, i.e., tumor plus margin plus regions of possible subclinical disease, such as nodes (red contours). The white outline encompasses the target with an approximately 1-cm margin and thus corresponds to the shape of the appropriate irradiation field from this perspective. Therefore, it can be used as a guide in the delineation of the block. The three icons on the right help the viewer visualize the location of the isocenter and the position of the radiation source.

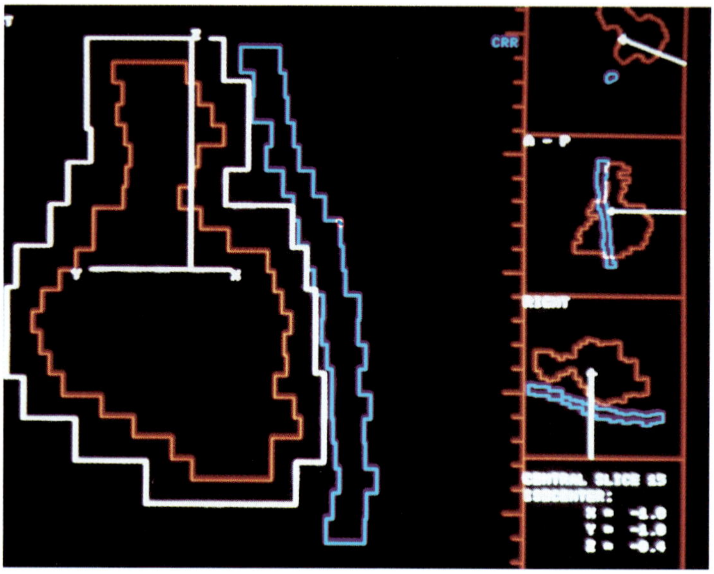

Fig. 27–2. Beam's eye view of the target (red) and spinal cord (blue) of the same patient from the same perspective as in Figure 27–1. The outlines indicate the largest extent of the projection, laterally, of the corresponding contour at each CT slice level, joined in a stepwise manner. The white outline is the same as in Figure 27–1 and it clearly avoids the cord.

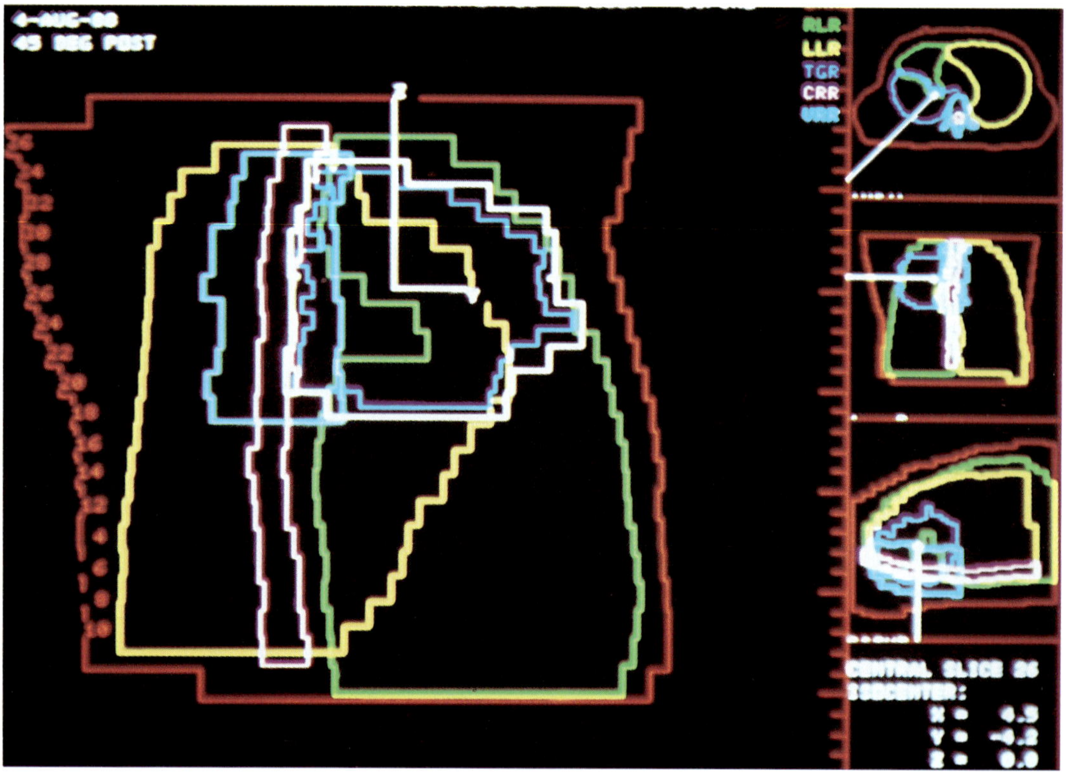

Fig. 27–3. Beam's eye view, from a 45-degree right posterior oblique perspective, of a patient with adenocarcinoma in the posterior aspect of the superior lobe of the right lung, with extension into the pleura. Shown are outlines of the external contours (red), right lung (green), left lung (yellow), target (dark blue), spinal cord (purple), and vertebrae (light blue). The white outline frames the target with an 0.5-cm margin, yet it barely clears the cord.

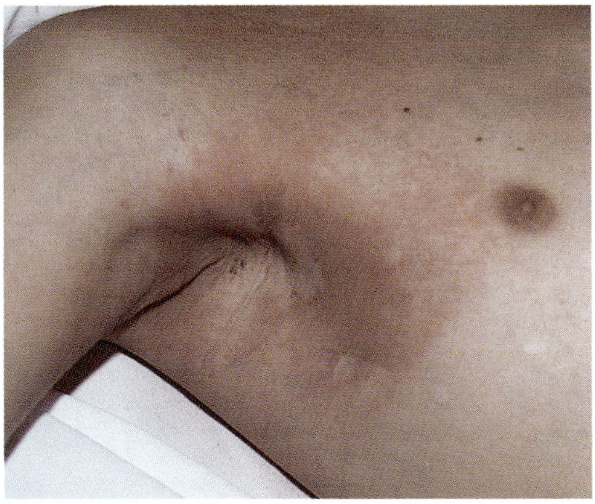

A

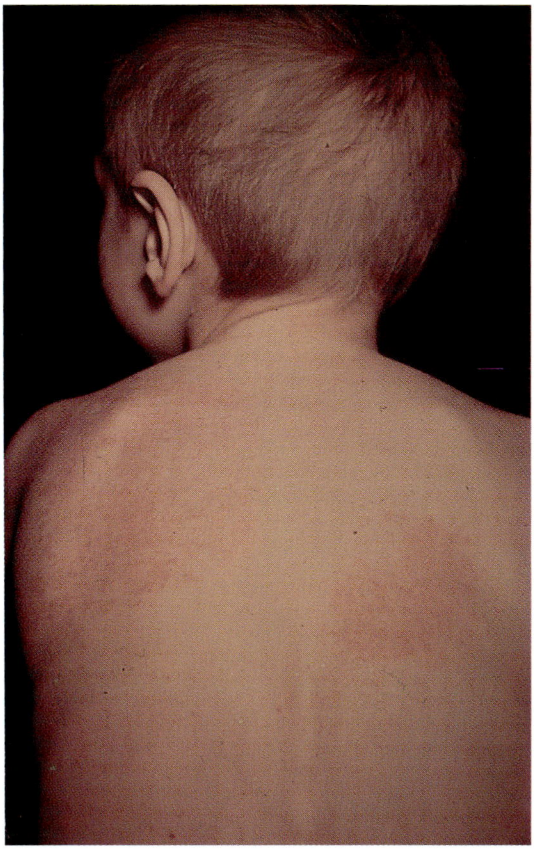

B

Fig. 36–1. This 7-year-old boy with metastatic rhabdomyosarcoma developed discrete erythema in the area of radiotherapy given several weeks prior to a dose of Actinomycin D. B. This 4-year-old boy received RT and Actinomycin D for left midlung and right pericardiac metastases from Wilms' tumor. (From D'Angio GJ. Am J Roentgen Rad Ther Nuc Med 87:106, 1962.)

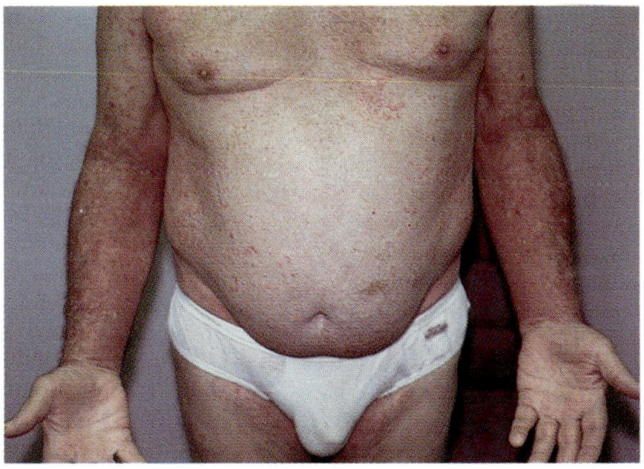

A

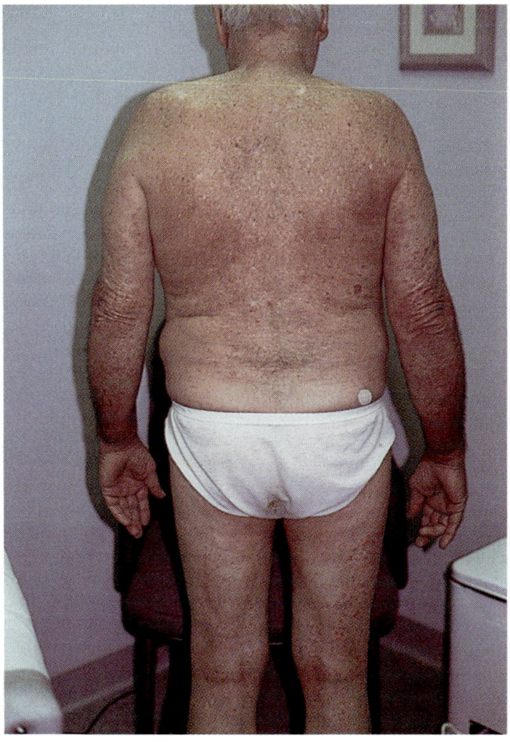

B

Fig. 36–2. This 69-year-old male with non-small-cell lung cancer received IV methotrexate and developed a generalized erythematous, papillary rash 2 days later, suggesting a hypersensitivity or allergic reaction.

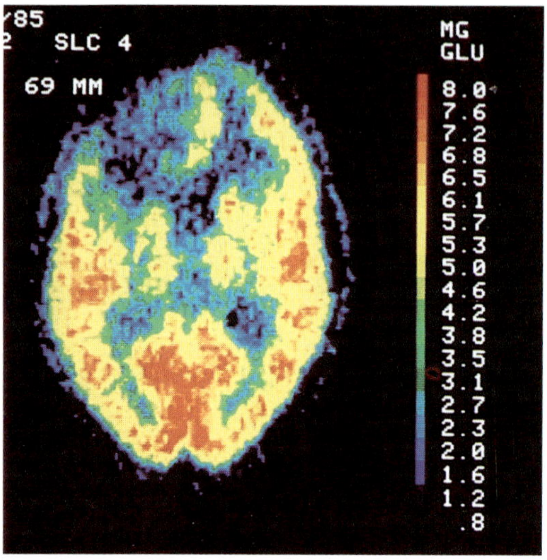

Fig. 40–3. Cerebral positron emission tomography (PET) with ^{18}F-deoxyglucose (FDG) in a 43-year-old man harboring a butterfly, bifrontal glioblastoma multiforme. Tumor had been treated with external beam radiotherapy (6300 cGy). CT shows a large bilateral frontal mass, which enhances with contrast. PET-FDG reveals marked hypometabolism in both prefrontal areas, larger on the left. Note selective sparing of interhemispheric gray matter, which is displaced toward the right. Color scale indicates range of metabolic values expressed in mg/glucose/100 g/min. (On PET scans, right side of patient is on right side of images.) Conclusion: Radiation necrosis. (Courtesy of Dr. Giovanni DiChiro, National Cancer Institute, Bethesda, Maryland.)

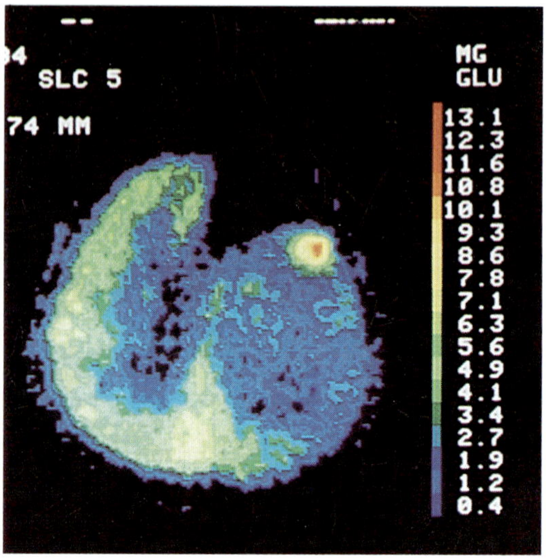

Fig. 40–4. PET-FDG scan in young female patient with a brain tumor treated with radiation plus chemotherapy. Note discrete area of intense hypermetabolism in right frontal region, behind wedge-like defect caused by previous surgery. The hypermetabolic focus indicates recurrent tumor. Vast, hypometabolic (blue) areas, most likely related to chemoradiation injury, are seen in ipsilateral as well as contralateral hemispheres. Conclusion: Radiation necrosis and recurrent tumor, which was not suspected on CT or MRI images. (Courtesy of Dr. Giovanni DiChiro, National Cancer Institute, Bethesda, Maryland.)

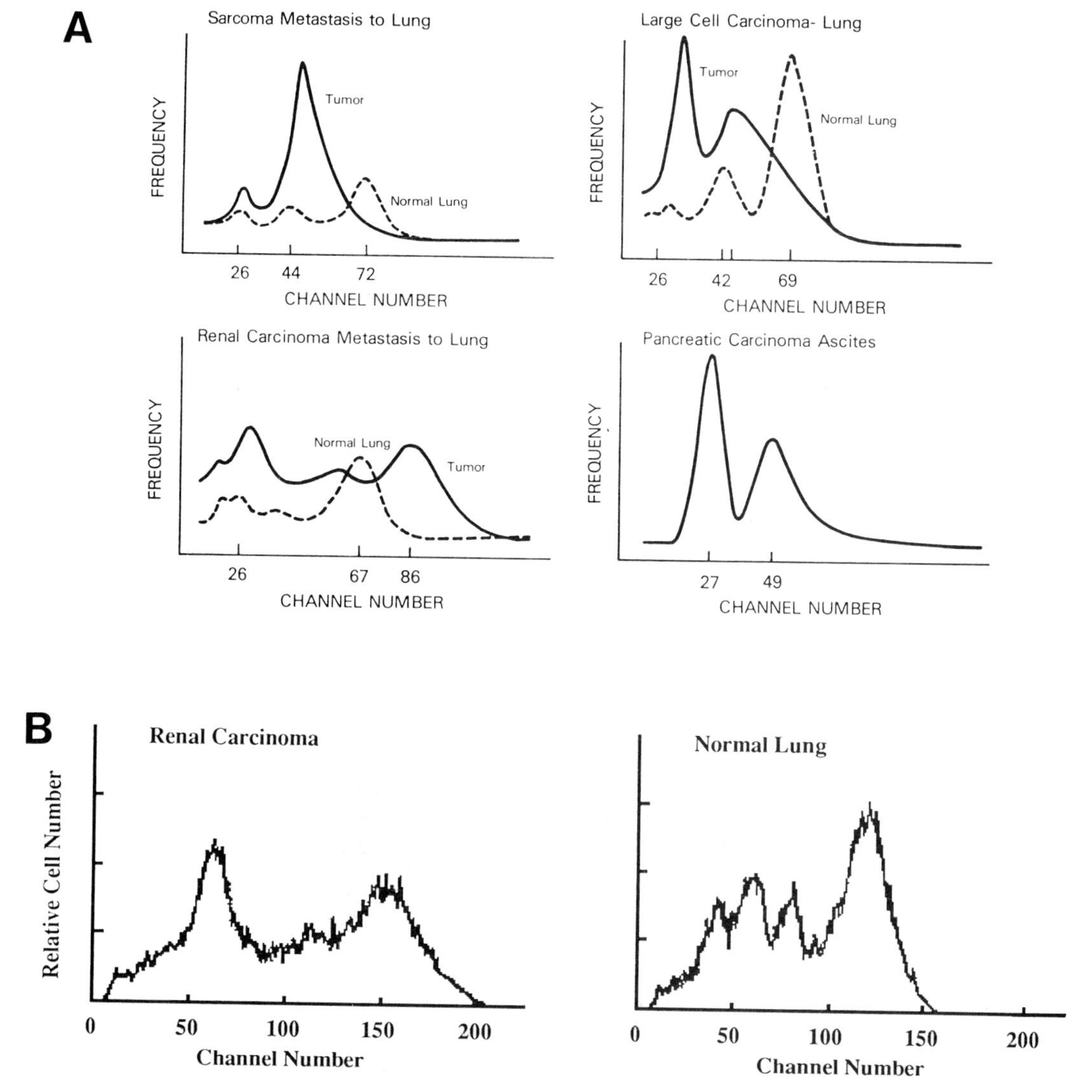

Fig. 13–9. Two examples of tumor and normal tissue heterogeneity. A. Volume distribution (as measured by a particle data counter) of various tumors and their corresponding normal tissue. To obtain these results, tumor and normal tissue biopsies were enzymatically digested and single cells were isolated. B. Heterogeneity with regard to glutathione content. Tumor and normal single cell suspensions were labeled for 1 hour with 1 μM monochlorobimane. Monochlorobimane is a GSH-specific probe that, upon conjugation to GSH, goes from a nonfluorescent to a fluorescent state with the magnitude of fluorescence being proportional to the intracellular glutathione content (131). The fluorescence from the cells was analyzed using an Epics V cell sorter with increasing channel number representing increased glutathione content.

due to the development of resistance, generally through genetic means. Undoubtedly, this will prove to be an important component in cancer treatment. However, heterogeneity in cell-cycle properties, environmental factors, and tumor drug levels will also prove to be vital components in the drive for tailoring treatments to individual patients. Already new technology is developing that can both rapidly and accurately identify properties specific to individual patients in time for the treating physician to choose from alternate protocols. It will require the combined effort of both researchers in the cancer treatment field and the practicing oncologist to verify the usefulness of these assays and their clinical importance. Hopefully, in the near future, continued research and cooperation between clinical and laboratory researchers will bring cancer treatment protocols closer to the needs of the individual patient.

REFERENCES

1. Phillips TL, Fu KK. Quantification of combined radiation therapy and chemotherapy effects on critical normal tissues. Cancer 37:1186, 1976.
2. von der Maase H. Experimental studies on interactions of radiation and cancer chemotherapeutic drugs in normal tissues and a solid tumour. Radiother Oncol 7:47, 1986.
3. Tubiana M. The combination of radiotherapy and chemotherapy: A review. Int J Radiat Oncol Biol Phys 55:497, 1989.
4. Young RC. Drug resistance: The clinical problem. *In:* Drug Resistance in Cancer Therapy. Ozols RF (Ed). Boston, Kluwer Academic, 1989, p. 1.
5. Durand RE. Keynote address: The influence of microenvironmental factors on the activity of radiation and drugs. Int J Radiat Oncol Biol Phys 20:253, 1991.
6. Puck TT, Markus PI. Action of x-rays on mammalian cells. J Exp Med 103:653, 1956.
7. Okada S. Radiation biochemistry. *In:* Radiation Biochemistry. Altman KI, Gerber GB, Okada S (Eds). New York, Academic Press, 1970, p. 1.
8. Senn JS, McCulloch EA. Radiation sensitivity of human bone marrow cells measured by a cell culture method. Blood 35:56, 1977.
9. Bromer RH, Mitchell JB, Soares N. Response of human hematopoietic precursor cells (CFUc) to hyperthermia and radiation. Cancer Res 42:1261, 1982.
10. Withers HR. The dose-survival relationship for irradiation of epithelial cells of mouse skin. Br J Radiol 40:187, 1967.
11. Withers HR, Elkind MM. Microcolony survival assay for cells of mouse intestinal mucosa exposed to radiation. Int J Radiat Oncol Biol Phys 17:261, 1970.
12. Fertil B, Malaise EP. Intrinsic radiosensitivity of human cell lines is correlated with radioresponsiveness of human tumors: Analysis of 101 published survival curves. Int J Radiat Oncol Biol Phys 11:1699, 1985.
13. Sklar MD. The ras oncogenes increase the intrinsic resistance of N 3T3 cells to ionizing radiation. Science 239:645, 1988.
14. McKenna WG, Weiss MC, Endlich B, et al. Synergistic effect of the v-myc oncogene with H-ras on radioresistance. Cancer Res 50:97, 1990.
15. Sklar MD. Increased resistance to cis-diamminedichloroplatinum (II) in NIH 3T3 cells transformed by ras oncogenes. Cancer Res 48:793, 1988.
16. Sklar MD, Prochownik EV. Modulation of cisplatinum resistance in Friend erythroleukemia cells by c-myc. Cancer Res 51:2188, 1991.
17. Kasid UN, Weichselbaum RR, Brennan T, et al. Sensitivities of NIH/3T3-derived clonal cell lines to ionizing radiation: Significance of gene transfer studies. Cancer Res 49:3396, 1989.
18. Munro TR. The relative radiosensitivity of the nucleus and cytoplasm of the Chinese hamster fibroblasts. Radiat Res 42:451, 1970.
19. Hofer KG, Harris CR, Smith JM. Radiotoxicity of intracellular 67Ga, 125I, and 3H. Nuclear versus cytoplasmic radiation effects in murine L1210 leukaemia. Int J Radiat Oncol Biol Phys 28:225, 1975.
20. Radford IR. Evidence for a general relationship between the induced level of DNA double-strand breakage and cell-killing after X-irradiation of mammalian cells. Int J Radiat Oncol Biol Phys 49:611, 1986.
21. Speth PAJ, van Hoesel QGCM, Haanen C. Clinical pharmacokinetics of doxorubicin. Clin Pharm 15:15, 1988.
22. Elkind MM, Sutton H. X-ray damage and recovery in mammalian cells in culture. Nature 184:1293, 1959.
23. Utsumi H, Elkind MM. Potentially lethal damage versus sublethal damage: Independent repair processes in actively growing Chinese hamster cells. Radiat Res 77:346, 1979.
24. Elkind MM, Whitmore GF. Chromosome damage and other cytological effects. *In:* The Radiobiology of Cultured Mammalian Cells. New York, Gordon & Breach, 1967, p. 383.
25. Kohn KW. Interstrand cross-linking of DNA by 1,3-bis(2-chloroethyl)-1-nitrosourea and other 1-(2-haloethyl)-1-nitrosoureas. Cancer Res 37:1450, 1977.
26. Mehta JR, Ludlum DB, Renard A, Verly WG. Repair of O^6-ethyguanine in DNA by a chromatin fraction from rat liver: Transfer of the ethyl group to an acceptor protein. Proc Natl Acad Sci USA 78:6766, 1981.
27. Wiestler O, Kleihues P, Pegg AE. O^6-alkylguanine-DNA alkyltransferase activity in human brain and brain tumors. Carcinogenesis (Lond) 5:121, 1984.
28. Downes CS, Johnson RT. DNA topoisom-

erases and DNA repair. Bioessays 8:179, 1988.
29. Miller MR, Chinault DN. The roles of DNA polymerases alpha, beta, and gamma in DNA repair synthesis induced in hamster and human cells by different DNA damaging agents. J Biol Chem 257:10204, 1982.
30. Ikegami S, Taguchi T, Ohashi M, et al. Aphidicolin prevents mitotic cell division by interfering with the activity of DNA polymerase alpha. Nature 275:458, 1978.
31. Spadari S, Pedrali-Noy G, Focher F, et al. DNA polymerases in DNA topoisomerases as targets for the development of anticancer drugs. Anticancer Res 6:935, 1986.
32. Bohr VA, Wassermann K. DNA repair at the level of the gene. Trends Biochem Sci 13:429, 1988.
33. Sancar A, Sancar GB. DNA repair enzymes. Annu Rev Biochem 57:29, 1988.
34. Dalrymple GV, Lynch TJ, Hardin JW. Deinococcus radiodurans DNA increases the radiation resistance of Escherichia coli. Radiat Res 120:532, 1989.
35. Barrows LR. Evidence for the cloning of Deinococcus radiodurans DNA fragments that render Escherichia coli radiation resistant. Radiat Res 120:537, 1989.
36. Stamato TD, Weinstein R, Giaccia A, Mackenzie L. Isolation of cell cycle-dependent gamma ray-sensitive Chinese hamster ovary cell. Somat Cell Mol Genet 9:165, 1983.
37. Jeggo PA, Kemp LM. X-ray-sensitive mutants of Chinese hamster ovary cell line. Isolation and cross-sensitivity to other DNA-damaging agents. Mutat Res 112:313, 1983.
38. Stamato TD, Peters B, Patil P, et al. Isolation and characterization of bleomycin-sensitive Chincsc hamstcr ovary cells. Cancer Res 47:1588, 1987.
39. Rubin JS, Joyner AL, Berstein A, Whitmore GF. Molecular identification of a human DNA repair gene following DNA-mediated gene transfer. Nature 306:206, 1983.
40. MacInnes MA, Bingham JM, Thompson LH, Strniste GF. DNA-mediated cotransfer of excision repair capacity and drug resistance into Chinese ovary mutant cell line UV-135. Mole Cell Biol 4:1152, 1984.
41. Benet LZ, Sheiner LB. Pharmacokinetics: The dynamics of drug absorption, distribution, and elimination. *In:* The Pharmacological Basis of Therapeutics. Gilman AG, Goodman LS, Rall TW, Murad F (Eds). New York, Macmillan Publishing Co., 1985, p. 3.
42. Ivy SP, Tulpule A, Fairchild CR, et al. Altered regulation of P-450IA1 expression in a multidrug-resistant MCF-7 human breast cancer cell line. J Biol Chem 263:19119, 1988.
43. Meister A: Selective modification of glutathione metabolism. Science 220:472, 1983.
44. Meister A, Anderson MA. Glutathione. Annu Rev Biochem 52:711, 1983.
45. Jakoby WB, Habig WH. Glutathione transferases. *In:* Enzymatic Basis of Detoxification. Jakoby WB (Ed). New York, Academic Press, 1980.
46. Russo A, Mitchell JB, McPherson S, Friedman N. Alteration of bleomycin cytotoxicity by glutathione depletion or elevation. Int J Radiat Oncol Biol Phys 10:1675, 1984.
47. Reed DJ, Fariss MW. Glutathione depletion and susceptibility. Pharmacol Rev 36:25S, 1984.
48. Arrick BA, Nathan CF. Glutathione metabolism as a determinant of therapeutic efficacy: A review. Cancer Res 44:4224, 1984.
49. Mitchell JB, Russo A. The role of glutathione in radiation and drug induced cytotoxicity. Br J Cancer 55(Suppl):96, 1987.
50. Griffith OW. Mechanism of action, metabolism, and toxicity of buthionine sulfoximine and its higher homologs, potent inhibitors of glutathione synthesis. J Biol Chem 257:13704, 1982.
51. Williamson JM, Boettcher B, Meister A. Intracellular cysteine delivery system that protects against toxicity by promoting glutathione synthesis. Proc Natl Acad Sci USA 79:6246, 1982.
52. Anderson ME, Powrie F, Puri RN, Meister A. Glutathione monoethyl ester: Preparation, uptake by tissues, and conversion to glutathione. Arch Biochem Biophys 239:538, 1985.
53. Mitchell JB, Russo A, Biaglow JE, McPherson S. Cellular glutathione depletion by diethyl maleate or buthionine sulfoximine: No effect of glutathione depletion on the oxygen enhancement ratio. Radiat Res 96:422, 1983.
54. Russo A, DeGraff W, Friedman N, Mitchell JB. Selective modulation of glutathione levels in human normal versus tumor cells and subsequent differential response to chemotherapy drugs. Cancer Res 46:2845, 1986.
55. Green JA, Vistica DT, Young RC, et al. Potentiation of melphalan cytoxocity in human ovarian cancer cell lines by glutathione depletion. Cancer Res 44:5427, 1984.
56. Batist G, Tulpule A, Sinha B, et al. Overexpression of a novel anionic glutathione transferase in multidrug-resistant human breast cancer cells. J Biol Chem 261:15544, 1986.
57. Phillips TL, Mitchell JB, DeGraff W, et al. Variation in sensitizing efficiency for SR-2508 in human cells dependent on glu-

tathione content. Int J Radiat Oncol Biol Phys 12:1627, 1986.
58. Mitchell JB, Phillips TL, DeGraff W, et al. The relationship of SR-2508 sensitizer enhancement ratio to cellular glutathione levels in human tumor cell lines. Int J Radiat Oncol Biol Phys 12:1143, 1986.
59. Carmichael J, Mitchell JB, Friedman N, et al. Glutathione and related enzyme activity in human lung cancer cell lines. Br J Cancer 58:437, 1988.
60. Hamilton TC, Lai G, Rothenberg ML, et al. Mechanisms of resistance to cisplatin and alkylating agents. *In:* Drug Resistance in Cancer Therapy. Ozols RF (Ed). Boston, Kluwer Academic, 1989, p. 151.
61. Mitchell JB, Russo A, Carmichael J, Glatstein E. Glutathione as a predictor of tumor response. *In:* Prediction of Tumor Treatment Response. Chapman JD, Peters LJ, Withers HR (Eds). New York, Pergamon Press, 1988, p. 157.
62. Greenstein JP. Biochemistry of Cancer. New York, Academic Press Inc., 1954.
63. Goldie JH, Coldman AJ, Gudauskas GA. Rationale for the use of alternating non-cross-resistant chemotherapy. Cancer Treat Rep 66:439, 1982.
64. Ling V, Kartner N, Sudo T, et al. Multidrug-resistance phenotype in Chinese hamster ovary cells. Cancer Treat Rep 67:869, 1983.
65. Kartner N, Ling V. Multidrug resistance in cancer. Sci Am 260:44, 1989.
66. Gerlach JH, Bell DR, Karakousis C, et al. P-glycoprotein in human sarcoma: Evidence for multidrug resistance. J Clin Oncol 5:1452, 1987.
67. Goldstein LJ, Galski H, Fojo A, et al. Expression of a multidrug resistance gene in human cancers. J Natl Cancer Inst 81:116, 1989.
68. Rothenberg M, Ling V. Multidrug resistance: Molecular biology and clinical relevance. J Natl Cancer Inst 81:907, 1989.
69. Salmon SE, Grogan TM, Miller T, et al. Prediction of doxorubicin resistance in vitro in myeloma, lymphoma, and breast cancer by p-glycoprotein staining. J Natl Cancer Inst 81:696, 1989.
70. Naito M, Tsuruo T. Competitive inhibition by verapamil of ATP-dependent high affinity vincristine binding to the plasma membrane of multidrug-resistant K562 cells without calcium ion involvement. Cancer Res 49:1452, 1989.
71. Dalton WS, Grogan TM, Meltzer RJ, et al. Drug-resistance in multiple myeloma and non-Hodgkin's lymphoma: detection of p-glycoprotein and potential circumvention by addition of verapmil to chemotherapy. J Clin Oncol 7:415, 1989.
72. Schimke RT. Gene amplification in cultured cells. J Biol Chem 263:5989, 1988.
73. Rice GC, Hoy C, Schimke RT. Transient hypoxia enhances the frequency of dihydrofolate reductase gene amplification in Chinese hamster ovary cells. Proc Natl Acad Sci USA 83:5978, 1986.
74. Rowley JD. Chromosome abnormalities in leukemia. J Clin Oncol 6:194, 1988.
75. Belli JA, Harris JR. Adriamycin resistance and radiation response. Int J Radiat Oncol Biol Phys 5:1231, 1979.
76. Wallner K, Li GC. Adriamycin resistance, heat resistance, and radiation response in Chinese hamster fibroblasts. Int J Radiat Oncol Biol Phys 12:829, 1986.
77. Wallner KE, Li GC. Effect of cisplatin resistance on cellular radiation response. Int J Radiat Oncol Biol Phys 13:587, 1987.
78. Mitchell JB, Gamson J, Russo A, et al. Chinese hamster pleiotropic multidrug-resistant cells are not radioresistant. NCI Monogr 6:187, 1988.
79. Louie KG, Behrens BC, Kinsella TJ, et al. Radiation survival parameters of antineoplastic drug-sensitive and resistant human ovarian cancer cell lines and their modification by buthionine sulfoximine. Cancer Res 45:2110, 1985.
80. Lehnert S, Greene D, Batist G. Radiation response of drug-resistant variants of a human breast cancer cell line. Radiat Res 118:568, 1989.
81. Russo A, Mitchell JB. Radiation response of Chinese hamster cells after elevation of intracellular glutathione levels. Int J Radiat Oncol Biol Phys 10:1243, 1984.
82. Vos O, Roos-Verhey WSD. Endogenous versus exogenous thiols in radioprotection. Pharmacol Ther 39:169, 1988.
83. Hopwood LE, Moulder JE. Radiation induction of drug resistance in RIF-1 tumors and tumor cells. Radiat Res 120:251, 1989.
84. Sharma RC, Schimke RT. Enchancement of the frequency of methotrexate resistance by gamma radiation in Chinese hamster ovary and mouse 3T6 cells. Cancer Res 49:3861, 1989.
85. Osmak M, Perovic S. Multiple fractions of gamma rays induced resistance to cis-dichlorodiammineplatinum (II) and methotrexate in human HeLa cells. Int J Radiat Oncol Biol Phys 16:1537, 1989.
86. Habraken Y, Lavel F. Enhancement of 1,3-bis(2-chloroethyl)-1-nitrosourea resistance by g-irradiation or drug pretreatment in rat hepatoma cells. Cancer Res 51:1217, 1991.

87. Hill BT, Deuchars K, Hosking LK, et al. Overexpression of p-glycoprotein in mammalian tumor cell lines after fractionated X irradiation in vitro. J Natl Cancer Inst 82:607, 1990.
88. Howard A, Pelc S. Synthesis of deoxyribonucleic acid in normal and irradiated cells and its relation to chromosome breakage. Heredity 6:261, 1953.
89. Mendelsohn ML. Chronic infusion of tritiated thymidine into mice with tumors. Science 135:213, 1962.
90. Mendelsohn ML. Autoradiographic analysis of cell proliferation in spontaneous breast cancer of C3H mouse. III. Growth fraction. J Natl Cancer Inst 28:1015, 1962.
91. Terasima R, Tolmach LJ. X-ray sensitivity and DNA synthesis in synchronous populations of HeLa cells. Science 140:490, 1963.
92. Sinclair WK. Hydroxyurea: Differential lethal effects on cultured mammalian cells during the cell cycle. Science 150:1729, 1965.
93. Krakoff IH. Inhibition of ribonucleoside diphosphate reductase by hydroxyurea. Cancer Res 28:1559, 1968.
94. Sinclair WK. The combined effect of hydroxyurea and x-rays on Chinese hamster cells in vitro. Cancer Res 28:198, 1968.
95. Elkind MM, Redpath JL. Molecular and cellular biology of radiation lethality. *In:* Cancer: A Comprehensive Treatise. Becker FF (Ed). New York, Plenum Publishing Corp., 1977, p. 51.
96. Gillette EL, Withers HR, Tannock IF. The age sensitivity of epithelial cells of mouse small intestine. Radiology 96:639, 1970.
97. Madoc-Jones H, Mauro F. Age responses in x-rays, vinca alkaloids, and hydroxyurea of murine lymphoma cells synchronized in vivo. J Natl Cancer Inst 45:1131, 1970.
98. Hermens AF, Barendsen GW. Changes of cell proliferation characteristics in a rat rhabdomyosarcoma before and after x-irradiation. Eur J Cancer 5:173, 1969.
99. Durand RE, Vanderbyl SL. Tumor resistance to therapy: A genetic or kinetic problem? Cancer Commun 1:277, 1989.
100. Painter RB, Drew RM. Studies on deoxyribonucleic acid metabolism in human cancer cell cultures (HeLa). 1. The temporal relationships of deoxyribonucleic acid synthesis to mitosis and turnover time. Lab Invest 8:278, 1959.
101. Quastler H, Sherman FG. Cell population kinetics in the intestinal epithelium of the mouse. Exp Cell Res 17:420, 1959.
102. DeVita VT, Young RC. Cell cycle characteristics of human solid tumors. Cell Tissue Kinet 3:285, 1970.
103. Gratzner H. Monoclonal antibody against 5-bromo- and 5-iododeoxyuridine: A new reagent for detection of DNA replication. Science 218:474, 1982.
104. Mortyn G, Pyke K, Gardner J, et al. Immunohistochemical identification of proliferating cells in organ culture using bromodeoxyuridine and a monoclonal antibody. J Histochem Cytochem 34:697, 1986.
105. Gray JW, Dolbeare F, Pallavicini MG, et al. Cell cycle analysis using flow cytometry. Int J Radiat Biol Phys 49:237, 1986.
106. Gerdes J, Schwab U, Lemke H, Stein H. Production of a mouse monoclonal antibody reactive with a human nuclear antigen associated with cell proliferation. Int J Cancer 31:13, 1983.
107. Nakamura H, Morita T, Masaki S, Yoshida S. Intracellular localization and metabolism of DNA polymerase alpha in human cells visualized with monoclonal antibody. Exp Cell Res 151:123, 1984.
108. Shapiro HM. Practical Flow Cytometry. New York, Alan R. Liss, 1985.
109. Inoue S. Ideo Microscopy. New York, Plenum Press, 1987.
110. Thomlinson RH, Gray LH. The histological structure of some human lung cancers and the possible implications for radiotherapy. Br J Cancer 9:539, 1955.
111. Powers WE, Tolmach LJ. A multicomponent x-ray survival curve for mouse lymphosarcoma cells irradiated in vivo. Nature 197:710, 1963.
112. Adams GE, Stratford IJ. Hypoxia-mediated nitro-heterocyclic drugs in the radio- and chemotherapy of cancer. Biochem Pharmacol 35:71, 1986.
113. Teicher BA, Lazo JS, Sartorelli AC. Classification of antineoplastic agents by their selective toxicities toward oxygenated and hypoxic tumor cells. Cancer Res 41:73, 1981.
114. Gupta V, Costanzi JJ. Role of hypoxia in anticancer drug-induced cytotoxicity for Ehrlich ascites cells. Cancer Res 47:2407, 1987.
115. Siemann DW, Chapman M, Beikirch A. Effects of oxygenation and pH on tumor cell response to alkylating chemotherapy. Int J Radiat Oncol Biol Phys 20:287, 1991.
116. Chapman JD, Franko AJ, Sharplin J. A marker for hypoxic cells in tumors with potential clinical applicability. Br J Cancer 43:546, 1981.
117. Hodgkiss RJ, Jones G, Long A, et al. Flow cytometric evaluation of hypoxic cells in solid experimental tumours using fluorescence immunodetection. Br J Cancer 63:119, 1991.

118. Roos A, Boron WF. Intracellular pH. Physiol Rev 61:296, 1981.
119. Warburg OH. Colon Metabolism Tumors. London, Constable Publ., 1930.
120. Weinhouse S. On respiratory impairment in cancer cells. Science 124:267, 1956.
121. Calderwood SK, Dickson JA. A pH and tumor response to hyperthermia. Adv Radiat Biol 10:135, 1983.
122. Thistlethwaite AJ, Leeper DB, Moylan DJ, Nerlinger RE. pH distribution in human tumors. Int J Radiat Oncol Biol Phys 11:1647, 1985.
123. Tannock IF, Rotin D. Acid pH in tumors and its potential for therapeutic exploitation. Cancer Res 49:4373, 1989.
124. Eagle H. The effect of environmental pH on the growth of normal and malignant cells. J Cell Physiol 82:1, 1973.
125. Tannock IF. Experimental chemotherapy and concepts related to the cell cycle. Int J Radiat Oncol Biol Phys 49:335, 1986.
126. Musgrove E, Seaman M, Hedley D. Relationship between cytoplasmic pH and proliferation during exponential growth and cellular quiescence. Exp Cell Res 172:65, 1987.
127. Vaupel P, Okunieff P, Kallinowshi F, Neuringer LJ. Correlations between 31P-NMR spectroscopy and tissue O_2 tension measurements in a murine fibrosarcoma. Radiat Res 120:477, 1989.
128. Li GC, Hahn GM. Ethanol-induced tolerance to head and adriamycin. Nature (London) 274:699, 1978.
129. Cook JA, Fox MH. Effects of chronic pH 6.6 on growth, intracellular pH, and response to 42/C hyperthermia of Chinese hamster ovary cells. Cancer Res 48:2417, 1988.
130. Rice GC, Bump EA, Shrieve DC. Quantitative analysis of cellular glutathione by flow cytometry utilizing monochlorobimane: Some applications to radiation and drug resistance in vitro and in vivo. Cancer Res 46:6105, 1986.
131. Sinclair WK: Hydroxyurea revisited: A decade of clinical effects studies. Int J Radiat Oncol Biol Phys 7:631, 1981.
132. Cook JA, Pass H, Russo A. Use of monochlorobimane for glutathione measurements in hamster and human tumor cell lines. Int J Radiat Oncol Biol Phys 16:1321, 1989.

Part III

CLINICAL APPLICATIONS

Chapter 14

HEAD AND NECK

SAMUEL G. TAYLOR AND ANANTHA K. MURTHY

EPIDEMIOLOGY

It is estimated that cancer of the upper aerodigestive tracts afflicted 42,800 Americans in 1992, and over 11,600 patients died (1). Approximately 60% of patients with cancer of the upper aerodigestive tract present with advanced disease. The characteristically late presentation of this cancer occurs despite the frequent history of physician contact within the preceding year. Many such patients have had illnesses relating to alcohol and/or tobacco abuse, leading them to medical consultation. A brief oral inspection, mirror examination, and palpation of the oropharyngeal area of such high-risk patients would undoubtedly lead to early diagnosis and treatment. Unfortunately, few internists and family practice physicians are trained to do this. Until the medical profession insists upon such screening, earlier diagnosis of these cancers is unlikely.

More than 95% of cancers of the head and neck are of squamous histology. These are commonly cancers developing after a long history of alcohol and tobacco abuse. Epidemiologic studies support the need for combined alcohol and tobacco use for maximal carcinogenic effect, in contrast to cancers of the lung or esophagus, which appear primarily dependent on only tobacco or alcohol exposure, respectively (2). Another contributing factor is poor dentition, presumably due to chronic irritation and infection. Sinus and paranasal cancers are an exception to this general rule; exposure to wood dust and heavy metal fumes appears to be an occupational hazard that plays a role in the carcinogenesis of these tumors.

Nasopharyngeal cancers are well recognized for their common occurrence in the Orient. Here, an association with consumption of smoked fish products at an early age may be important (3). Less well recognized in the United States is the common occurrence of these cancers in the middle eastern regions. These cancers have a high prevalence of the Epstein-Barr viral genome in epithelial cells. In North America, monitoring such patients with the IgA antiviral capsid antigen (VCA) appears to be most specific, with 83% of patients with nonkeratinizing carcinomas having positive serum tests (4).

Another endemic upper aerodigestive tract cancer is squamous cell carcinoma of the oral cavity in India. These cancers characteristically involve the buccal mucosa or anterior tongue. They are well differentiated and slow to metastasize, even to regional nodes. Their etiology is based on the local population's habits of placing various concoctions of betel nut and/or tobacco quid in the mouth, often to be left for several days at a time, as well as the use of inverse smoking along with poor nutrition and dental caries.

It should be appreciated that while the above considerations account for the overwhelming majority of patients with head and neck cancer, these cancers can occur without such history or risk factors. In the United States, such cancers tend to occur in younger individuals or as isolated events, usually involving the tongue or oropharynx. They generally carry a poor prognosis, at least in part because of the absence of suspicion by physicians and consequent late diagnosis.

CONVENTIONAL TREATMENT APPROACHES

Stage I and II cancers of the upper aerodigestive tracts are usually treated by radiation or surgery; cure rates are in the 60 to 90% range. Choice of treatment and results are dependent on the site of origin of the cancer and the expertise of the radiation oncologist and surgeon. Exceptions to the generally good prognosis of Stage I and II head and neck cancers are Stage II cancers involving the tongue, hypopharynx (especially the posterior wall), and nasopharyngeal carcinomas having squamous differentiation. These cancers usually have survival rates of less than 70% with single-modality therapy. More advanced cancers have progressively worse results, even with combined-modality therapy. The Radiation Therapy Oncology Group (RTOG) registry provides a resource for expected survival data based on TNM staging and performance status (5).

For regionally advanced head and neck cancer, results of treatment come from numerous reports of combined surgery and radiation or Phase II studies of chemotherapy with surgery and radiation. Unfortunately, these comprise clearly distinct patient populations that make cross-comparison impossible. Most series, including Stage III and IV patients, have median survivals of approximately 18 months. Randomized Phase III studies may be more representative, even though they often involve highly selected patient populations. Median survivals of most randomized trials range from 8 to 18 months, with worse survival in series that include unresectable cancers.

A major limitation of treatment in this patient population is the unwillingness or inability of these patients to complete the planned treatment. Multimodality therapy in sequence leads to up to 30% dropout rates for each subsequent modality (6,7). Such considerations must temper future treatment programs.

CHEMORADIATION EXPERIENCE

Head and neck cancers are a fascinating model to study the interaction of chemotherapy and radiation. These cancers are predominantly regional problems. Whether surgery is deemed a part of treatment or not, virtually all regionally advanced (Stage III and IV, M_0) cancers are treated with radiation therapy. Chemotherapy has been added in every conceivable schedule to attempt to improve results over regional therapy alone. While innumerable Phase II or pilot studies have been performed to test the feasibility and promise of one approach or another, the recognition of the real merits or deficiencies of a therapy are best derived from controlled comparative clinical trials.

Since its first use as an adjuvant treatment in head and neck cancer in the early 1960s, chemotherapy has been used either combined with radiation (simultaneous treatment) or given prior to regional therapy (induction therapy). Two separate expectations have been articulated over the years. The first hope is that chemotherapy might improve survival (cure) of such patients; the second is that chemotherapy might lessen the toxicity of treatment by limiting surgery. The results of sequential and concurrent chemoradiation must be reviewed in light of these two expectations, to guide the development of future strategies in the treatment of advanced head and neck cancers.

Induction Chemotherapy

Survival Impact

It is well recognized that response to induction chemotherapy correlates with subsequent prognosis. This is true of single-agent or combination chemotherapy. The significance of this observation, however, has been subject to misinterpretation. In order to understand the impact of chemotherapy on survival, one needs to evaluate the results of induction chemotherapy in all patients in each trial. For example, in the Wayne State experience, complete responders to chemotherapy had an excellent survival of 37 months (double the expected survival with surgery and radiation alone) (8). However, patients with a partial response had only an 8-month median survival and nonresponders had a 6-month survival. While the results in complete responders are considerably better than expected from regional treatment alone, the results in the remaining patients are worse than expected, even for unresectable patients. As overall survival reflects a composite of all of these response categories, it is not clear from uncontrolled trials whether chemotherapy improves, worsens, or has no overall treatment effect.

Independent of any impact by induction chemotherapy on treatment results, the observation that good responders to induction chemotherapy do much better than expected while poor responders do worse indicates that chemotherapy response successfully identifies a favorable patient population. This selection may be made by identifying patients with cancers that are particularly radiation responsive. Indeed, studies with cisplatinum and radiation suggest cross-sensitivity and cross-resistance (9,10). This may also explain the poor response to radiation observed in nonresponders to cisplatinum-based drug combinations (11).

Figure 14–1 summarizes the impact of induction chemotherapy on survival in randomized trials (6,7,12–20). Methotrexate is the only drug to have been tested in a randomized study design as a single agent with survival results. One trial indicated significant benefit for intra-arterial methotrexate, due to benefit in early-stage oral cavity lesions but not in Stage III and IV disease (13). Other trials show no (or very limited) advantage to neoadjuvant methotrexate in an

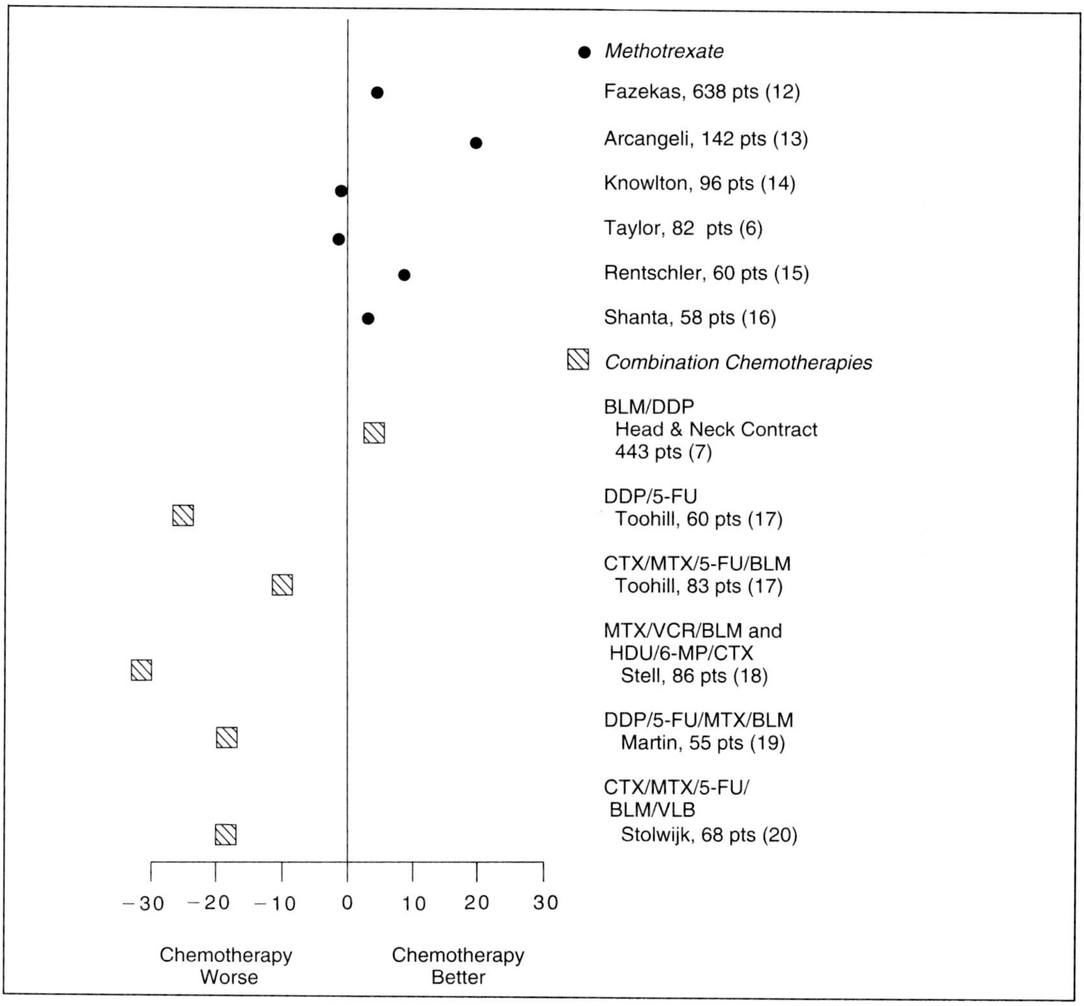

Fig. 14–1. The difference between the percentage survival of patient groups treated with induction chemotherapy minus that of their controls in randomized trials testing various induction chemotherapy regimens that have reported survival results.

apparently random distribution. Results with multidrug combinations, whether cisplatinum-, bleomycin-, or methotrexate-based, have unfortunately been consistently worse than controls (Fig. 14–1). These results indicate that neoadjuvant chemotherapy in its current form cannot be expected to improve survival of advanced head and neck cancers.

Limiting Surgery

One early rationale for giving chemotherapy prior to regional treatment (induction chemotherapy) was to cause tumor shrinkage that might enable resection of a previously unresectable cancer or that might reduce the extent of surgery. It was quickly realized, however, that while often dramatic, tumor shrinkage did not involve a predictable centripetal destruction of tumor cells. Compromise on surgical margins was consequently thought to be detrimental despite the response to induction chemotherapy.

This rationale was recently modified on the basis of the observation that a major response to induction chemotherapy may allow excellent disease control with radiation alone, avoiding all surgery. We attribute the first reference to this possibility to Ervin et al, who noted that responders to chemotherapy, with less than 3 cm of residual tumor bulk, appeared to have no additional benefit from including surgery as a part of regional treatment; however, patients with larger residual tumor masses did appear to benefit from surgical resection in addition to radiation therapy (21). Clearly, radiation therapy would be expected to have a higher sterilization potential with smaller residual tumor bulk. This fact alone would suggest that chemotherapy responders might be more likely to be controllable with radiation therapy due to downstaging. Ensley et al provided a further rationale for this selection criteria. They noted that 42 of 43 patients with a partial response to chemotherapy subsequently had further response to radiation, compared to only 1 of 18 nonresponders to induction chemotherapy (11). Thus, response to chemotherapy appears to indicate an increased sensitivity by the cancer to radiation.

Jacobs et al piloted this concept by prospectively treating all complete responders to induction chemotherapy with radiation alone, avoiding surgery in 40% of their series (22). The 2-year survival of all operable patients was 53%. Those patients who had a complete response and avoided surgery had a 2-year survival of 70%. The survival was not stated for patients with a lesser response who underwent surgery.

The larynx and tongue are crucial to speech and swallowing. Avoiding resection of these structures can be an enormous functional benefit to patients. One study specifically directed to preservation of laryngeal function has been the Veterans Administration Cooperative Group study, which randomized patients to traditional surgery and radiation or to two cycles of induction cisplatinum plus 5-fluorouracil (5-FU) chemotherapy followed by reassessment (23). Responders proceeded to a third cycle followed by radiation with surgical salvage. Nonresponders proceeded to surgery and radiation. Preliminary results showed that only 15% of patients randomized to induction chemotherapy initially failed to respond, requiring immediate surgery. Preservation of the larynx with subsequent follow-up has occurred in 64% of the chemotherapy group, with similar overall failure rates (25% with surgery and 31% with chemotherapy). Two-year survival was identical (68%). These results indicate that while induction chemotherapy has failed to improve survival, it may identify a subset of patients able to avoid surgery and thus improve the toxicity of treatment, at least in that subset.

Concurrent/Alternating Chemoradiation

Chemotherapy has been integrated into radiation treatment by either giving it simultaneously with radiation or by alternating both treatments, with the course of radiation interrupted for short cycles of chemotherapy. Both schedules have demonstrated benefit over radiation alone or induction chemotherapy plus radiation in randomized trials. While combined chemotherapy and radiation programs have been less well studied as ways for limiting surgery, improved regional control would logically be expected to enable a reduction in ablative surgery.

Survival Impact

Several single agents have been used concomitantly with radiation in comparison with radiation alone. Positive studies with improved disease-free status have been reported with bleomycin (16,24), methotrexate (25), 5-FU (26,27), and mitomycin C (28). A summary of findings is shown in Figure 14–2 (16,24–27,29–37). For bleomycin, methotrexate, and 5-FU, positive results were obtained when some compromise in the therapy was made either by reducing the dose or frequency of administration.

Both bleomycin and methotrexate improved disease control and tended to benefit survival when given at a dosage that would not be anticipated to have any independent antineoplastic effect. Methotrexate was used at a dose of 50 mg/m^2 for two treatments, spaced 2 weeks apart, on days 0 and 14 of radiation. Much higher dose-intense regimens, given prior to radiation, had no effect (see Figure 14–1). Bleomycin given at a dose of 5 u/m^2 twice weekly caused little increase in toxicity or interruption in the radiation course but appeared to act as a radiation enhancer (24), while higher dosages caused more toxicity without benefit (29).

With mitomycin C, full-dose therapy of both chemotherapy and radiation was possible (28). This trial included several patient subgroups of inoperable and postoperative disease status. Regional disease control was improved with the addition of mitomycin C (75% vs. 55%, $p < 0.01$). Survival was not

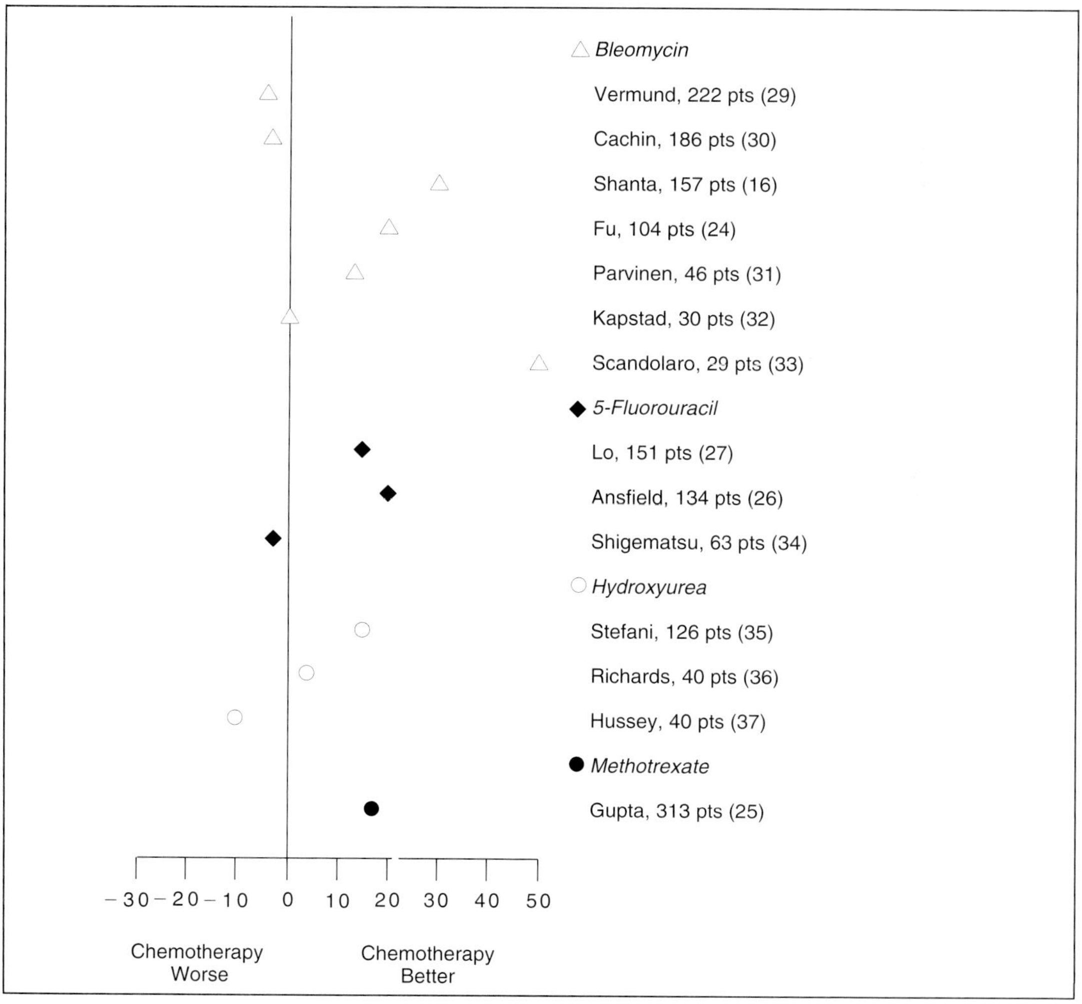

Fig. 14–2. The difference between the percentage survival of patient groups treated with concomitant chemotherapy and radiation therapy minus that of their control groups given radiation alone in randomized trials that have reported survival results.

significantly affected, however (48% vs. 40%) (28).

Recently, cisplatinum has shown benefit when given concomitantly with radiation postoperatively to high-risk patients (38). Eighty-eight patients with extracapsular nodal spread of cancer were given cisplatinum (50 mg weekly) plus radiation or radiation alone. With a 36-month median follow-up, 2-year disease-free survival was 65% and 41%, respectively ($p < 0.01$), and disease-related survival was 75% and 44% ($p < 0.05$). While this study used a fixed-dose regimen, it was a higher total dose than that used by the American intergroup study of cisplatinum (20 mg/m^2 weekly) plus radiation. That latter study has never been reported but has been described as negative by its study chairman (39). These two studies, as well as encouraging results from a pilot study of cisplatinum (100 mg/m^2 every 3 weeks) (40), suggest that the dose of cisplatinum may be important for its interaction with radiation.

Misonidazole is the only radiation sensitizer that has completed testing in head and neck cancers (41–43). All randomized studies have failed to show a benefit in over 1000 cases treated. New studies are ongoing with second-generation agents.

Alternating chemotherapy and radiation has also demonstrated superiority over the same chemotherapy given as induction treatment prior to conventional, uninterrupted radiation (44,45). Merlano recently published 4-year survival results of their randomized study of 116 patients given induction vinblastine, bleomycin, and methotrexate for four cycles, followed by 7000 cGy radiation or the same four cycles of chemotherapy with 2000 cGy of radiation over 2 weeks, given following the second, third, and fourth cycles (6000 cGy total). The difference in 4-year survival, favoring the alternating regimen (10% versus 22%), was significant ($p < 0.02$) (44). These results and those of a similarly designed trial from the South East Cooperative Oncology Group (SECOG) in England (45) are shown in Table 14–1.

While most radiation oncologists are reluctant to have planned interruptions in radiation, these studies show that such interruptions, when integrated with chemotherapy, improve efficacy over conventional radiation alone. The favorable results from these studies should open the way for further exploration of interrupted radiation schedules and other means of optimally integrating chemotherapy with radiation.

Since 1981, we have used a combination of cisplatinum, 5-FU infusion, and radiation given concomitantly on a split-course basis. Radiation was given only during chemotherapy, and both were given for 5 days with one week of rest. The actual schedule was cisplatinum (60 mg/m^2) on day 1, 5-FU (800 mg/m^2) continuous infusion on days 1 to 5 (120 hours), and radiation (200 cGy) on days 1 to 5, all given every other week for a total of seven cycles (7000 cGy) (46). This schedule was based on one developed by Byfield et al to integrate 5-FU with radiation (47). They had previously found that giving 5-FU in high doses and at an exposure for 24 hours after each radiation treatment was im-

Table 14–1. Induction Versus Alternating Chemotherapy and Radiation

Study	Number Patients	Survival (%) Disease Free		Overall	
Merlano (43)					
BVM × 4→7000 cGy	55	4	p<0.04	10	p<0.02
BVM→(BVM→2000 cGy) × 3	61	12		22	
SECOG (42)					
BOM × 2→6000 cGy→BOM × 2	131	14	p=0.02	32	NS
(BOM→2000 cGy) × 3→BOM	136	24		33	

Abbreviations: B = bleomycin, V = vinblastine, M = methotrexate, O = vincristine, NS = not significant.

portant for synergistic effect (48). Some kind of interrupted radiation schedule had first been suggested as an outgrowth of a randomized trial with 5-FU and radiation (49). The authors noted better survival with combined treatment in base-of-tongue lesions, despite more radiation interruptions and lower total dose delivered, and suggested that future combined treatment programs should use planned interruptions.

Toxicity from this treatment was primarily mucosal toxicity occurring during the "off" week. This usually subsided by the start of treatment the next week and was controllable by adjusting the 5-FU dosage. Residual painful soreness or a white blood cell count less than 2,000 required a treatment delay of an additional week. Weight loss was substantial, with a mean loss of 10% of initial weight. This was due to a combination of radiation effects plus nausea and anorexia from cisplatinum and 5-FU mucosal toxicity. Approximately 10% of patients required some intervention with forced-feeding procedures. However, we have found this weight loss not to be significantly different from sequential treatment in our ongoing randomized study.

Our results in 53 inoperable patients (15% Stage III and the rest Stage IV or recurrent) followed for a median of over 4 years showed that all patients responded, with the exception of one patient who developed a stroke during his second cycle and was not reevaluated (46). Although 43% of patients had a partial response by clinical assessment, the residual abnormality did not represent persistent disease in many of these patients, as survival of partial responders was not substantially different from that of complete responders. Only 25% of patients have had any regional failure. The median survival of all patients was 37 months. This overall survival was equal to the survival of those patients in the Wayne State series (8) who had a complete response to induction cisplatinum and 5-FU.

We regard the composite of randomized trials in the literature as showing convincing evidence that integration of chemotherapy with radiation achieves superior survival results over radiation alone. While trials establishing this have used single drugs with radiation, integration of currently active drug combinations such as cisplatinum and 5-FU have even greater potential promise. In order to successfully integrate such drug combinations, however, modification of both radiation scheduling and drug dosage for acceptable toxicity appears crucial. This requires substantial cooperation and trust between radiation oncologists and medical oncologists.

Limiting Surgery

Concomitant chemotherapy and radiation regimens have normally been used in unresectable patients and have only recently been analyzed as a technique for preserving speech or swallowing function. We have examined our pilot study of concomitant chemotherapy and radiation to evaluate its effect on preservation of tongue and laryngeal function and subsequent survival. As our patients were all considered inoperable, this analysis is hypothetical. Because they were inoperable and included hypopharyngeal and locally advanced (T3 and 4) tongue lesions, they would consequently be expected to have a considerably worse prognosis than the VA study patients described above (23). There were 28 patients who fulfilled the criteria of either requiring more than a hemiglossectomy (12 T3 or T4 tongue lesions) or requiring laryngectomy (6 T3 or T4 larynx and 10 T3 or T4 hypopharyngeal lesions) to encompass the tumor surgically. Two of these patients subsequently underwent surgery, with a limited partial glossectomy in one patient who had presented with a T4 base-of-tongue lesion, and a laryngectomy in another patient with a T4 hypopharyngeal lesion. Two more patients have had subsequent laryngectomies: one for an incompetent larynx due to local tissue destruction from a T4 supraglottic laryngeal cancer, and one due to recurrence at 18 months. Thus, 86% of patients had preservation of speech and/or swallowing function. There were seven (25%) regional failures, including one patient who was surgically salvaged. Median survival of the 28 patients, based on a Kaplan Meier estimate, was 45 months.

Evaluating these results another way, 17 of the 53 patients had Stage III or IV disease but did not have T4 or N3 disease. None of these patients had surgery; only two experienced recurrence, while an additional three patients died of a cerebral occlusion, emphysema, and a cardiac event, respectively. Survival is 71% with minimum 2-year follow-up (median 4 years).

These results indicate that chemotherapy and radiation should be at least as effective as surgery and radiation in resectable head and neck cancers. While a trial comparing surgery plus radiation therapy vs. chemotherapy and radiation is likely to be years away, current information indicates that the justification for such a trial is at hand.

CONCLUSIONS

Controlled clinical trials have shown various chemotherapy agents, given concomitantly with radiation, to be superior to radiation alone. These trials suggest that the main effect of chemotherapy is due to enhancement effects from interaction with radiation rather than due to additive antineoplastic effect:

1. Marked dose modification of chemotherapy to nontherapeutic levels has resulted in significant benefit with methotrexate (25) and bleomycin (24).
2. Giving more intensive chemotherapy combinations immediately prior to radiation (induction chemotherapy) has failed to produce any such benefit.
3. The benefit from concomitant treatment has been predominantly on regional control and not on the incidence of metastatic disease.

A further possibility is that the incidence of distant metastases may be reduced by adjuvant treatment given after regional therapy (7). While true adjuvant chemotherapy has had poor acceptance by both physicians and patients after regional treatment, such evidence would suggest that this approach may be promising. Outcome of the current randomized intergroup study testing cisplatinum and 5-FU after surgery will be important in defining this possibility.

Upper aerodigestive tract cancer remains predominantly a local problem, however, both in the risk of treatment failure and in treatment-related toxicity. Consequently, further exploration of concomitant treatment seems the most fruitful means of impacting both regional control and reduced regional toxicity by reducing the need for surgical intervention. Clearly, positive benefit found in randomized trials extending over the past two decades indicates that the addition of chemotherapy to regional treatment with radiation alters cure rates and thus survival in head and neck cancers.

REFERENCES

1. Boring CC, Squires TS, Tong T. Cancer Statistics, 1992. CA 42(1):19, 1992.
2. Blot WJ, McLaughlin JK, Winn DM, et al. Smoking and drinking in relation to oral and pharyngeal cancer. Cancer Res 48:382, 1988.
3. Yu MC, Ho JHC, Lai SH, Henderson BE. Cantonese-style salted fish as a cause of nasopharyngeal carcinoma: Report of a case-control study in Hong Kong. Cancer Res 46:956, 1986.
4. Pearson GR, Weiland HL, Neel HB III, et al. Application of Epstein-Barr virus (EBV) serology to the diagnosis of North American nasopharyngeal carcinoma. Cancer 51:260, 1983.
5. Pajak TF, Fazekas JT, Davis LW, Marcial VA. Analysis of Radiation Therapy Oncology Group head and neck database: Identification of prognostic factors and the re-evaluation of American Joint Committee staging system. *In:* Head and Neck Cancer. Vogl SE (Ed). New York, Churchill, Livingston Publishers, 1988, p. 41.
6. Taylor SG IV, Applebaum E, Showel JL, et al. A randomized trial of adjuvant chemotherapy in head and neck cancer. J Clin Oncol 3:672, 1985.
7. Head and Neck Contracts Program: Adjuvant chemotherapy for advanced head and neck squamous carcinoma: Final report of the Head and Neck Contracts Program. Cancer 60:301, 1987.
8. Jacobs JR, Weaver A, Ahmed K, et al. Protochemotherapy in advanced head and neck cancer. Head Neck 10:93, 1987.
9. Louie KG, Behrens BC, Kinsella TJ, et al. Radiation survival parameters of antineoplastic drug-sensitive and resistant human ovarian cancer cell lines and their modification by buthione sulfoximine. Cancer Res 45:2110, 1985.
10. Wallner KE, Li GC. Effect of cisplatin resistance on cellular radiation response. Int J Radiat Oncol Biol Phys 13:587, 1987.
11. Ensley JR, Jacobs JR, Weaver A, et al. Correlation between response to cisplatinum-combination chemotherapy and subsequent radiotherapy in previously untreated patients

with advanced squamous cell cancers of the head and neck. Cancer 545:811, 1984.
12. Fazekas JT, Sommer C, Kramer S. Adjuvant intravaneous methotrexate or definitive radiotherapy alone for advanced squamous cancers of the oral cavity, oropharynx, supraglottic larynx, or hypopharynx. Int J Radiat Oncol Biol Phys 6:533, 1980.
13. Arcangeli G, Nervi C, Righini R, et al. Combined radiation and drugs: The effect of intraarterial chemotherapy followed by radiotherapy in head and neck cancer. Radiother Oncol 1:101, 1983.
14. Knowlton AH, Percarpio B, Bobrow S, Fischer JJ. Methotrexate and radiation therapy in the treatment of advanced head and neck tumors. Radiology 116:709, 1975.
15. Rentschler RE, Wilbur DW, Petti GH, et al. Adjuvant methotrexate escalated to toxicity for resectable stage III and IV squamous head and neck carcinomas—a prospective randomized study. J Clin Oncol 5:278, 1987.
16. Shanta V, Krishnamurthi S. Combined bleomycin and radiotherapy in oral cancer. Clin Radiol 31:617, 1980.
17. Toohill RJ, Duncavage JA, Malin TC, et al. The effects of delay in standard treatment due to induction chemotherapy in two randomized prospective studies. Laryngoscope 97:407, 1987.
18. Stell PM, Dalby JE, Strickland P, et al. Sequential chemotherapy and radiotherapy in advanced head and neck cancer. Clin Radiol 34:463, 1983.
19. Martin M, Mazeron JJ, Glaubiger D, et al. Neoadjuvant polychemotherapy of head and neck cancer: Preliminary results of a randomized study. Proc Am Soc Clin Oncol 5:141, 1986.
20. Stolwijk C, Wagener DJ, VanDenBroek P, et al. Randomized adjuvant chemotherapy trial for advanced head and neck cancer. Neth J Med 28:347, 1983.
21. Ervin TJ, Weichselbaum RR, Fabian RL, et al. Advanced squamous carcinoma of the head and neck. Arch Otolaryngol Head Neck Surg 110:241, 1984.
22. Jacobs C, Goffinet DR, Goffinet L, et al. Chemotherapy as a substitute for surgery in the treatment of advanced head and neck cancer. Cancer 60:1178, 1987.
23. Wolf GT, Fisher SG, Hong WK, et al for The Department of Veterans Affairs, Laryngeal Cancer Study Group. Induction chemotherapy plus radiation compared to surgery plus radiation in patients with advanced laryngeal cancer. N Engl J Med 324:1685, 1991.
24. Fu KK, Phillips TL, Silverberg IJ, et al. Combined radiotherapy and chemotherapy with bleomycin and methotrexate for advanced inoperable head and neck cancer: Update of a Northern California Oncology Group randomized trial. J Clin Oncol 5:1410, 1987.
25. Gupta NK, Pointon RCS, Wilkinson PM. A randomized clinical trial to contrast radiotherapy with radiotherapy and methotrexate given synchronously in head and neck cancer. Clin Radiol 38:575, 1987.
26. Ansfield FJ, Ramirez G, Davis HL Jr, et al. Treatment of advanced cancer of the head and neck. Cancer 25:78, 1970.
27. Lo TCM, Wiley AL Jr, Ansfield FJ, et al. Combined radiation therapy and 5-fluorouracil for advanced squamous cell carcinoma of the oral cavity and oropharynx: A randomized study. Am J Roentgenol 126:229, 1976.
28. Weissberg JB, Son YH, Papac RJ, et al. Randomized clinical trial of mitomycin-C as an adjunct to radiotherapy in head and neck cancer. Int J Radiat Oncol Biol Phys 17:3, 1989.
29. Vermund H, Kaalhus O, Winther F, et al. Bleomycin and radiation therapy in squamous cell carcinoma of the upper aero-digestive tract: A phase III clinical trial. Int J Radiat Oncol Biol Phys 11:1877, 1985.
30. Cachin Y, Jortay A, Sanchco H, et al. Preliminary results of a randomized E.O.R.T.C. study comparing radiotherapy and concomitant bleomycin, to radiotherapy alone in epidermoid carcinomas of the oropharynx. Eur J Cancer Clin Oncol 13:1389, 1977.
31. Parvinen LM, Parvinen M, Nordman E, Kortekangas AE. Combined bleomycin treatment and radiation therapy in squamous cell carcinoma of the head and neck region. Acta Radiol 24:487, 1985.
32. Kapstad B, Bang G, Rennaes S, Dahler A. Combined preoperative treatment with cobalt and bleomycin in patients with head and neck carcinoma—A controlled clinical study. Int J Radiat Oncol Biol Phys 4:85, 1978.
33. Scandolaro L, Bertoni F. Tolleranza cutanea e mucosa e risposte cliniche a breve termine nella associazione tra radioterapia e bleomycin a per tumori del distretto cervico-cefalico. Acta Otorhinolaryngol Ital 2:213, 1982.
34. Shigematsu Y, Sakai S, Fuchihata H. Recent trials in the treatment of maxillary sinus carcinoma with special reference to the chemical potentiation of radiation therapy. Acta Otolaryngol 71:63, 1971.
35. Stefani S, Eells RW, Abbate J. Hydroxyurea and radiotherapy in head and neck cancer. Radiology 101:391, 1971.
36. Richards GJ Jr, Chambers RG. Hydroxyurea in the treatment of neoplasms of the head and neck. Am J Surg 126:513, 1973.
37. Hussey DH, Abrams JP. Combined therapy in advanced head and neck cancer: Hydrox-

yurea and radiotherapy. Prog Clin Cancer 6:79, 1975.
38. Bachaud JM, David JM, Boussin G, Daly N. Combined postoperative radiotherapy and weekly cisplatin infusion for locally advanced squamous cell carcinoma of the head and neck: Preliminary report of a randomized trial. Int J Radiat Oncol Biol Phys 20:243, 1991.
39. Haselow RE. Personal communication, 1990.
40. Al-Sarraf M, Pajak TF, Marcial VA, et al. Concurrent radiotherapy and chemotherapy with cisplatin in inoperable squamous cell carcinoma of the head and neck. Cancer 59:259, 1987.
41. MRC Working Party on Misonidazole in Head and Neck Cancer. A study of the effect of misonidazole in conjunction with radiotherapy for the treatment of head and neck cancer. Br J Radiol 57:585, 1984.
42. Sealy R, Cridland S, Barry L, Norris R. Irradiation with misonidazole and hyperbaric oxygen: Final report on a randomized trial in advanced head and neck cancer. Int J Radiat Oncol Biol Phys 12:1343, 1986.
43. Lee DJ, Pajak TF, Stetz J, et al. A phase I/II study of the hypoxic cell sensitizer misonidazole as an adjunct to a high fractional dose radiotherapy in patients with unresectable squamous cell carcinoma of the head and neck: An RTOG randomized study (#79-04). Int J Radiat Oncol Biol Phys 16:465, 1989.
44. Merlano M, Rosso R, Sertoli MR, et al. Randomized comparison of two chemotherapy, radiotherapy schemes for stage III and IV unresectable squamous cell carcinoma of the head and neck. Laryngoscope 100:531, 1990.
45. Clifford P, Durden-Smith DJ, Peto J. A randomized trial of combined multidrug chemotherapy and radiotherapy in advanced squamous cell carcinoma of the head and neck. An interim report from the SECOG participants. Eur J Surg Oncol 12:289, 1986.
46. Taylor SG, Murthy AK, Caldarelli DD, et al. Combined simultaneous cisplatin/5-FU infusion chemotherapy and split course radiation in head and neck cancer. J Clin Oncol 17:846, 1989.
47. Byfield JE, Sharp TR, Frankell SS, et al. Phase I and II trial of five-day infused 5-fluorouracil and radiation in advanced cancer of the head and neck. J Clin Oncol 2:406, 1984.
48. Byfield JE, Calabro-Jones PM, Klisak I, et al. Pharmacologic requirements for obtaining sensitization of human tumor cells in vitro to combined 5-fluorouracil or ftorafur and x-rays. Int J Radiat Oncol Biol Phys 8:1923, 1982.
49. Wiley AL Jr, Ramirez G, Johnson RO, et al. Treatment of carcinoma of base of tongue with radiation therapy and 5-fluorouracil. Acta Radiol 18:235, 1979.

Chapter 15

MALIGNANT GLIOMAS

MOSHE H. MAOR AND VICTOR A. LEVIN

EPIDEMIOLOGY AND SURVIVAL STATISTICS

An estimated 16,900 new cases of primary central nervous system (CNS) tumors were diagnosed in the United States in 1992. CNS tumors constitute 1.5% of all new invasive cancers and account for 11,800 deaths or 2.3% of all cancer deaths (1). The largest group of primary CNS tumors are gliomas (Table 15–1), of which astrocytomas at various grades of malignancy are the most prevalent. Cerebral astrocytomas are subdivided into categories or grades based on the degree of tumor anaplasia.

Noninfiltrating astrocytomas, such as juvenile pilocytic and subependymal astrocytomas, are relatively slow-growing tumors and occur more frequently in childhood. The 5-year survival rate for patients with these tumors is approximately 50 to 60%. Infiltrating astrocytomas fall into three groups of increasing malignancy: well to moderately differentiated anaplastic astrocytoma, anaplastic astrocytoma, and glioblastoma multiforme. The 5-year survival of these groups currently is 41 to 49%, 18 to 48%, and 0 to 10%, respectively (2–5). For simplicity, anaplastic astrocytoma and glioblastoma multiforme are grouped together and called **malignant gliomas.**

Table 15–1. A Working Classification of Gliomas

- I. Astrocytic tumors
  - A. Noninfiltrating
    - 1. Juvenile pilocytic
    - 2. Subependymal
  - B. Infiltrating
    - 1. Well-differentiated mild and moderately anaplastic astrocytoma
    - 2. Anaplastic astrocytoma
    - 3. Glioblastoma multiforme
- II. Ependymal tumors
  - A. Myxopapillary ependymoma
  - B. Well-differentiated ependymoma
  - C. Anaplastic ependymoma
  - D. Ependymoblastoma
- III. Oligodendroglial tumors
  - A. Well-differentiated oligodendroglioma
  - B. Anaplastic oligodendroglioma
- IV. Mixed tumors
  - A. Mixed astrocytoma-ependymoma
  - B. Mixed astrocytoma-oligodendroglioma
  - C. Mixed astrocytoma-ependymoma-oligodendroglioma

Since malignant gliomas are relatively common and have a poor prognosis, much effort has been devoted in the last 20 years to finding better therapies for these tumors through clinical trials. This chapter will be devoted to a review of these trials.

Malignant gliomas occur predominantly in the fifth and sixth decades of life and are slightly more common in men (4–7). No etiologic factors are known for malignant gliomas, although three rare genetic conditions are associated with a high rate of gliomas: neurofibromatosis, tuberous sclerosis, and Turcot syndrome.

The prognosis for patients with malignant gliomas is determined by the tumor's histologic type and grade, its postoperative size and extent, and the patient's age, performance status, and duration of symptoms (2–7). These tumors are rarely cured by surgery alone; some of the lower-grade tumors may be cured with surgery and radiotherapy, but the remainder are incurable and require surgery, radiation, and chemotherapy for maximal palliation. Because of the multiple prognostic factors, clinical trials should be controlled randomized studies or should at least follow rigorous criteria for comparison with data bases from institutional or cooperative trials.

CURRENT CONVENTIONAL TREATMENT APPROACHES

Even though the longterm outlook for cure in patients with malignant glioma is bleak, surgery and radiotherapy are effective in palliating symptoms and prolonging life. They are considered the standard treatment for these tumors.

Surgery

Surgery for these tumors plays a dual role of providing a biopsy specimen for diagnosis and debulking the tumor. A diagnostic biopsy is mandatory to exclude other processes and to establish the diagnosis of malignant glioma and its grade.

Despite the advances in radiographic tumor localization and surgical techniques, curative resection for malignant astrocytoma remains elusive. Nevertheless, a maximal resection without compromising function provides immediate palliation of symptoms. Optimal surgery reduces the tumor cell burden and improves the changes for successful radiotherapy, chemotherapy, or both. Tumor debulking improves blood perfusion and oxygenation to the residual tumor. Because the natural removal of dead cells in the brain occurs slowly, surgical tumor debulking facilitates this process. Necrotic tumors occupy space, produce edema, and are a major cause of neurologic symptoms. For these reasons, it is not surprising that patient survival is inversely related to the amount of residual tumor after surgery (8).

Radiotherapy

Based on the natural history of malignant gliomas, they should be best suited for treatment with radiotherapy. These tumors rarely metastasize, and patients invariably die of progressive local disease. Nevertheless, longterm experience has shown that even after effective surgery, radiotherapy is rarely capable of curing high-grade astrocytomas.

To assess whether radiation has value in the treatment of malignant glioma, the United States Brain Tumor Study Group (BTSG) initiated a postoperative prospective randomized multi-institutional trial for adult patients with malignant glioma (9). The study had four postsurgical arms: supportive therapy that included corticosteroids; carmustine (BCNU), 80 mg/m^2, on three successive days every 6 to 8 weeks; radiotherapy, 5000 to 6000 cGy to the whole brain at 170 to 200 cGy/day, in five fractions/week; and the combination of radiotherapy with BCNU. There were 222 evaluable patients, 90% with glioblastoma multiforme and 9% with anaplastic astrocytoma. Patients were stratified by prognostic factors such as age, degree of tumor resection, and performance status. Median survivals were 14 weeks for supportive care only, 18.5 weeks for BCNU, 36 weeks for radiotherapy, and 35 weeks for radiotherapy plus BCNU. The two treatment arms that received radiotherapy showed significantly longer survivals ($p = 0.001$) compared to those who received supportive care or BCNU alone. Although the median survival was not prolonged by the addition of BCNU to radiotherapy, 19% of 72 patients who were treated with radiotherapy and BCNU were alive, compared with 4% of 68 patients who were treated only with radiotherapy at 18 months.

The value of radiotherapy was demonstrated in another randomized trial by the Scandinavian Glioma Study Group (SGSG) (10); 118 patients were randomly assigned to receive either supportive care, 4500 cGy radiation to the whole brain given over 5 weeks, or the same radiotherapy combined with bleomycin. Median survival was 10.8 months for the two radiation groups and 5.2 months for the group receiving only supportive therapy.

These important studies established the usefulness of radiotherapy for malignant gliomas, making it the standard treatment following surgery. The question remains, however, regarding whether the delivery of the radiation can be improved to yield even better results. Walker et al examined the relationship between increasing doses of radiation and survival in 621 patients who were entered into three BTSG protocols between 1966 and 1975 (11). Median survival was 18 weeks for patients who received no therapy,

13.5 weeks for those who received less than 4500 cGy radiation, 28 weeks for those who received 5000 cGy, 36 weeks for 5500 cGy, and 43 weeks for 6000 cGy. The group that received less than 4500 cGy contained patients whose condition deteriorated rapidly and who could not complete the treatment. The difference in survival between the 6000-cGy and 5000-cGy groups was statistically significant. It should be noted, however, that in these protocols, patients were not prospectively randomized to receive the different radiation dose levels.

In a joint study conducted by the Radiation Therapy Oncology Group (RTOG) and the Eastern Cooperative Oncology Group (ECOG), patients were randomized to receive either 6000 cGy radiation to the whole brain or the same dose plus a boost dose of 1000 cGy to the tumor area (12). The median survival for 148 patients treated with 6000 cGy was 9.9 months, compared to 8.4 months for 88 patients treated with 7000 cGy. The inability to achieve any tumor control or significant prolongation of survival with the higher dose used shows that even 7000 cGy may still be on the early, flat part of the theoretical tumor control probability curve. Higher doses of external radiation increase the risk of necrosis in the surrounding brain to an unacceptable level.

To overcome this limitation of external beam radiation, interstitial brachytherapy was attempted in a study at the University of California, San Francisco (UCSF) (13). The Phase II protocol developed by the Northern California Oncology Group (NCOG) consisted of limited-field external beam radiation to 6000 cGy plus concomitant chemotherapy with oral hydroxyurea, followed by a 5000-cGy boost, with a high-intensity, removable ^{125}I interstitial implant. After radiotherapy, the patients received combination chemotherapy with lomustine (CCNU), procarbazine, and vincristine. Patient selection was based on performance status and tumor size, configuration, location and contrast enhancement on CT scanning. Previous experience with recurrent glioma patients showed that approximately 50% needed surgery for removal of tumor-induced necrosis sometime after ^{125}I implantation (14). Because of the frequency of reoperation, patients with deep or midline tumors were not candidates for this Phase II protocol. A total of 107 patients were entered in the protocol, 67 of whom had glioblastoma multiforme. Thirty-eight patients did not receive the implant, mostly because of tumor progression in the glioblastoma group. Median survival was 15.5 months for glioblastoma patients and 20.3 months for patients with anaplastic astrocytoma. The authors conclude that brachytherapy boost has no value for patients with anaplastic astrocytoma but may be valuable for some patients with glioblastoma.

CHEMORADIATION

To improve the results with radiotherapy, chemotherapy and radiosensitizers were added and the results of these studies are summarized in Tables 15–2 and 15–3.

Nitrosoureas

Chloroethylnitrosoureas are the agents most widely used with radiation for adjuvant chemotherapy for malignant gliomas. The nitrosoureas cross easily into the CNS, are active against glial neoplasms, and have no obvious overlapping CNS toxicity with radiation. Thus, radiotherapy and chloroethylnitrosourea chemotherapy can be given concurrently at full doses.

The first BTSG trial (#6901) suggested an improvement in the 18-month survival rate when BCNU was given in addition to radiation (9). The next trial (#7201) had four arms: semustine (MeCCNU), 220 mg/m^2, every 6 to 8 weeks; radiotherapy, 6000 cGy in 30 to 35 fractions; radiotherapy plus MeCCNU; and radiotherapy plus BCNU. Median survivals were 24, 36, 42, and 51 weeks, respectively (4). The survival difference between groups who received radiotherapy with or without BCNU was not significant ($p = 0.11$). The study also suggested that BCNU is superior to MeCCNU when given in combination with radiation. The third BTSG trial (#7501) compared radiotherapy plus either BCNU; procarbazine, 150 mg/m^2/day over 4 weeks every 8 weeks; methylprednisone, 400 mg/m^2 per day for 7 days every four weeks; or BCNU with methylprednisolone (15). Significantly longer survivals were experienced by patients receiving BCNU or procarbazine compared to patients receiving methylprednisolone. The addition of this

Table 15–2. Randomized Clinical Trials with Radiotherapy and Chemotherapy for Malignant Glioma

Author/Study (Reference)	Total Evaluable Patients	Treatment by Study Arm	Median Survival (Months) or Partial Regression (%)	Comments
Walker et al/ BTSG 6901 (9)	222	1. Surgery only 2. BCNU 3. RT 4. RT/BCNU	3.2 4.3 8.3 8.0	RT significantly better than surgery only or BCNU. More survivors at 18 mo. with RT/BCNU than RT alone.
Walker et al/ BTSG 7201 (4)	358	1. MeCCNU 2. RT 3. RT/MeCCNU 4. RT/BCNU	5.5 8.3 9.7 11.8	RT vs. RT/BCNU, p = 0 .11
Green et al/ BTSG 7501 (15)	557	1. RT/BCNU 2. RT/PCZ 3. RT/MePred 4. RT/BCNU/MePred	11.5 10.8 9.2 9.5	RT/PCZ as effective as RT/BCNU. MePred had no effect on survival.
Chang et al/ RTOG/ECOG (12)	535	1. RT (6000 cGy) 2. RT (7000 cGy) 3. RT (6000 cGy)/BCNU 4. RT (6000 cGy)/ MeCCNU/DTIC	9.9 8.4 10.0 9.8	For patients 40–60 yr, BCNU added significantly to survival (p = 0.01).
Shapiro et al/ BTSG 8301 (16)	183	1. RT/iv BCNU 2. RT/IA BCNU	Worse survival for IA group (p = 0.11)	Severe toxicity with IA administration.
Eyre et al/SWOG (17)	115	1. RT/CCNU 2. RT/CCNU/PCZ	13.8 12.5	PCZ had no additional effect over RT/CCNU.
Ushio et al (18)	82 87	1. RT 2. RT/ACNU 1. RT/ACNU 2. RT/ACNU/Tegafur	15 partial re- 48 gression (%) 34 41	RT/ACNU significantly better than RT alone. Tegafur did not enhance the effect of RT/ACNU.
EORTC (19)	116	1. RT/VM-26/CCNU 2. RT	13.4 14.0	Patients received chemotherapy upon disease progression.
Ushio et al (20)	60	1. RT 2. RT/Bleomycin 3. RT/MeCCNU 4. RT/Bleomycin/MeCCNU	7.2 10.8 12.0 16.8	Small study. RT/MeCCNU effective. Bleomycin did not add significantly to RT or RT/ MeCCNU.
Levin et al (21)	99	1. RT/BCNU 2. RT/HU/BCNU	7.2 to pro- 9.7 gression	Results only for the 62 patients with glioblastoma.
Green et al/ BTSG 8001 (22)	571	1. RT/BCNU 2. RT/BCNU/PCZ 3. RT/BCNU/HU/PCZ/ VM-26	11.4–13.9	No advantage of combination chemotherapy over RT/BCNU.
Kristiansen et al (10)	118	1. No treatment 2. RT 3. RT/Bleomycin	5.2 10.8 10.8	Bleomycin ineffective.
Afra et al (25)	84	1. RT 2. RT/DBD 3. RT/DBD/BCNU	9.2 13.2 13.8	Dibromodulcitol effective in prolonging survival. BCNU did not have an additional benefit.
Levin et al/ NCOG 6G61 (24)	GM 60 GM AA 73 AA	1. RT/HU/BCNU 2. RT/HU/PCV 1. RT/HU/BCNU 2. RT/HU/PCV	13.2 11.5 19.0 36.2	For glioblastoma, p = 0.51. For anaplastic gliomas, p = 0.02.

RT = radiotherapy; PCZ = procarbazine; DBD = dibromodulcitol; iv = intravenous; IA = intra-arterial; MePred = methylprednisolone; HU = hydroxyurea; GM = glioblastoma multiforme; AA = anaplastic astrocytoma.

corticosteroid to BCNU therapy did not prolong survival.

In the joint RTOG and ECOG study (12), the four treatment arms were radiation alone at 6000 cGy (control), radiation alone at 7000 cGy, radiation at 6000 cGy with BCNU, or radiation at 6000 cGy with MeCCNU and dacarbazine (DTIC), 150 $mg/m^2/day$ re-

Table 15–3. Randomized Clinical Trials with Radiotherapy and Hypoxic Cell Sensitizers

Author/Study (Reference)	Total Evaluable Patients	Treatment by Study Arm	Median Survival (Months)/Survival	Comments
Urtasun et al (34)	36	1. RT 2. RT/Metronidazole	3.5 6	Small number of patients. Low hypofractionated radiation dose. Poor results with RT only.
Urtasun et al (35)	66	1. RT 2. RT/Metronidazole 3. RT/Miso	6 4.4 6.2	No advantage of sensitizers when compared to conventional RT.
Green et al/ BTSG 7702 (36)	557	1. RT/BCNU 2. RT bid/BCNU 3. RT/Miso 4. RT/Streptozocin	9.2–10.4	No significant difference between the four groups.
Bleehen et al/ MRC (37)	384	1. RT/Miso 2. RT/Placebo	25% at 12 mo 28% at 12 mo	Identical survival curves.
Sack et al (38)	102	1. RT/Miso 2. RT/Placebo	No difference	
EORTC (39)	163	1. RT/Miso 2. RT/Placebo	10.3 10.6	Hypofractionated RT.
Horiot et al/ EORTC (40)	340	1. RT 2. RT tid 3. RT tid/Miso	11 11 10.4	No survival difference between the three arms.
Fulton et al (41)	128	1. RT 2. RT tid 3. RT tid/Miso	7 10.4 11.5	No survival difference between the three arms.
Hatlevoll et al/ Scandinavian Glioblastoma Study Group (42)	244	1. RT 2. RT/Misonidazole 3. RT hypo-frac 4. RT hypo-frac/Miso	No difference	
Nelson et al/ RTOG 7918 (43)	293	1. RT/BCNU 2. RT/Miso	12.7 10.6	Hypofractionated RT with Miso worse for anaplastic astrocytoma (p = 0.17).

RT = radiotherapy; Miso = misonidazole; bid = two times/day; tid = three times/day.

peated every 4 weeks. Overall, no treatment option was significantly better than the control group. However, further evaluation of patients between 40 and 60 years of age revealed that treatment with BCNU and radiation resulted in significantly increased survival compared to radiation alone ($p = 0.01$). Similarly, radiation plus MeCCNU and DTIC was more effective than radiation alone ($p = 0.08$) in the same age group.

The BTSG attempted to improve the results with BCNU by administering it intra-arterially (16). Patients received radiation plus BCNU either intravenously or intra-arterially by randomization. In the intra-arterial group, survival was shorter ($p = 0.11$) and associated with severe CNS and retinal toxic effects. The Southwest Oncology Group (SWOG) attempted to improve the results obtained with a nitrosourea by the addition of procarbazine (17). Patients were randomly assigned to receive 6000 cGy radiation in 7 weeks plus CCNU, 130 mg/m^2 every 6 weeks, or the same radiation plus CCNU, 75 mg/m^2, and procarbazine, 100 mg/m^2 on days 1 to 14 every 6 weeks. Median survivals were 55 and 50 weeks for the two groups, respectively.

In Japan, a cooperative clinical trial evaluated nimustine hydrochloride (ACNU) and ACNU plus tegafur (Ftorafur) as additions to radiotherapy for malignant gliomas (18). In the first trial, patients were randomly assigned to receive radiotherapy or radiotherapy plus concomitant chemotherapy with ACNU, 100 mg/m^2 on days 1 and 42. Partial regression of the tumor was observed in 15 and 47.6% of patients treated with radiation and radiation plus ACNU, respectively ($p = 0.005$). In a second trial, patients received either radiation plus ACNU or radiation plus ACNU and tegafur, 400 mg/m^2 for 8 weeks.

Partial regression was seen in 41% of patients who received radiation plus ACNU and in 34% of patients who received radiation plus ACNU and tegafur (p value not significant).

The European Organization for Research on Treatment of Cancer (EORTC) evaluated CCNU plus teniposide (VM-26) in combination with radiotherapy (19). Patients with disease progression who initially received only radiation were given CCNU or VM-26 plus CCNU, and patients who initially had chemotherapy received procarbazine. The combination of drugs and radiation did not prolong survival. In a small randomized study by Ushio et al, MeCCNU plus radiation significantly prolonged the survival of patients ($p = 0.05$) (20). Bleomycin did not prolong survival when added to radiation or to radiation plus MeCCNU.

In summary, the addition of a nitrosourea during postoperative irradiation for a malignant glioma confers a small but significant advantage. Although the widest experience is with BCNU, the other nitrosoureas seem to be just as effective. The combination of radiation plus nitrosourea is considered therefore, the best available treatment and the standard against which further improvements or developments must be measured.

The first drug that was found to enhance the effect of a nitrosourea plus radiotherapy was hydroxyurea (21). In this randomized trial by the now defunct Western Cancer Study Group and the Brain Tumor Research Center, UCSF, patients received either radiation plus BCNU (BR) or radiation plus BCNU and hydroxyurea (BHR). Patients were stratified by histologic findings and extent of tumor resection. Radiation consisted of 5000 cGy to the whole brain plus a 1000-cGy boost. BCNU, 80 mg/m^2, was given on the 3 days prior to radiation. In the BHR group, hydroxyurea (275 mg/m^2) was given every 6 hours on alternate days of radiotherapy. For patients with glioblastoma, the median time to tumor progression was 42 weeks on BHR therapy, compared to 31 weeks on BR therapy ($p = 0.04$). For patients who had other malignant gliomas, time to progression was longer in the BR group, but this difference was not significant because of the small number of patients with this histologic type in the study. Survival data are not provided in this paper.

In another trial (#8001), the BTSG included one treatment arm with BCNU and hydroxyurea alternating with procarbazine and VM-26 (22). Patients in the other arms received BCNU or BCNU plus procarbazine. All treatments were combined with 6020 cGy radiation. The preliminary analysis of this study has not shown any differences in results between the three chemotherapy groups.

Many of the aforementioned studies lumped glioblastoma multiforme and anaplastic astrocytoma patients together; in most studies, the majority of patients had glioblastoma multiforme. This inhomogeneity in the experimental population can sometimes present interpretive problems. For example, the first analysis of NCOG 6G61, a protocol that closed in 1983 and was reported in 1985 (23), the combination of post-radiation procarbazine, CCNU, and vincristine (PCV) did not demonstrate a significant benefit. This randomized trial compared BCNU with PCV combination after 6000 cGy radiation plus oral hydroxyurea, 400 mg/m^2 every 6 hours, in patients with glioblastoma multiforme or other anaplastic gliomas. A more recent analysis (24) showed that PCV produced a significantly longer survival and time to tumor progression than BCNU for the anaplastic glioma patients ($p = 0.02$). With PCV, time to progression and survival doubled for anaplastic glioma patients in the 50th and 25th percentiles. The median survival was 157 and 82 weeks with PCV and BCNU, respectively.

Other Chemotherapy Agents

There has been a dearth of studies evaluating the use of chemotherapy other than nitrosoureas during radiotherapy. In a randomized study reported by Afra (25), mitolactol (dibromodulcitol) added significantly to survival when combined with radiation, but the addition of CCNU to dibromodulcitol did not result in further improvement. These results are interesting because dibromodulcitol has not shown much activity against recurrent gliomas (26). The Scandinavian Glioblastoma Study Group showed that the addition of bleomycin to radiation did not improve survival (10). The value of cisplatinum with radiation remains unknown; it was administered intravenously

(27) and intra-arterially (28) in separate studies, neither of which was controlled and randomized. Finally, results of pilot studies with aziridinylbenzoquinone (29) and 5-fluorouracil (30) used in conjunction with radiotherapy have been reported, but little benefit can be inferred from these results.

HYPOXIC CELL SENSITIZATION

Since identification of necrosis in malignant gliomas connotes the histologic diagnosis of glioblastoma multiforme, there is little doubt that hypoxic tumor cells exist. Whether the hypoxic cells are biologically important in gliomas awaits verification. It has been theorized that the relative resistance of malignant gliomas to conventional radiation is due to the survival of hypoxic clonogenic tumor cells. Eradication of these cells may require three times the radiation dose that would be needed (if the same cells existed) in a well oxygenated environment.

Nondrug Sensitization

In an effort to overcome radioresistance due to hypoxia, the use of neutron radiation and radiation with hyperbaric oxygen has been studied. Neutron radiotherapy was studied because neutrons are only minimally dependent on oxygen as a sensitizer. In an RTOG randomized study of 166 patients, the whole brain was given 5000 cGy conventional radiation followed by an additional boost of 1500 cGy with photons or a neutron equivalent. There was no difference in survival (31). Autopsies were performed in 12 cases in each arm. In 9 of 12 autopsies of patients treated with neutrons, no space-occupying lesion or infiltrating tumor could be identified, but significant necrosis and gliosis were identified at the primary tumor site. In contrast, all autopsy patients treated with photons alone had an infiltrating viable tumor mass. Similar results were reported by Catterall et al, in a randomized trial (32): five patients treated with neutrons showed progressive dementia without signs of tumor recurrence. Even though neutrons seem to be more effective against malignant gliomas than photons, the vulnerability of the normal brain to neutrons precludes its routine use.

Chang (33) studied the use of hyperbaric oxygen radiotherapy. Patients irradiated under hyperbaric oxygen had a median survival of 38 weeks, compared to 31 weeks for patients irradiated in air. However, this study was nonrandomized and therefore has little relevance. The difficulties associated with hyperbaric oxygen administration discouraged larger, well designed studies.

Drug Sensitization

The theoretical consideration that oxygen may be quickly metabolized on its way to the hypoxic cell encouraged the search for electron-affinic compounds that mimic the radiosensitization of oxygen but reach the hypoxic tumor cells more readily than oxygen does. Most clinical activity has focused on the nitroimidazoles (Table 15–3). The first clinical trial of such drugs for malignant glioma was conducted by Urtasun et al using metronidazole (Flagyl) (34). In that study, 36 patients with glioblastoma multiforme received 3000 cGy radiation in 9 equal fractions given 3 times a week over 19 days. Half the patients received metronidazole, 6 g/m^2 4 hours before each radiation treatment. Median survival of the radiation alone group was 15 weeks, compared to 26 weeks for the patients receiving the sensitizer. Drawbacks of the study were the small number of patients, lack of stratification for prognostic factors, low overall radiation dose, and small number of fractions. The inferior radiation schedule used resulted in a low survival rate in the control group. Nevertheless, the study suggested that metronidazole could potentiate the cell-killing effect of radiation in glioblastoma multiforme.

Unfortunately, in a second study by Urtasun et al, the results were negative (35). Sixty-six patients stratified by functional level and tumor grade were randomly assigned to three treatment arms: 5800 cGy in 30 daily fractions over 6 weeks, 3900 cGy in nine equal fractions given 3 times a week preceded by 6 g/m^2 of metronidazole, or the same hypofractionated radiation dose with the more efficient sensitizer misonidazole at 1.25 g/m^2. The respective median survivals in the three treatment arms were 26, 19, and 27 weeks. In this better designed study, higher doses of radiation given with either sensitizer were unable to improve the results obtained with conventional daily radiotherapy.

A large BTSG study (77-02) randomly assigned patients to one of four treatment arms: 6000 cGy at 200 cGy once daily plus BCNU, 6600 cGy at 110 cGy twice daily plus BCNU, 6000 cGy at 200 cGy once daily plus misonidazole twice weekly at 1.5 g/m^2 followed by BCNU, or 6000 cGy at 200 cGy once daily plus streptozotocin. After analysis of the results in 557 patients, 86% of whom had glioblastoma multiforme, no significant difference in survival was noted among the four treatment arms (36). Neither increased radiation fractionation nor the misonidazole conferred a survival advantage. In this study, streptozotocin seemed to be as effective as BCNU.

Like most hypoxic cell sensitizers, radiation enhancement with misonidazole is directly related to the amount of drug administered before each radiation fraction. The toxicity seems most closely related to the total amount of sensitizer administered; in most trials, drug dosage is limited to 12 to 18 g/m^2, depending on the overall time of administration. To maximize the enhancement ratio of misonidazole, some investigators have modified the fractionation of radiotherapy to give as much radiation as possible after a few large doses of misonidazole, when the concentration of the drug in the serum is at its highest. Other studies divided the total tolerable amount into daily doses to be given before conventional radiotherapy. The latter approach reduces the enhancement ratio but has the advantage of not abandoning the well tested concept of fractionated irradiation.

In Britain, the Medical Research Council conducted a large double-blind study on 436 patients with Grades 3 and 4 astrocytoma (37). All patients were treated with 4500 cGy radiation given in 20 daily fractions. Patients were randomly assigned to receive either 0.6 g/m^2 misonidazole 4 hours before irradiation or placebo; 384 patients were eligible for analysis. The survival rate at 12 months was 25% for patients receiving misonidazole and 28% for patients receiving placebo. The survival curves up to 3 years were almost identical for the two groups.

A similar study with small daily doses of misonidazole was conducted in Germany (38). Patients were treated with 4000 cGy radiation to the whole brain followed by a boost to the tumor region. Patients randomly received either 0.4 g/m^2 misonidazole before each of the 30 fractions or a placebo. No improved survival was seen with the sensitizer.

The EORTC Brain Tumor Group also evaluated misonidazole in a randomized double-blind study (39). Radiotherapy was hypofractionated so that larger doses of misonidazole could be administered before each fraction. The radiation consisted of nine fractions of 350 cGy given every other day to the whole brain or to large fields, followed by a boost of six fractions of 300 cGy to the tumor site with a 2-cm margin, for a total dose of 4950 cGy in 15 fractions over 5 weeks. Misonidazole, 1.3 g/m^2, or placebo was given 4 hours before each of the first nine fractions of radiation. Results for 163 patients were analyzed. The mean survivals were 10.3 months (44.5 weeks) for the misonidazole group and 10.6 months (46.1 weeks) for the placebo group; the survival curves were almost identical. After this negative result, the EORTC carried out a randomized study comparing three treatments; conventional radiation (6000 cGy in 30 fractions over 6 weeks) radiation given in multiple fractions per day (3000 cGy at 200 cGy per fraction, 3 times daily for 5 days and repeated after a 2-week interval), or the latter radiotherapy combined with 1.2 g/m^2 misonidazole every treatment day (40). A total of 335 patients were entered into this study. Median survivals were 47, 48, and 45 weeks (approximately 12 months) for the three groups, respectively.

Another study employing multiple daily radiation fractions with misonidazole was reported on by Fulton et al (41). Patients were randomly assigned to receive either conventional fractionation of 5800 cGy in 30 fractions over 6 weeks, thrice-daily fractionation (each 89 cGy) for a total of 6140 cGy in 69 fractions over 4-½ weeks, or the same thrice-daily fractionation plus 1.25 g/m^2 misonidazole three times weekly for the first 3 weeks. Median survivals were 29, 45, and 50 weeks (7, 11, and 12.5 months) for the three groups, respectively. Survival was significantly improved for patients treated with multiple fractionation ($p < 0.002$), but the addition of misonidazole to this regimen did not result in further improvement in survival.

The Scandinavian Glioblastoma Group conducted a randomized study to test the effectiveness of misonidazole with conventional radiation fractionation (5000 cGy over 5 weeks) or with hypofractionation (4000 cGy in 10 fractions twice weekly over 5 weeks) (42). Before each treatment, half of the patients treated conventionally were given 0.45 g/m^2 misonidazole orally and the other half treated with hypofractionation was given 1.2 g/m^2. The four treatment groups were further subdivided into eight groups by addition of CCNU 3 months after surgery to half the patients in each group. Median survival was identical in all eight treatment groups.

In the United States, the RTOG evaluated misonidazole-radiosensitized radiotherapy in the treatment of malignant gliomas in a large randomized study (43). Patients in the control arm received 6000 cGy of whole-brain irradiation, 5 days/week with fractions of 170 to 200 cGy. BCNU (80 mg/m^2) was given on days 3, 4, and 5 of the first week of radiotherapy and repeated every 8 weeks for 2 years if tolerated. In the experimental arm, the fractionation of radiation was altered to enhance the effect of misonidazole. These patients received 400 cGy on Mondays and 150 cGy on Tuesdays, Thursdays, and Fridays for a total dose of 5400 cGy in 6 weeks. An additional 900 cGy was given in the seventh week in equally divided fractions of 180 cGy. Misonidazole was given on Mondays during the first 6 weeks of radiotherapy at a dose of 2.5 g/m^2, 4 hours before the 400 cGy was administered. BCNU was given the same way as in the control group. Results of 293 patients were analyzed. The median survival of the control group was 12.7 months compared with 10.6 months for the misonidazole group ($p = 0.12$). While there was no difference between treatment groups for patients with glioblastoma multiforme, the survival for patients with anaplastic astrocytoma treated with misonidazole was shortened to 13 months compared with 30 months in the control group ($p = 0.17$).

The NCOG evaluated daily misonidazole (0.5 g/m^2) given before conventional radiation fractions to a total dose of 6000 cGy (44). In this study, patients also received CCNU and 5-fluorouracil prior to radiotherapy, hydroxyurea during radiotherapy, and postradiation CCNU, procarbazine, BCNU, and vincristine. No difference in time to tumor progression was noted between this seven-drug protocol and the NCOG 6G61 protocol (radiation plus hydroxyurea followed by PCV).

Halogenated Deoxyuridines

The negative results with hypoxic cell sensitizers caused renewed interest in the halogenated deoxyuridines as radiosensitizers for rapidly dividing cells. Only limited pilot studies are available for this mode of sensitization.

The pioneering clinical work for gliomas was done by Hasino and Sano (45). They used intra-arterial BUdR at doses of 0.6 to 1.0 g/m^2/day to a total dose of 25 to 45 g. The radiation dose was 6000 cGy in daily fractions of 150 to 200 cGy. Although their study was not controlled, the authors' results for 107 patients with malignant gliomas revealed a 2-year survival rate of 72% for anaplastic astrocytoma and 44% for glioblastoma multiforme patients. The authors believed that their therapy was more effective than surgery and standard radiotherapy, but the morbidity of the intra-arterial approach precluded widespread use of the technique.

Preliminary results with intra-arterial BUdR have recently been reported by Hegarty et al (46). BUdR treatment (400 to 600 mg/m^2/day) was started 2 weeks before radiation treatment and continued during radiation for a total of 8.5 weeks. Focal beam radiotherapy (5940 cGy at 180 cGy/day) was used. All patients had ipsilateral forehead dermatitis, blepharitis, and conjunctivitis. In 18 patients whose tumors were classified as Grade 4 astrocytoma, 62% of patients were alive at a median follow-up of 12 months.

In November 1987, the NCOG closed a protocol 6G82-1 in which patients with glioblastoma received BUdR (0.8 g/m^2) intravenously for 4 days prior to and during radiation for 6 weeks. Radiation was given to a limited field for a total dose of 6000 cGy at 170 to 180 cGy/day. Following radiation, the patients received PCV. A total of 160 of 173 patients entered were evaluable. Patients had to have a Karnofsky performance $\geqq 70$. Mean survival was 12.9 months and time to failure was 8 months for the evaluable group.

The authors did not consider these results a significant improvement.

CONCLUSIONS

Even though the longterm prognosis for patients with malignant gliomas remains grim, a great deal has been learned in the controlled clinical trials reviewed in this chapter.

Surgery with maximal tumor resection continues to be the initial step in the treatment of all gliomas. It provides a histologic diagnosis, palliates symptoms by removing the space-occupying lesion, and facilitates ensuing therapies. With the development of new neuroimaging techniques and equipment, better neuroanesthesia, and better neurosurgical equipment in the past 20 years, surgery can now be performed more safely and effectively.

Radiotherapy has unequivocally been shown to prolong survival significantly in a number of trials, but even with the highest radiation doses tolerated by the brain, it is impossible to control the tumor permanently. If one presumes that persistent hypoxia is the major cause of radioresistance for glioblastoma multiforme and anaplastic astrocytoma, radiation doses will have to be increased threefold, to a level of 18,000 to 20,000 cGy, to have a reasonable probability of tumor control. Such high doses cannot be delivered with external beam irradiation given the present technology. An important step toward delivery of significantly higher doses of radiation was made with interstitial irradiation. Doses in the range of 11,000 to 12,000 cGy are currently delivered in some protocols. Although regional symptomatic necrosis may occur at these doses, neurosurgeons and radiation therapists have become more accustomed to reoperation for removal of necrotic tissue. It would be helpful, however, if means were developed to minimize the volume of irradiated normal brain that surrounds the tumor and thereby limit or reduce the necrosis.

To overcome the possible role of hypoxia, various clinical experiments have been performed. The use of hyperbaric oxygen was not pursued because of disappointing results, cumbersome administration procedures, and theoretical considerations related to oxygen's rapid metabolism, thus limiting its availability to hypoxic tumor cells. The experience with external neutron irradiation was interesting. Although survival was not prolonged, autopsy findings in some patients showed apparent tumor control concurrent with unacceptable brain toxicity.

Hypoxic-cell sensitizers are not as attractive as they once were. All trials with misonidazole, the best radiosensitizer available at the time, were negative regardless of treatment schedule. Although these negative results do not refute the role of hypoxia in the treatment of high-grade gliomas, they raise questions regarding its use. Physical limitations on incremental and total doses of misonidazole imposed by its neurotoxicity support a potential clinical radiation enhancement ratio of 1.2 (48). Under these ideal conditions, the addition of misonidazole will have the same effect as an increase in radiation dose of 20%. A demonstrable clinical benefit with misonidazole, therefore, can only be expected in a tumor system in which such an increase in dose will lead to a quantifiable improvement. In glioblastoma multiforme, a significant degree of sensitization with the doses used will go undetected since the threshold of a steep increase in tumor control with increasing dose is much higher (49).

Proponents of hypoxic-cell sensitization have produced more effective and less toxic new drugs by modifying the side chain in position 1 of the nitroimidazole group. The effectiveness of these drugs is yet to be demonstrated. Regardless of the drug chosen, the highest degree of radiosensitization is expected with maximal tolerable drug dosage in conjunction with each fraction of radiation.

The use of radioprotectors such as WR2721 to improve the therapeutic ratio for radiation by protecting the normal brain around the tumor has not been fruitful because the drug does not differentially concentrate in the normal brain surrounding the tumor.

If hypoxia is less important than other radioresistant mechanisms in gliomas, then chemotherapeutic agents active against oxygenated cells may offer the best hope for the future. The addition of chemotherapy, notably nitrosoureas and nitrosourea-based drug combinations, to radiotherapy has slightly but perceptibly prolonged survival. In most studies, it is difficult to sort out drug-radiation interactions because many of the drugs are also given following the completion of radiotherapy. In any case, no current evidence suggests that the combined effectiveness of radiotherapy plus chemotherapy is more than additive.

Oxygenated cycling cells can be sensitized with halogenated pyrimidines. For optimal utilization of these drugs, the same recommendation for radiotherapy administration as for hypoxic-cell sensitizers, should be followed. Since the halogenated pyrimidines and the nitroimidazoles address different types of radioresistance and act on different subpopulations of tumor cells, administration of both agents simultaneously or sequentially is feasible. By altering radiation schedules, it is possible to restudy many of the chemotherapy agents of proven value in high-grade gliomas and possible radiosensitizing effects of others, such as platinum derivatives.

Unfortunately an hypoxic environment not only reduces radiosensitivity but operates to increase resistance to chemotherapy by hampering drug distribution and increasing the number of noncycling G_0 cells. In addition, the limited number of drugs with activity against glial neoplasms has severely restricted the task of developing more effective chemotherapies (50).

In future studies, different modes of radiation administration with drug potentiators must be explored. External radiation should be accelerated by giving more than the conventional five fractions a week so that all treatments, including the implant, can be given with the drug. Individual fractions larger than 200 cGy should be avoided because they produce worse late effects on CNS tissue and necessitate reduction in the total radiation dose. The combination of radiosurgery with concurrent chemotherapy or sensitizer also deserves study.

REFERENCES

1. Boring CC, Squires TS, Tong T. Cancer Statistics, 1992. CA 42(1):30, 1992.
2. Nelson JS, Tsukada Y, Schoenfeld D, et al. Necrosis as a prognostic criterion in malignant supratentorial, astrocytic gliomas. Cancer 52:550, 1983.
3. Burger PC, Vogel, FS, Green SB, Strike TA. Glioblastoma multiforme and anaplastic astrocytoma. Pathologic criteria and prognostic implications. Cancer 56:1106, 1985.
4. Walker MD, Green SB, Byar DP, et al. Randomized comparisons of radiotherapy and nitrosoureas for the treatment of malignant glioma after surgery. N Engl J Med 303:1323, 1980.
5. Levin VA, Sheline GE, Gutin PH. Neoplasms of the central nervous system. *In:* Cancer: Principles and Practice of Oncology. 3rd Ed. DeVita VT Jr, Hellman S, Rosenberg SA (Eds). Philadelphia, JB Lippincott, 1989, p. 1557.
6. Roth JG, Elvidge AR. Glioblastoma multiforme: A clinical survey. J Neurosurg 17:736, 1960.
7. Leibowitz U, Alter M. Tumors of the nervous system: Incidence and population selectivity. Neurology 19:292, 1969.
8. Levin VA, Hoffman WF, Heilbron DC, et al. Prognostic significance of the pretreatment CT scan on time to progression for patients with malignant gliomas. J Neurosurg 52:642, 1980.
9. Walker MD, Alexander E Jr, Hunt WE. Evaluation of BCNU and/or radiotherapy in the treatment of anaplastic glioma: A cooperative clinical trial. J Neurosurg 49:333, 1978.
10. Kristiansen J, Hagen S, Kollevoid T. Combined modality therapy of operated astrocytomas grade III and IV: Confirmation of the value of postoperative irradiation and lack of potentiation of bleomycin on survival time. A prospective multicenter trial of the Scandinavian Glioblastoma Study Group. Cancer 47:649, 1981.
11. Walker MD, Strike TA, Sheline GE. An analysis of dose-effect relationship in the radiotherapy of malignant gliomas. Int J Radiat Oncol Biol Phys 5:1725, 1979.
12. Chang CH, Horton J, Schoenfeld D, et al. Comparison of postoperative radiotherapy and combined postoperative radiotherapy and chemotherapy in the multidisciplinary management of malignant gliomas. A Joint Radiation Therapy Oncology Group and Eastern Cooperative Oncology Group Study. Cancer 52:997, 1983.
13. Gutin PH, Prados MD, Phillips TL, et al. External irradiation followed by an interstitial high activity iodine-125 implant "boost" in the initial treatment of malignant gliomas. NCOG 6G-82-2. Int J Radiat Oncol Biol Phys 21:601, 1991.
14. Gutin PH, Leibel SA, Wara WM, et al. Recurrent malignant gliomas: Improved survival

following interstitial brachytherapy with high activity iodine-125 sources. J Neurosurg 67:864, 1987.

15. Green SB, Byar DP, Wapker MD, et al. Comparisons of carmustine and high-dose methylprednisolone as additions to surgery and radiotherapy for the treatment of malignant glioma. Cancer Treat Rep 67:121, 1983.
16. Shapiro WR, Green SB, Burger PC, et al. A randomized comparison of intra-arterial (IA) vs. intravenous (IV) BCNU for patients with malignant glioma (Study 8301): Interim analysis demonstrating lack of efficacy for IA BCNU (abstract). Proceedings of the American Society of Clinical Oncology 6(A268):69, 1987.
17. Eyre JH, Quagliana JM, Eltringham JR, et al. Randomized comparisons of radiotherapy and CCNU versus radiotherapy, CCNU plus procarbazine for the treatment of malignant gliomas following surgery. A Southwest Oncology Group Report. J Neurooncol 1:171, 1983.
18. Ushio Y, Abe H, Suzuki J, et al. Evaluation of ACNU alone and combined with tegafur as additions to radiotherapy of the treatment of malignant gliomas—A cooperative clinical trial. No To Shinkei 37:999, 1985.
19. European Organization for Research on Treatment of Cancer (EORTC) Brain Tumor Group. Evaluation of CCNU, VM-26 plus CCNU, and procarbazine in supratentorial brain gliomas. Final evaluation of a randomized study. J Neurosurg 55:27, 1981.
20. Ushio T, Hayakawa T, Hasegawa H, et al. Chemotherapy of malignant gliomas. Neurosurg Rev 7:3, 1984.
21. Levin VA, Wilson CB, Davis R, et al. A phase III comparison of BCNU, hydroxyurea, and radiation therapy to BCNU and radiation therapy for treatment of primary malignant gliomas. J Neurosurg 51:526–532, 1979.
22. Green, SB, Byar DB, Strike TA, et al. Randomized comparisons of single or multiple drug chemotherapy combined with either whole brain or whole brain plus coned-down boost radiotherapy for the postoperative treatment of malignant gliomas (Study 8001) (abstract). Proceedings of the American Society of Clinical Oncology 5:A527, p. 135, 1986.
23. Levin, VA, Wara WM, Davis RL, et al. Phase III comparison of chemotherapy with BCNU and the combination of procarbazine, CCNU and vincristine administered after radiation therapy with hydroxyurea to patients with malignant gliomas. J Neurosurg 63:218, 1985.
24. Levin VA, Silver P, Hannigan J, et al. NCOG 6G61 final report: Superiority of post-radiotherapy adjuvant chemotherapy with CCNU, procarbazine, and vincristine (PCV) over BCNU for anaplastic gliomas. Int J Radiat Oncol Biol Phys 18:321, 1990.
25. Afra D, Kocsis B, Dobay JR, et al. Combined radiotherapy and chemotherapy with dibromodulcitol and CCNU in the postoperative treatment of malignant gliomas. J Neurosurg 59:106, 1983.
26. Levin VA, Edwards MSB, Gutin PH, et al. Phase II evaluation of dibromodulcitol in the treatment of recurrent medulloblastoma, ependymoma, and malignant astrocytoma. J Neurosurg 61:1063, 1984.
27. Feun LG, Stewart DJ, Maor MH, et al. A pilot study of cis-diamminedichloroplatinum and radiation therapy in high grade astrocytomas. J Neurooncol 1:109, 1983.
28. Lehane D, Moiel R, Bryan N, et al. Adjuvant therapy for malignant gliomas using intra-arterial cis-platinum radiation therapy and CCNU (abstract). Proceedings of the Fourth International Conference on the Adjuvant Therapy of Cancer, Tuscon 1984, p. 41.
29. Tapazolou E, Lee M, Simpson J, et al. Concurrent aziridinylbenzoquinone (AZQ) chemotherapy and radiotherapy (RT) in patients with malignant gliomas: RTOG study (abstract). Proceedings of the American Society of Clinical Oncology 7:A329, p. 86, 1988.
30. Adelstein DJ, Likavec MJ, Sharan VM, et al. Intravenous 5-fluorouracil infusion and simultaneous radiotherapy in glioblastoma multiforme (abstract). Proceedings of the American Journal of Clinical Oncology, 6(A274): 71, 1987.
31. Griffin TW, Davis R, Laramore G, et al. Fast neutron radiation therapy for glioblastoma multiforme. Results of an RTOG study. Am J Clin Oncol 6:661, 1983.
32. Catterall M, Bloom HJ, Ash DV, et al. Fast neutrons compared with megavoltage x-rays in the treatment of patients with supratentorial glioblastoma: A controlled pilot study. Int J Radiat Oncol Biol Phys 6:261, 1980.
33. Chang CH. Hyperbaric oxygen and radiation therapy in the management of glioblastoma. NCI Mongr 46:163, 1977.
34. Urtasun RC, Band P, Chapman JD, et al. Radiation and high-dose metronidazole in supratentorial glioblastoma. N Engl J Med 294:1364, 1976.
35. Urtasun R, Feldstein ML, Partington T. Radiation and nitroimidazoles in supratentorial high grade gliomas: A second clinical trial. Br J Cancer 46:101, 1982.
36. Green SB, Byar DP, Strike TA, et al. Randomized comparisons of BCNU, streptozotocin, radiosensitizer, and fractionation of radiotherapy in the postoperative treatment of ma-

lignant glioma (abstract). Proceedings of the American Society of Clinical Oncology 3(A1018):260, 1984.
37. Bleehen NM, Adams GE, Ayoub MA, et al, in a report from the MRC. A study of the effect of misonidazole in conjunction with radiotherapy for the treatment of grades 3 and 4 astrocytomas. Br J Radiol 56:673, 1983.
38. Sack HJ, Capcanis A, Godehardt E, et al. Postoperative radiotherapy of astrocytomas grade 3 and 4 with the radiosensitizer misonidazole. End results of a multicenter controlled German study. Strahlentherapie 158:466, 1982.
39. EORTC Brain Tumor Group. Misonidazole in radiotherapy of supratentorial malignant brain gliomas in adult patients. A randomized double-blind study. Eur J Cancer Clin Oncol 19:39, 1983.
40. Horiot JC, van den Bogaert W, Ang KK, et al. European organization for research on treatment of cancer trials using radiotherapy with multiple fractions per day. Front Radiat Ther Oncol 22:149, 1988.
41. Fulton DS, Urtasun RC, Shin KH, et al. Misonidazole combined with hyperfractionation in the management of malignant glioma. Int J Radiat Oncol Biol Phys 10:1709, 1984.
42. Hatlevoll R, Lindegaard KF, Hagen S, et al. Combined modality treatment of operated astrocytomas grade 3 and 4: A prospective and randomized study of misonidazole and radiotherapy with two different radiation schedules and subsequent CCNU chemotherapy. Stage II of a prospective multicenter trial of the Scandinavian Glioblastoma Study Group. Cancer 56:41, 1985.
43. Nelson DF, Diener-West M, Weinstein AS, et al. A randomized comparison of misonidazole sensitized radiotherapy plus BCNU and radiotherapy plus BCNU for treatment of malignant glioma after surgery: Final report of an RTOG study. Int J Radat Oncol Biol Phys 12:1793, 1986.
44. Levin VA, Wara WM, Davis RL, et al. Response to treatment with radiation therapy and seven drug chemotherapy in patients with glioblastoma multiforme. Cancer Treat Rep 70:739, 1986.
45. Hoshino T, Sano K. Radiosensitization of malignant brain tumours with bromouridine (thymidine analogue). Acta Radiol 8:15, 1969.
46. Hegarty TJ, Thornton AF, Diaz RF, et al. Intraarterial bromodeoxyuridine radiosensitization of malignant gliomas Int J Radiat Oncol Biol Phys 19:421, 1990.
47. Phillips TL, Levin VA, Ahn DK, et al. Evaluation of bromodeoxyuridine in glioblastoma multiforme. A Northern California Cancer phase II study. Int J Radiat Oncol Biol Phys 21:709, 1991.
48. Phillips TL, Wasserman TH, Stetz J, Brady LW. Clinical trials of hypoxic cell sensitizers. Int J Radiat Oncol Biol Phys 8:327, 1982.
49. Maor MH, Peters LJ. Selection of appropriate studies for phase III trials of radiosensitizers. Int J Radiat Oncol Biol Phys 9:271, 1983.
50. Levin VA. Chemotherapy of primary brain tumors. Neurol Clin 3:855, 1985.

Chapter 16

SOFT-TISSUE SARCOMAS

REY RODRIGUEZ AND TIMOTHY J. KINSELLA

INTRODUCTION

Soft-tissue sarcomas are malignant neoplasms that arise from mesodermally derived tissues. They are relatively uncommon, with an incidence of 5,900 cases (0.5% of new cancer cases) estimated for 1992 in the United States (1). Because of widespread distribution of soft tissues, sarcomas can arise in a variety of anatomic sites. These tumors have a wide spectrum of histologic types, classified on the basis of the putative cell of origin, but they are usually considered together because of similar behavioral characteristics (2). Treatment and prognosis are based on factors other than histologic subtype. Independent prognostic factors include malignancy grade, tumor size, intratumor vascular invasion, and DNA aneuploidy (3–5).

In about 90% of cases, sarcomas present as an apparently localized soft-tissue mass with no evidence of metastasis. However, these tumors expand locally, creating a pseudocapsule of the compressed adjacent normal tissue. The pseudocapsule is virtually always invaded by tumor cells (6,7), with spread along muscle and fascial planes, blood vessels, and nerves. Because of this, a local recurrence can develop at a surprising distance from the original tumor. High-grade tumors have a propensity for early systemic dissemination, particularly to the lung (8). These factors account for a substantial mortality (3,300 estimated deaths in 1992 in the United States) (1). Clinical advances in the treatment of soft-tissue sarcomas have been hampered by the difficulty of accruing adequate numbers of patients for prospective, randomized therapeutic trials and by the multiple tumor sites that influence the treatment options. However, evolution of management during the past decades has resulted in substantial improvement in local control and longterm survival. These improved results are related to more thorough staging, precise radiotherapeutic techniques, and the use of aggressive combined modality therapy.

SOFT-TISSUE SARCOMAS OF THE EXTREMITIES

Approximately 60% of soft-tissue sarcomas occur in the extremities; lower-extremity lesions predominate in a ratio of 3:1 compared to upper-extremity tumors (9). As these tumors have a pseudocapsule, it often appears that minimal surgical procedures would be sufficient for achieving local control. Historically, many patients were treated with limited excision. However, various reports demonstrated unacceptable high local failure rates (50 to 93%) (10–15) and these practices were abandoned. Therefore, a trend developed toward more aggressive surgery with amputation or radical compartmental excision being adopted as the procedures of choice. These surgical procedures resulted in marked improvement in local failure rates (2 to 34%) (10–18). Unfortunately, significant functional and cosmetic impairment were observed.

With the emergence of megavoltage radiotherapy, this modality was used to enhance treatment of sarcomas. Initial results were disappointing because tumors often regressed slowly or incompletely after radiation. These tumors gained the reputation of being radioresistant. Residual masses, however, often never changed or regressed gradually long after treatment and, under microscopic examination, would be shown to be sterilized of tumor (19). Interest returned after it was realized that the tumors were not truly radioresistant, but most were simply too large and bulky to be treated with radiation alone without exceeding normal tissue tolerance. Since the pioneering work of Cade (20) in the 1950s, radiation therapy plus limited surgical resection has been used to improve local control. Surgery is used to remove the primary tumor mass and the radiation to treat microscopic tumor extension. This combined approach yields better functional and cosmetic results with local control rates comparable to or better than those achieved by radical surgery.

A number of approaches have been proposed for combined modality therapy. These include preoperative radiation, postoperative radiation, preoperative radiation with regional chemotherapy, and adjuvant chemotherapy. Although these general strategies are now well established, the precise technique to best obtain tumor control while minimizing normal tissue morbidity is under active investigation.

Preoperative Radiotherapy

There is currently good rationale for preoperative irradiation. Even when treating a large tumor mass, preoperative radiation to a dose of 4500 to 5000 cGy may inactivate greater than 99% (up to two logs of cell kill) of the tumor cells. This will decrease the likelihood of tumor implantation during surgery. With preoperative radiation, the oncologist needs to treat only tissues thought to be at risk for tumor involvement, and radiation fields need not encompass areas to be manipulated by the surgeon, as in the case of postoperative therapy. The greatest potential advantage in the use of preoperative radiation is that some patients, who would have needed an amputation if surgery were done initially, may become eligible for conservative treatment. Radiation therapy administered preoperatively may allow the surgeon to decrease the extent of the surgical procedure and to perform a limb-preserving operation. Even if the tumor mass does not decrease in size after irradiation, the tumor may consist pathologically of necrotic debris with little viable tumor. A potential difficulty with preoperative radiation is delayed healing of the surgical wound, although if good surgical and radiotherapeutic techniques are used, primary healing should occur (21,22). There are several series that demonstrate that planned preoperative radiation therapy in patients with high-grade sarcoma can yield excellent results with 5-year disease-free survival of 56 to 74% and local control rates of 83 to 95% (23–25).

Postoperative Radiotherapy

There are several theoretical advantages of postoperative radiotherapy. These include immediate surgery, avoiding radiation-induced delays in wound healing, and a large specimen available for histopathologic investigation with definite interpretation of tumor size and extension. However, with this technique, the initial postoperative treatment volume should include the wound, which is usually a larger volume than would have been treated preoperatively. Several retrospective, single-institution series have been reported utilizing this approach (6,26–28). The 5-year results include a disease-free survival of 60 to 68% and a local control rate of 78 to 92%. The National Cancer Institute conducted a randomized, prospective trial evaluating limb-sparing surgery with postoperative radiation compared with amputation in patients with high-grade extremity sarcomas (29). The local control rate was somewhat better for the amputation arm; however, this was not reflected in survival rates, with similar disease-free and overall survival observed between groups. In the limb-sparing group, 85% of patients maintained a functional limb.

Preoperative Radiotherapy with Regional Chemotherapy

The discovery and clinical application of doxorubicin (Adriamycin, ADR) significantly modified the treatment of soft-tissue sarcomas. Since 1974, Eilber and associates at UCLA have used preoperative intra-arterial ADR and radiation for the management of extremity sarcomas (30–33). The rationale for this approach was to regionally deliver an active chemotherapeutic agent that had direct cytotoxicity and potential radiosensitization. A total of 344 patients with high-grade extremity soft-tissue sarcomas were treated in sequential protocols. The first protocol consisted of intra-arterial ADR 30 mg/day for 3 consecutive days, followed by radiation therapy to a dose of 3500 cGy at 350 cGy per fraction, followed by surgical resection. Of the 77 patients treated, the local recurrence rate was 4% with a minimum follow-up of 7 years. However, the complication rate in this protocol was 35%. These complications consisted mainly of bone fractures and wound sloughs.

In order to reduce complications, a second protocol was conducted. This protocol involved 137 patients treated with intra-arterial ADR at the same doses followed by 1750 cGy of radiation delivered at 350 cGy per fraction. Although the complication rate decreased, the local recurrence rate increased to 13%. Therefore, in a third protocol, patients were treated with preoperative ADR, followed by radiation to a dose of 2800 cGy. The recurrence rate decreased to 7%, with a similar rate of complications. In addition, this protocol randomized patients to intra-arterial vs. intravenous doxorubicin. There was no difference in the local recurrence rate. Therefore, these protocols showed that there was a dose-response relationship to radiation and that intra-arterial infusion was not superior to the intravenous route.

A recent protocol utilized cisplatinum (120 mg/m^2) followed by ADR infusion and radiation to 2800 cGy. The preliminary results showed an improved local recurrence rate of 4% (34). Overall, the limb salvage rate of these protocols was greater than 96% and the local tumor control was 91%. Similar results were reported by Denton and associates (35) using an approach similar to the UCLA group.

Although randomized studies comparing the UCLA approach to standard radiation therapy given pre- or postoperatively are not available, the neoadjuvant approach with preoperative ADR and radiation allows excellent local tumor control and functional results in the majority of patients. Whether this will translate into improved longterm survival rates and local control is a question that will have to await further follow-up for an answer.

Adjuvant Chemotherapy

Despite adequate local control, a significant proportion of patients (40 to 60%) with high-grade soft-tissue sarcomas will ultimately have recurrences and die from metastatic disease, usually in the lung. Adjuvant chemotherapy has been proposed in an effort to eradicate micrometastasis; several trials have evaluated its role. Only randomized prospective studies will be presented because the survival in the control arms of randomized studies has been superior to those of historical controls.

There is controversy regarding whether single-agent (Adriamycin) or multiagent chemotherapy is superior (36–39), Gherlinzoni et al at the Instituto Orthopedica Rizzoli randomized patients to receive ADR (45 mg/m^2) in the adjuvant arm versus observation after primary treatment. With a median follow-up of 28 months in 59 patients, the disease-free survival was 79.1% in the adjuvant group and 54.3% in the control arm (40). A subsequent report confirmed the disease-free advantage (68% vs. 41.5%, $p < 0.02$) and noted a survival advantage as well (87.5% vs. 67.5%, $p < 0.02$) (41).

However, other randomized trials of adjuvant ADR in patients with high-grade extremity soft-tissue sarcomas have failed to demonstrate either a significant survival or disease-free survival benefit. At UCLA, Eilber et al randomized 119 patients with Grade III extremity sarcoma to ADR (450 mg/m^2) versus observation given over five monthly cycles after preoperative intra-arterial ADR and radiation therapy. No difference was noted in disease-free survival (58% vs. 54%) and overall survival (85% vs. 80%) after a median follow-up of 18 months. There was a slightly higher frequency of local recurrences in the control group, but this was not statistically significant (33).

The Scandinavian sarcoma group randomized 240 patients with resectable, localized high-grade sarcomas to adjuvant ADR (60 mg/m^2 for nine cycles) and observation after primary therapy. With a median follow-up of 40 months, there was no significant difference in overall or disease-free survival between groups (42).

Trials conducted at Dana Farber Cancer Institute/Massachusetts General Hospital and Eastern Cooperative Oncology Group (ECOG) also showed no survival or disease-free survival benefit in the Adriamycin group (43–45). At the M.D. Anderson Tumor Institute, 47 patients with high-grade sarcoma were randomized to observation versus combination chemotherapy with cyclophosphamide, Adriamycin, vincristine, and Actinomycin-D for seven cycles. Primary therapy included conservative surgical excision and postoperative radiotherapy. The disease-free survival in the chemotherapy group was 85% at 2 years, 60% at 5 years, and 55% at 10 years; this was significantly superior to that of the observation group, which experienced disease-free survivals of 57%, 35%, and 35%, respectively. However, overall survival was not significantly improved (46).

At the National Cancer Institute, 67 patients with extremity sarcomas were randomized to observation versus combination chemotherapy with cyclophosphamide, Adriamycin, methotrexate, and leucovorin rescue after treatment of their primary sarcoma. At 7.1 years median follow-up, the 5-year disease-free survival and overall survival were 75% and 82% in the chemotherapy group, which was superior to that seen in the observation group of 54% and 60%, respectively (47,48). The high dose of ADR utilized in this trial was associated with significant cardiac toxicity. A subsequent trial comparing the same chemotherapy regimen with a reduced ADR dose and no methotrexate regimen showed no difference in disease-free or overall survival between the two arms. Importantly, treatment-related cardiotoxicity was reduced in the low-dose regimen (47).

Edmonson and co-workers, from the Mayo Clinic, randomized patients to eight cycles of ADR, vincristine, and Actinomycin-D after complete excision. No radiation therapy was utilized. They noted no survival advantage for the chemotherapy group, although these patients experienced some delay in the development of distant metastases and required fewer salvage surgical procedures for excision of metastases (49). Local failure was 70% in the two arms of this study, underscoring the need for adjuvant irradiation.

The European Organization for Research on Treatment of Cancer (EORTC) conducted a multi-institutional study randomizing 225 patients to observation vs. combination chemotherapy with CYVADIC (cyclophosphamide, vincristine, ADR, and DTIC) for eight cycles. All patients received postoperative irradiation. The 3-year disease-free survival was 67% for the chemotherapy group vs. 52% for the control patients. However, overall survival was not significantly improved (50).

In summary, the value of adjuvant chemotherapy for patients with high-grade soft-tissue sarcomas of the extremity is unresolved. While some trials showed a disease-free survival advantage, other trials have not confirmed these findings (Table 16–1). Prolonged survival benefit has not been observed with extended follow-up in any randomized study.

NONEXTREMITY SARCOMAS

Approximately 40% of soft-tissue sarcomas occur in nonextremity sites. The surgical approach to these tumors is tempered by the inability to perform an ablative (amputation) or, in some cases, a radical procedure (compartmental resection). Adjacent vital structures often constrain the surgeon to local excision with limited margins of resection. Because of the difficulty in obtaining wide negative margins, adjuvant therapy is often recommended.

Since 1977, the NCI has conducted a randomized prospective study of patients with high-grade sarcoma of the head and neck, breast, and trunk. Thirty-one patients were randomized after surgical resection and postoperative radiotherapy to adjuvant combination chemotherapy (Adriamycin, cyclophosphamide, and methotrexate) versus observation. The results revealed a 3-year actuarial disease-free survival in the chemotherapy arm of 77% compared to 49% in the control group ($p = 0.075$). There was no significant benefit in overall survival. Subset analysis demonstrated that the group of patients with sarcoma of the trunk demonstrated the greatest benefit from chemotherapy (51).

Retroperitoneal tumors are more difficult to manage. Most of these tumors are large (greater than 10 cm) and locally advanced at diagnosis. They surround vital structures, often precluding satisfactory wide excision. In addition, adjacent radiosensitive organs, particularly the bowel and kidneys, limit the delivery of postoperative radiotherapy. At the NCI, combined modality studies were performed with resectable soft-tissue sarcomas of the retroperitoneum. After surgical resection and high-dose postoperative radiation, 15 patients were randomized to receive or

Table 16–1. Selected Randomized Series of Adjuvant Chemotherapy for High-Grade Soft-Tissue Sarcomas

Author	No. of Patients	Drug(s)	5-year Survival (%) Disease-Free	Overall	Comments
1. Picci et al (41)	33	ADR	68	87.5	38% received RT
	44	Control	41.5 ($p < 0.02$)	67.5 ($p < 0.02$)	
2. Rosenberg et al (48)	37	ADR, CPM, MTX	73	84	Drugs given ± RT
	28	Control	53 ($p < 0.04$)	60 ($p < 0.04$)	
3. Bramwell et al (50)	173	CPM, VCR, ADR, DTIC	67*	79*	45% of patients received RT as well as chemotherapy—reduced local recurrence
	185	Control	52* ($p = 0.01$)	74* ($p = 0.12$)	
4. Benjamin et al (46)	20	VACA	60	75	All patients in treatment arm received 6500 cGy in 6.5 weeks
	23	Control	35 ($p = 0.05$)	61 ($p > 0.05$)	

*3-year survival
ADR = Adriamycin, doxorubicin
CPM = Cyclophosphamide, cytoxan
MTX = Methotrexate
VCR = Vincristine
VACA = VCR + ADR + CPM + Actinomycin-D

not receive adjuvant Adriamycin, cyclophosphamide, and methotrexate. The 2-year actuarial survival, disease-free survival or locoregional control was not improved in the chemotherapy arm. In addition, there was significant morbidity, primarily related to bowel injury (52).

In an attempt to improve locoregional control and reduce bowel injury associated with external beam radiation, a randomized prospective trial was carried out comparing postoperative conventional high-dose external beam radiation therapy (5000 to 5500 cGy) versus intraoperative radiation (2000 cGy) plus low-dose external beam radiation (3500 to 4000 cGy). Intraoperative radiation was used at the time of surgery and permitted a high single dose of electron beam therapy to be delivered directly to the tumor bed after moving as many incidental organs and tissues as possible out of the radiation field. The therapy in the intraoperative arm was better tolerated with less acute toxicity. At 5-year follow-up, there was a trend toward an improved in-field local control in the experimental arm. However, no improvement in disease-free or overall survival was seen (53).

UNRESECTABLE SARCOMAS

When soft-tissue sarcomas are judged to be technically unresectable or when the patient is medically inoperable, such patients are treated with palliative intent by many physicians. The rationale behind this strategy is partially based on the traditional belief that soft-tissue sarcomas are radioresistant. In 1951, Sir Stanford Cade was among the first to report encouraging results in the treatment of sarcoma by radiation therapy alone (20). Subsequently, others have shown that radiation therapy alone can achieve local control in patients with sarcomas. Tepper and Suit treated 36 patients with radiation alone (54). The 5-year overall survival rate was 28% and local control was 44%. There was an inverse relationship between tumor size and the ability to obtain tumor control. It was concluded that local control can be achieved by radiation alone but usually requires aggressive treatment with high doses of radiation, which carry significant risk of adverse sequelae.

At the NCI, in an attempt of improving tumor response and minimizing late radiation-induced complications, patients with unresectable sarcomas were treated with hyperfractionated, high-dose external beam radiation (6500 to 7500 cGy in twice daily fractions over 7 to 9 weeks) combined with continuous infusion of iododeoxyuridine (IUdR), a nonhypoxic radiosensitizer. Of the 28 patients treated, five had complete tumor response, 14 had a partial objective response, and in six patients the tumor size remained stable. Local tumor control that lasted for the patients' remaining life was achieved in 17 of 28 patients (61%) (55,56). It seems that radiotherapy alone for selected patients with unresectable (or inoperable) sarcoma can result in local control. Although preliminary results of external beam radiation and radiosensitizers are encouraging, their definite role awaits the results of controlled, randomized trials that are just beginning (55–57).

SUMMARY

Soft-tissue sarcomas include a wide variety of tumors arising from various primary sites but have fairly homogenous natural histories. The primary concern in their management is the prevention of local recurrence. Consequently, surgical excision is usually combined with radiotherapy, preoperatively or postoperatively, in the treatment of soft-tissue sarcomas. Potential advances in the delivery of radiotherapy include the use of hyperfractionation and intraoperative radiotherapy, particularly in nonextremity, retroperitoneal, and unresectable sarcomas.

High-grade soft-tissue sarcomas show a proclivity for distant metastases. Combination chemotherapy, usually Adriamycin-based, have been used in tandem with surgery and radiotherapy for these high-grade tumors and those that exhibit characteristics that herald a high rate of recurrence. Table 16–2 is a meta-analysis of series utilizing preoperative and postoperative radiotherapy and adjuvant chemotherapy following surgery with or without radiotherapy. Although several Phase II studies show an apparent survival advantage with the addition of chemotherapy, no such advantage has been established in randomized Phase III studies. It appears certain, however, that systemic therapy will continue to be used in high-risk subgroups of patients with soft-tissue sarcomas in an attempt to improve cure rates, as well as to define the optimal drug combinations and doses.

Table 16–2. Meta-Analysis of Preoperative, Postoperative, and Adjuvant Chemotherapy ± Radiotherapy for High-Grade Soft-Tissue Sarcomas

Treatment	Local Control (%)	5-year Disease-free Survival (%)
Preoperative RT (23–25)	83–95	56–74
Postoperative RT (6,26–28)	78–92	60–68
Adjuvant chemotherapy* ± RT (41,46,48,50)	80–90	67

*25–40% of this group had local recurrence following surgery at presentation.
RT = radiotherapy

REFERENCES

1. Boring CC, Squires TS, Tong T. Cancer statistics 1991. CA 42(1):19, 1992.
2. Trojani M, Contesso G, Coindre JM, et al. Soft-tissue sarcoma of adults: Study of pathological, prognostic variables and definition of a histopathological grading system. Int J Cancer 33:37, 1984.
3. Alvegard RA, Berg NO, Baldetorp B, et al. Cellular DNA content and prognosis of high grade soft tissue sarcoma: The Scandinavian Sarcoma Group experience. J Clin Oncol 8:538, 1990.
4. Potter DA, Kinsella T, Glatstein E, et al. High-grade soft tissue sarcomas of the extremities. Cancer 58:190, 1986.
5. Rooser B, Attewell R, Berg NO, Rydholm A. Prognostication in soft tissue sarcoma. A model with four risk factors. Cancer 61:817, 1988.
6. Bowden L, Booher RJ. The principles and techniques of resection of soft parts for sarcoma. Surgery 44:963, 1958.
7. Enzinger FM, Weiss SW. Soft Tissue Tumors. St. Louis, C.V. Mosby Co., 1983.
8. Potter DA, Glenn J, Kinsella T, et al. Patterns of recurrence in patients with high grade soft tissue sarcoma. J Clin Oncol 3:353, 1985.
9. Chang AE, Rosenberg SA, Glatstein EJ, Antman KH. Sarcomas of soft tissue. *In:* Cancer: Principles and Practice of Oncology. DeVita VT, Hellman S, Rosenberg SA (Eds). Philadelphia, JB Lippincott Co., 1989, p. 1345.
10. Simon MA, Enneking WF. The management of soft tissue sarcoma of the extremities. J Bone Joint Surg 58:317, 1976.
11. Gerner RE, Moore GE, Pickren JW. Soft tissue sarcomas. Ann Surg 181:803, 1975.
12. Shiu MJ, Castro FB, Hajdu SI, et al. Surgical treatment of 297 soft tissue sarcomas of the lower extremity. Ann Surg 182:597, 1975.
13. Cantin J, McNeer GP, Chu FC, et al. The problem of local recurrence after treatment of soft tissue sarcoma. Ann Surg 168:47, 1968.
14. Clark RL Jr, Martin RG, White EC, Old JW. Clinical aspects of soft tissue tumors. AMA Arch Surg 74:859, 1957.

15. Shieber W, Graham P. An experience with sarcomas of the soft tissue in adults. Surgery 52:295, 1962.
16. Martin RG, Butler JJ, Albores-Saaverdra J. Soft tissue tumors: Surgical treatment and results. *In:* Tumors of Bone and Soft Tissue. Chicago, Year Book Medical, 1965, p. 333.
17. Collin C, Hadju SI, Godbold J, et al. Localized, operable soft tissue sarcoma of the lower extremity. Arch Surg 121:1425, 1986.
18. Karakousis CP, Emrich LJ, Rao U, et al. Feasibility of limb salvage and survival in soft tissue sarcomas. Cancer 57:484, 1986.
19. Suit HD, Russell WO. Radiation therapy of soft tissue sarcomas. Cancer 36:759, 1975.
20. Cade SS. Soft tissue tumors: Their natural history and treatment. Proc R Soc Med 19:19, 1951.
21. Suit H, Proppe K, Mankin M, et al. Preoperative radiation therapy for sarcoma of soft tissue. Cancer 47:2269, 1981.
22. Tepper JE. Role of radiation therapy in the management of patients with bone and soft tissue sarcomas. Semin Oncol 16:281, 1989.
23. Suit HD, Mankin MJ, Schiller AL, et al. Results of treatment of sarcoma of soft tissue by radiation and surgery at Massachusetts General Hospital. Cancer Treat Symp 3:43, 1985.
24. Lindberg R. Treatment of localized soft tissue sarcomas in adults at M.D. Anderson Hospital and Tumor Institute (1960–1981). Cancer Treat Symp 3:59, 1985.
25. Enneking WF, McAuliffe JA. Adjunctive preoperative radiation in treatment of soft tissue sarcoma: A preliminary report. Cancer Treat Symp 3:37, 1985.
26. Lindberg RD, Martin RG, Romsdahl MM, et al. Conservative surgery and postoperative radiotherapy in 300 adults with soft tissue sarcomas. Cancer 47:2391, 1981.
27. Leibel SA, Transbaugh RF, Wara WM, et al. Soft tissue sarcomas of the extremities. Survival patterns of failure with conservative surgery and postoperative irradiation compared to surgery alone. Cancer 50:1076, 1982.
28. Suit HD, Mankin HJ, Wood WC, et al. Preoperative, intraoperative, and postoperative radiation in the treatment of primary soft tissue sarcomas. Cancer 55:2659, 1985.
29. Rosenberg SA, Tepper J, Glatstein E, et al. Prospective randomized evaluations of (1) limb-sparing surgery plus radiation therapy compared with amputation and (2) the role of adjuvant chemotherapy. Ann Surg 196:305, 1982.
30. Eilber FR, Mirra JJ, Grant TT, et al. Is amputation necessary for sarcomas? Ann Surg 192:431, 1980.
31. Eilber FR, Morton DL, Eckhardt T, et al. Limb salvage for skeletal and soft tissue sarcomas: Multidisciplinary preoperative therapy. Cancer 53:2579, 1984.
32. Eilber FR, Guiliano AE, Muth J, et al. Limb salvage for high grade soft tissue sarcomas of the extremity: Experience at the University of California, Los Angeles. Cancer Treat Symp 3:49, 1985.
33. Eilber FT, Guiliano AE, Huth JF, Morton DL. A randomized prospective trial using postoperative adjuvant chemotherapy (Adriamycin) in high grade extremity soft tissue sarcoma. Am J Clin Oncol 11:39, 1988.
34. Eilber FR, Huth J, Rosen G. Neo-adjuvant therapy for extremity soft tissue sarcoma: Intra-arterial chemotherapy and radiation followed by surgical resection. Workshop on progress in Regional Cancer Therapy I, Vienna, Austria, 1988.
35. Denton JW, Dunham WK, Salter M, et al. Preoperative regional chemotherapy and rapid fraction irradiation for sarcomas of the soft tissue and bone. Surg Gynecol Obstet 158:545, 1984.
36. Borden EC, Amato DA, Rosenbaum C, et al. Randomized comparison of three adriamycin regimens for metastatic soft tissue sarcomas. J Clin Oncol 5:840, 1987.
37. Omura GA, Major FJ, Blessing JA, et al. A randomized study of adriamycin with and without dimethyl trazenomidazole carboxamide in advanced uterine sarcoma. Cancer 52:626, 1983.
38. Schoenfeld D, Rosenbaum C, Horton J, et al. A comparison of adriamycin versus vincristine, adriamycin and cyclophosphamide for advanced sarcomas. Cancer 50:2757, 1982.
39. Muss HB, Bindy B, Disaia PJ, et al. Treatment of recurrent or advanced uterine sarcoma: A randomized trial of doxorubicin versus doxorubicin and cyclophosphamide (a phase III trial of the Gynecologic Oncology Group). Cancer 55:1648, 1985.
40. Gherlinzoni F, Bacci G, Picci P, et al. A randomized trial for the treatment of high grade soft-tissue sarcomas of the extremities: Preliminary observations. J Clin Oncol 4:552, 1986.
41. Picci P, Bacci G, Gherlinzoni F, et al. Results of a randomized trial for the treatment of localized soft tissue tumors (STS) of the extremities in adult patients. *In:* Recent Concepts in Sarcoma Treatment. Ryan JR, Baker LO (Eds). Boston, Kluwer Academic, 1988, p. 144.
42. Alvergard TA, Sigurdsson H, Mouridsen H, et al. Adjuvant chemotherapy with doxorubicin in high-grade soft tissue sarcoma: A random-

ized trial of the Scandinavian Sarcoma Group. J Clin Oncol 10:1504, 1989.
43. Antman K, Suit H, Amato D, et al. Preliminary results of a randomized trial of adjuvant doxorubicin for sarcomas: Lack of apparent difference between treatment groups. J Clin Oncol 2:601, 1984.
44. Lerner HJ, Amato DA, Savlov Ed, et al. Eastern Cooperative Oncology Group: A comparison of adjuvant doxorubicin and observation for patients with localized soft tissue sarcoma. J Clin Oncol 5:613, 1987.
45. Wilson RE, Wood WC, Lerner HL, et al. Doxorubicin chemotherapy in the treatment of soft tissue sarcoma. Arch Surg 121:1354, 1986.
46. Benjamin RS, Terjanian TO, Fenoglio CJ, et al. The importance of combination chemotherapy for adjuvant treatment of high-risk patients with soft tissue sarcomas of the extremities. *In:* Adjuvant Therapy of Cancer V. Orlando, Grune and Stratton, 1987, p. 735.
47. Chang AE, Kinsella T, Glatstein E, et al. Adjuvant chemotherapy for patients with high grade soft tissue sarcomas of the extremity. J Clin Oncol 6:1491, 1988.
48. Rosenberg SA, Chang AE, Glatstein E. Adjuvant chemotherapy for treatment of extremity soft tissue sarcomas: Review of the National Cancer Institute experience. Cancer Treat Symp 3:83, 1985.
49. Edmonson JH, Fleming TR, Ivins JC, et al. Randomized study of systemic chemotherapy following complete excision of nonosseous sarcomas. J Clin Oncol 2:1390, 1984.
50. Bramwell V, Rousse J, Steward W, et al. European experience of adjuvant chemotherapy for soft tissue sarcoma: Interim report of a randomized trial of CYVADIC versus control. *In:* Recent Concepts in Sarcoma Treatment. Ryan JR, Baker LO (Eds). Boston, Kluwer Academic, 1988, p. 156.
51. Glenn J, Kinsella T, Glatstein E, et al. A randomized prospective trial of adjuvant chemotherapy in adults with soft tissue sarcomas of the head and neck, breast and trunk. Cancer 55:1206, 1985.
52. Glenn J, Sindelar WF, Kinsella T, et al. Results of multi-modality therapy of resectable softtissue sarcomas of the retroperitoneum. Surgery 97:316, 1985.
53. Kinsella TJ, Sindelar WF, Lock E, et al. Preliminary results of a randomized study of adjuvant radiation therapy in resectable adult retroperitoneal soft tissue sarcomas. J Clin Oncol 6:18, 1988.
54. Tepper JE, Suit HD. Radiation therapy of soft tissue sarcomas. Cancer 55:2273, 1985.
55. Kinsella TJ, Glatstein E. Clinical experience with intravenous radiosensitizers in unresectable sarcomas. Cancer 59:908, 1987.
56. Tochner Z, Kinsella TJ, Rowland J, et al. Treatment of unresectable sarcomas of adults with hyperfractionated irradiation and iododeoxyuridine. BIR Report 19:107, 1989.
57. Rosenthal CJ, Rotman M. Concomitant continuous infusion Adriamycin and radiation: Evidence of synergistic effects in soft tissue sarcomas. *In:* Concomitant Continuous Infusion Chemotherapy and Radiation. Rotman M, Rosenthal CJ (Eds). Berlin, Springer-Verlag, 1991, p. 271.

Chapter 17

PEDIATRIC TUMORS

GIULIO J. D'ANGIO

Some of the major successes in medicine during the past few decades have occurred in the field of pediatric oncology. Much of this is due to the effective collaboration among surgical, radiation, and medical oncologists (1). Each member of the team has adapted his strengths to those of his partners. This has meant assuming either a dominant role or, in some cases, a secondary position, deferring to another team member who carries the major burden of management. This cooperation and coordination has led to better survival rates and fewer iatrogenic complications. It has, for example, made possible the development of limb- and organ-sparing procedures rather than amputations and radical exenterative procedures, due, in part, to surgeons' increasing confidence in their colleagues in medical and radiation oncology to control residual disease. Radiation oncologists have lowered doses and decreased irradiated volumes because systemic anticancer drugs have been shown to suppress not only distant micrometastases but residual local disease as well.

This chapter will focus on specific instances in which better control of circumscribed tumor volumes results from combined chemoradiation. In most of these instances, true potentiation of radiation effects has not been established. Instead, converging cytotoxicity nearly on an additive basis seems to be the case.

No attempt will be made to cover the many examples of chemotherapeutic efficacy in the control of primary, metastatic, or recurrent neoplasms when radiotherapy (RT) has not been or is not part of the initial management program.

LEUKEMIA

Radiation therapy has a restricted role in children with leukemia. It is used almost exclusively for treatment of **sanctuary sites;** i.e., organs and structures that are sheltered from effective control by systemically administered antileukemic drugs. The leptomeninges are the sanctuary sites of most importance.

Acute Lymphoblastic Leukemia (ALL)

Leptomeninges

Prevention of meningeal leukemia has been one of the important advances made in the management of children with leukemia. Much of this work has been accomplished in patients with ALL.

Three decades ago, it became clear as remission rates climbed that meningeal leukemia was being seen with increasing frequency (2). Evans et al showed that it is possible to suppress the disease by giving intrathecal (IT) methotrexate (MTX) monthly to asymptomatic patients (3). St. Jude investigators pioneered the development of RT methods that accomplish the same goal (4). Craniospinal RT of 2400 cGy reduced the incidence of CNS leukemia from $> 50\%$ to $< 10\%$ (5). This form of therapy became the standard against which alternate treatments were measured. It is beyond the scope of this discussion to detail those interesting trials, which entailed RT to the brain and/or the spinal cord at different dose levels, intrathecal medications (MTX $\pm$ cytarabine and prednisone), variations of systemic drugs (mainly high doses of MTX), and various combinations of these. Several effective regimens have been developed, some without a RT component. Of interest here is the demonstration that cranial irradiation plus IT/MTX was as protective as craniospinal RT (6). Lowering the dose to 1800 cGy and failure to include the base of the skull did not seem to compromise that result, although objections to the latter conclusion have been voiced (7,8). This suggests that MTX concentrations in the cerebrospinal fluid and flow patterns to the basilar cisterns bathe the meninges efficiently, as they do in the spinal canal, but do not attain the same protective levels elsewhere in the cranial vault. The two treatment methods, therefore, are truly complementary.

The neuropsychologic adversities that develop in the cranially irradiated children are discussed in Chapter 38. These problems have led to wider use of methods that do not entail RT, which is reserved for patients with high-risk prognostic features at diagnosis and for those who develop meningeal disease.

Testes

A Children's Cancer Study Group (CCSG) randomized clinical trial confirmed the testes as a sanctuary site (6). A dose of 1200 cGy to the testes at the time of remission induction reduced the frequency of testicular involvement during maintenance therapy to zero. However, it did not affect the later testicular relapse rate and did not impact eventual survival. Therefore, RT is used only when testicular leukemia is manifest, either at diagnosis or thereafter. Doses of 2400 cGy are commonly employed. Here again, RT is used to fill a "gap" left by chemotherapy, which is the mainstay of treatment for these children.

Other Sanctuary Sites

Enlarged kidneys, liver, spleen, and thymus secondary to cellular infiltrates are not uncommon at the time of diagnosis (9). RT is seldom used, except in children with nephromegaly and impaired renal function, in an attempt to reverse the pathophysiology. This usually is caused by uric acid nephropathy rather than the leukemia infiltrate, which is not destructive. The cells tend to infiltrate between nephrons, preserving the functional unit in most instances. Nonetheless, RT is often requested while other medical measures are instituted. Doses in the range of 1000 to 1500 cGy can be tried.

Central Nervous System (CNS) Relapse

Although this chapter concerns the primary treatment of pediatric tumors, an exception will be made here in discussing management of recurrent disease. Children with ALL can develop meningeal leukemia despite RT or other prophylaxis at the time of diagnosis (7). This often entails cranial irradiation, with its known deleterious neuropsychologic sequelae, so that reirradiation of the brain is viewed with some alarm. The severity of longterm CNS damage after a certain dose seems to be inversely related to the size of the individual fractions used to achieve that total dose (10). Also, Considine et al reported good results using widely spaced small-fraction radiation for CNS prophylaxis, e.g., 100 to 120 cGy q 10 wks for 3 years (11).

These observations were used to fashion a combined intermittent IT chemotherapy + RT regimen for babies for prophylaxis (when only the head is irradiated) and for therapy of those who develop CNS leukemia when craniospinal RT is given (12). This regimen entails the delivery of 600 cGy to the designated volume as 150 cGy/day × 4 or 200 cGy/day × 3. Thereafter, 100 cGy is added monthly for 1 year, for a total of 1800 cGy. The monthly treatments are given 24 to 48 hours before the IT medications. This is done for two reasons: to use RT as an adjuvant drug following the chemotherapy schedule, and to lyze any heaped-up leukemic cells that might block free flow of the IT drugs through the subarachnoid pathways and down the perivascular spaces of Virchow. The IT drugs used are MTX, cytarabine, and hydrocortisone.

The details regarding RT doses and the chemotherapy used for reinduction and the results of a pilot study using this system were reported recently (12). Three babies developed bone marrow relapse and died. Nine of 10 patients treated in first CNS relapse, however, remained in CNS and bone marrow remission after reinduction systemic chemotherapy and the intermittent RT and IT chemotherapy described. The minimum follow-up period was 2 years. Two of the nine patients developed testicular relapses, which were treated successfully, and one of the 10 developed acute myelomonocytic leukemia (AMML) and died. Only one of eight patients treated after two or more episodes of CNS leukemia remained in complete remission.

There are other successful ways of salvaging patients (13,14). The above method has been detailed because it uses RT in an unconventional manner, with the twofold purpose described. It meanwhile seeks to avoid neuropsychologic damage through the use of low single fractions, as originally conceived by the Detroit group (11).

Nonlymphoblastic Leukemia (NLL)

In addition to what has been said for ALL sanctuary sites, patients with granulocytic leukemia can develop cellular infiltrates, forming localized plaques or frank masses (chloromas or granulocytic sarcomas) in the skin or deeper organs (15). They can be present at diagnosis or can develop thereafter, and RT is usually added to systemic chemotherapy under those circumstances. Doses of 2400 cGy are recommended when the CNS is involved (16).

LYMPHOMAS

Hodgkin's Disease (HD)

Management of children with HD remains in flux, but it is becoming increasingly clear that multidrug regimens will play a major role (17,18). A full exposition of the many and complex issues involved that balance means of controlling disease vs. treatment-related adversities would not be germane to this discussion; for more information, see Chapter 38. Chemotherapy already is substituting for 3600- to 4000-cGy large-field RT for Stage III patients, and fields and doses are being reduced toward zero for these patients as confidence in the efficacy of chemotherapy builds (19).

The search for effective disease control with the least troublesome longterm sequelae has extended to early-stage HD, in which chemotherapy with or without low-dose local-field RT, and local-field RT alone are being explored (17,21). Each has its proponents, but until these issues are resolved, most patients, especially prepubertal children, will receive chemoradiation therapy. This typically contains multidrug chemotherapy based on Nitrogen *m*ustard, *o*ncovin, *p*rednisone, *p*rocarbazine (MOPP) and *A*driamycin, *b*leomycin, *v*inblastine, *da*carbazine (ABVD) and their modifications and combinations, plus moderate-dose RT (e.g., 2000 cGy) to volumes containing bulky disease (variously defined) (22,23). RT is given to reduce the incidence of relapses in the areas of bulky disease. The evidence that RT is needed for this purpose is tenuous (17,19). It is not clear that combined therapy will have a place in the initial management of children once drug regimens evolve further. Such chemotherapy regimens will have to yield high disease-control rates and low incidences of therapy-related infertility and cancer. Then, chemotherapy alone will be the treatment of choice. A possible exception would be the infrequent child with disease high in the neck, who is eligible for RT alone. In summary, combined therapy is fading from the picture and may soon disappear (23).

Non-Hodgkin's Lymphoma (NHL)

Much of what has been stated regarding HD applies to the spectrum of malignant disease considered non-Hodgkin's lymphoma. Relatively specific and very successful multidrug regimens have been developed for small- and large-cell lymphomas* (24,25). The pioneering LSA_2L_2 regimen from Memorial Hospital in New York included RT, which the initial reports suggested was needed to reduce recurrence in sites of bulky disease and the CNS (26). Doses of 2400 to 3000 cGy were being used. The indications for RT have been refined, and it is usually omitted from the care of these children, all of whom are given multiagent chemotherapy appropriate to the NHL type (27).

BRAIN TUMORS

There have been many attempts to improve survival in children with brain tumors.

*The cytohistologic constellation once termed "non-African Burkitt's lymphoma" is now rarely used. It is no longer considered a separate entity and is included in the large-cell NHL designation.

Recent successes with the malignant gliomas and medulloblastoma encourage further exploration. Here, a true interplay between RT and chemotherapy can be documented.

Malignant Gliomas

A group-wide study by the CCSG has documented the efficacy of prednisone, lomustine (CCNU), and vincristine (VCR) added to 5580-cGy local RT in improving the outlook of children with high-grade astrocytomas; i.e., anaplastic astrocytomas and glioblastomas multiforme (28). RT alone in these children gave a 18% 5-year event-free survival; combined therapy resulted in 46% survival. These encouraging results are being pursued in various centers, using different drug combinations. The CCSG trial is employing the "8-in-one" drug regimen, for example (29). Parenthetically, some investigators believe that the entire neuroaxis should be irradiated, especially in children with posterior fossa primaries. They report a high risk of leptomeningeal dissemination in such patients (30).

Medulloblastoma (MBL)

The traditional term "medulloblastoma" will be used for this discussion because some relevant studies antedated the advent of the new nosology, primitive neuroectodermal tumor (PNET)* (31).

Two major cooperative group trials were conducted in the 1970s and 1980s, one was by the International Society of Pediatric Oncology (SIOP) (32), the other was an intergroup trial encompassing the CCSG and the Radiation Therapy Oncology Group (RTOG) (33). The two designs were similar except that the CCSG/RTOG chemotherapy regimen added prednisone to CCNU and VCR. Both the SIOP and the CCSG/RTOG trial used similar doses of these two drugs. In the SIOP trial, the doses and timing were as follows: VCR 1 mg/m^2/week × 8 during RT; 4 to 6 weeks rest; then VCR 1.5 mg/m^2 on days 1, 8, and 15, plus 100 mg/m^2 oral CCNU on day 1 of courses that were cycled q 6 weeks for 1 year. The CCSG/RTOG trial added prednisone (40 mg/m^2/day × 14) during the initial course, when the VCR dose was 1.5 mg/m^2/week × 8. The SIOP RT doses were 3500 to 4500 cGy (whole brain), 5000 to 5500 cGy (posterior fossa), and 3000 to 3500 cGy (spinal cord). The CCSG/RTOG doses were 3500 to 4000 cGy (whole brain and spinal cord) and 5000 to 5500 cGy (posterior fossa).

The 5-year event-free survival rates for the RT only and RT + chemotherapy groups were about 42% and 57%, respectively, for the SIOP trial. In the same order, the results for CCSG/RTOG were 50% and 59%. Neither of the differences between the RT ± CT arms were statistically significant. Thus, no benefit could be demonstrated for chemotherapy, except in certain subsets. These were defined in the SIOP trial as patients with subtotal tumor removal, brain stem involvement, and larger tumors (Chang T_3, T_4) at diagnosis (Table 17–1). Patients with larger tumors also seemed to benefit in the CCSG/RTOG study, as did those with evidence of spinal dissemination at diagnosis.

These early trials gave encouragement to the use of adjuvant chemotherapy, even though they had been overtaken by better imaging and other diagnostic methods, better surgical techniques, and more promising chemotherapeutic agents. The major advance, however, has been from the addition of cisplatinum (CDDP) to the armamentarium.

Lefkowitz et al initiated a pilot study of CDDP added to VCR and CCNU in children with posterior fossa PNETs in relapse (34). Definite responses were obtained, and these three drugs were employed as adjuvants to postoperative RT in children with high-risk PNETs. These were defined as tumors that were biopsied only or partially resected, tumors that infiltrated the brain stem, and/or tumors that had evidence of dissemination (i.e., Chang Stage M1, M2, or M3) (Table 17–1). Neither age nor histologic type were considered to be risk factors, but children under 18 months of age were excluded (35).

The doses and timing of chemotherapy were similar to the CCSG/RTOG trial described, except that the CCNU dose was reduced to 75 mg/m^2, and 68 mg/m^2 of CDDP was added on the first day of the eight 6-week cycles given after irradiation. RT doses for most children were 3600 cGy to the craniospinal axis and 5580 cGy to the

*The term "PNET," when applied to the posterior fossa, includes those tumors previously called medulloblastomas, pure or with ependymal elements.

Table 17–1. Chang Staging System for Posterior Fossa Primitive Neuroectodermal Tumor/Medulloblastoma

Stage	Definition
Tumor	
T_1	Tumor < 3 cm in diameter and limited to the midline position in the vermis, roof of the fourth ventricle, and (less frequently) to the cerebellar hemispheres.
T_2	Tumor ≧ 3 cm in diameter, further invading one adjacent structure or partially filling the fourth ventricle.
T_3	
T_{3a}	Tumor invading two adjacent structures or completely filling the fourth ventricle with extension into the aqueduct of Sylvius, foramen of Magendie, or foramen of Luschka, thus producing marked internal hydrocephalus.
T_{3b}	Tumor arising from the floor of the fourth ventricle or brain stem and filling the fourth ventricle.
T_4	Tumor further spreading through the aqueduct of Sylvius to involve the third ventricle or midbrain, or tumor extending to the upper cervical cord.
Metastasis	
M_0	No evidence of gross subarachnoid or hematogeneous metastasis.
M_1	Microscopic tumor cells found in cerebrospinal fluid.
M_2	Gross nodular seedings demonstrated in the cerebellar, cerebral subarachnoid space, or in the third or lateral ventricles.
M_3	Gross nodular seedings in the spinal subarachnoid space.
M_4	Extraneural metastasis.

posterior fossa. Variations from this basic scheme are specified in the report by Packer et al that updates the results of this trial (36). The 5-year relapse-free and overall survival rates for 42 patients were 92%, with an apparent plateau at 18 months. This result was significantly better ($p = 0.001$) than that of 18 historical controls in which the survival curve flattened at about 30% after 5-½ years. By contrast, the projected 5-year event-free survival rate for 10 standard-risk patients who were treated with RT alone was, at best, 52% and was not statistically significantly different from results in 18 historical controls also treated with RT alone. Cisplatinum-related nephrotoxicity was not a major problem reported by Packer et al, but ototoxicity was more pronounced than would be expected after cisplatinum alone (37).

Other researchers have explored the use of lower doses of craniospinal RT in MBL patients (38–40). Most recently, a randomized clinical trial comparing standard to reduced doses has been aborted because of excess failures in the low-dose arm (41).

Tentative conclusions can be drawn from these disparate data. First, CDDP appears to have a role in the management of MBL patients; secondly, both standard-dose RT and a CDDP-containing regimen (or one equally effective) are needed for best control of high-risk MBL/PNET children. It may be that low-risk MBL/PNET patients receiving chemotherapy (e.g., CDDP) can be given reduced doses of craniospinal RT, but it first must be demonstrated that the drug(s) used improve the results after standard RT techniques. This is because there must be objective evidence of a supplementary gain by the chemotherapy. Otherwise, patients are put at both the risk of a higher relapse rate and the notable ototoxicity experienced by children having cranial RT plus CDDP (see Chapter 38). Any such study must also include careful neuropsychiatric evaluation to establish whether the lower RT dose decreases the cognitive adversities associated with standard RT methods and doses (42).

In order to decrease these difficulties in younger children, attempts have been made by several investigators to delay RT by giving chemotherapy initially. Various drug regimens have been employed for this purpose, including MOPP (43–45). Gratifying responses have been reported. It remains to be demonstrated that RT can be delayed for the many months or years needed for the child to become at least 6 years old, which is the chronologic age when neuropsychologic sequelae become less obvious, albeit not negligible (see Chapter 38).

Gliomas of the Optic Nerve and Chiasm

Gliomas of the optic nerve and chiasm are often found in young children, in whom the adversities of RT are prounounced (46). With a rationale similar to that noted above, Rosenstock et al attempted to suppress tumor growth delay or at least obviate the need for RT (47). They employed dactinomycin (AMD) and VCR. The natural course of these tumors is notoriously unpredictable. A recent update of experience using this approach (48) reported a 45% progression-free survival rate at 5 years after chemotherapy alone. How much can be ascribed to the chemotherapy vs. innate tumor/host interplays cannot be established with certainty. It also is not clear whether both AMD and VCR are needed to obtain these results (if real) or whether another drug regimen might be superior. Suffice it to say here that the AMD + VCR regimen is relatively well tolerated and is not known to be associated with major longterm disabilities. Therefore, it is still in use. Although not truly a chemoradiation regimen, because the RT is kept in therapeutic reserve, it demonstrates how the two modalities can be used with restraint to achieve a desired result.

NEUROBLASTOMA (NBL)*

Neuroblastoma is a tumor that remains an enigma. There is spontaneous resolution on the one hand, and inexorable disease progression despite therapy on the other (24). Considerable progress has been made, however, in identifying prognostic factors. Age and stage (Table 17–2) have long been known; cytohistologic pattern and biologic indices have been added more recently (49–51). Elevated serum ferritin values, NBL cell hyperdiploidy and hypotetraploidy, and 10 or more MYCN copy numbers are associated with a poor outcome (52–55). A formula for calculating probable survival has recently been published by Silver et al (56).

The foregoing is a preamble to the statement that surgery, RT, and chemotherapy play relatively small roles in determining outcome (53,57,58). The biology of the tumor/host relationship is such a dominating factor that it is impossible to establish which surgery-RT-drug combination is best or whether any at all is needed. Matthay et al reviewed 156 Stage II patients entered in Children's Chemotherapy Study Group trials (59). They found that neither surgery nor chemoradiation had an influence on survival when compared with controls. The same holds true for the other stages. Good results can be anticipated for Stages I and IV-S, and poor outcome can be expected for Stages III and IV. A possible exception is Stage III disease, in which total surgical removal and postoperative RT have each been reported to be of benefit (60–62). Analyses are confounded because different staging systems have been used and because of unconscious bias introduced by powerful biologic discriminating factors that were unknown or not obtained systematically when these children were being treated. There could well be a subset of patients with Stage III disease who have more favorable features, such as better circumscribed tumors that lend themselves to complete excision. The better result would then improperly be ascribed to the operation rather than intrinsic factors.

The improved results after RT reported by the Pediatric Oncology Group (POG) investigators were based on patients with POG Stage C disease (62), which encompasses both Stages IIB and III in the International Neuroblastoma Staging System (INSS) (Table 17–2). Most of the patients in the POG study were Stage III/INSS, and it can be inferred that the betterment applies to this larger of the two subsets. Firm conclusions await the analysis underway by Castleberry et al, who state that they will reexamine their data according to the INSS criteria. There will remain, even then, the uncertainties occasioned by the unknown distributions of patients according to biologic discriminants, as discussed regarding RT. Universal use of the INSS will eliminate one of these problems; agreement regarding which biologic indices to record is also needed (63).

In summary, children with favorable staging and biologic features will fare well, with an 80 to 100% expectation of survival regardless of therapy, and 80% or more of those with unfavorable features will not survive despite therapy (56). The exception to the latter statement is intensive treatment followed by allogeneic or autologous bone based on bone-marrow transplant (BMT) methods, including marrow rescue (see following).

Encouragement for the BMT approach is provided by the results after doses of combined chemoradiation short of the lethal levels used in BMT. It is described briefly here because it serves as another example of how large-field RT is explored in pediatric oncology as an extension of the concepts inherent in the use of systemic chemotherapy (see the ALL and Ewing's Sarcoma sections of this

*The Children's Cancer Study Group (Evans) staging system is used in this discussion unless otherwise specified.

Table 17–2. Neuroblastoma Staging Systems

Children's Cancer Study Group	Pediatric Oncology Group	International Neuroblastoma Staging System
Stage I Tumor confined to the organ of structure of origin.	Stage A Complete gross resection of primary tumor, with or without microscopic residual. Intracavitary lymph nodes, not adhered to and removed with primary (nodes adhered to or within tumor resection may be positive for tumor without upstaging patient to Stage C) histologically free of tumor. If primary in abdomen or pelvis, liver histologically free of tumor.	Stage 1 Localized tumor confined to the area of origin; complete gross excision, with or without microscopic residual disease; identifiable ipsilateral and contralateral lymph nodes negative microscopically.
Stage II Tumor extending in continuity beyond the organ or structure of origin but not crossing the midline. Regional lymph nodes on the ipsilateral side may be involved.	Stage B Gross unresected primary tumor. Nodes and liver same as Stage A.	Stage 2A Unilateral tumor with incomplete gross excision; identifiable ipsilateral and contralateral lymph nodes negative microscopically.
Stage III Tumor extending in continuity beyond the midline. Regional lymph nodes may be involved bilaterally.	Stage C Complete or incomplete resection of primary tumor. Intracavitary nodes not adhered to primary histologically positive for tumor. Liver as in Stage A.	Stage 2B Unilateral tumor with complete or incomplete gross excision; with positive ipsilateral regional lymph nodes; identifiable contralateral lymph nodes negative microscopically.
Stage IV Remote disease involving the skeleton, bone marrow, soft tissue, and distant lymph node groups, etc. (see Stage IV-S).	Stage D Any dissemination of disease beyond intracavitary nodes, i.e., extracavitary nodes, liver, skin, bone marrow, bone.	Stage 3 Tumor infiltrating across the midline with or without regional lymph node involvement or unilateral tumor with contralateral regional lymph node involvement or midline tumor with bilateral regional lymph node involvement. Stage 4 Dissemination of tumor to distant lymph nodes, bone, bone marrow, liver, and/or other organs (except as defined in 4S).
Stage IV-S Patients who would otherwise be Stage I or II, but who have remote disease confined to liver, skin, or bone marrow (without radiographic evidence of bone metastases on complete skeletal survey).		Stage 4S Localized primary tumor as defined for Stage 1 or 2 with dissemination limited to liver and/or skin.

chapter). Low doses of total body irradiation (TBI) (e.g., 50 cGy/day × 2–3) given in 3-week courses were added to routine chemotherapy [cyclophosphamide (CP) + VCR + dacarbazine] for children with Stage IV disease (64). Prompt complete responses were obtained in all 14 children so treated. The pilot study was stopped because of life-threatening thrombocytopenia (two deaths due to intracranial hemorrhage), a problem that can be solved by restitution of stored bone marrow as is done for BMT.

In conclusion, there is little convincing evidence that any form of standard therapy, including chemoradiation, has had a major impact on the outcome for NBL patients once all prognostic factors are taken into account.

KIDNEY TUMORS

Wilms' Tumor (WT)

Not long ago, routine postoperative RT was given to all children with WT (65). This continued even after the advent of effective chemotherapy in the form of AMD and VCR (66). Systematic studies by cooperative study groups have now narrowed the indications according to histologic type and stage of disease (Table 17–3). The series of clinical trials conducted by the National Wilms' Tumor Study (NWTS) helped to define and separate two types of WT from two other entities previously considered WT variants (67). The two WT types are the favorable histology (FH) and anaplastic (Ana) forms. The two non-WT entities are the clear cell sarcoma of the kidney (CCSK) and the rhabdoid tumor of the kidney (RTK).

Table 17–3. The National Wilms' Tumor Study Staging System

STAGE:	
I	Tumor limited to kidney and completely excised. The surface of the renal capsule is intact. Tumor was not ruptured before or during removal. There is no residual tumor apparent beyond the margins of resection.
II	Tumor extends beyond the kidney but is completely excised. There is regional extension of the tumor, i.e., penetration through the outer surface of the renal capsule into perirenal soft tissues. Vessels outside the kidney substance are infiltrated or contain tumor thrombus. The tumor may have been biopsied or there has been local spillage of tumor confined to the flank. There is no residual tumor apparent at or beyond the margins of excision.
III	Residual nonhematogenous tumor confined to abdomen. Any one or more of the following occur:
	a. Lymph nodes on biopsy are found to be involved in the hilus, the periaortic chains, or beyond.
	b. There has been diffuse peritoneal contamination by tumor such as by spillage of tumor beyond the flank before or during surgery or by tumor growth that has penetrated through the peritoneal surface.
	c. Implants are found on the peritoneal surface.
	d. The tumor extends beyond the surgical margins either microscopically or grossly.
	e. The tumor is not completely resectable because of local infiltration into vital structures.
IV	Hematogenous metastases. Deposits beyond Stage III; e.g., lung, liver, bone, and brain.
V	Bilateral renal involvement at diagnosis. An attempt should be made to stage each side according to the above criteria on the basis of extent of disease prior to biopsy.

Favorable Histology (FH)

Favorable histology WT, as its name implies, has cytohistologic features associated with a good therapeutic outcome (67,68). The NWTS trials are based on postoperative therapies and have included RT questions. Results of the first three NWTS trials indicate that effective chemotherapy can suppress not only distant metastases but also residual microscopic disease in the operative bed in FH Stage I and FH Stage II patients and thus replace RT. The trials also indicated that a drug, in this case doxorubicin (Adriamycin, ADR), provides local control to a degree that appears to be equivalent to about 1000 cGy of RT to the operative bed (69–71). The evidence for these statements is as follows. All Stage I patients in the first NWTS (NWTS-1) were given AMD only and then randomized between those who were and those who were not to receive local RT.* The RFS rate was better for the irradiated children over 2 years of age, but equal for the younger sample (69). The relapse-free survival (RFS) rate for Stage I patients in NWTS-2 exceeded that of NWTS-1, regardless of age (70). NWTS-2 used both AMD and VCR but gave no local RT to these patients. NWTS-3 children were stratified by histology before randomization; four Stage II/FH groups became available for analysis (72). The overall 4-year disease-free survival (DFS) rate was about 88%, without outcome differences for patients given AMD + VCR ± ADR ± 2000 cGy. There also were four Stage III/FH groups with a higher but not statistically significant number of infradiaphragmatic relapses found in those given AMD + VCR + 1000 cGy than in the other three samples receiving AMD + VCR + 2000 cGy vs. AMD + VCR + ADR + 1000 cGy ± 1000 cGy. The overall 4-year DFS rate was nearly 80%.

*Stage I patients were not stratified by histology in NWTS-1 or NWTS-2. The outcomes are the same for Stage I/FH and Stage I/Ana; therefore, the conclusions were not biased by this consideration.

Past and current SIOP trials support the findings of the NWTS trials (72,73). SIOP data are based on preoperative therapy and therefore cannot be compared directly with NWTS results.

Stage IV/FH and unfavorable histology (UH) patients with pulmonary metastases provide additional information. NWTS-3 patients were given 1200 cGy + AMD + VCR + ADR ± CP (VAC) with a 4-year DFS rate of 76% (71). SIOP investigators have given AMD + VCR + ADR but without RT for initial management, and de Kraker et al also reported a DFS of 75% with similar treatment (74). Stage is assigned by means of initial chest x-ray examinations in both studies; therefore, pre- vs. postoperative therapy is not a factor here. Chemoradiation would not appear to produce a better DFS probability, and eventual survival also seems equivalent in the two studies. Four-year survival results for the NWTS and SIOP patients were both 83% (71,73).

de Kraker et al pointed out that only four of their 30 surviving children required pulmonary RT, compared to 100% of NWTS children, in whom there has been an important toxicity rate, including iatrogenic death (74,75).

The excellent SIOP results have not been duplicated by others who have used chemotherapy only for metastatic WT (76). Should others confirm the good outcomes recorded by SIOP, then it could be inferred that 1200 cGy added to the three drugs is not needed in all patients for the control of pulmonary lesions. Higher RT doses are not advisable, given the toxicity associated with 1200 cGy and the results recorded by Tefft, in which 1400 cGy was used with only two drugs (AMD + VCR), not including the RT enhancer and reactivator ADR (77).

Because the SIOP trial was not a randomized prospective study but collected experience reported by cooperating institutions and because the results of NWTS-3 therapy are the best recorded in the NWTS series,* it is prudent to continue combined modality therapy for Stage IV patients.

In summary, there are enough accumulated comparative data to indicate where chemoradiation management of WT patients can be expected to produce best control of local and distant disease.

*Two-year survival for Stage IV/FH + UH histology in NWTS-2 and NWTS-3 was about 50% and 78%, respectively.

Anaplastic (Ana) WT

No comparable systemic studies of the role of RT have been conducted for the anaplastic form of WT except for Stage I/Ana WT, for which it has been shown that RT is not needed (71). Chemoradiation is used with indifferent results insofar as both local and distant disease is concerned. The 4-year DFS for Stages II to IV is 55% (71). The NWTS-4 design does not deal with RT issues but aims to determine whether added VAC will improve the results procured by AMD + VCR + ADR + RT given in age-adjusted doses escalating from 1260 to 3780 cGy for children aged 1 to 41 months (71).

Other Primary Malignant Renal Tumors

No comparative RT data are available for other primary malignant renal tumors, which include the clear cell sarcoma, rhabdoid tumor, and renal cell carcinoma. Routine postoperative RT is given to patients with rhabdoid tumor in doses similar to the case of Ana WT (see below). The outlook for patients with clear cell sarcoma has improved greatly (4-year survival for all stages of about 75%) with the use of AMD + VCR + ADR, and infradiaphragmatic recurrences are uncommon (71). It is considered prudent to give all of these children 1000 cGy to the tumor bed, although it is not known whether RT truly is necessary. The course of renal cell carcinoma in children appears similar to that in adults, so that routine tumor-bed RT is not used. Chemotherapy for rhabdoid tumor and renal cell carcinoma has been disappointing.

In summary, empiricisms rules, and the correct place of chemoradiation, if any, for these tumors remains to be defined.

RHABDOMYOSARCOMA (RMSa)

Much of the information regarding the role of radiation therapy in children with RMSa is derived from the systematic studies of the Intergroup Rhabdomyosarcoma Study (IRS), which included undifferentiated soft-tissue sarcoma and extraosseous Ewing's tumor in its clinical trials (78). RMSa in children is divided into three types: **embryo-**

nal, alveolar, and **pleomorphic.** The last is also termed "the adult type;" as this implies, it is rare in the pediatric age group and therefore is not included in the discussion that follows.

Embryonal RMSa (ERMSa)

The IRS grouping method has been widely adopted (Table 17–4) (78). The first IRS showed that Group I children treated with VCR, AMD, and CP (VAC) did not require postexcisional RT (78). The 5-year event-free survival rates for VAC ± RT were compatible, at about 80%.

Data concerning the role for RT were derived from the study of subsets of Group II and Group III patients, who were randomized between pulse VAC ± ADR. The details regarding these regimens are given by Mauer et al (78). All patients were irradiated after 6 weeks of chemotherapy. The doses were 4000 cGy to children under 3 years of age and 5000 to 6000 cGy for older children, at a rate of 900 to 1200 cGy/week. Findings relevant to chemoradiation include the following.

Parameningeal Primaries

ERMSa arising from sites adjacent to the base of the skull tend to infiltrate the adjacent bony and soft-tissue structures. Seeding via the cerebrospinal pathways, as well as frank invasion of the brain, can result (79). Parameningeal sites are defined by the IRS as the nasal cavity, nasopharynx, mastoid, middle ear, maxillary, ethmoid and sphenoid sinuses, the pterygopalatine-infratemporal fossa, and the parapharyngeal region (80). The orbit is not included. The first IRS (IRS-1) found a 35% meningeal seeding rate

Table 17–4. The Intergroup Rhabdomyosarcoma Study Grouping System

Group I:	*Localized disease, completely resected* (Regional nodes not involved—lymph node biopsy or dissection is required, except for head and neck lesions). (a) Confined to muscle or organ of origin (b) Contiguous involvement—infiltration outside the muscle or organ of origin, as through fascial planes. Notation: This includes both gross inspection and *microscopic confirmation of complete resection.* Any nodes that may be inadvertently taken with the specimen must be negative. If the latter should be involved microscopically, then the patient is placed in Group II b or c. (See below.)
Group II:	*Total gross resection with evidence of regional spread.* (a) *Grossly resected tumor with microscopic residual disease.* (Surgeon believes that he/she has removed all of the tumor, but the pathologist finds tumor at the margin of resection *and* additional resection to achieve clean margins is not feasible.) No evidence of gross residual tumor. *No evidence of regional node involvement.* Once radiotherapy and/or chemotherapy have been started, reexploration and removal of the area of microscopic residual does not change the patient's group. (b) *Regional disease with involved nodes, completely resected with no microscopic residual.* Notation: Complete resection with microscopic confirmation of no residual disease makes this different from Groups IIa and IIc. Additionally, in contrast to Group IIa, regional nodes (which are completely resected, however) are involved, but the most distal node is histologically negative. (c) *Regional disease with involved nodes, grossly resected, but with no evidence of microscopic residual and/or histologic involvement of the most distal regional node (from the primary site) in the dissection.* Notation: This presence of microscopic residual disease makes this group different from Group IIb, and nodal involvement makes this group different from Group IIa.
Group III:	*Incomplete resection with gross residual disease.* (a) After biopsy only. (b) After gross or major resection of the primary tumor (> 50%).
Group IV:	*Distant metastatic disease present at onset* (Lung, liver, bones, bone marrow, brain, and distant muscle and nodes). Notation: The above excludes *regional* nodes and adjacent organ infiltration, which places the patient in a more favorable grouping (as noted above under Group II).

in this subgroup of ERMSa patients and a poor outlook (10% survival despite local RT in the doses described) (79). The incidence was reduced in IRS-2, in which local RT was given earlier and was coupled with IT chemotherapy and craniospinal RT in the intensive treatment of patients considered to be at risk for meningeal involvement. Risk was defined as evidence of cranial nerve palsy, cranial base erosion, and/or intracranial extension (80). The local RT fields in all patients, whether at risk for meningeal disease or not, were designed to include the primary site plus 2 cm of the adjacent skull base (80). The doses were 4000 to 6000 cGy in 5 to 6 weeks. Patients at risk had cranial RT starting on day 0, and 3000 cGy was given to the whole brain, along with IT chemotherapy consisting of methotrexate (12 mg/m^2) starting on day 0. This was repeated at weeks 2, 4, 8, 14, and then every 2 months for 18 months. This combined therapy approach was modified for the few children with positive cerbrospinal fluid at diagnosis and for those who presented with a spinal cord block.

Systemic chemotherapy was randomized by group: VA (VCR + AMD) 1 year vs. pulse VAC for 2 years for Group II; pulse VAC for 2 years vs. pulse VAC-VA + doxorubicin for 2 years for Group III (80). The meningeal/CNS relapse rate was reduced to 6% using these methods. The IRS investigators point out that these better results cannot be attributed with certainty to the more intensive approach. Tefft et al had noted that 42% of the children in IRS-1 who developed meningeal disease had received doses of less than 4000 cGy in 5 weeks, and 58% had not had a 2-cm margin to include the meninges superiorly (79). More adequate local RT fields and doses, instituted earlier in patients having more precise imaging studies at diagnosis, are factors that could account for the better control rates. The need for craniospinal irradiation and intrathecal drugs remains unproven and has been called into doubt by Gasparini et al (81). The transverse myelopathies encountered with the intensive regimen give importance to these issues, although the frequency of this complication has been reduced by curtailing the number of courses of the IT medications (82).

The facts remain that patients with meningeal involvement have a worse outlook than those without (3-year tumor-free survival and survival being 51% vs. 81% and 57% vs. 90%, respectively) and the IRS has successfully reduced the frequency of meningeal involvement from 28 to 6%, a betterment they attribute to RT given early and accurately in adequate volume and dose (79). These conclusions are consonant with earlier observations made by Chan et al (83). Meanwhile, the overall outcome was improved in patients receiving the more intensive chemotherapy and other protocol changes. Three-year tumor-free survival and survival were 57% and 68%, respectively, versus 33% and 41% for Group II patients (80). In summary, better results are obtained in these patients by more effective chemotherapy, providing better systemic control and possibly contributing to local control complemented by appropriate RT locally.

Acral and Truncal Primaries

IRS-1 established in a randomized study that postoperative RT is not beneficial in Group I patients who also received VAC chemotherapy (78). A subsequent analysis by Hays et al suggests that some Group I patients were actually occult Group IIa (84). Hays et al found that Stage IIa patients who had prompt reexcisions after inadequate primary removal fared better than those who did not, even though the RT doses ranged from 4000 cGy for children under 3 years to 5000 to 6000 cGy for older patients. Data presented by Mandell et al indicating that doses of 4000 cGy suffice are based on patients with different stages and sites of disease treated by different chemotherapy regimens (85). Therefore, those results cannot be applied to children such as those discussed by Hays et al. They comprise about half of the patients with extremity primaries, for instance.

The best means of employing combined surgery and chemoradiation for cure of pelvic ERMSa remains to be defined. Pilot studies both in single institutions and the IRS have been aimed at preservation of organs and function, and these were followed by a large-scale IRS trial (86,87). IRS II enrolled 109 patients with gross residual tumors (after biopsy) of the prostate (43 patients), bladder (43 patients), vagina (20 patients), and uterus (3 patients) (88). They received

VAC chemotherapy followed by RT and/or surgery for residual disease. This approach did not compromise survival expectancy (about 75%) but also did not improve the bladder salvage rate. These disappointing results have been duplicated by others who have attempted bladder salvage, but a more encouraging note is sounded by de Kraker et al (89). Five of the 12 children treated for tumors of the bladder and prostate survived free of disease for periods ranging from 14 to 172 months; a sixth patient survived for an apparently shorter time after relapse. These six patients reportedly retained normal bladder capacity and continence. The regimen consisted of chemotherapy with AMD, VCR, and CP (later replaced by ifosfamide) followed by surgery for residual disease. The relapse rate was high (59%) despite an initial complete response (CR) rate of 92%; and tumors recurred in the RT field in four of five patients who were irradiated for salvage. The survival rate was 58% (time not specified) and was lower than that reported by the IRS.

Thus, it can be seen that primary chemotherapy in various drug combinations can achieve a high complete response rate in these children, but the local relapse rate also is high when surgery ± RT is needed (88,89). It is not yet clear how many patients will survive with organs and function spared using these approaches. More work is needed; so far, combined chemoradiation for these purposes cannot be said to be entirely successful. It may be that procedures based on BMT will prove more promising.

These attempts have been more rewarding for girls with ERMSa of the distal genital tract (90). The IRS series of trials indicate that the several chemotherapy regimens employed achieved striking responses but not complete tumor ablation. Local excisions sufficed for local control, however, and pelvic exenterations were virtually eliminated in the later trials. RT has a minor role in producing these results, as it is reserved for salvage. The longterm survival has been good, especially when doxorubicin was added to the three mainstay drugs.

While not so critical as in neuroblastoma, there are also important variables at the biologic level for ERMSa. First, general agreement is needed to establish histopathologic criteria for the separate forms of soft-tissue sarcoma (91). It is generally, but not universally, agreed that the alveolar rhabdomyosarcoma has a worse prognosis than ERMSa. Yet, there was important nonconcordance in reaching such a diagnosis when expert pediatric pathologists reviewed the same slides. Tumor-cell ploidy has recently been reported to have prognostic value (92). These and other features must be taken into account when treatment results are evaluated.

Orbital ERMSa

Local RT or orbital exenteration gave good survival results before the advent of chemotherapy (93). Currently, RT is used universally in orbital ERMSa, with preservation of vision in a high proportion of patients. Four-year survivals of 85 to 90% are reported in patients with locoregional disease at diagnosis. The part that chemotherapy plays in yielding these results is questionable.

Other Sarcomas

Other forms of soft-tissue sarcomas are rare in childhood. Evaluation of the role of combined therapy by subtype is therefore impossible. A recent report by Horowitz et al exemplifies the problem (94). They record their results in 62 patients with non-rhabdomyosarcomatous tumors of various types; e.g., neurofibrosarcoma, hemangiopericytoma, and malignant fibrous histiocytoma. Their conclusion is that surgical excision plays the major role in control and survival and that the value of chemoradiation is marginal. A more aggressive approach for high-risk sarcomas is described below under Ewing's sarcoma.

BONE TUMORS

The two most common malignant bone tumors of childhood are osteogenic sarcoma and Ewing's sarcoma.

Osteogenic Sarcoma

In the prechemotherapy era, 15 to 20% survival rates were recorded by surgery alone. Since then, notable successes have been recorded for chemotherapy in the management of these patients and confirmed by randomized trials (95–97). Multiagent regimens, especially those that include ADR, high doses of methotrexate with citrovorum rescue and cisplatinum, have increased the 5-year relapse-free survival rates in patients free of metastases at diagnosis to the 50 to 60% range. The results of several trials have been tabulated by Link and Eilber (98). More recently, ifosfamide has been found to be active (99). A detailed review of the various combined chemotherapy regimens that have been shown to have promise is beyond the scope of this discussion, which is concerned with chemoradiation effects. RT has not affected life expectancy either before or after the advent of chemotherapy, nor is there a defined role for RT in multimodal therapy.

Ewing's Sarcoma (ES)

RT has always played an important role in ES. Ewing himself described the radioresponsiveness of this tumor in his original publication (100). Since then, control of the primary tumor was expected in two of three cases or more after doses in the 6000- to 7000-cGy range delivered to the entire affected bone (101). This figure is extremely uncertain. Reports in the prechemotherapy era were based on relatively few patients gathered over long periods in single institutions. Many confounding disparities are possible under such circumstances, especially in an ill-defined entity like ES. These and allied issues are discussed at greater length elsewhere (102,103). While surgery ± postoperative RT could be considered when an expendable bone (e.g., rib fibula) was affected, the radioresponsiveness of ES provided a suitable alternative to ablative surgery when nonexpendable bones (e.g., tibia, femur, humerus) were involved* (101,103).

Distant metastases present at diagnosis or after primary management all too often defeated either approach and resulted in a 5-year survival expectancy of less than 20% (101–104). An innovative approach, exploiting the radioresponsiveness of the tumor, was that of Jenkin et al, who added 300 cGy TBI to local RT and, later, the adjuvants VCR and CP (103). They concluded that the toxicity of TBI delayed chemotherapy, which was producing impressive gains, and they therefore abandoned this approach. A modification of large-field RT was tested by the Intergroup Ewing's Sarcoma Study (IESS) (105). The first IESS trial incorporated a specific RT question: is prophylactic irradiation of the lung with 1200 cGy + VAC chemotherapy effective in reducing the incidence of pulmonary metastases in patients given 6000 cGy to the primary site? Comparison was made to control groups given systemic chemotherapy using VAC with or without ADR. The best relapse-free survival results were obtained in patients with nonpelvic primary tumors who received adjuvant chemotherapy that included ADR. The 5-year survival was 60% for those patients, versus 24% for patients receiving VAC alone and 44% for patients receiving VAC and lung RT (105). However, the radiation-enhancing drugs AMD and ADR used in such chemotherapy regimens augment the anticipated local radiation damage in the high-dose regions. This can be so severe, in some cases, that amputations are necessary (106). Like the Intergroup Rhabdomyosarcoma Study, this experience demonstrates the considerable morbidity that can be encountered when high doses of RT are used with certain anticancer drugs.

The shrinking-field method has been used with good control of the primary tumor, for example, the entire bone is given 4000 to 4500 cGy. The field is then reduced to encompass the bone and soft-tissue components, as visualized on the original imaging studies plus a 3- to 5-cm margin, and another 500 cGy is given. The field may again be reduced to include only the tumor as originally seen, and a final 500 cGy is administered. This method, first made prominent by Suit, achieves satisfactory control without undue morbidity (107). It also suggests that effective chemotherapy adds to the control of local disease and reduces the frequency of distant metastases. In fact, the need to irradiate the entire bone has been questioned (108). Most relapses have been reported in distant sites. This was true historically and remains so, more recently in the era of multiple-agent chemotherapy, in which good local tumor control has been obtained after irradiation of the lesion with an appropriate margin. It thus promises to make it possible to reduce the RT field and dose to the primary. This impression is strengthened by the data reported by Fernandez et al in the era before

*High doses of RT to growing bones in young children lead to unacceptable deformity. Surgical intervention (e.g., amputation) is preferable because rehabilitation is more successful.

effective chemotherapy. Relapses even then occurred at the primary site, not at the ends of long bones (100). Further support is provided by Perez et al, who found fewer relapses in bone in ADR-treated IESS-1 patients who did not have the entire marrow cavity irradiated (109).

Other approaches, still under study, include biopsy of the bone and soft-tissue after RT with local excisions of residual tumor so identified ± RT, often at reduced doses. Only preliminary reports of these disparate approaches are available (110,111).

Evaluation of results of therapy for ES is difficult because of inherent prognostic factors at diagnosis, such as age and site (105). Older patients and those with large tumors and pelvic primaries have a worse prognosis. The picture is further clouded because of the occasional aberrant clinical course of ES, and it has become more so recently because of new histopathologic evidence. It has long been known that some ET patients can develop metastases 5 or more years after apparent complete control of the local lesion (102). This indicates that there is at least a biologically distinct subgroup within the ES nosology. The number of patients of this type might have been included by chance within clinical studies is impossible to estimate. Their inclusion would color the results. Moreover, what may or may not prove to be a distinct entity, the peripheral neuroectodermal tumor (PerNET), has been identified within the ES spectrum (112). The diagnosis of ES has often been one of exclusion, so that tumors of differing histopathologic patterns were accepted as ES variants as long as certain fundamental morphologic criteria were met. Better discrimination is now possible through immunochemistry and electron microscopy; nonetheless, the differential diagnosis often remains a problem (112). There is increasing evidence that ES is of neuroectodermal origin, so that the current distinction between ES and PerNET may prove illusory on further study. Cytogenetic characterization shows similar changes for both ES and PerNET. Ambros et al reported t(11;22) (q 23–24; q 11–12) or the chromosome 22 deletion, del 22 (q11–12), in the ES and PerNET tumors and cell lines they analyzed (113). The clinical evolution of ES and PerNet also appears similar. At this time, however, it remains unclear whether the already complex evaluation of ES treatment results is further confounded by the PerNET admixture.

In any case, distant metastases remain the major cause of death in high-risk patients. This has led to the use of aggressive therapies based on BMT methods that include TBI. Stea et al reported the results of pilot studies in 23 patients with local or metastatic Ewing's sarcoma (8 patients), ERMSa (7 patients), malignant peripheral neuroepithelioma (3 patients), and undifferentiated sarcoma (5 patients) (114). The intensive combined modality therapy began with five cycles of VCR, ADR, and CP (VADRIAC) together with 5500 to 6000 cGy to the primary lesion and 4500 to 5000 cGy to areas of gross metastatic disease (criteria not defined). The 22 patients* achieving a complete response then had 400 cGy/day × 2 total body irradiation, followed by VADRIAC chemotherapy and "rescue" by stored autologous bone marrow. Persistent local control was achieved in all patients, but nine developed systemic relapses. Seven of these nine were among the 13 who had metastatic disease upon entry into the study, and all seven died; the other two were alive after retrieval therapies, as were the remaining eight of the 10 without metastases when first treated. Kinsella et al reported the longterm results of ES patients using a similar regimen (115). Their 5-, 10-, and 15-year survivals were 51%, 39%, and 34%, respectively, among 80 patients without metastases. Although almost all relapses occurred before the fifth year, the need for prolonged surveillance before recording survival data is obvious. Marcus et al used local RT (120 cGy b.i.d. to 5040 to 6000 cGy) + pulmonary RT (100 to 150 cGy/day to 1000 to 1500 cGy) for those with lung lesions + VCR + ADR + CP for preparation (116). This was followed by 400 cGy/day × 2 TBI + VCR + ADR + CP before marrow reinfusion. They report 80% 2-year disease-free survival. Longer follow-up with more patients is needed, but the results compare favorably, with about 20% survival in patients treated earlier and less aggressively by the same group.

In summary, there are indubitable advantages to chemoradiation for many ES pa-

*Two of the 22 required intraoperative RT to achieve complete response.

tients. It remains to be found how best to use the two potent component modalities.

BONE-MARROW TRANSPLANTATION (BMT)

Chemoradiation has been used extensively in BMT regimens. A comprehensive review of autologous BMT methods for children with solid tumors has appeared recently, along with reports from single institutions and small groups using this approach (117–119). Some centers have explored the use of high-dose chemotherapy alone for both the leukemias and certain solid tumors, apparently with success, and the need for TBI has been called into question (120,121). This discussion will be concerned with combined therapy regimens, however, and will concentrate on the two conditions in which the most experience has been accumulated in children. They are acute lymphoblastic leukemia (ALL) and neuroblastoma. There seems to be a consensus that TBI is not needed in children with acute nonlymphoblastic leukemia.

The objectives of the preparative chemoradiation regimens are to procure maximum cytoreduction of malignant cells with acceptable toxicity, to provide immunosuppression when allogeneic marrow is to be infused, and to provide room for the infused marrow (121). Most of the reported regimens achieve the second and third of these goals because failure of bone marrow to engraft in children is rare. Much more needs to be done to achieve the first aim; toxicity and relapse remain major problems.

Leukemia

Various conditioning and cytoreductive chemotherapy regimens have been used in conjunction with total body irradiation prior to BMT. The original Seattle regimen was based on high-dose CP (60 mg/kg/day × 2) and 1000 cGy TBI in a single session (122). This has been modified over the years in several centers to fractionation of total body irradiation TBI and the use of more than one drug. Thomas has recently reviewed the various TBI regimens in use (122). In Seattle, 200 cGy/day × 6 (1200 cGy total) has been shown to be superior to 1000-cGy single dose and less toxic than 225 cGy/day × 7 (1575 cGy total), the CP chemotherapy being kept a constant. Thomas did not believe that other TBI variations would produce major alterations in event-free survival. Brochstein et al adopted TBI given in 11 t.i.d. doses of 120 cGy each (with lung shielding) to a total of 1320 cGy (123). Unlike most other investigators, they give TBI before chemotherapy, which is based on CP (60 mg/kg/day × 2). Good survival is reported by Brochstein et al, whose 5-year disease-free survival rates range from 64 to 75% for ALL in second remission and ANLL in first or second remission. They postulate that the t.i.d. fractionation may be instrumental in the good results they report through partial synchronization of the leukemia cells and greater protection of the normal tissues. Kamani et al explored the same RT-drug sequence in 16 children with acute leukemia but gave 1200 cGy TBI in 200 cGy b.i.d. fractions (124). High-dose cytarabine followed (12 doses of 3 gm/m^2 every 12 hours), starting 12 hours after completion of TBI. The cytarabine was delivered as an intravenous infusion over 3 hours. All 14 of the 16 children (88%) who survived the acute post-transplant toxicity were alive free of leukemia for periods ranging from 8 to 56 months (median: 29 months), eight of them longer than 2 years. Woods et al used a similar TBI/cytarabine sequence and noted no advantage over their 60% 3-year relapse-free survival results using TBI/CP (125). However, they gave TBI as a single 850-cGy dose at 25 cGy/min. Kamani et al also note the evidence that chemotherapy (e.g., alkylators) given prior to RT may protect malignant as well as normal cells (126). They suggest that the sequence reversal may avoid this problem and thus add another explanation to those advanced by Brochstein et al. Kamani and colleagues tentatively conclude that high-dose cytarabine-containing regimens plus fractionated TBI give good results, sequencing may play a role, and there is little to choose between t.i.d. and b.i.d. TBI.

In summary, there are extremely important interplays between the drugs used, their doses, and their sequencing in relation to TBI. These require further study. Practical disadvantages aside, the putative radiobiologic advantages of multiple daily TBI fractions remain to be proven.

Neuroblastoma

Early research used high-dose chemotherapy (melphalan) alone in the treatment of neuroblastoma (127). The methods employed for the BMT of leukemia were, however, soon adapted to this solid tumor, and an early report from Philadelphia gave encouraging results (118). Because of the long follow-up available after multimodality therapy as part of BMT for a solid tumor, it will be reviewed briefly and updated here. Patients with a less than 20% chance for cure were selected; all 26 had relapsed after chemotherapy ± radiotherapy. For BMT, patients were given both local RT and TBI as well as high-dose chemotherapy. August et al fractionated TBI, giving 333 cGy/day × 3. Allogeneic and autologous marrow was used for rescue, mostly the latter. It was screened for the presence of NBL cells, and if positive, was purged using the magnetic bead method (128). Bulky disease, defined as any lesion measuring more than 5 cm in greatest diameter present at diagnosis or thereafter, was prepared with 1000 cGy (200 cGy/day × 5 or 250 cGy/day × 4) prior to TBI and BMT. Soft-tissue lesions amenable to surgical excision were removed, and these regions were irradiated, usually with 1000 cGy. The chemotherapy regimen included melphalan + teniposide ± ADR. Doses were melphalan, 140 + 70 mg/m^2 on successive days, and teniposide, 180 mg/m^2 × 2.

ADR also was given (45 mg/m^2 × 2) to children not having had more than 300 mg/m^2 as prior therapy. Seven of the 26 patients (26%) treated in this way survived for 6-½ to 12 years. None who relapsed did so later than 20 months post-transplant, although one child developed AML 8 months after BMT and died free of neuroblastoma 7 months thereafter. The Philadelphia experience with this protocol does not duplicate the results reported by others in which late relapses occurred (129). Six of 23 patients survived 2 to 5-½ years after treatment in Philadelphia, using a different protocol (melphalan became unavailable). No relapses after 20 months have been encountered in these 23 patients. Seeger et al recently recorded comparable results in patients treated before disease progression using a similar treatment regimen to which cisplatinum was added (130). The contribution of combined therapy to these results is inferential, because no direct randomized comparison of chemotherapy + surgical excision ± local RT has been made. A recent analysis of the Philadelphia results by Ikeda et al suggests that local RT after surgical debulking of infradiaphragmatic sites improves the outlook (131). It is also not clear whether TBI is needed. In fact, Hartmann et al report good results using only chemotherapy (carmustine, melphalan, and teniposide) as do Kushner et al, with a regimen based on cisplatinum, carmustine, etoposide, and either thiotepa or melphalan (132,133). Firm conclusions about the best procedure cannot be drawn from the available data, including the results of a POG trial reported by Graham-Pole and colleagues (117,134). Management of the local lesions, the drug regimens, and the patient populations all differ. Eligibility continues to change as more precise prognostic criteria are identified and used in the selection process, and patients are transplanted earlier in the clinical course. The experience with cyclic low-dose TBI and nonlethal doses of chemotherapy cited above under neuroblastoma suggests that the two modalities are complementary in producing earlier complete responses (64). That experience cannot be extended to this setting nor can the complete response rate be equated with survival expectancy.

Only a properly designed clinical trial will resolve these issues. Until then, surgery plus chemotherapy combined with RT (both local and TBI) seems a reasonable albeit emperic approach to the BMT of children with NBL.

CONCLUSION

The traditional roles of chemotherapy and radiation therapy overlap in pediatric oncology. In the past, the function of chemotherapy was thought to lie chiefly in the ablation of distant micrometastases, while radiation therapy has been considered to be instrumental in providing local control. For chemosensitive lesions, it is now clear that drugs can contribute to local control and that RT in the form of total body irradiation can help to eliminate disseminated disease. Moreover, RT can complement the effectiveness of chemotherapy by eliminating microscopic and gross disease in body areas that are not penetrated well by systemically administered anticancer drugs. It would appear that these important interplays can be made most effective by timing and sequencing of the two modalities and of the third (surgery) as well.

Much has been done to make multimodal therapy successful in pediatric oncology. More remains to be accomplished before the objective—cure of cancer without lasting damage to normal tissues—is attained.

REFERENCES

1. Hammond GD. The cure of childhood cancers. Cancer 58(Suppl):407, 1986.
2. Evans AE, Gilbert ES, Zandstra R. The increasing incidence of central nervous system leukemia in children. Cancer 26:404, 1970.
3. Evans AE, D'Angio GJ, Mitus A. Central nervous system complications of children with acute leukemia. J Pediatr 64:94, 1964.
4. Aur RJA, Simone JV, Hustu HO, et al. Central nervous system therapy and combination chemotherapy of childhood lymphocytic leukemia. Blood 37:272, 1971.
5. Hustu HO, Aur RJA, Verzosa MS, et al. Prevention of central nervous system leukemia by irradiation. Cancer 32:585, 1973.
6. Nesbit ME, Sather H, Robison LL, et al. Sanctuary therapy: A randomized trial of 724 children with previously untreated acute lymphoblastic leukemia. Cancer Res 41:674, 1982.
7. Nesbit ME Jr, Sather HN, Robison LL, et al. Presymptomatic central nervous system therapy in previously untreated childhood acute lymphoblastic leukaemia: Comparison of 1800 rad and 2400 rad. A report for Childrens Cancer Study Group. Lancet 1:461, 1981.
8. Elyan SJ, Williams MV. The role of cranial irradiation in low risk ALL. Int J Radiat Oncol Biol Phys 16:284, 1989.
9. Hammond GD, Sather H, Bleyer WA, Coccia P. Stratification by prognostic factors in the design and analysis of clinical trials for acute lymphoblastic leukaemia. Haematology and blood transfusion. *In:* Acute Leukemias. Buchner T, Schellong G, Hiddemann W, Urbanitz D, Ritter J (Eds). Berlin, Springer-Verlag, 1987, p. 161.
10. D'Angio GJ, Rorke LB, Packer R, Sutton L. Key problems in the management of children with brain tumors. Int J Radiat Oncol Biol Phys 18:805, 1990.
11. Considine B Jr, Cook JJ, Zuelzer WW, Ravindranath Y, et al. Repetitive low-dose radiation therapy for acute stem-cell leukemia. Int J Radiat Oncol Biol Phys 2:257, 1977.
12. Belasco JB, Rate W, Mancini A, Paolucci G. Intermittant low-dose central nervous system radiation for high-risk pediatric leukemia patients: Preliminary results. Med Pediatr Oncol 19:106, 1991.
13. Nesbit M, Sather H, Ortega J, et al. Effect of isolated central nervous system leukaemia on bone marrow remission and survival in childhood acute lymphoblastic leukaemia. Lancet 1:1386, 1981.
14. Steinherz P, Jereb B, Galicich J. Therapy of CNS leukemia with intraventricular chemotherapy and low-dose neuroaxis radiotherapy. J Clin Oncol 3:1217, 1985.
15. Evans AE. Central nervous system involvement in children with acute leukemia. A study of 921 patients. Cancer 17:256, 1964.
16. Pui CH, Dahl GV, Kalwinsky DK, et al. Central nervous system leukemia in children with acute nonlymphoblastic leukemia. Blood 66:1062, 1985.
17. Ekert H, Waters KD, Smith PJ, et al. Treatment with MOPP or ChIVPP chemotherapy only for all stages of childhood Hodgkin's disease. J Clin Oncol 6:1845, 1988.
18. Bubman I, Kirchoff LV, Morioka H, et al. Treatment of Hodgkin's disease Stages I and II with chemotherapy alone. Med Pediatr Oncol 14:208, 1986.
19. Dionet C, Oberlin O, Habrand JL, et al. Initial chemotherapy and low-dose radiation in limited fields in childhood Hodgkin's disease: Results of a joint cooperative study by the French Society of Pediatric Oncology (SFOP) and Hospital Saint-Louis, Paris. Int J Radiat Oncol Biol Phys 15:341, 1988.
20. Jereb B, Tan C, Bretsky S, et al. Involved field irradiation with or without chemotherapy in the management of children with Hodgkin's disease. Med Pediatr Oncol 12:325, 1984.
21. Barrett A, Crennan E, Barnes J, et al. Treatment of clinical Stage I Hodgkin's disease by local radiation therapy alone. Cancer 66:670, 1990.
22. Jenkin RDT, Chan H, Freedman M, et al. Hodgkin's disease in children: Treatment results with MOPP and low-dose extended field irradiation. Cancer Treat Rev 66:949, 1982.
23. Donaldson SS, Link MP. Combined modality treatment with low-dose radiation and MOPP chemotherapy for children with Hodgkin's disease. J Clin Oncol 5:742, 1987.

24. Weinstein HJ, Lack EE, Cassady JR. APO therapy for malignant lymphoma of large cell "histiocytic" type of childhood: Analysis of treatment for 29 patients. Blood 62:422, 1984.
25. Hvizdala EV, Berard C, Callihan T, et al. Lymphoblastic lymphoma in children. A randomized trial comparing LSA_2-L_2 with the A-COP + therapeutic regimen. A Pediatric Oncology Group Study. J Clin Oncol 6:26, 1988.
26. Wollner N, Burchenal JH, Leiberman PH, et al. Non-Hodgkin's lymphoma in children: A comparative study of two modalities of therapy. Cancer 37:123, 1976.
27. Anderson JR, Wilson JF, Jenkin RD, et al. Childhood non-Hodgkin's lymphoma: The results of a randomized therapeutic trial comparing a 4-drug regimen (COMP) with a 10-drug regimen (LSA_2-L_2). N Engl J Med 308:559, 1983.
28. Sposto R, Ertel IJ, Jenkin RDT, et al. The effectiveness of chemotherapy for treatment of high grade astrocytoma in children: Results of a randomized trial. J Neurooncol 7:165, 1989.
29. Pendergrass TW, Milstein JM, Geyer RJ, et al. Eight drugs in one day chemotherapy for brain tumors: Experience in 107 children and rationale for preradiation chemotherapy. J Clin Oncol 5:1221, 1987.
30. Packer RJ, Siegel KR, Sutton LN, et al. Leptomeningeal dissemination of primary central nervous system tumors of childhood. Ann Neurol 18:217, 1985.
31. Rorke LB. The cerebellar medulloblastoma and its relationship to primitive neuroectodermal tumors. J Neuropathol Exp Neurol 42:1, 1983.
32. Tait DM, Thornton-Jones H, Bloom HJG, et al. Adjuvant chemotherapy for medulloblastoma: The first multi-centre control trial of the International Society of Paediatric Oncology (SIOP). Eur J Cancer 26:464, 1990.
33. Evans AE, Jenkin RDT, Sposto R, et al. The treatment of medulloblastoma. Results of a prospective randomized trial of radiation therapy with and without CCNU, vincristine, and prednisone. J Neurosurg 72:572, 1990.
34. Lefkowitz IB, Packer RJ, Siegel KR, et al. Results of treatment of children with recurrent primitive neuroectodermal tumors-medulloblastoma (PNET/MB) with CCNU, cisplatinum (CPDD) and vincristine (VCR). Cancer 65:412, 1990.
35. Packer RJ, Siegel KR, Sutton LN, et al. Efficacy of adjuvant chemotherapy for patients with poor-risk medulloblastoma: A preliminary report. Ann Neurol 24:503, 1988.
36. Packer RJ, Sutton LN, Goldwein JW, et al. Improved survival with the use of adjuvant chemotherapy in the treatment of medulloblastoma. J Neurosurg 74:433, 1991.
37. Granowetter L, Rosenstock JG, Packer RJ. Enhanced cisplatinum neurotoxicity in pediatric patients with brain tumors. J Neurooncol 1:293, 1983.
38. Halberg FE, Wara WM, Fippin LF, et al. Low-dose craniospinal radiation therapy for medulloblastoma. Int J Radiat Oncol Biol Phys 20:651, 1991.
39. Hughes EN, Shillito J, Sallan SE, et al. Medulloblastoma at the Joint Center for Radiation Therapy between 1968 and 1984. The influence of radiation dose on the patterns of failure and survival. Cancer 61:1992, 1988.
40. Tomita T, McLone DG. Medulloblastoma in childhood: Results of radical resection and low-dose neuraxis radiation therapy. J Neurosurg 64:238, 1986.
41. Kun LE, Constine LS. Medulloblastoma. Caution regarding new treatment approaches. Int J Radiat Oncol Biol Phys 20:897, 1991.
42. Packer RJ, Sutton LN, Atkins TE, et al. A prospective study of cognitive function in children receiving whole brain radiotherapy and chemotherapy: 2-year results. J Neurosurg 70:707, 1989.
43. van Eys J, Cangir A, Coady D, Smith B. MOPP regimen as primary chemotherapy for brain tumors in infants. J Neurooncol 3:237, 1984.
44. Loeffler JS, Kretschmar CS, Sallan SE, et al. Pre-radiation chemotherapy for infants and poor prognosis children with medulloblastoma. Int J Radiat Oncol Biol Phys 15:177, 1988.
45. Kovnar EH, Kelli SJ, Horowitz ME, et al. Preirradiation cisplatin and etoposide in the treatment of high risk medulloblastoma and other malignant embryonal tumors of the central nervous system: A phase II study. J Clin Oncol 8:330, 1990.
46. Duffner PK, Cohen ME, Thomas PRM, Lansky SB. The long-term effects of cranial irradiation on the central nervous system. Cancer 56:1841, 1985.
47. Rosenstock JG, Packer RJ, Bilaniuk LT, et al. Chiasmatic optic glioma treated with chemotherapy. A preliminary report. J Neurosurg 63:862, 1985.
48. Packer RJ, Sutton LN, Bilaniuk LT, et al. Treatment of chiasmatic/hypothalamic gliomas of childhood with chemotherapy: An update. Ann Neurol 23:79, 1988.
49. Breslow N, McCann H. Statistical estimation of prognosis for children with neuroblastoma. Cancer Res 31:2098, 1971.
50. Shimada H, Chatten J, Newton WA Jr, Sachs

N. Histopathologic prognostic factors in neuroblastic tumors: Definition of subtypes of ganglioneuroblastoma and an age-linked classification of neuroblastomas. J Natl Cancer Inst 73:405, 1984.

51. Evans AE, D'Angio GJ, Propert K, et al. Prognostic factors in neuroblastoma. Cancer 59:1853, 1987.
52. Hann H-WL, Levy HM, Evans AE. Serum ferritin as a guide to therapy in neuroblastoma. Cancer Res 40:1411, 1980.
53. Hayashi Y, Kanda N, Inaba T, et al. Cytogenetic findings and prognosis in neuroblastoma with emphasis on marker chromosome 1. Cancer 63:126, 1989.
54. Look AT, Hayes FA, Shuster JJ, et al. Clinical relevance of tumor cell ploidy and N-myc gene amplication in childhood neuroblastoma: A Pediatric Oncology Group Study. J Clin Oncol 9:581, 1991.
55. Brodeur GM, Seeger RC, Schwab M, et al. Amplification of N-myc in untreated human neuroblastomas correlates with advanced disease stage. Science 224:1121, 1984.
56. Silber JH, Evans AE, Fridman M. Models to predict outcome from childhood neuroblastoma: The role of serum ferritin and tumor histology. Cancer Res 51:1426, 1991.
57. Evans AR, Brand W, de Lorimier A, et al. Results in children with local and regional neuroblastoma managed with and without vincristine, cyclophosphamide, and imidazolecarboxamide. Am J Clin Oncol 6:3, 1984.
58. Evans AE, D'Angio GJ, Koop CE. The role of multimodal therapy in patients with local and regional neuroblastoma. J Pediatr Surg 19:77, 1984.
59. Matthay KK, Sather HN, Seeger RC, et al. Excellent outcome of Stage II neuroblastoma is independent of residual disease and radiation therapy. J Clin Oncol 7:236, 1989.
60. O'Neill JA, Littman P, Blitzer P, et al. Neuroblastoma: Influence of age at diagnosis, stage, tumor site and sex on prognosis. Cancer 46:1896, 1980.
61. Haase GM, Wong KY, de Lorimier A, et al. Improvement in survival after excision of primary tumor in Stage III neuroblastoma. J Pediatr Surg 24:194, 1989.
62. Castleberry RP, Kun LE, Shuster JJ, et al. Radiotherapy improves the outlook for patients older than 1 year with Pediatric Oncology Group Stage C neuroblastoma. J Clin Oncol 9:789, 1991.
63. Brodeur GM, Seeger RC, Barrett A, et al. International criteria for diagnosis, staging, and response to treatment in patients with neuroblastoma. J Clin Oncol 6:1874, 1988.
64. D'Angio GJ, Evans AE. Cyclic, low-dose total body irradiation for metastatic neuroblastoma. Int J Radiat Oncol Biol Phys 9:1961, 1983.
65. Gross RE, Neuhauser EBD. Treatment of mixed tumors of the kidney in childhood. Pediatrics 6:843, 1950.
66. Aron BS. Wilms' tumor. A clinical study of 81 patients. Cancer 33:637, 1974.
67. Beckwith JB, Palmer N. Histopathology and prognosis of Wilms' tumor. Results from the first National Wilms' Tumor Study. Cancer 41:1937, 1978.
68. Beckwith JB. Wilms' tumor and other renal tumors of childhood: An update (The John Littimer Lecture). J Urol 126:320, 1986.
69. D'Angio GJ, Evans AE, Breslow N, et al. The treatment of Wilms' tumor: Results of the National Wilms' Tumor Study. Cancer 38:633, 1976.
70. D'Angio GJ, Evans A, Breslow N, et al. The treatment of Wilms' tumor: Results of the Second National Wilms' Tumor Study. Cancer 47:2302, 1981.
71. D'Angio GJ, Breslow N, Beckwith JB, et al. Treatment of Wilms' tumor. Results of the Third National Wilms' Tumor Study. Cancer 64:347, 1989.
72. Lemerle J, Voute PA, Tournade MF, et al. Preoperative versus postoperative radiotherapy, single versus multiple courses of actinomycin D, in the treatment of Wilms' tumor. Cancer 38:647, 1976.
73. Lemerle J, Voute PA, Turnade MF, et al. Effectiveness of preoperative chemotherapy in Wilms' tumor: Results of an International Society of Paediatric Oncology (SIOP) clinical trial. J Clin Oncol 1:604, 1983.
74. de Kraker J, Lemerle J, Voute PA, et al. Wilms' tumor with pulmonary metastases at diagnosis. The significance of primary chemotherapy. J Clin Oncol 8:1187, 1990.
75. Green DM, Finklestein JZ, Tefft ME, Norkool P. Diffuse interstitial pneumonitis after pulmonary irradiation for metastatic Wilms' tumor. A report from the National Wilms' Tumor Study. Cancer 63:450, 1989.
76. Pritchard J. Personal communication. October 1991.
77. Tefft M. Radiation related toxicities in National Wilms' Tumor Study No. 1. Int J Radiat Oncol Biol Phys 2:455, 1977.
78. Maurer HM, Beltangady M, Gehan EA, et al. The Intergroup Rhabdomyosarcoma Study-I. A final report. Cancer 61:209, 1988.
79. Tefft M, Fernandez C, Donaldson M, et al. Incidence of meningeal involvement by rhabdomyosarcoma of the head and neck in children. Cancer 42:253, 1978.
80. Raney RB Jr, Tefft M, Newton WA, et al. Im-

proved prognosis with intensive treatment of children with cranial soft tissue sarcomas arising in nonorbital parameningeal sites. Cancer 59:147, 1987.

81. Gasparini M, Lombardi F, Gianni MC, et al. Questionable role of CNS radioprophylaxis in the therapeutic management of childhood rhabdomyosarcoma with meningeal extension. J Clin Oncol 8:1854, 1990.

82. Raney RB, Tefft M, Newton WA, et al. Ascending transverse myelitis in patients with parameningeal sarcoma treated intensively on Intergroup Rhabdomyosarcoma Studies (IRS) (Abstract No. 1129). Proc Am Soc Clin Oncol 9:291, 1990.

83. Chan RC, Sutow WW, Lindberg RD. Parameningeal rhabdomyosarcoma. Radiology 131:211, 1979.

84. Hays DM, Lawrence W Jr, Wharam M, et al. Primary reexcision for patients with microscopic residual tumor following initial excision of sarcomas of trunk and extremity sites. J Pediatr Surg 24:5, 1989.

85. Mandell L, Ghavimi F, Peretz T, et al. Radiocurability of microscopic disease in childhood rhabdomyosarcoma with radiation doses less than 4000 cGy. J Clin Oncol 8:1536, 1990.

86. Mahesh-Kumar AP, Wrenn EL Jr, Fleming ID, et al. Combined therapy to prevent complete pelvic exenteration for rhabdomyosarcoma of the vagina or uterus. Cancer 37(1):118, 1976.

87. Ortega JA. A therapeutic approach to childhood pelvic rhabdomyosarcoma without pelvic exenteration. J Pediatr 94(2):205, 1979.

88. Raney RB Jr, Gehan EA, Hays DM, et al. Primary chemotherapy with or without radiation therapy and/or surgery for children with localized sarcoma of the bladder, prostate, vagina, uterus, and cervix. Cancer 66:2072, 1990.

89. de Kraker J, Russel IMB, Voute PA. Rhabdomyosarcoma of bladder and prostate. Pediatr Hematol Oncol 5:253, 1988.

90. Hays DM, Shimade H, Raney RB Jr, et al. Clinical staging and treatment results in rhabdomyosarcoma of the female genital tract among children and adolescents. Cancer 16:1893, 1988.

91. Newton WA Jr, Soule EH, Hamoudi AB, et al. Histopathology of childhood sarcomas, Intergroup Rhabdomyosarcoma Studies I and II: Clinicopathologic correlation. J Clin Oncol 6:67, 1988.

92. Shapiro DN, Parham DM, Douglass EC, et al. Relationship of tumor-cell ploidy to histologic subtype and treatment outcome in children and adolescents with unresectable rhabdomyosarcoma. J Clin Oncol 9:159, 1991.

93. Cassady JB, Sagerman RH, Tretter P, Ellsworth RM. Radiation therapy for rhabdomyosarcoma. Radiology 91:116, 1968.

94. Horowitz ME, Pratt CB, Webber BL, et al. Therapy for childhood soft-tissue sarcomas other than rhabdomyosarcoma: A review of 62 cases treated at a single institution. J Clin Oncol 4:559, 1986.

95. Jaffe N, Frei E III, Traggis D, Bishop Y. Adjuvant methotrexate and citrovorum-factor treatment of osteogenic sarcoma. N Engl J Med 291:994, 1974.

96. Link MP, Goorin AM, Miser AW, et al. The effect of adjuvant chemotherapy on relapse-free survival in patients with osteosarcoma of the extremity. N Engl J Med 314:1600, 1986.

97. Eilber G, Giuliano A, Eckardt J, et al. Adjuvant chemotherapy for osteosarcoma: A randomized prospective trial. J Clin Oncol 5:21, 1987.

98. Link MP, Eilber F. Osteosarcoma. *In:* Principles and Practice of Pediatric Oncology. Pizzo PA, Poplack DG (Eds). Philadelphia, JB Lippincott Company, 1989, p. 704.

99. Marti C, Kroner T, Remagen W, et al. High-dose ifosfamide in advanced osteosarcoma. Cancer Treat Rev 69:115, 1985.

100. Ewing J. Diffuse endothelioma of bone. Proc NY Pathol Soc 21:17, 1921.

101. Fernandez CH, Lindberg RD, Sutow WW, Samuels ML. Localized Ewing's sarcoma. Treatment and results. Cancer 34:143, 1974.

102. D'Angio GJ. Bone tumours, radiation therapy. *In:* Bone Tumours and Soft-Tissue Sarcomas. D'Angio GJ, Evans AE (Eds). London, Edward Arnold Ltd, 1985, p. 157.

103. Jenkin RDT, Rider WD, Sonley MJ. Ewing's sarcoma. Adjuvant total body irradiation, cyclophosphamide and vincristine. Int J Radiat Oncol Biol Phys 1:407, 1976.

104. Dahlin DC, Coventry MD, Scanlon PW. Ewing's sarcoma. A critical analysis of 165 cases. J Bone Joint Surg 43:185, 1961.

105. Nesbit ME Jr, Gehan EA, Burgert EO Jr, Vietti TJ. Multimodal therapy for the management of primary, nonmetastatic Ewing's sarcoma of bone: A long-term follow-up of the first Intergroup Study. J Clin Oncol 8:1664, 1990.

106. Tefft M, Lattin PB, Jereb B, et al. Acute and late effects on normal tissues following combined chemo-radiotherapy for childhood rhabdomyosarcoma and Ewing's sarcoma. Cancer 137(Suppl):1201, 1976.

107. Suit H. Role of therapeutic radiology in cancer of bone. Cancer 35:930, 1975.
108. Donaldson S, Shuster J, Andreozzi C, et al. The Pediatric Oncology Group experience in Ewing's sarcoma of bone. Proc SIOP 17:283, 1989.
109. Perez CA, Tefft M, Nesbit M, et al. The role of radiation therapy in the management of non-metastatic Ewing's sarcoma of bone. Report of the Intergroup Ewing's Sarcoma Study. Int J Radiat Oncol Biol Phys 7:141, 1981.
110. Wilbur JR, King OY, Ho L. Chemotherapy and segmental resection without radiation therapy in the treatment of Ewing's sarcoma of bone. Proc SIOP 17:283, 1989.
111. Winkelmann W, Vysocanska A, Dunst D, et al. The role of surgery in Ewing's sarcoma: Results of the GPO-Cooperative Ewing's Sarcoma Studies. Proc SIOP 17:282, 1989.
112. Miser JS, Triche TJ, Pritchard DJ, Kinsella T. Ewing's sarcoma and the nonrhabdomyosarcoma soft tissue sarcomas of childhood. *In:* Principles and Practice of Pediatric Oncology. Pizzo PA, Poplack DG (Eds). Philadelphia, JB Lippincott Company, 1989, p. 661.
113. Ambros PF, Ambros IM, Strehl S, et al. Cytogenetic and immunological characterization of Ewing's tumor. Proc SIOP 17:284, 1989.
114. Stea B, Kinsella TJ, Triche TJ, et al. Treatment of pelvic sarcomas in adolescents and young adults with intensive combined modality therapy. Int J Radiat Oncol Biol Phys 7:141, 1981.
115. Kinsella TJ, Miser JS, Waller B, et al. Long-term follow-up of Ewing's sarcoma of bone treated with combined modality therapy. Int J Radiat Oncol Biol Phys 20:389, 1991.
116. Marcus RB Jr, Graham-Pole JR, Springfield DS, et al. High-risk Ewing's sarcoma: End-intensification using autologous bone marrow transplantation. Int J Radiat Oncol Biol Phys 15:53, 1988.
117. Yaniv I, Bouffet E, Irle C, et al. Treatment of advanced neuroblastoma with supralethal chemotherapy, radiation and allogeneic or autologous marrow reconstitution. J Clin Oncol 2:609, 1984.
118. August CS, Serota FT, Koch PA, et al. Treatment of advanced neuroblastoma with supralethal chemotherapy, radiation and allogeneic or autologous marrow reconstitution. J Clin Oncol 2:609, 1984.
119. Emminger W, Emminger-Schmidmeier W, Hawliczek R, et al. High-dose melphalan, etoposide ± carboplatin (MEC) combined with 12-Gray fractionated total-body irradiation in children with generalized solid tumors. Pediatr Hematol Oncol 8:13, 1991.
120. Santos GW, Tutschka PJ, Brookmeyer R, et al. Marrow transplantation for acute nonlymphocytic leukemia after treatment with busulfan and cyclophosphamide. N Engl J Med 309:1347, 1983.
121. Gale RP, Butturini A, Bortin MM. What does total body irradiation do in bone marrow transplants for leukemia? Int J Radiat Oncol Biol Phys 20:631, 1991.
122. Thomas ED. Total body irradiation regimens for marrow grafting. Int J Radiat Oncol Biol Phys 19:1285, 1990.
123. Brochstein JA, Kernan NA, Groshen S, et al. Allogeneic bone marrow transplantation after hyperfractionated total body irradiation and cyclophosphamide in children with acute leukemia. N Engl J Med 317:1618, 1987.
124. August CS, Kamani N, Bunin N, et al. Fractionated total-body irradiation preceding high-dose cytosine arabinoside as a preparative regimen for bone marrow transplantation in children with acute leukemia. Med Ped Oncol 20:436, 1992.
125. Woods WB, Ramsay NKC, Weisdork DJ, et al. Bone marrow transplantation for acute lymphocytic leukemia utilizing total body irradiation followed by high doses of cytosine arabinoside: Lack of superiority over cyclophosphamide-containing conditioning regimens. Bone Marrow Transplant 6:9, 1990.
126. Miller JL, Stephens TC, Wist EA. An explanation for the ability of cytotoxic drug pretreatment to reduce bone marrow related lethality of total body irradiation. Int J Radiat Oncol Biol Phys. 8:581, 1982.
127. Pritchard J, McElwain TJ, Graham-Pole J. High dose melphalan with autologous bone marrow rescue for treatment of advanced neuroblastoma. Br J Cancer 48:86, 1982.
128. Kemshead JT, Treleaven JG, Gibson FM, et al. Monoclonal antibodies and magnetic microspheres for the depletion of malignant cells from bone marrow. *In:* Proceedings of the First International Symposium on ABMT. Dicke K, Spitzer G, Zander AR (Eds). Vol 1. Houston, University of Texas, 1985, p. 409.
129. Philip T, Armitage J, Cahn JY, et al. Pilot study of the DHAP rescue protocol and of a new conditioning regimen in responding NHL at relapse. Bone Marrow Transplant 3(Suppl 1):81, 1988.
130. Seeger RC, Moss TJ, Feig SA, et al. Bone marrow transplantation for poor prognosis neuroblastoma. *In:* Advances in Neuroblastoma Research. Evans AE, D'Angio GJ, Knudson AG (Eds). New York, A. Liss, 1988, p. 203.
131. Ikeda H, August CS, Goldwein JW, et al. Sites

of relapse in patients with neuroblastoma following bone marrow transplantation relation to preparatory "de-bulking" treatments. J Pediatr Surg 27:1438, 1992.

132. Hartmann O, Benhamou E, Beaujean F, et al. Repeated high-dose chemotherapy followed by purged autologous bone marrow transplantation as consolidation therapy in metastatic neuroblastoma. J Clin Oncol 5:1205, 1987.

133. Kushner BH, O'Reilly RJ, Mandell LR, et al. Myeloablative combination chemotherapy without total body irradiation for neuroblastoma. J Clin Oncol 9:274, 1991.

134. Graham-Pole J, Gee AP, Gross S, et al. Bone marrow transplantation for advanced neuroblastoma: A multicenter POG pilot study. *In:* Advances in Neuroblastoma Research. Evans AE, D'Angio GJ, Knudson AG (Eds). New York, A. Liss, 1988, p. 215.

Chapter 18

BONE MARROW TRANSPLANTATION

NELSON J. CHAO, RICHARD T. HOPPE, STEPHEN J. FORMAN, AND KARL G. BLUME

INTRODUCTION

The first use of bone marrow to rescue patients following drug exposure was performed in 1939, when a young woman with gold-induced aplasia was given marrow intravenously from her brother with identical blood group antigens (1). Engraftment did not occur and the patient died 5 days later. The modern era of transplantation began in the 1950s, with the demonstration of the protective effect from lethal irradiation in the recipient. This protection was mediated through the delivery of new, normal donor-derived hematopoietic precursors (2,3). Animals were deliberately irradiated to prepare (condition) the recipient to receive donor marrow. Since then, total body irradiation (TBI), in conjunction with chemotherapy, has been considered an integral component of preparative regimens for bone marrow transplantation (BMT) in patients with hematological malignancies. Pioneer work by Thomas and co-workers at Seattle demonstrated prolonged disease-free survival in a significant number of patients, even though they generally had relapsed advanced leukemias or multiply transfused aplastic anemia (4). Recent data, however, suggest that preparatory regimens consisting only of high-dose chemotherapy may be similarly effective (5,6).

The aim of preparative regimens vary according to the disease for which BMT is being employed. For hematologic malignancies, the conditioning regimen is intended to achieve at least three purposes. The first goal is to create space. The new donor marrow must replace the host's hematopoietic system. Unless there is an area for these new cells to settle, the new bone marrow may not grow. This is in contrast to patients with aplastic anemia, in which sufficient marrow space is present. The success of autologous bone marrow in rescuing lethally treated animals suggests that sufficient space could be created (7).

The second purpose of a conditioning regimen is to decrease or remove host resistance to transplantation—to immunosuppress the host. Host cells (T cells and NK cells) are present and capable of rejecting the graft. The allogeneic graft is clearly foreign to the host, and the host defense mechanisms are designed specifically to recognize allogeneic differences and to remove foreign cells. This host resistance to the donor graft can be seen by the increase in the number of cells required for successful transplantation. Fourfold more cells are required for a major histocompatibility complex (MHC) identical allogeneic transplant than for a autologous or syngeneic transplant to be successful, even following TBI. When MHC mismatched grafts are used, the number of bone marrow cells required increases 10-fold from the MHC matched setting (7). Experiments in dogs using single agents for conditioning prior to BMT suggest that TBI is the most effective preparatory agent in MHC identical pairs (8,9). Cyclophosphamide (CP) or dimethylmyleran are less effective, leading to mixed chimerism (containing both host and donor cells) in MHC identical donor recipient pairs (10–12). Chemotherapeutic agents have less of an impact in eliminating host resistance or in immunosuppressing the host sufficiently to prevent graft rejection. This has been well documented in aplastic anemia patients, in whom the use of CP alone is related to a higher incidence of graft rejection. The addition of TBI decreases the risk of graft rejection in aplastic anemia patients. However, this benefit is obtained at a cost of greater toxicity and has no impact in overall survival (13,14).

The third purpose of the conditioning regimen in the therapy of malignant diseases is to eradicate the tumor cells. The efficacy of the conditioning regimen depends on the sensitivity of the tumor cells to those agents. The advantages of TBI are that there are no sanctuary sites and that nondividing cells will be equally affected. The disadvantage is that a single fraction of TBI or fractionated TBI (FTBI) is limited in the tumor log cell kill. In vitro and in vivo studies document that the use of more frequent and higher doses of radiation results in optimal tumor cell kill (15). The dose of TBI, however, is limited due to other organ toxicity, especially the lungs (interstitial pneumonia) and the gastrointestinal tract (16,17). The use of high-dose chemotherapy such as CP or busulfan is more effective in the number of log tumor cell kill (18,19). An overall schema for BMT is illustrated in Figure 18–1.

TECHNIQUE

Historically, TBI has been administered as a single dose to attain the three goals described above. Frequently, patients were ill at the time of transplantation and a single fraction was more technically practical and medically feasible (20). Thomas and coworkers demonstrated in dogs that exposure to 800 cGy TBI at a low dose rate permitted successful engraftment in some animals, whereas a 1000-cGy dose was sufficient to permit consistent engraftment (20–22). The commonly employed technique delivers a single midplane dose of around 1000 cGy, at less than 10 cGy per minute (23). Low dose rate has several disadvantages, such as prolonged treatment time and the development of radiation sickness during exposure. Use of high-dose-rate exposure using a linear accelerator has been the recommended technique. Furthermore, use of fractionated TBI appears to be more radiobiologically sound, in that greater tumor cell kill can be achieved and normal tissue toxicity is less severe (23,24).

The optimal size of dose per fraction to maximize the therapeutic ratio is the highest tolerated dose. Essentially, all lung damage results from irreparable single-hit events.

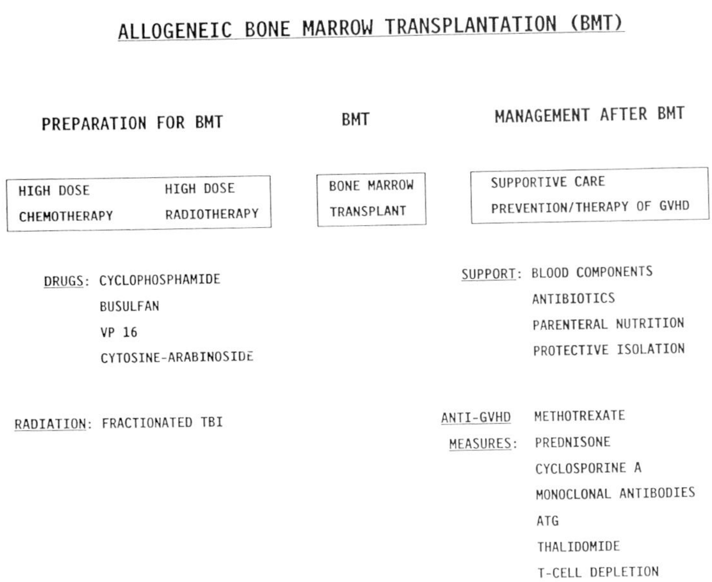

Fig. 18–1. Overall schema for an allogeneic bone marrow transplantation (BMT).

Fractionation of radiation can aid in tissue recovery between doses with minimal repair or tumor cells. Lung tolerance (i.e., less than 5% probability of pneumonitis) is usually considered to be in the range of 2500 cGy in 20 fractions over 4 weeks (25–27). The influence of dose fractionation and overall treatment time on lung damage has been investigated using LD_{50} for respiratory death in mice (28,29). The results suggest that the number of dose fractions is more critical than the overall time of treatment. A dose-rate reduction from 10 cGy/min to 5 cGy/min increases the acutely tolerated dose of TBI 1.2 to 1.4 times (30). The incidence of interstitial pneumonia appears to be related to the dose rate at which TBI is given, especially if the total lung dose exceeds 800 cGy (31). Thus, the total doses of radiation and the radiation dose rate are related in a complex manner, and their individual contribution to lung damage is not clearly defined (32,33). Furthermore, in larger animals and in humans, the factor of radiation absorption of tissues becomes relatively more important due to the variation in dose rates.

A regimen for cytoreduction is illustrated in Figure 18–2. The radiotherapy technique was developed at Memorial Sloan-Kettering Cancer Center (34,35). Patients were simulated in the treatment position and both anterioposterior (AP) and posteroanterior (PA) diagnostic quality radiographs were taken for the design of individually contoured lung blocks. The lung blocks were cast from cerrobend, a low-melting-point alloy, and were one half-value layer thick (approximately 2.8 cm). Body-thickness measurements were taken at representative points along the midline vertical axis of the patient in order to construct a compensator, which provided for a dose of ± 5% for all calculated points compared to the prescribed dose at the central axis of the beam.

Patients were treated with 15 MV photons produced by a linear accelerator at a dose rate of 17 cGy/min. FTBI treatments are administered alternatively AP and PA, 120 cGy per fraction, two or three fractions per day, for a total dose of 1320 cGy in 3-1/2 days. This higher total dose has been associated with improved outcome in allogeneic transplantation for leukemia (35,36). Since the anterior and posterior chest walls (and ribs) are partially shielded by the 50% transmission lung blocks, additional chest wall boost treatment is required. Computerized tomographic scans are used to determine chest-wall thickness at representative horizontal planes. Using computerized treatment-planning programs, an appropriate energy of electrons is chosen to treat the chest wall (and rib marrow), while limiting the dose to the underlying lung to about 10% of the chest-wall dose. Chest-wall electron therapy is delivered on the first 2 days of treatment, 300 cGy per fraction for two fractions, or a total dose of 600 cGy. With this technique, the dose to the midplane of the lungs is no greater than 730 to 780 cGy.

TBI is used in conjunction with a single chemotherapeutic agent, either CP, etoposide (VP-16), or cytosine arabinoside (Ara-C). More recently, combinations of TBI and two chemotherapeutic drugs are being explored. The drugs are given prior to or following TBI. Bone marrow infusion is given usually one to two days following the completion of therapy. Preparative regimens using combination chemotherapy without TBI are also used. These include busulfan and CP for the treatment of leukemias and carmustine, VP-16 and CP for the therapy of lymphomas.

TOXICITY*

The acute toxicity of the preparatory regimen will vary according to the method of

*The reader is referred to Chapter 38 for additional material related to BMT toxicity in pediatrics.

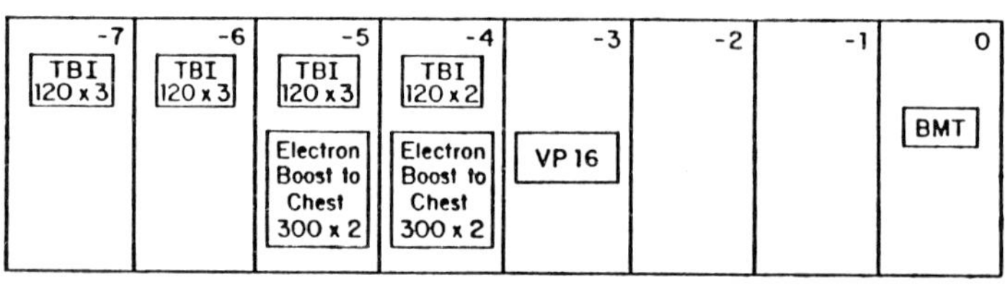

Fig. 18–2. A cytoreduction regimen of fractionated total body irradiation (TBI) and chemotherapy prior to BMT.

radiation and to the combinations used. All regimens, however, will cause severe hematologic toxicity, as evidenced by the disappearance of lymphocytes, monocytes, platelets, and granulocytes in the peripheral blood. Depending on how radiotherapy is administered (single fraction versus fractionated), the rate of disappearance of these cells will vary. Single-fraction TBI is associated with a rapid drop in the numbers of lymphocytes. Granulocytes and platelets decrease at a slower rate. FTBI is associated with a more gradual decrease of the hematopoietic cell lines.

Lung

The most important potential complication of TBI is interstitial pneumonitis. Numerous studies indicate that irradiation dose, fractionation, presence of graft-versus-host disease (GVHD), and preexisting pulmonary disease are risk factors for the development of this complication. Shank et al analyzed the risk of interstitial pneumonitis in their series of hyperfractionated TBI compared to their previous experience with single-dose TBI (34). Of 48 patients treated with hyperfractionation, 16 (33%) developed interstitial pneumonitis and 11 (23%) died of pulmonary toxicity. With single-fraction TBI, 14 of 20 patients (70%) had interstitial pneumonitis and 10 of 20 (50%) died of this toxicity in their TBI experience. It is important to note, however, that in the hyperfractionated group, 50% lung shielding was employed as well.

Cossett et al compared two TBI programs used at the Institute Gustave-Roussy. Thirty-one patients received single-fraction TBI of 1000 cGy (lungs received 800 cGy), and 23 patients were treated with hyperfractionated TBI to 1320 cGy (lungs were treated to 900 cGy) (37). In the single-fraction TBI group, 55% experienced treatment-related toxicity, including 45% bilateral interstitial pneumonitis and 26% lethal interstitial pneumonitis. In the hyperfractionated TBI group, only 26% experienced treatment-related toxicity. This included bilateral interstitial pneumonitis in 13% and lethal interstitial pneumonitis in 4%, both of which were significantly less ($p = 0.02$ and 0.008) than in the single-fraction TBI group. These differences in rate of interstitial pneumonitis were significant, even when adjusted for differences in GVHD and age in the two different treatment groups.

Pino y Torres et al, at Johns Hopkins, investigated the risk factors for development of interstitial pneumonitis in 161 patients receiving allogeneic transplants for leukemia or aplastic anemia (38). Risk was related to dose in patients who received single-dose TBI. The rate was 27.2% for patients receiving 600-cGy TBI and 80% or greater for patients receiving single-fraction TBI of 800 cGy or greater. The rate was 39% in patients who did not receive TBI. In general, the presence of GVHD increased the risk for interstitial pneumonitis twofold for any given dose of irradiation. In the absence of GVHD, the relative risk of interstitial pneumonitis was 1.00 if no irradiation was administered, 3.44 with single-fraction TBI of 800 to 1000 cGy, 1.5 for two fractions of 400 cGy, and 0.9 for three fractions of 300 cGy.

Deeg et al reported that the risk of idiopathic interstitial pneumonitis was greater in the presence of preexisting pulmonary disease (39). They also reported that abnormalities in pulmonary function following the administration of TBI may be reversible in longterm follow-up. CP can sensitize tissues to radiotherapy. In experimental animals, as well as in humans, CP alone can cause lung damage (40,41).

Cataracts

Deeg et al reported on the risk of cataract development among patients treated for aplastic anemia or hematologic malignancy (42). The risks were 19% for 96 patients prepared with chemotherapy alone, 18% for 76 patients treated with fractionated TBI (1200 to 1575 cGy) plus chemotherapy, and 80% for 105 patients treated with single-fraction TBI (1000 cGy) plus chemotherapy. The proportional hazards model revealed that the risk of developing cataracts after single-fraction TBI was 4.7 times the risk after preparation with fractionated TBI or no TBI. The other important risk factor for developing cataracts was chronic steroid use.

Liver

Deeg et al also reported their experience on hepatic toxicity (43). Six of 22 patients treated with single-fraction TBI (920 cGy) developed veno-occlusive disease of the liver compared to 14 of 27 patients treated with 1000 cGy. However, only 5 of 26 patients given 600 cGy × 2 developed this complication. The difference between those given a single fraction and those given FTBI was significant ($p = 0.02$).

Growth and Development

Considerations of growth and development are complicated by previous cranial irradiation and chronic GVHD. Sanders et al reviewed 142 patients between the ages of 1 to 17 years who underwent TBI (44). All had received prior chemotherapy and 55 had received prior CNS irradiation. The TBI schedules varied and included single-fraction treatments of 920 to 1000 cGy and fractionated TBI with 200 to 225 cGy fractions for total doses of 1200 to 1575 cGy. Impaired growth was influenced by the presence of GVHD and single-fraction TBI. Growth disturbances were most apparent, with follow-up exceeding 3 years. Males treated with single-fraction TBI were significantly shorter in height than those treated with fractionated TBI ($p < 0.03$). In females, the trend was the same, but the difference was not significant. These effects on height were greater than those observed in aplastic anemia patients of similar age treated with chemotherapy alone.

In the same report, the frequency of abnormal thyroid function studies was high (39%). The authors emphasize the importance of monitoring patients routinely to assess thyroid function. Growth hormone deficiency (partial or complete) was identified in 21 of 25 (84%) patients who had received previous cranial irradiation and in 6 of 18 (33%) patients without previous cranial irradiation. The use of human growth hormone in such patients is currently under investigation.

In prepubertal children, there was delayed development of secondary sexual characteristics in 68%, and this was associated with hypergonadotrophic hypogonadism. However, not all prepubertal children experienced irreversible gonadal damage. Nearly all postpubertal children experienced gonadal failure. In all postpubertal males, TBI had an adverse effect on fertility but Leydig cell function was spared. Effects on fertility were more notable in this group than in a group of patients of similar age treated with chemotherapy alone.

Blood Cell Kinetics

Dutriex et al reviewed the experience at Institut Gustave-Roussy using single-fraction (1000 cGy in 4 hours) or hyperfractionated TBI (120 cGy × 11 in 4 days) (45). Following single-fraction TBI, there was an initial increase in granulocyte levels, followed by a return to normal 44 hours following completion of TBI and a decrease to 25 to 40% of normal levels at 68 hours post-TBI. Lymphocyte numbers decreased to 40 to 70% of normal at the completion of the 4-hour course of TBI, to less than 30% of baseline values at 44 hours after completion, and to 6 to 15% of normal at 68 hours. Platelets and red blood cell counts were in the normal range throughout the 72-hour observation period (until just before the initiation of high-dose chemotherapy). With hyperfractionated TBI, the lymphocyte counts were reduced to 58% of normal just before the administration of the second 120-cGy fraction. Lymphocyte counts were reduced to 25% following the sixth fraction and 10% following the eleventh fraction of TBI. In this analysis, there was no indication that fractionation enhanced lymphocyte survival. No difference in relative radiosensitivity of T cells versus B cells or OKT4 versus OKT8 subsets was detected.

Central Nervous System

Leukoencephalopathy can also be encountered especially in patients with known central nervous system leukemia who receive intensive local drug administration and radiation (46).

Second Malignancies

Second malignancies have always been a serious concern following treatment of the first cancer. Second cancers may be secondary because of the primary therapy or may be related to the genetic predisposition or underlying immunodeficiency in the patient. These second(ary) malignancies have been a concern with the use of high doses of chemotherapy and radiation. An analysis of

1,926 patients transplanted for hematologic malignancies described 35 patients who developed second(ary) malignancies (47). A significant risk associated with this has been the use of antithymocyte globulin or anti-CD3 monoclonal antibody and TBI. The overall risk has been 1.2 cases of malignancy observed per 100 exposure years during the first year post-transplant and 0.5 cases for the ensuing years. The International Bone Marrow Transplant Registry lists 109 patients developing new malignancies from 9,732 patients transplanted (48). That incidence is calculated to be approximately 0.6 per 100 person years. It is important to keep these numbers in perspective. The possibility of second malignancies following conventional therapy, such as for Hodgkin's disease, is not unlike that described with the experience following BMT. Tucker et al reported 83 second cancers among 1,507 patients with Hodgkin's disease treated at Stanford University Medical Center since 1968 (49). There was a 17.6% cumulative risk of all second cancers, with the probability of leukemia reaching a plateau of 3.3% at 10 years. Similar observations have also been described by Kaldor et al, who noted a higher relative risk of secondary leukemias following treatment of Hodgkin's disease at 6.6% at 6 to 8 years (50). Moreover, the occurrence of secondary malignancies following standard chemotherapy treatment for acute lymphoblastic lymphoma again suggests a similar incidence of second(ary) leukemias, with a relative risk of 2.5% at 15 years after diagnosis in one study and 3.8% at 6 years in a second study (51,52). Although these data remain disturbing and a better understanding of second(ary) malignancies must be pursued, the observance of similar rates of second(ary) malignancies with the preparatory regimens associated with the BMT preparative regimens as compared to standard chemotherapy are reassuring, in that there does not seem to be any additional increase in the incidence of second(ary) malignancies following BMT.

RESULTS*

Preparatory regimens for the therapy of malignant disease have consisted of TBI (single or fractionated dose) given with one chemotherapeutic agent, such as cyclophosphamide, VP-16, or Ara-C. Data from animal and human experiments suggest that the marrow-limiting dose of radiation therapy alone is insufficient for eradication of leukemias (53). Although chemoradiation regimens can achieve cures, the toxicity varies for each of the chemotherapy components added to the radiotherapy. High-dose CP (60 mg/kg/day × 2) is sometimes associated with cardiac injury and hemorrhagic cystitis. High-dose VP-16 (60 mg/kg) is limited by mucositis and hepatitis. High-dose Ara-C (3 g/m^2 q 12 hours × 12 doses) is limited by central nervous system toxicity and mucositis. There are ongoing prospectively randomized studies comparing one regimen versus another for the therapy of malignant diseases. These studies are still at early stages. In aplastic anemia, addition of TBI to CP is associated with a decrease in incidence of graft rejection but with a higher incidence of toxicity (interstitial pneumonitis), resulting in no difference in overall survival. However, recent data suggest that the addition of thoracoabdominal irradiation for patients with aplastic anemia is associated with a high incidence of second malignancies (54).

Acute Lymphoblastic Leukemia (ALL)

Longterm disease-free survival (DFS) or cure can be achieved in patients, depending on the timing of the transplant in relation to the status of the disease. Patients transplanted in first complete remission of acute leukemia can enjoy up to a 60% chance of cure (5,6,55,56). Figure 18–3 illustrates the survival of 53 patients with acute lymphoblastic leukemia in first complete remission who received high-dose chemoradiation followed by a matched histocompatible sibling bone-marrow transplant at the City of Hope National Medical Center and at Stanford University Medical Center. Sixty percent of patients were alive and free of disease past the 10-year mark, with a 14% relapse rate over the same period. Most of these patients were likely to be cured of their disease.

Direct comparison of efficacy of one regimen to another is difficult due to small series and overall numbers of patients treated. A recent review of marrow transplant results with TBI (single or fractionated dose) in

*Additional data on BMT in children are available in Chapter 17.

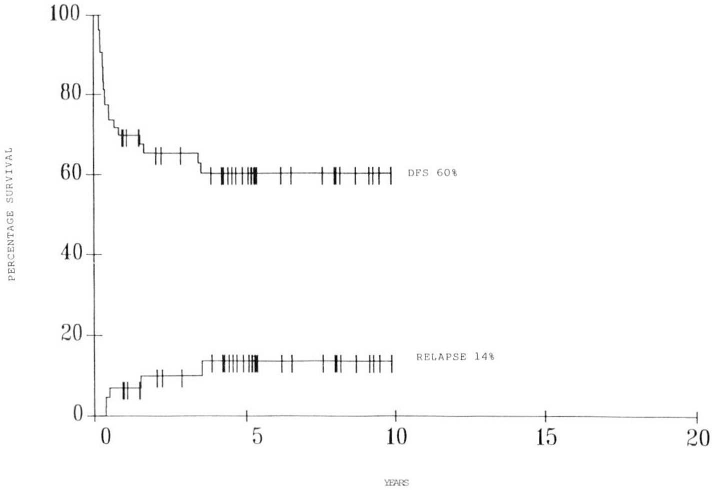

Fig. 18–3. Disease-free survival (DFS) of 53 patients with acute lymphoblastic leukemia in first complete remission following BMT.

combination with CP from six American BMT Centers, from European Bone Marrow Transplant Groups (EBMTG), and from the International Bone Marrow Transplant Registry (IBMTR) indicated the following treatment outcome for patients with acute lymphoblastic leukemia. Approximately 40 to 65% of the patients treated in first complete remission (CR) obtained a DFS lasting 2 or more years, and most of these patients (90%) were expected to be cured of their malignancy (Table 18–1). For patients transplanted in second CR, DFS ranged from 25 to 65% (mean 40%), with more favorable data coming from pediatric BMT recipients. For patients in their third CR, the DFS ranged from 30 to 40%. The least favorable patients were those treated in fourth CR, in relapse or with primary or reinduction failure, in whom DFS is only in the range of 15 to 25% (57).

Table 18–1. Disease-Free Survival Following Allogeneic BMT: Effect of Pretransplant Remission Status

	ANLL	ALL	CML
First CR or first and second chronic phase	45–65%	40 – 65%	55–75%
Second CR or first relapse and accelerated phase	20–45%	25–65%	20–40%
Third and subsequent CR, or advanced relapse, and blastic phase	10–25%	15 – 40%	5–15%

FTBI in combination with high dose CP has been explored by various centers. The results are variable (range of 20 to 50%); children tolerated this preparatory regimen significantly better.

Acute Nonlymphoblastic Leukemia (ANLL)

The largest experience that has been accumulated with CP (60 mg/kg/day × 2) and TBI was developed by Deeg et al. The dose of TBI is either a single fraction of 920 to 1000 cGy or multiple daily fractions of 200 to 225 cGy, to a total dose of 1200 to 1575 cGy. The 5-year DFS for matched allogeneic bone marrow transplant patients in first CR is 50%. For patients in first relapse or second CR, there is a 27% DFS, and there is a 20% DFS for patients in resistant relapse (Table 18–1) (53,58–61). In a prospective randomized study conducted at the Royal Marsden, melphalan-TBI was reported to be equivalent to CP-TBI for patients in first CR (62). Other combinations, such as Ara-C–TBI has yielded similar results to CP-TBI (63). The use of FTBI and VP-16 resulted in a 43% DFS among patients with ANLL not in first CR, which is an improvement over a historical control group who had been treated with CP-TBI (single dose) (64).

Chronic Myelogenous Leukemia (CML)

The largest group of patients treated for CML has again been using the regimen consisting of CP followed by 920 to 1075 cGy TBI. For patients transplanted in chronic phase, the projected DFS in 5 years is 63%. If a patient enters an accelerated phase, the survival rate decreases to 22% and further, down to 16% if patients are transplanted in the blastic phase (65–67). Other important factors that predict poor DFS include the presence of splenomegaly, a time interval from diagnosis to transplant longer than 1 year, and age over 30 years. Newer preparatory regimens such as FTBI/VP-16 are currently being evaluated for CML.

Other Malignancies

TBI has been used in various combinations for other malignancies, such as Hodgkin's and non-Hodgkin's lymphoma, and other solid tumors followed by allogeneic or autologous bone marrow transplantation (ABMT) (Table 18–2) (68–70). The number of patients, however, is too small to allow definitive conclusions. In lymphomas, the use of TBI has been associated with improved DFS (71). Investigators in Nebraska and M.D. Anderson found results for ABMT and non-Hodgkin's lymphoma to be superior when irradiation was included in the preparatory regimen, compared with chemotherapy alone (72). Patients with Hodgkin's disease present a particularly difficult group for consideration of TBI, as a significant group of patients have had previous mantle radiotherapy, which includes significant lung exposure. The addition of TBI to the preparatory regimen of such patients may result in prohibitive and fatal pulmonary toxicity. Other approaches, such as increased cytoreduction using involved field radiotherapy prior to a chemotherapy-based preparatory regimen for BMT or consolidative radiotherapy following BMT, are being investigated.

Table 18–2. Disease-Free Survival Following Autologous BMT: Effect of Pretransplant Remission Status

	Hodgkin's Disease	Non-Hodgkin's Lymphoma
"Good" risk/sensitive relapse	60–70%	65–70%
"Poor" risk/resistant relapse	15–20%	10–15%

FUTURE DIRECTIONS

Over the past 20 years, BMT has evolved to an acceptable and successful therapy for certain diseases. However, current preparatory regimens still lack specificity in eradicating the malignant clones. This lack of specificity results in multiple organ toxicity, with associated morbidity and potential mortality. Toxicities such as mucositis, enteritis, hemorrhagic cystitis, myocarditis, veno-occlusive hepatic disease, and interstitial pneumonitis are related to the aggressive nature of combination regimens.

Research concerning the addition of two chemotherapeutic agents with TBI will hopefully lower the rate of relapse for leukemias without excessive toxicity compared to current regimens. There are new strategies for enhancing tissue resistance to such toxicity. Use of radioprotective agents that are currently in clinical trials, tissue-selective irradiation such as with radiolabeled monoclonal antibodies, lung shielding and eye protection during total body irradiation for certain malignant and nonmalignant conditions, as well as chemoprotectants currently under investigation, should decrease acute and delayed complications and improve the quality of life for surviving patients. As the understanding of human immunology and cellular communication mechanisms improves, this knowledge may be of added value to current preparatory regimens. Thus, therapeutic modalities that may be more tissue selective in their destructive capacities, such as immune targeting, lymphokine-activated killer cells, or tumor-infiltrating lymphocytes, could provide improved results with less overall normal-tissue destruction. Finally, although delayed complications are seen with BMT, these complications must be weighed against the excellent disease-free survival in certain cohorts of patients and the acceptable quality of life following this procedure as judged by the patients themselves.

REFERENCES

1. Osgood EE, Riddle MC, Matthews TJ. Aplastic anemia treated with daily transfusions and in-

travenous marrow: Case report. Ann Intern Med 13:357, 1939.
2. Vos O, Davids JAG, Weyzen WWH, van Bekkum DW. Evidence for the cellular hypothesis in radiation protection by bone marrow cells. Acta Physiol Pharmacol Neerl 4:482, 1956.
3. Ford CE, Hamerton JL, Barnes DWH, Loulit JF. Cytological identification of radiation chimeras. Nature 177:452, 1963.
4. Thomas ED, Buckner CD, Banaji M, et al. One hundred patients with acute leukemia treated by chemotherapy, total body irradiation and allogeneic marrow transplantation. Blood 49:511, 1977.
5. Santos GW, Tutschka PJ, Brookmeyer R, et al. Marrow transplantation for acute nonlymphoblastic leukemia after treatment with busulfan and cyclophosphamide. N Engl J Med 309:1347, 1983.
6. Tutschka PJ, Copelan EA, Klein JP. Bone marrow transplantation for leukemia following a new busulfan and cyclophosphamide regimen. Blood 70:1382, 1987.
7. Vriesendorp HM, van Bekkum DW. Role of total body irradiation in conditioning for bone marrow transplantation. Hematol Blood Transfusion 25:349, 1981.
8. Vriesendorp HM, Bijen AB, Zurcher C, van Bekkum DW. Donor selection and bone marrow transplantation in dogs. *In:* Histocompatibility Testing 1975. Kissmeyer-Neilson F (Ed). Copenhagen, Munksgaard, 1975, p. 963.
9. Weiden PL, Storb R, Graham TC, Sale GE, Thomas ED. Resistance to DLA-nonidentical marrow grafts in lethally irradiated dogs. Transplant Proc 9:285, 1977.
10. Kolb HJ, Storb R, Weiden PL, et al. Immunologic, toxicological and marrow transplantation studies in dogs given dimethylmyleran. Biomedicine 20:341, 1974.
11. Rieder I, Kolb HJ, Schaffer E, et al. Leukocyte transfusions for the modification of host-versus-graft reactions in dogs. *In:* Experimental Hematology Today. Baum SJ, Ledney GD (Eds). New York, Springer, 1978.
12. Storb R, Weidern PL, Graham TC, et al. Hemopoietic grafts between DLA-identical canine littermates following dimethylmyleran. Transplantation 24:349, 1977.
13. Ramsay NKC, Kim T, Nesbit ME, et al. Total lymphoid irradiation and cyclophosphamide as preparation for bone marrow transplantation in severe aplastic anemia. Blood 55:344, 1980.
14. Champlin RE, Horowitz MM, van Bekkum DW, et al. Graft failure following bone marrow transplantation for severe aplastic anemia: Risk factors and treatment results. Blood 73:606, 1989.
15. Whitmore GF, Till JE. Quantitation of cellular radiobiological responses. Ann Rev Nuclear Sci 14:347, 1964.
16. Bortin MM, Kay HEM, Gale RP, Rimm AA. Factors associated with interstitial pneumonitis after bone marrow transplantation for acute leukemia. Lancet 1:437, 1982.
17. Neiman PE, Thomas ED, Reeves WC, et al. Opportunistic infection and interstitial pneumonitis following marrow transplantation for aplastic anemia and hematologic malignancy. Transplant Proc 7:663, 1976.
18. Santos GW, Owens AH Jr. Syngeneic and allogeneic marrow transplants in the cyclophosphamide pretreated rat. Adv Transplant 28:431, 1968.
19. Sharkis SJ, Santos GW. Bone marrow transplantation in a BN rat model of acute myelogenous leukemia (AML). Leuk Res 1:251, 1977.
20. Thomas ED, Storb R, Buckner CD. Total body irradiation in preparation for marrow engraftment. Transplant Proc 8:591, 1976.
21. Storb R, Thomas ED. Bone marrow transplantation in randomly bred animal species and in man. *In:* Proceedings of the Sixth Leukocyte Culture Conference. Schwarz MR (Ed). New York, Academic Press, 1972, p. 805.
22. Thomas ED, Ashley CA, Lochte HL Jr, et al. Homografts of bone marrow in dogs after lethal total body irradiation. Blood 14:720, 1959.
23. Peter LJ, Withers HR, Cundiff JH, Dicke KA. Radiobiological considerations in the use of total-body irradiation for bone-marrow transplantation. Radiology 131:243, 1979.
24. Serota FT, Burkey ED, August CS, D'Angio GJ. Total body irradiation as preparation for bone marrow transplantation in treatment of acute leukemia and aplastic anemia. Int J Rad Oncol Biol Phys 9:1941, 1983.
25. Newton KA, Spittle MF. An analysis of 40 cases treated by total thoracic irradiation. Clin Radiol 20:19, 1969.
26. Phillips TL, Margolis L. Radiation pathology and clinical response of lung and esophagus. *In:* Frontiers of Radiation Therapy and Oncology, Radiation Effect and Tolerance, Normal Tissue. Vaeth JM (Ed). Vol 6. Basel, Switzerland, S. Karger, 1972, p. 254.
27. van der Werf-Messing B. The treatment of pulmonary metastases of malignant teratoma of the testis. Clin Radiol 24:121, 1973.
28. Wara WM, Phillips TL, Margolis LW, et al. Radiation pneumonitis: A new approach to the derivation of time-dose factors. Cancer 32:547, 1973.
29. Field SB, Hornsey S, Kutsutani Y. Effects of fractionated irradiation on mouse lung and a

phenomenon of slow repair. Br J Radiol 49:700, 1976.
30. Deeg HJ, Storb R, Weiden PL, et al. High dose total body irradiation and autologous marrow reconstitution in dogs: Dose rate related acute toxicity and fractionation dependent long term survival. Radiat Res 88:385, 1981.
31. Barrett A. Total body irradiation (TBI) before bone marrow transplantation in leukemia: A co-operative study from the European Group for Bone Marrow Transplantation. Br J Radiol 55:562, 1982.
32. Bortin MM, Rimm AA. Interstitial pneumonitis: Dose rate vs. total dose of radiation. Int J Radiat Oncol Biol Phys 8:1815, 1982.
33. Keane TJ, van Dijk J, Rider WD. Interstitial pneumonitis: Dose rate vs. total dose of radiation. Int J Radiat Oncol Biol Phys 8:1816, 1982.
34. Shank B, Hopfan S, Kim JH, et al. Hyperfractionated total body irradiation for bone marrow transplantation. I. Early results in leukemia patients. Int J Radiat Oncol Biol Phys 7:1109, 1981.
35. Shank B, Chu FCH, Dinsmore R, et al. Hyperfractionated total body irradiation for bone marrow transplantation. Results in seventy leukemia patients with allogeneic transplants. Int J Radiat Oncol Biol Phys 9:1607, 1983.
36. Scarpati D, Frassoni F, Vitale V, et al. Total body irradiation in acute myeloid leukemia and chronic myelogenous leukemia: Influence of dose and dose-rate on leukemia relapse. Int J Radiat Oncol Biol Phys 17:547, 1989.
37. Cosset JM, Baume D, Pico JL, et al. Single dose versus hyperfractionated total body irradiation before allogeneic bone marrow transplantation. A non-randomized comparative study of 54 patients at the Institut Gustave-Roussy. Radiother Oncol 15:151, 1989.
38. Pino y Torres JL, Bross DS, Lam W-C. Risk factors in interstitial pneumonitis following allogeneic bone marrow transplantation. Int J Radiat Oncol Biol Phys 8:1301, 1982.
39. Deeg HJ, for the Seattle Marrow Transplant Team. Acute and delayed toxicities of total body irradiation. Int J Radiat Oncol Biol Phys 9:1933, 1983.
40. Trask CWL, Joannides T, Harper PG, et al. Radiation-induced lung fibrosis after treatment of small cell carcinoma of the lung with very high-dose cyclophosphamide. Cancer 55:57, 1985.
41. Collis CH, Wilson CM, Jones JM. Cyclophosphamide-induced lung damage in mice: Protection by a small preliminary dose. Br J Cancer 41:901, 1980.
42. Deeg HJ, Flournoy N, Sullivan KM, et al. Cataracts after total body irradiation and marrow transplantation: A sparing effect of dose fractionation. Int J Radiat Oncol Biol Phys 10:957, 1984.
43. Deeg HJ, Sullivan KM, Buckner CD. Marrow transplantation for acute non-lymphoblastic leukemia in first remission: Toxicities and long term follow-up of patients conditioned with single dose of fractionated total body irradiation. Bone Marrow Transplant 1:151, 1986.
44. Sanders JE, Pritchard S, Mahoney P. Growth and development following marrow transplantation for leukemia. Blood 68:1129, 1986.
45. Dutriex J, Girinsky T, Cosset JM. Blood cell kinetics and total body irradiation. Radiother Oncol 9:119, 1987.
46. Thompson CB, Sanders JE, Flourno N, et al. The risks of central nervous system relapse and leukoencephalopathy in patients receiving marrow transplants for acute leukemia. Blood 67:195, 1986.
47. Witherspoon RP, Fisher LD, Schoch G, et al. Secondary cancers after bone marrow transplantation for leukemia or aplastic anemia. N Engl J Med 321:784, 1989.
48. Socie G, Kolb HJ, Ljungman P. Malignant diseases after allogeneic bone marrow transplantation: The case for assessment of risk factors. Br J Haematol 80:427, 1992.
49. Tucker MA, Coleman CN, Cox RS, et al. Risk of second cancers after treatment for Hodgkin's disease. N Engl J Med 318:76, 1988.
50. Kaldor JM, Day NE, Clarke EA, et al. Leukemia following Hodgkin's disease. N Engl J Med 322:7, 1990.
51. Neglia JP, Meadows AT, Robinson LL, et al. Second neoplasms in acute lymphoblastic leukemia in childhood. N Engl J Med 325:1330, 1991.
52. Pui C-H, Ribeiro RL, Hancock ML, et al. Acute myeloid leukemia in children treated with epipodophyllotoxins for acute lymphoblastic leukemia. N Engl J Med 325:1682, 1991.
53. Thomas ED, Storb R, Clift RA, et al. Bone marrow transplantation. N Engl J Med 292:832, 1975.
54. Socie G, Heury-Amar M, Cosset JM, et al. Increased incidence of solid malignant tumors after bone marrow transplantation for severe aplastic anemia. Blood 78:277, 1991.
55. Thomas ED, Buckner CD, Clift RA, et al. Marrow transplantation for acute nonlymphoblastic leukemia in first remission. N Engl J Med 301:597, 1979.
56. Chao NJ, Forman SJ, Schmidt GM, et al. Allogenic bone marrow transplantation for high

risk acute lymphoblastic leukemia during first complete remission. Blood 78:1923, 1991.

57. Blume KG. Marrow transplantation for acute lymphoblastic leukemia. New preparative regimens. *In:* Bone Marrow Transplantation. Current Controversies. Gale RP, Chaplin RE (Eds). New York, Alan R. Liss, Inc., 1989, p. 47.
58. Appelbaum FR, Clift RA, Buckner CD, et al. Allogeneic marrow transplantation for acute nonlymphoblastic leukemia after first relapse. Blood 61:949, 1983.
59. Clift RA, Buckner CD, Thomas ED, et al. The treatment of acute non-lymphoblastic leukemia by allogeneic marrow transplantation. Bone Marrow Transplant 2:242, 1987.
60. Champlin RE, Ho WG, Gale RP, et al. Treatment of acute myelogenous leukemia. Ann Intern Med 102:285, 1985.
61. Blume KG, Forman SJ, Snyder DS, et al. Allogeneic bone marrow transplantation for acute lymphoblastic leukemia during first complete remission. Transplantation 43:389, 1987.
62. Helenglass G, Powles RL, McElwain TJ, et al. Melphalan and total body irradiation (TBI) versus cyclophosphamide and TBI as conditioning for allogeneic matched sibling bone marrow transplants for acute myeloblastic leukaemia in first remission. Bone Marrow Transplant 3:21, 1988.
63. Appelbaum FR, Petersen FB, Buckner CD, et al. New preparative regimens prior to marrow transplantation for acute nonlymphoblastic leukemia. *In:* Bone Marrow Transplantation: Current Controversies. Gale RP, Chaplin RE (Eds). New York, Alan R Liss, Inc., 1989, p. 107.
64. Blume KG, Forman SJ, O'Donnell MR, et al. Total body irradiation and high-dose etoposide: A new preparatory regimen for bone marrow transplantation in patients with advanced hematologic malignancies. Blood 69:1015, 1987.
65. Thomas ED, Clift RA, Fefer A, et al. Marrow transplantation for the treatment of chronic myelogenous leukemia. Ann Intern Med 104:155, 1986.
66. Martin PJ, Clift RA, Fisher LD, et al. HLA-identical marrow transplantation during accelerated-phase chronic myelogenous leukemia: Analysis of survival and remission duration. Blood 72:1978, 1988.
67. Goldman JM, Gale RP, Horowitz MM, et al. Bone marrow transplantation for chronic myelogenous leukemia in chronic phase. Increased risk for relapse associated with T-cell depletion. Ann Intern Med 108:806, 1988.
68. Appelbaum FR, Herzig GP, Ziegler JL, et al. Successful engraftment of cryopreserved autologous bone marrow in patients with malignant lymphoma. Blood 52:85, 1978.
69. Phillips GL, Herzig RH, Lazarus HM, et al. Treatment of resistant malignant lymphoma with cyclophosphamide, total body irradiation and transplantation of cryopreserved autologous marrow. N Engl J Med 310:1557, 1984.
70. Phillips GL, Wolff SN, Herzig RH, et al. Treatment of progressive Hodgkin's disease with intensive chemoradiotherapy and autologous bone marrow transplantation. Blood 73:2086, 1989.
71. Takvorian T, Canellos GP, Ritz J, et al. Prolonged disease-free survival after autologous bone marrow transplantation in patients with non-Hodgkin's lymphoma with a poor prognosis. N Engl J Med 316:1499, 1987.
72. Jagannath S, Armitage JD, Dicke KA, et al. Prognostic factors for response and survival after high dose cyclophosphamide, carmustine and etoposide with autologous bone marrow transplantation for relapsed Hodgkin's disease. (Abstract). Blood 68:274a, 1986.

Chapter 19

MALIGNANT LYMPHOMAS

SANDRA J. HORNING AND C. NORMAN COLEMAN

INTRODUCTION

The lymphoid malignancies, Hodgkin's disease and non-Hodgkin's lymphomas, have served as a model for the development of combined modality therapy and for the assessment of toxicity related to such treatment. A large proportion of patients with malignant lymphoma experience prolonged survival and many are cured of their disease by the initial treatment. Although these diseases occur in patients of all ages, Hodgkin's disease tends to occur in a younger population. As will be detailed below, age may be an important factor in late toxicity. Optimal therapy is based upon a number of significant variables, including histology, stage, and tumor burden. The chemotherapeutic agents chosen for a given clinical setting vary, such that this group of patients has a wide range of potential drug exposures that allow the assessment of longterm effects of the specific drugs. Similarly, the dose and volume of radiotherapy vary, allowing assessment of chronic toxicity related to this modality.

The purpose of this chapter is to review the role of combined modality (CM) therapy, specifically chemoradiation in the treatment of adults with lymphoid malignancies. It is not a comprehensive review of the extensive literature on the subject but rather a discussion of selected studies that illustrate important principles. While a major emphasis has been placed on randomized trials, data from nonrandomized studies have been included as well. Treatment results for the same general clinical setting vary among institutions. These differences reflect a number of variables, including histologic interpretation, staging procedures, selection of chemotherapeutic agents, doses and schedules, subtleties of radiation technique, and sequencing of treatment modalities. The experience with Hodgkin's disease will be emphasized because it includes a more homogeneous group of patients and thus lends itself more readily to analysis.

HODGKIN'S DISEASE

Stage I and II

The early stages of Hodgkin's disease (HD) have been treated successfully using radiation therapy (RT) alone, chemoradiation, or chemotherapy alone. The first two treatments have been more extensively tested in randomized trials. There are relatively less data available using drugs alone in the adult population. The evolution and summary results of the Stanford randomized trials, which have been in existence since 1962, have been summarized (1). The initial series of Stanford trials defined the pattern of spread of HD and demonstrated the necessity of appropriate staging procedures, including the use of the lymphogram and the introduction of the staging laparotomy with splenectomy. Meanwhile, DeVita and colleagues developed the successful combination chemotherapy program, MOPP [nitrogen *m*ustard, vincristine (*O*ncovin), *p*rocarbazine, *p*rednisone], for advanced stage disease (2). Following the stepwise standardization of a staging system (3,4) and the development of successful multidrug chemotherapy, the Stanford investigators embarked on a second series of randomized trials initiated in 1967. Patients with Stage I and IIA HD were randomized to involved-field (IF) RT or extended-field RT. In this study, males received total lymphoid irradiation (TLI) and females received subtotal lymphoid irradiation (STLI), omitting the pelvic field. Those with Stage I and IIB received either TLI or TLI with six courses of MOPP chemotherapy.

Table 19–1 describes the results of the Stanford clinical trials in Stage I and II HD from 1967 through 1988. The actuarial results at 20 years favor extended-field irradiation over IF RT for asymptomatic patients with a significantly superior freedom from progression (FFP) ($p < 0.0001$) although there was no survival advantage, given the efficacy of secondary treatment with MOPP chemotherapy. The results in symptomatic patients were excellent in both arms; no benefit is seen for the CM arm. The next series of studies was initiated in 1974 and continued through 1980. Patients with pathologic Stage I–IIA HD randomly received IF RT plus six courses of MOP(P) (the prednisone was omitted after mediastinal irradiation) or STLI. Data at 15 years (Table 19–1) indicated no significant difference in the treatment arms. This study, when combined with the earlier one, demonstrated that MOP(P) can substitute extended-field irradiation in this setting. However, as will be discussed below, the price paid for MOPP was high compared with the toxicity of STLI, suggesting that for Stage I and II disease one should use RT alone or, if using drugs in lieu of STLI or TLI, one should consider a combination of drugs with less acute and chronic toxicity than that associated with MOPP.

Such considerations led to a subsequent randomized trial initiated in 1980 for favorable Stage I/II and IIIA HD at Stanford. Patients received either STLI/TLI or IF + six cycles of a novel chemotherapy combination (5). It was anticipated that VBM (*v*inblastine, *b*leomycin, *m*ethotrexate) would have acceptable acute toxicity, little adverse effect on fertility, and a minimal risk of leukemogenesis. With a median follow-up of 7 years, the data indicate that VBM can substitute extended-field irradiation, similar to the results

Table 19–1. Results of Treatment for Stage I and II Hodgkin's Disease

Stage	Number of Patients (N)	Treatment	Years of Follow-up	Freedom From Progression (%)	Freedom From Progression (p)	Survival (%)	Survival (p)	Ref.
			STANFORD SERIES					
PS	(28)	IF RT	20	25	(< 0.0001)	40	(NS)	*
I-IIA	(35)	STLI, TLI		80		65		
PS	(27)	TLI	20	75	(NS)	78	(NS)	*
I-IIB	(27)	TLI + MOPP		76		50		
PS	(35)	STLI	15	80	(NS)	80	(NS)	*
I,IIA	(36)	IF + MOPP		77		70		
PS	(38)	STLI, TLI	10	72	(0.02)	91	(NS)	*
I, IIA/B IIIA	(34)	IF + VBM		97		100		
			CHEMOTHERAPY SERIES					
NCI:								
PS I-IIA	(51)	STLI	10	60**	(0.009)	76	(0.05)	21
	(54)	MOPP		86		92		
ITALY:								
PS I-IIA	(45)	STLI	5	74	(NS)	94	(NS)	22
	(44)	MOPP		66		88		

*Updated by author for this publication, see text for additional references.
**Results not significant when patients with large mediastinal masses are excluded.
Abbreviations: PS = pathological stage; IF = involved field; RT = radiation therapy; TLI = total lymphoid irradiation; STLI = subtotal lymphoid irradiation; MOPP = nitrogen mustard, vincristine (Oncovin), procarbazine, prednisone; VBM = vinblastine, bleomycin, methotrexate; NS = not significant.

obtained with IF + MOP(P) discussed above (Table 19–1). In fact, the CM arm is superior, with an actuarial FFP at 10 years of 97% with IF + VBM and 72% with STLI/TLI ($p = 0.02$). As anticipated, VBM had relatively little adverse effect on male or female fertility. No hospitalization was required among the VBM patients, before or after treatment. Pulmonary function analysis showed no significant difference in the treatment arms. Patients with large mediastinal masses were excluded from this study; however, patients with systemic symptoms and favorable IIIA (see below) were included. The results of this study are encouraging, and VBM + RT is currently under study in clinically staged patients with favorable HD.

A series of randomized trials for the treatment of early-stage HD was initiated in 1964 by the European Organization for Research and Treatment of Cancer (EORTC). These results have been summarized by Tubiana et al (6). As with the Stanford trials, the early studies asked predominantly RT questions, treating patients with clinical stage (CS) I or II with regional RT, either a mantle or an inverted Y, with no prophylactic RT being given to the noninvolved side of the diaphragm. The RT dose of 4000 cGy was similar to that used by Stanford investigators. Patients were then randomized to receive weekly vinblastine for 2 years or no further therapy. This interesting study demonstrated that RT + vinblastine produced a statistically superior 10-year FFP, 61% vs. 38% ($p < 0.001$), and a borderline survival advantage, 70% vs. 60% ($p = 0.08$). The benefit was limited to patients with mixed cellularity (MC) histology. Of the MC patients with supradiaphragmatic presentations treated with a mantle alone, 40% relapsed in para-aortic nodes. This observation was consistent with the data being derived from the Stanford staging laparotomy series (7).

Based on the results of this study, a second trial was initiated by the EORTC, in which 300 patients with supradiaphragmatic CS I or II disease were randomized to undergo splenic irradiation, or laparotomy and splenectomy, all receiving para-aortic lymph node irradiation (no pelvic node irradiation was given). Patients with the unfavorable histologies (MC or lymphocyte depleted) were randomized to receive two years of chemotherapy with either vinblastine or vinblastine plus procarbazine. Splenectomy and splenic irradiation were equally effective in terms of relapse-free survival and survival. The presence of splenic disease was correlated with an increased incidence of relapse at 7 years (80% FFP for spleen negative vs. 57% for spleen positive, $p < 0.01$), primarily in extranodal and nonirradiated nodal sites. In this trial and in the earlier study, the negative prognostic significance of the presence of systemic symptoms and of an elevated erythrocyte sedimentation rate was noted. However, there was no difference in survival between patients with similar prognostic factors. There was no advantage to one chemotherapy arm vs. the other, but it must be remembered that only the unfavorable histologies received chemotherapy and only one or two drugs were employed (6).

A subsequent study of early-stage HD performed by the EORTC was begun in 1977 and concluded in 1982, after accruing 471 patients (8). This study stratified patients into a good prognostic group based on histology (nodular sclerosis or lymphocyte predominance), age < 40, Erythrocyte Sedimentation Rate (ESR) < 70, CS I, and CS II mediastinal positive; the poor prognostic group either did not meet these prelaparotomy criteria or had a positive (PSIII) staging laparotomy. After the good prognostic group underwent staging laparotomy, those with negative explorations were randomized to receive mantle RT vs. mantle plus para-aortic RT. The unfavorable group received TLI or CM therapy: MOPP × 3 → mantle → MOPP × 3. The selected favorable group had an FFP of 72% at 6 years in both arms of the study, suggesting that in well selected patients who are laparotomy-staged, mantle RT is adequate treatment. In the unfavorable group, the 6-year results favor CM therapy, with an FFP of 73% (TLI) vs. 89% (CM), $p = 0.01$. A substantial subset of patients (48%) did not receive TLI, as the pelvic field was omitted. A decreased FFP (p = NS) was observed in patients receiving STLI compared with TLI; however, the survival was comparable. The overall survival at 6 years is significantly higher ($p = 0.05$) in the CM arm (89%) as compared with TLI (82%) in the unfavorable patients. This trend in favor of the CM group was not appreciated in prior reports of this study. The patients who derived the greatest benefit from CM treatment were those with the poorest prognostic factors, particularly age > 40. Indeed, patients under age 40 had no statistically significant increased benefit from CM vs. TLI for either FFP or survival parameters.

More recent studies from the EORTC have randomized 578 CS I–II supradiaphragmatic HD patients in a strategy tailored to prognostic features (9). Favorable patients were randomized to STLI or a staging laparotomy. If laparotomy was negative, treatment consisted of mantle RT or STLI. If positive, patients were randomized together with unfavorable patients to MOPP or ABVD (*A*driamycin, *b*leomycin, *v*inblastine, *d*acarbazine) (10) in combination with RT. Disease-free survival among the favorable patients favored those who underwent surgical staging (91% vs. 80%, p = 0.02), while survival was identical. Among the unfavorable patients, results with either of the two CM treatments were excellent and not different.

In addition to the features noted in the EORTC studies outlined above, massive intrathoracic disease, defined as tumor mass > one-third the maximum intrathoracic diameter is considered unfavorable due to a relapse probability of 50 to 60% when treated with radiotherapy alone (11–15). This compares with about 20 to 25% for combined modality. Even so, there is no survival benefit for the use of initial CM therapy in this clinical setting due to the efficacy of MOP(P) chemotherapy at relapse (13,15). Initial use of chemotherapy is preferred because it allows a smaller volume of RT, sparing normal tissues, and significantly reduces the probability of relapse. Recent data from the National Cancer Institute (NCI) indicate that a high rate of relapse is seen in patients with massive mediastinal HD treated with MOPP alone, making the case for a CM approach (16). Therefore, the nature of the optimal chemotherapy in the CM therapy of massive intrathoracic HD is still a major question.

A large controlled trial was conducted by the Milan group, randomizing 232 Stage IIB and III patients to three cycles of MOPP or ABVD, followed by STLI, followed by three additional cycles of chemotherapy (17). The 7-year results are statistically significant in favor of ABVD/RT (FFP 81% vs. 63% with MOPP/RT). This study included a subset of 100 patients with large mediastinal masses. In a randomized trial conducted on a smaller group of 47 patients, all with locally extensive disease, the Stanford group has had excellent results, finding no difference in outcome between patients receiving *p*rocarbazine + *A*lkeran or phenylalanine mustard + *Ve*lban or vinblastine (PAVe) or ABVD × 3 → mantle RT → PAVe or ABVD × 3 (18). FFP was in excess of 75% on both arms of this study. Staging laparotomy was omitted in the Stanford trial and discontinued midway through the Milan trial. Given the greatly different spectrum of toxicity associated with these chemotherapeutic programs (see below), the major issue becomes that of the acute and chronic morbidity of therapy.

In contrast, Hoppe has reported the clinical outcome of 13 patients with unfavorable mediastinal masses who had treatment selected and planned based on CT findings of mass size and location and staging laparotomy (19). The 83% 2-year actuarial freedom from relapse suggests that highly selected patients with large mediastinal masses and pathologically staged, limited disease may be treated with RT alone. Thus, the configuration of the mass, as well as the size, may influence the choice of primary therapy.

There are relatively less data available regarding the use of primary chemotherapy alone in early-stage HD. A Cancer and Leukemia Group B (CALGB) trial 7751, compared six cycles of CVPP (*C*CNU, *v*inblastine, *p*rocarbazine, *p*rednisone) chemotherapy alone vs. involved field RT + 6 CVPP cycles for 55 poor-risk Stage I or II patients (20). These patients were poor risks by virtue of having B symptoms, MC or lymphocyte depleted histology, large mediastinal masses, or age > 40 years. The combined modality group had a statistically significant improved complete remission rate (95% vs. 61%, p = 0.04), with the advantage limited to those with B symptoms. Insufficient data are available regarding survival. NCI reported results of a study in 136 PS-I-II HD patients who were randomized to receive STLI or six cycles of MOPP (Table 19–1) (21). This study excluded favorable patients with peripheral IA disease. The projected 10-year disease-free survival significantly favors MOPP over STLI (86% vs. 60%, p = 0.009) and survival also favors the chemotherapy arm (92% vs.

76%). When patients with massive mediastinal disease were excluded, there were no significant differences between the treatments. As expected, the toxicity profile between the two arms was very different. Another randomized study of MOPP vs. extended-field RT for PS I-IIA patients has been conducted by Cimino et al (Table 19–1) (22). No significant difference in survival or disease-free survival was observed. However, the early treatment-related complications were more severe in the MOPP group.

The routine use of staging laparotomy in the management of Stage I and II HD has become a controversial subject. It is clear that the risk of finding disease at laparotomy is related to a number of presenting variables (23). There are clinical presentations associated with such a low likelihood of the presence of disease at laparotomy [i.e., disease limited to intrathoracic sites (24)] that they may be treated by RT alone after clinical staging. Patients who receive chemotherapy because of massive intrathoracic disease or other reasons do not require surgical staging. Omitting laparotomy but retaining more minimal therapy (mantle/STLI) in supradiaphragmatic CS I and II will result in a somewhat higher relapse rate. This may be justified if the secondary therapy is both successful, as judged by a lack of difference between the survival curves, and not unduly toxic. However, relapse rates in excess of 40 to 50% in early-stage HD are not considered acceptable.

Stage IIIA

While many patients with Stage I and II Hodgkin's disease are candidates for primary radiotherapy, treatment results in Stage III and IV disease make chemotherapy, or perhaps CM treatment, the more appropriate choice. Selection of treatment for Stage IIIA disease has been based on the clinical/pathologic situation below the diaphragm. In this discussion, it is assumed that the supradiaphragmatic presentation is such that this does not require CM therapy, as opposed to the case with massive intrathoracic disease.

As a consequence of treatment results, a number of authors have proposed that Stage III disease be subdivided. In the Cotswald staging system, the subdivision is into Stage III_1, which includes disease in the upper abdomen only (spleen, splenic hilar nodes, celiac nodes, and/or portal nodes), and III_2, which involves paraortic, iliac, or mesenteric nodes (25–27). The report from Desser et al showed that patients with III_1 disease fared better in terms of survival and freedom from relapse compared to those with stage III_2 disease (25). The presence of B symptoms was not a major predictor of outcome once substage was taken into account. Stein et al, in a somewhat smaller series, demonstrated that patients with III_2 disease had a freedom from relapse statistically inferior to those with III_1 disease (13% vs. 73%), but there was no statistically significant difference in survival (65% vs. 100%), although the trend was in favor of the III_1 group (26). There were insufficient numbers of patients to comment specifically on the efficacy of CM therapy. However, in both of these studies, the use of radiation alone was sufficient in the III_1 group and chemotherapy was an important addition to the treatment of the III_2 group (25,26). Mauch et al, in a series of patients not treated in a randomized trial, reported that survival using CM therapy was superior to that for patients with Stage III_2 [66% vs. 44%, $p = 0.04$], III_1 [97% vs. 73%, $p = 0.05$], and Stage III with extensive splenic involvement as defined below [77% vs. 58%, $p = 0.02$] (28).

In the Stanford randomized trials, patients with Stage IIIA disease receiving CM therapy enjoyed an improved FFP (80% vs. 70%, $p = 0.07$) and survival (92% vs. 68%, $p = 0.05$) compared to those treated with TLI alone (1). Hoppe further analyzed factors that predicted for treatment outcome (29). The strongest variable was the degree of splenic involvement, with extensive splenic disease (five or more nodules of Hodgkin's disease) being an adverse factor. Anatomic substaging into stage III_1 vs. III_2 was not useful in predicting treatment outcome. Despite the improvement in FFP using CM therapy for a number of prognostic subsets, in no case did CM offer a statistically significant improvement in survival, which was in the range of 80 to 90% for all subsets (29).

MOPP or MOPP-like chemotherapy is also effective therapy for patients with Stage IIIA disease. From the original MOPP series, 94% of 23 asymptomatic patients with Stage III (7) or IV (16) HD remained disease-free at 5 years (30). Lister et al reported a FFP of 96%

among 32 patients receiving MVPP (vinblastine substituted for vincristine in MOPP) at a median follow-up of 5.5 years (31). In a randomized study of 56 patients with Stage IIIA disease, Crowther et al found no benefit by adding 3000 cGy of irradiation to selected disease sites to MVPP chemotherapy in terms of freedom from relapse or survival, the latter being approximately 85% (32). In their more recent trials, the Stanford group has treated patients with Stage $IIIA_2$ HD and extensive splenic disease with CM therapy or MOPP-ABVD (1). Similarly, other groups have tested various chemotherapy regimens (MOPP, ABVD, MOPP, alternating with ABVD, MOPP-ABV hybrid) in Stage $IIIA_2$ HD. The mature results of these large multi-institutional studies employing chemotherapy only for Stage IIIA will provide an important contribution to the existing literature.

Stages IIIB and IV

Chemotherapy is critical to the curative treatment of patients with Stage IIIB and IV HD (Table 19–2). MOPP chemotherapy, as delivered at the NCI, ultimately cures about 50% of patients (33). A number of alternative drug combinations has been employed in the treatment of advanced HD. One group

Table 19–2. Comparative Efficacy of Selected Combination Chemotherapy Regimens in Advanced Hodgkin's Disease

Stage	Number of Patients (N)	Treatment	Freedom from Progression (%)	(p)	Survival (%)	(p)	Ref.
		ACTUARIAL RESULTS AT 8 YEARS					
Milano Study:							
IV*	(43)	MOPP	36	(< 0.005)	64	(< 0.06)	36
	(45)	MOPP/ABVD	65		84		
		ACTUARIAL RESULTS AT 10 YEARS					
NCI Series:							
II, III, IV*	(188)	MOPP	54		50		33
		ACTUARIAL RESULTS AT 4 YEARS					
Canadian Study:							
IIIB, IV, or radiotherapy failures	(146)	MOPP/ABV	62	(NS)	84	(NS)	41
		MOPP/ABVD	57		84		
		ACTUARIAL RESULTS AT 4 YEARS					
ECOG Study:							
IIIA, IIIB, IV	(305)	BCVPP	57	(0.39)	74	(0.14)	38
		MOPP/ABVD	60		81		
		BCVPP + RT	62		74		
		ACTUARIAL RESULTS AT 3 YEARS					
CALGB Study:							
IIIA, IIIB, IV*	(275)	ABVD	64	(0.004)	~79	(NS)	37
		MOPP/ABVD	64		~79		
		MOPP	48		~79		

*Includes radiotherapy failures.
See text for descriptions of treatment.
~ Denotes extrapolation from published actuarial curves.
Abbreviations: MOPP = nitrogen mustard, vincristine (Oncovin), procarbazine, prednisone; ABVD = Adriamycin, bleomycin, vinblastine, dacarbazine; NCI = National Cancer Institute; ABV = Actinomycin D, bleomycin, and vincristine; ECOG = Eastern Cooperative Oncology Group; BCVPP = BCNU (bischloroethylnitrosourea), cyclophosphamide, vinblastine, procarbazine, prednisone; RT = radiation therapy; CALGB = Cancer and Leukemia Group B; NS = not significant.

is the MOPP-like combinations, which include alkylating agents, procarbazine, vinca alkaloids, and corticosteroids, and another group includes drugs that are intended to be noncross-resistant. The prototype of this latter group is ABVD, which was initially designed to treat patients whose disease relapsed following treatment with MOPP (17). The MOPP-like regimens such as BCVPP [*B*CNU, *c*yclophosphamide, *v*inblastine, *p*rocarbazine, *p*rednisone] (34), ChlVPP (*chlo*rambucil, *v*inblastine, *p*rocarbazine, *p*rednisone) (35) and PAVe (*p*rocarbazine, *A*lkeran, *v*inblastine used in conjunction with RT) appear to be as efficacious as MOPP and less acutely toxic (1). They are interesting as alternatives.

Primary chemotherapy incorporating seven or more drugs has been widely employed in the last decade. In a randomized trial of 12 months of MOPP vs. 12 months of alternating MOPP and ABVD (six cycles of each), the combination produced a superior freedom from relapse (77% vs. 44%, $p < 0.004$) and a superior 7-year survival (82% vs. 61%) in Stage IV patients (36) (Table 19–2). This alternating program has been tested in two large cooperative trials and the preliminary results have been presented. The CALGB study randomly assigned patients with Stage $IIIA_2$, IIIB, and IV HD to ABVD, MOPP, or alternating MOPP/ABVD after stratification for age, stage, and previous RT (37). Of interest, the FFP data at 3 years favored both ABVD alone (64%) and MOPP/ABVD (64%) over MOPP alone (48%), $p = 0.004$. The ECOG (Eastern Cooperative Oncology Group) study randomly assigned Stage $IIIA_2$, IIIB, and IV patients to BCVPP, MOPP/ABVD, or BCVPP followed by low-dose consolidative RT (38). The results at 4 years are similar: FFP is 57% for BCVPP, 60% for MOPP/ABVD, and 62% for BCVPP-RT. These interesting studies require more complete analysis as the data mature. An innovative study from Vancouver combined these drugs in a hybrid fashion, such that MOPP/ABV was given within a single 28-day cycle (39). While the early results from this trial were outstanding, the results have not been sustained with mature data (40). In a large randomized trial conducted in Canada, MOPP-ABV hybrid and MOPP alternating with ABVD yielded identical preliminary results (41). Bonadonna also incorporated MOPP/ABVD into a single cycle (M/A) for treatment of advanced-stage HD (42). As in the Canadian trial, the hybrid and alternating regimens were equivalent.

The role of CM therapy in advanced-stage HD is less certain. Data supporting the theoretic use of radiation therapy plus chemotherapy come from the NCI analysis of the patterns of relapse in patients treated with MOPP (43). Of those who relapsed, 92% did so in previously involved sites (71% exclusively); the majority relapsed in nodal sites. As noted above, the relapse rate was particularly prominent among those with massive mediastinal disease (16). A discussion of the relative merits of chemotherapy alone or a CM approach requires careful analysis of the drug components and the dose and volume of RT, in addition to the sequence of treatment.

In a series of randomized trials conducted at Stanford from 1974 to 1980, patients with Stage IIIB disease received alternating chemotherapy (MOPP or PAVe for six cycles) and TLI in order to optimize the doses of both (1). The actuarial results at 10 years, 70% FFP and 75% survival, are very similar to the best chemotherapy data and apparently superior to the NCI MOPP results. In a subsequent study, patients with extensive splenic Stage IIIA, IIIB, and IV HD were randomly assigned to chemotherapy (MOPP/ABVD) or PAVe/TLI (17). While the patient numbers in each arm are relatively small, the 5-year actuarial results are identical—76% FFP in both arms. The RT used in these trials was a standard 4000 cGy.

A lower dose of RT (2000 cGy) has been used by the Yale group as a consolidation to chemotherapy with very successful results (44). This principle has been employed in sequential randomized trials performed by ECOG (38,45). A total of 1476 patients with Stage IIIB and IV HD received six cycles of MOPP-bleomycin and were then randomized to either low-dose RT (1500 to 2000 cGy) or ABVD. At 7 years, the freedom from progression (62% vs. 45%, $p = 0.07$) and overall survival (87% vs. 65%, $p = 0.05$) favored ABVD over RT consolidation. The more recent trial described above did not show a benefit to low-dose RT when used as a consolidation to BCVPP. These results suggest that the dose and sequence of RT may be important in the CM treatment of advanced-stage HD, but the usual cautions regarding the comparisons between institutions and across treatment arms must be exercised.

Intensity of chemotherapy, including rate of drug delivery and total amount of drug, is also a consideration in the interpretation of treatment results. Carde et al showed the importance of delivering optimal doses of MOPP according to schedule in the treatment of patients who relapsed following radiotherapy (46), a principle which is also supported by the findings of others in the initial management of advanced-stage disease (47,48). The concept of intensity of therapy, as related to both drugs and RT, provides the rationale for the use of marrow-ablative chemotherapy and radiotherapy in combination with bone marrow transplantation (BMT) for refractory or recurrent Hodgkin's disease, as discussed below. Hematopoietic growth factors are currently used to optimize treatment and allow further intensification of therapy for selected high-risk patients in the future.

Treatment of Relapses

One of the features that makes interpretation of the efficacy of primary therapy in early-stage HD difficult is the ability of chemotherapy to salvage RT failures. Following relapse after primary radiotherapy, Portlock et al reported that MOPP can effectively salvage about half of the patients, with the 2-year freedom from further progression being 73% for nodal relapse, 40% for nonmarrow extranodal relapse, and 20% for marrow relapse (although almost all patients with marrow relapse eventually progressed) (49). Perhaps due to the lesser bulk of disease present, it appears that salvage chemotherapy is more effective than primary therapy (50). The ability to salvage the relapses explains the similarity in survival of patients who received widely disparate primary therapy and emphasizes the need for careful follow-up examinations. However, patients with less favorable prognoses after failure of RT, particularly those who fail in multiple sites and are symptomatic at relapse, can be identified (51).

The situation in advanced-stage disease is quite different. Despite the fact that ABVD can produce complete remissions in almost 60% of patients with recurrent disease after MOPP, only about 20% have durable control of their disease (17). The experience of others using ABVD or alternative second-line regimens indicates that fewer than 25% of patients will be cured by salvage therapy (52). These data have led to the use of intensive cytoreductive therapy followed by BMT in high-risk HD.

Jagannath et al reported on a relatively large experience of 61 patients receiving intensive chemotherapy—CBV (*c*yclophosphamide, *B*CNU, *V*P-16) followed by autologous bone marrow transplantation (ABMT) in patients failing two or more combination chemotherapy regimens (53). With a minimum follow-up of 2 years, 38% were alive, free of disease. Adverse risk factors for survival included failure of more than two chemotherapy regimens and a poor performance status. Additional data from University College in London and the University of Nebraska indicate that results of high-dose therapy depend on the extent of prior therapy and that longterm follow-up will be necessary for proper interpretation of results (54,55).

The NCI group updated their results on retreatment with MOPP, demonstrating the importance of the duration of initial remission on complete remission rate and disease-free survival (56). The Italian group has also reported that duration of remission to primary chemotherapy is a key variable to the success of salvage therapy. Their data suggest that a significant subset of patients who relapse after 1 year enjoy long remissions and, perhaps, cures with secondary chemotherapy (57). A recent series from Vancouver confirms these results (58). Thus, the role and timing of high-dose therapy and ABMT should be considered in the context of the result of primary chemotherapy. Adequate follow-up of published and ongoing studies and randomized trials are necessary to better define optimal treatment of relapses.

Very few studies have evaluated the role of radiotherapy in salvaging chemotherapy failures, but two recent series have suggested that highly selected patients, who initially responded to chemotherapy with a remission duration > 12 months and relapsed in nodal sites only, may have a cure rate as high as 50% (59,60).

Trends and Future Directions

Before leaving the discussion of treatment results for HD, it is worth noting overall trends in outcome over various periods of time. Figure 19–1 shows the results of the four major study periods from Stanford. There is a trend toward improvement in freedom from relapse from the early 1960s to the late 1970s. Survival, on the other hand, improved from the first to the second time period but appears to have stabilized. Favorable, early-stage HD is highly curable, such that attention should be directed at reducing or preventing the complications of treatment, as will be elaborated below. The data suggest that some improvements have been made in the treatment of advanced-stage disease, but further refinement of treatment—increased efficacy for selected subgroups and lower morbidity for others—is needed. The proper role of intensified treatment with growth factors or BMT requires definition. With each of these, it is important that treatments are properly conducted and methodically analyzed, with careful attention given to adequate statistical power and length of follow-up. The latter is particularly important, given the long natural history of the disease.

NON-HODGKIN'S LYMPHOMA

Non-Hodgkin's lymphomas are far more heterogeneous than HD. They have been subdivided into three categories based on morphology according to the Working Formulation for Clinical Usage (61). The categories define the survival characteristics of these lymphomas according to therapy prior to 1975, which, by definition, is not current. The low-grade lymphomas are usually disseminated at presentation, have a relatively long natural history, and are not readily curable. The low-grade lymphomas comprise small lymphocytic (morphologically consistent with CLL), follicular, small cleaved-cell lymphomas or follicular, mixed large and small cleaved-cell lymphomas. Intermediate-grade lymphomas include follicular, large-cell lymphoma and the diffuse small cleaved, mixed, or large-cell lymphomas. This group, in general, has a plateau on the disease-free survival curve of about 40 to 60% and is, therefore, felt to be curable with aggressive therapy. The three high-grade lymphomas are large-cell immunoblastic, lymphoblastic, and small noncleaved-cell lymphomas. Current treatment regimens have produced promising cure rates in these rapidly proliferating subtypes. It should be noted that some of the newer immunohistochemical and molecular techniques have allowed investigators to study the cell of origin (B or T cell), determine clonality, and identify molecular markers, such as bcl-2, that may ultimately give clinicians a better understanding of the etiology, natural history, and appropriate treatment of the non-Hodgkin's lymphomas.

Low-Grade Lymphomas

Longterm, disease-free status has been obtained in some patients with limited disease.

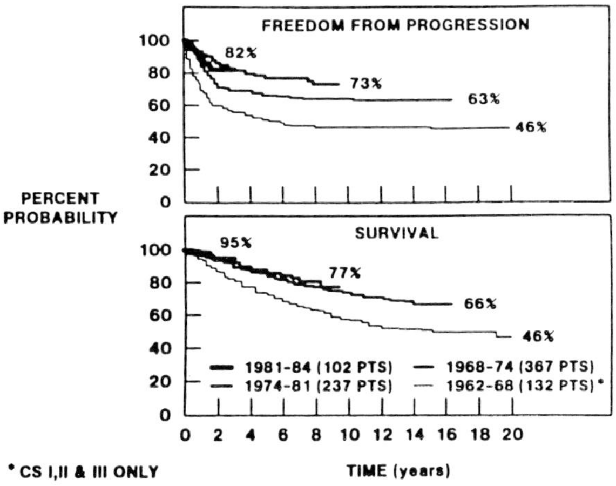

Fig. 19–1. Overview of treatment results over time, from the Stanford Hodgkin's Disease Trials (1). (From Int J Radiat Oncol Biol Phys 11:5, 1985.)

Paryani et al (62) reviewed the Stanford patients with Stage I or II disease at a follow-up of 17 years and found that radiotherapy produced an FFP curve that appeared to flatten at approximately 50%. For patients under 40 years of age, the FFP and survival curves reached a plateau at over 80%. In a small subset of laparotomy-staged patients who were part of a randomized trial, there was no difference between treatment with IF/RT and TLI. Thus, for early-stage low-grade lymphomas, radiotherapy appears to be the treatment of choice; there are insufficient data on which to base field size. However, these patients may, indeed, have a favorable natural history; therefore, the impact of treatment cannot be stated with certainty. Given new aggressive approaches such as high-dose therapy and ABMT, the design of RT fields should consider future options for treatment of relapse.

The treatment of the more advanced stages of the low-grade lymphomas is generally felt to be palliative in nature, as most patients will eventually relapse. Selected patients with Stage III disease may benefit from therapy with curative intent, however. Paryani et al (63) from Stanford reported on treatment results for patients with Stage III follicular lymphoma who received total lymphoid irradiation (4000-cGy dose) or whole body irradiation (150 cGy) followed by a boost of 2000 to 3000 cGy to involved lymph nodes sites. A small subset of 16 patients randomly received no further treatment or CVP (*c*yclophosphamide, *v*incristine, and *p*rednisone) following TLI. There was no benefit from chemotherapy in this study. Since the freedom-from-relapse curve had a plateau after 10 years, the authors concluded that TLI may be curative in some patients with Stage III nodular lymphoma, particularly for a favorable subgroup. This subgroup had fewer than five sites of involvement, as defined by the Ann Arbor staging system (4), and had no areas of disease larger than 10 cm in diameter. The favorable group had an 88% FFP, and the remaining patients had a 32% FFP at 15 years ($p = 0.05$). The favorable group also had a 10-year survival advantage (100% vs. 30%, $p = 0.02$). It must be emphasized that the favorable group makes up a small subset of Stage III patients, and it is possible that the excellent results are merely due to selecting the most favorable patients. However, as is the case with Stages I and II, radiotherapy may indeed be curing patients. McLaughlin et al have combined TLI with CHOP (cyclophosphamide, doxorubicin, vincristine, prednisone) chemotherapy for Stage III patients (64). They report a 43% FFP at 5 years and suggest that some patients may be cured. There are insufficient numbers of these lower-stage patients available to answer the question of curability in a single-institution randomized trial, especially with the long follow-up that would be required. The designation of cure is further compounded in the low-grade lymphomas, which are usually without constitutional symptoms, and occult disease in the marrow or abdomen may be undetected for long periods of time.

In considering the results of treatment for the majority of the patients with low-grade lymphomas, i.e. those with Stage IV or unfavorable Stage III, one must take into account the long natural history of this disease. There are many nonrandomized trials that cannot be covered in any detail. Rosenberg presented an overview of low-grade lymphomas (65). Overall, at 10 years, the survival in the Stanford randomized trials was approximately 50% and the FFP was approximately 20%. Due to the indolent nature of the disease and the apparent lack of curability, a number of patients were observed rather than treated when initially seen; treatment was reserved for those who had progressive disease (66). Overall, half of the patients required some therapy by 3 years; the median time to therapy was 16.5 months for the follicular mixed histology, 48 months for the follicular, small cleaved subtype, and 72 months for the patients with the diffuse, small lymphocytic type. Further confounding the assessment of the effect of treatment in the low-grade lymphomas was the observation of spontaneous regression, which occurred in about 25% of the patients (66).

Varied treatment plans have been tested in the low-grade lymphomas. The Stanford group conducted randomized trials, which included CVP chemotherapy alone, CVP plus TLI, and whole body irradiation plus boost (as described above) (65), and single-agent chemotherapy. Although the number of patients on these studies was small (17 to 40 per arm), there was no difference in FFP and survival among the various treatment groups. Although one-third of the patients had not progressed at 10 years, there was a continual downward trend in the freedom-from-relapse curve, suggesting a lack of curability. About half of the patients remained alive at 10 years.

The use of more aggressive combinations of drugs has also been tried. Longo and coworkers, from the NCI (67), reported on the results of treatment using a number of regimens including CVP, C-MOPP (*c*yclophosphamide, nitrogen *m*ustard, *v*incristine (*O*ncovin), *p*rocarbazine, and *p*rednisone), and various other regimens, some of which included doxorubicin. As seen in almost all studies, the complete remission rate was high (approximately 75%). The authors noted that patients with the nodular mixed histology (follicular, mixed in the Working Formulation) (61) had a suggestion of a plateau on the relapse-free survival curve; such a plateau was not observed for follicular, small cleaved-cell lymphoma patients. Despite the observation that relapses were seen up to 8 years after diagnosis, the authors concluded that prolonged initial remissions can be obtained in patients with the mixed histology. Glick et al reported on the results of an Eastern Cooperative Oncology Group randomized trial for patients with Stage III or IV follicular mixed lymphoma (68). Fifty-two patients were randomized to one of three drug regimens: CP (*c*yclophosphamide, *p*rednisone), COPP (*c*yclophosphamide, *O*ncovin, *p*rocarbazine, *p*rednisone), or BCVP (BCNU, plus the drugs in CVP). No difference was observed among the groups and, in contrast to the data reported by Longo and co-workers (67), there was no evidence of longterm remission.

The NCI has conducted an interesting trial randomizing patients with Stage III and IV low-grade lymphoma to no initial therapy or an aggressive, immediate-treatment approach with ProMACE-MOPP (*p*rednisone, *m*ethotrexate, *A*driamycin, *c*yclophosphamide, *E*toposide + MOPP) and low-dose TLI, which has been successfully employed in intermediate-grade lymphomas (69,70). Patients randomized immediately to ProMACE-MOPP/TLI had a higher complete remission rate (76%) compared with those who crossed over from watchful waiting (44%) at a later date. Despite a longer CR duration compared with historical controls, which included patients with bulky tumor or with systemic symptoms necessitating immediate therapy, there is no survival benefit to the more aggressive treatment to date. The outcome of this study will be of particular interest because it may provide evidence that aggressive combination therapy can cure advanced low-grade lymphomas.

The Vancouver group is studying a 12-week chemotherapy program: VACOP-BP (*V*P-16, *A*driamycin, *c*yclophosphamide, *O*ncovin, *p*rednisone, *b*leomycin, cis*p*latinum) and total lymphoid irradiation (71). Preliminary results indicate a high rate of complete response. Investigators at Stanford and the Dana Farber Cancer Center are studying the role of high-dose chemoradiation and ABMT in selected, advanced-stage patients who are in first remission. Nadler and colleagues have published interesting papers that suggest that the ability to purge the autograft of residual lymphoma cells, as detected by molecular analyses, is correlated with early relapse (72,73).

Levy and colleagues have pioneered a series of studies in which tumor-specific (anti-idiotype) antibodies were developed and used to treat patients with low-grade B-cell lymphomas (74). They have also immunized patients with the tumor-specific, surface immunoglobulin (idiotype) and induced immune responses (75). These novel approaches allow a CM approach in which cytotoxic therapy is preceded by immunotherapy.

At the present time, for Stage III and IV low-grade lymphomas, there is no compelling evidence that any therapy, including deferred therapy, radiotherapy, a wide variety of drug regimens, or CM therapy is superior to any other in terms of cure or survival.

Intermediate-Grade Lymphomas

In the Working Formulation, the intermediate-grade lymphomas include follicular large cell (Rappaport nodular histiocytic lymphoma), the diffuse lymphomas—large-cell (Rappaport diffuse histiocytic), mixed, and small cleaved-cell types. Although diffuse immunoblastic lymphoma is included in the high-grade group, this category has been included with the Rappaport diffuse histiocytic group in most clinical studies. As most of the current treatment regimens include immunoblastic lymphoma with diffuse large cell and studies have indicated no significant difference in progression, it is included with the intermediate-grade histologies. The majority of patients with intermediate-grade lymphomas will have diffuse large-cell lymphoma and, therefore, most of the discussion in this section will relate to patients with this subtype.

There is an extensive literature discussing the treatment of large-cell lymphoma in particular, since there are many different drug regimens. This review will cite a limited number in order to present the general concepts involved in treatment selection. Single institutions have reported superior outcomes with the more aggressive regimens, but definitive randomized trials have failed to confirm them.

Historically, the treatment for Stage I and II disease was radiation therapy. In comparing studies, one must try to account for a number of prognostic factors, such as Stage I vs. II, the presence of an extranodal lesion ("E") (4), the bulk of the disease, the number of involved sites, the presence of constitutional symptoms, and, in some cases, the site of involvement. The results of treatment by the Stanford group, using radiotherapy alone initially or with adjuvant chemotherapy, provide an important historical perspective (76). For the 148 patients with Stage I or II disease in this study, the 5-year freedom from relapse was approximately 45% and survival was 50% (Table 19–3). In addition to the pretreatment prognostic factors

Table 19–3. Treatment of Limited-Stage, Intermediate-Grade Lymphomas

Stage	Number of Patients (N)	Treatment	Freedom From Progression (%) (p)	Survival (%) (p)	Ref.
		ACTUARIAL RESULTS AT 5 YEARS			
Stanford Radiotherapy Series					
I	(57)	Primary RT*	62 (0.0008)	56 (0.13)	76
II	(91)	Primary RT*	38	48	
I, II	(68)	IF/EF	25 (0.0001)	35 (0.0005)	
	(47)	STLI/TLI	67	67	
		ACTUARIAL RESULTS AT 5 YEARS			
Stanford Combined Modality Series					
I	(24)	CT + RT*	81 (0.31)	78 (0.71)	86
II	(70)	CT + RT*	72	70	
		ACTUARIAL RESULTS AT 5 YEARS			
Tucson and Vancouver Studies					
I, II	(142)	Primary CHOP ± RT	81	80	83
I	(61)		~90 (0.16)	~90 (0.003)	
II	(81)		~70	~78	
I, II	(34)	CHOP only	~75 (0.2)	NA	
	(108)	CHOP + RT	~84	NA	
		ACTUARIAL RESULTS AT 5 YEARS			
National Cancer Institute Series					
I	(47)	ProMACE–MOPP + RT	~96	~94	84

*See text for description of treatment.
~ denotes extrapolation from published actuarial curves.
NA = not available.
Abbreviations: RT = radiation therapy; IF = involved field; EF = extended field; STLI = sub-total lymphoid irradiation; TLI = total lymphoid irradiation; CT = chemotherapy; CHOP = cyclophosphamide, hydroxydaunorubicin or doxorubicin, vincristine (Oncovin), prednisone; ProMACE = prednisone, methotrexate, Adriamycin, cyclophosphamide, etoposide; MOPP = nitrogen mustard, vincristine (Oncovin), procarbazine, prednisone; NA = not available.

(stage, bulk, number of sites and presence of extranodal disease), the extent of RT was also quite important. The 5-year FFP was 25% for involved-field/extended-field RT (to only one side of the diaphragm) was 67% for STLI/TLI, and 65% for radiation therapy (any extent) with adjuvant chemotherapy following RT. The level of significance for the difference was p = 0.001 between the IF/EF and STLI/TLI groups and p = 0.0006 between the IF/EF and RT plus chemotherapy groups. These significant differences persisted even after removing early relapses from analysis. Patients could be retrospectively grouped into a favorable subset, with < 3 sites of involvement and bulk < 10 cm, and into an unfavorable subset, which lacked one or both of these factors. Omitting patients that had limited radiation alone, the favorable group had a 5-year freedom from relapse of 85% compared to 55% for the unfavorable group. Obviously, there is potential bias in the retrospective definition of prognostic groups. However, in comparing the results of primary RT with primary chemotherapy, one must consider the pretreatment composition of the group and the extent of RT, particularly if RT was the only initial treatment. Of interest is a subset of patients included in this retrospective analysis who were participants in a randomized study that demonstrated no benefit to adjuvant chemotherapy following TLI; however, the patient numbers are small and the sequence of therapy and drug combination were not optimal.

Monfardini and co-workers, from Milan (77), reported on a randomized trial of patients with Stage I and II, diffuse or nodular non-Hodgkin's lymphomas, in which 96 patients were evaluable. RT was administered to sites on one side of the diaphragm followed by no further treatment or six cycles of CVP. For patients with diffuse lymphomas, there was an advantage to the CM therapy at 5 years in freedom from relapse (76% vs. 45%, p = 0.007) with a borderline survival advantage of 80% vs. 52%, p = 0.09). As noted above, the radiation as given in this study was inferior to more extensive irradiation, probably accounting for some of the advantage conferred by the CVP chemotherapy.

Two small series have described excellent results in treating selected, laparotomy-staged Stage I or II large-cell lymphoma patients with primary RT (78,79). Levitt et al (78), from the University of Minnesota, administered radiation to contiguous, uninvolved transdiaphragmatic sites, as did Vokes et al (79), from the University of Chicago. All 10 patients in the Levitt series were free of disease. In the University of Chicago report, the FFP was 94% for Stage I patients and 56% for those with Stage II disease.

Miller and Jones were the first to report on the primary treatment of patients with localized large-cell lymphoma (Stage I or II) with CHOP [cyclophosphamide, *h*ydroxydaunorubicin or doxorubicin, vincristine (*On*covin), *p*rednisone] chemotherapy (80). They reported on 45 patients who received primary CHOP: 28 received chemotherapy alone, 17 were also given radiotherapy. It must be noted that the radiotherapy was given to those who required a reduction in dose rate of chemotherapy or those who failed to achieve a complete response after three courses of initial chemotherapy. Therefore, it appears that they were a less favorable group. Overall, 44 of 45 patients achieved a CR status, the one failure being in the combined modality group. Five of the 28 chemotherapy-only patients relapsed from CR status, compared to one of 16 given the CM treatment. The 5-year survival was approximately 90% for the CM group and 80% for the chemotherapy-only group. Approximately two-thirds of the patients had Stage II disease, and one-third had bulky disease > 7 cm. Of interest is that the combined modality group did at least as well as the chemotherapy-only group. Since this was a group of patients with either poor tolerance or response to initial chemotherapy, one might infer that radiation added to the efficacy of the chemotherapy. Cabanillas et al also reported that primary chemotherapy produced excellent results with Stage I patients (5-year freedom from relapse 100%), while Stage II patients had a 5-year survival of 75% with a FFP of 66% (81).

Connors et al reported on a series of 78 patients with favorable, limited-stage diffuse large-cell or mixed lymphoma who received brief chemotherapy (three cycles of CHOP) and involved-field irradiation (82). All patients had nonbulky tumor (< 10 cm) and no constitutional symptoms. The FFP was 83% in this group at 4 years, with a median follow-up of 30 months. Clinical data from Vancouver and the University of Arizona have been combined to allow analysis of prognostic features (83). The 5-year FFP in 142 patients was 82%; survival at 5 years was 80%. Only stage of disease (I vs. II) emerged as a prognostic indicator of FFP. It is important to keep in mind that there were differences in the two patient populations. All Vancouver patients received CM therapy; symptomatic patients and those with bulky disease were excluded. In Tucson, as described above, treatment was individualized. These factors make it impossible to definitively address any potential advantage of combined therapy over chemotherapy alone in this two-center analysis. However, there was a higher relapse-free survival among the 108 combined therapy patients compared to the 34 chemotherapy-only patients, but this was not statistically significant (86% vs. 76%, p = 0.2, at 5 years).

The optimal drug combination and whether more intensive regimens should be used in selected clinical settings are yet unanswered questions in the management of limited-stage intermediate-grade lymphomas. Longo et al have reported 96% FFP (median follow-up 42 months) in 47 CS/I and IE patients with diffuse, aggressive lymphoma who received four cycles of ProMACE-MOPP chemotherapy followed by 4000 cGy IF/RT (84). Bulky disease (> 10 cm) was present in two patients, constitutional symptoms in one patient, and elevated lactic dehydrogenase (LDH) in three patients. These adverse prognostic features highly correlate with stage and help to explain the findings in the previous study, in which Stage I vs. Stage II was the only independently significant variable. These results are not superior to those in patients treated with CHOP alone or with IF/RT in CS I (described above).

Mauch et al (85) reported on the retrospective analysis of treatment with patients with the diffuse lymphomas (histiocytic and undifferentiated, the latter being included in the high-grade category of the Working Formulation) (61). He considered minimal disease to be that involving no more than two contiguous disease sites with bulk < 10 cm. In both the minimal and extensive disease groups, the addition of RT to chemotherapy, which included BACOP, CHOP, CMOPP, COPP, CVP, or M-BACOD (see below for regimens) enhanced freedom from relapse and survival. Most patients received RT to one side of the diaphragm. For minimal disease, the 4-year freedom from relapse was 81% for the CM group and 52% for the radiation group (p = 0.03). For extensive disease, the CM group had far superior FFP (40% vs. 9%, p = 0.001). A statistically significant survival advantage was present as well for both groups. As noted above (76), more extensive radiation therapy would probably have improved the result of the radiation-alone group (76).

The Stanford group published their combined modality results in limited-stage diffuse large-cell lymphoma (86). Patients were treated with Adriamycin-containing chemotherapy and involved-field irradiation in one of three sequences: C-RT-C, C-RT, or RT-C. The "sandwich" approach was associated with better overall results in this retrospective, nonrandomized report. Overall, with a median follow-up of 33 months, the 72% FFP and 74% survival at 5 years were superior to the historical results employing RT alone as discussed above. Large tumor bulk and elevated lactic dehydrogenase were found to be negative prognostic factors in multivariate analysis.

In summary, for Stage I and II intermediate-grade lymphomas, primary chemotherapy has proven to be the optimal initial therapy for most patients. For selected patients, especially those unable to tolerate chemotherapy, primary radiotherapy may be adequate. The use of radiation following full-dose, primary chemotherapy may be advantageous for selected patients and has allowed the use of abbreviated chemotherapy. The role of consolidative RT is currently being addressed in large multi-institutional randomized trials. It is probable, as in HD, that the thrust of future efforts will be to minimize the toxicity of therapy for favorable CS I and to address the question of optimal, intensive therapy for unfavorable Stage II disease, which is often combined in clinical trials with advanced-stage disease (as discussed below).

There are a number of chemotherapy regimens available for treatment of the intermediate-grade lymphomas. The early regimens have been considered to be less intensive than some of the newer ones. Early combinations included CHOP, C-MOPP, BACOP (bleomycin and the drugs in CHOP but in a more continuous schedule), and COMLA [*c*yclophosphamide, *O*ncovin, *m*ethotrexate with *l*eucovorin, cytosine *a*rabinoside] (87). The complete remission rates for these regimens were 40 to 55%; 37 to 48% of the treated patients were in longterm remission. Regimens introduced in the last 15 years include the same drugs in varied doses and schedules, with the addition of antimetabolites and the effective single agent, etoposide. These include ProMACE-MOPP [discussed above], ProMACE-CytaBOM [includes cytarabine] (88), M-BACOD/m-BACOD [methotrexate in high or moderate dose with leucovorin rescue and bleomycin] (89); COP-BLAM [similar drugs to M-BACOD plus procarbazine, alternate scheduling] (90); and MACOP-B [unique, weekly scheduling for 12 weeks; same drugs as M-BA COD] (91). The complete remission rate using these regimens is in the range of 70 to 80%; about 60 to 70% of the treated patients remained disease free.

A large-scale, randomized comparative study has been conducted to determine whether these newer regimens are superior to the earlier ones (92). Patients with bulky Stage II, III, and IV intermediate- or high-grade lymphoma were randomized to receive CHOP, M-BACOD, MACOP-B, or Pro-MACE-CytaBOM. At 4 years, with 1138 patients entered, the FFP figures were not significantly different (34 to 45%) and survival also was not different. These results indicate that new strategies are indicated for these patients. The Milan group introduced high-dose sequential chemoradiation with stem-cell transplant and, in a randomized trial, the preliminary results are superior to MACOP-B (93). Other groups have used consolidative ABMT in high-risk patients (94,95). An international study was conducted recently to address a major concern for a uniform definition of high-risk patients (96).

The role of the addition of radiation therapy to combination chemotherapy has not been addressed in high-risk disease. The use of consolidative radiotherapy in advanced-stage disease is complicated by the fact that relapses do not necessarily occur in previously bulky sites (97). Furthermore, residual masses frequently contain no viable tumor (98). While radiation therapy may be useful for patients who do not have a complete response in a site suitable for irradiation, and possibly for bulky disease, this remains to be proven.

High-Grade Lymphomas

For the sake of completeness, the two remaining high-grade lymphomas will be briefly discussed. Coleman et al have reported the results of two sequential studies of lymphoblastic lymphoma in a total of 44 patients (99). The studies involved intensive regimens, including multi-agent chemotherapy and CNS prophylaxis with cranial irradiation and intrathecal methotrexate, modeled after those used successfully for patients with acute lymphoblastic leukemia. Overall, about half of the patients were cured of this once uniformly fatal disease (99,100). The authors defined a favorable group, which included patients with Ann Arbor Stages I to III or Stage IV with nonmarrow, non-CNS disease and with serum LDH < 1.5 times the normal level. Almost all of the patients in the latter Stage IV subset had a cytologically positive pleural effusion. The freedom from relapse for the favorable group of 19 patients was in excess of 90%. The remaining 25 patients had advanced disease and, depending on the definition of lymphoma vs. leukemia, many investigators would have considered this group to have acute lymphoblastic leukemia. The cure rate for this group was 20%, using the regimens reported by Coleman et al, implying that more aggressive therapy, possibly including BMT, might be part of the planned primary therapy. These studies are currently in progress.

There is a paucity of data available for the treatment of adults with diffuse undifferentiated lymphomas. A few patients were included in the M-BACOD study and were not noted to behave differently than those with diffuse histiocytic lymphoma. Bernstein et al (101) reported on the results of treatment from Stanford for 18 adult patients with small noncleaved-cell lymphoma. The staging system used is that for Burkitt's lymphoma, initially described by Ziegler (102). The therapy was an intensive multidrug regimen, including central nervous system prophylaxis. Some of the patients with advanced abdominal disease received twice-daily radiotherapy to a dose of approximately 1500 cGy as part of their induction treatment. All nine patients with the earlier stages were in sustained complete remission. Five of the remaining nine patients died, all had Stage D disease (abdominal plus extra-abdominal); one died of a toxic death during induction and the others expired with progressive disease. Thus, as is the case with lymphoblastic lymphoma, one subset of patients is curable, while a poor-risk subpopulation requires more aggressive treatment. Overall, the actuarial survival and freedom from relapse were approximately 70%. The freedom from relapse was 100% for the patients without Stage D disease and 41% for those with Stage D disease. Therefore, with aggressive treatment, many patients with high-grade lymphomas can be cured. Successful strategies for high tumor burden have yet to be described for adults, but curative treatments for pediatric patients with bone marrow involvement have been reported. Many investigators are treating high-tumor-burden patients in complete remission with ablative therapy plus allogeneic or autologous marrow transplantation.

COMPLICATIONS OF TREATMENT*

With improvements in longterm survival, as a result of the development of successful initial or subsequent therapy, increasing late effects of treatment can be observed. They are important in that considerable efforts should be made to avoid them, but it should be remembered that the curability of the disease cannot be compromised merely to avoid a possible late effect. In some cases, as described in the section on treatments in this chapter, one modality can be used, after which a percentage of patients will have a disease recurrence. The disease can then be treated successfully in a certain proportion of the relapses. Thus, the freedom from relapse of the initial treatment may be significantly lower than the ultimate cure rate. For instance, the choice between an initial approach with CM therapy vs. primary RT with salvage chemotherapy for the relapses in early-stage HD should be made not only on basis of the FFP of the first treatment but also upon the ultimate cure rate and overall morbidity. The same line of reasoning is applicable to a choice between various drug combinations or initial CM versus chemotherapy alone. Integral to decision-making is the success rate of subsequent therapies, some of which (i.e., intensive chemoradiation and BMT) are still under investigation. Thus, the risk of complications and the ultimate cure rate must be considered in decision making.

With the vast array of treatments used in lymphoid malignancies—various chemotherapeutic agents, different drug schedules and duration of therapy, various radiotherapy ports and doses, and numerous permutations of chemotherapy—it is difficult to tabulate all of the toxic interactions. In general terms, there is no organ system that cannot be damaged by a selected chemotherapeutic agent or by a sufficient dose of irradiation. Acute injury or toxicity occurs with a much higher frequency than late toxicity. In general, acute toxicity is not predictive of late toxicity. With the radiation and chemotherapy regimens and doses that are used conventionally in the lymphomas, organs that are infrequently damaged permanently include the skin, central nervous system, liver, kidney, bladder, and gastrointestinal tract. This report will focus on the toxicity to the reproductive, cardiac, and pulmonary systems; on the risk of infection with herpes zoster; and on the development of secondary malignant tumors. This discussion will be limited to patients with HD.

It is known that anthracyclines are toxic to the heart and bleomycin is toxic to the lung. The lung is an extremely radiosensitive organ; permanent lung damage occurs in about 5% of patients given a whole-lung dose in the range of 1500 to 2000 cGy. Likewise, a dose of 4500 cGy can permanently damage the heart in about 5% of patients. The combination of radiation to the heart and doxorubicin administration can lead to an increased risk of cardiac damage (103). **Cardiopulmonary sequelae** of radiation are dependent upon a number of factors, including total dose, fractionation, and technique (anterior and posterior weighting, shielding of lungs, pericardium, and subcarinal region). The methodology of damage assessment and the time elapsed from completion of therapy are also important. A report from Stanford measured static pulmonary function

*For additional material, the reader is referred to Chapter 38 on pediatric toxicity.

and oxygen consumption with maximal exertion, in order to assess subtle abnormalities in function in patients receiving modern mantle RT (104). All patients had normal resting pulmonary function tests. Patients receiving a large mantle field for extensive mediastinal disease, followed by MOPP or PAVe, had a peak oxygen consumption 15% below predicted (considered to be borderline low by conventional criteria). Gomez assessed heart size and function after radiation therapy to the mediastinum, finding that the ratio of cardiac to intrathoracic diameter as measured on chest x-ray was decreased in patients with extensive mediastinal disease compared to those with moderate or no mediastinal disease (105). First-pass left ventricular ejection fraction was significantly lower in patients who had received mediastinal irradiation.

Santoro et al reported on a comparison of cardiac and pulmonary function parameters in patients given CM therapy with radiation plus MOPP or ABVD (17). As discussed above, the therapeutic results were superior in the ABVD group. There was no difference in cardiac function, as assessed by left ventricular ejection fraction. Pulmonary function testing was expressed as a reduction from the predicted normal. Despite greater evident decrease in mean values following ABVD, neither vital capacity nor forced expiratory volume was significantly different between the two groups. The dose to the mantle was 3458 cGy in patients treated with MOPP and 3691 cGy in those treated with ABVD. Results of cardiopulmonary sequelae from ongoing trials at Stanford and the EORTC, using different RT techniques and total doses in the mantle irradiation, are awaited with interest.

Gonadal dysfunction has been reported in patients with HD both before and after receiving chemotherapy (106,107). Chapman et al reported that 16 of 37 men (43%) were functionally subfertile before therapy, primarily due to inadequate semen, with adequate defined as 50 million or more sperm per ejaculate with > 40% motility (108). Multi-agent chemotherapy, such as MOPP and MVPP, leads to azoospermia in all males shortly after the initiation of therapy. Recovery of any degree of sperm production is uncommon. The induction of azoospermia is related to the number of cycles of MOPP-like therapy received. DaCunha et al reported recovery of sperm production in seven of seven males (five normospermic, two oligospermic) treated with just two cycles of MOPP and no pelvic irradiation (109). The ABVD regimen has much less gonadal toxicity. Viviani et al compared gonadal function of 25 males given six cycles of ABVD and 31 males given MOPP (110). Azoospermia developed in 97% of males given MOPP and 36% of those given ABVD; an additional 20% of the ABVD-treated patients developed oligospermia. Furthermore, of those studied, only 22% of patients given MOPP recovered, compared to 100% of patients with ABVD. The time to recovery was also more abbreviated with ABVD. Pedrick and Hoppe (111) studied spermatogenesis in 43 males given pelvic irradiation and no chemotherapy. A sperm count above 20 million was considered to be a fertile level. While < 20% of patients were fertile within 18 months of completing treatment, two-thirds were fertile when studied 19 to 26 months post-treatment, and 88% of those > 26 months post-therapy had fertile sperm levels (111).

Horning et al, from Stanford, reported on female reproductive potential following treatment for HD (112). Patients were placed into the chemotherapy group if they had received chemotherapy (MOPP or PAVe) but no pelvic irradiation (they might have received para-aortic irradiation), the TLI group if they received TLI but no chemotherapy, and the TLI plus chemotherapy group if they received both treatments. The probability of regular menses decreased with increasing age, particularly as age 30 approached. The incidence of amenorrhea was similar for chemotherapy without pelvic irradiation or TLI without chemotherapy but was markedly enhanced in women receiving both. Only about 20% of patients in the latter group had regular menses. The probability of regular menses was also found to be related to age by the NCI group, who reported that 80% of women under age 25 continued menstruating after treatment with MOPP chemotherapy (113). As in males, the adverse effects of MOPP-like chemotherapy in females are contingent upon the total dose of the alkylating agent received. Similarly, ABVD chemotherapy has had essentially no permanent adverse effects in females (110). As mentioned previously, the VBM adjuvant tested by the Stanford group was not found to be associated with chronic male or female reproductive toxicity (5).

The data from the prospective studies currently in progress are needed to best understand the effects of HD and its various forms of treatment on gonadal function. Abnormally low sperm counts have been reported prior to treatment (108). Males and females can remain fertile after pelvic irradiation (111,112), but the gonadal dose can vary based on shielding techniques and portal arrangement. Female gonadal failure may take the form of premature menopause; therefore, longterm studies are needed. Offspring of parents treated for HD have been reported to have no increased incidence of birth defects or developmental abnormalities, but these and additional children need to be monitored to determine any risk of malignancy and to evaluate their own fertility (112). The above results indicate that, in general, CM therapy is likely to have more adverse effects than single modality therapy but the nature and duration of the effects will depend on the specifics of the treatments themselves.

Prior to discussing the most serious late effect, that of secondary malignancy, the risk of herpes zoster and varicella (HZ-V) infections will be mentioned. Reboul et al studied the incidence of HZ-V infections in 181 children treated for HD at Stanford (114). The incidence increased according to the treatment received: limited-field RT 2/18 (11.1%), extended-field RT 16/67 (23.8%), and extended-field RT and chemotherapy 19/34 (56%). The incidence increased with the stage of disease, but this may have reflected intensity of treatment. Splenectomy did not influence the incidence of infection.

The most serious late effect seen in longterm survivors of HD is the development of **secondary malignancy.** There have been many reports discussing this late effect, only a few of which will be discussed here. The second malignancies may be conveniently discussed as secondary leukemias, lymphomas, and solid tumors. Alkylating agents have been shown to be leukemogenic in patients treated for a variety of cancers, with the risk directly correlated to total drug exposure (115). In general, secondary leukemia has been associated with MOPP-like chemotherapy for HD, with an increased incidence (but not relative risk) among patients over 40 to 50 years of age at treatment (116). The actuarial risk appears to plateau between 7 and 10 years following treatment (117). The reported actuarial incidence of acute leukemia following MOPP-like chemotherapy has varied from < 2% to > 10% (116–119). Problems in the analysis include the small number of events from a given institution or cooperative group, the heterogeneity of initial or relapse treatment, the variable classification of preleukemia or myelodysplasia, correction for patient age, and method of analysis. The incidence of acute leukemia following therapeutic RT is increased over that of the general population, but the 10-year actuarial risk is < 1% (116,119). Some reports have indicated that CM therapy, particularly when the irradiation is extensive, greatly enhances the incidence of secondary leukemia (120,122). Other factors thought to increase the risk include splenectomy and the total dose of the alkylating agent used (119,123,124). A recent case-control study involving over 26,000 patients concluded that the risk of secondary acute myelogenous leukemia is related to total alkylating agent exposure with a relative risk of 9 compared to primary radiotherapy and no increased risk associated with CM therapy (119). Advanced stage of disease and splenectomy increased the risk twofold. ABVD chemotherapy has not yet been associated with the increased risk of secondary leukemia seen with MOPP (120). A note of caution must be raised by recent reports of acute leukemia after etoposide, particularly when combined with alkylating agents (125,126). Secondary leukemia after etoposide, which has a characteristic cytogenetic abnormality, requires further characterization.

The occurrence of secondary non-Hodgkin's lymphomas in longterm survivors of HD was initially reported by Krikorian et al to be 4.4% (127). Subsequent reports have described a lower incidence with a 15-year actuarial risk of approximately 1% (116). The risk is equal in patients given radiation alone and in those given CM treatment. Secondary lymphoma may be a consequence of the immune defects due to the disease, otherwise related to the development of HD, or due to the oncogenicity of the treatment. Unlike the uniform fatality of treatment-induced leukemias, about half of the secondary lymphomas and secondary solid tumors are curable.

The occurrence of secondary solid tumors following treatment with RT is increasing. In absolute numbers, solid tumors outnumbered leukemias even in the earlier reports. However, these reports indicated that the development of leukemias in irradiated patients exceeded its incidence in the general population. The latency period for solid tumors following radiation is longer than for secondary leukemia, and there is no apparent plateau of risk (Fig. 19–2). Lung cancer is the most common secondary cancer and has occurred in nonsmokers as well as smokers. Gastric cancer, soft-tissue sarcomas, and bone sarcomas have been seen with a greater incidence than expected. One particularly interesting observation by Tucker et al was the pattern of occurrence of malignant melanoma, a malignancy that is not felt to be related to ionizing radiation (128). Tucker noted that the patients who developed melanoma had evidence of the dysplastic nevus syndrome, which predisposes patients to the development of melanomas. The risk of solid tumors appeared higher after adjuvant chemotherapy in the most recent Stanford analysis, but the difference was not significant (116). No significant difference in the risk of secondary tumors was related to the extent of RT. The actuarial risk of secondary cancers from the Stanford series is shown in Figure 19–2. Table 19–4 describes the relative risk of secondary cancers, according to follow-up interval. The increasing relative risk of secondary solid tumors, according to latency period, is demonstrated. The use of chemotherapy does not appear to be critical to the development of secondary solid tumors, although this entire phenomenon may be better understood when more time is available for observation.

CONCLUSIONS AND FUTURE DIRECTIONS

Hodgkin's Disease

Stages I and II, Favorable

Patients with favorable, early-stage HD have a high rate of cure following careful staging, including laparotomy and primary RT. The role of laparotomy and splenectomy will continue to be questioned, and current randomized trials are addressing this issue. For older patients, the relative risks of subdiaphragmatic disease or relapse after primary RT must be balanced against the morbidity of laparotomy and splenectomy. Additional evaluation of cardiopulmonary sequelae from radiotherapy (alone or in combination with chemotherapy) and the risk of lung cancer will certainly have an impact on treatment selection. Insights into carcinogenesis and DNA repair following irradiation and/or chemotherapy from a molecular viewpoint may allow better patient selection. The ongoing development of rela-

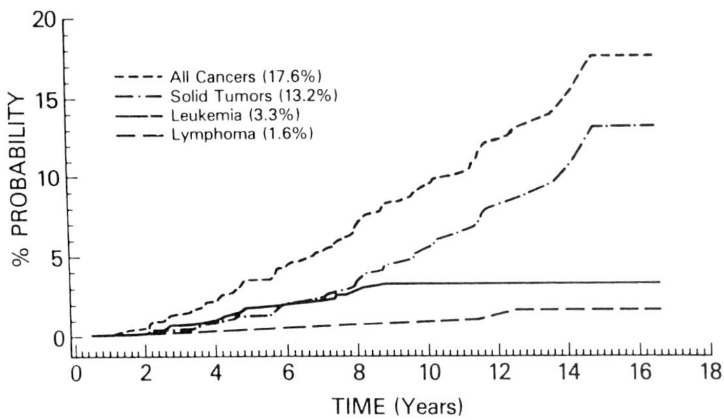

Fig. 19–2. Actuarial risk of second cancers in 1,507 patients with Hodgkin's disease (98). The percentages in parentheses indicate the actuarial risk at 15 years. (From N Engl J Med 318:76, 1988.)

Table 19–4. Relative Risk of Secondary Solid Tumors According to Follow-Up Interval—Stanford Data

	Latency Period (Years of Follow-up)					
	1–4 years (5654):		5–9 years (2789):		10+ years (796):	
Type	No. Observed	Observed/Expected (95% CI)	No. Observed	Observed/Expected (95% CI)	No. Observed	Observed/Expected (95% CI)
ALL	13	1.9 (0.9–2.9)	22	4.9 (2.8–6.7)	11	6.3 (2.9–10.5)
Lung	1	0.9 (0.01–5.2)	7	9.7 (3.3–16.9)	6	21 (7.7–45.9)
Stomach	0		3	24 (4.9–70.9)	1	20 (0.3–112.4)
Melanoma	4	13 (3.4–32.4)	0		0	
Bone	2	44 (4.9–157.8)	0		0	
Connective Tissue	0		1	23 (0.3–128.3)	1	69 (0.9–383.1)

CI = confidence level

tively nontoxic chemotherapy may eventuate in the use of primary chemotherapy for favorable disease. It is clear that the evolution of therapy is dependent upon careful clinical research efforts directed toward both efficacy and toxicity endpoints. Deviation from time-honored, effective treatments must be done with caution.

Stages I and II, Unfavorable

By definition, this subgroup of patients, with apparently early Stage I and II disease, are unfavorable for cure with radiotherapy or chemotherapy alone, usually by virtue of locally extensive disease. The major issue is how to optimally combine these modalities. In general, if chemotherapy is to be used, it precedes radiotherapy, although the precise number of cycles is not yet defined. There is a choice of chemotherapeutic options, and the superior efficacy of one over another in combined therapy is unclear. However, the spectrum of toxicities is very different, in that the results of prospective monitoring of cardiopulmonary and other toxicities in current randomized trials are of great interest. It is important to keep in mind that these results may require a long period of follow-up to evaluate fully. The choice of optimal treatment may be influenced by additional patient characteristics such as family history of cardiovascular disease, smoking history, or serum cholesterol. Similarly, patient variability in drug disposition or tissue-repair mechanisms may eventually influence the choice of therapy.

Stages III and IV

Clinical trials to date have demonstrated that primary chemotherapy is critical to successful treatment in advanced-stage HD. Ongoing clinical trials are attempting to define the optimal combination of drugs and, possibly, the optimal CM approach. Patients with locally extensive disease should generally be considered for the latter. It is probable that in future studies, some patients with advanced stages of the disease will be considered favorable, for whom efforts should be made to reduce toxicity, or unfavorable, for whom more successful therapy would be required. These efforts will be influenced by increased understanding of chronic toxicity and the emergence of new biotechnology.

New biotechnology includes hematopoietic growth factors that allow intensification of many chemotherapeutic agents. Clinical research with these agents holds the promise of improved outcome for poor-risk patients, but the caveats regarding secondary leukemia and other toxic effects discussed above must be heeded. Also, the proper use of BMT must be defined. It is expected that secondary tumors will emerge as a consequence of this therapy, thereby adding to the risk of prior treatment in the overall risk analysis. In contrast to acute leukemias and aggressive lymphomas, recurrence of HD may be more subtle; a longer period of surveillance is required to determine the rate of cure.

Improved understanding of the molecular genetics of secondary malignancy may eventually translate into better patient selection for therapy or management of complications. Most secondary leukemias related to alkylating agents have cytogenetic abnormalities involving chromosomes 5 and 7 (128). A critical region consisting of band 5 q31 (that is uniformly deleted in del [5q]) is often deleted in de novo myelodysplasia and acute myelocytic leukemias. This region has a remarkable cluster of genes, including those for GM-CSF, IL-3, IL-4, IL-5, and CSF-1.

The therapeutic success enjoyed with HD is extraordinary given our relative lack of understanding of etiology or even the characteristics of the neoplastic cell. Increased knowledge of the biology of HD may eventually allow strategies geared toward prevention.

Non-Hodgkin's Lymphoma

Low Grade

There is no obvious curative therapy for patients with advanced or recurrent low-grade lymphoma. Since the disease has a long natural history, aggressive therapies must be cautiously studied. The prognostic features in patients with low-grade lymphoma have received insufficient attention. Patients with a less favorable natural history may be identified and approached with intensive treatment, such as marrow ablative cytoreduction prior to BMT. In this basically radiosensitive disease, which is associated with durable remissions in early stages, marrow transplantation affords an opportunity to deliver more intensive whole body irradiation. As fractionated total body irradiation is given in combination with chemotherapy, which is also very active in low-grade lymphoma, such intensive chemotherapy represents the ultimate combined modality therapy. The application of molecular markers for minimal disease, taking advantage of the 14;18 chromosomal translocation and the polymerase chain reaction to amplify DNA, allows close scrutiny in these neoplasms, which may be otherwise occult (130). Therapeutic use of lymphoma-specific or generic monoclonal antibodies, alone or conjugated with irradiation or toxins, are under active investigation. Current strategies to enhance the efficacy of these approaches include CM therapy with other biologicals, chemotherapy, or irradiation.

Intermediate and High Grade

Half or more of the new cases of the diffuse, aggressive lymphomas are currently curable. The next decade will allow a further appreciation of the sequelae of therapy. Prognostic factors in the intermediate and high-grade lymphomas clearly separate patients into favorable and unfavorable categories. Strategies to offer dose-intensified therapy with growth factors and hematopoietic stem cells are currently under study. Challenges to be faced in the future include effective treatment of the elderly and treatment of the patient who develops lymphoma in the setting of acquired immunodeficiency. Future efforts will be made to understand and perhaps to control growth of these rapidly proliferating neoplasms at the molecular level.

The malignant lymphomas are a fascinating, heterogeneous group of neoplasms that have often served as paradigms for clinical and laboratory research in oncology. Certainly, this has been true in the application of chemoradiation. It is critical to continue to study patients in careful therapeutic trials with sufficient follow-up and proper statistical analyses to assess the endpoints of response, curability, and acute and chronic toxicity as our colleagues conduct further basic research in the lymphomas.

REFERENCES

1. Rosenberg SA, Kaplan HS. The evolution and summary results of the Stanford randomized clinical trials in the management of Hodgkin's disease. 1962–1984. Int J Radiat Oncol Biol Phys 11:5, 1985.
2. DeVita VT, Serpick AA, Carbone PP. Combination chemotherapy in the treatment of advanced Hodgkin's disease. Ann Intern Med 73:881, 1970.
3. Rosenberg SA. Report of the committee on the staging of Hodgkin's disease. Proc Am Assoc Cancer Res 10:19, 1966.
4. Carbone PP, Kaplan HS, Mushoff K, et al. Report of the committee on Hodgkin's disease staging classification. Cancer Res 31:1860, 1971.
5. Horning SJ, Hoppe RT, Hancock SL, et al. Vinblastine, bleomycin, and methotrexate. An effective adjuvant in favorable Hodgkin's disease. J Clin Oncol 12:1822, 1988.
6. Tubiana M, Hayat M, Burgers M, et al. The EORTC treatment of early stages of Hodg-

kin's disease. The role of radiotherapy. Int J Radiat Oncol Biol Phys 10:197, 1984.
7. Glatstein E, Guernsey JM, Rosenberg SA, et al. The value of laparotomy and splenectomy in the staging of Hodgkin's disease. Cancer 24:709, 1969.
8. Carde P, Burgers JMV, Henry-Amar M, et al. Clinical stages I and II Hodgkin's disease. A specifically tailored therapy according to prognostic factors. J Clin Oncol 6:239, 1988.
9. Carde P, Meerwaldt JH, Monconduit M, et al. EORTC controlled trials in clinical stage (CS) I-II Hodgkin's disease (HD): First report on the results of a randomized staging laparotomy (Sx) in favorable cases and of a randomized MOPP versus ABVD with combined radiotherapy (RT) modality in unfavorable cases. (Abstr 985). Proc Am Soc Clin Oncol 9:254, 1990.
10. Bonadonna G. Chemotherapy strategies to improve the control of Hodgkin's disease. The Richard and Linda Rosenthal Foundation Award Lecture. Cancer Res 42:4309, 1982.
11. Levi JA, Wiernik PH, O'Connell MJ. Patterns of relapse in stage I, II and IIA Hodgkin's disease. Influence of initial therapy and implications for the future. Int J Radiat Oncol Biol Phys 2:853, 1977.
12. Mauch P, Goodman R, Hellman S. The significance of mediastinal involvement in early stage Hodgkin's disease. Cancer 42:1039, 1978.
13. Hoppe RT, Coleman CN, Cox RS, et al. The management of stage I-II Hodgkin's disease with irradiation alone or with combined modality therapy. The Stanford experience. Blood 59:455, 1982.
14. Prosnitz LR, Curtis AM, Knowlton AH, et al. Supradiaphragmatic Hodgkin's disease. Significance of large mediastinal masses. Int J Radiat Oncol Biol Phys 6:809, 1980.
15. Mauch P, Hellman S. Supradiaphragmatic Hodgkin's disease. Is there a role for MOPP chemotherapy in patients with bulky mediastinal disease? Int J Radiat Oncol Biol Phys 6:947, 1980.
16. Longo D, Russo A, Duffey P, et al. Treatment of advanced stage massive mediastinal Hodgkin's disease. The case for combined modality treatment. J Clin Oncol 9:227, 1991.
17. Santoro A, Bonadonna G, Valagussa P, et al. Long-term results of combined chemotherapy-radiotherapy approach in Hodgkin's disease. Superiority of ABVD plus radiotherapy versus MOPP plus radiotherapy. J Clin Oncol 5:27, 1987.
18. Hoppe RT, Horning SJ, Hancock SL, et al. Current Stanford clinical trials for Hodgkin's disease. *In:* Recent Results in Cancer Research. Diehl V (Ed). New York, Springer-Verlag, 1989, p. 182.
19. Hoppe RT. The management of stage II Hodgkin's disease with a large mediastinal mass. A prospective program emphasizing irradiation. Int J Radiat Oncol Biol Phys 11:349, 1985.
20. Bloomfield CD, Pajak TF, Glicksman TS, et al. Chemotherapy and combined modality therapy for Hodgkin's disease. A progress report on Cancer and Leukemia Group B studies. Cancer Treat Rep 66:835, 1982.
21. Longo D, Glatstein E, Young R, et al. Radiation therapy versus combination chemotherapy in the treatment of early-stage Hodgkin's disease. Seven-year results of a prospective randomized trial. J Clin Oncol 9:906, 1991.
22. Cimino G, Biti G, Anselmo A, et al. MOPP chemotherapy versus extended-field radiotherapy in the management of pathological stage I-IIA Hodgkin's disease. J Clin Oncol 7:732, 1989.
23. Liebenhaut MH, Hoppe RT, Efron B, et al. Prognostic indicators of laparotomy findings in clinical stage I-II supradiaphragmatic Hodgkin's disease. J Clin Oncol 7:81, 1989.
24. Johnson DW, Hoppe RT, Cox RS, et al. Hodgkin's disease limited to intrathoracic sites. Cancer 52:8, 1983.
25. Desser RK, Golomb HM, Ultmann JE, et al. Prognostic classification of Hodgkin's disease in pathologic stage III, based on anatomic considerations. Blood 4:883, 1977.
26. Stein RS, Hilbarn RM, Flexner JM, et al. Anatomical substages of stage III Hodgkin's disease. Cancer 42:429, 1978.
27. Lister TA, Crowther D, Sutcliffe SB, et al. Report of a committee convened to discuss the evaluation and staging of patients with Hodgkin's disease. Cotswolds meeting. J Clin Oncol 7:1630, 1989.
28. Mauch P, Goffman T, Rosenthal DS, et al. Stage III Hodgkin's disease. Improved survival with combined modality therapy as compared with radiation therapy alone. J Clin Oncol 3:1166, 1985.
29. Hoppe RT. The definitive management of limited and intermediate stages of Hodgkin's disease with radiation therapy alone. *In:* Controversies in the Management of Lymphomas. Bennett JM (Ed). Boston, Martinus Nijhoff Publishers, 1983, p. 129.
30. DeVita VT Jr, Simon RM, Hubbard SM, et al. Curability of advanced Hodgkin's disease with chemotherapy. Ann Intern Med 92:587, 1980.

31. Lister TA, Doree MS, Faux M, et al. The treatment of stage III Hodgkin's disease. J Clin Oncol 1:745, 1983.
32. Crowther D, Wagstaff J, Deakin D, et al. A randomized study comparing chemotherapy alone with chemotherapy followed by radiotherapy in patients with pathologically staged IIIA Hodgkin's disease. J Clin Oncol 2:892, 1984.
33. Longo DL, Young RC, Wesley M, et al. Twenty years of MOPP therapy for Hodgkin's disease. J Clin Oncol 4:1295, 1986.
34. Bakemeier RF, Anderson JR, Costello W, et al. BCVPP chemotherapy for advanced Hodgkin's disease. Evidence for greater duration of complete remission, greater survival, and less toxicity than with a MOPP regimen. Ann Intern Med 104:477, 1984.
35. Dady PJ, McElwain TJ, Austin DE, et al. Five years' experience with ChIVPP. Effective low toxicity combination chemotherapy for Hodgkin's disease. Br J Cancer 45:851, 1982.
36. Bonadonna G, Valgussa P, Santoro A. Alternating non-cross-resistant combination chemotherapy or MOPP in stage IV Hodgkin's disease. A report of 8-year results. Ann Intern Med 104:739, 1986.
37. Canellos GP, Propert K, Cooper R, et al. MOPP vs. ABVD vs. MOPP alternating with advanced ABVD in Hodgkin's disease. A prospective randomized CALGB trial. Proc Am Soc Clin Oncol 7:230, 1988.
38. Glick J, Tsiatis A, Chen M, et al. A randomized ECOG trial of alternating MOPP-ABVD vs. BCVPP vs. BCVPP plus radiotherapy (RT) for advanced Hodgkin's disease (HD). Proc Am Soc Clin Oncol 7:223, 1988.
39. Klimo P, Connors JM. MOPP/ABV hybrid program. Combination chemotherapy based on early introduction of seven effective drugs for advanced Hodgkin's disease. J Clin Oncol 3:1174, 1985.
40. O'Reilly SF, Hoskins P, Klimo P, et al. MACOP-B and VACOP-B in diffuse large cell lymphomas and MOPP/ABV in Hodgkin's disease. Ann Oncol 2:17, 1991.
41. Connors JM, Klimo P, Adams G, et al. MOPP/ABV hybrid versus alternating MOPP/ABV for advanced Hodgkin's disease. Proc Am Soc Clin Oncol (Abstr 1073) 11:317, 1992.
42. Viviani S, Bonadonna G, Santora A, et al. Alternating versus hybrid MOPP-ABVD in Hodgkin's disease. The Milan experience. Ann Oncol 2:55, 1991.
43. Young RC, Canellos GP, Chabner BA, et al. Patterns of relapse in advanced Hodgkin's disease treated with combination chemotherapy. Cancer 42:1001, 1978.
44. Farber JR, Prosnitz LR, Cadman EC, et al. Curative potential of combined modality therapy for advanced Hodgkin's disease. Cancer 46:1509, 1980.
45. Glick JH, Barnes JM, Bakemeier RF, et al. Treatment of advanced Hodgkin's disease. 10-year experience in the Eastern Cooperative Oncology Group. Cancer Treat Rep 66:855, 1982.
46. Carde P, MacKintosh FR, Rosenberg SA. A dose and time response analysis of the treatment of Hodgkin's disease with MOPP chemotherapy. J Clin Oncol 1:146, 1983.
47. DeVita VT Jr, Hubbard SM, Longo DL. The chemotherapy of lymphomas. Looking back moving forward—The Richard and Hinda foundation award lecture. Cancer Res 47:5810, 1987.
48. van Rijswijk R, Haanen C, Dekker AW, et al. Dose intensity of MOPP chemotherapy and survival in Hodgkin's disease. J Clin Oncol 7:1776, 1989.
49. Portlock CS, Rosenberg SA, Glatstein E, et al. Impact of salvage treatment on initial relapses in patients with Hodgkin's disease, stages I-III. Blood 51:825, 1978.
50. Cooper MR, Pajak TF, Gottlieb AJ, et al. The effects of prior radiation therapy and age on the frequency and duration of complete remission among various four-drug treatments for advanced Hodgkin's disease. J Clin Oncol 2:748, 1984.
51. Roach M, Brophy J, Cox R, et al. Prognostic factors for patients relapsing after radiotherapy for early-stage Hodgkin's disease. J Clin Oncol 8:623, 1990.
52. Harker WG, Kushlan P, Rosenberg SA. Combination chemotherapy for advanced Hodgkin's disease after failure of MOPP: ABVD and B-CAVe. Ann Intern Med 101:440, 1981.
53. Jagannath S, Armitage JO, Dicke KA, et al. Prognostic factors for response and survival after high-dose cyclophosphamide, carmustine, and etoposide with autologous bone marrow transplantation for relapsed Hodgkin's disease. J Clin Oncol 7:179, 1989.
54. Gribben D, Linch D, Singer C, et al. A successful treatment of refractory Hodgkin's disease by high-dose combination chemotherapy and autologous bone marrow transplantation. Blood 73:340, 1989.
55. Armitage JO, Bierman PJ, Vose JM. Autologous bone marrow transplantation for patients with relapsed Hodgkin's disease. Am J Med 91:605, 1991.
56. Longo DL, Duffey PL, Young RC, et al. Conventional-dose salvage chemotherapy in patients relapsing with Hodgkin's disease after

combination chemotherapy. The low probability for cure. J Clin Oncol 10:210, 1992.
57. Vivani S, Santoro A, Negretti E, et al. Salvage chemotherapy in Hodgkin's disease. Results in patients relapsing more than twelve months after first complete remission. Ann Oncol 1:123, 1990.
58. Lohri A, Barnett M, Fairey R, et al. Outcome of Hodgkin's disease (HD) relapsing after chemotherapy (CT) induced complete remission (CR) time to first relapse (TTR) is still crucial. Am Soc Clin Oncol 9:257, 1990.
59. Roach M, Kapp DS, Rosenberg SA, et al. Radiotherapy with curative intent. An option in selected patients relapsing after chemotherapy for advanced Hodgkin's disease. J Clin Oncol 5:550, 1987.
60. Mauch P, Tarbell N, Skarin A, et al. Widefield radiation therapy alone or with chemotherapy for Hodgkin's disease in relapse from combination chemotherapy. J Clin Oncol 5:544, 1987.
61. The non-Hodgkin's Lymphoma Pathologic Classification Project. National Cancer Institute sponsored study of classifications of non-Hodgkin's lymphomas. Summary and description of a working formulation for clinical usage. Cancer 49:2112, 1982.
62. Paryani SB, Hoppe RT, Cox RS, et al. Analysis of non-Hodgkin's lymphomas with nodular and favorable histologies, stages I and II. Cancer 52:2300, 1983.
63. Paryani SB, Hoppe RT, Cox RS, et al. The role of radiation therapy in the management of stage III follicular lymphomas. J Clin Oncol 2:841, 1984.
64. McLaughlin P, Fuller LM, Velasquez WS, et al. Stage III follicular lymphoma. Durable remissions with a combined chemotherapy-radiotherapy regimen. J Clin Oncol 5:867, 1987.
65. Rosenberg SA. The low-grade non-Hodgkin's lymphomas. Challenges and opportunities—Karnofsky Memorial Lecture. J Clin Oncol 3:299, 1985.
66. Horning SJ, Rosenberg SA. The natural history of initially untreated low grade non-Hodgkin's lymphomas. N Engl J Med 311:1471, 1984.
67. Longo DL, Young RC, Hubbard SM, et al. Prolonged initial remission in patients with nodular mixed lymphoma. Ann Intern Med 100:651, 1984.
68. Glick JH, Barnes JM, Ezdinli EZ, et al. Nodular mixed lymphoma. Results of a randomized trial failing to confirm prolonged disease-free survival with COPP chemotherapy. Blood 58:920, 1981.
69. Young RC, Longo DL, Glatstein E, et al. Watchful-waiting (WW) vs. aggressive combined modality therapy (Rx) in the treatment of stage III-IV indolent non-Hodgkin's lymphoma. Proc Am Soc Clin Oncol 6:200, 1987.
70. Fisher RI, DeVita VT Jr, Hubbard SM, et al. Diffuse aggressive lymphomas. Increased survival after alternating flexible sequences of ProMACE and MOPP chemotherapy. Ann Intern Med 98:34, 1983.
71. Klasa RJ, Hoskins PJ, O'Reilly SE, et al. BP-VACOP and extensive lymph node irradiation (RT) for advanced stage low grade lymphoma. Proc Am Soc Clin Oncol (Abstr 1117) 11:328, 1992.
72. Freedman E, Rakvorian T, Anderson K, et al. Autologous bone marrow transplantation in B-cell non-Hodgkin's lymphoma. Very low treatment-related mortality in 100 patients in sensitive relapse. J Clin Oncol 8:784, 1990.
73. Gribben JG, Freedman AS, Neuberg D, et al. Immunologic purging of marrow assessed by PCR before autologous bone marrow transplantation for B-cell lymphoma. N Engl J Med 325:1525, 1991.
74. Brown SL, Miller RA, Levy R. Antiidiotype antibody therapy of B-cell lymphoma. Semin Oncol 16:199, 1989.
75. Kwak L, Campbell M, Czerwinski D, et al. Induction of immune responses in patients with B-cell lymphoma against the surface immunoglobin expressed by their own tumors. N Engl J Med (Submitted 1992)
76. Kaminski MS, Coleman CN, Colby TV, et al. Factors predicting for survival in adults with stage I and II large cell lymphoma treated with primary radiation therapy. Ann Intern Med 104:744, 1986.
77. Monfardini S, Banfi A, Bonadonna G, et al. Improved five year survival after combined radiotherapy-chemotherapy for stage I-II non-Hodgkin's lymphoma. Int J Radiat Oncol Biol Phys 6:125, 1980.
78. Levitt SH, Bloomfield CD, Frizzera G, et al. Curative radiotherapy for localized diffuse histiocytic lymphoma. Int J Radiat Oncol Biol Phys 6:115, 1980.
79. Vokes EE, Ultman JE, Golomb JM, et al. Long-term survival of patients with localized diffuse histiocytic lymphoma. J Clin Oncol 3:1309, 1985.
80. Miller TP, Jones SE. Initial chemotherapy for clinically localized lymphomas of unfavorable histology. Blood 62:413, 1983.
81. Cabanillas F, Bodey GP, Freireich EJ. Management with chemotherapy only of stage I and II malignant lymphoma of aggressive histologic types. Cancer 46:2356, 1980.

82. Connors JM, Klimo P, Fairey RN, et al. Brief chemotherapy and involved field radiation therapy for limited-stage histologically aggressive lymphoma. Ann Intern Med 107:25, 1987.
83. Jones SE, Miller TP, Connors JM. Long-term follow-up and analysis for prognostic factors for patients with limited-stage diffuse large-cell lymphoma treated with initial chemotherapy with or without adjuvant radiotherapy. J Clin Oncol 7:1186, 1989.
84. Longo DL, Glatstein E, Duffey PL, et al. Treatment of localized aggressive lymphomas with combination chemotherapy followed by involved-field radiation therapy. J Clin Oncol 7:1295, 1989.
85. Mauch P, Leonard R, Skarin A, et al. Improved survival following combined radiation therapy and chemotherapy for unfavorable prognosis stage I-II non-Hodgkin's lymphomas. J Clin Oncol 3:1301, 1985.
86. Prestidge BR, Horning SJ, Hoppe RT. Combined modality therapy for stage I-II large cell lymphoma. Int J Radiat Oncol Biol Phys 15:633, 1988.
87. Gaynor ER, Ultmann JE, Golomb HM, et al. Treatment of diffuse histiocytic lymphoma (DHL) with COMLA (cyclophosphamide, oncovin, methotrexate, leucovorin, cytosine arabinoside): A 10-year experience in a single institution. J Clin Oncol 3:1596, 1985.
88. Fisher RI, Miller TP, Dana BW, et al. Southwest Oncology Group clinical trials for intermediate-high grade non-Hodgkin's lymphoma. Semin Hematol 24:21, 1987.
89. Canellos GP, Skarin AT, Klatt MM, et al. The m-BACOD combination chemotherapy regimen in the treatment of diffuse large cell lymphoma. Semin Hematol 24:2, 1987.
90. Coleman M, Gerstein G, Topilow A, et al. Advances in chemotherapy for large cell lymphoma. Semin Hematol 24:8, 1987.
91. Klimo P, Connors JM. MACOP-B chemotherapy for the treatment of diffuse large-cell lymphoma. Ann Intern Med 102:596, 1985.
92. Fisher RI, Gaynor E, Dahlberg S, et al. A Phase III comparison of CHOP vs. m-BACOD vs. ProMACE-CytaBOM vs. MACOP-B in patients with intermediate or high-grade non-Hodgkin's lymphoma. Preliminary results of SWOG 8516's (Intergroup 0067). The National High Priority Lymphoma Study. Proc Am Soc Clin Oncol (Abstr 1067)11:315, 1992.
93. Gianni AM, Bregni S, Siena C, et al. Prospective randomized comparison of MACOP-B vs. rhGM-CSF-supported high-dose sequential myeloablative chemoradiotherapy in diffuse large cell lymphomas. Proc Am Soc Clin Oncol (Abstr 951)10:274, 1991.
94. Gulati S, Shank B, Black P, et al. Autologous bone marrow transplantation for patients with poor prognosis lymphoma. J Clin Oncol 6:1303, 1988.
95. Nademanee AP, Schmidt GM, O'Donnell MR, et al. High dose therapy and autologous BMT as a consolidation therapy during first CR in patients with poor-risk aggressive lymphoma. A pilot study. Blood 80:1130, 1992.
96. Shipp MA, Harrington D, Anderson J, et al. Development of a predictive model for aggressive lymphoma. The international NHL prognostic factors project. Proc Am Soc Clin Oncol (Abstr 1089)11:319, 1992.
97. Shipp MA, Klatt MM, Yeap B, et al. Patterns of relapse in large-cell lymphoma patients with bulk disease. Implications for the use of adjuvant radiation therapy. J Clin Oncol 7:613, 1989.
98. Surbane A, Longo DL, DeVita VT Jr, et al. Residual abdominal masses in aggressive non-Hodgkin's lymphoma after combination chemotherapy. Significance and management. J Clin Oncol 6:1832, 1988.
99. Coleman CN, Picozzi VJ Jr, Cox RS, et al. Treatment of lymphoblastic lymphoma in adults. J Clin Oncol 4:1628, 1986.
100. Slater DE, Mertelsmann R, Koziner B, et al. Lymphoblastic lymphoma in adults. J Clin Oncol 4:57, 1986.
101. Bernstein JI, Coleman CN, Strickler JG, et al. Combined modality therapy for adults with small non-cleaved cell lymphoma (Burkitt's and non-Burkitt's types). J Clin Oncol 4:847, 1986.
102. Ziegler JL. Burkitt's lymphoma. N Engl J Med 305:559, 1981.
103. Torti FM, Bristow MR, Howes AE, et al. Reduced cardiotoxicity of doxorubicin delivered on a weekly schedule. Assessment by endomyocardial biopsy. Ann Intern Med 99:745, 1983.
104. Watchie J, Coleman CN, Raffin T, et al. Minimal long-term cardiopulmonary dysfunction following treatment for Hodgkin's disease. Int J Radiat Oncol Biol Phys 13:517, 1987.
105. Gomez GA, Park JJ, Panahon AM, et al. Heart size and function after radiation therapy to the mediastinum in patients with Hodgkin's disease. Cancer Treat Rep 67:1099, 1983.
106. Schilsky RL, Lewis BJ, Sherins RJ, et al. Gonadal dysfunction in patients receiving chemotherapy for cancer. Ann Intern Med 93:109, 1980.
107. Chapman RM. Effect of cytotoxic therapy on

sexuality and gonadal function. Semin Oncol 9:84, 1982.
108. Chapman RM, Sutcliffe SB, Malpas JS. Male gonadal dysfunction in Hodgkin's disease. JAMA 245:1323, 1981.
109. DaCunha MF, Meistrich ML, Fuller LM, et al. Recovery of spermatogenesis after treatment for Hodgkin's disease. Limiting dose of MOPP chemotherapy. J Clin Oncol 2:571, 1984.
110. Viviani S, Santoro A, Ragni G, et al. Gonadal toxicity after combination chemotherapy for Hodgkin's disease. Comparative results of MOPP vs. ABVD. Eur J Cancer Clin Oncol 21:601, 1985.
111. Pedrick TJ, Hoppe RT. Recovery of spermatogenesis following pelvic irradiation for Hodgkin's disease. Int J Radiat Oncol Biol Phys 12:117, 1986.
112. Horning SJ, Hoppe RT, Kaplan HS, et al. Female reproductive potential after treatment for Hodgkin's disease. N Engl J Med 304:1377, 1981.
113. Schilsky RL, Sherins RJ, Hubbard SM, et al. Long term follow-up of ovarian function in women treated with MOPP chemotherapy for Hodgkin's disease. Am J Med 71:552, 1981.
114. Reboul F, Donaldson SS, Kaplan HS. Herpes zoster and varicella infections in children with Hodgkin's disease. Cancer 41:95, 1978.
115. Canellos GP. Therapy-related leukemia. A necessary complication of successful systemic chemotherapy? J Clin Oncol 2:1077, 1984.
116. Tucker MA, Coleman CN, Cox RS, et al. Risk of second cancers after treatment for Hodgkin's disease. N Engl J Med 318:76, 1988.
117. Blayney DW, Longo DL, Young RC. Decreasing risk of leukemia with prolonged follow-up after chemotherapy and radiotherapy for Hodgkin's disease. N Engl J Med 316:710, 1987.
118. Coltman CA, Dixon DO. Second malignancies complicating Hodgkin's disease. A Southwest Oncology Group 10-year follow-up. Cancer Treat Rep 66:1023, 1982.
119. Kaldor JM, Day NE, Clark EA, et al. Leukemia following Hodgkin's disease. N Engl Med 322:7, 1990.
120. Valagussa P, Santoro A, Kenda R, et al. Second malignancies in Hodgkin's disease. A complication of certain forms of treatment. Br Med J 280:216, 1980.
121. Mauch PM, Canellos GP, Rosenthal DS, et al. Reduction of fatal complications from combined modality therapy in Hodgkin's disease. J Clin Oncol 3:501, 1985.
122. Andrieu JM, Ifrah N, Payen C, et al. Increased risk of secondary acute nonlymphocytic leukemia after extended-field radiation therapy combined with MOPP chemotherapy for Hodgkin's disease. J Clin Oncol 8:1148, 1990.
123. van der Velden JW, van Putten WL, Guinee VR, et al. Subsequent development of acute non-lymphocytic leukemia in patients treated for Hodgkin's disease. Int J Cancer 42:252, 1988.
124. van Leeuwen FE, Somers R, Hart AA. Splenectomy in Hodgkin's disease and second leukemias. Lancet 2:210, 1987.
125. Pui C, Behm F, Raimondi S, et al. Secondary acute myeloid leukemia in children treated for acute lymphoid leukemia. N Engl J Med 321:136, 1989.
126. Pederson-Bjergaard J, Daugaard G, Hansen S, et al. Increased risk of myelodysplasia and leukemia following etoposide and cisplatin from germ cell tumors. Proc Am Soc Clin Oncol 10:221, 1991.
127. Krikorian JG, Burke JS, Rosenberg SA, et al. Occurrence of non-Hodgkin's lymphoma after therapy for Hodgkin's disease. A study of 21 patients. N Engl J Med 300:452, 1979.
128. Tucker MA, Misfeldt D, Coleman CN, et al. Cutaneous malignant melanoma after Hodgkin's disease. Ann Intern Med 102:37, 1985.
129. Le Beau MM, Albain KS, Larson RA, et al. Clinical and cytogenetic correlations in 63 patients with therapy-related myelodysplastic syndromes and acute nonlymphocytic leukemia. Further evidence for characteristic abnormalities of chromosomes no. 5 and 7. J Clin Oncol 4:325, 1986.
130. Nagan BO, Jamison N, Cleary ML. Detection of chromosomal translocation t(14;18) within the minor cluster region of *bcl*-2 by polymerase chain reaction and direct genomic sequencing of the enzymatically amplified DNA in follicular lymphomas. Blood 73:1759, 1989.

Chapter 20

BREAST

SEWA S. LEGHA AND MARSHA D. MCNEESE

INTRODUCTION

Breast cancer is the most common malignancy affecting Caucasian women and has been gradually increasing in incidence. In North America, it is estimated that one of every nine women will develop breast cancer during her lifetime. Breast cancer is projected to affect 181,000 women in 1992 and be responsible for approximately 46,300 deaths. The incidence of breast cancer increases with advancing age; the median age at diagnosis is 55 years. Approximately one-third of the women with breast cancer are premenopausal and two-thirds are postmenopausal at the time of diagnosis. The 5-year survival for breast cancer ranges from 70 to 75%; however, the disease recurs beyond 5 years in a substantial number of patients, such that the mortality from breast cancer does not level off until approximately 15 years after diagnosis. Although the exact etiology of breast cancer is unknown, the disease is more common in Caucasian women compared to non-Caucasians. Dietary fat intake is considered to be a potential contributing factor in its etiology although other causative agents, particularly the estrogens, play a key role as shown by the fact that breast cancer can be completely prevented by elimination of ovarian hormones during the prepubertal years. The incidence of breast cancer is higher in nulliparous women; pregnancy at a younger age has a protective effect. Breast cancer also has a familial predilection, with a significant increase in incidence in first-degree relatives of women with breast cancer.

NATURAL HISTORY

The most commonly used staging system categorizes breast cancer into four stages. Stage I includes patients with tumor size of 2 cm or less without involvement of the regional lymph nodes. Patients with a tumor size of > 2 cm to 5 cm and/or those with metastases to the axillary lymph nodes are categorized as Stage II. Stage III includes tumors of > 5 cm in size or those with fixation to the overlying skin or underlying muscles or advanced stages of nodal disease in the axilla with matting of the lymph nodes. Involvement of the supraclavicular lymph nodes, classified under Stage III in the past, is currently grouped as M1 and, therefore, shifted into the Stage IV category, which primarily includes patients with distant metastases.

The survival of patients with breast cancer is clearly related to the stage at diagnosis. When treated with local therapy alone, patients with Stage I have a survival of 70 to 75% at 10 years; those with Stage II are at a high risk of relapse with a disease-free survival of only 25 to 30% at 10 years. Patients with Stage III breast cancer do poorly and have a 5-year survival ranging from 10 to 30%, depending on whether they are operable (Stage III-A) or inoperable (Stage III-B) at the time of diagnosis. Patients with metastatic breast cancer are generally incurable and have a median survival of 2 years although approximately 10 to 15% may live for 5 years after diagnosis.

TREATMENT OF BREAST CANCER

Treatment of breast cancer requires a multidisciplinary approach involving surgery, radiotherapy, and chemotherapy, depending on the stage of the disease. During the past two decades, there has been a conceptual transformation in the approach to the treatment of operable breast cancer, which includes Stages I, II, and III-A. In the past, the standard approach to the treatment of these patients involved radical or modified radical mastectomy, which included total removal of the breast and axillary lymph nodes, usually followed by postoperative radiation therapy. A better understanding of the biology of breast cancer has revealed the systemic nature of the disease, based on the existence of micrometastases in a majority of patients by the time the primary tumor is diagnosed and removed surgically (1). Consequently, radical surgery and radiotherapy are not always justifiable because they do not improve the survival of patients with breast cancer (1). These concepts have evolved into the modern approach to the treatment of breast cancer, which is less radical in terms of local therapy but places more emphasis on systemic therapy directed at the micrometastases. The contemporary role of each modality of treatment in different stages of breast cancer, along with interactions of chemotherapy and radiotherapy, are discussed later in this chapter.

Role of Surgery

For many years, the standard surgical approach to operable breast cancer was radical mastectomy, as popularized by Halstead. This operation required removal of the breast, along with the pectoralis major and minor muscles, and a complete removal of the axillary lymph nodes. For some time, extended radical mastectomy requiring removal of internal mammary lymph nodes was also practiced. However, the lack of improvement in survival of more radically treated patients led to a series of prospective trials comparing radical surgery to less extensive surgery, which produced similar survival regardless of the extent of surgery (2,3). Consequently, the modern concept of conservative surgery in the form of simple mastectomy, or excision of tumor (lumpectomy) combined with breast irradiation, was introduced (2,3). It has been established that complete removal of the primary tumor with negative surgical margins is the basic requirement of surgical therapy of early breast cancer. Additionally, removal of ipsilateral axillary lymph nodes is necessary because of the therapeutic as well as prognostic value. Based on a multitude of recent trials, the concept of the systemic nature of breast cancer has gained solid ground; consequently, breast conservation has become the standard approach to the treatment of early breast cancer. This involves removal of the primary tumor, either by removing a quadrant of the breast or by a segmental resection or "lumpectomy," in which the primary tumor is removed along with a 1-cm margin of surrounding normal tissue. Removal of the axillary lymph nodes, usually through a separate incision, is carried out in order to properly stage the disease as well as to guide the need for adjuvant therapy for the control of micrometastases. Breast conservation is usually possible in patients with a single tumor that is $\leq$ 4 cm in size and has not involved the nipple, the overlying skin, or the structures deeper in the breast (4). Patients treated with lumpectomy require irradiation of the whole breast to control the microscopic residual disease around the primary tumor as well as to control other subclinical foci of cancer, which is based on the frequent multifocal nature of primary breast cancer. Patients with larger tumors or those with small breasts may not be suitable candidates for breast conservation, depending on the tumor size in relation to the breast size, because of the poor cosmetic outcome as a result of removal of a large portion of the breast.

Simple mastectomy with axillary dissection is the treatment of choice for patients with tumors measuring 5 cm or greater or in patients in whom the cosmetic result from lumpectomy would be less than satisfactory. However, most of these patients have Stage III breast cancer, which is best treated initially with chemotherapy followed subsequently by local therapy with surgery and/or irradiation of the breast and regional lymphatics (5). In patients responsive to chemotherapy, surgery may play an important complementary role in elimination of the residual tumor, which is expected to be relatively resistant to chemotherapy. When the primary tumor is unresponsive to chemotherapy, surgery may be the best method of tumor control, if technically feasible, although preoperative radiotherapy is sometimes used to convert patients to resectability and/or make it easier to obtain negative surgical margins. Surgery is rarely used for Stage IV disease, except in circumstances in which recurrence of tumor is limited to the chest wall or regional lymph nodes and the tumor is easily resectable.

Role of Radiotherapy

Although radiation therapy was once used routinely as postoperative therapy, it has recently become obvious that most patients with early breast cancer treated with mastectomy do not benefit from postoperative radiation therapy (6). The primary purpose of postoperative radiotherapy is to control the microscopic residual tumor and eliminate the risk of local recurrence following mastectomy. Once the prognostic factors predicting local recurrences were elucidated, it became clear that most patients with Stage I and II breast cancer treated with total mastectomy did not need radiotherapy because of the low risk (5 to 10%) of chest wall recurrence. Since the incidence of local or locoregional recurrences is significantly higher for tumors that are larger than 5 cm (T3 or T4), as well as in patients with four or more axillary lymph node metastases, such patients are prime candidates for postoperative radiation therapy, which has been shown to reduce the risk of locoregional recurrence from 20 to 30% to 5 to 10% (7,8). Adjuvant chemotherapy, although useful in reducing the risk of local and systemic relapse, has not been sufficiently effective in preventing locoregional relapses. Therefore, high-risk patients should be given the benefit of locoregional radiotherapy (9,10). This is well illustrated in a retrospective analysis of patients treated at the M.D. Anderson Cancer Center from 1971 to 1982, in which the incidence of locoregional recurrence was reduced to 10% by postoperative radiotherapy alone and to 12% by adjuvant chemotherapy. But the best results were obtained in patients who received both modalities of treatment; their recurrence rate was reduced to 5% (10).

During the past decade, the predominant role of radiation therapy has shifted from postoperative usage to one of primary radiation therapy to the breast following lumpectomy; it has thus become an integral component of breast conservation therapy (4). Patients undergoing lumpectomy require whole-breast irradiation in order to prevent local recurrences from residual microscopic tumor. Unless four or more positive nodes are found on axillary dissection, they usually do not require treatment to the regional lymphatics. Without whole-breast radiotherapy, these patients have a 5-year relapse rate of 25 to 30% (37% at 8 years) in the breast; with radiotherapy this relapse rate is reduced to 8 to 10% (3). The risk of relapse does increase with longer follow-up and may be as high as 15 to 20% at 10 years after lumpectomy (11). The occurrence of relapse in the irradiated breast should be treated with salvage mastectomy, which can control the disease in 50 to 60% of patients and therefore does not have the same connotation of bad prognosis as in patients who relapse in the chest wall after a previous mastectomy (12,13).

In patients with locally advanced breast cancer (Stage III-B or IV), including inflammatory carcinoma, who are initially treated with primary chemotherapy, radiation therapy has been used as consolidation therapy (14–18). Although there is no significant difference in the survival based on whether the local therapy, following initial chemotherapy, is radiation therapy or surgery, it is clear that the gross residual tumor cannot be sterilized with standard dose schedules (5000 to 6500 cGy) of radiation therapy in a majority of the patients (16). On the other hand, when treated with surgery alone, such patients have a high risk of chest wall recurrence and should be treated with postoperative radiation therapy to reduce the risk of local relapse (15). Overall, the risk of local recurrence is in excess of 30% following either surgery or radiotherapy alone; the sequential use of both modalities lowers the risk to less than 15% (15). In more recent trials, a proportion of patients with Stage III breast cancer who have achieved a good response to induction chemotherapy have subsequently undergone lumpectomy and whole-breast irradiation and have been able to avoid mastectomy by virtue of an effective downstaging of their disease (19).

Radiotherapy is also indicated in patients previously treated with mastectomy who later relapse with local or regional disease, if it can be excised, and the patient is otherwise free from distant metastases. Since these patients are at high risk for systemic relapse, they should also receive adjuvant systemic therapy (20). For patients with metastatic breast cancer, radiotherapy has a limited but important palliative role, largely for the treatment of brain or spinal cord metastases, which are usually not responsive to chemotherapy or endocrine therapy. Radiotherapy is also useful for pain relief from bone metastases, not responding to systemic therapy, and for prevention of pathologic fractures in weight-bearing bones when involved by lytic bone metastases.

Role of Systemic Therapy

Systemic therapy consisting of chemotherapeutic agents and endocrine therapy plays an important role in the treatment of metastatic breast cancer. The anticancer drugs active against breast cancer include cyclophosphamide (C), methotrexate (M), 5-fluorouracil (F), Adriamycin (A), vinblastine, mitoxantrone, and mitomycin-C. Combinations of three drugs, such as CMF and FAC, are effective in inducing objective response in 60 to 70% of patients with metastatic disease. Although a majority of responses are partial, complete response is achievable in 15 to 20% of patients. Complete responses last longer and are sometimes quite durable. The average duration of response varies from 9 to 12 months; nearly all patients ultimately fail and require backup chemotherapy, which usually consists of vinblastine and mitomycin-C alone or in combination. Patients with extensive disease and those with visceral metastases involving liver or brain are best treated with combination chemotherapy initially.

Hormonal therapy plays an important palliative role and is generally used before chemotherapy if the tumor burden is small and the metastases are limited to bone, soft tissues, or lungs. Although patients with estrogen and progesterone receptor positive tumors are commonly treated with hormonal therapy, only 50% respond to endocrine therapy. Chemotherapy is equally effective, regardless of the hormone-receptor status of the tumor. Although in the past hormonal therapy consisted of ablation of endocrine glands in the form of oophorectomy, adrenalectomy, and hypophysectomy, modern endocrine therapy is largely medical in nature, making use of a variety of drugs. Tamoxifen is commonly used as the first choice, and progestational agents such as megestrol acetate (megace) or medroxyprogesterone acetate are used as secondary choice; both choices are equally effective and can be used in the reverse sequence. Aminoglutethimide is another alternative that is frequently useful in patients who have previously responded to tamoxifen and/or megace.

Adjuvant Therapy

Although chemotherapy and endocrine therapy were once commonly used as palliative treatments for metastatic disease, the past two decades have witnessed an important shift in the use of chemotherapy and hormonal therapy as adjuvant treatments for early stages of breast cancer (21–24). Accordingly, systemic therapy is an important component of management of patients with primary breast cancer (Stages II and III) because of the high probability of relapse when local therapy is used alone. Adjuvant chemotherapy has been particularly useful in increasing the survival of premenopausal women with axillary lymph node metastases, with a lesser degree of benefit in postmenopausal women (21–23). In postmenopausal women, adjuvant therapy with tamoxifen has resulted in a significant increase in the disease-free and overall survival, and it has become a standard component of treatment for nearly all women with Stage II breast cancer (24–26).

Since the risk of relapse for women with Stage I breast cancer is low (< 30%), adjuvant therapy is not routinely used for these patients. However, subsets of patients with Stage I breast cancer who are at high risk of relapse have recently been treated with adjuvant chemotherapy or hormonal therapy with a demonstrated reduction in the rate of recurrence and death (27–29). For estrogen-receptor positive tumors, adjuvant therapy with tamoxifen has proven useful both in premenopausal and postmenopausal women (29). Patients with hormone-receptor negative tumors experienced a significant increase in disease-free survival when treated with combination chemotherapy (CMF or

MF) for 6 to 9 months (27,29). Although there is no significant increase in survival of patients with Stage I breast cancer treated with adjuvant therapy, longer follow-up is needed to determine the overall impact of adjuvant treatment in this group of patients.

MULTIMODAL THERAPY FOR LOCALLY ADVANCED BREAST CANCER

Although 80 to 85% of patients with breast cancer in the United States have Stage I or II disease at the time of diagnosis, the remaining patients present with locally advanced disease or with metastatic disease (Stage IV) at the time of diagnosis. Locally advanced breast cancer includes a heterogeneous group of patients in whom the disease is characterized by extensive primary or nodal disease in the absence of demonstrable distant metastases. Some of these patients have large primary tumors, which are operable (Stage III-A); others present with signs of tumor invasion into the skin or deeper structures ("grave signs") or with spread to the supraclavicular lymph nodes and are clearly inoperable (often categorized as Stage III-B) (30). Patients with inflammatory carcinoma of the breast are also included in the latter group for therapeutic considerations.

During the past two decades, a number of clinical trials have been carried out in an attempt to define the relative role of surgery, radiotherapy, and chemotherapy in the treatment of locally advanced breast cancer (5,14–18). Patients with Stage III-A have a better prognosis, 5-year survival ranges from 30 to 45% when treated with surgery and/or radiotherapy. Patients with Stage III-B do poorly with local therapy alone and have a 5-year survival in the range of 10 to 30% (5). Consequently, systemic therapy was introduced as a component of the management of Stage III-B breast cancer and has been used either as initial or induction therapy or as adjuvant therapy for operable patients (31). Induction chemotherapy using FAC or CMF results in objective response in 80 to 90% of patients after three to four courses of treatment administered over a period of 2 to 4 months. Patients who respond to chemotherapy are subsequently treated with local therapy consisting of either surgery and/or radiation therapy. The results of selected trials in the management of locally advanced breast cancer are summarized in Table 20–1. Although the results of prospectively randomized studies have not shown a significant increase in the survival of patients treated with combined chemotherapy and local therapy (32,33), several recent trials have reported a doubling of survival when compared to historical controls treated with local therapy alone (5,30,36).

Although surgery and radiotherapy appear to be equivalent in their efficacy, surgery is the preferred mode of local therapy because it causes the least amount of delay in resumption of systemic therapy as opposed to radiation therapy, which frequently requires an

Table 20–1. Results of Combined Modality Treatment in Locally Advanced Breast Cancer

Reference	Treatment	Number of Patients	Median Survival (Mo)	5-Yr Survival (%)
Schaake-Konig, et al (32)	RT	45	42	37
	RT+CT	34	45	37
	CT+RT+CT	39	50	35
Valagussa, et al (34)	CT+RT	72	30	20
	CT+RT+CT	126	42	36
	CT+S+CT	79	58	49
Rubens, et al (33)	RT	91	42*	35*
	RT+CT	88	34*	30*
Perloff, et al (35)	CT+RT+CT	44	39	NA
	CT+S+CT	43	39	NA
Hortobagyi, et al (5)	CT+RT/S+CT	174	66	55
Jacquillat, et al (36)	CT+RT	94	60	60
Swain, et al (37)	CT+RT/S+CT	107	50	NA

* Approximate survival determined from graph in the publication.
RT = radiation therapy; S = surgery with mastectomy; CT = chemotherapy; NA = not available.

8 to 10-week interruption of systemic therapy that may be detrimental because of the systemic nature of disease in most cases (16,34). Moreover, radiotherapy has limited efficacy against grossly palpable tumors, which, although responsive, often show incomplete regression and tend to recur locally in a majority of patients after a variable period of time. Because radiotherapy is more effective against microscopic disease, it is most effective in preventing postsurgical locoregional relapse and, therefore, should be considered for nearly all patients with locally advanced breast cancer. However, radiation can be safely delayed and carried out at the conclusion of chemotherapy, particularly in patients who have shown good response to chemotherapy (16,38).

Inflammatory carcinoma of the breast is best managed with a combined modality treatment approach, as outlined above for the treatment of locally advanced breast cancer. When treated with either surgery or radiotherapy alone, the median survival of patients with this disease has ranged from 12 to 18 months, and the 5-year survival ranged from 5 to 10% (39). These results initially led to the abandonment of surgery as a useful therapy more than two decades ago. Radiotherapy alone was used for some time, until it was realized that the disease was nearly always disseminated at the time of diagnosis and local therapy alone would be futile. Accordingly, primary chemotherapy was tested and produced response rates of 60 to 70%, although most patients required additional local therapy to control the residual tumor. Recent results using combined modality approaches to the management of this disease are summarized in Table 20–2. Using induction chemotherapy with FAC or CMF followed by local therapy, several groups have reported substantial improvements in survival ranging from 36-48 months (41–43). These studies have also shown that chemotherapy alone is not capable of eradicating the primary tumor in most patients, leading to the incorporation of local consolidation therapy using radiotherapy and/or surgery.

Our experience at the M.D. Anderson Cancer Center indicates that inflammatory carcinoma of the breast is best managed by utilization of a multimodal approach consisting of initial chemotherapy followed by mastectomy in responding patients. Surgery appears to be more efficient in providing local control, by removing the gross residual tumor, in comparison to radiotherapy, which has been used alone by some investigators (41,44). Radiotherapy, which can be done at the conclusion of chemotherapy, is also necessary for maximizing local control by eradicating the microscopic disease and thus allows locoregional control of disease in 70 to 80% of cases, depending on response to chemotherapy (44). Hence, in the management of inflammatory breast cancer, there is need for all three modalities of treatment as is the case with locally advanced breast cancer (45). A judicious use of all therapies has resulted in a significant improvement in the 5-year survival of patients with inflammatory carcinoma of the breast, which currently ranges from 30 to 40% (40,42–44).

CHEMORADIATION INTERACTIONS

Since both chemotherapy and radiation therapy play important roles in the management of breast cancer, there has been continuing debate about their individual contributions as well as the sequence in which

Table 20–2. Recent Trials in the Treatment of Inflammatory Breast Carcinoma

Reference	Number of Patients	Treatment*	Median Survival (Mo)	5-Yr Survival (%)
Rouësse, et al (40)	230	RT (60)	30	28
		CT+RT (170)	60	66
Fields, et al (41)	107	RT±S (47)	21	13
		CT+RT (23)	33	27
		CT+S+RT (37)	47	44
Maloisel, et al (42)	43	CT+S+RT (43)	46	48
Koh, et al (43)	106	CT+RT (40)	39	37
		CT+S+RT (66)	51	48

*Number in parentheses = number of patients in the respective treatment categories.

they should be used when both modalities are utilized. Although radiotherapy is effective in improving the local control, it is most effective in controlling microscopic disease and does not effectively control a gross or palpable tumor unless high doses (> 8000 cGy) are given. Such doses can sterilize up to 75% of palpable tumors but frequently result in serious late sequelae in the form of necrosis or fibrosis of the normal tissues (46). Therefore, it is most useful for patients who are at increased risk of local recurrence from microscopic residual disease after the bulk of the tumor has been removed either with surgery (37,47) or controlled with chemotherapy (19). Because of the local nature of its biologic effects, there is clear evidence in the literature that postoperative radiotherapy following mastectomy does not increase the survival of patients with breast cancer and should not be used routinely for all patients (6,48). Some reports in the literature suggest that radiotherapy may be detrimental and could compromise the survival of patients, particularly when used as a routine postoperative therapy for early breast cancer (49,50). However, these data are largely derived from the orthovoltage era in which cardiovascular complications of radiotherapy may have contributed to increased mortality.

Radiotherapy can cause significant local toxicity, including skin and subcutaneous tissue injury, which is proportional to dosage and fractionation, varying degrees of injury to the underlying lung, radiation-induced rib fractures, frequent development of lymphedema of the arm on the affected side of those patients treated with radiotherapy to the axilla and secondary malignancies (sarcoma) (46,51). The incidence of these side-effects, without exception, is increased by the addition of surgery and chemotherapy. With the exception of second malignancies, these toxicities can be minimized by attention to radiation technique in delivery, dose, and fractionation.

In addition, radiotherapy may compromise the ability to tolerate full-dose chemotherapy because of its bone marrow toxicity (52–56). Although only a limited area of flat bones is included in the field of radiation, whole-breast irradiation as a component of breast conservation therapy may increase the marrow toxicity of adjuvant chemotherapy. This is more likely to occur if regional lymphatics are included in the field. Such patients frequently require a 20 to 25% reduction in chemotherapy dosage (Table 20–3). A decrease in the dose intensity of chemotherapy following radiotherapy could theoretically reduce the overall antitumor effect. However, there is no clinical evidence of compromise in survival of patients treated in this manner. Radiation recall, manifest by ex-

Table 20–3. Effect of Breast Irradiation on Tolerance to Adjuvant Chemotherapy in Breast Cancer

Reference	Primary Local Therapy	Chemotherapy Regimen	Outcome
Lippman, et al (53)	Mastectomy vs. lumpectomy + RT	A+C	Patients receiving RT required dose reduction more often, 17% vs. 9% ($p > 0.1$)
Weiss, et al (54)	Mastectomy vs. lumpectomy + RT	CMF or CMF + A	Increased frequency of leukopenia in RT group (33% vs. 10%, $p < 0.02$) leading to dose reduction in 13% vs. 4%, ($p < 0.01$) of patients
Perloff, et al (35)	Mastectomy vs. radiotherapy	CAFVP	Increased incidence of severe leukopenia in RT group, 42% vs. 20% in mastectomy group
Coppin, et al (55)	Mastectomy + RT vs. mastectomy	CMF	Myelosuppression-related reduction in dose intensity from 89 to 81% ($p < 0.001$) in patients receiving RT
Habibollahi, et al (56)	Mastectomy vs. lumpectomy + RT	CMF	RT compromised the delivered chemotherapy dose to 71% of the planned dose vs. 85% ($p < 0.05$) in the mastectomy group

A = Adriamycin; C = cyclophosphamide; M = methotrexate; F = fluorouracil; V = vincristine; P = prednisone; RT = radiotherapy.

acerbation of toxicity to the skin, esophagus, lung, and heart, particularly in patients treated with Adriamycin, which is commonly used in the treatment of breast cancer, are additional concerns in patients who have been treated with radiotherapy (51).

Timing Considerations

Simultaneous chemotherapy and radiotherapy have been used, both in patients treated with lumpectomy and breast irradiation (54,57,58) as well as in locally advanced breast cancer (59–62). The commonly used drugs for breast cancer, such as cyclophosphamide, methotrexate, and 5-fluorouracil, have no major negative interactions with radiotherapy and can be used simultaneously (54), however, the dosage of all drugs may have to be reduced by 25% in order to reduce the risk of bone marrow toxicity, and the dosage of methotrexate may have to be reduced by 50% in order to reduce skin toxicity. Simultaneous administration of Adriamycin and radiotherapy is clearly hazardous and should not be used outside the setting of a research protocol. Simultaneous use may have some merit for patients with locally advanced breast cancer (Stages III-B or IV), but there is no clear evidence that the concurrent use of Adriamycin and radiotherapy is superior to the sequential use of both modalities of treatment even for local control (61–64). Certainly, a delay of 2 to 3 months in starting adjuvant chemotherapy following radiotherapy did not compromise the survival of patients in one such trial (65). However, because the dosage of chemotherapy is compromised by prior or concurrent radiotherapy, it may be advantageous to delay radiotherapy, particularly when it is used postmastectomy, to the end of treatment after the planned course of chemotherapy is completed. This is not likely to compromise radiation therapy in any significant way and allows the patient to receive the maximum benefit from both modalities of treatment. This approach is quite reasonable for patients who have had mastectomy and require postoperative radiotherapy due to the high risk for local recurrence.

Whether primary radiotherapy used as a component of breast-conserving therapy can be delayed until after adjuvant chemotherapy has been completed in part or total is a matter of debate (66,67). In a trial reported by Recht et al (66), delaying primary radiotherapy to the breast resulted in a significantly high rate (15%) of local recurrence. More recently, McCormick et al have reported their experience in which a delay in radiotherapy until after three to six courses of adjuvant chemotherapy did not compromise the local control rate (67). Because of these conflicting reports, it is prudent that the standard practice of up front completion of primary radiotherapy to the breast be followed and that adjuvant chemotherapy be used either simultaneously or immediately following completion of radiation.

SUMMARY

Treatment of breast cancer has changed drastically during the past two decades. The routine use of radical mastectomy followed by postoperative radiotherapy was clearly excessive as local therapy in most patients and is no longer acceptable for early breast cancer in which breast conservation is possible with lumpectomy and whole-breast irradiation. Adjuvant therapy with combinations of cytotoxic agents or tamoxifen is essential in most patients in order to control the micrometastases that are responsible for recurrence of disease when local therapy is used alone. For locally advanced breast cancer, the order of therapy has been reversed to systemic therapy first, which succeeds in downstaging the tumor and provides the needed systemic effect without the delay that can occur if local therapy is used initially. Moreover, surgery alone would be too mutilating and radiotherapy alone would not be successful in eradicating gross disease. Induction chemotherapy, followed by surgery and relegating radiotherapy to the last, is a preferred strategy. For metastatic cancer, currently available drugs, although quite useful as palliative treatment, are not curative in 95 to 99% of the patients. This has led to evaluation of high-dose chemotherapy with autologous bone marrow or stem-cell support as a means of dose intensification and as a means of increasing the complete response rate and the chance for cure. A similar strategy is under study for adjuvant therapy in high-risk patients with

10 or more lymph node metastases at the time of initial diagnosis.

REFERENCES

1. Fisher B, Redmond C, Fisher ER, participating NSABP investigators. The contribution of recent NSABP clinical trials of primary breast cancer therapy to an understanding of tumor biology—An overview of findings. Cancer 46:1009, 1980.
2. Veronesi U, Saccozzi R, del Vecchio M, et al. Comparing radical mastectomy with quadrantectomy, axillary dissection and radiotherapy in patients with small cancers of the breast. N Engl J Med 305:6, 1981.
3. Fisher B, Redmond C, Poisson R, et al. Eight-year results of a randomized clinical trial comparing total mastectomy and lumpectomy with or without radiation in the treatment of breast cancer. N Engl J Med 320:822, 1989.
4. Danoff BF, Haller DG, Glick JH, et al. Conservative surgery and irradiation in the treatment of early breast cancer. Ann Intern Med 102:634, 1985.
5. Hortobagyi GN, Ames FC, Buzdar AU, et al. Management of stage III primary breast cancer with primary chemotherapy, surgery and radiation therapy. Cancer 62:2057, 1988.
6. Cuzick J, Stewart H, Petro R, et al. Overview of randomized trials of postoperative adjuvant radiotherapy in breast cancer. Cancer Treat Rep 71:15, 1987.
7. Fowble B, Glick J, Goodman R. Radiotherapy for the prevention of local-regional recurrence in high risk patients post mastectomy receiving adjuvant chemotherapy. Int J Radiat Oncol Biol Phys 15:627, 1988.
8. Fowble B, Gray R, Gilchrist K, et al. Identification of a subgroup of patients with breast cancer and histologically positive axillary nodes receiving adjuvant chemotherapy who may benefit from postoperative radiotherapy. J Clin Oncol 6:1107, 1988.
9. Sykes HF, Sim DA, Wong CJ, et al. Local-regional recurrence in breast cancer after mastectomy and adriamycin-based adjuvant chemotherapy. Evaluation of the role of postoperative radiotherapy. Int J Radiat Oncol Biol Phys 16:641, 1989.
10. Buzdar AU, McNeese MD, Hortobagyi GN, et al. Is chemotherapy effective in reducing the local failure rate in patients with operable breast cancer? Cancer 65:394, 1990.
11. Stotter AT, McNeese MD, Ames FC, et al. Predicting the rate and extent of locoregional failure after breast conservation therapy for early breast cancer. Cancer 64:2217, 1989.
12. Osborne MP, Ormistron N, Harmer CL, et al. Breast conservation in the treatment of early breast cancer—A 20-year follow-up. Cancer 53:349, 1984.
13. Recht A, Schnitt SJ, Connolly JL, et al. Prognosis following local or regional recurrence after conservative surgery and radiotherapy for early stage breast carcinoma. Int J Radiat Oncol Biol Phys 16:3, 1989.
14. DeLena M, Varini M, Zucali R, et al. Multimodal treatment for locally advanced breast cancer. Cancer Clin Trials 4:229, 1981.
15. Montague ED, Fletcher GH. Local regional effectiveness of surgery and radiation therapy in the treatment of breast cancer. Cancer 55:2266, 1985.
16. Montague ED. Radiation therapy and breast cancer—past, present and future. Am J Clin Oncol 8:455, 1985.
17. Fastenberg NA, Buzdar AU, Montague ED, et al. Management of inflammatory carcinoma of the breast—A combined modality approach. Am J Clin Oncol 8:134, 1985.
18. Fields JN, Perez CA, Kuske RR, et al. Inflammatory carcinoma of the breast. Treatment results on 107 patients. Int J Radiat Oncol Biol Phys 17:249, 1989.
19. Hortobagyi GN, Frye D, Ames F, et al. Quantitation of downstaging after neoadjuvant chemotherapy for primary breast cancer. Proc Am Soc Clin Oncol 8:23, 1989.
20. Janjan NA, McNeese MD, Buzdar AU, et al. Management of locoregional recurrent breast cancer. Cancer 58:1552, 1986.
21. Glick JH, Abeloff MD, Brown BW, et al. Adjuvant chemotherapy for breast cancer. JAMA 254:3461, 1985.
22. Bonadonna G, Valagussa P, Tancini G, et al. Current status of Milan adjuvant chemotherapy trials for node-positive and node-negative breast cancer. NCI Monogr 1:45, 1986.
23. Buzdar A, Hortobagyi G, Smith T, et al. Ten year results of FAC adjuvant chemotherapy trial in operable breast cancer. Proc Am Soc Clin Oncol 6:63, 1987.
24. Legha SS. Tamoxifen in the treatment of breast cancer. Ann Intern Med 109:219, 1988.
25. Henderson IC, Mouridsen H, Abe O, et al. Effects of adjuvant tamoxifen and of cytotoxic therapy on mortality in early breast cancer. N Engl J Med 319:1681, 1988.
26. Love RR. Tamoxifen therapy in primary breast cancer. Biology, efficacy and side effects. J Clin Oncol 7:803, 1989.
27. Fisher B, Redmond C, Dimitrov NV, et al. A randomized clinical trial evaluating sequential methotrexate and fluorouracil in the treatment of patients with node-negative

breast cancer who have estrogen receptor-negative tumors. N Engl J Med 320:473, 1989.
28. Mansour EG, Gray R, Shatila AH, et al. Efficacy of adjuvant chemotherapy in high-risk node-negative breast cancer. N Engl J Med 320:485, 1989.
29. Fisher B, Costanitino J, Redmond C, et al. A randomized clinical trial evaluating tamoxifen in the treatment of patients with node-negative breast cancer who have estrogen-receptor-positive tumors. N Engl J Med 320:479, 1989.
30. Swain SM, Lippman ME. Systemic therapy of locally advanced breast cancer. Review and guidelines. Oncology 3(1):21, 1989.
31. Klefström P, Gröhn P, Heinonen E, et al. Adjuvant postoperative radiotherapy, chemotherapy and immunotherapy in stage III breast cancer. Cancer 60:936, 1987.
32. Schaake-Koning C, van der Linden EH, Hart G, Engelsman E. Adjuvant chemo- and hormonal therapy in locally advanced breast cancer. A randomized clinical study. Int J Radiat Oncol Biol Phys 11:1759, 1985.
33. Rubens RD, Bartelink H, Engelsman E, et al. Locally advanced breast cancer. The contribution of cytotoxic and endocrine treatment to radiotherapy. Eur J Cancer Clin Oncol 25:667, 1989.
34. Valagussa P, Zambetti M, Bignami P, et al. T_{3b}-T_4 breast cancer. Factors affecting results in combined modality treatments. Clin Exp Metastasis 1:191, 1983.
35. Perloff M, Lesnick GJ, Korzun A, et al. Combination chemotherapy with mastectomy or radiotherapy for stage III breast carcinoma. A cancer and leukemia group B study. J Clin Oncol 6:261, 1988.
36. Jacquillat C, Weil M, Baillet F, et al. Results of neoadjuvant chemotherapy and radiation therapy in the breast-conserving treatment of 250 patients with all stages of infiltrative breast cancer. Cancer 66:119, 1990.
37. Swain SM, Sorace RA, Bagley CS, et al. Neoadjuvant chemotherapy in the combined modality approach of locally advanced nonmetastatic breast cancer. Cancer Res 47:3889, 1987.
38. Griem K, Henderson IC, Gelman R, et al. Postoperative radiation therapy (XRT) after adjuvant chemotherapy (CTX) in breast cancer patients. Results of a randomized trial. Proc Am Soc Clin Oncol 5:68, 1986.
39. Sherry MM, Johnson DH, Page DL, et al. Inflammatory carcinoma of the breast. Am J Med 79:355, 1985.
40. Rouësse J, Friedman S, Sarrazin D, et al. Primary chemotherapy in the treatment of inflammatory breast carcinoma. A study of 230 cases from the Institut Gustav-Roussy. J Clin Oncol 4:1765, 1986.
41. Fields JN, Kuske RR, Perez CA, et al. Prognostic factors in inflammatory breast cancer. Cancer 63:1225, 1989.
42. Maloisel F, Dufour P, Bergerat JP, et al. Results of initial doxorubicin, 5-fluorouracil, and cyclophosphamide combination chemotherapy for inflammatory carcinoma of the breast. Cancer 65:851, 1990.
43. Koh EH, Buzdar AU, Ames FC, et al. Inflammatory carcinoma of the breast. Results of a combined-modality approach—M.D. Anderson Cancer Center experience. Cancer Chemother Pharmacol 27:94, 1990.
44. Thomas WW, McNeese MD, Fletcher GH, et al. Multimodal treatment for inflammatory breast cancer. Int J Radiat Oncol Biol Phys 17:739, 1989.
45. Montague ED, Fletcher GH. The need for every modality of treatment to prevent catastrophic local and regional failures in advanced breast cancer. Int J Radiat Oncol Biol Phys 9:419, 1983.
46. Spanos WJ Jr, Montague ED, Fletcher GH. Late complications of radiation only for advanced breast cancer. Int J Radiat Oncol Biol Phys 6:1473, 1980.
47. Manji M, Ragaz J, Worth A, et al. Is mastectomy (M) indicated in patients with stage III breast cancer treated with preoperative (neoadjuvant) therapy (PT)? Proc Am Soc Clin Oncol 7:36, 1988.
48. Lipsett MB. Postoperative radiation for women with cancer of the breast and positive axillary lymph nodes. Should it continue? N Engl J Med 304:112, 1981.
49. Stjernsward J. Decreased survival related to irradiation postoperatively in early operable breast cancer. Lancet 2:1285, 1974.
50. Holland JF, Glidewell O, Cooper RG. Adverse effect of radiotherapy on adjuvant chemotherapy of breast cancer. Surg Gynecol Obstet 150:817, 1980.
51. Hrafnkelsson J, Nilsson K, Soderberg M. Tolerance of radiotherapy combined with adjuvant chemotherapy in breast cancer. Acta Oncol 26:269, 1987.
52. Levine JF, Coleman CN, Cox RS, et al. The effect of postoperative and primary radiation therapy on delivered dose of adjuvant cyclophosphamide, methotrexate, and 5-fluorouracil (CMF) chemotherapy in breast cancer. Cancer 53:237, 1984.
53. Lippman ME, Lichter AS, Edwards BK, et al. The impact of primary irradiation treatment of localized breast cancer on the ability to administer systemic adjuvant chemotherapy. J Clin Oncol 2:21, 1984.

54. Weiss RB, Valagussa P, Moliterni A, et al. Adjuvant chemotherapy after conservative surgery plus irradiation versus modified radical mastectomy. Am J Med 83:455, 1987.
55. Coppin C, Ragaz J, Nordahl K, Jackson S. The impact of radiotherapy on adjuvant chemotherapy delivery for node positive breast cancer. Proc Am Soc Clin Oncol 7:36(A-139), 1988.
56. Habibollahi F, Fentiman IS, Chaudary MA, et al. Influence of radiotherapy on the dose of adjuvant chemotherapy in early breast cancer. Breast Cancer Res Treat 13:237, 1989.
57. Borger JH, Keijser AH. Conservative breast cancer treatment. Analysis of cosmetic results and the role of concomitant adjuvant chemotherapy. Int J Radiat Oncol Biol Phys 13:1173, 1987.
58. Ray GR, Fish VJ, Marmor JB, et al. Impact of adjuvant chemotherapy on cosmesis and complications in stages I and II carcinoma of the breast treated by biopsy and radiation therapy. Int J Radiat Oncol Biol Phys 10:837, 1984.
59. Perez CA, Presant C, Philpott G, Ratkin G. Phase I-II study of concurrent irradiation and multi-drug chemotherapy in advanced carcinoma of the breast. A pilot study by the Southeastern Cancer Study Group. Int J Radiat Oncol Biol Phys 5:1329, 1979.
60. Meek AG, Order SE, Abeloff MD, et al. Concurrent radiochemotherapy in advanced breast cancer. Cancer 51:1001, 1983.
61. Olson JE, Gray R, Sponzo RW, et al. Management of nonresectable locally advanced (stage III) breast cancer. An ECOG trial. Breast Cancer Res Treat 8:109, 1986.
62. Piccart MJ, de Valeriola D, Paridaens R, et al. Six-year results of a multimodality treatment strategy for locally advanced breast cancer. Cancer 62:2501, 1988.
63. Hansen R, Erickson B, Komaki R, et al. Concomitant adjuvant chemotherapy and radiotherapy for high risk breast cancer patients. Breast Cancer Res Treat 17:171, 1990.
64. Denham JW. Synchronous radiation and chemotherapy for locally-advanced cancer. Is it the answer? Med J Aust 147:590, 1987.
65. Buzdar AU, Smith TL, Powell KC, et al. Effect of timing of initiation of adjuvant chemotherapy on disease-free survival in breast cancer. Breast Cancer Res Treat 2:163, 1982.
66. Recht A, Come SE, Gelman RS, et al. Integration of conservative surgery, radiotherapy, and chemotherapy for the treatment of early-stage, node-positive breast cancer: Sequencing, timing, and outcome. J Clin Oncol 9:1662, 1991.
67. McCormick B, Hakes T, Yahalom J, et al. Breast conserving surgery and radiation: The delay of primary radiation after adjuvant chemotherapy does not influence local control. Proc Am Clin Oncol 11:55, 1992.

ORGAN-SPECIFIC APPLICATIONS

Chapter 21

ESOPHAGUS

MADHU J. JOHN AND MARSHALL S. FLAM

INTRODUCTION

Although cancer of the esophagus is relatively uncommon in North America, it is the leading cause of cancer-related deaths in several parts of Asia and Africa (1,2). A wide geographical and racial variation in incidence and mortality exists. The Asian "esophageal cancer belt" cuts an uneven swath through the Turkmenia province in the erstwhile USSR, China, the Gonbad provinces of Iran, Afghanistan, the vale of Kashmir in India, and Singapore. The disease is also endemic in parts of France, the Transkei region of South Africa, and Rhodesia. Decreasing mortality rates from esophageal carcinoma (ECA) in countries such as England and Japan are offset by the increasing incidence rates of ECA in specific subpopulations in the United States and Canada (2,3). The overall yearly incidence of 11,000 new cases of ECA in the United States overshadows the high incidence of squamous cell carcinoma of the esophagus in African–American men in the cities of Detroit and San Francisco (2). The incidence of adenocarcinoma of the esophagus has been steadily increasing in Caucasian men at a rate of 45 to 110% in several regions in the United States (4).

The major known risk factors associated with ECA are combinations of cigarette smoking and alcohol consumption, along with certain genetic, dietary, and environmental factors (5–7). However, there are obviously unknown culpable factors that have yet to be ascertained. Adenocarcinoma has been described as developing in Barrett's esophagus in a multistep process from metaplasia, dysplasia, and early adenocarcinoma onto invasive and metastatic disease (8). Human papillomavirus infections (types 16/18) have been implicated in the development of squamous cell cancer of the esophagus (9). The possibility of decreasing the incidence of ECA in high-risk groups exists with increasing public awareness of the risk factors involved. However, no practical large-scale screening procedure for early diagnosis exists.

The natural history of ECA is characterized by extensive local contiguous growth and lymph node metastases culminating eventually in distant metastases. These features are facilitated by unique anatomic and physiologic factors (10,11). The proclivity for ECA to spread through submucosal lymphatics results in "skip areas" in which the extent of the primary tumor is grossly underestimated on endoscopy and barium contrast studies. Also, the lack of serosa permits the facile involvement of adjacent vital structures, especially in the middle esophagus. The esophagus has the inherent capability to adjust to regurgitation or subobstruction; therefore, a tumor must be almost circumferential before the patient experiences dysphagia. These three reasons result in the presence of extensive local disease and lymphatic spread in most patients at the time of diagnosis. In fact, some of these features are responsible for the 20 to 85% incidence of local recurrence following definitive surgery or radiotherapy (6,12,13). Although several autopsy series show a 70 to 90% incidence of distant metastases, the distant failure rate in several surgery/radiation series is between 15 and 70% and generally presents simultaneously with local disease (6,12–15).

Fifty years after the first surgical resection was performed and two decades after Pearson's landmark treatise on the radiotherapeutic management of ECA, oncologists still face the task of managing a disease with an accrued death rate of over 93% (16–18). ECA remains a most appalling disease, with a mortality and morbidity exceeding almost all cancers. As stated above, the major risk factors of ECA have been identified and the potential for prevention of the disease exists. This is of particular import to people in various parts of the world where ECA is endemic and where incidence rates can approach up to 200 cases per 100,000 population. The need for local control is paramount. The possibility of decreasing overall failure is directly related to local control, notwithstanding the probability that distant metastases may eventually develop in some patients whose locoregional disease has been eradicated.

TRADITIONAL MANAGEMENT APPROACHES

Surgery

Definitive

Although the first successful resection of the thoracic esophagus was reported by Torek in 1913, it was only after the first one-stage resection and reconstruction for an esophageal cancer was conducted at Memorial Hospital in New York about 50 years ago that surgery became the mainstay of management in ECA (16,19). Even so, it is estimated that less than 5% of all ECA patients may be truly appropriate candidates for definitive surgery (20).

There is a vast discrepancy in the criteria used for operability (21–27), including the patients' general condition, evidence of nodal involvement, extra-esophageal spread, or distant metastases. The wide variations in operability and resectability rates in various surgical series imply that the methods employed in preoperative assessment of patients are not uniformly used in the surgical community. Cytologic screening in high-risk endemic areas in China have yielded large numbers of patients with preclinical lesions who have been cured by surgical resection (30% 5-year survival) (25). If strict criteria of resectability are used by experienced surgeons, a 20 to 30% 5-year survival rate is possible (24,26,28). On the other hand, if all cancers are included in any series, the operative mortality can range from 15 to 45% and 5-year survival rates ranges from 2 to 9% (21–23,29). The Earlam and Cunha-Melo study of 83,783 surgically treated patients covered the literature between the years 1960 and 1979 (21). There is no evidence in subsequent large surgical series suggesting that these survival figures have changed significantly (22,29,30). As surgeons became more selective and anesthesiological procedures became more refined, the surgical mortality rates have declined perceptibly from around 30 to about 10% (24–26,30). For example, over a period of 30 years, the operative mortality for ECA at the Massachusetts General hospital fell from 30.5 to 10.4% (30).

Palliative

Procedures employed for palliation include the standard esophagectomy followed by its replacement by the stomach, jejunum, colon, or synthetic tube although such drastic procedures are rarely used.

The surgical procedure of transhiatal (without thoracotomy) esophagectomy (THE) has been revived lately, particularly following preoperative chemoradiation. It must be remembered that THE is a debulking procedure and does not allow the removal of extra-esophageal tumor and can still be followed by major complications (32).

Other procedures include the placement of a cervical stoma, a gastrostomy, peroral dilatation of the malignant stricture by rubber/balloon dilators, endoscopic intubation, and, more recently, laser therapy (31,33–36).

Radiotherapy

Radiotherapy in the form of intraluminal radium application, super voltage external radiotherapy (RT), or radon seed implantation preceded surgical resection as the treatment of choice for esophageal carcinoma by about 30 years (16). From 1940, when the first thoracic esophagectomy (with cervical esophagostomy and gastrostomy) was done, until 1980, surgical management (both definitive and palliative) was the preferred form of management through most of the world. As far as can be ascertained, there was no call made for a randomized prospective trial to compare radiotherapy and surgery during those years, despite the sizable surgical mortality rate that prevailed. The patient referred for definitive or palliative radiotherapy was generally one with more extensive local and regional disease, with preexisting medical conditions, or with a performance status that precluded surgical intervention (37).

In 1980, when Earlam and Cunha-Melo undertook critical reviews of surgery (20 years, 1960 to 1979, 122 publications, 83,783 patients) and radiotherapy (25 years, 1954 to 1979, 49 publications, 8489 patients) for ECA, neither modality got rave reviews (21,37). What emerged from these studies, however, was the fact that although most patients had been referred by surgeons as unfit for operation in the radiotherapy series, there was no significant advantage for surgery over radiotherapy in terms of 1-year (18% vs. 18%), 2-year (9% vs. 8%) and 5-year (4% vs. 6%) survival rates. Moreover, the 29% mean surgical mortality rate was a statistic that may have persuaded surgeons to operate only on patients with early disease after using the strictest of medical, surgical, and staging criteria.

Preoperative and Postoperative Radiotherapy

Because the results of treatment with resection alone and radiotherapy alone were equally dismal, it was logical that attempts be made to combine the two predominant modalities.

The rationale for preoperative radiotherapy was an increased curative resection rate. Akakura et al described an increase of resectability from 29 to 65% when preoperative radiotherapy was employed (38). Thus, patients entered on these studies had more advanced disease than pure surgical series.

Two major findings resulted from these preoperative studies.

1. High-dose preoperative regimens such as 4000 cGy in 1 to 1½ weeks (Launois et al) or 6600 cGy in 6½ to 7 weeks (Doggett et al) resulted in 25 and 33% operative mortality rates, respectively, and marked morbidity (39,40).
2. The survival benefits of preoperative radiotherapy when used in modest doses, such as 2000 cGy in 4 to 5 days by Nakayama and Kinoshita or 4000 cGy in 4 weeks by van Andel, were marginal (41,42).

Recently, Morrison et al reported a 24% 5-year overall survival in selected patients receiving preoperative hyperfractionated radiotherapy (43). A postoperative irradiation study by Kasai et al has also suggested a marginal but definite improvement in survival rates in those patients whose resected mediastinal nodes were not involved by metastatic disease (44). No other postoperative radiotherapy series have substantiated this finding, however.

CURRENT MANAGEMENT APPROACHES COMBINING LOCAL AND SYSTEMIC MODALITIES

Rationale

The rationale for attempting therapy other than surgery or radiotherapy in ECA was based on several coincident but unrelated factors. The major reason for concern was that the predominant regional modalities of surgery and radiotherapy had virtually no impact on the life span of most patients who develop esophageal cancer. Seventy-five to 85% of patients with ECA died within 12 months, irrespective of modality used. It was also evident that whatever treatment modality was used, the major site of failure was locoregional in the esophagus itself or in the mediastinal and upper abdominal nodes (12–15).

The record of chemotherapy (CT) in ECA was, in most regards, poor. In 1974, for example, Rubin categorically stated that no discussion of CT for ECA was warranted, since the value of this approach had not been significant (45). Rider was even more harsh and described adjunctive chemotherapy in ECA as "pathetic" (46). Ten years later, Kelsen was slightly more optimistic and noted that 9 of 10 adequately tested drugs had "modest-moderate" activity in ECA and that combined modality approaches, including chemotherapy, were possible (47).

Nevertheless, the poor results of surgery and radiotherapy, the marginal improvements when the two were used together, and the concept of multimodality therapy, which came into vogue in the late 1970s and early 1980s, formed the milieu for investigators to use drugs in combination with the locoregional modalities of surgery and/or radiation. Theoretically, chemotherapy could reduce tumor volume and thereby increase the effectiveness of surgery/radiotherapy; some drugs could potentially enhance the local radiotherapeutic effect and perhaps eliminate occult systemic disease as well.

Chemotherapy

Kelsen has described in considerable detail the history of most single chemotherapeutic agents and their combinations in ECA (47). Single-agent activity is summarized in Table 21–1. Vindesine, mitomycin C, and cisplatinum (CDDP) have the most activity, ranging from 22 to 32%, although for modest time periods. Of interest is that several patients tested for vindesine activity had previously received CDDP chemotherapy.

Because combined chemotherapy is generally more effective than single agents, several drug combinations have been utilized in several trials. Most of these combinations included CDDP. Response rates in patients with regional disease were in the range of 50 to 60%, including 1 to 5% complete responses (48).

Since the mid-1970s, a few studies, primarily from Memorial Sloan-Kettering Cancer Center, employing induction chemotherapy followed by esophagectomy and reconstruction were reported. Since 1980, there have been many reports from single institutions of Phase II in-house protocols using drugs, generally 5-fluorouracil (5-FU) and CDDP or 5-FU and mitomycin C, concurrently with external radiotherapy (generally 3000 to 5000 cGy). Many of these reports have followed the chemoradiation regimen with esophagectomy built into the treatment schema.

An equal number of reported studies have avoided esophagectomy altogether, often because the patients were thought to be inoperable at initial presentation due to extensive locoregional disease, poor performance status, or preexistent medical problems. Some earlier studies employed single drugs, but in the last 5 years, multiple-drug combinations were used concurrently with radiotherapy.

Due to the uniformly poor results obtained by using either local modality of surgery or radiation (or both) and despite the limited activity of chemotherapeutic drugs in general against ECA, the last two decades were noteworthy for the increasing use of a systemic modality (chemotherapy) with surgery or radiotherapy. Preoperative chemotherapy was used either alone or with radiotherapy in several series. When surgery was not used, drugs were used either singly or in combination with radiotherapy.

Four distinct categories of chemotherapy use are available; these are elaborated separately below and are summarized in Tables 21–2 through 21–5.

Table 21–1. Single-Agent Activity in Esophageal Carcinoma

Drugs	Response Rate (%)	Duration in Months
1. Bleomycin	15	1–4
2. Mitomycin C	26	3
3. Adriamycin	15	2–3
4. 5-Fluorouracil	15	2–4
5. Methotrexate	12	2–4
6. Lomustine	16	NS
7. Methyl-GAG	22	2–3
8. Cisplatinum	22	2–3
9. Vindesine	32	3–4
10. Etoposide	7	NS

NS = Not stated
Extracted from Kelsen D. Semin Oncol 11(2):159, 1984.

Preoperative Chemotherapy Series

A small group of investigators explored the use of induction chemotherapy prior to esophagectomy (Table 21–2) (25,49–52). All have used CDDP-based combinations of chemotherapy with either bleomycin and vindesine or 5-FU for about two to three cycles prior to surgery. The patients in these studies were screened extensively; resultant resectability rates averaged 80%, the operative mortality averaged 5%, and a pathologic complete response rate of about 5% was noted. Consequently, at least four of these studies mention the use of varying doses of RT and/or CT postoperatively. For these 109

Table 21–2. Selected Preoperative Chemotherapy Studies in Esophageal Carcinoma

Series	Number of Patients	Preoperative Chemotherapy	Surgical Mortality (%)	Postoperative RT (cGy)	Survival Median (mos)	1 Yr (%)	2 Yr (%)
Kelsen, et al (50) 1983	34	CDDP + VDS + BLM × 2	9	5500/5 weeks	16	55	43
Kelsen, et al (51) 1986	14	CDDP + VDS + MGBG × 2	7	5500/5–6 weeks	26	50	NS
Kies, et al (49) 1987	9	5-FU + CDDP × 3	0	4500–5000	25	89	56
Roth, et al (52) 1988	17	CDDP + VDS + BLM × 2	11	None	9	48	25
Hilgenberg, et al (25) 1988	35	5-FU + CDDP × 2	4	5000–5400	NS	80	60

NS = Not stated.
RT = Radiotherapy; CDDP = cisplatinum; VDS = vindesine; BLM = bleomycin; MGBG = mitoguozone; 5-FU = 5-fluorouracil.

patients (predominantly Stage I and II), an average median survival of 19 months and a 2-year survival rate of 46% were obtained (Table 21–2).

Preoperative Chemoradiation

In 1981, Steiger and co-workers, from Wayne State University, reported remarkable results when they used either 5-FU + mitomycin C or 5-FU + CDDP concurrently with radiotherapy prior to esophagectomy (53). This multimodality regimen was based on their success with epidermoid cancers of the anal canal. Since then, multiple institutions took up preoperative chemoradiation protocols and reported fairly consistent results (Table 21–3) (54–61).

Most studies used cycles of 5-FU and CDDP with 3000 cGy of concomitant radiotherapy in patients with Stage II to III disease who had no contraindications for surgery. A second course of the same drugs was usually given after completion of the RT course. Esophagectomy followed in about 3 weeks in 55 to 100% of patients. A large number of patients in some studies refused surgery because they were symptomatically better after the chemoradiation course; in other series, patients who did not undergo surgery were not included in result analysis at all. Postoperative radiotherapy, usually in the range of 2000 to 5000 cGy, was delivered in select cases in which surgical margins were positive or when microscopic or gross disease was present in resection margins.

Table 21–3. Selected Preoperative Chemoradiation Studies for Esophageal Carcinoma

Series	Number of Patients	Chemotherapy	RT Dose (cGy)	Surgical Mortality (%)	Survival Median (mos)	1 Yr (%)	2 Yr (%)
Steiger, et al (53) 1981	35	5-FU + Mitomycin C or 5-FU + CDDP × 2	3000	8.5	NS	52	30
Franklin, et al (54) 1983	30	5-FU + Mitomycin C × 2	3000	30	19	53	13
Leichman, et al (55) 1984	21	5-FU + CDDP × 2	3000	27	18	57	42
Poplin, et al (56) 1987	113	5-FU + CDDP × 2	3000	11	12	50	28
Richmond, et al (57) 1987	15	5-FU + CDDP × 3	5600–6000	20	13	57	38
Seydel, et al (RTOG) (58) 1988	27	5-FU + CDDP × 1	3000–5000	4	13	44	15
Herskovic, et al (59) 1988	89	5-FU + CDDP	3000–5000	NS	10	38	18
Parker, et al (60) 1989	33	5-FU + Mitomycin C × 1	3000	12	NS	NS	33
Orringer, et al (61) 1990	41	5-FU + VBL + CDDP	4500	2*	29	72	60

*Transhiatal esophagectomy done in this series.
RT = radiotherapy; 5-FU = 5-fluorouracil; CDDP = cisplatinum, VBL = vinblastine.

A meta-analysis of these nine studies shows that preoperative chemoradiation in 394 patients achieved an average median survival of 16 months and 1- and 2-year survival of 53% and 31%, respectively. The surgical mortality again ranged from 0 to 30%, with a mean of 13%. The percentage of patients who had no evidence of disease in the surgical specimen ranged from 0 to 35% (mean: 21%). With few exceptions, only those patients with a pathologic complete response at esophagectomy have a good chance at cure. Similarly, the life span of patients with limited disease, microscopic or gross in the esophagectomy specimen, appeared limited.

The study by Orringer et al is noteworthy, in that the addition of vinblastine to 5-FU and CDDP to moderate doses of RT followed by debulking surgery (transhiatal esophagectomy) yielded apparently superior median and 2-year survivals with no significant morbidity (61).

Definitive Chemoradiation Using Single Drug

Reports of the use of a single drug concurrently with RT in patients with ECA are tabulated in Table 21–4. Kolaric and co-workers, from Yugoslavia, described the administration of bleomycin and Adriamycin (separately) to patients with locally advanced ECA in conjunction with an average of 4500 cGy of thoracic RT (62,63). Complete response rates were 25% and 26% respectively, on the basis of esophagoscopy.

An Eastern Cooperative Oncology Group study of bleomycin with concurrent RT was published in 1980 (64). The results did not match the earlier Kolaric study, with the same combination, with discouraging 1- and 2-year survival rates of 24% and 12%, respectively.

Byfield et al (1980) described the use of infusional (20 mg/day/24 hrs) 5-FU alone with radiotherapy and noted a high complete response rate of 83% (65). More recently, Lokich described the use of higher doses (300 mg/m^2/24 hrs) of 5-FU and RT in 13 patients, with more impressive results of 73% survival at 1 year and 22% at 3 years (66). Both authors noted rapid and sustained palliation of dysphagia, a distinct feature of several chemoradiation therapy studies, in comparison with pure radiotherapy studies, in which the relief from dysphagia is of gradual onset, often erratic and frequently reversed.

What could be derived from these studies was that some chemotherapeutic drugs, particularly 5-FU, could be given concurrently with fairly standard doses of radiotherapy with little addition to morbidity and that commendable (if only short term) palliative results could be obtained in locally advanced esophageal cancer.

Definitive Chemoradiation Using Multiple Drugs

With some exceptions, most patients who received chemoradiation (without esophagectomy) were considered clinically inoperable due to advanced disease or had coexistent medical conditions that made surgery inadvisable (Table 21–5) (57,67–72). Consequently, these patients generally had ei-

Table 21–4. Selected Series of Definitive Chemoradiation (Single Drug) in Esophageal Carcinoma*

Series	Number of Patients	Chemotherapy/ Cycles/Dose	RT Dose in cGy	Survival Median (mos)	Survival 1 Yr (%)	Survival 2 Yr (%)
Kolaric, et al (63) 1977	15	ADR × 3	4500–5200	9	NS	NS
Kolaric, et al (62) 1976	24	BLM biweekly	4000–5000	9	52	NS
Earle, et al (ECOG) (64) 1980	40	BLM daily for 14 days	5000–6000	6	24	12
Byfield, et al (65) 1980	6	5-FU × 6	6000	NR	50	—
Lokich, et al (66) 1987	13	5-FU × 6	4400–6900	16	77	22**

*No treatment related mortality reported in any series.
**At 3 years.
NR = Not reached; NS = Not stated; ADR = Adriamycin; BLM = bleomycin; 5-FU = 5-fluorouracil.

Table 21–5. Select Series of Definitive Chemoradiation (Without Surgery) in Esophageal Carcinoma

Series	Number of Patients	Chemotherapy/ No. of Cycles	RT (cGy)	Treatment Mortality (%)	Survival Median (mos)	Survival 1 Yr (%)	Survival 2 Yr (%)
Marcial, et al (67) 1980	25	VCR, BLM, MTX × 1 or 2	5000 in 4 weeks	0	11	48	20
Keane, et al (68) 1985	35	5-FU + Mito C × 1 or 2	4500–5000 continuous or split course	3	12	47	28
Richmond, et al (57) 1987	25	5-FU + CDDP × 3	5600–6000	4	12	55	37
Coia, et al (69) 1987	30*	5-FU + Mitomycin C × 2	6000 continuous	2	24	68	47
Leichman, et al (70) 1987	20	5-FU, CDDP, Mitomycin C + BLM	5000 split course	0**	22	75	35
John, et al (71) 1989	30	5-FU, Mitomycin C, CDDP, MTX, LVR	3000–5040	3	11	51	29
Seitz, et al (72) 1990	35	5-FU, CDDP × 2	4000 split course	3	17	55	41

*Stage I and II cases only.
**Treatment-related morbidity considered "prohibitive."
RT = radiotherapy; VCR = vincristine, BLM = bleomycin; MTX = methotrexate; 5-FU = 5-fluorouracil, CDDP = cisplatinum, LVR = leucovorin

ther more locally advanced disease or poorer performance status than the patients that underwent esophagectomies following chemotherapy or chemoradiation (21,37).

The two most commonly used drug combinations are 5-FU + mitomycin C and 5-FU + CDDP. While most institutions, research groups, and medical oncologists seem to prefer the 5-FU + CDDP combination, purportedly due to increased pulmonary toxicity seen with mitomycin C and RT interaction or superimposed action, both the Canadian and Fox Chase experiences were contrary (68,69). Despite using 5-FU and mitomycin C exclusively, less than 1% mortality in their studies was attributable to radiation pneumonitis or the acute respiratory distress syndrome (ARDS). In our series of 30 cases, in which we preferred to alternate CDDP with mitomycin C (both with 5-FU), theoretically to reduce their individual toxicities, only one possible case of ARDS was noted (71).

The RT doses in these reports ranged from 3000 to 6000 cGy, with at least three studies suggesting a dose-survival relationship (57,68,71). Radiation treatment techniques were virtually identical; the combination of a single anterior field and two wedged posterior oblique fields was the most commonly used technique. Lung inhomogeneity corrections in dose calculations are either not generally used or mentioned in these reports. John et al used nontraditional RT fields with 3-cm margins in the craniocaudal plan and 6.5-cm-wide fields in general and treated the supraclavicular region only on gross nodal involvement or with upper thoracic/cervical primaries. Lung inhomogeneity corrections were also used. No appreciable increase in marginal failure was noted (1 in 30 cases) (71,73).

The median survival in these selected seven reports averaged 16 months. The mean 1-year and 2-year survival rates were 57% and 34%, respectively. The overall treatment mortality averaged 2%. Even though most patients in these reports involve Stage III inoperable patients, these survival figures are comparable to those obtained by preoperative chemoradiation in patients with less advanced disease. A more equitable comparison of patients with similar disease would involve Coia's study of predominantly Stage I and II patients (69) and the preoperative chemoradiation therapy studies (53–61). As flawed as it may be, such a comparison would make a compelling case against esophagectomy in patients receiving definitive chemoradiation therapy.

Much of the criticism of the multiple Phase II protocols employing chemotherapy with the regional modalities of surgery or radiotherapy or both was based on the premise that no prospective randomized trial had been undertaken to compare such a combination with either regional modality alone. The Radiation Therapy Oncology Group (RTOG) undertook such a Phase III trial comparing radiotherapy alone versus chemoradiation for locoregionally confined ECA. Herskovic et al reported its results on 121 patients recently (74). Radiation-treated patients had a median survival of 9 months compared to 12.5 months in chemoradiation-treated patients. One- and 2-year survival rates for single and combined modality groups were 50% vs. 33% and 35% vs. 10%, respectively ($p < 0.001$). A decreased incidence of local and distant failure was noted in the chemoradiation group, which also experienced increased Grade 3 and 4 side effects.

TREATMENT SEQUELAE OF CHEMORADIATION IN ECA

The side effects or complications of treating ECA with either surgery, radiotherapy, or chemotherapy are well established. The effects of chemoradiation in relation to the esophagus are described in Chapter 32; in this chapter, we will only discuss the specific complications that are peculiar to the combination of the systemic modality of chemotherapy with either of the two modalities (surgery or radiotherapy) during the treatment of ECA.

Myelotoxicity

When standard radiation fields are used for ECA, approximately 10 to 20% of active bone marrow may be irradiated. This would generally have minimal additional impact on the myelotoxicity secondary to chemotherapy. In our own experience, there was a 5% incidence of transient leukopenia and/or thrombocytopenia with radiotherapy alone, which increased to 16% when drugs were combined with radiotherapy (71,73). Although no deaths secondary to such myelotoxicity have been described in the literature, it is nevertheless a point of concern and should be monitored carefully in such drug-RT combinations.

In the series of reports on induction chemotherapy prior to surgery, no specific mention of myelotoxicity is made. Moreover, the mortality rate of 0 to 11% is no different from esophagectomy series. This, coupled with the observation of low rates of complete responses (average 5%), suggests that unless more vigorous drug regimens are used and the concept of intraoperative chemotherapy is not exploited, there is probably no need for concern with myelotoxicity in this scenario of preoperative induction chemotherapy.

Pulmonary Toxicity

Pulmonary toxicity manifested by respiratory failure or by ARDS is the single most important complication of chemoradiation in ECA. There is some evidence that this complication may actually increase in incidence when surgical resection is added to chemoradiation. For example, of 23 patients who underwent surgery following 5-FU and mitomycin C chemotherapy and 3000 cGy radiotherapy in the original Wayne State study (92), three postoperative deaths (13%) were attributed to histologically proven toxic pneumonitis related to the chemotherapy, radiotherapy, and oxygen toxicity. The incidence of pneumonitis in pure chemoradiation studies is usually reported to be between 0 and 6%, but fatal pneumonitis or death secondary to respiratory failure is reported to be between 0 and 5% and averages 1% (62–72). ARDS is characterized by progressive dyspnea, pulmonary infiltrates within and without radiation fields, and occasional response to steroids.

The etiology of ARDS in chemoradiation studies may be related to lung damage caused by radiotherapy, mitomycin C, and forced O_2 ventilation during anesthesia for surgery. These three factors could possibly have an attenuated effect on pulmonary tissues as a result of their interaction. The incidence of this side effect could be drastically reduced by modifying each of these factors. Radiotherapy fields could be drastically reduced without compromising results (71,73). We initially use 3-cm margins beyond known disease craniocaudally and restrict field width to 6.5 cm or 1 cm beyond gross mediastinal disease. Also, our wedged posterior oblique fields come in through more acute angles in order to minimize dose to lung tissue not included in the anterior-posterior fields. As for concerns regarding mitomycin C, we alternate combinations of 5-FU + mitomycin C with 5-FU + CDDP in our chemotherapy protocol to reduce mitomycin C + CDDP toxicity. Finally, we utilize surgical resection only in $T_1N_0M_0$ cases that do not have medical contraindications to surgery. Seydel et al reported the potential for decreasing pulmonary toxicity by reducing O_2 tension during respiratory support in anesthesia given during esophagectomy (58).

Respiratory Fistula

Fistula formation involving the respiratory tract during treatment of ECA is generally the result of tumor lysis in anatomic structures contiguous to the esophagus (75,76). The overall incidence of respiratory fistula in ECA is said to be between 5 and 10%.

There is a questionable perception among some investigators that chemoradiation or perhaps chemotherapy alone may reduce the incidence of fistula formation caused by tumor sloughing off during treatment. The incidence of respiratory fistula in the entire chemoradiation series averages 2%. In our own experience, we have successfully treated two patients with biopsy-proven tracheal involvement adjacent to esophageal cancer. One patient died with distant metastases 1 year after treatments, without symptoms of mediastinitis or other local symptoms; the other is alive disease-free 5 years after treatment. Kelsen also reports bronchoscopically proven healing of histologically proven invasion of trachea without fistula formation after treatment with a CDDP, vindesine, and bleomycin combination (50).

FUTURE DIRECTIONS

Intraluminal Treatment

Radium bougienage as a form of intraluminal therapy for ECA was actively attempted as a palliative measure in 1909 by Giuzer (77). Such treatment techniques received intermittent periods of attention and neglect through the years; there were no appreciable changes in cure rates and only some subjective and undocumented improvement in palliation. Rider reported on the Canadian experience with combined external radiotherapy and radium bougienage and reported a 37% 3-year survival in a select group of patients with early disease (46,78). Reports of combined external radiotherapy and intraluminal iridium or Cobalt-60 (low, intermediate, and high-dose rates) have indicated good palliation and significant local control (79–83).

While Syed et al used external radiotherapy followed by minimal doses of 5-FU infusion with intraluminal brachytherapy (83), the UCSF–Fresno group used concurrent chemotherapy with 5-FU, mitomycin C, CDDP, methotrexate, and leucovorin with both external and intraluminal high-dose rate (HDR) brachytherapy in locally advanced ECA (84,85). Although follow-up was relatively short for the HDR brachytherapy group, the complete response rate by endoscopy-biopsy is 88%, and 1-year and 2-year disease-free survival rates were 63% and 43%, respectively.

The emerging modality of hyperthermia has found its way into external and intraluminal treatment regimens for ECA in various combinations with surgery, radiotherapy, and chemotherapy (86–89). While these techniques are noteworthy and intriguing attempts at increasing local control of ECA, several inconsistencies in heat delivery require clarification and results are preliminary.

Radiobiologic Strategies

The theoretical advantage of using large radiation fractionation to increase cell kill in the relatively radioresistant "shoulder" portion of cell survival curves has been tested in uncontrolled clinical studies in ECA with no advantage being noted over conventional fractionation regimens (77).

The use of multiple daily fractions of radiotherapy or hyperfractionation has been reported to show significant advantage over conventional fractionation in terms of increased disease-free survival in advanced head and neck cancer (90,91). This method could be used to exploit the dose-survival relationships in ECA by increasing total nominal radiation dose without increasing side effects. Morrison et al reported the M.D. Anderson Hospital experience in 33 patients with ECA treated with preoperative b.i.d. or t.i.d. RT to doses of 3000 to 4600 cGy (43).

A 29% 5-year survival was obtained in those receiving t.i.d. RT.

Chemoprevention

Two major problems have occurred with the management of ECA: the 25 to 85% incidence of local and marginal recurrence rate, and the 25% risk of developing a second aerodigestive tract malignancy at 5 years (12,92). Laboratory and clinical data suggest that a synthetic vitamin A, called cis-retinoic acid, has the potential for reversing dysplastic mucosa to normalcy (93,94). This forms the basis of a current multigroup prospective randomized cancer control study of cis-retinoic acid (or placebo) given to patients who have no evidence of disease after treatment for upper aerodigestive tumors, including those of the esophagus.

Intensification of Chemoradiation Therapy

Chemoradiation protocols for ECA appear to have fairly consistently increased the 1-year, 2-year, and perhaps the 5-year survival figures twofold or threefold compared to either surgery or radiotherapy alone. Toxicity of these regimens does not appear to be excessive and may even be less than either modality alone, probably due to several factors.

1. Most chemoradiation studies employ about 5000 cGy total RT dose, approximately 15% less than conventional RT doses.
2. Several centers have used split-course RT allowing for better normal tissue tolerance.
3. The use of reduced RT fields and the alternating use of effective drugs may be responsible for reduced pulmonary toxicities.

These chemoradiation protocols, with or without esophagectomy, appear to have reached a nadir in terms of 2-year survivals at around 30%. For further improvement, one must intensify both the RT and CT doses without significantly increasing toxicity.

Radiotherapy

With the recognition of the essential heterogeneity of tumor population, it may be worthwhile to use different fractionation schemes within a single treatment schedule. This may entail the use of larger fractions per day for about 1 week, hyperfractionation or accelerated fractionation for another week, and the use of intraluminal boosts with moderate-dose-rate or high-dose-rate units.

Chemotherapy

There are several drugs and drug combinations (Table 21–1) that have moderate activity against ECA and that have yet to be exploited in a chemoradiation regimen. The theoretical advantages of using several drugs in such a regimen include the following.

1. To reduce the incidence of drug resistance.
2. To exploit different mechanisms of action against different cell subpopulations in a heterogeneous tumor by synchronization and direct cell kill.
3. To reduce overall toxicity by interspersing drugs with differential toxicity.

There are also potential theoretic advantages of using chemotherapeutic agents in the perioperative setting, which would be similar to using a systemic agent simultaneously with a local modality such as RT. Intensive induction chemotherapy would potentially increase the resectability rate in a manner similar to preoperative radiotherapy. This approach would address the potential problem of tumor spill and dissemination during surgery.

SUGGESTED TREATMENT AND RESEARCH APPROACHES

It is recommended that all patients with biopsy-proven ECA be staged clinically with endoscopy, biopsy, CT scan of mediastinum and upper abdomen, blood chemistries including liver profile, and radioisotopic scans as necessary. No specific recommendations are being made for adenocarcinomas because no significant difference in outcome has been noted in any recent radiotherapy, surgical, or chemoradiation series. A clinical staging system, such as those suggested by John et al (71) or Coia (76), is recommended. These systems take into consideration that most ECA do not undergo surgical staging, maintain overt resemblance with the 1975 American Joint Committee on Cancer (AJCC) Staging System (with regard to T classification), and are based on clinical and radiologic studies readily available in most countries.

Stage I ($T_1N_0M_0$) Middle and Lower Third Esophagus

The treatment options suggested for patients with early Stage I disease include radical esophagectomy and en-bloc resection of the posterior mediastinum or a definitive chemoradiation regimen. The option of choice should depend primarily on the physician's familiarity and interest in either modality. It is recommended that the surgical option be exercised only by surgeons who have a special interest in these patients and preferably by those who have significant experience with this difficult surgical procedure and the specialized postoperative care that is required to prevent perioperative and late complications.

The option of chemoradiation therapy is apparently more innocuous and is not associated with a significant mortality rate. However, there is potential for significant pulmonary morbidity and even mortality when the two modalities are combined. The opportunity for surgical salvage exists and should be considered in select patients.

Stage I ($T_1N_0M_0$) Upper Third (Cervical Esophagus) Stage II and III Middle and Lower Third Esophagus

For patients with locally advanced Stage II and III disease the recommended course of action is a fairly intense multiple drug–RT concurrent treatment similar to those detailed in Table 21–5. It is preferred, of course, that patients be entered through a recognized protocol that is studying the proper administration of drugs and RT. This recommendation is based on consistent 1- and 2-year survival rates obtained by chemoradiation protocols that are superior to those obtained by surgery or RT alone.

The second option suggested would be a combination of perioperative chemotherapy and surgery. The induction chemotherapy used in such protocols has been comparatively ineffective. It is suggested, therefore, that intensification of chemotherapy be undertaken and consideration be given to employing infusional drug therapy during the surgical procedure and that maintenance chemotherapy and/or chemoradiation measures be undertaken postsurgery.

Stage IV and Recurrent Tumors

Despite the short expected duration of life in patients with Stage IV and recurrent tumors, there is hope for prolonged palliation in some of these patients. Syed et al, for example, reported a 25-month mean survival for 10 patients who presented with recurrent esophageal carcinoma (83). Palliative treatment approaches in these patients, therefore, must be of short duration with few, if any, side effects. Consequently, any number of newer chemotherapeutic drugs could be used in these patients in conjunction with brief courses of local RT or bypass surgical procedures. Such an approach would serve the need for the study of newer drugs in this disease, help define their interaction with RT and surgery, and provide local palliation of the most common and distressing symptom of dysphagia.

Adenocarcinoma of the Esophagus

Adenocarcinomas of the esophagus are generally considered to be uncommon. However, as previously discussed, its incidence in the Caucasian population appears to be increasing (4).

Most previous reports of chemoradiation in ECA have suggested that no difference exists in the outcome between squamous cell carcinoma and adenocarcinomas of the esophagus. Coia et al indicated that adenocarcinomas of the esophagus are adequately treated by definitive chemoradiation and that esophagectomy may not be necessary (69,95).

Forastiere and co-workers, at the University of Michigan, reported a systematic approach to esophageal adenocarcinomas. Urba et al initially reported on 48 patients treated by THE alone (96). The 62% 1-year survival rate and the 48% 2-year survival rate were not improved by subsequent trials using single and multiple drug regimens and nonstandard RT fractionations (97–99). Their rationale for using THE is to document the histologic response to various chemoradiation combinations (99). Ajani and colleagues, at M.D. Anderson Cancer Center, treated 35 patients with esophageal adenocarcinoma with three to four courses of 5-FU, CDDP, and etoposide (VP-16) preoperatively and reported just one complete pathologic response and a median survival of 23 months (100). Both groups are engaged in Phase II and III prospective trials involved in refining preoperative chemoradiation or comparing it to THE alone.

CONTROVERSIES IN MANAGEMENT OF ECA

The current optimal treatments for nonmetastatic ECA is a concurrent combination of chemotherapy and radiotherapy delivered preoperatively or as definitive treatment. Unless a dramatic breakthrough occurs, as in immunologic therapy, oncologists are faced by the following two questions.

1. What is the role of esophagectomy in the curative approach to ECA?
2. What constitutes the best chemoradiation combination for ECA?

Role of Esophagectomy

Table 21–6 is a composite metaanalysis of various definitive treatment options involving chemotherapy that have been and continue to be used in nonmetastatic ECA.

It can be seen that preoperative chemotherapy alone can achieve prolonged survival in a very select group of patients. Since four of five studies in this group (Table 21–2) used RT postoperatively, one could argue that RT can be restricted to those patients who have residual disease at surgery. Kelsen et al reported on 48 patients who received two cycles of CDDP, bleomycin, and vindesine preoperatively (and RT postoperatively) (101). A median survival of 10.4 months and a 4-year actuarial survival of 10% was noted. They suggested that chemotherapy was as effective as RT in treating local tumors and that induction preoperative chemotherapy should be a continued avenue of investigation for ECA. However, the 6 to 10% operative mortality rate in these studies should be considered. The chemoradiation studies, particularly with combinations of drugs, achieve similar median and 2-year survivals without the treatment mortality associated with the surgical studies.

Even for early ECA, there are some indications suggesting that chemoradiation can supplant radical esophagectomy and thereby avoid the mortality associated with the latter. Coia reported a local relapse-free rate of

Table 21–6. Results of Chemotherapy—Aided Combined Modality Management of Esophageal Carcinoma

Series	Number of Reports (Patients)	RT Dose (cGy)	Chemotherapy Drugs/ No. of Cycles	Surg/Tx Mortality	Survival Median (mos)	Survival 1 Yr (%)	Survival 2 Yr (%)
Preoperative Chemotherapy	5(109)	4500–5500 in 4 series*	5-FU, CDDP, BLM, VDS, MGBG (2 cycles)	6	19	64	46
Preoperative Chemoradiation	9(404)	3000–6000	5-FU + Mito C, 5-FU + CDDP ± VBL (1-2 cycles)	14	16	53	31
Chemoradiation (single drug)	5(98)	4000–6900	5-FU, BLM, ADR (3-9 cycles)	0	10	51	17
Chemoradiation (multiple drugs)	7(200)	3000–6000	5-FU, CDDP, MTX, Mito C, BLM, LVR, VCR (2-5 cycles)	2	16	57	34

RT = radiotherapy; 5-FU = 5-fluorouracil; CDDP = cisplatinum; BLM = bleomycin; VDS = vindesine; MGBG = mitoguozone; VBL = vinblastine; ADR = Adriamycin; VCR = vincristine.
*Radiotherapy given postoperatively in 4/5 series.

100% at 1 year for Stage I tumors (76). The question of whether esophagectomy has a role following chemoradiation is debatable and requires quick resolution in the interest of progress. If surgery follows chemoradiation, then serious consideration must be given to altering the currently used preoperative chemoradiation regimen, with the possibility of excluding RT altogether and using more intensive chemotherapy regimens in the preoperative period. If surgery does not follow chemoradiation, then one can proceed with the gradual escalation of both chemotherapy and radiation doses in progressively aggressive chemoradiation protocols, without the apprehension of increased morbidity/mortality that would certainly accompany esophagectomy.

The pros and cons of esophagectomy following chemoradiation therapy are as follows.

One of the major reasons why surgery would be useful in ECA is the accurate staging possible. In fact, the 1988 AJC Staging System has changed the preexisting T classification to accommodate the prognostic factor of depth of tumor invasion, which can only be gauged by surgical staging. On the other hand, neither the 1978 nor the 1988 AJC Staging System takes into consideration the fact that most patients with ECA will simply not be surgically staged. This is a reflection of the locally advanced and/or distal disease status in most patients, coupled with the inordinate cachexia and poor performance status frequently associated with ECA.

The Chinese experience of about 86% 5-year survival rates in asymptomatic patients with primary tumors measuring less than 2 cm without muscular wall penetration or lymph node metastases is frequently cited as another reason why esophagectomy should be continued as an integral part of treatment for ECA (11,26). Skinner has advocated radical mediastinectomy as part of an en-bloc resection of the esophagus and adjacent structures when regional nodes are involved and muscle penetration exists (27). Even so, in his series of 181 patients, only 80 (44%) were suitable for radical treatment (in this case, surgery). In these select 80 patients, the 1-, 2-, and 5-year actuarial survival rates were 52%, 33%, and 18%, respectively. This is apparently no better (or worse) than the 68%, 45%, and 32% survival rates reported in a group of 22 inoperable/unresectable patients by John et al (85). The Chinese example is not duplicable because fewer patients with far more advanced disease are diagnosed in the United States.

Esophagectomy, even with radical mediastinectomy, may not be consistently or more frequently effective due to the inherent anatomical restrictions endowed by the lymphatic drainage of the middle and lower third of the esophagus (10). A rich plexus of lymphatic capillaries in the mucosal and submucosal layers communicates more freely in the long axis of the esophagus than in the circumferential direction. They drain into the paraesophageal nodes that occupy the posterior mediastinum. Most of the nodes draining the upper third of the esophagus drain into the jugular nodes in the neck. The middle third paraesophageal nodes drain into another level of nodes lying between the aorta and the esophagus. The portion of the esophagus below the bifurcation of the trachea drain into subdiaphragmatic nodes, the celiac chain, and then the para-aortic chain. According to Skinner, a radical resection of the posterior mediastinum would remove "both pleural surfaces, the pericardium, the esophageal mesentery, azygous vein, thoracic duct, aortic arterial branches and adjacent lymphatic and fibrofatty tissue" —a formidable task indeed (27).

Finally, the major factor correlated with longterm survival in most preoperative studies is whether the patient has been rendered tumor-free at the time of surgery. The presence of disease in the esophagectomy specimen is tantamount to treatment failure. Because there is a new wealth of evidence suggesting that clearance of ECA is both radiation dose dependent and chemotherapy dose related, it is evident that more aggressive chemoradiation protocols must be undertaken. The Leichman study (1987) was a step in this direction, using moderate doses of radiotherapy and several active drugs (70). Unfortunately, while the survival and quality of survival were superior in this series and although no toxicity-related death was reported, the toxicity of the drug regimen was excessive and "prohibitive."

Therefore, if the reader agrees that more intensive chemoradiation protocols are the logical means of progress in this disease, then the place for esophagectomy in ECA is suspect for the following reasons.

1. The addition of esophagectomy has had no impact on survival in patients treated with chemoradiation protocols.
2. The perioperative mortality rates may have decreased significantly in the last decade but still approximate 9%, a figure that is unacceptable in most other surgical procedures.
3. The overall morbidity of treating ECA is bound to increase as radiation and chemotherapy doses are increased; the addition of esophagectomy in this scenario would only increase morbidity and further worsen perioperative mortality statistics.

The second question regarding the nature of the optimal chemoradiation regimen is equally debatable. The central aim should be to use the most effective RT and chemotherapy combinations in the shortest period of time (see Chapter 5). Compared to current chemoradiation regimens, this may entail the use of hyperfractionated external RT, intraluminal RT, alternating various effective drugs (using them for longer maintenance periods), and biologic modifiers and radioprotectors.

CONCLUSION

Table 21–7 is a composite meta-analysis of the use of surgery, radiotherapy, and chemoradiation in ECA. It clearly indicates that chemoradiation has provided a remarkable improvement, if not a quantum leap, in the treatment results of ECA. There may be some disagreements regarding the specific roles of surgery, chemotherapy, and radiation in a multimodality approach to ECA. However, after 70 years of stagnant cure rates and relentless morbidity that characterized the management of ECA, the last decade has clearly marked the advent and consolidation of the role of chemoradiation in this disease. It undoubtedly represents the first ray of hope for sizable cure rates in the future.

REFERENCES

1. Schottenfeld D. Epidemiology of cancer of the esophagus. Semin Oncol 11(2):92, 1984.
2. Frank-Stromborg M. The epidemiology and primary prevention of gastric and esophageal cancer. A worldwide perspective. Cancer Nurs 12(2):53, 1989.
3. Ayiomamitis A. Epidemiology of cancer of the esophagus in Canada 1931–1984. Gastroenterology 94:374, 1988.
4. Blot WJ, Devesa SS, Kneller RW, Fraumeni JF Jr. Rising incidence of the adenocarcinoma of the esophagus and gastric cardia. JAMA 265(10):1287, 1991.
5. Wynder EL, Mabuchi K. Etiological and environmental factors. *In:* Cancer of the gastrointestinal tract. B. Esophagus. Detection and diagnosis. Current concepts in cancer. Rubin P (Ed). JAMA 226(13):1546, 1973.
6. Fisher SA, Brady LW. Carcinoma of the esophagus. *In:* Principles and Practices of Radiation Oncology. Perez CA, Brady LW (Eds). Philadelphia, WB Saunders Co., 1987, p. 700.
7. Khuroo MS, Zargar SA, Mahajan R, Banday MA. High incidence of oesophageal and gastric cancers in Kashmir in a population with

Table 21–7. Meta-analysis of Results of Treatment of Esophageal Carcinoma by Three Major Methods

Modality	Number of Patients (Reports)	Treatment Mortality	Survival 2-Yr (%)	Survival 5-Yr (%)
Surgery (21,22,29)	67,885 (124)	33⁺	12	6
Radiotherapy (37,101)	8,933 (50)	0	8	6
Chemoradiation** (± surgery)	811 (26)	5.5*	32	25⁺⁺

⁺Surgical mortality in smaller recent reports average < 10%
⁺⁺Based on two reports (71,102)
*10% mortality in surgical series; 1% in nonsurgical series
**From Table 21–6

special personal and dietary habits. GUT 33(1):11, 1992.
8. Reid BJ. Barrett's esophagus and esophageal adenocarcinoma. Gastroenteral Clin North Am 20(4):817, 1991.
9. Benamouzig R, Pigot F, Quiroga G, et al. Human papillomavirus infection in esophageal squamous cell carcinoma in western countries. Int J Cancer 50(4):549, 1992.
10. Weinberg JA. Esophagus. *In:* Lymphatics in Cancer. Haagensen CD, Feind CR, Herter FP, Slanetz CA, Weinberg JA (Eds). Philadelphia, WB Saunders Co., 1972, p. 245.
11. Skinner DB. Surgical treatment for esophageal carcinoma. Semin Oncol 11(2):136, 1984.
12. Aisner J, Forastiere A, Aroney R. Patterns of recurrence for cancer of the lung and esophagus. *In:* Cancer Treatment Symposia: Proceedings of the Workshop on Patterns of Failure After Cancer Treatment. Vol. 2. Wittes RE (Ed). Washington, US Dept of Health and Human Services, 1983, p. 87.
13. Elkon D, Lee MS, Hendrickson FR. Carcinoma of the esophagus. Sites of recurrence and palliative benefits after definitive radiotherapy. Int J Radiat Oncol Biol Phys 4:615, 1978.
14. Mandard AM, Chasle J, Marnay J, Villedieu B, et al. Autopsy findings in 111 cases of esophageal cancer. Cancer 48:329, 1981.
15. Mantravadi RVP, Thomas L, Briele H, et al. Carcinoma of the esophagus: Sites of failure. Int J Radiat Oncol Biol Phys 8:1897, 1981.
16. Goodner JT. Surgical principles of resection and reconstruction. *In:* Cancer of the Gastrointestinal Tract. Esophagus: Treatment–localized and advanced. Current concepts in cancer. Rubin P (Ed). JAMA 227(2):176, 1974.
17. Pearson JG. The value of radiotherapy in the management of esophageal cancer. Am J Roentgenol 105:500, 1969.
18. Boring C, Squires TS, Tong T. Cancer Statistics 1992. CA 42(1):19, 1992.
19. Torek F. The first successful case of resection of the thoracic portion of the esophagus for carcinoma. Surg Gynecol Obstet 16:614, 1913.
20. Pearson JG. The present status and future potential of radiotherapy in the management of esophageal cancer. Cancer 39:882, 1977.
21. Earlam R, Cunha-Melo JR. Oesophageal squamous cell carcinoma. I. A critical review of surgery. Br J Surg 67(6):381, 1980.
22. Lam KH, Wong J, Lim STK, Ong GB. Surgical treatment of carcinoma of the upper third of the esophagus. *In:* Medical and Surgical Problems of the Esophagus. Stipa S, Belsey RHR, Moraldi A (Eds). New York, Academic Press Inc., 1981, p. 353.
23. Borst HG, Dragojevic C, Peck W. Carcinoma of the esophagus. Results of resection and reconstruction. *In:* Medical and Surgical Problems of the Esophagus. Proceedings of the Serono Symposium. Vol. 43. Stipa S, Belsey RHR, Moraldi A (Eds). New York, Academic Press Inc., 1981, p. 345.
24. Endo M, Kinoshita Y, Yamada A, et al. Surgical treatment of thoracic esophageal cancer, including clinical evaluation of early esophageal cancer. *In:* Cancer of the Esophagus. Vol. II. Pfeiffer CJ (Ed). Boca Raton, FL, CRC Press Inc., 1982, p. 57.
25. Hilgenberg AD, Carey RW, Wilkins EW, et al. Preoperative chemotherapy, surgical resection, and selective postoperative therapy for squamous cell carcinoma of the esophagus. Ann Thorac Surg 45:357, 1988.
26. Huang KC. Diagnosis and surgical treatment of early esophageal carcinoma. *In:* Medical and Surgical Problems of the Esophagus. Proceedings of the Symposium. Stipa S, Belsey RHR, Moraldi A (Eds). New York, Academic Press Inc., 1981, p. 296.
27. Skinner DB. Mediastinectomy for esophageal carcinoma. *In:* Medical and Surgical Problems of the Esophagus. Proceedings of the Serono Symposium. Stipa S, Belsey RHR, Moraldi A (Eds). 1981, p. 331.
28. Skinner DB. En-bloc resection for neoplasms of the esophagus and cardia. J Thorac Cardiovasc Surg 85:59, 1983.
29. Giuli R, Gignoux M. Treatment of carcinoma of the esophagus. Retrospective study of 2,400 patients. Ann Surg 192(1):44, 1980.
30. Katlic MR, Wilkins EW Jr, Grillo HC. Three decades of treatment of esophageal squamous carcinoma of the Massachusetts General Hospital. J Thorac Cardiovasc Surg 99(5):929, 1990.
31. Boyce HW. Palliation of advanced esophageal carcer. Semin Oncol 11(2):186, 1984.
32. Shakian DM, Neptune WB, Ellis FH, et al. Transthoracic versus extrathoracic esophagectomy, mortality, morbidity and long-term survival. Ann Thorac Surg 41:237, 1986.
33. der Hartog Jagern FCA, Bartelman JFWM, Tygat GN. Palliative treatment of obstructing esophagogastric malignancy by endoscopic positioning of a plastic prosthesis. Gastroenterology 77:1008, 1979.
34. Hagenmuller F, Sander C, Ries G, Classen M. Laser and endoluminal 192-Iridium radiation. Endoscopy 19:16, 1987.
35. Bown SG, Hawes R, Matthenson K, et al. Endoscopic laser palliation for advanced malignant dysphagia. GUT 28:799, 1987.

36. Krasner N, Barr H, Skidmore C, Morris AI. Palliative laser therapy for malignant dysphagia. GUT 28:799, 1987.
37. Earlam R, Cunha-Melo JR. Oesophageal squamous cell carcinoma: I. A critical review of radiotherapy. Br J Surg 67(7):457, 1980.
38. Akakura I, Nakamura Y, Kakegawa T, et al. Surgery of carcinoma of the esophagus with preoperative radiotherapy. Chest 57:47, 1970.
39. Launois B, Delarue D, Campion JP, Kerbaol M. Preoperative radiotherapy for carcinoma of the esophagus. Surg Gynecol Obstet 153:690, 1981.
40. Doggett RLS, Guernsey JM, Bagshaw MA. Combined radiation and surgical treatment of carcinoma of the thoracic esophagus. Radiation Ther Oncol 5:147, 1970.
41. Nakayama K, Kinoshita Y. Surgical treatment combined with preoperative concentrated irradiation. *In:* Cancer of the gastrointestinal tract. Esophagus: Treatment–local and advanced. JAMA 227(2):178, 1974.
42. van Andel JG, Dees J, Dijkhuis M, et al. Carcinoma of the esophagus. Results of treatment. Ann Surg 190(6):684, 1979.
43. Morrison WH, Rich TA, Quong G, et al. Accelerated hyperfractionated, preoperative radiation therapy for esophageal carcinoma. Proceedings of the 33rd Annual ASTRO Meeting (Abstract 121). 21(Suppl):179, 1991.
44. Kasai M, Mori S, Watanabe T. Follow up results after resection of thoracic esophageal carcinoma. World J Surg 2:543, 1978.
45. Rubin P. Introduction. *In:* Cancer of the gastrointestinal tract. B. Esophagus: Treatment–localized and advanced. JAMA 227(2):175, 1974.
46. Rider WD. Innovations in radiation therapy. *In:* Cancer of the gastrointestinal tract. B. Esophagus: Treatment–localized and advanced. JAMA 227(2):183, 1974.
47. Kelsen D. Chemotherapy of esophageal cancer. Semin Oncol 11(2):159, 1984.
48. Kelsen DP. Chemotherapy for loco-regional and advanced esophageal cancer. Cancer Updates 2(10):1, 1988.
49. Kies MS, Rosen ST, Tsang TK, et al. Cisplatin and 5-fluorouracil in the primary management of squamous esophageal cancer. Cancer 60:2156, 1987.
50. Kelsen D, Hilaris B, Coonley C. Cisplatin, vindesine and bleomycin chemotherapy of local-regional and advanced esophageal carcinoma. Am J Med 75:645, 1983.
51. Kelsen DP, Fein R, Coonley C, et al. Cisplatin, vindesine and mitoguozone in the treatment of esophageal cancer. Cancer Treat Rep 70(2):255, 1986.
52. Roth JA, Pass HI, Flanagan M, et al. Randomized clinical trial of preoperative and postoperative adjuvant chemotherapy with cisplatin, vindesine and bleomycin for carcinoma of the esophagus. J Thorac Cardiovasc Surg 96:242, 1988.
53. Steiger Z, Franklin R, Wilson RF, et al. Complete eradication of squamous cell carcinoma of the esophagus with combined chemotherapy and radiotherapy. Am Surg 47:95, 1981.
54. Franklin R, Steiger Z, Vaishampayan G, et al. Combined modality therapy for esophageal squamous cell carcinoma. Cancer 51:1062, 1983.
55. Leichman L, Steiger Z, Seydel HG. Preoperative chemotherapy and radiation therapy for patients with cancer of the esophagus. A potentially curative approach. J Clin Oncol 2(2):75, 1984.
56. Poplin E, Fleming T, Leichman L, et al. Combined therapies for squamous cell carcinoma of the esophagus, a Southwest Oncology Group Study (SWOG-8307). J Clin Oncol 5:622, 1987.
57. Richmond J, Seydel HG, Bae Y, et al. Comparison of three treatment strategies for esophageal cancer within a single institution. Int J Radiat Oncol Biol Phys 13:1617, 1987.
58. Seydel HG, Leichman L, Byhardt R, et al. The Radiation Therapy Oncology Group. Preoperative radiation and chemotherapy for localized squamous cell carcinoma of the esophagus. A RTOG study. Int J Radiat Oncol Biol Phys 14:33, 1987.
59. Herskovic A, Leichman L, Lattin P, et al. Chemoradiation with and without surgery in the thoracic esophagus. The Wayne State experience. Int J Radiat Oncol Biol Phys 15:655, 1988.
60. Parker EF, Marks RD, Kratz J, et al. Chemoradiation therapy and resection for carcinoma of the esophagus. Short term results. Ann Thorac Surg 40(2):121, 1985.
61. Orringer MB, Forastiere AA, Perez-Tamayo C, et al. Chemotherapy and radiation therapy before transhiatal esophagectomy for esophageal carcinoma. Ann Thorac Surg 49(3):348, 1990.
62. Kolaric K, Maricic Z, Dujmovic I, Roth A. Therapy of advanced esophageal cancer with bleomycin, irradiation and combination of bleomycin with irradiation. Tumori 62:255, 1976.
63. Kolaric K, Maricic Z, Roch A, Dujmovic I. Adriamycin alone and in combination with

radiotherapy in the treatment of inoperable esophageal cancer. Tumori 63:485, 1977.
64. Earle JD, Gelber RD, Moertel CG, Hahn RG. A controlled evaluation of combined radiation and bleomycin therapy for squamous cell carcinoma of the esophagus. Int J Radiat Oncol Biol Phys 6:821, 1980.
65. Byfield JE, Barone R, Mendelsohn J, et al. Infusional 5-fluorouracil and x-ray therapy for non-resectable esophageal cancer. Cancer 45:703, 1980.
66. Lokich JJ, Shea M, Chaffey J. Sequential infusional 5-fluorouracil followed by concomitant radiation for tumors of the esophagus and gastroesophageal junction. Cancer 60:275, 1987.
67. Marcial A, Velez-Garcia E, Cintron J, Ydrach AA. Radiotherapy preceded by multidrug chemotherapy in carcinoma of the esophagus. A pilot study of the Radiation Therapy Oncology Group. Can Clin Trials 3:127, 1980.
68. Keane TJ, Harwood AR, Elhaleim T, et al. Radical radiation therapy with 5-fluorouracil infusion and mitomycin C for oesophageal squamous carcinoma. Radiother Oncol 4:205, 1985.
69. Coia LR, Engstrom PF, Paul A. Nonsurgical management of esophageal cancer: Report of a study of combined radiotherapy and chemotherapy. J Clin Oncol 5:1783, 1987.
70. Leichman L, Herskovic A, Leichman CG, et al. Nonoperative therapy for squamous-cell cancer of the esophagus. J Clin Oncol 5(3):365, 1987.
71. John MJ, Flam MS, Mowry PA, et al. Radiotherapy alone and chemoradiation for nonmetastatic esophageal carcinoma. A critical review of chemoradiation. Cancer 63:2397, 1989.
72. Seitz JF, Giovannini M, Padant-Cesana J, et al. Inoperable nonmetastatic squamous cell carcinoma of the esophagus managed by concomitant chemotherapy (5-fluorouracil and cisplatin) and radiation therapy. Cancer 66:214, 1990.
73. John M, Flam M, Wittlinger P, Mowry PA. Inoperable esophageal carcinoma. Results of aggressive synchronous radiotherapy and chemotherapy. A pilot study. Am J Clin Oncol (CCT) 10(4):310, 1987.
74. Herskovic A, Martz K, Al-Sarraf M, et al. Combined chemotherapy and radiotherapy compared with radiotherapy alone in patients with cancer of the esophagus. N Engl J Med 326:1593, 1992.
75. Martini N, Goodner JT, D'Angio GJ, et al. Tracheo-esophageal fistulae due to cancer. J Thorac Cardiovasc Surg 59:319, 1970.
76. Coia LR. Esophageal cancer. Is esophagectomy necessary? Oncology. 3(4):101, 1989.
77. Hancock SL, Glatstein E. Radiotherapy of esophageal cancer. Semin Oncol 11(2):144, 1984.
78. Rider WD, Diaz-Menodz R. Some opinions on the treatment of cancer of the esophagus. Am J Roentgenol 105:514, 1969.
79. Bottrill DO, Plane JH, Newaishy GA. A proposed afterloading technique for irradiation of the oesophagus. Br J Radiol 52:573, 1979.
80. George FW. Radiation management in esophageal cancer. Am J Surg 139:795, 1980.
81. Abe M, Kitagawa T. Treatment of esophageal cancer with high dose rate intracavitary irradiation. Tohoku J Exp Med 134:159, 1981.
82. Moorthy CR, Nibhanupudy JR, Ashayeri E, et al. Intraluminal radiation for esophageal cancer. A Howard University technique. J Natl Med Assoc 74:261, 1982.
83. Syed AMN, Puthawala AA, Severeance S, Zamost B. Intraluminal irradiation in the treatment of esophageal cancer. Endocurietherapy/Hyperthermic Oncology. 3:105, 1987.
84. John MJ. Esophageal carcinoma. *In:* Concomitant Continuous Infusion Chemotherapy and Radiation. Rotman M, Rosenthal CJ (Eds). Berlin, Springer Verlag, 1991, p. 247.
85. John M, Flam M. Curative treatment approaches for esophageal cancer. *In:* Radiotherapy/chemotherapy interactions in cancer therapy. Front Radiat Ther Oncol 26:83, 1992.
86. Li DJ, Hon BS. Preliminary report on the treatment of esophageal cancer by intraluminal microwave hyperthermia and chemotherapy. Cancer Treat Rep 71(11):1013, 1987.
87. Petrovich Z, Astrahan M, Lam K, et al. Intraluminal thermoradiotherapy with teletherapy for carcinoma of the esophagus. Endocuritherapy/Hyperthermia Oncol 4:155, 1988.
88. Astrahan MA, Sapozink MD, Luxton G, et al. A technique for combining microwave hyperthermia with intraluminal brachytherapy of the oesophagus. Int J Hyperthermia 5(1):37, 1989.
89. Astrahan MA, Sapozink MD, Luxton G, et al. A technique for combining microwave hyperthermia with intraluminal brachytherapy of the oesophagus. Int J Hyperthermia 5(1):37, 1989.
90. Wang CC. Local control of oropharyngeal carcinoma after two accelerated hyperfractionation radiation therapy schemes. Int J Radiat Biol Phys 14(6):1143, 1988.

91. Million RR, Parsons JT. The University of Florida experience with two fractions per day for head and neck cancer. Front Radiat Ther Oncol 22:79, 1988.
92. Fogel TD, Harrison LB, Yung HS. Subsequent upper aerodigestive malignancies following treatment of esophageal cancer. Cancer 55:1882, 1981.
93. Goodman DS. Vitamin A and retinoids in health and disease. N Engl J Med 310:1023, 1984.
94. Meyskens FL, Gilmartin E, Alberts DS, et al. Activity of isotretinoin against squamous cell cancers and preneoplastic lesions. Cancer Treat Rep 66:1315, 1982.
95. Coia LR, Paul AR, Engstrom PF. Combined radiation and chemotherapy as primary management of adenocarcinoma of the esophagus and gastroesophageal junction. Cancer 61:643, 1988.
96. Urba SG, Orringer MB, Perez-Tamayo C, et al. Concurrent preoperative chemotherapy and radiation therapy in localized esophageal adenocarcinoma. Cancer 69(2):285, 1992.
97. Forastiere AA, Gennis M, Orringer MB, Agha FA. Cisplatin, vinblastine and mitoguazone chemotherapy for epidermoid and adenocarcinoma of the esophagus. J Clin Oncol 5:1143, 1987.
98. Forastiere AA, Orringer MB, Perez-Tamayo C, et al. Concurrent chemotherapy and radiation therapy followed by transhiatal esophagectomy for local-regional carcinoma of the esophagus. J Clin Oncol 8:119, 1990.
99. Urba SG, Orringer MS, Perez-Tamayo G, et al. Concurrent preoperative chemotherapy and radiation therapy in localized esophageal adenocarcinoma. Cancer 69(2):285, 1972.
100. Ajani JA, Roth JA, Ryan B, et al. Evaluation of pre and postoperative chemotherapy for resectable adenocarcinoma of the esophagus or gastroesophageal junction. J Clin Oncol 8:1231, 1990.
101. Kelsen DP, Minsky B, Smith M, et al. Preoperative therpay for esophageal cancer. A randomized comparison of chemotherapy versus radiotherapy. J Clin Oncol 8:1352, 1990.
102. Newaishy GA, Read GA, Duncan W, Kerr GR. Results of radical radiotherapy of squamous cell carcinoma of the esophagus. Clin Radiol 33:347, 1982.
103. Coia LR, Engstrom PF, Paul AR, et al. Long-term results of infusional 5-FU, mitomycin C and radiation as primary management of esophageal carcinoma. Int J Radiat Oncol Biol Phys 20(1):29, 1991.

Chapter 22

STOMACH, PANCREAS, BILIARY SYSTEM

TYVIN A. RICH AND JAFFER A. AJANI

INTRODUCTION

In 1992, cancers of the stomach and the pancreaticobiliary tract accounted for approximately 67,700 new cases in the United States, approximately 50,600 (83%) of which will have progressive disease regardless of the administered therapy (1). Although precise figures are not available, a reasonable estimate is that about one-half of the total patients will die with symptomatic uncontrolled local disease as a component of the failure pattern (2,3,4). Another estimate is that an additional one-third will also have asymptomatic locoregional disease in conjunction with distant metastases. Surgical techniques and postoperative care have improved over the past decades, but this has resulted in only a small increase in cure rate, mainly for those with early-stage disease. Radiation therapy (RT) and chemotherapy have been used for palliation of local symptoms, an alternative curative therapy for selected patients unfit for surgery, and as an adjuvant to surgery in those with pathologically determined cancer extending beyond the confines of the organ. This chapter emphasizes the use of chemotherapy combined concurrently with RT for tumors arising in these locations. Sequential chemotherapy treatment before or after RT will be mentioned when these data further the understanding of the interaction between these modalities.

BACKGROUND

The details of the radiobiologic and pharmacologic basis of the combination of chemotherapeutic agents plus RT are beyond the scope of this chapter. The reader is referred to the introductory chapters of this text concerning the rationale for temporal cooperation between simultaneously administered chemotherapy and RT. It is important, however, to examine some of the basic scientific findings that led to the early clinical trials regarding halogenated pyrimidines and concomitant RT. Laboratory studies by Heidelberger showed that 5-fluorouracil (5-FU) plus RT was additive or, in some cases, synergistic at dosages of each modality that were not curative by themselves (5). Clinical trials using a combination of 5-FU plus RT were started, and by 1963, there was a compendium of over 30 clinical trials reported in the North American literature (6). Initially, 5-FU was given as a bolus administration with RT; however, more recently, a rationale for its use by continuous venous administration has emerged. The reader is referred to sources that review this subject in greater detail (7,8).

The landmark clinical trials of 5-FU plus RT for gastrointestinal cancers were performed at Mayo Clinic in the 1960s and 1970s. In the first study on 42 patients with advanced gastrointestinal cancers, a maximum dose of 15 mg/kg/day of 5-FU administered by bolus intravenous injection was determined to be tolerable for three successive days (9). The use of longer 5-FU treatment schedules resulted in unacceptable acute complications, including moderate to severe leukopenia, stomatitis, and some fatal toxicity. There was no correlation between toxicity and the radiation dosage (220- to 550-cGy fractions), field size (< 200 cm^2), or field location. This study determined that 5-FU in total doses of 40 to 50 mg/kg at the beginning of radiotherapy was tolerated and that higher doses were associated with unacceptable side effects.

A follow-up controlled, randomized study was undertaken at the Mayo Clinic to confirm the apparent value of concomitant 5-FU plus RT for the patient with advanced gastrointestinal cancer (10). Patients with advanced, unresected stomach, pancreas, and colon cancers were randomized to receive 5-FU or placebo for the first three days of radiotherapy (3500 to 4000 cGy). The results showed a significant improvement in survival for all patients treated with 5-FU plus RT. The duration of palliation of local symptoms was also improved (11 vs. 17 months) in favor of those receiving combined modality therapy.

STOMACH CANCER

Postsurgical Residual/Unresectable Disease

In 1982, the Gastrointestinal Tumor Study Group (GITSG) reported the results of a prospective, randomized trial of chemotherapy alone versus chemotherapy plus RT for locally advanced gastric cancer (11). All patients had residual tumor ranging from microscopic residual disease (44 to 51%) to gross unresected disease. The chemotherapy treatment consisted of 5-FU (325 mg/m^2 on days 1 to 5, and days 36 to 40, intravenously) plus methyl-CCNU (150 mg/m^2 day 1, orally) given every 5 weeks for 18 months. The chemoradiation arm used the same systemic chemotherapy schedule plus radiation: 5-FU (500 mg/m^2) intravenously during days 1 to 3 of RT, administered twice during an interrupted radiotherapy treatment schedule of 5000 cGy given in a total of 8 weeks. The results initially favored patients treated with chemotherapy alone, in whom the 1-year survival was 68% versus 44% for chemoradiation. This large survival difference involved 14 deaths in the chemoradiation group versus five deaths with chemotherapy alone encountered in the first 26 weeks of the study. The acute gastrointestinal toxicity of chemoradiation treatment can be formidable in patients who have undergone gastrectomy or in those with upper GI dysfunction secondary to disease. As late follow-up became available, the eventual superiority of the chemoradiation arm over the chemotherapy arm became evident. With follow-up of 2 to 4 years, 8 of 45 patients who received chemoradiation were alive and free of disease, compared to 3 of 45 patients who received chemotherapy alive. At 48 months, the actuarial survival for the chemoradiation group was 25% and ~10% for the resected and nonresected subgroups, respectively. These trends favoring surgical resection were also seen for patients treated with chemotherapy alone.

The importance of the total radiation dose can be inferred from the GITSG trial and by comparison with other trials (Table 22–1). First, there appears to be better survival with concurrent chemoradiation when compared to the data from the prospective randomized trial from Cape Town, South Africa reported by Dent et al in 1979 (12). In the latter trial, 5-FU (500 mg/day × 4 days) was given prior to low-dose RT. The actuarial survival at 140 weeks was 35 to 40% for all patients treated with curative surgery; however, this result primarily reflects the favorable outcome in T_1–T_2 N_O patients. The need for adequate total radiation dose is relevant because the Cape Town study limited the RT dose to 2000 cGy (^{60}Co irradiation). Only 5% survived beyond 110 weeks in those with residual or unresectable disease. The finding of a 20 to 25% survival at 4 years in the GITSG study in comparison indicates a marginal but real improvement in results with the additional chemotherapy (MeCCNU) and chemoradiation when higher external beam radiotherapy doses were used.

In 1985, the Eastern Cooperative Oncology Group (ECOG) reported a prospective, randomized study comparing 5-FU alone (31 patients) versus 5-FU plus RT (26 patients) (13). In this case, the total radiation dose was 4000 cGy given over 4 weeks with 600 mg of 5-FU given intravenously as a bolus. There was no difference in median survival or time to treatment failure for either group. Although the dose of irradiation was moderate, there were two fatal toxicities (2/26 = 1.5%) in the chemoradiation arm as well as one fatal toxicity in the control arm.

In summary, the randomized studies using chemoradiation are conflicting at best, regarding the utility of routine postoperative RT for patients with unresected gastric cancer. The question of routine use of RT for

Table 22–1. Chemoradiation for Postsurgical Residual/Unresectable Stomach Cancer

Study/ Year	No. of Patients	Chemo/Radiation	Pre/Post Chemo	Local Tumor Control	Survival	Acute Toxicity and Comments
Dent et al (12) 1979	50	2000 cGy; start: day 5	5-FU 500 mg, days 1–4	N/A	T_1–T_2 N_O:100% T_1–T_4, N1-M1: <10%	Randomized (surgery ± 5-FU/RT). Acute hematologic 31–78%, acute GI toxicity 22–60%.
GITSG (11) 1982	45	2550 cGy+5-FU × 2, 5-FU 500 mg/m², IV bolus, days 1–3, 5000 cGy/8-week split course	375 mg/m² 5-FU, days 1–5 q 36–40 days MeCCNU 150 mg/m² day 1	N/A	Resected: 25 mo Unresected: 7 mo	Randomized 5-FU, MeCCNU ± RT. 3 deaths related to RT nutritional complications, 3 deaths from sepsis.
ECOG (13) 1985	57	4000 cGy/4 wks + 600 mg/m² 5-FU IV bolus	5-FU 600 mg/m² IV bolus wkly	N/A	Median survival: 5-FU = 9.3 mo; 5-FU + RT = 8.2 mo.	Randomized (5-FU ± RT) 3 fatal toxicities. 1 – 5-FU, 2 – 5-FU + RT
Douglass (17) 1988	91	4320 cGy/4½ wks	5-FU 325 mg/m² days 1–5, 36–40; ADR 40 mg/m² day 1, 36; methyl CCNU 10 mg/m² day 1 (repeat q wks)	N/A "No difference in patterns"	FAMe + RT = 20% FAMe = 28% (2-yr survival)	Randomized (FAMe ± RT)
Haas et al (15) 1980	12	4500 cGy/10 wks	1. 5-FU-500 mg/m² day 29 2. ADR 30 mg/m² day 29 3. mito-C8mg/m² day 8 (repeat q 8 wks)	N/A	6/12 alive, NED 97–311 days	Early stopping: 1 pt. Cessation of RT: 4 pts.
Asakawa et al (19) 1982	133	5000 cGy min. 37: 5-FU 500 mg IV bolus × 2/wk; 62: Tegafur; 34: FAMT or FMC	None	N/A	5-yr survival T_1: 32, T_2: 17, T_3: 16, T_4: O (5-yr survival of all those completing treatment = 13%)	*Acute:* bleeding: 6.7% perforation: 1.5% treatment interruption: 67% *Late:* hemorrhagic gastritis: 1.9% chronic ulcer: 3.7%
Gunderson et al (16)	46	5-FU IV bolus days 1–3, 4500–5200 cGy 5–5½ weeks	FAM	15/27	14–24 mo. (median survival)	Hematologic (WBC) acceptable, nausea
Mayo (18) 1985	14	5-FU IV bolus days 7–9, 4300 cGy/2 wks	5-FU/ADR	7/8	Time to progression 19 weeks (median)	Toxicity 6/14 prolonged N/V, 3/6 WBC < 2500 "excessive toxicity"

RT = radiation therapy; F, 5-FU = 5-fluorouracil; A, ADR = Adriamycin; Me = methyl CCNU; T = toyomycin; C = cytosine-arabinoside; M, mito C = mitomycin C; NED = no evidence of disease; FAMe = 5-FU + Adriamycin + methyl CCNU; N/A = not available; FAM = 5-FU + Adriamycin + Mitomycin C.

patients with advanced disease is still, unfortunately, not resolved. When RT with or without 5-FU is used, the doses of 4000 to 4500 cGy given in fractions of 180 to 200 cGy per day must be used with caution.

Subsequent reports have been generally nonrandomized studies that have focused investigation in several areas.

1. RT plus more aggressive chemotherapy regimens mainly containing doxorubicin (Adriamycin, ADR).
2. More aggressive RT in the form of accelerated fractionation (possibly of value in tumors with short doubling times).
3. Higher doses of external beam irradiation in combination with concomitant 5-FU–based treatment schedules.
4. Chemoradiation using a low-dose, continuous-infusion 5-FU schedule.

Four trials have assessed RT/5-FU chemoradiation for treatment of advanced, unresectable disease with a combination of systemic ADR-based chemotherapy, sandwiched before or after irradiation (14–17). This systemic chemotherapy combination was chosen because of the initial reports of a 50% objective response rate with FAM (5-*F*U, Adriamycin, and *m*itomycin C) found on patients with advanced gastric cancer (14). Two reports (15,16) indicate the feasibility of combining sequential FAM with RT alone (15) or with 5-FU plus RT (Table 22–1) (16). Median survival varied from 14 to 24 months in the Massachusetts General Hospital (MGH) trial. The Southwest Oncology Group (SWOG) reported 50% survival, but follow-up was limited to less than 1 year. Acute hematologic and gastrointestinal toxicity in both reports were increased compared to historic controls treated with RT only. More recently, a prospective trial comparing FAMe (5-*F*U + Adriamycin + *m*ethyl CCNU) with or without local RT (4320 cGy/24 fractions) showed no difference in local relapse patterns or survival (17). In this latter study, the radiation dose was limited to 4320 cGy and RT was used alone.

The study by Gunderson and co-workers at MGH is one of the largest single institutional trials from North America using 5-FU–based chemoradiation ± systemic therapy (16). In a study of 46 gastric cancer patients, there was a low incidence of toxicity compared to the experience in the GITSG or ECOG trial and others (Table 22–1). The use of "tailored" radiation portals and the use of multiple fields may account for the reduced toxicity. The chemoradiation treatment followed two sequences: RT plus 3 days of bolus 5-FU followed by maintenance 5-FU with or without other drugs in 26 patients; and single-course FAMe or 5-FU and bis-chloronitrosourea (BCNU) followed by RT (± 5-FU) and maintenance combination chemotherapy in 14 patients. The radiation dose varied between 4500 to 5200 cGy in 25 to 29 fractions over 5 to 6 weeks. Only 9% (4 patients) had poor acute tolerance to this treatment. The median survival for those with unresectable/gross residual varied between 14 and 15 months. In those that had tumor debulking and only microscopic residual, the median time to progression was 18.6 months (1/8, 13% infield recurrence) and the median survival was 24 months.

Using the rationale that gastric cancer is frequently poorly differentiated and, therefore, potentially a rapidly proliferating cancer, Gunderson later reported on the use of accelerated irradiation (4300 cGy/2 wks) plus 3 days of intravenous (IV) bolus 5-FU (500 mg/m^2) (18). This regimen, in contrast to conventional fractionation schedules, resulted in increased acute reaction (nausea, vomiting) requiring a reduction of chemotherapy or RT in a majority of patients. Local control was reported in seven of eight patients, but the median time to disease progression was only 19 weeks. Accelerated radiation fractionation schedules, when given alone or in combination with chemotherapy, are limited by the heightened acute response. These altered radiation fractionation schedules must be used with extreme caution in patients with cancers arising in the abdominal cavity.

The report published in 1982 by Asakawa et al is the best example of the effort to use chemoradiation when conventionally fractionated RT doses have routinely exceeded 5000 cGy (19). This interesting study indicates that there is a possibility of curing a small percentage of patients with unresected T_{1-3}, M_0 tumors. All 133 patients received at least 5-FU with RT, 62 patients had Tegafur (Ftorafor), which is an analog of 5-FU, and 34 patients received FaMT (5-FU, cyclophosphamide, mitomycin, toyomycin) or FMC (5-FU, mitomycin, cytosine-arabinoside) with RT. Eighty-one patients completed the prescribed therapy; of these, 13% survived 5 years, and the median survival was 15 months. Perhaps the most important aspect illustrated by this study is the use of higher doses of RT than are generally acceptable in radiotherapeutic practices in the west. Indeed, all but one of the seven 5-year survivors was treated to doses > 5700 to 6250 cGy given in conventional or hypofractionated schedules. Four of the seven longterm survivors had a complete pathologic response based on endoscopic material obtained post-treatment. Complications were reported to be acceptable: 6.7% acute bleeding, 1.5% perforation. All patients had radiation gastritis with doses > 3000 cGy, and 61% required variable treatment interruptions. Late reactions (2 to 6 months after RT) were 1.9% hemorrhagic gastritis, 3.7% chronic ulceration, and 0.9% radiation necrosis of the transverse colon.

In summary, the use of external beam irradiation for gastric cancer has been disappointing because of the difficulty in demonstrating conclusive improvement in local tumor control or survival. There are both acute and late side effects of treatment that can be a formidable problem for patients who have had gastric resection or who have upper gastrointestinal tract dysfunction from surgery or tumor bulk. However, when high doses of RT (> 5000 cGy) are used, some patients achieve longterm palliation, especially those with early disease. This should be kept in mind for the medically inoperable patient, who should be offered this alternative of a potentially curative therapeutic modality.

Completely Resected Disease

If RT does play a role in reducing local recurrence in the patient with unresected disease or poor prognosis because of extensive local infiltration of adjacent organs, are there possible benefits from local adjuvant irradiation for the patient with completely resected gastric cancer? The first randomized study that evaluated adjuvant 5-FU–based chemoradiation for gastric cancer patients was performed at the Mayo Clinic, beginning in 1965. The results showed a potential benefit for those receiving adjuvant chemoradiation, but the study did not show any superiority of treatment over surgical controls (Table 22–2) (16).

More recently, Gez et al reported on the use of adjuvant chemoradiation for advanced gastric cancer in 27 patients (20). The treatment schedule used a split-course radiotherapy sequence to an initial dose of 2000 cGy (200- to 250-cGy fractions) followed by a 2-week treatment break. A second course of treatment used an additional total dose of 3000 cGy with spinal cord shielding added

Table 22–2. Postoperative Chemoradiation for Completely Resected Gastric Cancer

Series	No. of Patients	Disease Status	Chemoradiation	Pre/Post Chemo	Local Control	Survival (Mos)	Complications
Gunderson et al (16)	12	Resected, high risk	5-FU 500 mg/m^2 IV bolus days 1–3; 4500–5000 cGy/ 5–6 weeks	9 patients, maintenance 5-FU, 12 patients, 5-FU + nitrosourea	12/14	Resected 24 mo, microresidual 14 mo	No fatal toxicity
Gez et al (20)	27	Resected, high risk	5-FU 500 mg IV bolus days 1–3 (2500 cGy + 5-FU) × 2. 5000 cGy/7 wks	5-FU 500 mg/q wk, × 12 mo.	24/27	Median 27 mo, resected high risk 23.5 mo, positive margin 28 mo	No fatal toxicity
Rich et al (7)	9	Resected, high risk	5-FU 300 mg/m^2 continuous infusion 4500–5000 cGy/5–5½ wks	(No systematic use of chemotherapy)			No fatal toxicity; treatment stopped in 1 patient (severe nausea)

after 4000 cGy. The total treatment time was 7 weeks. 5-FU was given by bolus IV administration in doses of 500 mg for the first 3 days of each RT course and continued for 1 year at weekly intervals in the same dosage. All patients had undergone surgical resection, and 24 of 27 had lymph node involvement on pathologic examination. There were 16 specimens with negative surgical margins: 8 were positive and 3 were unknown. The median survival was 27 months; 6 patients were free of disease at a median of 62 months. There was no significant difference in median survival time for the following patient or tumor characteristics (age, sex, tumor histology, lymph node involvement, or surgical margin status), although there was a difference based on the location of the tumor in the stomach. There was also a difference in survival based on bone marrow suppression as measured by the white blood cell count (WBC). For patients having (5-FU–induced) WBCs below 3000/mm^3, the median survival was 42 months, but the median survival was only 19 months for those with WBCs greater than 3000/mm^3. The toxicity during chemoradiation treatment was acceptable and fatal toxicity was not encountered. Although this entire treatment was not given strictly in the adjuvant setting, there is a striking similarity between the median survival achieved in this study and that reported by Gunderson for 12 patients receiving adjuvant chemoradiation (16) (Table 22–2).

In 1985, we reported the feasibility of adjuvant chemoradiation using 4500 to 5000 cGy given in conventional RT fractionation (180 cGy/day, 5 days per week) in conjunction with low-dose continuous infusion of 5-FU (7). 5-FU doses generally varied between 7.5 to 28.4 grams given over 9 to 44 days. Most patients, however, were able to tolerate up to 4½ to 5 weeks of treatment. Among the total 41 patients reported in this pilot study, the nine patients with gastric cancer had the most severe weight loss (average of 4.6% of pretreatment body weight loss) despite careful nutritional support and the use of tailored irradiation portals. Further trials are needed to determine the value of adjuvant continuous-infusion 5-FU plus concomitant RT with or without other systemic chemotherapy for gastric cancer patients.

PANCREATIC CANCER

The utility of chemoradiation for patients with advanced, unresectable pancreas cancer or in those with resected cancers has been demonstrated in a variety of nonrandomized and randomized trials over the last two decades (Table 22–3). The enthusiasm for chemoradiation can be traced back to the Mayo Clinic trial mentioned earlier (10). Briefly, this report by Moertel et al in 1969 showed that the use of 5-FU (15 mg/kg) for 3 successive days, combined with radiotherapy (3500 to 4000 cGy), improved the survival of 32 patients with unresectable pancreas cancer compared to placebo-treated controls ($p = 0.05$). One criticism of this study relates to the question of whether the benefit in the chemoradiation arm was related to only 5-FU. This is unlikely because the therapeutic effect of a single 3-day course of 5-FU alone is probably negligible.

In an effort to expand the question of whether chemotherapy alone for unresectable, localized pancreatic cancer is of value and whether it is as good or better than chemoradiation, medical oncologists have tested a variety of chemotherapeutic regimens built around 5-FU treatment. The results of a Phase II trial using SMF (*s*treptozocin, *m*itomycin C, and 5-*F*U) treatment in 17 patients with advanced pancreatic cancer indicated potential superiority over irradiation alone or 5-FU chemoradiation (21). A trial was undertaken by the GITSG, therefore, to compare SMF with 5-FU given for the first and last 3 days of treatment during radiation. The results of this study showed a survival benefit in favor of the chemoradiation arm versus SMF alone (41 vs. 19% 1-year survival) (22). Although ultimate survival is still very poor in both treatment arms, at face value, this prospective randomized trial supports the notion that 5-FU chemoradiation should be maintained as the community standard for treatment of patients with localized unresectable pancreatic cancer.

Radiation oncologists have attempted to improve the local control of unresectable pancreas cancer by using the following approaches.

1. Increasing total radiation dose solely through external beam treatment techniques.

Table 22–3. Selected Chemoradiation Series in Pancreatic Cancer

Study/Year	No. of Patients	Chemotherapy and Dose	RT (cGy)	Survival	Comments
Moertel et al (10) 1969	25	5-FU	3500–4000	2-yr: 14%	Minimal 5-FU dose
	33	Placebo	Same	2-yr: 0% ($p < 0.01$)	Randomized study
GITSG (22) 1988	21	SMF	None	1-yr: 19%	Randomized study
	22	RT + 5-FU	5400	1-yr: 41% ($p < 0.02$)	
Gunderson et al (27) 1987	49	5-FU: 500 mg/m^2/IV push × 3 days or 1 gm/m^2 infusion × 3 days	4500–5000 external + 2000 IORT	1-yr: 46% 2-yr: 8%	20% 2-year survival when "widefield" irradiation used
Komaki et al (29) 1988	16	5-FU: 500 mg/m^2 days 1–3, 29–31 then weekly maintenance 1 year	6120 in 7 weeks Hepatic RT: 2340 in 2½ weeks	1-yr: 66.7% 2-yr: 46.7% (disease free)	4-yr. survival: 13.3%

FAM = 5-FU + Adriamycin + mitomycin C; SMF = Streptozotocin + mitomycin C + 5-FU; 5-FU = 5-fluorouracil; IORT = Intra-operative radiotherapy.

2. Altered radiation fractionation schedules with or without chemotherapy.
3. Altered methods of administration of 5-FU using either short (4 to 5 days) or prolonged (more than 30 days) infusion schedules.
4. The use of wide-field irradiation techniques to include the primary cancer, the regional lymph nodes, and the whole liver.
5. Intraperitoneal chemotherapy plus chemoradiation.

In 1975, Cavanaugh demonstrated that radiation therapy doses of 6000 cGy given by split course over 8 weeks could be used in the upper abdomen to relatively confined treatment volumes (23). In 1981, the GITSG reported on a prospective randomized trial that assessed the utility of radiation alone using a split-course approach compared to chemoradiation for unresectable pancreatic cancer (24). The three treatment arms were radiation therapy alone (6000 cGy) versus 5-FU chemoradiation to doses of 4000 or 6000 cGy. The radiation-alone arm of 6000 cGy was soon abandoned because of the demonstrated inferiority to the chemoradiation treatment. In the chemoradiation arms, median time to progression was 33.7 weeks for the 6000-cGy arm and 23.2 weeks for the 4000-cGy arm. This improvement was also associated with a better median survival of 49.4 versus 36.5 weeks for the high- and low-dose chemoradiation arms, respectively. In summary, this trial demonstrated that survival could be improved marginally with the use of higher total doses of irradiation.

In the last decade, several alternate methods for the delivery of high-dose irradiation to the pancreas have been assessed. Trials utilizing external beam and interstitial implants have been able to achieve radiation doses in excess of 6000 cGy using conventionally fractionated nonsplit-course treatment techniques. Reports by Dobelbower et al using chemoradiation with such high-dose irradiation have demonstrated some gain in local control and survival, but the median survival remains 15 months (25).

Potentially curative doses of irradiation for unresected tumors have been attempted by the use of external beam treatment with concurrent 5-FU chemotherapy and **intraoperative electron beam boost (EB-IORT).** The initial trials at the Massachusetts General Hospital (MGH), (26) and the Mayo Clinic (27,28) have reported favorable results for selected patients. In general, the therapeutic plan employs a surgical exploration for the determination of resectability with EB-IORT given at the initial surgical staging procedure. Patients with peritoneal disease and distant metastasis have been excluded from most trials, although EB-IORT alone may be reasonably effective for the palliation of local symptoms. Gunderson et al reported on a study of 49 primary unresectable pancreatic patients treated with EB-IORT and 5-FU chemoradiation (27). Eighteen patients received chemoradiation using 5-FU in doses of 500 mg/m^2 IV × 3 days at the beginning of radiotherapy, and 10 patients received 1000 mg/m^2 infusion × 3 days. Precise survival and local control data regarding the two different chemotherapy regimens were not given. An analysis of all EB-IORT patients showed that the local control was 84% at 1 year. This appeared to be an improvement over the local control achieved with external beam with or without concomitant 5-FU treatment from historical controls at the Mayo Clinic. The report from MGH showed a median survival of 16.5 months with the use of EB-IORT with or without chemoradiation, which also supports the theory that improved local control can be achieved with higher radiation doses (26).

In a later and larger retrospective analysis of all patients with unresectable pancreatic cancer treated at the Mayo Clinic, those who received 5-FU had poorer local control at 1 and 2 years than those not receiving 5-FU; however, this was not statistically significant (log rank test) (28). Selection factors may have accounted for poor prognosis in patients treated with chemotherapy and radiotherapy. Survival and local control appear to be marginally improved with high total radiation doses given by external beam and intraoperative techniques from these nonrandomized studies.

The use of **wide field irradiation** for pancreatic cancer has been fostered by the success with whole abdominal irradiation for ovarian cancer. Since the pattern of tumor spread for pancreatic cancer includes peritoneal seeding, regional lymph nodes, and liver metastasis, there is a rationale for the use of upper abdominal or whole abdominal treatment for patients at high risk for failure. At the Mayo Clinic, a sequential pilot study investigated the use of upper abdominal irradiation alone in conjunction with localized fields with chemotherapy (27). In the second phase of the investigation, 5-FU was given by continuous infusion of 1000 mg/m^2/24 hrs for 3 days during the first and fifth weeks of external irradiation. Two of these latter 10 patients also received intraperitoneal 5-FU. Analysis of the data revealed no difference in median survival or survival rate at 1 year compared to conventional RT ± 5-FU. There was an improvement in 2-year survival when those treated with wide field RT were compared to local irradiation alone (20% vs. 6.5% 2-year survival rate, respectively). More recently, the investigators at the Medical College of Wisconsin have reported on the use of regional irradiation to the pancreas and surrounding lymph nodes combined with prophylactic hepatic irradiation (29). The dosage to the pancreas was 6120 cGy in 34 fractions over 7 weeks. Treatment to the liver began 4 weeks after commencing pancreatic irradiation and delivered 2340 cGy in 13 fractions over 2½ weeks. The entire liver was encompassed within the irradiation portal as determined by CT scan. The irradiation was given with concomitant IV 5-FU in a dosage of 500 mg/m^2/day on days 1 through 3 of the pancreatic irradiation. A second course of IV 5-FU was administered at the commencement of hepatic irradiation on days 30 through 32. Results of this trial also show an improvement over the best treatment arm in GITSG or when compared to the results of previous radiotherapy alone at the Medical College of Wisconsin. The 2-year disease-free survival rate was 46.7% (13.3% at 4 years). Median survival, however, was still 60 weeks, which is a marginal improvement over the prior study cited. These two nonrandomized trials suggest the possibility of further improvement of median survival and possibly longterm survival for a small subpopulation of patients with pancreatic cancer treated with more aggressive doses to the local tumor as well as prophylactic upper abdominal therapy to the area or liver.

The value of an alternate method of 5-FU administration by low-dose, continuous-infusion 5-FU administration with conventionally fractionated irradiation has been tested at the M.D. Anderson Cancer Center (MDACC) (30,31). We have used low-dose continuous-infusion 5-FU in dosages of 250 to 300 mg/m^2/day during an entire course of external beam irradiation to the pancreas tumor and surrounding lymphatics. Irradiation dose in our pilot study was generally 5500 cGy in 5½ weeks given at 180 cGy per fraction. Patients are treated with portable Travenol infusor pumps, which are managed in the outpatient setting. We treated 15 patients with localized pancreatic cancer with a combination intraperitoneal 5-FU infusion in doses ranging from 1 to 2 grams/24 hrs × 5 days. Following intraperitoneal 5-FU infusion, RT was given in doses of 5500 cGy over 34 days with continuous infusion 5-FU administered at 300 mg/m^2/24 hrs delivering a median total dose of 16.77 grams. Acute toxicities were acute nausea (74%), diarrhea (65%), and vomiting (42%). These gastrointestinal side effects were due to a combination of chemotherapy and irradiation. However, 30% of patients experienced mucositis and 15% had the hand/foot syndrome, both of which are related to continuous-infusion 5-FU administration. These side effects as well as leukopenia, which occurred in 24%, were managed by medications or treatment interruption of 5-FU in approximately one-third of the patients. Treatment interruption varied from 3 to 7 days. 5-FU was discontinued more frequently than radiotherapy. Fifteen percent were hospitalized for 3 to 27 days (median = 4 days). The acute toxicity was not related to treatment site, RT dose, or 5-FU dose. Late effects did not appear to be increased. The actuarial local tumor control for patients with pancreatic cancer was 32% at 22 months, and 35% of the patients were surviving at 22 months. Intraperitoneal 5-FU infusion followed by chemoradiation using low-dose continuous-infusion 5-FU is feasible, although acute complications are definitely increased over those compared with conventionally fractionated irradiation alone.

In summary, the data available so far regarding 5-FU chemoradiation show that modest improvement in local control and survival over surgical bypass alone has been gained by the use of 5-FU with radiotherapy for unresectable pancreatic cancer. Alternate forms of 5-FU administration by the infusion technique may improve local control over radiotherapy alone. However, substantially higher doses of radiotherapy than can be achieved with external beam techniques alone may be necessary to achieve permanent tumor eradication. Patients with unresectable pancreatic cancer are also at risk for distant disease. Improved methods for systemic management as well as regional (intraperitoneal chemotherapy) and wide field RT will need to be investigated in future trials.

Adjuvant Chemoradiation for Resected Pancreatic Cancer

Locoregional tumor recurrence after pancreatic resection by the Whipple procedure or after total pancreatectomy can occur in 50% of patients (3). The use of adjuvant radiotherapy with or without chemotherapy has been used in nonrandomized (32) and randomized (33,34) trials in order to improve local control and survival. The GITSG reported on a prospective randomized study employing surgery alone versus surgery plus adjuvant chemoradiotherapy for resected pancreas cancer (33). Forty-nine patients were randomized, 20 of whom received adjuvant therapy consisting of two courses of 2000 cGy, each separated by an interval of 2 weeks for a total dose of 4000 cGy. 5-FU was given concurrently during the first 3 days of each 2-week course of irradiation. 5-FU was given in doses of 500 mg/m^2 by IV bolus injection.

The results comparing surgery alone to adjuvant chemoradiotherapy showed a significant improvement in survival throughout the follow-up period ($p = 0.03$). Disease-free recurrence at 2 years was 15% for the control group and 42% for the adjuvant chemoradiation group.

An additional 30 patients were registered to this protocol after the preliminary report; they demonstrated continued beneficial effect of adjuvant chemoradiation. The median survival time in the 30 patients was 18 months and the 2-year actuarial survival was 46% (34).

BILE DUCT CANCER

The optimal management of patients with biliary tract cancer has not been established because the prognosis for most patients is still as dismal as that for unresectable pancreatic cancer. There are some patients with distal common bile duct or periampullary tumors that may enjoy up to a 35% 5-year survival after complete resection. Two reports indicate the use of chemotherapy in the management of patients with biliary tract cancer. The first, from Kopelson in 1977, reported six patients who received 5-FU as adjuvant chemotherapy (35). Three patients were treated with 5-FU during the first 3 days of radiotherapy, but dosages are not given. Based on small numbers, it is impossible to determine any benefit achieved in these patients. A report by Mittal et al reported on another six patients who received 5-FU with or without mitomycin C or methyl CCNU in the management of biliary tract cancer (36). Again, details of the chemotherapy are not sufficient to conclude whether this combined modality treatment is superior to that of radiation alone.

Over the past decade, there have been numerous reports indicating the utility of high-dose external radiotherapy in the management of patients with biliary tract cancer (37–40). Median survivals were reported, ranging from 11 to 16 months for patients treated with external beam radiotherapy and transcatheter Iridium^{192} intraluminal boost. Although median survival was improved modestly and, therefore, palliation for patients with unresected disease was prolonged, nearly all patients in these radiotherapy studies died and many had local progression. Therefore, further improvement in local and systemic management of these patients is warranted.

At MDACC, we reported on the preliminary results of 5-FU chemoradiation for patients with advanced biliary tract cancer (30,31). Our initial results showed a 20+ month median survival for a group of patients with microscopic or residual or unresected cancer following surgery treated with postoperative chemoradiation. 5-FU was given in doses of 300 mg/m^2 as a continuous infusion during the course of radiotherapy. External beam doses generally varied between 4500 and 5000 cGy, and a boost either by an arch wedge technique or through transcatheter iridium wire implantation was given. Complications occurred in four patients who included duodenal bleeding, ulceration, and fistula. Three patients were managed conservatively with antacids and H-2 blockers with gradual improvement unless patients had concurrent tumor regrowth in the same area.

These data indicate the potential usefulness for the combination of fluoropyrimidine therapy plus external beam radiation therapy. The best method of delivery of 5-FU or related compounds is uncertain. It may be feasible to deliver intra-arterial chemotherapy in order to achieve a high concentration of drug in the tumor with concurrent radiotherapy. Furthermore, the ability of the liver to extract 5-FU on the first pass after venous administration and the potential for concentration of parent or active metabolites in the biliary tract could possibly also yield higher tumor cell drug concentrations via a shared regional blood supply. New protocols to explore these possibilities are warranted in order to improve the survival for these patients.

SUMMARY

There are a plethora of interesting data indicating the potential usefulness of fluoropyrimidine chemotherapy given concurrently with external beam irradiation. For gastric cancer, selected subpopulations of patients at high risk for local-regional progression should be studied further in properly designed trials. The impact of a radical course of chemoradiation on local control and survival for the patient who is medically unfit for surgery and in whom disease is confined to the organ or local-regional area requires assessment. Systemic chemotherapy administration, including Adriamycin-containing regimens, has been demonstrated to be tolerated by patients receiving 5-FU–based chemoradiation. For pancreatic cancer, 5-FU chemoradiation can be considered standard management. Further improvements in the care of these patients may include the continued use of high-dose radiation treatment techniques either with external beam or preferably with intraoperative electron beam boost. Whole upper abdominal irradiation or chemotherapeutic peritoneal cavity treatment would seem likely choices for future experimental protocols in order to reduce the failure rates below the diaphragms and to possibly improve survival. Finally, the expanded use of chemoradiation for biliary tract cancer would seem to be a logical extension of current clinical research and is supported by preliminary work. The use of high radiotherapy doses to this site, in combination with 5-FU infusion, has been demonstrated to be feasible and appears to improve local control and survival.

REFERENCES

1. Boring CC, Squires TS, Tong T. Cancer statistics, 1992. CA 42:19, 1992.

2. Gunderson LL, Sosin H. Adenocarcinoma of the stomach: Areas of failure in a reoperation series (second or symptomatic looks). Clinicopathologic correlation and implications for adjuvant therapy. Int J Radiat Oncol Biol Phys 8:1, 1982.
3. Tepper JE, Nardi GE, Suit HD. Carcinoma of the pancreas. Review of MGH experience from 1963 to 1973. Cancer 37:1519, 1976.
4. Buskirk SJ, Gunderson LL, Adson MA, et al. Analysis of failure following curative irradiation of gallbladder and extrahepatic bile duct carcinoma. Int J Radiat Oncol Biol Phys 10:2013, 1984.
5. Heidelberger C, Griesbach L, Montag BJ, et al. Studies on fluorinated pyrimidines II. Effects of trans-planted tumors. Cancer Res 18:305, 1958.
6. Hodnett EM. Radiosensitization by radiotherapy and 5-fluorouracil. Cancer Chemother Rep 32:55, 1963.
7. Rich TA, Lokich JJ, Chaffey JT. A pilot study of protracted venous infusion of 5-fluorouracil and concomitant radiation therapy. J Clin Oncol 3:402, 1985.
8. Byfield JE. The clinical use of 5-fluorouracil and other halopyrimidines as radiosensitizers in man. *In:* Cancer Chemotherapy by Infusion. Lokich JJ (Ed). Chicago, Precept Press, 1987, p. 479.
9. Moertel CG, Reitemeier RJ, Childs DS, et al. Advanced gastrointestinal cancer. Mayo Clinic Proceedings 39:767, 1964.
10. Moertel CG, Childs DS, Reitemeier RJ, et al. Combined 5-fluorouracil and supervoltage radiation therapy of locally unresectable gastrointestinal cancer. Lancet 1:865, 1969.
11. Gastrointestinal Tumor Study Group. A comparison of combination chemotherapy and combined modality therapy for locally advanced gastric carcinoma. Cancer 49:1771, 1982.
12. Dent DM, Werner ID, Novis B, et al. Prospective randomized trial of combined oncological therapy for gastric carcinoma. Cancer 44:385, 1979.
13. Klaassen DJ, MacIntyre JM, Catton GE, et al. Treatment of locally unresectable cancer of the stomach and pancreas. A randomized comparison of 5-fluorouracil alone with radiation plus concurrent and maintenance 5-fluorouracil—An Eastern Cooperative Oncology Group Study. J Clin Oncol 3:373, 1985.
14. MacDonald JS, Schein PS, Wolley PV, et al. 5-FU, doxorubicin, and mitomycin (FAM) combination for advanced gastric cancer. Ann Intern Med 93:533, 1980.
15. Haas L, Vaitkevicius V, Bukowski R, et al. Southwest Oncology Group (SWOG) pilot study of radiotherapy + 5-fluorouracil + adriamycin + mitomycin-C in patients with minimal gastric cancer (abstract). Proc Am Soc Clin Oncol 21:342, 1980.
16. Gunderson LL, Hoskins RB, Cohen AC, et al. Combined modality treatment of gastric cancer. Int J Radiat Oncol Biol Phys 9:965, 1983.
17. Douglass HO Jr, Stablein DM, Stemmerman G, et al for the Gastrointestinal Tumor Study Group (GITSG). Therapy of locally advanced, surgically incurable gastric cancer with postoperative chemotherapy of 5-fluorouracil (F), Adriamycin (A) and Methyl-CCNU (Me) with or without external beam radiation therapy (RT). Proc Am Soc Clin Oncol 7:96, 1988.
18. O'Connell MJ, Gunderson LL, Moertel CG, Kvols LK. A pilot study to determine clinical tolerability of intensive combined modality therapy for locally unresectable gastric cancer. Int J Radiat Oncol Biol Phys 11:1827, 1985.
19. Asakawa H, Otawa H, Yamada S, Matsumota K. Combination therapy of gastric carcinoma with radiation and chemotherapy. Tohoku J Exp Med 137:445, 1982.
20. Gez E, Sulkes A, Peretz T, Weshler Z. Combined 5-fluorouracil and radiation therapy following resection of locally advanced gastric carcinoma. A 5-year follow-up. Recent Results Cancer Res 110:52, 1988.
21. Smith FP, Stablein D, Korsmeyer S, et al. Combination chemotherapy for locally advanced pancreatic cancer. Equivalence to external beam irradiation and implication for future management. J Clin Oncol 1(7):413, 1983.
22. Gastrointestinal Tumor Study Group. Treatment of locally unresectable carcinoma of the pancreas. Comparison of combined-modality therapy (chemotherapy plus radiotherapy) to chemotherapy alone. J Natl Cancer Inst 80(10):751, 1988.
23. Cavanaugh PJ. Considerations appropriate to a clinical trial of definitive radiation therapy in adenocarcinoma of the pancreas. J Surg Oncol 7:135, 1975.
24. Moertel CG, Frytak S, Hahn RG, et al. Therapy of locally unresectable pancreatic carcinoma. A randomized comparison of high dose (6000 rads) radiation alone, moderate dose radiation (4000 rads + 5-fluorouracil), and high dose radiation + 5-fluorouracil. Cancer 48:1705, 1981.
25. Dobelbower RR Jr, Merrick HW III, Ahuja R, Skeel RT. ^{125}I interstitial implant, precision high-dose external beam therapy, and 5-FU for unresectable adenocarcinoma of pancreas and extrahepatic biliary tree. Cancer 58:2185, 1986.
26. Shipley WU, Wood WC, Tepper JE, et al. In-

traoperative electron beam irradiation for patients with unresectable pancreatic carcinoma. Ann Surg 200:289, 1984.
27. Gunderson LL, Martin JK, Kvols LK, et al. Intraoperative and external beam irradiation ± 5-FU for locally advanced pancreatic cancer. Int J Radiat Oncol Biol Phys 13:319, 1987.
28. Roldan GE, Gunderson LL, Nagorney DM, et al. External beam versus intraoperative and external beam irradiation for locally advanced pancreatic cancer. Cancer 61:1110, 1988.
29. Komaki R, Hansen R, Cox JD, et al. Phase I-II study of prophylactic hepatic irradiation with local irradiation and systemic chemotherapy for adenocarcinoma of the pancreas. Int J Radiat Oncol Biol Phys 15:1447, 1988.
30. Rich TA, Ajani JA, Goudeau R, Ende K. High dose radiotherapy RT with protracted venous 5-fluorouracil (PV 5-FU) radiosensitization for advanced gastrointestinal cancer. Proc Am Soc Clin Oncol 6:79, 1987.
31. Rich T. Protracted (continuous 5-fluorouracil) infusion with concomitant radiation therapy. Indications and results. *In:* Concomitant Continuous Infusion Chemotherapy and Radiation. Rotman M, Rosenthal CM (Eds). Berlin, Springer-Verlag, 1991, p. 181.
32. Rich TA. Radiation therapy for pancreatic cancer. Eleven year experience at the JCRT. Int J Radiat Oncol Biol Phys 11:759, 1985.
33. Kalser MH, Ellenberg SS. Pancreatic cancer adjuvant combined radiation and chemotherapy following curative resection. Arch Surg 120:899, 1985.
34. Gastrointestinal Tumor Study Group. Further evidence of effective adjuvant combined radiation and chemotherapy following curative resection of pancreatic cancer. Cancer 59:2006, 1987.
35. Kopelson G, Harisiadis L, Tretter P. The role of radiation therapy in cancer of the extrahepatic biliary system. An analysis of thirteen patients and a review of the literature of the effectiveness of surgery, chemotherapy, and radiotherapy. Int J Radiat Oncol Biol Phys 2:883, 1977.
36. Mittal B, Deutsch M, Iwatsuki S. Primary cancers of extrahepatic biliary passages. Int J Radiat Oncol Biol Phys 11:849, 1985.
37. Hishikawa Y, Shimada T, Miura T, Imajyo Y. Radiation therapy of carcinoma of the extrahepatic bile ducts. Radiology 146:787, 1983.
38. Fletcher MS, Brinkley D, Dawson JL, et al. Treatment of hilar carcinoma by bile drainage combined with internal radiotherapy using ^{192}iridium wire. Br J Surg 70:733, 1983.
39. Johnson DW, Safai C, Goffinet DR. Malignant obstructive jaundice. Treatment with external-beam and intracavitary radiotherapy. Int J Radiat Oncol Biol Phys 11:411, 1985.
40. Fields JN, Emami B. Carcinoma of the extrahepatic biliary system: Results of primary and adjuvant radiotherapy. Int J Radiat Oncol Biol Phys 13:331, 1987.

Chapter 23

LIVER

J. MICHAEL HAMILTON, STACY R. NERENSTONE, AND MICHAEL A. FRIEDMAN

LIVER METASTASES

Background

Considered together, primary liver carcinoma and metastatic liver tumors are exceedingly common events. Metastatic liver tumors occur 40 times more frequently than primary hepatic neoplasms. Of the one million patients diagnosed with cancer each year in the United States, 41% will have metastases of the liver during the course of their illness (1). For some specific histologies, liver involvement characterizes the malignant nature of the tumor. For example, liver metastases are initially present in 15 to 25% of the 156,000 patients diagnosed each year with colorectal cancer (2,3,4); more than 50% of these patients will eventually develop hepatic metastases.

The basic processes of tumor metastases have been reviewed elsewhere (5–8). The liver is a preferred metastatic site in part because of the high blood flow through its capillary bed. Perfusion by both the portal and the systemic circulations delivers 25 to 30% of the body's total blood volume to the liver each minute. The liver can receive circulating tumor cells from either the systemic or the portal circulations. Liver metastases occur in up to 64% of patients with breast cancer, 53% of leukemias and lymphomas, and 43% of nonsmall-cell lung tumors. Malignant cells transported from intra-abdominal primary sites directly to the liver via the portal circulation cause liver metastases in more than half of all cases of pancreatic, biliary, and gastric cancer (9). Features of the intrahepatic vessels may facilitate metastatic tumor adherence, invasion, and growth. In vitro model systems indicate that specific cellular receptors within the hepatic vasculature promote tumor adherence and invasion and that there is a near absence of basement membrane in the hepatic vessels (10,11).

Although dissemination of cancer to the liver is common, it is rarely the only site of metastatic disease. It is more typically the sole site of recurrence with intra-abdominal primary tumors than with extra-abdominal cancers. These facts must be considered when local-regional therapy is planned for a patient with liver metastases. Moreover, death primarily attributable to hepatic failure occurs in only about 10% of all patients. Most patients have additional extrahepatic disease. Clearly, in such patients, even with an effective means for controlling local disease, the results of that treatment could only have a modest impact on survival. For some primary sites, such as colorectal cancers, the opportunity for regional treatment success is greater. In patients with colorectal cancer, hepatic failure causes one-fourth of all deaths, and in those patients with liver only disease, death is directly attributable to those metastases in roughly 80% (12). Consequently, most trials that evaluate local therapies of liver metastases, including surgery, infusional chemotherapy, and irradiation, are restricted to or heavily weighted toward patients with colorectal primaries.

The lethal potential of hepatic tumors is related to their overall size, number, and location within the liver. Among all patients with liver metastases, single tumors are found in 6 to 14%, tumors limited to a single lobe or segment are found in 13%, and multiple deposits are found in 70 to 75% (13).

The average survival for all patients with clinically evident liver metastases is about 5 months (14,15) but patients with solitary hepatic metastases and no extrahepatic malignant disease may have an extended survival (4). Isolated cases, representing 0.5 to 5% of large patient studies, have been observed to survive for 3 to 10 years with no specific treatment of the hepatic metastases (2,15,16,17). Other patient selection factors and/or patterns of care are associated with apparent increases in survival and are not directly related to treatment of the metastatic disease. Goslin's study of 125 "natural history" patients described a median survival of 12.5 months, which is more than double the average survival of similar, untreated patients seen at other institutions. These long-term survivors must be recalled when published reports cite uncontrolled data or the occasional patient with prolonged survival as a proof of treatment effectiveness.

The number and distribution of metastases within the liver not only influence treatment options but also have a direct bearing on survival (regardless of the treatment administered). Staging of hepatic involvement is essential for appropriate treatment planning and for evaluating the relative effectiveness of any therapy (see Table 23–1). Several preoperative and intraoperative staging systems have been proposed. Most systems assess the quantity of intrahepatic tumor and/or the functional status of the liver. Other factors, such as patient performance status, the presence or absence of extrahepatic tumor, and the primary histology, must also be considered in selecting patients for treatment and in interpreting reported therapeutic results. As demonstrated in Table

Table 23–1. Staging of Liver Metastases

Author/Reference	Treatment	Staging Criteria	Survival
Jaffe et al, 1968, (15)	Natural history	Single metastasis	136 days median
		Multiple metastases, 1 lobe	93 days
		Multiple metastases, 2 lobes	72 days
Wood et al, 1976 (4)	Natural history	Single metastasis	16.7-month mean
		Multiple metastases, 1 lobe	10.6 months
		Multiple metastases, 2 lobes	3.1 months
Wagner et al, 1984 (18)	Natural history	Single metastasis	24-month median
		Multiple metastases, 1 lobe	18 months
		Multiple metastases, 2 lobes	12 months
Fortner et al, 1981 (19)	Liver resection	Tumor-free margins, no vascular or biliary invasion	79% 2-year
		Any residual tumor or invasion	0%
August et al, 1985 (45)	Liver resection	1–3 metastases	44-month median
		≥ 4 metastases	20 months
		Unilobar disease	54 months
		Bilobar disease	23 months
Cady et al, 1974 (20)	Chemotherapy infusion	<25% liver replaced by tumor	16-month median
		25–50% liver replaced	13 months
		>50% liver replaced	8 months
Pettavel et al, 1978 (125)	Chemotherapy infusion	Normal liver size and function	15-month mean
		Abnormal liver size or function	4.7 months
		Abnormal liver size and function	1.4 months
Goslin et al, 1982 (12)	Various treatments	<3 metastases on scan, normal liver size and LFTs, normal performance status	18–24 month median
		≥ 4 metastases on scan, hepatomegaly, abnormal LFTs, less than normal performance, or >10% weight loss, poorly differentiated histology of primary	6–10 month median
Lahr et al, 1983 (21)	Various treatments	1–4 metastases, unilobar	12-month median
		>4 metastases, bilobar	4.5 months
		Normal bilirubin & alkaline phosphatase	8 months
		≥1–5X elevated bilirubin or >2X elevated alkaline phosphatase	2.5 months

23–1, even in untreated patients, the extent of tumor affects survival. In Jaffe's series of 390 patients (15), for example, median survival for all patients was 75 days, and 1-year survival was 7%. Survival of patients with a single metastasis was roughly twice that of those with widespread intrahepatic disease. In Wagner's more recent review of untreated patients (18), the overall survival is superior to that seen by Jaffe. However, a similar doubling of survival is noted for those with a single tumor deposit compared to those with widespread disease.

These staging criteria have prognostic import. As seen in Fortner's patients undergoing major hepatic resection for metastatic colorectal cancer (19), disease confined to the resected specimen (without vascular or biliary invasion—Stage I) was associated with a greater than 70% 3-year survival. By contrast, no patients with a tumor that was incompletely resectable or invasive (Stages II and III) survived longer than 2 years. In Cady's report of patients receiving hepatic arterial chemotherapy (20), median survival was 16 months for those with less than 25% of the liver replaced by tumor, compared to 8 months for those with greater than 50% of the liver involved. Multifactorial analyses from Lahr (21) support the correlation of survival with the number and extent of metastases and with liver function.

The biologic explanation for the prognostic importance of these staging systems is debated. The systems may simply reflect the influence of "tumor burden" on survival or may indirectly reveal the intrinsic aggressiveness of the primary tumor, i.e., more malignant tumors produce earlier, multiple metastases (22). Table 23–1 points out staging systems that are based on clinical information that can be obtained preoperatively and that can help direct treatment planning for the individual patients (ranging from surgical resection, regional chemotherapy, irradiation, to systemic therapy). Staging information that requires surgical exploration can provide more precise data and can assist in understanding the outcome of therapy but, obviously, is limited to patients undergoing laparotomy. Staging information is an essential part of the data collection and interpretation of reported results of treatment of liver metastases.

Treatment

Surgery

Attempts to obliterate liver metastases surgically date back to a report by Keene in 1899 (23). Even surgical studies from 50 years ago noted 5-year postresection survivals up to 50% and cure rates up to 20% in patients with colorectal tumors (24–27). These figures are confirmed by current experience (28–30).

Surgical options for unresectable liver metastases include vascular manipulation procedures. Devascularization procedures have achieved tumor necrosis after **hepatic arterial ligation** (32,33,34), **arterial embolization** (35,36), and other techniques of vascular occlusion (37) with or without an accompanying infusion of chemotherapy. However, these approaches are associated with toxicity, are generally considered to be palliative, and are of short-term benefit only.

Hepatic resection, on the other hand, currently represents the only curative approach to metastatic disease. It is generally recognized that only about 5% of all patients with liver metastases could be cured by surgery (38,39). That is, resection of hepatic metastases in cases of colorectal primary cancers is possible in only about 25 (18,40) to 30% (41) of patients. Cure rates of 20 to 30% are achieved with such surgery, yielding a longterm benefit of about 5%. Patients with primary cancers other than colorectal carcinoma have a much lower resectability rate and are cured only half as often (40). Both cure and palliative benefit must be balanced against a surgical morality rate of about 4 to 5% and serious, nonlethal complication rate of 25 to 50% (42,43,44). These postoperative complications include perihepatic hematomas, wound infections, subphrenic abscesses, pneumonia, pleural effusions, intestinal obstruction, and hepatic insufficiency. Surgical techniques will continue to advance, reducing the complications of resection, but the percentage of patients cured by the procedure without the addition of other cytotoxic therapy is unlikely to change greatly.

Prognostically, some patients would benefit from postoperative therapy. Hughes et al

(29) identified patients who have undergone incomplete liver resection for bilobar disease as high-risk candidates for recurrence. They would possibly benefit from additional local-regional or systemic therapy. August et al (45) also advocated adjuvant chemotherapy for specific subsets of patients after hepatic metastases resection as a means of improving cure rates.

Chemotherapy

As noted earlier, the bulk of experience with treatment of liver metastases is in patients with colorectal cancer, although limited numbers of patients treated for hepatic metastases from other specific histologies have been reported (46,47). In more general reviews of overall results with systemic chemotherapy, relatively chemoresponsive cancers, such as breast or small-cell lung cancer, show response rates for intrahepatic disease roughly that are one-half to two-thirds of those seen in the primary tumor (or in other metastatic sites, excluding the central nervous system) (48,49). For less sensitive solid tumors, such as colorectal cancer, gastric cancer, or nonsmall-cell lung cancer, the response rate in the liver is roughly similar to the overall response rate, averaging 20 to 30% (50). Generally, with the development of superior therapies, control of intrahepatic disease has increased. This generalization holds for colorectal cancer as newer therapies have improved overall response rates. Prior to the 1980s, no treatment for metastatic colorectal cancer was superior to the 12 to 20% response rate achieved with single-agent 5-fluorouracil (5-FU) therapy. Since that time, several biochemical modulations of 5-FU have yielded apparent therapeutic advance. These modulations include combining 5-FU with folinic acid (51,52), with PALA (53), or with alpha interferon (54) or prolonged infusion of 5-FU (55). These regimens have produced objective response rates in metastatic colorectal cancer of 28 to 43%.

While these improvements represent an advance over single agents, systemic 5-FU regional infusion of chemotherapy to the liver can achieve an even higher local response rate. Intrahepatic tumor shrinkage after liver perfusion has been seen in as many as 83% of patients (56); response rates average about 44% (57), even in patients who have previously failed systemic 5-FU (58,59).

The basic rationale for regional chemotherapy is that higher concentrations of a cytotoxic agent can be delivered to tumor and/or there will be lower systemic exposure to drug toxicity (60). To realize the advantages of regional therapy, the site of drug delivery cannot be the site of dose-limiting toxicity with systemic administration and the drug must remain at the site of local therapy (e.g., a body cavity) or must be rapidly metabolized to minimize effects after leaving that site. The liver, in fact, is a model organ for infusion therapy and fluoropyrimidines are favorable agents for local hepatic delivery. The liver has a dual vascular supply; the predominant blood supply to grossly detectable metastatic lesions is via the hepatic artery (61,62), but adequate blood supply to the liver parenchyma can be maintained through the portal vein. The liver has the capacity to extract and metabolize a high percentage of many agents that circulate through it on first pass, effecting a high local clearance of those compounds with minimal systemic exposure. The liver possesses moderate functional excess or redundancy, thereby tolerating some degree of injury by tumor or treatment. In addition, the liver itself is relatively resistant to cell-cycle-specific chemotherapy because it has a low rate of cell division, while retaining the ability to regenerate after injury. The fluoropyrimidines (5-FU and FUdR) have among the highest target-to-systemic, regional delivery advantages of any chemotherapy. The ratio of increased concentrations achievable in the liver with hepatic artery infusion is 10 to 250 times depending on the volume of hepatic arterial flow (60). First-pass extraction of these agents has been shown to be 90%, with a fourfold concentration superiority seen after regional compared to systemic infusion of FUdR (63) and a two- to sixfold (64) benefit for 5-FU. Uptake of FUdR by tumor tissue is about one-half as efficient as extraction by normal liver after hepatic artery infusion (65), but the regional to systemic advantage still produces higher intratumor concentrations of drugs.

The initial attempts to control metastatic disease with arterial chemotherapy infusion was with nitrogen mustard in 1950 (66,67) and predated the introduction of fluoropyrimidine in about 1955 (68). Investigations of hepatic artery therapy with 5-FU began in the early 1960s, and even these early trials produced remissions in about 45 to 60% of patients (69–72). Criteria for these responses were somewhat less stringent than those currently employed but were similar to those criteria that assigned a 20% response rate to intravenous 5-FU (73). Despite promising preliminary findings, general enthusiasm was limited because of the technical difficulties associated with maintenance of the infusional systems. The hepatic arterial catheters could be directly placed at the time of laparotomy (74) or transcutaneously under fluoroscopic guidance through the femoral (75) or brachial (72) arteries. Until the introduction of totally implantable infusional systems, each of these catheters had to pass through the skin and employed a bulky extracorporeal pump and drug reservoir. Although the brachial arterial approach was utilized to accomplish prolonged outpatient infusions, catheter displacement was common. The other approaches were limited to short-term applications because they required hospitalization and severely restricted patient activities. The need to maintain a percutaneous foreign body and/or the requirement for repeated reinsertion of the catheters limited their use for chronic therapy and longterm control of disease. With the introduction of fully implantable pump and reservoir systems in the early 1980s (76,77), the cost, inconvenience, infection rate, and many of the vascular complications of therapy were reduced while the high local response rates were preserved (56).

Several agents have been tested for hepatic arterial infusion, including the fluoropyrimidines, mitomycin-C, cisplatinum, Adriamycin, and BCNU. However, because of its pharmacologic properties, high extraction rate by the liver, and superior response rate, FUdR remains the agent most commonly employed (78,79). An estimated 20,000 implantable infusion systems have been placed in the last 5 years (80). Despite the popularity of this therapy, the precise value of regional therapy compared to systemic therapy remains undefined.

The first attempt to conduct a randomized comparison of hepatic arterial and intravenous chemotherapy was by Grage and colleagues (81), who administered either IV or percutaneous intra-arterial 5-FU to 61 evaluable patients. The arterial therapy was limited to a 21-day infusion, after which any further therapy was administered intravenously. The response rate for the intra-arterial patients was slightly higher (34% versus 23%) and the median survival was somewhat shorter (13.5 versus 15.4 months), but neither of these differences was statistically significant. Kemeny and associates (82) tested repetitive regional therapy of FUdR via an implantable system versus systemic therapy in 99 colon cancer patients. They noted a significantly superior response rate for intra-arterial therapy (50% versus 20%) but also an increased rate in progression of extrahepatic disease (56% versus 37%) and a statistically insignificant advantage in survival (17 versus 12 months). Chang et al (83) conducted a similar randomized comparison of FUdR therapy in 50 patients and also observed a significant advantage for intra-arterial therapy in response (62% versus 17%) but not in survival. Finally, Hohn and colleagues' trial (84) of basically similar design but larger size (115 eligible patients) confirmed a superior response rate for regional therapy (42% versus 10%) but failed to demonstrate a meaningful survival difference (a median survival of 503 days for arterial therapy and 484 days for intravenous therapy). These few randomized, comparative trials of the two modes of therapy have been difficult to conduct because of the technical expertise required and the recognized difficulty in conducting trials in which patients and physicians accept random assignment of divergent therapies (i.e., surgery versus no surgery). The size of the trials has been small and stratification for prognostic factors, such as those discussed earlier, has been incomplete. In addition, the ability of the individual trials to identify important differences between the routes of administration has been limited by specific design factors in each study, such as short duration of regional infusion (Grage) and crossover of patients at the time of progression (Kemeny and Hohn). Furthermore, benefit must be balanced against cost and toxicity. The acute side effects from aggressive systemic therapy of metastatic solid tumors are commonly encountered and well known, resulting in hospitalization in about 30% of patients and occasional toxic deaths. The toxicity associated with intra-arterial therapy has been reviewed (85,86). Ignoring the technical aspects of inability to establish or maintain arterial vascular access, the common, serious toxicities are chemical hepatitis in 50 to 70%, gastric ulcer formation in approximately 20%, and biliary sclerosis in 8 to 20% of patients.

While the analysis of response rates, survival, side effects, and social/economic costs of systemic and regional chemotherapy leave the preferred treatment in doubt, determination of the better of the two modes of drug delivery may not be an important clinical consideration. Just as the combination of radiation and chemotherapy attempts to achieve at least additive effects, perhaps the comparison of real interest is a combination of intra-arterial and intravenous therapy versus systemic therapy. Such a combination, particularly in patients with liver metastases from colorectal cancer, could maximize control of intrahepatic and extrahepatic disease.

Radiation Therapy

Successful treatment of liver metastases with irradiation has been limited by the relative radioresistance of the tumors, by the relatively low radiation tolerance of the normal hepatocytes, and by the opportunity to effect only palliative results. The threshold dose for liver injury is 2500 to 3500 cGy (87–89). The liver is at increased risk for radiation injury when it is regenerating after a previous insult such as surgery. The radiation dose that can be tolerated is inadequate for cytotoxic therapy, except for the most sensitive leukemias, lymphomas, and germ cell tumors. If these tumors involve the liver, they are most likely to require and respond to systemic chemotherapy. Coupled with suboptimal dosage, one is also faced with the clinical setting in which liver metastases may represent only a portion of the tumor burden. The real intent of therapy then becomes palliation.

Palliative control of hepatic metastases with radiation therapy has been attempted since 1954 (90). Several uncontrolled series have demonstrated that liver capsular pain, nausea and vomiting, fever, and night sweats could be reduced in 50 to 90% of patients. Small studies utilizing doses of external beam irradiation of 2500 to 3100 cGy (91,92) showed that the approach was useful in controlling symptoms without significant toxicity but appeared to have no impact on patient survival. In Sherman's report (93) of hepatic irradiation in 55 patients, most of whom also received one of 14 individual chemotherapeutic agents, an excellent palliative benefit was seen in 54 to 63% of cases, including some patients with extensive hepatic involvement. Median survival was still only 4.5 months but, not surprisingly, median survival for patients enjoying an excellent response was twice that. In Borgelt's study (94), one-half of 109 patients with symptomatic liver metastases had improved pain control within 2 weeks of treatment but, again, median survival was very short (11 weeks). The patients with the smallest volume of metastatic disease are the ones more likely to demonstrate disease control by irradiation, but they are also the ones likely to have fewer symptoms from their hepatic disease and, therefore, have less potential to be palliated. The argument can be made that external beam irradiation accomplishes results equivalent to regional chemotherapy with less difficulty. No direct comparisons of these treatment modalities have been made, although Friedman and colleagues performed a comparative trial of external beam radiation versus combined chemoradiation (123). This trial is discussed in the following section.

The second major means of delivering hepatic irradiation is the injection of **radioactive isotopes** or particulates. A third, minor method of radiating hepatic metastases is **interstitial therapy** (95). External beam irradiation provides a roughly uniform and restricted area of exposure. Arterially injected radiation sources are theoretically delivered just to the target organ but have the same technical and pharmacologic limitations as regional chemotherapy and tend to cause more systemic (e.g., bone marrow) toxicity than either external beam irradiation or intra-arterial chemotherapy. Arterially directed radiation therapy takes advantage of tumor vascular characteristics and total doses of 5,000 to 10,000 cGy to the liver (96) and 20,000 cGy may be delivered without excessive toxicity to tumor (97,98). Several methods for administering internal radiation have been attempted including Yttrium-90–labeled microspheres (99–101), colloidal gold-198 (102), P-32 chromium phosphate colloid (103,104), and Iodide-131–labeled Lipiodol (105). Since colloidal gold and phosphorous are taken up by hepatic Kupffer's cells, their investigational use has been limited to the adjuvant setting, that is, the prevention of hepatic metastases. The preliminary results with the Iodine-131 product demonstrate palliation of pain in three of eight patients with liver metastases but not objective tumor responses. A future role for treatment of established hepatic metastases for any of these isotopes is questionable.

Taking advantage of the presence of capillary proliferation within tumors (106,107), it has been observed that microspheres of various composition (averaging 15 micra in diameter) will lodge preferentially in tumor tissue and, when labeled with radioactive Yttrium-90, will provide a 3 to 4 times differential in cellular radiation dose. The collective response rate for liver metastases after Yttrium-90 therapy in the three studies cited above is 50 to 60%. This response rate is consistent with that achieved with external beam irradiation or regional chemotherapy. Just as a direct comparison of systemic and intra-arterial chemotherapy is of limited interest, the actual ranking of the several radiation techniques is an unsatisfactory exercise. Determining a method of administering a maximally effective multimodality treatment is the key. Perhaps linking to monoclonal or polyclonal antibodies can improve the therapeutic index.

Chemoradiation

The rationale for developing combination therapy is that while individual therapies are less than curative, they can be combined to provide benefit without a corresponding increase in toxicity. Byfield has reviewed some of the biologic and methodologic considerations for multimodality therapy of hepatic metastases (108). The clinical experience with chemoradiation therapy of liver metastases has shown that, in general, full doses of both modalities result in an increase in toxicity over that associated with the individual modalities. However, overall survival has remained short, obscuring the observation of subacute toxicity. Haddad (109) observed patients who were longterm survivors after hepatic exposure to radiation and systemic Adriamycin/nitrosourea chemotherapy. Seven of 20 patients showed clinically evident liver damage, but all of these patients had received 3000 to 4000 cGy of radiation to at least half of the liver. In a colon cancer adjuvant setting, where prolonged observation is possible, McCraken (110) provided further data on serious liver toxicity and myelosuppression after combined hepatic therapy. In that trial, two cycles of standard-dose regional 5-FU and mitomycin were coupled with 1950 cGy external beam irradiation in 13 fractions. Only two of 13 patients did not experience liver function abnormalities. Eight patients continued to experience liver function abnormalities 119 to 684 days after therapy, and one individual died on fulminant hepatic failure at 90 days with no evident cancer at autopsy.

Thirteen trials of cytotoxic chemotherapy plus radiation are summarized in Table 23–2. For hepatic metastases, chemoradiation has included integration of both systemic and intra-arterial cytotoxic drugs with standard fraction, external beam irradiation (111–119) with altered fraction irradiation (120), and with Yttrium microspheres (121,122). With the possible exception of the two trials from Ariel with Yttrium microspheres, the results from these several reports are disappointing and consistent with those achieved with either modality alone. Only a single trial was of randomized design, comparing chemoradiation to radiation alone, and it failed to show a substantial benefit for combined treatment (123). The addition of the hypoxic cell sensitizer (misonidazole) to 2100 cGy whole liver irradiation has been tested in a randomized trial and similarly has been found to be of no significant benefit in amelioration of pain, improving performance status, reducing liver size, or improving survival (124). Table 23–2 presents the collective experience with 370 evaluable patients who received combined chemoradiation. The overall response rate is 42%. Except for three possible complete responses from Smith (118), all of the responses were incomplete. For the 260 patients in whom survival is reported, the median survival is 12.4 months. If the unusually high survival figures from Ariel are excluded by assessing only the 155 patients

Table 23–2. Chemoradiation Trials in Patients with Hepatic Metastases

Author/Reference	Patients: Eval/Total	Therapy RT (Total dose in cGy)	Responses	Median Survival (mos)
Herbsman, 1978 (111)	11/13	FUdR IA + RT 2500–3000	82%	16.2
Webber, 1978 (112)	18/25	FUdR IA + RT 2500	72%	12.5
Friedman, 1979 (113)	21/22	5-FU/ADR/RT 2100	48%	4+ mos.
Lokich, 1981 (114)	16	5-FU or FUdR/RT 3000	60%	N/A
Volberding, 1982 (115)	21/27	5-FU/ADR/MTX/RT 2100	33%	6.5
Barone, 1982 (116)	18	5-FU or FUdR/RT 2000–3000	56%	8
Byfield, 1984 (117)	27/28	FUdR IA + RT 2000–3000	N/A	15
Smith, 1984 (118)	31	DTIC/MITO-C/RT 1500	3%	5.5
Rotman, 1986 (119)	23/27	5-FU CI + RT 2700–3200	65%	7.5
Raju, 1987 (120)	12	5-FU or FUdR/RT 2100 (BID fractionation)	67%	14
Ariel, 1978 (121)	65	5-FU IA + Yt-90 IA	38%	13
Ariel, 1982 (122)	40	5-FU IA + Yt-90 IA	N/A	28
Friedman, 1988 (123)	51	5-FU IV + ADR/MITO-C + RT 2100	18%	N/A
		VS		
		5-FU IA + ADR/MITO-C – RT 2100	14%	
		VS.		
		RT 2100	17%	

IA = intra-arterial; IV = intravenous; Yt-90 = Yttrium-90; N/A = not available.

who received external beam irradiation, the median survival is 8.4 months.

PRIMARY HEPATOCELLULAR CANCER

Background

Primary hepatocellular carcinoma (HCC), or hepatoma, is a relatively rare tumor in the United States. Less than 10,000 new cases are reported annually, so HCC comprises less than 2% of the total malignancies (126). Other areas of the world, such as Northern Europe and South America, have a similar disease incidence. However, in parts of Africa and Asia, it is the most commonly diagnosed malignant tumor. In certain areas in Mozambique, this tumor accounts for more than 50% of all tumors in men (127). Worldwide, HCC may be responsible for between 250,000 and 1,250,000 deaths per year.

The development of HCC is epidemiologically associated with chronic hepatic injury, particularly hepatitis B virus (HBV) infection (128). In endemic areas of HCC, the chronic carrier rates of HBV are very high. More importantly, prospective studies have shown that carriers of HBV are at a much higher risk of developing HCC than age and sex matched, noninfected controls (129). Investigators have also found integration of HBV viral DNA into the hepatic cells of HCC patients.

Other causes of chronic hepatic injury (such as hemochromatosis, alpha-I-antitrypsin deficiency, alcoholic cirrhosis, steroid use, and perhaps naturally occurring carcinogens such as nitrosamines and aflatoxicins) have also been associated with an increased incidence of HCC, but the epidemiologic association is not as strong as with HBV.

Treatment Options

Only patients eligible for complete surgical resection may be cured of this tumor. However, less than 5% of the total number of patients presenting with this disease will be appropriate surgical candidates. By the time clinical symptoms arise, most patients have a locally unresectable tumor (e.g., the tumor involves both lobes of the liver, the portal vein, or vena cava or the patient already has metastatic disease) or insufficient hepatic reserve to withstand a major liver resection (e.g., advanced cirrhosis with clinically apparent ascites, jaundice, low albumin, abnormal bleeding parameters, etc.). The median survival of symptomatic patients is approximately 4 months. In contrast, a mass screening program of a population with a high risk of HCC in China has uncovered subclinical HCC cases (130). There, the 5-year survival rate may be over 50%.

The various treatment options of HCC have been extensively reviewed (131). The most active chemotherapeutic agent to date is the anthracycline derivative doxorubicin (Adriamycin). However, in examining the published study of doxorubicin-treated HCC patients, only approximately 20% of patients will respond to therapy, with significant treatment related morbidity and mortality (131). The weighted-average median survival in nine studies in which survival information was given was calculated to be 4 months. As this is the same as the survival of untreated patients, it is not clear that chemotherapy was beneficial.

Other single agents, such as 5-FU, mechlorethamine, etoposide, cisplatinum, and the anthracycline analogs mitoxantrone, idarubicin, and epirubicin have also been given intravenously, with minimal activity reported. Combination chemotherapy, while adding to the toxicity of treatment, has likewise not improved response rates or survival in this refractory tumor (131).

Intra-arterial administration of chemotherapeutic agents has also been extensively studied. HCC is a good model for intra-arterial therapy; the liver has a dual blood supply, with normal hepatocytes supplied mainly from the portal vein, while HCC derives most of its blood supply from the hepatic artery. Despite theoretical advantages of increased local drug concentrations to the tumor and lessened systemic side effects, neither single agents nor combinations when given intra-arterially have produced striking tumor responses.

Other methods of localized drug delivery, including intra-arterial injection of degradable starch microspheres and foreign material impregnated with chemotherapeutic agents, remain unproven.

Radiation therapy alone has not been an effective modality in the treatment of HCC patients. Early experience showed that low doses of external irradiation (2000 to 3000 cGy) were not effective in controlling the primary site of disease, while larger doses could cause radiation injury of the liver, with a high risk of hepatic failure in patients both with and without underlying hepatic dysfunction. Pathologically, venous occlusion of small hepatic vessels with parenchymal fibrosis can be produced when the hepatic tolerance dose is exceeded.

Chemoradiation

Combined modality treatment with radiation therapy and chemotherapy has not been widely tested. Cochrane reported a small Phase III trial of 18 hepatoma patients (133) randomly assigned to receive quadruple chemotherapy (5-FU, cytoxan, mitomycin-C, vincristine) or whole liver radiation (200 cGy/day × 15) followed by the same chemotherapy. Only two of the eight patients who received radiation therapy survived long enough to receive chemotherapy. The median survival was 5 months in the chemotherapy group and 3 months in the radiotherapy group, while none of the 18 patients had an objective response to therapy.

Two pilot studies of concomitant chemotherapy with radiotherapy were reported in the late 1970s. A Phase I/II pilot study of 13 hepatoma patients treated with intra-arterial 5-FU and doxorubicin with 300 cGy/day × 5 to 7 days produced responses in six of 13 patients (134). Nine of 20 HCC patients also had partial responses when treated with similar chemotherapy and additional methotrexate with leucovorin or mitomycin-C, along with the same dose and schedule of hepatic radiation (135). However, few responses were seen in a randomized trial comparing RT alone with concomitant IV or intra-arterial therapy in patients with HCC (123). There was no significant advantage to adding either intra-arterial or IV chemotherapy to the hepatic radiation, although the number of HCC patients in the study was small.

A more recent Phase II trial using doxorubicin (12 mg/m^2/day × 5 days) by continuous infusion with concomitant radiotherapy (150 cGy/day × 5 days) yielded four partial responses among the 11 patients studied (137). All patients had moderate bone-marrow suppression, while three patients developed catheter-induced sepsis. Whether the resulting toxicity warrants the combined modality approach in these patients remains to be proven.

Future Trends

Internal radiotherapy is a recent approach that is being explored in a variety of research centers. Using several different techniques and isotopes, the goal is to deliver high doses of radioactivity directly to the tumor, sparing normal liver parenchyma.

Order and colleagues, at Johns Hopkins University, developed radioactive isotopes directed against tumor-associated antigens for use in unresectable hepatoma patients. They showed that the tumor-associated protein ferritin was found in high concentrations both surrounding the tumor cells and in the stroma of hepatomas and thus could be made the target for specific antibody-mediated radiotherapy. In initial clinical studies, patients received sequential treatment with external beam radiation therapy, systemic chemotherapy using doxorubicin plus 5-FU, and then several courses of (Iodine-131) IgG antiferritin antibodies raised from differing animal species (rabbit, pig, monkey, and cow) (138). Data from 66 patients who were evaluated via CT scan by tumor volumetric measurements demonstrated that 30 had a response (defined as at least a 30% decrease in tumor volume) after the antiferritin antibody infusion. They described four patients who had apparent complete remission.

The Radiotherapy Therapy Oncology Group conducted a randomized trial in unresectable hepatoma patients, comparing the use of doxorubicin and 5-FU with and without Iodine-131 antiferritin antibodies, given after external beam radiation therapy with chemotherapy induction (139); 183 patients were entered in the trial, but only 98 were randomized. Similar response rates were seen in the randomized patients; 23% of those receiving radiolabeled antibody and 28% of chemotherapy-treated patients achieved a partial response. Median survial for both treatments was 6 months. Of interest, median survival was twice as long (10 versus 5 months) for patients with a normal alpha feto-protein (AFP) titer in contrast to patients with an elevated titer. Also noted was a partial response rate of 63% (7 of 11) in AFP normal patients who progressed after chemotherapy and were crossed over to antibody treatment.

Yttrium-90 labeled antiferritin is also being piloted by the Johns Hopkins group in an effort to find an isotope with more energetic beta particle emission compared to Iodine-131 (140). Yttrium-90 microspheres have also been intra-arterially administered to small numbers of patients, with anecdotal responses noted in hepatoma patients (101,141).

A number of investigators have been interested in the use of fatty acid esters, used in the past as contrast agents in lymphographic studies, as agents to carry radiation directly to hepatomas. Japanese researchers showed that when directly injected in the hepatic artery, the iodized oil selectively remains in hypervascular tumors for as long as several days. These agents have been used in therapeutic protocols, mixed with a variety of chemotherapeutic agents and gelatin sponge particles, or labeled with Iodine-131. Recent dosimetry studies show that the Iodine-131 ethiodol is accumulated in vascular hepatomas, the liver, and lungs during the first pass of the agent (142). The concentration of the isotope was an order of magnitude greater than normal tissue surrounding the tumor, with a 20 to 25% longer half-life in the tumors compared to normal liver. Thus, large radiation doses could be delivered to hepatomas with acceptable radiation doses to the liver, lungs, and total body. Pilot studies (143,144) have demonstrated that toxicity is minimal; successful palliation of pain, reduction of ascites, decreases in AFP, and actual tumor shrinkage in patients with advanced disease have all been seen when Iodine-131–labeled iodized oil was injected intra-arterially alone or with embolization of polyvinyl sponges or intra-arterial chemotherapy. Larger Phase II studies are under way to confirm these encouraging results. Additional trials may use Yttrium-90 for more effective cytotoxicity.

REFERENCES

1. Pickren JW, Tsukada Y, Lane WW. Liver metastases: Analysis of autopsy data. *In:* Liver Metastasis. Weiss L, Gilbert HA (Eds). Boston, GK Hall Medical Publishers, 1982, p. 2.
2. Bengmark S, Hafstrom L. The natural history of primary and secondary malignant tumors of the liver. Cancer 23:198, 1969.
3. Oxley EM, Ellis H. Prognosis of carcinoma of the large bowel in the presence of liver metastases. Brit J Surg 56:149, 1969.
4. Wood CB, Gilles CR, Blumgart LH. A retrospective study of the natural history of patients with liver metastases from colorectal cancer. Clin Oncol 2:285, 1976.

5. Nicholson GL. Cancer metastases. Organ colonization and the cell surface properties of malignant cells. Biochem Biophys Acta 695:113, 1982.
6. Nicholson GL, Poste G. Tumor implantation and invasion at metastatic sites. Int Rev Exp Pathol 25:77, 1983.
7. Schirrmacher V. Cancer metastases. Experimental approaches. Theoretical concepts, and impacts for treatment strategies. Adv Cancer Res 43:1, 1981.
8. Liotta LA. Tumor invasion and metastases—Role of the extracellular matrix. Rhoads Memorial Lecture. Cancer Res 45:1, 1986.
9. Cameron GR. The liver as a site and source of cancer. Br Med J 1:347, 1954.
10. Warren BA. Ultrastructural aspects of the invasion of liver by cancer cells. *In:* Liver Metastasis. Weiss L, Gilbert HA (Eds). Boston, GK Hall Medical Publishers, 1982, p. 40.
11. Roos E. Invasion of the liver by tumor cells. *In:* Liver Metastases: Basic Aspects, Detection, and Management. Van de Vilde CJH, Sugarbaker PH (Eds). Boston, Martinus Nijhoff Publishers, 1984, p. 1.
12. Goslin R, Steele G, Zamcheck N, et al. Factors influencing survival in patients with hepatic metastases from adenocarcinoma of the colon or rectum. Dis Colon Rect 8:749, 1982.
13. Wood CB. Natural history of liver metastases. *In:* Liver Metastases: Basic Aspects, Detection, and Management. Van deVilde CJH, Sugarbaker PH (Eds). Boston, Martinus Nijhoff Publishers, 1984, p. 47.
14. Pestana C, Reitemeir RJ, Moertel CG, et al. The natural history of the carcinoma of the colon and rectum. Am J Surg 108:826, 1964.
15. Jaffe BM, Donegan WL, Watson F, et al. Factors influencing survival in patients with untreated hepatic metastases. Surg Gynecol Obstet 127:1, 1968.
16. Galanta M, Dunphy JE, Fletcher WS. Cancer of the colon. Ann Surg 165:732, 1967.
17. Baden H, Andersen B. Survival of patients with untreated liver metastases from colorectal cancer. Scand J Gastroenterol 10:221, 1975.
18. Wagner JS, Adson MA, van Heerden JA. The natural history of hepatic metastases from colorectal cancer. A comparison with resective treatment. Ann Surg 199:502, 1984.
19. Fortner JS, MacLean BJ, Kim DK, et al. The seventies evolution in liver surgery for cancer. Cancer 47:2162, 1981.
20. Cady B, Oberfield RA. Regional infusion chemotherapy of hepatic metastases from carcinoma of the colon. Am J Surg 127:220, 1974.
21. Lahr CJ, Soong SJ, Cloud G, et al. A multifactorial analysis of prognostic factors in patients with liver metastases from colorectal carcinoma. J Clin Oncol 1:720, 1983.
22. Cady B, McDermott MV. Major hepatic resection for metachronous metastases from colon cancer. Ann Surg 201:204, 1985.
23. Keene W. Report of a case of resection of the liver for the removal of a neoplasm. With a table of seventy-six cases of resection of the liver for hepatic tumors. Ann Surg 30:267, 1988.
24. Woodington GF, Waugh JM. Results of resection of metastatic tumors of the liver. Am J Surg 105:24, 1963.
25. Foster JH. Survival after liver resection for cancer. Cancer 26:493, 1970.
26. Wanebo HH, Semoglou C, Attujeh F, et al. Surgical management of patients with primary operable colorectal cancer and synchronous liver metastases. Am J Surg 135:81, 1978.
27. Wilson SM, Adson MA. Surgical treatment of hepatic metastases from colorectal cancer. Arch Surg 111:330, 1976.
28. Hughes KS, Sugarbaker PH. Treatment of metastatic liver tumors. *In:* Treatment of Metastatic Cancer. Rosenberg SA (Ed). Philadelphia, JB Lippincott, 1987. p. 110.
29. Hughes KS, Simon R, Songhorabodi S, et al. Resection of the liver for colorectal carcinoma metastases. Surg 100:278, 1986.
30. Iwatsuki S, Starzl TE. Personal experience with 411 hepatic resections. Ann Surg 208:421, 1988.
31. Nilsson LAV. Therapeutic hepatic artery ligation in patients with secondary liver tumors. Rev Surg 23:374, 1966.
32. Murry-Lyon IM, Parsons VA, Blendis LM, et al. Treatment of secondary tumors by ligation of hepatic artery and infusion of cytotoxic drugs. Lancet II:172, 1970.
33. Almersjo O, Bengmark S, Rudenstam CM, et al. Evaluation of hepatic dearterialization in primary and secondary cancer of the liver. Am J Surg 124:5, 1972.
34. Evans JT. Hepatic artery ligation in hepatic metastases from colon and rectal malignancies. Dis Colon Rect 22:370, 1979.
35. Lindell B, Aronsen KF, Nosslin B, et al. Studies in pharmacokinetics and tolerance of substance temporarily retained in the liver by microsphere embolization. Ann Surg 187:95, 1978.
36. Aronsen KF. Controlled blocking of hepatic artery flow with enzymatically degradable microspheres combined with oncolytic drugs. Eur Surg Res 11:99, 1979.
37. Persson B, Jeppson B, Puntis MCA, et al. The

use of an implantable vascular occluder in the treatment of nonresectable hepatic malignancies. Recent Results Cancer Res 110:178, 1988.
38. Raven RW. Hepatectomy. Proc Int Soc Surg 16:1099, 1955.
39. Flanagan L, Foster JH. Hepatic resection for metastatic tumors. Am J Surg 113:551, 1967.
40. Foster JH. Survival after liver resection for secondary tumors. Am J Surg 135:389, 1978.
41. Fortner JG, Silva JS, Golbey RB, et al. Multivariate analysis of a personal series of 247 consecutive patients with liver metastases from colorectal cancer. I. Treatment by hepatic resection. Ann Surg 199:306, 1984.
42. Hanks JB, Meyers WC, Filston HC, et al. Surgical resection for benign and malignant liver disease. Ann Surg 191:584, 1980.
43. Bengmark S, Hafstrom L, Jeppsson B, et al. Metastatic disease in the liver after colorectal cancer. An appraisal of liver surgery. World J Surg 6:61, 1982.
44. Ekberg H, Tranberg K, Anderson R, et al. Pattern of recurrence in liver resection for colorectal secondaries. World J Surg 11:541, 1987.
45. August DA, Sugarbaker PH, Ottow RT, et al. Hepatic resection of colorectal metastases. Ann Surg 201:210, 1985.
46. Carrasco CH, Wallace S, Charnsangavej C, et al. Treatment of hepatic metastases in ocular melanoma. Embolization of the hepatic artery with polyvinyl sponge and cisplatin. JAMA 255:3152, 1986.
47. Ajani JA, Carrasco CH, Jackson DE, et al. Combination of cisplatin plus fluoropyrimidine chemotherapy effective against liver metastases from carcinoma of the anal canal. Am J. Med 87:221, 1989.
48. George SL, Hoogstraten B. Prognostic factors in the initial response to therapy by patients with advanced breast cancer. J Natl Cancer Inst 60:731, 1978.
49. Ihde DC, Deisseroth AB, Lichter AS, et al. Late intensive combined modality therapy followed by autologous bone marrow infusion in extensive-stage small-cell lung cancer. J Clin Oncol 4:1443, 1986.
50. Kemeny N. The systemic chemotherapy of hepatic metastases. Semin Oncol 10:148, 1983.
51. Grem JL, Hoth DF, Hamilton JM, et al. Overview of current status and future directions of clinical trials with 5-fluorouracil in combination with folinic acid. Cancer Treat Rep 71:1249, 1987.
52. O'Connell MJ. A phase III trial of 5-fluorouracil and leucovorin in the treatment of advanced colorectal cancer. A Mayo Clinic/North Central Cancer Treatment Group Study. Cancer 63:1026, 1989.
53. Grem JL, King SA, O'Dwyer PJ, et al. Biochemistry and clinical activity of N-(phosphonacety)-L-aspartate. A review. Cancer Res 48:4441, 1988.
54. Wadler S, Lyver A, Goldman M, et al. Therapy with 5-fluorouracil and recombination alpha-2a-interferon in refractory GI malignancies. Proc ASCO 8:99, 1989.
55. Lokich JJ, Ahlgren JD, Gullo JJ, et al. A prospectively randomized comparison of continuous infusion fluorouracil with a conventional bolus schedule in metastatic colorectal carcinoma. A Mid-Atlantic Oncology Program study. J Clin Oncol 7:425, 1989.
56. Niederhuber JE, Ensminger WD, Gyves JW, et al. Regional chemotherapy of colorectal cancer metastatic to the liver. Cancer 53:1336, 1984.
57. Kemeny N. Role of chemotherapy in the treatment of colorectal carcinoma. Semin Surg Oncol 3:190, 1987.
58. Patt YZ, Peters RE, Chuang VP, et al. Effective retreatment of patients with colorectal cancer and liver metastases. Am J Med 75:237, 1983.
59. Buroker T, Samson M, Correa J, et al. Hepatic artery infusion of 5-FUdR after prior 5-fluorouracil. Cancer Treat Rep 60:1277, 1976.
60. Collins JM. Pharmacologic rationale for regional drug delivery. J Clin Oncol 2:498, 1984.
61. Bierman HR, Byron RL, Kelly KH, et al. Studies in blood supply of tumors in man, III. Vascular patterns of liver by hepatic arteriography in vitro. J Natl Cancer Inst 12:107, 1951.
62. Breedis C, Young C. The blood supply of neoplasms in the liver. Am J Pathol 30:969, 1954.
63. Ensminger WD, Rosowsky A, Raso A, et al. A clinical-pharmacologic evaluation of hepatic arterial infusions of 5-fluoro-2′-deoxyuridine and 5-fluorouracil. Cancer Res 38:3784, 1978.
64. Wagner JH, Gyves JW, Stetson PL, et al. Steady-state nonlinear pharmacokinetics of 5-fluorouracil during hepatic arterial and intravenous infusions in cancer patients. Cancer Res 46:1499, 1986.
65. Sigurdson ER, Ridge JA, Daly JM, et al. Fluorodeoxyuridine uptake by human colorectal hepatic metastases after hepatic artery infusion. Surg 100:285, 1986.
66. Bierman HR, Byron RL Jr, Miller ER, et al. Effects of intraarterial administration of nitrogen mustard (Abst). Am J Med 8:535, 1950.

67. Klopp CT, Bateman J, Berry N, et al. Fractionated regional cancer chemotherapy (abst). Cancer Res 10:229, 1950.
68. Heidelberger C, Chaudhari NK, Danneberg P, et al. Fluorinated pyrimidines. A new class of tumour-inhibitory compounds. Nature 1798:663, 1957.
69. Rochlin DB, Smart CR. An evaluation of fifty-one patients with hepatic artery infusion. Surg Gynecol Obstet 123:535, 1966.
70. Burrows JH, Talley RW, Drake EH, et al. Infusion of fluorinated pyrimidines in hepatic artery for treatment of metastatic carcinoma of the liver. Cancer 20:1886, 1967.
71. Fortuny IE, Theologies A, Kennedy BJ. Cancer of the liver. Minn Med 55:197, 1972.
72. Ansfield FJ, Ramire G, Skibba JL, et al. Intrahepatic arterial infusion with 5-fluorouracil. Cancer 28:1147, 1971.
73. Zubrod CG. The limited usefulness of 5-fluorouracil (5-FU) and 5-fluorodeoxyuridine (5-FUdR) in the management of patients with adenocarcinoma. *In:* Controversy in Internal Medicine. Inglefinger FJ, Relman AS, Finland M (Eds). Philadelphia, WB Saunders, 1966, p. 591.
74. Labelle JJ, Lucas RJ, Eisenstein B, et al. Hepatic artery catheterization for chemotherapy. Arch Surg 96:683, 1968.
75. Tandon RN, Bunnell L, Cooper RG. The treatment of metastatic carcinoma of the liver by the percutaneous selective hepatic artery infusion of 5-fluorouracil. Surg 73:118, 1973.
76. Gonzalez ER. Implantable pump concentrates chemotherapy for the liver. JAMA 246:925, 1981.
77. Ensminger W, Neiderhuber J, Dakhill S, et al. Totally implanted drug delivery system for hepatic arterial chemotherapy. Cancer Treat Rep 65:393, 1981.
78. Friedman MA. Hepatic interarterial chemotherapy. Current status and future prospects. J Cancer Chemother 10:1209, 1983.
79. Stagg RJ, Lewis BJ, Friedman MA, et al. Hepatic arterial chemotherapy for colorectal cancer metastatic to the liver. Ann Intern Med 100:736, 1984.
80. Ensminger W. Hepatic arterial chemotherapy for primary and metastatic liver cancers. Cancer Chemother Pharmacol 23(Suppl):S68, 1989.
81. Grage TR, Vassilopoulos PP, Shingleton WW, et al. Results of a prospective randomized study of hepatic artery infusion with 5-fluorouracil versus intravenous 5-fluorouracil in patients with hepatic metastases from colorectal cancer. A Central Oncology Group Study. Surg 86:550, 1979.
82. Kemeny N, Daly J, Reichman B, et al. Intrahepatic or systemic infusion of fluorodeoxyuridine in patients with liver metastases from colorectal cancer. Ann Intern Med 107:459, 1987.
83. Chang AE, Schneider PD, Sugarbaker PH, et al. A prospective randomized trial of regional versus systemic continuous 5-fluorodeoxyuridine chemotherapy in the treatment of colorectal liver metastases. Ann Surg 206:685, 1987.
84. Hohn DC, Stagg RJ, Friedman MA, et al. A randomized trial of continuous intravenous versus intraarterial floxuridine in patients with colorectal cancer metastatic to the liver. The Northern California Oncology Group Trial. J Clin Oncol 7:1646, 1987.
85. Hohn D, Rayner AA, Economous JS, et al. Toxicities and complications of implantable pump hepatic arterial and intravenous floxuridine infusion. Cancer 47:465, 1986.
86. Hohn D, Melnick J, Stagg R, et al. Biliary sclerosis in patients receiving hepatic arterial infusions of floxuridine. J Clin Oncol 3:98, 1985.
87. Ingold JA, Reed GB, Kaplan HS, et al. Radiation hepatitis. Am J Roentgenol 93:200, 1965.
88. Wharton JT, Declos L, Gallagher S, et al. Radiation hepatitis induced by abdominal irradiation with the cobalt 60 moving strip technique. Am J Roentgenol Rad Ther Nucl Med 117:73, 1973.
89. Kaplan HS, Bagshaw MA. Radiation hepatitis. Possible prevention by combined isotopic and external beam therapy. Radiology 91:7214, 1968.
90. Phillips R, Karnofsky DA, Hamilton JD, et al. Roentgen therapy of hepatic metastases. Am J Roentgenol Rad Ther Nuc Med 71:826, 1954.
91. Turek-Maischeider M, Kazem I. Palliative irradiation for liver metastases. JAMA 232:625, 1975.
92. Prasad B, Lee MS, Hendrickson PR. Irradiation of hepatic metastases. Int J Radiat Oncol Biol Phys 2:129, 1977.
93. Sherman DA, Weichselbach R, Order SE, et al. Palliation of hepatic metastases. Cancer 41:2013, 1978.
94. Borgelt BB, Gelber R, Brady LW, et al. The palliation of hepatic metastases. Results of the Radiation Therapy Oncology Group pilot study. Int J Radiat Oncol Biol Phys 7:587, 1981.
95. Dritschilo A, Grant EG, Harter KW, et al. Interstitial radiation therapy for hepatic metastases. AJR 147:275, 1986.

96. Boos G, Thirlwell M, Blanchard R, et al. Phase I-II study of hepatic arterial infusion of yttrium-90 (Yt-90) glass microspheres in cancer of the liver. Proc Am Soc Clin Oncol 8:103, 1989.
97. Houle S, Yip T-CK, Shephard FA, et al. Pilot trial of y-90 glass microspheres in the treatment of primary hepatocellular carcinoma. Radiology 165:98, 1987.
98. Herba MJ, Illescas FF, Thirwell MP, et al. Hepatic malignancy. Improved delivery methods for the treatment with intraarterial Y-90. Radiology 165:181, 1987.
99. Ariel IM. Treatment of inoperable primary pancreatic and liver cancer by the intraarterial administration of radioactive isotope (Y90 radiating microspheres). Ann Surg 162:267, 1965.
100. Grady ED. Internal radiation therapy of hepatic cancer. Dis Colon Rectum 22:371, 1979.
101. Mantravadi RVP, Spigos DG, Grady ED, et al. Treatment of hepatic malignancies by intravascular administration of radioisotopes. *In:* Nuclear Medicine in Clinical Oncology. Winkler C (Ed). Berlin, Springer-Verlag, 1986, p. 365.
102. Alfonso A, Hassan A, Gardner B, et al. Prevention of hepatic metastases by intravenous radioactive gold. Cancer Res 38:2740, 1978.
103. Mantravadi RVP, Spigos DG, Karesh SM, et al. Work in progress. Intraarterial P-32 chromic phosphate for prevention of postoperative liver metastases in high-risk colorectal cancer patients. Radiology 148:555, 1983.
104. Grady ED. Adjuvant therapy of Duke's C colon cancer by intraarterial P-32 colloid for internal radiation therapy of the liver. Am Surg 50:488, 1984.
105. Bretagne JF, Raoul J, Bourguet P, et al. Hepatic arterial injection of I-131-labeled Lipiodol. Radiology 168:547, 1988.
106. Sundqvist K, Hafstrom L, Persson B. Measurements of total and regional blood tumor blood flow and organ blood flow using Tc99m labelled microspheres. Eur J Surg Res 10:433, 1978.
107. Gyves J, Ziessman HA, Ensminger WD, et al. Definition of hepatic tumor microcirculation by single photon emission computerized tomography (SPECT). J Nuc Med 25:972, 1983.
108. Byfield JE. Combined use of drugs and radiation in the treatment of liver metastases. Recent Results Cancer Res 100:298, 1986.
109. Haddad E, Le Bourgeois J, Kuentz M, et al. Liver complications in lymphomas treated with a combination of chemotherapy and radiotherapy. Preliminary results. Int J Radiat Oncol Biol Phys 9:1313, 1983.
110. McCracken JD, Weatherall TJ, Oishi N, et al. Adjuvant intrahepatic chemotherapy with mitomycin and 5-FU combined with hepatic irradiation in high-risk patients with carcinoma of the colon. A Southwest Oncology Group phase II pilot study. Cancer Treat Rep 69:129, 1985.
111. Herbsman H, Hassan A, Gardner B, et al. Treatment of hepatic metastases with a combination of hepatic arterial infusion chemotherapy and external beam radiotherapy. Surg Gynecol Obstet 147:13, 1978.
112. Webber BM, Soderberg CH, Leone LA, et al. A combined treatment approach to management of hepatic metastases. Cancer 42:1087, 1978.
113. Friedman MA, Cassidy M, Levine M, et al. Combined modality therapy of hepatic metastasis. Cancer 44:906, 1979.
114. Lokich L, Kinsella T, Perri J, et al. Concomitant hepatic radiation and intraarterial fluorinated pyrimidine therapy. Cancer 48:2569, 1981.
115. Volberding PA, Friedman MA, Resser KJ, et al. Therapy of liver tumors metastatic from colorectal cancer with whole-liver radiation combined with 5-FU, adriamycin, and methotrexate. Cancer Chemother Pharmacol 9:127, 1982.
116. Barone RM, Byfield JE, Goldfarb PB, et al. Intraarterial chemotherapy using an implantable infusion pump and liver irradiation for colon carcinoma metastatic to the liver. Cancer 50:850, 1982.
117. Byfield JE, Barone RM, Frankel SS, et al. Treatment with combined intraarterial 5-FUdR infusion and whole liver radiation for colon carcinoma metastatic to the liver. Am J Clin Oncol 7:319, 1984.
118. Smith BJ, Evans M, Hellman K, et al. Inefficacy of dacarbazine, mitomycin C and hepatic irradiation in patients with metastatic adenocarcinoma of the gastrointestinal tract. J Clin Oncol 6:578, 1984.
119. Rotman M, Kuruvilla AM, Choi K, et al. Response of colorectal hepatic metastases to concomitant radiotherapy and intravenous infusion 5-fluorouracil. Int J Radiat Biol Phys 12:2179, 1986.
120. Raju PI, Maruyama Y, DeSimone P, et al. Treatment of liver metastases with a combination of chemotherapy and hyperfractionated external radiation therapy. Am J Clin Oncol 10:41, 1987.
121. Ariel IM, Padula G. Treatment of symptomatic metastatic cancer to the liver from primary colon and rectal cancer by intraarterial

administration of chemotherapy and radioactive isotopes. J Surg Oncol 20:327, 1978.
122. Ariel IM, Padula G. Treatment of asymptomatic metastatic cancer to the liver from primary colon and rectal cancer by intraarterial administration of chemotherapy and radioactive isotopes. J Surg Oncol 20:151, 1982.
123. Friedman MA, Phillips TL, Hannigan JF, et al. Phase III trial of irradiation plus chemotherapy for patients with hepatic metastases and hepatoma. Experience of the Northern California Oncology Group. NCI Monogr 6:259, 1988.
124. Liebel SA, Pajak TF, Massullo V, et al. A comparison of misonidazole sensitized radiation therapy to radiation alone for the palliation of hepatic metastases. A Radiation Therapy Oncology Group prospective randomized trial. Int J Radiat Oncol Biol Phys 13:1057, 1987.
125. Pettavel J, Morgenthales F. Protracted arterial chemotherapy of liver tumors. An experience of 107 cases over a 12 year period. *In:* Progress in Clinical Cancer. Ariel IM (Ed). New York, Grune and Stratton, 1978, p. 217.
126. Silverberg E. Cancer statistics 1985. CA 35:19, 1985.
127. Kew M. Clinical, pathologic, and etiologic heterogeneity in hepatocellular carcinoma. Evidence from southern Africa. Hepatology 1:366, 1981.
128. Nerenstone S, Friedman M, Ihde D. Primary liver cancer. *In:* Comprehensive Textbook of Oncology. 2nd Ed. Kaplan R, Schimpff S, Moossa A, Robson M (Eds). Baltimore, Williams & Wilkins, 1991, p. 948.
129. Beasley R. Hepatitis B virus. The major etiology of hepatocellular carcinoma. Cancer 61:1942, 1988.
130. Tang Z. Subclinical hepatocellular carcinoma—Historical aspects and general considerations. *In:* Hepatocellular Carcinoma. Tang Z (Ed). New York, Springer-Verlag, 1985, p. 1.
131. Nerenstone S, Ihde D, Friedman M. Clinical trials in primary heptocellular carcinoma. Current status and future directions. Cancer Treat Rev 15:1, 1988.
132. Lai E, Choi T, Tong S, et al. Treatment of unresectable hepatocellular carcinoma. Results of a randomized controlled trial. World J Surg 10:501, 1986.
133. Cochrane A, Muray-Lyon I, Brinkley D, Williams R. Quadruple chemotherapy versus radiotherapy in treatment of primary hepatocellular carcinoma. Cancer 40:609, 1977.
134. Friedman M, Volberding P, Cassidy M, et al. Therapy for hepatocellular cancer with intrahepatic arterial adriamycin and 5-fluorouracil combined with whole-liver irradiation: A Northern California Oncology Group Study. Cancer Treat Rep 63:1885, 1979.
135. Friedman M, Volberding P, Cassidy M, et al. Therapy of hepatocellular cancer with combined intrahepatic arterial chemotherapy and whole liver irradiation. Ann Acad Med 9:260, 1980.
136. Friedman M, Phillips T, Hannigan J, Carter S. Phase III trial of irradiation plus chemotherapy for patients with hepatic metastases and hepatoma. Experience of the Northern California Oncology Group. NCI Monogr 6:259, 1988.
137. Ohri A, Rosenthal C, Stark R, et al. Adriamycin (A) by continuous infusion (CI) and concomitant radiation therapy in hepatocellular carcinoma. (Abstr.) Proc Am Soc Clin Oncol 6:93, 1987.
138. Order S, Stillwagon G, Klein J, Leichner P, et al. Iodine 131 antiferritin, a new treatment modality in hepatoma. A Radiation Therapy Oncology Group Study. J Clin Oncol 3:1573, 1985.
139. Order S, Pajak T, Leibel S, et al. A randomized prospective trial comparing full dose chemotherapy to ^{131}I antiferritin: an RTOG study. Int J Radiat Oncol Biol Phys 20:953, 1991.
140. Leichner P, Yang N, Frenkel T, et al. Dosimetry and treatment planning for $_{90}$Y-labeled antiferritin in hepatoma. Int J Radiat Oncol Biol Phys 14:1033, 1988.
141. Boos G, Thirlwell M, Blanchard R, et al. Phase I-II study of hepatic arterial infusion of yttrium-90 (Y-90) glass microspheres in cancer of the liver. (Abstr.) Proc Am Soc Clin Oncol 8:103, 1989.
142. Madsen M, Park C, Thakur M. Dosimetry of Iodine-131 Ethiodol in the treatment of hepatoma. J Nucl Med 29:1038, 1988.
143. Park C, Suh H, Yoo H, et al. Treatment of hepatocellular carcinoma (HCC) with radiolabeled Lipiodol. A preliminary report. Nucl Med Commun 8:1075, 1987.
144. Bretagne J, Raoul J, Bourguet P, et al. Hepatic artery injection of I-131-labeled Lipiodol—Part II. Preliminary results of therapeutic use in patients with hepatocellular carcinoma and liver metastases. Radiology 168:547, 1988.

Chapter 24

COLON AND RECTUM

JAFFER A. AJANI AND TYVIN A. RICH

INCIDENCE AND NATURE OF THE PROBLEM

Carcinomas of the colon and rectum continue to pose a significant health problem. These malignancies are the second most common cause of cancer death in the United States (1). It is estimated that 156,000 persons will be diagnosed with colon or rectal carcinoma and approximately 58,300 patients will succumb to these neoplasms in 1992 (1). While 70 to 80% of patients at presentation have potentially curable tumors, surgical resection has lead to cures of approximately 50% of patients presenting with colorectal carcinomas. Therefore, a significant proportion of patients after curative resection remains at high risk for the development of systemic metastases or local recurrence. Currently available therapies offer little hope of cure for patients who have distant metastases; occasionally, successful resection of isolated metastases has resulted in longterm survival (2,3). Similarly, a local or regional (peritoneal) relapse of carcinoma presents a difficult management problem. Surgical removal of the locally recurrent carcinoma offers the only chance of potential cure, however, a curative resection of the recurrent tumor is possible in only a small fraction of patients due to invasion of nerves, adjacent viscera, blood vessels, and bony structures. Therefore, more effective therapies are needed to reduce the risk of local and systemic relapse and to increase the resectability rate in patients with local recurrence.

PROGNOSTIC FACTORS AND NATURAL HISTORY

It is important to recognize that there are a number of characteristics of the primary carcinoma that determine the clinical course of patients with colorectal carcinoma. Unfortunately, clinical methods of assessing the extent of the primary carcinoma to date are much less efficient than desired. The prognostic factors are defined most precisely by examining the resected specimen. In the future, endoscopic ultrasonography and understanding of biologic markers in the biopsy specimen will certainly enhance our ability to improve clinical staging of these tumors.

Clinical and pathologic factors established as prognostic factors are listed in Table 24–1. Many biologic characteristics of the carcinoma, such as specific genetic abnormalities and DNA contents of the tumor cells, are currently being studied to determine their value in predicting patients' survival. Of interest is a recent report describing chromosomal abnormality in the malignant tissues as a reliable predictor of prognosis (4). In this study, the clinical and pathologic features associated with molecular genetic alterations were studied in 83 patients with colorectal carcinoma. Fractional allelic loss and allelic deletions of specific chromosomal arms (the short arm of 17 and long arm of 18) each provided independent prognostic information by a multivariate

Table 24–1. Prognostic Factors of Colorectal Carcinoma

1. Depth of penetration
2. Adjacent organ invasion
3. Lymph node metastases
4. Lymphatic and blood vessel invasion
5. Site of the primary tumor
6. Histologic grade
7. Age at diagnosis
8. Serum level of CEA at diagnosis

analysis when compared individually with traditional Dukes' classification. This study exemplifies the emerging value of biologic study to better understand the natural course of these illnesses and apply appropriate therapies. The factors listed in Table 24–1 have been studied more extensively. The most important factors are the depth of penetration of bowel wall, number of lymph node metastases, and serum level of carcinoembryonic antigen (CEA) at diagnosis. Many studies are now in progress to assess whether molecular and genetic determinants might supercede more traditional prognostic factors. Nonetheless, it is essential that a treating physician assess all traditional prognostic factors in a patient prior to recommending longterm therapy (e.g., adjuvant therapy).

In addition to identification of the prognostic factors, a staging system is necessary in order to group them. An ideal staging system that can do justice to all independent prognostic factors does not exist currently. However, the Astler-Coller modification of Dukes' classification system remains the most popular and practical staging system (5). In addition, some investigators have also used the Gunderson-Sosin modification of the Astler-Coller system (6).

The incidence of local recurrence of rectal carcinoma is dependent on the stage of the primary carcinoma. For instance, it ranges from only 5 to 10% if the primary carcinoma is confined to the muscularis propria with no lymph node metastases, i.e. modified Astler-Coller Dukes' B_1 (7). However, the rate of local relapse increases dramatically, reaching up to 75% with increasing penetration of bowel wall and adjacent structures and with metastases to the lymph nodes in patients with Gunderson-Sosin's modified Dukes' Stages B_2/B_3 and C_2/C_3. Therefore, it is essential to develop better adjuvant treatments for patients at the highest risk.

This chapter will summarize approaches to adjuvant therapy of colon and rectal carcinoma and strategies used to control local recurrences in patients with carcinoma of the rectum.

ADJUVANT THERAPY OF COLORECTAL CARCINOMA

In the late 1960s, investigators at the Mayo Clinic reported a survival advantage in patients with locally advanced gastrointestinal malignancies when treated with the combination of chemotherapy and radiotherapy when compared to patients who were treated with radiotherapy alone (8). These data led to numerous subsequent studies. In addition, substantial preclinical data exist suggesting that the radiosensitivity of cancer cells increases with the addition of radiosensitizing agents such as 5-fluorouracil (5-FU) (9,10).

Rectal Carcinoma

Patterns of local and regional recurrence of rectal carcinoma are distinct from those of colon carcinoma, although the frequency of systemic metastases appears similar (11). The incidence of local recurrence remains much higher in rectal carcinoma than colon carcinoma while intraperitoneal failure is more frequent in patients with colon carcinoma. The emphasis of adjuvant strategies to counter local as well as systemic relapse is, therefore, obvious.

Radiotherapy Alone

The effect of radiation therapy alone in reducing the rate of local recurrence has been reported in randomized (12–15) and nonrandomized studies (16). A number of nonrandomized studies summarized by Rich (16) demonstrate that recurrence rates following postoperative radiation therapy varied between 4 and 11% compared to a range between 20 and 75% in a similar group of patients treated with surgical resection alone. This conclusion, however, is not substantiated by the results of three representative randomized trials that are described in Table 24–2 (15,17–19). We can conclude that radiotherapy alone is ineffective in reducing the rate of local recurrence, prolonging disease-free interval, or increasing the overall survival of patients with Dukes' B and C rectal carcinoma.

Chemoradiation

In the past decade, studies have also utilized a combination of systemic chemotherapy and postoperative chemoradiation to control local recurrences. Representative studies are summarized in Table 24–3 (12,15,17,18).

Table 24–2. Representative Studies Utilizing Radiotherapy Alone as a Surgical Adjuvant in Rectal Carcinoma

Group (Reference)	Regimen Used	No. of Patients	Results
GITSG (17,18)	Control vs. radiotherapy	108	No difference in LR or OS with radiotherapy.
NSABP (15)	Control vs. radiotherapy vs. chemotherapy	555	Reduction in LR (0.06) with radiotherapy but no improvement in DFS or OS.
Balslev et al (19)	Control vs. radiotherapy	988	No difference in LR and no improvement in OS.

LR = local recurrence; DFS = disease-free survival; OS = overall survival.

In a study conducted by the Gastrointestinal Tumor Study Group (GITSG), 202 patients with rectal carcinoma (modified Astler-Coller Dukes' B_2 and C) were randomized to surgery alone (control group), postoperative radiation therapy alone, chemotherapy alone with 5-FU and methyl CCNU, or a combination of postoperative radiotherapy and chemotherapy (17). The median duration of follow-up has been more than 5 years, and an improvement in disease-free survival was reported in patients treated with combined modality therapy. Further follow-up revealed an overall survival benefit for patients who received chemotherapy plus radiotherapy (18). In this study, the incidence of local recurrence was not significantly reduced by radiotherapy alone possibly because of the employment of a lower radiotherapy dose. The local recurrence rate was 55% (32 of 58) for the surgery alone group; 46% (22 of 48) for chemotherapy alone group; 48% (24 of 50) for radiation alone group; and 33% (15 of 48) for the patients receiving combined modality therapy. It should be noted that these recurrence rates are higher than expected and serve to emphasize the need to develop even more effective therapies.

In another study, the North Central Cancer Treatment Group (NCCTG), utilizing a similar strategy, reported a decrease in local recurrences with combined modality therapy (12). In this study, 200 patients were randomized to receive radiotherapy or radiotherapy plus 5-FU and methyl CCNU. At a median follow-up duration of 3 years, an advantage in terms of disease-free survival was noted for patients who received the sandwich therapy with chemoradiation. The incidence of local recurrence was nearly one-half in the combined modality therapy group compared to radiation alone group.

It is also important to note that a number of differences exist in the duration of chemotherapy and sequencing of therapy in two randomized studies described above. The duration of chemotherapy was 18 months in the GITSG study and only 4 months in the NCCTG study. Chemoradiation preceded prolonged systemic chemotherapy in the GITSG study while it was sandwiched be-

Table 24–3. Representative Randomized Chemoradiation Trials for Patients with Dukes' B and C Rectal Carcinoma

Group (Reference)	Regimen Used	No. of Patients	Follow-up	Results and Comments
GITSG (17,18)	Surgery vs. 5-FU + methyl CCNU vs. radiotherapy vs. radiotherapy + 5-FU + methyl CCNU	202	80 months	Prolonged DFS and OS with combined modality therapy and decreased local recurrence.
NCCTG (12)	Radiotherapy vs. 5-FU + methyl CCNU + 5-FU + radiotherapy (sandwich)	200	> 48 months	Prolonged DFS and OS with combined modality therapy and decreased local recurrence.
NSABP (15)	No postoperative therapy vs. radiotherapy vs. 5-FU + methyl CCNU + vincristine	555	> 60 months	Prolonged DFS and OS with chemotherapy compared to surgery.

5-FU = 5-fluorouracil; DFS = disease-free survival; OS = overall survival.

tween brief systemic chemotherapy (2 months) in the NCCTG. Moreover, the survival advantage has not yet been demonstrated in the NCCTG study due to shorter follow-up (3 years). More mature analyses of this study are forthcoming.

Whether methyl CCNU contributed substantially in the reduction of local relapse rate and overall survival is a subject of an ongoing study. A multi-institutional study based at the Mayo Clinic is currently under way to determine the value of methyl CCNU in the adjuvant setting. Two different schedules of 5-FU (low-dose continuous infusion throughout the radiotherapy period or bolus 5-FU on the first and the last 3 days of radiotherapy) during chemoradiation are also being studied in a randomized fashion to determine the impact on local recurrence rate in patients with Dukes' B_2 and C rectal carcinoma.

Assessment of the current data suggests that the addition of chemotherapy to radiotherapy in the adjuvant treatment of patients with rectal carcinoma significantly reduces the incidence of local recurrence, thus exceeding what would be expected from radiotherapy alone. However, it is too early to conclude that this approach consistently prolongs survival of such patients. A number of questions remain unanswered; more effective therapies must be developed to increase the cure rate in this group of patients.

Colon Carcinoma

Stage per stage, rate of local relapse is significantly lower in patients with colon carcinoma compared to those with rectal carcinoma. The rate of local relapse is approximately 10%, and the rate of peritoneal seeding is approximately 12%. These patients most often succumb to overwhelming systemic metastases. Thus, the role of chemoradiation or intraoperative radiotherapy must be systemically evaluated in select groups of patients with Gunderson-Sosin's modified Dukes' C_3 lesions and in those cases in which the resection of the primary tumor is incomplete.

Recently, there have been significant developments in the postoperative adjuvant therapy of patients with Dukes' C colon carcinoma. Representative studies have been summarized in Table 24–4 (20–26). The most important study among these are those using the immunomodulator levamisole. The

Table 24–4. Representative Randomized Adjuvant Therapy Trials for Patients with Dukes' B and C Colon Carcinoma.

Group (Reference)	Regimen Used	No. of Patients	Follow-up	Results and Comments
GITSG (23)	No therapy control vs. MER vs 5-FU + methyl CCNU vs 5-FU + methyl CCNU + MER	621	> 60 months	No improvement in DFS or OS with therapy. Seven patients developed leukemia (all had MeCCNU).
NSABP (24)	No therapy control vs. 5-FU + methyl CCNU + vincristine vs. BCG	1166	> 70 months	Borderline improved DFS and OS (0.05) with chemotherapy vs. control. Improved OS with BCG vs. control but no DFS.
SWOG (25)	Control vs. 5-FU + methyl CCNU vs. 5-FU + methyl CCNU + BCG	628	> 60 months	No improvement in DFS or OS with therapy.
Intergroup (22)	Control vs. 5-FU + levamisole vs. levamisole	1296	36 months	Improved DFS and OS with chemoimmunotherapy vs. control for Dukes' C but not for Dukes' B.
Windle et al (20)	Control vs. 5-FU + levamisole vs. 5-FU	141	> 60 months	Improved OS with chemoimmunotherapy. One-third of the patients had rectal cancer.
VASOG (26)	Control vs. 5-FU + methyl CCNU	659	> 48 months	No improvement in DFS or OS.
NCCTG (21)	Control vs. levamisole vs. 5-FU + levamisole	401	> 80 months	Improved DFS and OS with chemoimmunotherapy vs. control for Dukes' C but not Dukes' B.

DFS = disease-free survival; OS = overall survival; 5-FU = 5-fluorouracil; MER = Methanol extraction residue at BCG; RT = Pelvic radiotherapy; BCG = Bacillus Calmette-Guerin vaccine.

benefit of this drug for patients with colorectal carcinoma was first demonstrated by a small European study (20), followed by the NCCTG study (21), suggesting significant improvement in overall survival for patients with Dukes' C colon carcinoma. A much larger Intergroup trial reported by Moertel et al confirmed a survival benefit to the patients treated with levamisole plus 5-FU compared to no therapy following surgery (22).

Previously, the National Surgical Adjuvant Breast Program (NSABP) study (24) had suggested only borderline statistically significant improvement in the survival of patients with Dukes' B and C colon carcinoma with combination chemotherapy (methyl CCNU, vincristine, and 5-FU) compared to no treatment following surgery. At present, 5-FU plus levamisole should be considered standard adjuvant therapy for patients with Dukes' C colon carcinoma. Notably, the NCCTG and Intergroup trials did not show any survival benefit for patients with Dukes' B colon carcinoma (21,22). Thus, until future studies are completed, there is no recommended adjuvant therapy for patients with Dukes' B colon carcinoma.

Advanced Primary Rectal Carcinoma

The possibility of achieving a curative resection is less than 5% if the rectal carcinoma is fixed to the surrounding structures at the time of digital examination performed with or without general anesthesia. Thus, the strategy of preoperative downstaging has the potential of offering surgical cures. At M.D. Anderson Cancer Center, we have conducted a series of studies utilizing radioenhancers (5-FU, cisplatinum, or both) to downstage the advanced carcinoma and explore patients following completion of chemoradiation. Early results are quite encouraging (unpublished data). The global strategy has incorporated the use of pelvic radiotherapy up to 4500 cGy along with the concurrent use of a radioenhancing drug followed by an attempt to resect the primary tumor. In addition, the potential contribution of intraoperative radiotherapy in this situation is being evaluated at M.D. Anderson and elsewhere.

Locally Recurrent or Residual Carcinomas

Despite currently available adjuvant therapies, approximately 15% of patients with rectal carcinoma (Gunderson-Sosin's modified Dukes' $B_{2/3}$ or $C_{2/3}$ will recur during their natural history. The rate of recurrence can be as high as 50% in some patients with rectal carcinoma who have curative resection but fail to receive postoperative adjuvant therapy. An isolated local relapse is more frequent in a patient with rectal carcinoma than in a patient with colon carcinoma. A small fraction of patients (perhaps between 5 and 10%) with rectal carcinoma has locally unresectable or residual carcinoma at the time of primary surgery.

Local recurrence or residual carcinoma is one of the most difficult clinical situations to manage. Recognizing that surgical resection provides the only chance for potential cure, our general philosophy has been to downstage recurrent or advanced primary carcinoma with the use of chemoradiation to render them surgically resectable. However, this strategy cannot be applied to carcinomas that have recurred in adequately irradiated areas. For previously adequately irradiated patients surgical resection should be considered. For previously unirradiated patients having local recurrence or residual carcinoma, an attempted downstaging would appear reasonable as preoperative therapy or palliative therapy. In addition, intraoperative radiotherapy could potentially effectively control the local recurrence (27). However, randomized studies would be necessary to determine the true value of intraoperative radiotherapy. For those patients who fail salvage attempts, their situation remains universally grim, resulting in increasing pelvic pain, renal insufficiency due to urinary tract obstruction, and subsequent death due to cancer-related causes. In general, the prognosis of these patients remains poor with a 5-year survival rate of approximately 10%. Newer methods such as intraoperative radiotherapy currently remain investigational and may have more to offer than current therapies.

RESEARCH TRENDS IN COLORECTAL CARCINOMA

Active research is under way to counter the risk of the development of metastatic carcinoma and to overcome established metastatic disease. Numerous strategies are incorporating the use of intraoperative radiotherapy, whole-abdominal radiotherapy with concurrent chemotherapy, use of radioprotectors, a variety of potential radioenhancers (cisplatinum, mitomycin-C, 5-FU, folinic acid), use of monoclonal antibodies for early detection of carcinoma as well its therapy, autoimmunization of patients with their own irradiated tumor cells, and a variety of chemotherapy combinations in the adjuvant setting. The future prospects of developing more effective therapy for patients with colorectal carcinoma have become more promising, and therapy-induced survival benefit to patients with various stages of colorectal carcinoma have become a real possibility.

CONCLUSIONS

Analyses of a number of trials conducted over the past 15 years suggest that there is good reason to change clinical practice for patients with Dukes' B_2 and C rectal carcinomas such that all patients with these stages should receive chemotherapy concurrently with radiotherapy. The role of additional systemic chemotherapy remains to be determined. However, all positive studies have utilized systemic chemotherapy along with chemoradiation. For patients with Dukes' B_2 colon carcinoma, no adjuvant standard therapy can be recommended at this time. However, all patients with Dukes' C colon carcinoma should either be entered into clinical protocols or treated with 5-FU and levamisole for a period of 1 year. In the future, of particular interest would be trials containing adjuvant chemotherapy with 5-FU and folinic acid. The results of these trials will become available shortly.

Strategies to down-stage carcinoma in an attempt to render it potentially resectable should be investigated thoroughly in all patients with locally advanced rectal primary or recurrent carcinoma. In addition, the role of intraoperative radiotherapy must be defined. Efforts are under way to determine the biologic determinants of prognosis that can be used to modify therapy of these patients.

REFERENCES

1. Boring CC, Squires TS, Tong T. Cancer Statistics, 1992. CA 42:19, 1992.
2. Adson MA. Natural history of liver metastases and resective treatment. *In:* Biology and Treatment of Colorectal Cancer Metastases. Mastromarino AJ (Ed). Boston, Martinus Nijhoff Publishing, 1986, p. 3.
3. Mountain CF, McMurtrey MT, Hermes KE. Surgery for pulmonary metastases. A 20 year experience. Ann Thorac Surg 38:323, 1984.
4. Kern SE, Fearon ER, Tersmette KW, et al. Allelic loss in colorectal carcinoma. JAMA 261:3099, 1989.
5. Astler VB, Coller FA. Prognostic significance of direct extension of carcinoma of the colon and rectum. Ann Surg 139:846, 1954.
6. Gunderson LL, Sosin H. Areas of failure found at reoperation (second or symptomatic look) following "curative surgery" for adenocarcinoma of the rectum. Clinicopathologic correlation and implications for adjuvant therapy. Cancer 34:1278, 1974.
7. Rich TA, Romsdahl MM, Brock WA. Adjuvant radiotherapy for cancer of the rectum. Cancer Bull 40:229, 1988.
8. Moertel CG, Childs DS, Reitemeier RJ, et al. Combined 5-fluorouracil and supervoltage radiation therapy of locally unresectable gastrointestinal cancer. Lancet 2:865, 1969.
9. Hondett EM. Radiosensitization of radiotherapy and 5-fluorouracil. Cancer Rep 32:55, 1963.
10. Byfield JE. The clinical use of 5-fluorouracil and other halopyrimidines as radiosensitizers in man. *In:* Cancer chemotherapy by infusion, Lokich JJ (ed), Precept Press, Chicago, 1987, p. 479.
11. Gunderson LL, Sosin H, Levitt S. Extrapelvic colon—Areas of failure in a reoperation series. Implications for adjuvant therapy. Int J Radiat Oncol Biol Phys 11:731, 1985.
12. Krook J, Moertel CG, Weiand H, et al. Radiation vs. sequential chemotherapy-radiation-chemotherapy. A study of North Central Cancer Treatment Group. Proc Am Soc Clin Oncol 5:82, 1986.
13. Gerard A, Berrod JL, Pene F, et al. Interim analysis of a phase II study on pre-operative radiation therapy in resectable rectal carcinoma. Cancer 55:2373, 1985.
14. Lise M, Gerard A, Arnaud JP, et al. EORTC clinical trials on adjuvant therapy of colorectal cancer. Proc 14th UICC Cancer Congress 3:1293, 1986.
15. Fisher B, Wolmark N, Rockette H, et al. Postoperative adjuvant chemotherapy or radiation therapy for rectal cancer. Results from NSABP Protocol R-01. J Natl Cancer Inst 80:21, 1988.
16. Rich TA. Adjuvant radiation therapy for colorectal cancer. *In:* Biology and Treatment of Colorectal Cancer Metastases. Mastromarino AJ (Ed). Boston, Martinus Nijhoff Publishing, 1986, p. 145.

17. Gastrointestinal Tumor Study Group. Prolongation of the disease-free interval in surgically treated rectal carcinoma. N Engl J Med 312:1465, 1985.
18. Douglass HO, Moertel CG, Mayer RJ, et al. Survival after postoperative combination treatment of rectal cancer. N Engl J Med 315:1294, 1986.
19. Balslev IB, Pedersen M, Teglbjaerg PS, et al. Postoperative radiotherapy in Dukes' B and C carcinoma of the rectum and rectosigmoid. A randomized multicenter study. Cancer 58:22, 1986.
20. Windle R, Bell PRF, Shaw D. Five year results of a randomized trial of adjuvant 5-fluorouracil and levamisole in colorectal cancer. Br J Cancer 74:569, 1987.
21. Laurie JA, Moertel CG, Fleming TR, et al. Surgical adjuvant therapy of large bowel carcinoma. An evaluation of levamisole and the combination of levamisole and 5-fluorouracil. A study of the North Central Cancer Treatment Group (NCCTG) and the Mayo Clinic. J Clin Oncol 7:1447, 1989.
22. Moertel CG, Fleming TR, MacDonald JS, et al. Levamisole and fluorouracil for adjuvant therapy of resected colon carcinoma. N Engl J Med 322:352, 1990.
23. Gastrointestinal Study Group. Adjuvant therapy of colon cancer. Results of a prospective randomized trial. N Engl J Med 310:737, 1984.
24. Wolmark N, Fisher B, Rockette H, et al. Postoperative adjuvant chemotherapy or BCG for colon cancer. Results from NSABP protocol C-01. J Natl Cancer Inst 80:30, 1988.
25. Penettiere FJ, Goodman PJ, Costanzi JJ, et al. Adjuvant therapy in large bowel adenocarcinoma. Long-term results of a Southwest Oncology Group study. J Clin Oncol 6:947, 1988.
26. Higgins GA, Amadio JH, McElhenney J, et al. Efficacy of prolonged intermittent therapy with combined 5-fluorouracil and methyl-CCNU following resection for carcinoma of the large bowel. Cancer 53:1, 1984.
27. Gunderson LL, Martin JK, Nagorney, et al. Intraoperative irradiation for gastrointestinal cancers. *In:* Gastrointestinal Cancer. Current Approaches to Diagnosis and Treatment. Levin B (Ed). Austin, U. T. Press, 1988, p. 177.

Chapter 25

ANAL CANAL

MARSHALL S. FLAM AND MADHU J. JOHN

Chemoradiation in the treatment of epidermoid carcinoma of the anus represents one of the most auspicious examples of the efficacy of combined therapy in the treatment of cancer. The evolution of combined radiation (RT) and chemotherapy (CT) programs in the treatment of cancer of the anal canal, over the past 15 years, has led to the displacement of radical surgery to a secondary role. Successful application of CT-RT regimens against anal cancer (including tumors of the anal canal and anal verge) has paved the way for clinical trials employing similar regimens against other epidermoid malignancies, including esophageal, cervical, and head and neck cancer.

HISTORICAL PERSPECTIVE

Prior to the introduction of chemoradiation in 1974, the accepted treatment of anal cancer was radical surgery consisting of abdominal-perineal resection (APR) including the rectovaginal septum (1,2). Reported 5-year survivals ranged from 24 to 62%, with an average of about 50% (3,4), and perioperative mortality ranged from 2 to 6% (5). When synchronous inguinal lymph node metastases were present, the 5-year survival rate after APR and lymphadenectomy was only 10 to 20% (4,6).

While epidermoid anal cancer is generally radiosensitive, the limited tolerance of the perineal area to radiation, especially in tumors extending close to the perineal skin, resulted in substantial morbidity, thereby limiting its effective application. The use of external radiation, interstitial radiation, and combinations of external and interstitial radiation regimens yielded 5-year survival rates of 30 to 50%, not substantially different than surgery (7). For example, Rousseau et al, delivering a total dose of 6000 to 7000 cGy over 6 to 7 weeks with a Co-60 unit, achieved a 5-year survival of 44%, a local failure rate of 42%, and a 20% incidence of serious complications (8). The survival rates in this and other radiation studies declined with increasing tumor size. Studies employing interstitial therapy demonstrated similar 5-year survival rates (32 to 47%) and high rates of serious complications often necessitating colostomy (7). Current results of interstitial therapy limited to specialized centers are more promising, particularly if applied to small lesions and tumors of the anal verge (9). The results of radiation therapy of surgical failures and of patients with inguinal lymph node metastases have been disappointing (10). Finally, complications including anal ulceration, perineal necrosis, and stricture developed frequently in patients treated with radiation necessitating colostomy or local excision of necrosis or stricture in 10 to 20% of patients (10).

CHEMORADIATION OF ANAL CANCER

In 1974, Nigro and associates (11), at Wayne State Medical Center, reported an attempt to overcome the biologic and anatomic restraints to surgical and radiotherapeutic cure of anal canal cancer by employing a preoperative regimen consisting of radiation therapy and concomitant chemotherapy with 5-fluorouracil (5-FU) infusion and mitomycin-C. At APR performed in six patients 6 weeks after chemoradiation, five patients were found to be pathologically free of tumor. Subsequently, these investigators and others (12–16) employed variations of this preoperative chemoradiation regimen with impressive results. Eventually, it was suggested that the frequency of complete local tumor clearance was adequate to consider chemoradiation of epidermoid anal malignancies as a definitive rather than a preoperative treatment regimen (17). In the past 5 years, chemoradiation has become the treatment of choice for most patients with anal cancer, with a 5-year survival rate projected to 80 to 90% in over 400 reported patients, as outlined in Table 25–1 (18–35). Radical surgery is now reserved for local treatment failures following chemoradiation and for small tumors arising at the anal verge, which can frequently be managed with limited resection (36).

The success of this combined-modality nonoperative approach is reflected not only in improved disease-free survival compared to patients treated in the past with surgery or radiation alone (20) but also in the significant reduction in late morbidity and in the preservation of anal sphincter and sexual function (25).

Acute toxicities of this regimen include diarrhea, proctitis, and perineal dermatitis in all patients. While these regional toxicities are often severe and occasionally require a brief interruption in therapy, they are usually short-lived and easy to manage. Cystitis, stomatitis, and alopecia occur in approximately one-half of the patients treated. Despite the concomitant use of pelvic radiation and chemotherapy, myelosuppression is rarely severe, with less than 10% Grade 4 leukopenia and/or thrombocytopenia, because significant radiation doses to the pelvis rarely exceed 3000 cGy due to the coning down of treatment fields to the central pelvis and perineum after a dose of 3000 cGy administered to the whole pelvis (37) (Fig. 25–1). Additionally, 5-FU given as a continuous infusion is rarely myelosuppresive (38). When mitomycin-C is administered with both courses of 5-FU, the degree of myelosuppression following the second cycle of chemotherapy is not significantly greater than after the first, although the time to recovery of blood counts is marginally longer (17, 25).

Tables 25–2 and 25–3 are representative of the toxicities observed in patients treated with combined-modality therapy when two cycles of both 5-FU and mitomycin-C are used concomitantly with 4100 to 4500 cGy supervoltage radiation (25).

Efficacy of Chemoradiation

The observed improvement in local disease control and in survival when radiation, 5-FU infusion, and mitomycin-C are employed concurrently clearly demonstrates the greater efficacy of the combination of treatment components compared with either radiation or chemotherapy employed alone. Additionally, rapid clearance of palpable tumor during the course of treatment is frequently observed (17). These observations suggest a synergistic interplay of treatment components in their combined attack on the neoplasm. Nevertheless, there are limited data regarding the relative importance of each component used in this regimen due to lack of comparative clinical trials of this program, which has evolved entirely as an empiric treatment.

The biologic observations that served as a foundation for the initial development and subsequent application of this combined-modality program are as follows.

Observations of Clinical Behavior of Anal Carcinoma

Direct extension and regional lymphatic spread of this neoplasm is much more common than hematogenous dissemination at the time of diagnosis. Even large and extensive lesions that infiltrate the perineal skin and/or rectovaginal septum are rarely associated with distant metastases at diagnosis, which is found in less than 10% of cases (7,39). Consequently, a regimen capable of eradicating the local tumor should be capable of exerting a significant impact on disease-free survival.

Limitations to Radiation Imposed by Normal Tissue Tolerance

Radiation efficacy is limited by anatomic constraints and narrow therapeutic index and not by tumor insensitivity. The delivery of doses greater than 5000 cGy or the use of dose fractionation schedules exceeding 200 cGy per fraction results in prohibitive normal tissue toxicity. Thus, methods of increasing the radiation effect against the tumor without increasing normal tissue effects

Table 25–1. Chemoradiation of Anal Cancer—Published Series Summary

Institution, Years (Reference)	No. of Patients	Chemotherapy Dose & Schedule: 5-FU Infusion ($mg/m^2/d$)	Chemotherapy Dose & Schedule: Mitomycin-C (mg/m^2)	Radiation Schedule (cGy)	Timing of XRT + CT	Local Control	Survival (% NED)
Wayne State, 1971–1984 (18)	45	1000 × 4 d 1 + 28	15 d 1	3000 at 200/fx	synchronous	38/45 (84%)	84
Memorial, 1973–1986 (19,20)	44	750 × 5d × 1	10–15 d 1	3000 at 200/fx start day 8	sequential	25/45 (59%)	73
U. Rochester 1976–1985 (21,22)	29	1000 × 4, d 2 + 28	10 d 2	4000–5000 at 170/fx pelvis, 4000 ing. nodes if neg., 5000 ing. nodes if positive 1000–1600 at 1 cm. over 48 hr.-implant for resid palpable nodularity	synchronous	26/29 (89%)	77
Princess Margaret Hospital, 1978–1983 (23,24)	16	1000 × 4d × 1	10 d 1	5000 at 250/fx—continuous	synchronous	15/16 (93%)	75
	14	1000 × 4 d 1 + 42	10 d 1 + 42	5000 at 250/fx-split course with 4-week break	synchronous	13/14 (93%)	
UCSF-Fresno, 1979–1987 (25)	30	1000 × 4 d 1 + d21 or 28	10–15 d 1 + d21 or d28	4140–4500 at 180/fx pelvis, 900 ing. nodes + skin if involved	synchronous	26/30 (87%)	100
Genova, Italy, 1979–1986 (26)	16	750 × 5d × 1 12 hr. per day	15 d 1	3000 at 200/fx start day 8	sequential	3/16 (19%)	63
U. Kentucky, 1979–1985 (27)	19	1000 × 4 d 1 + 29	15 d 1	3000 at 200/fx pelvis + ing. nodes if palpable	synchronous	16/19 (87%)	87
U. Geneva, 1980–1985 (28)	29	1000 × 5d × 1	15 d 1	3000–4000 at 200/fx Interstitial iridium^{192} implant week 6	synchronous	24/29 (82%)	93
Australia, 1981–1982 (29)	5	1000 × 4 d 1 + 28	10 d 1	5000–7000 at 200/fx	synchronous	5/5 (100%)	100
RTOG, 1983–1987 (30)	79	1000 × 4, d 2 + 28	10 d 2	4080 in 4–5 weeks, 4090 at 3 cm. ing. nodes	synchronous	71/79 (90%)	84
Lyon, France, 1977–1984 (31)	70	600 × 4d × 1	12 d 1	3500 at 175/fx interstitial iridium^{192} implant boost 2 mos. after ext. radiation	synchronous	80/89 (81%)	NOT STATED
M.D. Anderson, 1979–1987 (32)	25	300 × 32d	NONE	4500 at 180/fx pelvis + ing. nodes 7 pts. boost iridium^{192} implant	synchronous	18/24 (75%)	92
Sao Paulo, Brazil, 1982–1988 (33)	28	1000 × 4 d 1 + 29	15 d 1	3000–4500 at 180–200/fx	synchronous	20/28 (71%)	75
Washington, 1983–1988 (34)	14	1000 × 4 d 1 + 28	10 d 1	5440–5780 at 170/fx	synchronous	14/14 (100%)	71
Columbus, Ohio, (35)	20	1000 × 4 d 1 + 28	15 d 1	3000 at 200/fx; 2 pts. 4140 at 180/fx	synchronous	14/20 (70%)	95

were needed. The logical approach was the addition of a radioenhancing agent. If the radioenhancer also possessed activity against the tumor, additional therapeutic gain might be anticipated. 5-FU was the ideal radioenhancer in this case.

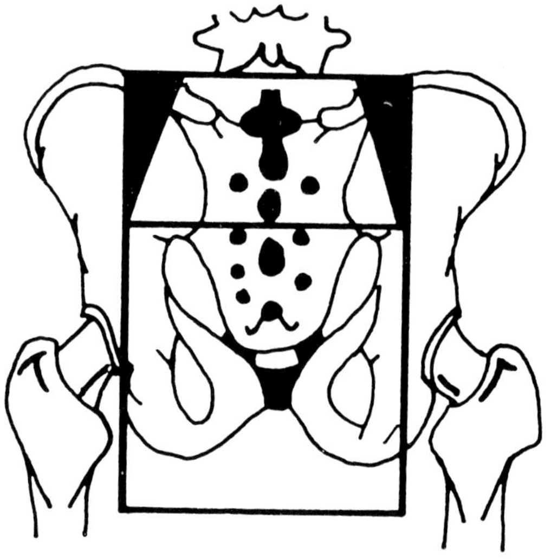

Fig. 25–1. Initial radiotherapy fields (AP/PA) used at UCSF-Fresno. The superior border is dropped to the lower border of the sacro-iliac joints after 3000 cGy.

Table 25–2. Acute Toxicity in 30 Patients Treated for Anal Cancer

Toxic Effect	No. of Patients (%)
Diarrhea	30 (100)
Proctitis	30 (100)
Dermatitis (Perineal)	30 (100)
Stomatitis	19 (63)
Urinary symptoms	13 (43)
Alopecia	9 (30)
Fever	8* (27)
Fluid-electrolyte	4 (13)
Wt. loss (> 10%)	3 (10)
Ileus	1 (3)
Neuropathy	1 (3)

*3/8 documented infectious episodes.

Clinical and In Vitro Observations of Radiation/5-FU Synergy

Clinical trials comparing radiation to radiation plus 5-FU in locally advanced gastrointestinal adenocarcinomas in the late 1960s demonstrated improved survival in the combined therapy group (40,41). These clinical trials were based on preclinical studies indicating that the survival curve of human epithelial tumor cells in culture was strongly influenced by coincident exposure to 5-FU (42,43). Scheduling studies by Vietti (44) demonstrated enhancement of tumor cell killing by this combination. In vitro studies by Byfield (45) demonstrated maximal radiosensitization when 5-FU was present for 24 hours or more following radiation exposure, while Looney (46) observed increased tumor growth delay greater than the additive effect of the two modalities given independently for schedules in which radiation was given from 4 days prior to 2 days after 5-FU. Recently, the use of chemotherapy with 5-FU infusion and mitomycin-C but without radiation has been reported by the Memorial group (36), who describes a subset of patients who relapsed following APR; 15 patients demonstrated disseminated disease at relapse, eight patients received 5-FU and mitomycin-C using a dose schedule similar to that employed in their combined-modality regimen (19), and one patient received 5-FU alone. Three partial responses and no complete remissions were observed. No effect of the chemotherapy on survival was noted. This limited experience suggests that the antineoplastic effect of the chemotherapy is not as important as its radioenhancing and possibly potentiating effect.

Demonstration of Improved Efficacy and Tolerance of 5-FU Infusion

In the early 1970s, clinical trials with 5-FU delivered by continuous infusion demon-

Table 25–3. Hematologic Toxicity in 30 Patients Treated for Anal Cancer

	Platelets		Leukocytes	
Median Values	Cycle 1	Cycle 2	Cycle 1	Cycle 2
Nadir counts (cells/mm^2)	104,000	86,000	2500	2000
No. of days to nadir	15.3	16.3	14.2	11.9
No. of days to recovery*	22.3	29.6	20.5	24.1

*From nadir: Platelets > 100,000; WBC > 3000 (Excluding patients with nadirs > above values)

strated a toxicity profile different than bolus 5-FU (38). As a bolus, 5-FU produces dose-limiting myelotoxicity, but as an infusion, dose-limiting gastrointestinal and epithelial toxicity is noted. Considerably higher doses of 5-FU were, consequently, clinically feasible when delivered by continuous infusion. Significant activity of infusional 5-FU was demonstrated in both gastrointestinal adenocarcinomas and a variety of squamous carcinomas. Thus, an infusion of 5-FU in doses of 750 to 1000 mg/m^2 over 96 to 120 hours could be expected to result in lessened bone-marrow toxicity and greater gastrointestinal toxicity, a possible independent effect against micrometastic disease outside of irradiated areas due to the use of a higher dose of drug, and an enhancement of irradiated tumor destruction due to the duration of exposure of the tumor to the drug when delivered by prolonged continuous infusion.

Mitomycin: The Unknown Quantity

The inclusion of mitomycin-C is the most empiric component of the combined-modality regimen. Its use as a single agent or in combination has not been reported in the treatment of metastatic anal cancer. Mitomycin is active against gastric and pancreatic carcinoma as a single agent or in combination with 5-FU and/or Adriamycin, and in squamous carcinoma of the lung, cervix, and transitional cell carcinoma of the bladder (47). The radioenhancing properties of mitomycin-C, however, were not reported until years following the introduction of the combined modality program (48). The issue of whether mitomycin-C is an essential and necessary component of this chemoradiation program is currently being addressed in a randomized Phase III trial sponsored by the Radiation Therapy Oncology Group (49) (Figure 25–2). If no difference in disease control and survival is demonstrated in the group receiving both 5-FU and mitomycin-C compared to the group receiving only 5-FU; mitomycin-C could be eliminated from the combined regimen with the expectation of a modest reduction in toxicity.

Recently, Cummings has reported significant improvement in local disease control in tumors greater than 2 cm in size, with radiation plus 5-FU and mitomycin-C (FUMIR) compared with either radiation alone or radiation and 5-FU (FUR), in a series of prospectively designed, sequential nonrandomized protocols (50). Primary tumor control was achieved in 32 of 57 (56%) with radiation alone; in 39 of 65 (60%) with radiation plus 5-FU, and 59 of 69 (86%) with radiation plus 5-FU and mitomycin-C. The 5-year cause-specific survival rates were not significantly different. Interestingly, the distant failure rate (41%)* and the distant plus local failure rate (60%)** in the group treated with mitomycin-C were considerably higher than in both the group treated with radiation alone (3.6% and 36%)*** and the group treated with 5-FU and radiation (9.7% and 26%)****. This would suggest that mitomycin-C is ineffective against micrometastatic disease and its impact on local control as a radioenhancer is considerably more important. If this is correct, chemotherapeutic agents with greater antitumor activity against this neoplasm (such as cisplatinum (51) or sequential methotrexate, 5-FU, and leucovorin) (52) could improve overall survival if employed either with 5-FU and radiation during the second cycle of chemoradiation or as consolidation following chemoradiation.

Management of Chemoradiation Failures

Despite the impressive results of combined-modality programs, there remains a cohort of patients with anal carcinoma who demonstrate residual local tumor following completion of treatment. The incidence of patients with persistent tumor can be accurately determined by post-treatment biopsies of any palpable residual scar or nodularity and ranges from 10 to 20% (Table 25–4) (25).

The highest reported incidence of residual tumor following chemoradiation reported in the Memorial and Genova studies (19,26) could possibly be attributed to the use of only one course of chemotherapy and to the sequential use of chemotherapy followed by radiation, rather than the simultaneous application of modalities as employed in all other

*% of distant failures of the total failures in the FUMIR group.

**% of distant plus local failures of the total failures in the FUMIR group.

***3.6% distant failure and 36% distant plus local failure of total failures in the radiation-alone group.

****9.7% distant failure and 26% distant plus local failure of total failures in the FUR group.

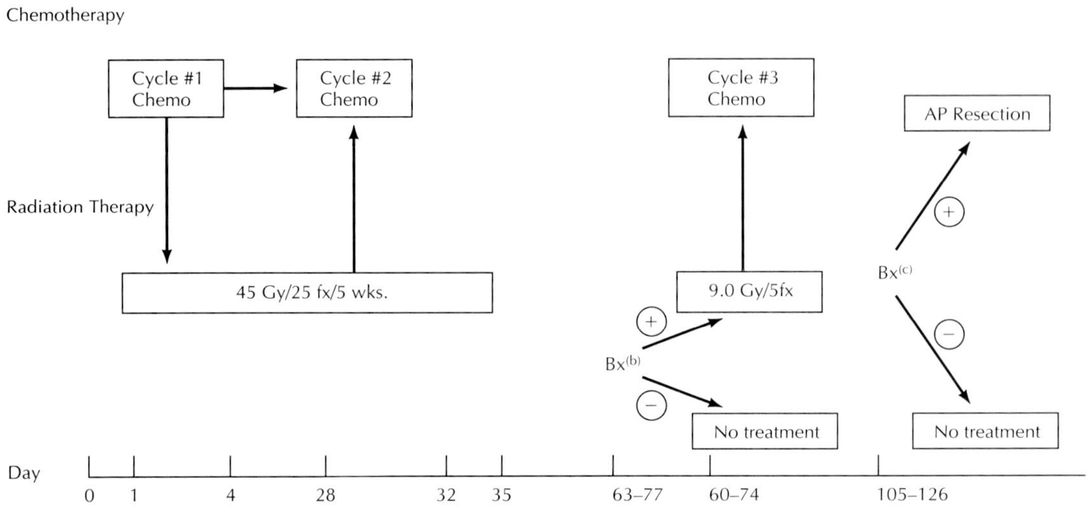

Radiation Therapy: 1.8 Gy daily 5 times per week for 5 weeks.
Reduced field at 30.60 Gy
For + inguinal nodes and/or local residual disease after 45 Gy proceed to 50.40 Gy with boost fields.

Chemotherapy: Cycles 1 & 2
ARM 1: 5-FU 1000 mg/m^2/24 hrs. continuous IV for 96 hours, Day 1 and Day 28 of RT
ARM 2: 5-FU as above + Mito C: 10 mg/m^2 IV bolus on day 1 of each 5-FU course (max 20 mgs per cycle)

Surgery:
a) Biopsy of palpable inguinal lymph nodes prior to treatment.
b) Full-thickness biopsy to be performed 4-6 weeks after completion of radiation and chemotherapy.
c) Repeat full-thickness biopsy for patients treated with salvage combined therapy 21–28 days after completion of salvage therapy.

Salvage Therapy:
Chemo (Cycle 3): 5-FU as above. Starting within 2 weeks of biopsy. CDDP 100 mg/m^2 IV over 6 hrs. on day 2 of RT (if creatinine < 50 substitute mito C).
Radiation: 9.00 Gy boost RT with electron/photon beam on perineum/inguinal nodes/both.

Fig. 25–2. Treatment schema of a phase III randomized study employing 5-fluorouracil and radiotherapy vs. 5-fluorouracil, mitomycin-C, and radiotherapy in carcinoma of the anal canal (RTOG 87-04/ECOG 1289).

reported series (18,22–25,27–35). The incidence of persistent local tumor (40 to 53% in the Memorial series and the 81% in the Genova series) is, therefore, not representative of a definitive nonsurgical, synchronous combined-modality approach (19,20,26).

The Rochester group employed the standard two cycles of chemotherapy simultaneous with external radiation but subsequently used an interstitial implant in patients with residual nodularity without prior biopsy of the residual nodularity (21,22). It is, therefore, not possible to determine their exact local failure rate prior to implantation and the estimated 31% (9 of 29) may be higher than the actual rate. Nevertheless, four of the nine patients implanted demonstrated residual local tumor employing this salvage method. The lowest local failure rate (10%) was reported by the Princess Margaret Hospital group, who employed a considerably higher dose of external radiation (5000 cGy in 250 fractions over 4 weeks) but experienced a high rate (17%) of serious late toxicity requiring surgical intervention (23). The subsequent adoption of split-course radiation with chemotherapy led to a reduction in late complications but may be responsible, in part, for the high incidence of distant failures (10 of 60) despite a low local failure rate (24). The Wayne State group reported a local failure rate of 15% in 45 patients following combined modality therapy and were unable to salvage any of these patients with APR (18). To date, most investigators employing combined modality therapy of anal carcinoma have resorted to APR for patients with residual pelvic tumor

Table 25–4. Initial Local Treatment Failures Employing Combined CT-RT in Carcinoma of the Anus: Survey of Published Series

Institution	No. of Patients	No. (%) Local Failure	Salvage Rx. of Local Failures	No. Dead in Local Failure Group	No. Alive With Disease	No. Salvaged	% NED (Entire Group)
Wayne State (18)	45	7 (15)	6 APR; 1 No Rx	7	0	0	84
U. Rochester (21,22)	29	9* (13)	9 interstitial implants	3	1	5	77
Memorial (19,20)	37	15 (40)	18 APR, 10 Loc Exc.	4	1	10	78
Princess Margaret (23,24)	60	6 (10)	5 APR	2	0	4	75**
		1 Loc Exc.					
U. Kentucky (27)	19	3 (16)	3 APR	0	0	3	100
U. Geneva (28)	29†	4† (14)	4 APR	1‡	1	3	84
UCSF-Fresno (17,25)	30	4 (13)	4 CT-RT	1‡	0	4	100
Grant-Ohio (35)	20	3 (15)	1 APR, 1 CT-RT, 1 RT	0	0	3	95

*9/27 demonstrated "residual nodularity" and were implanted without biopsy. Thus, actual local failure rate before implantation is unknown. Figures in table assume all patients with "residual nodularity" had residual tumor prior to implantation.
**10/60 failed with distant metastases; only 1 of 10 distant failures are in the local failure group.
†Patients treated with an interstitial iridium implant in lieu of 2nd cycle of 5-FU plus external radiation.
‡Dead of intercurrent disease free of cancer following salvage treatment.

(18,19,23,27,28,33,35). An analysis of published studies of patients failing definitive chemoradiation and subjected to either local excision or abdominoperineal resection reveals the attainment of initial tumor-free salvage in approximately one-third of patients (53). Nevertheless, the reported time of follow-up of these patients is relatively short or unknown. In addition, in the Wayne State study (18), in which the longest follow-up durations are reported, all patients with local persistence of tumor following combined therapy in whom salvage APR was employed have died.

The UCSF-Fresno group (25) employed a chemoradiation salvage regimen in their four local treatment failures (of 30 patients). An additional course of radiation was employed in conjunction with either 5-FU infusion and cisplatinum or with sequential methotrexate–5-FU–leucovorin (52). All patients achieved complete tumor eradication without additional late toxicity and without resorting to APR. Whether additional chemoradiation can salvage a significant proportion of patients with persistent local tumor is currently under evaluation by the RTOG (49).

The salvage of pelvic recurrences following APR has been evaluated by Greenall et al (36). Of 67 patients with recurrent anal cancer following APR, 32 (48%) recurred in the pelvis and/or perineum, 20 (30%) recurred in inguinal lymph nodes, and 15 (22%) recurred in viscera. Nine of the patients with pelvic perineal recurrence were treated with chemoradiation. Six patients received the identical program of mitomycin-C, 5-FU infusion, and radiation employed at Memorial Hospital preoperatively, followed by maintenance 5-FU infusion and mitomycin if a response was observed. No complete responses and three partial responses were observed, and the median survival of this group was 14 months. These results are considerably inferior to that observed when this combined regimen is employed initially.

INGUINAL LYMPH NODES

At diagnosis of epidermoid carcinoma of the anal canal, pelvic lymph node metastases are present in 30 to 43% of patients and inguinal node metastases (usually unilateral) in 15 to 36% (4). When synchronous inguinal lymph node metastases are present, the 5-year survival rate following APR with lymphadenectomy is only 10 to 20% (4,6). Prophylactic groin dissection is not recommended due to the high morbidity and mortality of the procedure (54). In patients treated with radiation, the late nodal recurrence rate was 15 to 25% if the inguinal areas were not treated electively (2,9).

Cummings has reported that elective radiation of the inguinal nodes greatly reduces the risk of late nodal failure and produces little morbidity (7,55). Most patients treated with combined modality therapy receive at least 3000 cGy to the medial inguinal nodes, which are included in the pelvic treatment field (18), although some groups have treated only palpable inguinal nodes (19,27). The Rochester Group routinely treats inguinal nodes to 4000 cGy and to more than 5000 cGy if clinically positive (21). The UCSF-Fresno group (37) employed 9 MeV elections to boost palpable inguinal nodes to a total dose of 5040 cGy. Recurrence in inguinal lymph nodes is infrequently reported in combined-treatment studies. Only one regional relapse was reported in a group of 78 patients treated in the RTOG multi-institutional study (30), but patients with involved nodes at presentation were excluded from this study. The current RTOG Study (87-04) stratifies patients upon entry into node-negative and positive groups, based on fine-needle aspiration biopsy of palpable inguinal nodes. The inguinal regions are routinely treated to 4500 cGy and boosted to 5040 cGy with electrons if positive upon entry into the study.

In contrast to synchronous (at initial presentation) lymph node metastases, metachronous inguinal relapses (following initial treatment) can be successfully salvaged by radical groin dissection; 5-year survival rates range from 50 to 75% (6,36).

CONCLUSIONS

The impact of combining radiation and radioenhancing chemotherapy in the treatment of epidermoid anal canal malignancies has radically improved survival while limiting the extent of surgical intervention to pretreatment and post-treatment biopsies in most patients with this cancer. The toxicity of radiation has also been considerably reduced due to the lower doses of radiation employed concomitantly with radioenhancing chemotherapy in the combined modality programs. The radioenhancing role of the chemotherapeutic components appears to be significantly more important to the efficacy of these regimens than their direct antitumor effect. The cosmetic and functional results are excellent in most patients treated. The value of salvage chemoradiation for patients with residual local tumor following treatment in further reducing the number of patients subjected to APR must be determined, along with the role of consolidation chemotherapy with additional agents to prevent late metastatic relapse.

Whether the combined modality regimens will be effective in homosexual men, who have recently been reported to have an increased incidence of anal cancer (56,57), and in adenocarcinoma of the anus must be determined.

REFERENCES

1. Dillard BM, Spratt JS Jr, Ackerman IV, et al. Epidermoid cancer of anal margin and canal: Review of 79 cases. Arch Surg 86:772, 1963.
2. Stearns MW Jr, Urmacher C, Sternberg C, et al. Cancer of the anal canal. Curr Probl Cancer 4:1, 1980.
3. Cortese AF. Surgical approach for treatment of epidermoid anal carcinoma. Cancer 36:1869, 1975.
4. Gordon PH. Squamous cell carcinoma of the anal canal. Surg Clin N Am 68(6):1391, 1988.
5. Bowman BM, Moertel CB, O'Connell MJ, et al. Carcinoma of the anal canal: A clinical and pathological study of 188 cases. Cancer 54:114, 1984.
6. Frost DB, Richards PC, Montague ED, et al. Epidermoid cancer of the anorectum. Cancer 53:1285, 1985.
7. Cummings BJ. The place of radiation therapy in the treatment of carcinoma of the anal canal. Cancer Treat Rev 9:125, 1982.
8. Rousseau J, Mathieu G, Fenton J, et al. Radiotherapie des cancers malpighiens de l'anus. J Radiol Electrol Med Nucl 54:622, 1973.
9. Papillon J. The responsibility of radiologists in the preservation of breast and rectum in cancer treatment. Clin Radiol 37:303, 1986.
10. Hintz BL, Charyulu KKD, Surdarsanam A. Anal carcinoma: Basic concepts and management. J Surg Oncol 10:141, 1978.
11. Nigro ND, Vaitkevicius VK, Considine B Jr. Combined therapy for cancer of the anal canal: A preliminary report. Presented at the American Proctologic Society, 1973. Dis Colon Rectum 17:354, 1974.
12. Buroker TR, Nigro N, Bradley G, et al. Com-

bined therapy for cancer of the anal canal: A follow-up report. Dis Colon Rectum 20:677, 1977.
13. Nigro ND, Vaitkevicius BJ, Buroker T, et al. Combined therapy for cancer of the anal canal. Dis Colon Rectum 24:73, 1981.
14. Newman HK, Quan SHQ. Multimodality therapy for epidermoid carcinoma of the anus. Cancer 37:12, 1976.
15. Sischy B, Remington JH, Sobel SH, et al. Treatment of carcinoma of the rectum and squamous carcinoma of the anus by combined chemotherapy, radiotherapy and operation. Surg Gynecol Obstet 151:369, 1980.
16. Cummings BJ, Rider WD, Harwood AR, et al. Combined radical radiation therapy and chemotherapy for primary squamous cell carcinoma of the anal canal. Cancer Treat Rep 66:489, 1982.
17. Flam MS, John M, Lovalvo L, et al. Definitive non-surgical therapy of epithelial malignancies of the anal canal. A report of 12 cases. Cancer 51:1378, 1983.
18. Leichman L, Nigro N, Vaitkevicius VK, et al. Cancer of the anal canal: Model for preoperative adjuvant combined modality therapy. Am J Med 78:211, 1985.
19. Michaelson RA, Magill GB, Quan SH, et al. Preoperative chemotherapy and radiation therapy in the management of anal epidermoid cancer. Cancer 51:390, 1983.
20. Enker WE, Heilwell M, Janov AJ, et al. Improved survival in epidermoid carcinoma of the anus in association with preoperative multidisciplinary therapy. Arch Surg 121:1386, 1986.
21. Sischy B. The use of radiation therapy combined with chemotherapy in the management of squamous cell carcinoma of the anus and marginally resectable adenocarcinoma of the rectum. Int J Radiat Oncol Biol Phys 11:1587, 1985.
22. Haghbin M, Sischy B, Hinson J. A long term follow up of definitive conservative therapy for anal canal carcinoma (Abst). Proc Am Soc Clin Oncol 4:81, 1985.
23. Cummings B, Keane T, Harwood A, et al. Results and toxicity of the treatment of anal canal carcinoma by radiation therapy or radiation therapy and chemotherapy. Cancer 54:2062, 1984.
24. Cummings BJ. Personal communication, 1987.
25. Flam MS, John MJ, Mowry PA, et al. Definitive combined modality therapy of carcinoma of the anus. A report of 30 cases including results of salvage therapy in patients with residual disease. Dis Colon Rectum 30(7):495, 1987.
26. Secco GB, Sertoli MR, Scarpati D, et al. Preoperative chemotherapy and radiotherapy in the management of epidermoid carcinoma of the anal canal. Tumori 73:151, 1987.
27. Meeker WR Jr, Sickie-Santanello BJ, Philpott G, et al. Combined chemotherapy, radiation and surgery for epithelial cancer of the anal canal. Cancer 57:525, 1986.
28. Pipard G, Peytremann R, Marti MC. Conservative multidisciplinary treatment of locally advanced epidermoid and cloacogenic cancer of the anal canal (Abst). Proc Am Soc Clin Oncol 5:268, 1986.
29. Tiver KW, Langlands O. Synchronous chemotherapy and radiotherapy for carcinoma of the anal canal-alterative to abdominoperineal resection. Aust NZ J Surg 54:101, 1984.
30. Sischy B, Krall J, Pazdur B, et al. Evaluation of RTOG 83-14 phase II study of the treatment of squamous cell basaloid carcinoma of the anal canal by radiation therapy and chemotherapy for sensitization followed by biopsy + surgery. Proc Am Soc Clin Oncol 7:93, 1988.
31. Papillon J, Montabaron JF, Gerard JP, et al. Interstitial curietherapy in the conservative treatment of anal and rectal cancers. Int J Radiat Oncol Biol Phys 17:1161, 1989.
32. Hughes LL, Rich TA, Delclos L, et al. Radiotherapy for anal cancer: Experience from 1979–1987. Int J Radiat Oncol Biol Phys 17:1153, 1989.
33. Habr-Gama A, DaSilva E, Sousa A, et al. Epidermoid carcinoma of the anal canal. Results of treatment by combined chemotherapy and radiation therapy. Dis Colon Rectum 32:773, 1989.
34. Knecht BH. Combined chemotherapy and radiotherapy for carcinomas of the anus. Am J Surg 159:518, 1990.
35. Cho CC, Taylor CW II, Padmanabhan A, et al. Squamous-cell carcinoma of the anal canal: Management with combined chemo-radiation therapy. Dis Colon Rectum 34:675, 1991.
36. Greenall MJ, Magill GB, Quan SHQ, et al. Recurrent epidermoid carcinoma of the anus. Cancer 57:1437, 1986.
37. John MJ, Flam M, Lovalvo L, et al. Feasibility of non-surgical definitive management of anal canal carcinoma. Int J Radiat Oncol Biol Phys 13:299, 1987.
38. Seifert P, Baker LH, Reed ML, et al. Comparison of continuously infused 5-Fluorouracil with bolus injection in treatment of patients with colorectal adenocarcinoma. Cancer 36:123, 1975.
39. Cummings BJ. Current management of epidermoid carcinoma of the anal canal. Gastroenterol Clin North Am 16:125, 1987.

40. Moertel CG, Childs DS, Rutermeier RT, et al. Combined 5-Fluorouracil and supervoltage radiation therapy of locally unresectable gastrointestinal cancer. Lancet 2:865, 1969.
41. Childs DS, Moertel CG, Holbrook MA, et al. Treatment of unresectable adenocarcinomas of the stomach with a combination of 5-Fluorouracil and radiation. Am J Roentgenol 102:541, 1968.
42. Bagshaw MA. Possible role of potentiators in radiation therapy. Am J Roentgenol 85:822, 1961.
43. Berry RJ. Effects of some metabolic inhibitors on x-ray dose response curves for survival of mammalian cells in vitro and on early recovery between fractionated x-ray doses. Br J Radiol 39:458, 1968.
44. Vietti T, Eggerding F, Valeriote F. Combined effects of x-irradiation and 5-Fluorouracil on survival of transplanted leukemic cells. J Natl Cancer Inst 47:865, 1971.
45. Byfield JE, Chan PYM, Seagren S. Radiosensitization by 5-Fluorouracil (5-FU): Molecular origons and clinical scheduling implications. Proc Am Assoc Cancer Res 18:74, 1977.
46. Looney WB, Hopkins HA, MacLeod MS, et al. Solid tumor models for the assessment of different treatment modalities. XII. Combined chemotherapy-radiotherapy: Variations of time interval between time of administration of 5-Fluorouracil and radiation and its effect on the control of tumor growth. Cancer 44:437, 1979.
47. Carter SK, Crook ST. Mitomycin-C Current Status and New Developments. San Diego, Academic Press, 1979.
48. Rockwell S, Kennedy K. Combined therapy with radiation and Mitomycin C. Preliminary results with EMT6 tumor cells in vitro and in vivo. Int J Radiat Oncol Biol Phys 5:1673, 1979.
49. Flam MS, John MJ, Russell A, et al. Radiation Therapy Oncology Group (RTOG) 87-04. A phase III randomized study employing 5-Fluorouracil and radiotherapy vs. 5-Fluorouracil, Mitomycin-C and radiotherapy in carcinoma of the anal canal. Submitted to Proc Amer Soc Clin Oncol, 1993.
50. Cummings BJ, Keane TJ, O'Sullivan, et al. Epidermoid anal cancer. Treatment by radiation alone or by radiation and 5-Fluorouracil with and without mitomycin-C. Int J Radiat Oncol Biol Phys 21:1115, 1991.
51. Brunet R, Sadek H, Vignoud J, et al. Cisplatin and 5-Fluorouracil, for the neoadjuvant treatment of epidermoid anal canal carcinoma. (Abst 402.) Proc Amer Soc Clin Oncol 9:104, 1990.
52. Gewirtz AM, Cadman E. Preliminary report on the efficacy of sequential Methotrexate and 5-Fluorouracil in advanced breast cancer. Cancer 47:2552, 1981.
53. Flam MS. Anal cancer: The non-surgical management of advanced disease. *In:* Cancer of the Colon, Rectum, and Anus. Cohen AM, Winawer SJ (Eds). New York, McGraw Hill. In press.
54. Stearns MW Jr, Quan SHQ. Epidermoid carcinoma of the anorectum. Surg Gynecol Obstet 131:953, 1970.
55. Cummings BJ, Thomas GH, Keane TJ, et al. Primary radiation therapy in the treatment of anal canal carcinoma. Dis Colon Rectum 25:778, 1982.
56. Mitchell EP. Carcinoma of the anal region. Semin Oncol 15(2):148, 1988.
57. Daling JR, Weiss NS, Hoffenstein LI, et al. Correlates of homosexual behavior and the incidence of anal carcinoma. JAMA 247:1988, 1982.

Chapter 26

SMALL-CELL CARCINOMA OF THE LUNG

ANDREW T. TURRISI III, DAVID H. JOHNSON, AND ROBERT L. COMIS

INTRODUCTION

Small-cell lung cancer (SCLC) used to be a death sentence. Surgeons abandoned operations in the 1960s because of systemic spread and short survival. A trial, conducted by the British Medical Research Council (MRC), randomized patients who were deemed fit for surgery to receive either surgery or radiotherapy. Despite selecting the best patients, only 48% of surgical patients were resected completely. Only 85% of patients randomized to radiotherapy received the full dose. Furthermore, the mean survival time for radiotherapy was 10 months versus 6 months for surgically treated patients ($p = 0.04$) (1). No patient randomized to surgery and only three patients randomized to radiotherapy survived for 5 years (1). However, in general, the median survival of patients with limited disease is only 3 months; for those with extensive disease the median survival was 5 weeks (2,3).

This poor survival after local modalities underscores the fact that SCLC is a systemic disease. Introducing active drugs for systemic disease increased survival. Cyclophosphamide plus radiotherapy significantly improved survival when compared to radiotherapy alone (4). Complete responses (CRs) and improvement in median survival and longterm survival have been reported with many multi-agent regimens. During the 1970s, most combinations were cyclophosphamide-based. The two most common regimens were CAV [cyclophosphamide, doxorubicin (Adriamycin, ADR), and vincristine] and CMC [cyclophosphamide, methotrexate, and lomustine (CCNU)], which produced similar results. These and other regimens of this era have been reviewed by Aisner and Comis (5,6). Perhaps the most active single agent is etoposide [VP-16, (E)] (7). Its optimal schedule and dose are not established. In previously untreated patients, a 24-hour infusion was compared to a daily administration for 5 days. The 5-day schedule was significantly more active than the infusion (8). The value of protracted oral etoposide has been reported in elderly patients and in previously untreated patients in Canada (9,10). Although cisplatinum (CDDP, P) by itself has only marginal activity (11), its testing was done on previously treated patients. Since carboplatinum has a high response rate (60 to 79%) in previously untreated patients (12,13), CDDP is likely to have a high response rate in patients without prior treatment. Platinum-etoposide (PE) is synergistic in murine systems (14). The Memorial group treated patients with PE with very encouraging results (15). However, no particular schedule of CDDP + VP-16 stands out as optimal treatment, but divided doses of VP-16 seem to be important.

The search for combined-modality programs acknowledges that unimodal approaches often fail. Facts about local control are hard to find from the early local-modality trials. Systemic therapy produces survival, which has plateaued at 12 to 24 months, but local failure occurs commonly at sites of initial bulk. Too many studies fail to provide data about the time and frequency of local failure. The problem of local failure provides the rationale to add local modalities to systemic therapy.

The categories of **limited** and **extensive** disease have prognostic value. Staging studies are imperfect—there are false clues suggesting advanced stage; for example, tussive fractures on bone scan or cystic disease of the liver on CT scans can be mistaken for extensive small cell cancer. On the other hand, some tests are insufficiently sensitive; distant disease may be missed or may escape detection by MRI. Nevertheless, the limited categorization allows the addition of local therapy to the bulk disease and identifies a set of patients with a chance for longterm survival. As long as resistant cells are confined to the chest, local therapy provides a chance to destroy the resistant subclone.

A functional definition of limited disease is disease that can fit into a reasonable radiotherapeutic portal. Many exclude pleural effusions found by routine chest x-rays prior to surgery, but until recently, the Southwest Oncology Group (SWOG) investigators continued to include them. Radiotherapy to the entire pleura, especially in conjunction with chemotherapy, may be risky. Whether supraclavicular disease should be classified as limited or extensive is also a point of controversy. Both subjects are debatable.

What constitutes an acceptable **staging work-up** remains controversial. Since small-cell carcinoma commonly involves the adrenal, brain, bone, bone marrow, liver, and lungs, imaging these organs and sampling bone marrow makes good sense. For clinical investigations, complete staging remains mandatory. Since combined-modality therapy is toxic, excluding patients with extensive disease is very much to the patient's benefit. Staging is an important variable from study to study, institution to institution, and from one era to another. These variations must be kept in mind and may explain differences between studies. In extensive disease, focusing on the chest with radiotherapy has not produced noteworthy results (16).

The case for local modalities in limited disease rests on the frequency of local failure after chemotherapy alone. For patients treated with chemotherapy alone, chest failure occurred in 80 to 100% (17,18). Since post-treatment relapses commonly have nonsmall-cell histology (19) and resist salvage therapy, surgery has had a resurgence of interest. Surgery's role seems to be confined to patients free of mediastinal nodal metastasis (18,20,21).

Steel defined the principles of combined-modality therapy (22). Although articulated a decade ago, these principles still apply (these are further elaborated by Phillips in Chapter 2). The principles of spatial cooperation, independent toxicity, enhancement of tumor response, and normal tissue protection all have particular pertinence in the management of SCLC. Sensitizers and protectors used to facilitate the administration of chemotherapy and radiotherapy have been reviewed in detail by Coleman and Turrisi (23) and in Chapter 45. Timing of modalities, selection of chemotherapeutic agents, and radiotherapy techniques, schedules, and fraction schemes all influence protection. These issues and a full discussion about combined-modality therapy are detailed elsewhere (24).

Pathobiologic features of SCLC may also provide information regarding prognosis and treatment. The light microscopic diagnosis of small-cell cancer obscures considerable heterogeneity. The role of oncogenes, tumor suppressor genes, chromosomal deletions, and growth factors is being unfolded. Carney has provided a clear overview of this exciting area of ongoing research (25). Clinical correlations with many of these new ideas must be performed. The morphologic **variant histology,** also known as mixed histology, probably has clinical importance (26,27); however, in one recent study of extensive disease patients, variant histology had no significant influence on response or survival (28).

RADIOTHERAPY FACTORS

Many factors obfuscate the role of radiotherapy. Simply looking at total radiation dose can be misleading. Other radiotherapeutic variables also require evaluation and control. The volume of irradiation for SCLC has not been standardized. Although some treat supraclavicular and contralateral hilar nodes, this policy is not firmly established. All trials of the past decade, and many current trials, attempt to protect the spinal cord with direct posterior shields, but that can inadvertently shield mediastinal tumor particularly in the subcarinal location. This technique is to be avoided. The edges of portals do not receive 100% of the dose. To accomodate this, many investigators have enlarged the length and width of irradiation portals, thereby increasing the treatment volume. However, with these expanded margins, adjacent structures such as the lung, heart, or esophagus receive an increased dose, which may increase toxicity.

Daily dose is an often neglected variable. More than 200 cGy per fraction causes more late damage to normal tissues, but many SCLC trials have employed these large fractions, which may increase late toxic effects. The total dose necessary for control is not established. Some have suggested a dose-response relationship, indicating better control with larger doses (29), but local control does not improve above 4000 to 4500 cGy. The biologic dose of combined modality may not be well expressed in centigray. Quite clearly, 4500 cGy in 5 weeks is less active than the same radiotherapy plus CAV or PE and shortening the time may increase effectiveness and acute toxicity. Continuous course is believed to be superior to split course because the split may permit proliferation of tumor between courses. Alternating modalities require split course but may abort proliferation of cancer cells between courses by strategic timing with chemotherapy.

TIMING AND INTEGRATION OF CHEMORADIATION

Sequential therapy gives all of one modality followed by the other modality. Sandwich therapy is a variation of this theme. When chemotherapy is used first, it causes the tumor to shrink prior to thoracic radiotherapy (TRT). This separation of the two modalities reduces the prospect of toxicity due to a disadvantageous interplay of modalities. There is less prospect of synergism between the two modalities. This strategy may allow for smaller radiotherapy (RT) volumes, but the use of postchemotherapy residual disease to determine RT volume must be tested against the treatment of initial tumor volume.

Concurrent therapy uses both modalities at the same time; it has also been called simultaneous or concomitant therapy. If the tumor has a subpopulation of cells resistant to either modality, concurrent therapy may provide a strategy to overcome resistance. Synergistic or additive interactions can occur in normal tissues and tumors. Cell-cycle effects synchronize cells in phases of the cell cycle, which may increase or decrease radiotherapy or chemotherapy effects. Counterbalancing these potential advantages are the prospect of synergistic toxicity to normal tissues within the RT portal.

Alternating therapy keeps both chemotherapy and radiotherapy in close temporal proximity but far enough apart to reduce toxicity. The radiotherapy is always given by split course. Chemotherapy is given in full doses, but the radiotherapy is administered either the week *before* chemotherapy or the week *after* chemotherapy. Thus, the modalities alternate, frequently with 1 or 2 weeks with no therapy, in order to allow recovery from the other modality's toxicity. Looney has tested this theory in the laboratory using rodent models, which demonstrated better than expected results in tumors resistant to various schedules of chemotherapy alone and radiotherapy alone (30). Cures were obtained using twice-daily irradiation followed a week later by chemotherapy.

CLINICAL TRIALS

In the early 1970s, the National Cancer Institute (NCI)-USA pioneered combined-modality trials with CAV plus concurrent and sequential radiotherapy schemes (31–33). This study employed six different methods of TRT in 71 patients. All therapy was completed within 4 months. The trial included both limited- and extensive-disease patients. Of the limited-disease patients, 81% achieved CR. Only 7% of extensive patients survived for 2 years, but nearly 40% of the limited-disease group survived 2 years. About 90% had white blood cell (WBC) nadirs $< 1,000$ cells/mm^3; this, along with esophagitis and pneumonitis, resulted in 17 deaths (24%). Reanalysis of this trial by Catane suggested that concurrent therapy for 3 weeks was optimal. Longer therapy resulted in excess toxicity; shorter therapy resulted in fewer CRs (34).

The attention provoked by these survival data was tempered by the incidence of complications and mortality. Table 26–1 displays the displays the state of the art as of 1983. We have labeled the trials as either sequential, concurrent, or alternating. The Danish, MRC, and NCI-USA studies were presented in preliminary form (35) and the Southeast Group (SEG) data detailed results

Table 26–1. Chemoradiation in SCLC Selected Trials—Early 1980s

Method and Group	Chemotherapy	Thoracic RT Dose (cGy)/Wks (Course)	Median Survival (mos)		2-Yr Survival (%)	
			Chemo	CR	Chemo	CR
Sequential:						
Denmark [35]	CMLoV	4000/4(S)	12	10.5	13	8
United Kingdom [36]	AV-CM	4000/4(C)	11	12.0	18	8
Concurrent:						
NCI-USA [39]	CMLo	4000/3(C)	12	17.0	15	32
Alternating:						
SEG [38]	CAV	4000/8(S)	12	17.0	12	18

KEY:

C = cyclophosphamide
V = vincristine
Lo = lomustine (CCNU)
A = doxorubicin (Adriamycin)
M = methotrexate
CR = chemoradiation
NCI = National Cancer Institute
SEG = Southeast Group
cGy = centigray (1 rad)
(S) = split course
(C) = continuous course
RT = radiation therapy

of only 199 patients (36). All of these trials employed cyclophosphamide and used 4000 cGy as the radiation dose. The median survival for chemotherapy alone was consistent at approximately 12 months. The dose per fraction of radiotherapy varied in each of these trials; the MRC trial used 200 cGy (standard fraction), but the Danish study used 400 cGy, the NCI-USA used 270 cGy, and the SEG used 300 cGy per fraction. The larger than 200 cGy fractions are probably more damaging to normal tissues and, therefore, are more toxic when combined with chemotherapeutic agents. None of these trials used concurrent ADR with radiotherapy. Most of the drugs had thoracic organ toxicity. Both the Danish and MRC trials reduced intensity by delaying chemotherapy for modest depressions in WBCs. In these two trials, the addition of radiotherapy caused no improvement in median or 2-year survival, which was in fact slightly worse than the chemotherapy control.

Table 26–2 outlines the results of more recent randomized trials of chemotherapy alone versus combined-modality therapy. These trials are also cyclophosphamide based. The TRT doses were mostly 4000 cGy, but the cooperative groups both used 5000 cGy.

Sequential Trials

The course length and treatment duration varied. Table 26–2 reflects the final reports from the Danish study (37) and the MRC study (38). The median survival approximated 1 year with chemotherapy alone and was ever so slightly altered by the addition of TRT. The Eastern Cooperative Oncology Group (ECOG) study (39) was the only sequential trial showing a statistically significant benefit to the addition of TRT. It randomized both responders and nonresponders but separated them for analysis. The ECOG results reflect only the CRs, but the modest improvement in median and 2-year survival was seen in other subsets as well.

In comparing the earlier reports (Table 26–1) with the final reports (Table 26–2), the 2-year survival of the chemotherapy-alone group decreases slightly and the bimodality group improves slightly. With more follow-up, the chemotherapy-alone group has done slightly worse and the combined-modality arms have done slightly better, emphasizing the need for both later endpoints and longer follow-up. Also, this emphasizes that median survival is not the most useful endpoint. The 2-year survival is a better endpoint to measure differences due to treatment. When selecting only complete responders for randomization to receive TRT, early progressors and nonresponders are eliminated. This selection produces data that cannot be compared to data from nonresponsive patients. Excluding patients with unfavorable factors makes the results look better but confuses comparisons to data collected from a permanent population.

Table 26–2. Summary of Completed Randomized Trials of Chemoradiation in SCLC

Method and Group	Chemotherapy	Thoracic RT Dose (cGy)/Wks (Course)	Median Survival (mos)		2-Yr Survival (%)	
			Chemo	CR	Chemo	CR
Sequential:						
Denmark [35]	CMLo-V	4000/4(S)	12	11	10	7
United Kingdom [36]	AV-CM	4000/4(C)	12	12	15	15
ECOG* [37]	CMLo	4000/5(C)	15	18	18	24
Alternating:						
SEG [38]	CAV	4000/8(S)	12	16	19	28
Concurrent:						
NCI-USA [39]	CM-Lo	4000/3(C)	12	15	10	28
CALGB [40]	CEV(A)	4000/5(C)	14	13(i) 15(d)	15	25(i) 30(d)

*Randomizes responders only to +/− TRT.

KEY:

C = cyclophosphamide
V = vincristine
Lo = lomustine (CCNU)
A = doxorubicin (Adriamycin)
M = methotrexate
E = etoposide (VP-16)
CR = chemoradiation
NCI = National Cancer Institute
SEG = Southeast Group
ECOG = Eastern Cooperative Oncology Group
CALGB = Cancer and Leukemia Group B
TRT = thoracic radiation therapy
cGy = centigray (1 rad)
(S) = split course
(C) = continuous course
(i) = immediate TRT
(d) = delayed treatment

Alternating Trials

The first SEG trial (40) typifies the alternating approach—it was designed to integrate radiotherapy without increasing toxicity. It avoided concurrent ADR and TRT. Two split-courses of 300 cGy, 5 times each week, were administered during weeks 5 and 8 and, subsequently, a 1000-cGy boost was administered during week 11. Chemotherapy was given during weeks 1, 4, 7, and 10. Cranial irradiation was given during the same weeks as the TRT (40). Toxicity was modest. This trial fits the chemoradiation model, subsequently termed "alternating therapy" after the model of Looney (30).

Concurrent Trials

Concurrent strategies have also been compared in randomized trials. Table 26–2 shows the two most recent studies. Both trials avoided the use of concurrent radiotherapy with doxorubicin; the NCI trial reported by Bunn (41) used the CMC regimen, and the Cancer and Leukemia Group B (CALGB) trial (42), substituting VP-16 (E) for Adriamycin during induction, used CEV. Bunn and colleagues delivered the concurrent therapy in 3 weeks. The TRT dose was 4000 cGy, using a daily dose of 266 cGy. This study excluded patients with variant histology, which was then called "mixed histology." The CALGB gave 5 weeks of concurrent therapy, using a dose of 5000 cGy as TRT, overlapping with two cycles of chemotherapy (42). This trial had two arms receiving radiotherapy. In one arm, the "immediate arm," the TRT began on day 1, cycle 1. In the other arm, the "delayed arm," the TRT was given after completing three full cycles of CEB. The delayed TRT was given concurrent with cycle 4 of CEV. Both TRT arms proved to be superior to the chemotherapy-alone arm, but the delayed TRT arm actually provided the best survival. However, the frequency of chemotherapy dose reduction was not balanced. After the first cycle, the immediate TRT arm received only 50% of the intended cyclophosphamide, VP-16, or doxorubicin doses. Either immediate TRT prevents the use of subsequent full-dose chemotherapy or the dose-reduction criteria may need modification if more intensive treatment is used.

Many assert that these two studies prove the need for TRT because of the slight but definite improvement in 2-year survival. However, VP-16 alone or in combination may provide similar survival. Two trials have added VP-16 to the CAV regimen, followed by TRT. The Piedmont Oncology Group used 3000 cGy in 2 weeks and randomized inclusion versus exclusion of VP-16 (43). The VP-16 arm produced significantly more responses, an insignificant improvement in median survival, and increased toxicity. A similar regimen was used at Arizona, but higher dose TRT (5000 cGy) was used after four cycles of CAV + E. This trial suggested excellent preliminary results but had short follow-up (44). A final report has not appeared. Equitoxic doses of CAV produced the same results. These trials added VP-16 but kept the CAV dose constant. VP-16 does not appear to produce the results desired.

The Role of Platinum

Because neither CDDP nor VP-16 have appreciable cardiac, esophageal, or pulmonary toxicity, they are ideal to add to TRT. CDDP sensitizes radiation and decreases radiation repair (45–47). CDDP-radiation interactions have been thoroughly reviewed by Dewit (48). The critical test depends on whether these synergistic effects are expressed more in tumor than in normal tissues. Lelieveld and colleagues successfully attempted to probe benefit versus toxicity in an elegant set of laboratory experiments (49). Using dose-effect factors, a measure of how much chemotherapy substitutes for radiotherapy, they demonstrated that CDDP's interaction with radiotherapy causes a net gain when the augmentation of its antitumor effects were balanced against the normal-tissue effects.

Platinum-Etoposide-Based Trials

Table 26–3 demonstrates trials using platinum-etoposide (PE). These trials were carried out during this decade with more sophisticated staging than earlier trials.

The Memorial trial exemplifies the sequential method. The Memorial trial provided four alternating cycles of CAV and PE, then TRT followed by maintenance chemotherapy. Sophisticated techniques to define target and critical normal tissue volumes were used for radiotherapy. This technique protected the spinal cord without using a posterior spinal cord block. This regimen produced 35% CRs after chemotherapy alone but increased the CR rate to 65% after TRT. The median survival was 21 months, and the 2-year survival was 46% (50).

The Institute Gustave Roussy has fostered an alternating approach with a somewhat complex 5-drug regimen. It included CDDP (100 mg/m^2 on day 2) and VP-16 (75 mg/m^2 on days 1, 2, and 3). The TRT was delayed to week 2 of the second, third, and fourth cycle of chemotherapy. The TRT gave 1000 to 2000 cGy course using 250-cGy fractions after the second and third cycles of chemotherapy and a third TRT course of 1500 cGy after the fourth cycle of chemotherapy. Each cycle lasted 28 days. When TRT was interdigitated, the cycle time lengthened to 32 to 34 days. A week of no treatment preceded and followed each course of TRT. Besides PE, doxorubicin, cyclophosphamide, and methotrexate were also used (all of the chemotherapy was given during days 1 to 6 of each cycle). This scheme attempted to eliminate resistant cells by using many active agents and TRT early in treatment, but it also tried to avoid chemoradiation toxicity interplay by timing and by flanking TRT with weeks of no chemotherapy. The TRT dose was escalated during the trial from 4500 to 5500 cGy by adding two treatments of 250 cGy to each of the first and second courses. The dose was increased because of 17% local failure rate observed at 1 year in the group receiving 4500 cGy. The median survival was 17 months, but with only 19 of 109 patients surviving more than 3 years. The actuarial projected survival at 2 years was about 30% and the third-year plateau was about 20%. Despite the avowed aim of toxicity reduction, three patients died of myelotoxicity and nearly 30% had life-threatening myelotoxicity. Although not detailed, esophageal toxicity was reported as mild and pulmonary toxicity reported as an infrequent occurrence (51). Arriagada et al recently updated this experience and reported that despite increasing the thoracic radiotherapy dose from 4500 to 5500 cGy and then to 6500 cGy, local failure remained a steady 30%. Thus, the alternating strategy, at least by the local control parameters, offered no improvement by increasing dose (52).

Table 26–3 sketches the highlighted results of concurrent trials employing PE. Both the University of Pennsylvania (Penn) and SWOG (Southwest Oncology Group) trials

Table 26–3. Selected Chemoradiation Trials Platinum + VP-16 and Chest Radiotherapy

Method and Institution	Chemotherapy	TRT Dose (cGy)/Wks (Course)	Median Survival (mos)	2-Yr Survival
Sequential:				
Memorial [48]	CAV-PE	4500/5(C)	21	46
Alternating:				
		4500/5(S)		
Gustave-Roussy [47]	AEMC ± P		17	30
		5500/6(S)		
Concurrent:				
Penn* [51]	PE-CAV	4500/3(C)	23	50
SWOG [50]	PE-V	4500/5(C)	18	42
			23 (+PE)	40 (+PE)
SEG** [54]	CAV ± PE	4500/7(S)		
			16 (−PE)	20 (−PE)

*Twice-daily radiotherapy.
**Responders randomized to +/− PE. Data on Responders to 6 weeks of CAV + concurrent RT.

KEY:

P = platinum
E = VP-16
C = cyclophosphamide
V = vincristine
Lo = lomustine (CCNU)
A = doxorubicin (Adriamycin)
M = methotrexate
E = etoposide (VP-16)
CR = chemoradiation

NCI = National Cancer Institute
SEG = Southeast Group
SWOG = Southwest Oncology Group
Penn = University of Pennsylvania
TRT = thoracic radiation therapy
cGy = centigray (1 rad)
(S) = split course
(C) = continuous course
RT = radiotherapy

use the PE combination concurrently with radiation. The SEG trial treated with an induction regimen that randomized half of the population to concurrent CAV plus TRT (using 300 cGy fractions and a planned split course) and the other half to CAV alone. Subsequently, a second randomization was made in responding surviving patients; they received additional PE or no further treatment.

The SWOG trial began in 1982 and closed in 1986. This trial entailed CDDP (50 mg/m^2 on days 1 and 8) and VP-16 (50 mg/m^2 on days 1 through 5) for three cycles. Vincristine was given during each 28-day cycle. The radiotherapy began on day 1 and continued for 5 weeks. The TRT dose was 4500 cGy using a daily dose of 180 cGy. The treatment volumes include the supraclavicular fossa, contralateral hilum, and 5 cm below the carina. The overall response rate was 83%, with a 56% CR. Remarkable toxicity included six patients dead of myelosuppression, two-thirds with life-threatening leukopenia, but < 10% thrombocytopenia. Roughly one-half of the patients had no esophagitis; the other half had mild to to moderate esophagitis, but only 5% were considered severe. Pneumonitis was infrequent. Median survival was 18 months, and the 2-year survival was 40% (53).

The Penn trial used twice-daily TRT, directed at the tumor bulk, administered concurrently with day 1 CDDP (60 mg/m^2) and VP-16 (120 mg/m^2) on days 4, 6, and 8 (54). TRT consisted of 150-cGy fractions, 4 to 6 hours apart each day, Monday through Friday. Technically, the initial week's treatment used the same portals for both morning and afternoon sessions; however, the afternoon treatment during weeks 2 and 3 was angled to avoid the spinal cord but included the subcarinal nodes and other mediastinal nodal areas. The TRT target was outlined by CT scan, which defined field size as well as the depth of the isocentric treatment point. Normal tissue margins were limited to 1.0 to 1.5 cm. All patients were staged using chest, brain, and abdominal CT scans, radionuclide bone scans, and bone marrow evaluation. The TRT and CDDP began within 24 hours of each other. This study entered 32 patients: four with variant histology and 28 with pure small-cell histology (i.e., oat cell, lymphocyte-like, polygonal, or fusiform). Toxicity was life-threatening in 25% and treatment clearly caused one death (3%). Myelotoxicity and esophagitis predominated, but there have been no permanent strictures and no problematic acute or chronic pulmonary reactions attributed to treatment. With a median follow-up of 40 months and a minimum follow-up of 1 year, 14 patients remain alive and disease-free. The median and 2-year survivals are 23 months and 50%, respectively. The four variant patients failed locoregionally and all died by 2 years. Only one pure small-cell patient failed locally, and at failure, variant histology was found. A multi-institutional pilot study of this regimen has been reported, but the data are confirmatory and a final analysis is in progress (55). A similar study reported comparable results at the NCI-Navy, Bethesda (56). Encouraged by these results, a randomized trial is nearing completion. The randomized trial compares the SWOG once-daily TRT approach to the Penn twice-daily TRT, both with concurrent PE and both using 4500 cGy.

In contrast to these concurrent PE trials, the second SEG trial used six cycles of CAV, concurrent with large fraction radiotherapy in randomized patients, then a second randomization to add PE or no further therapy (57). The TRT was administered concurrently with CAV, giving 3000 cGy on days 1 to 14 and a 1500-cGy boost concurrent with the third cycle of chemotherapy. Because of toxicity, the TRT randomization was stopped. TRT added no survival advantage. Table 26–3 reflects the results of a second randomization to PE, which produced significant gains in median and 2-year survivals. The second randomization was offered only to responders. Nevertheless, these results appear better than any other cooperative group. However, TRT concurrent with CAV was too toxic and did not improve survival, and patients who failed to respond to CAV induction were excluded from randomization to PE analysis (58).

The total duration and number of cycles of systemic chemotherapy are in flux. At this time, 1 or 2 years of chemotherapy appears excessive and does not improve survival. Two studies show that maintenance is not necessary (59,60), but no trial has established exactly how many cycles of PE, CMC, or CAV are necessary or what constitutes the best induction combination.

LOCAL FAILURE

Thoracic recurrence of SCLC may cause death even without disseminated disease (57,61). In a review of local control as a survival variable, there was poor survival when local control was not achieved and quite excellent survival when it was (57). In the studies tabulated above, local failure ranged between 32 and 85% for chemotherapy alone and between 0 and 60% with the addition of TRT. Although the sequential studies had higher local failure proportions and the concurrent and alternating studies had somewhat better local control, it is not clear what factors influence local control the most. Studies with poorer systemic therapy, poor patient selection, and shorter median survivals produce the appearance of local control. However, patients who die early of progressive disease may not manifest local failure.

Factors such as radiotherapy volume, dose, or schedule and the PE chemotherapy regimen may influence local control, but few studies address any of these issues. Lastly, the improved local results with concurrent and alternating regimens must be balanced against the prospect of increased toxicity. If the local modality compromises the intensity of systemic therapy, the better local control may be too costly if the compromised systemic therapy leads to poorer survival.

PROPHYLACTIC CRANIAL IRRADIATION

Prophylactic cranial irradiation (PCI) attempts to address the high frequency of brain relapse in SCLC. The central nervous system (CNS), with its blood-brain barrier (BBB), provides a sanctuary from chemotherapy for SCLC. In 1974, Newman and coworkers reported the high CNS metastatic frequency in SCLC (62). Chemotherapeutic agents (including those that cross the BBB) have been uniformly unsuccessful at reducing CNS relapse (63–65) but recent studies suggest some renewed interest in this strategy (66,67). Because small-cell tumors are exquisitely sensitive to irradiation, Hansen postulated that lower dose CNS irradiation might decrease CNS relapse (64). This prompted several trials evaluating PCI in SCLC (65–74). Although a variety of doses and fractionation schedules were administered, CNS relapse was reduced on average from 22% without PCI to 8% with PCI (65). No randomized trial has demonstrated improvement in overall survival. Nevertheless, these data lead most clinicians to employ PCI routinely.

The longterm toxicity of PCI in SCLC was underestimated until recently because few patients survived beyond 1 to 2 years. Currently, however, between 20 and 25% (or more) of limited-stage patients enjoy longterm disease-free survival (75). With better survival, late toxic effects have been manifest. Although the longterm effects of PCI in SCLC have not been fully elucidated, a number of studies report its effects in acute lymphoblastic leukemia (ALL) survivors (76–79). Some patients have reduced intelligence and gait, memory, or sensory-motor performance. Many have indicated cranial irradiation as the culpable factor in developing neurotoxicities; however, chemotherapy, its timing with PCI, and/or the disease or its accompanying infections have been implicated as well (see Chapter 38) (76–80). Some chemotherapy by itself is neurotoxic, viz lomustine, procarbazine, VP-16, and vincristine. Concurrent administration of these drugs with radiotherapy may augment this usually minor toxicity (81). Because radiotherapy may increase the permeability of the BBB, subsequent courses of chemotherapy may enter the CNS and produce unexpected additive damage.

Some longterm SCLC survivors have developed debilitating neurologic sequelae. Ellison et al (82) reported that four of 10 longterm, disease-free survivors, who developed CNS toxicity characterized by hemiparesis, confusion, organic brain syndrome, and ataxia, had received combination chemotherapy (CMC) plus PCI. They suggested that the neurotoxicities were probably caused by combining brain irradiation with nitrosourea chemotherapy. Catane et al noted that post-PCI brain CT scans often showed evidence of cortical atrophy (83). However, these changes were not correlated with pretherapy scans, and there were no reported neurologic deficits in the patients with abnormal CT scans.

Following the observations of Ellison and Catane, several groups have reported late neurotoxicities in longterm survivors (84–89). Generally, patients developed dementia with or without associated neurological signs, including confusion, aphonia, ataxia, psychomotor retardation, cerebellar dysfunction, optic neuropathy, and intellectual deficits. One group found that near 50% of their 5-year survivors had been unable to resume their pre-SCLC lifestyle presumably due to their neurotoxicity (88). The latter study also demonstrated subtle neurologic abnormalities in 12 of 14 patients, as determined by a battery of standard neuropsychologic tests (90).

Not every group reporting late-developing neurotoxicity has described treatment in detail. However, a majority of affected patients received cranial irradiation either prophylactically or therapeutically (usual dose 2400 to 3000 cGy in 8 to 10 fractions over 2 weeks). Some were also given methotrexate, procarbazine, and/or CCNU-containing chemotherapy regimens. These drugs cross the BBB and may themselves cause late neurotoxicity. However, neurotoxic sequelae were also detected in several patients who did *not* receive these lipophilic agents but did receive cranial irradiation (88,89). Thus, it appears very likely that cranial irradiation plays a major role in the etiology of the late complications of PCI. The PCI fraction size has been implicated as a cause of late neurologic effects. Most PCI regimens used 300-cGy fractions. Since these larger-than-200-cGy fractions cause damage to late-responding tissues, especially neurologic tissue, the schedule of 3000 cGy in fractions of 300 cGy has fallen out of favor.

The timing of PCI with chemotherapy is another variable to consider. If the PCI is intended to eliminate the "last" cell in a protected sanctuary, the PCI must have a rationale only for complete responders. If there is residual systemic disease, therapy directed at the cranium is illusory. If systemic disease is vanquished, the role for more systemic therapy vanishes. Subsequent courses of chemotherapy, crossing the BBB, may augment brain toxicity or inhibit its repair.

Interestingly, the Canadian trials have used even larger fractions: 400 cGy to a total dose of 2000 cGy. They have reported little neurologic sequelae. They do not use chemotherapy subsequent to PCI (91). A trial from Arizona reported 4000 cGy in 10 fractions following 4 cycles of induction chemotherapy. Although chemotherapy was suspended during PCI, maintenance therapy continued for 2 years. Two patients developed subacute CNS toxicity (44). Thus, there are some data showing the apparent safety of large-fraction PCI and other data showing the apparent toxicity of small-fraction PCI when followed by CAV-E chemotherapy.

Clinicians are left with unanswered questions—should SCLC patients routinely receive PCI, and if so, which patients? Are all SCLC patients candidates for PCI or should only completely responding patients receive it? We assert that only patients achieving a complete remission might benefit from PCI. Those with less than a CR might "reseed" the CNS, negating any benefit of PCI. On the other hand, CR patients may be the least likely group to benefit from PCI and the group at greatest risk for longterm neurotoxicity. None of the randomized PCI studies assess the influence of PCI on the rate of "primary" CNS relapse from complete remission, nor was the impact of PCI on the long-term survival of complete responders reported. General conclusions about the value of PCI in CR patients are difficult because crude rather than actual or actuarial relapse percentages were reported, because follow-up periods were short and autopsy data usually were not reported, and because timing, dose, and fractionation of the radiotherapy varied. Not surprising, these studies have led various authors to strikingly different conclusions regarding the use of PCI. Some experts believe that *no* patients should receive PCI, others believe *all* patients should receive PCI, while still others believe only completely responding patients should receive PCI (92).

Two recent studies attempted to evaluate the influence of PCI on the development of primary CNS relapse and its impact on survival in patients achieving a CR to initial systemic chemotherapy (93,94). In a retrospective analysis of the NCI experience, Rosen et al reported that among completely responding patients, those given PCI developed fewer CNS relapses (19% vs. 40%) and had longer survival than patients not receiving PCI (93). However, these differences were not statistically significant after adjusting for other prognostic features. There was, however, a significant reduction in the percentage of patients with primary and solitary CNS (17% vs. 0%), and the 2.5-year survival in limited-stage CR patients receiving PCI was > 30% vs. 14% for those not given PCI. The authors concluded that a randomized trial was needed to confirm the apparent beneficial results of PCI in patients in CR (93).

In a small randomized study, Aroney et al reported that PCI given within 14 days of an observed CR significantly delayed the time to CNS relapse (94). However, no significant survival benefit was seen. The frequency of primary and solitary CNS relapse was lower in patients receiving PCI compared to those not given PCI (0% vs. 15%; $p = 0.05$). The combined weight of these two studies suggests that primary CNS relapse in CR patients can be reduced with PCI.

The role of PCI is also controversial because of uncertainties regarding the value of therapeutic brain irradiation in patients experiencing a CNS relapse, particularly in those who have not received PCI. Several reports have shown high response rates (50 to 90%), and neurologic symptoms have been well controlled usually for the life span of such patients (63,68). However, other studies suggest lower response rates and neurologic deaths in patients not given PCI (95). Early diagnosis with the judicious use of CT and/or MRI scanning, early institution of high-dose corticosteroids, and expeditious cranial irradiation may alleviate these poor responses. There are no prospective studies detailing the value of corticosteroids and cranial irradiation in the amelioration of symptomatic CNS metastases.

COMPLICATIONS OF CHEMORADIATION

Chemoradiation trials reportedly cause more toxicity than trials using chemotherapy alone. The main incremental toxicities are myelosuppression and esophagitis. The nadirs caused by chemotherapy commonly limit dose and are titrated to be maximally tolerated. TRT infrequently increases major myelosuppression. Many have assumed that the combined-modality toxicity was due to TRT effects on bone marrow, which may not be so. Although the total WBC is depressed by TRT, it is not clear that the absolute granulocyte count is depressed at all. This may be due to the irradiation of the entire blood volume. Because the great vessels are in the irradiated fields, the cardiac output is probably irradiated twice—once from the pulmonary circuit and then again in the systemic circuit. Lymphocytes are very sensitive to irradiation and, like SCLC itself, without a radiobiologic shoulder. Thus, circulating lymphocytes are efficiently killed when TRT irradiates the blood volume. The WBC appears lower than usual, but the absolute granulocyte count may be relatively unchanged. None of the randomized trials report this. If an arbitrary WBC level is chosen to trigger dose-modification or delays, the chemoradiation arm may get less systemic treatment.

The other main toxicity is esophagitis. The endpoint for esophagitis is subjective and, as a consequence, it is quite difficult to compare reported frequencies of the acute reactions. When TRT is administered *without* chemotherapy, acute esophagitis is infrequently sufficient to cause interruption. Strictures are almost never seen. Chemoradiation programs clearly exacerbate the frequency of both esophagitis and strictures. A comparison of the two SEG trials demonstrates the importance of timing, at least with the Adriamycin-containing regimens. In the first SEG trial, the esophagitis was a minor issue after alternating therapy and the TRT arm had significantly improved survival (40). In the second SEG trial, the concurrent treatment toxicity was significantly greater than that occurring with chemotherapy alone. The esophagitis seen in the CDDP-based trials seems less in degree but equally frequent. Fewer strictures are reported, but in some trials the late-effect endpoints may not have had time to be expressed.

Field has reviewed the other complications of SCLC treatment (96). Pneumonitis, carditis, and dermatitis are less common. In the NCI-USA study, Bunn reported an incidence of deaths due to pulmonary toxicity when CMC was used (41). Each of these drugs are low-level pulmonary toxins. Therefore, when added to TRT, it is not surprising that unacceptable toxicity resulted. The PE-TRT studies report virtually no acute pulmonary reactions, carditis, and infrequent cutaneous reactions. The chronic events also seem to be much less.

CONCLUSION

With progress in the last decade, the outlook is much brighter for many patients with SCLC. Sufficient challenges remain, but the death sentence has been stayed for many.

REFERENCES

1. Fox W, Scadding JG. Medical research council comparative trial of surgery and radiotherapy for primary treatment of small-cell or oat-cell carcinoma of the bronchus. Lancet 2:63, 1973.
2. Roswit B, Patno ME, Rapp R, et al. The survival of patients with inoperable lung cancer. A large-scale randomized study of radiation therapy versus placebo. Radiology 90:688, 1968.
3. Wolf J, Patno ME, Roswit B. Controlled study of survival of patients with clinically inoperable lung cancer treated with radiation therapy. Am J Med 40:360, 1966.
4. Bergsagel D, Jenkin RD, Pringle JF, et al. Lung cancer: Clinical trial of radiotherapy alone versus radiotherapy plus cyclophosphamide. Cancer 30:621, 1972.
5. Aisner J, Alberto P, Bitran J. The role of chemotherapy in small cell lung cancer: A consensus report of the International Association for the Study of Lung Cancer Workshop. Cancer Treat Rep 67:37, 1983.
6. Comis RL. Small cell carcinoma of the lung. Cancer Treat Rev 9:237, 1982.
7. Morstyn G, Ihde DC, Lichter AS, et al. Small cell lung cancer 1973–1983: Early progress and recent obstacles. Int J Radiat Oncol Biol Phys 10:515, 1984.
8. Slevin ML, Clark PI, Osborne RJ, et al. A randomized trial to evaluate the effect of schedule on the activity of etoposide in small cell lung cancer. Proc Am Soc Clin Oncol 5:175, 1986.
9. Stewart DJ, Maroun J, Logan D, et al. Oral VP-16 and carboplatin for small cell lung cancer. Proc Am Soc Clin Oncol 10:247, 1991.
10. Shepherd F, Goss P, Evans W, et al. Treatment of small cell lung cancer (SCLC) in the elderly. Proc Am Soc Clin Oncol 10:241, 1991.
11. Dombernowsky P, Sorensen S, Aisner J, Hansen H. Cisdichlorodiammine platinum (II) in small cell anaplastic bronchogenic carcinoma: A phase II study. Cancer Treat Rep 4:543, 1979.
12. Smith LE, Harland SJ, Robinson BA, et al. Carboplatin: A very active new cisplatin analog in the treatment of small cell lung cancer. Cancer Treat Rep 69:43, 1985.
13. Jacobs RH, Bitran JD, Deutsch M, et al. Phase II study of carboplatin in previously untreated patients with metastatic small cell lung carcinoma. Cancer Treat Rep 71:311, 1987.
14. Schabel FM, Trader MW, Laster WJ Jr, et al.

Dichlorodiammine platinum (II): Combination chemotherapy and cross-resistance studies with tumors in mice. Cancer Treat Rep 63:1459, 1979.
15. Sierocki JS, Hilaris BS, Hopfan S, et al. Cis-diammine-dichloro-platinum (II) and VP-16-213. An active induction regimen for small cell carcinoma of the lung. Cancer Treat Rep 63:1593, 1979.
16. Eagan RT, Frytak S, Lee RE. No routine role for vincristine, adriamycin and cyclophosphamide (VAC) or thoracic radiation therapy in extensive stage small cell lung cancer. Am J Clin Oncol 10(2):141, 1987.
17. Salazar OM, Creech RH. The state of the art toward defining the role of radiation therapy and the management of small cell bronchogenic carcinoma. Int J Radiat Oncol Biol Phys 6:1103, 1980.
18. Comis RL. The role of surgery in small cell lung cancer: A reappraisal. *In:* Clinics in Oncology 4. Spiro SG (Ed). Philadelphia, WB Saunders Co., 1985.
19. Matthews MJ, Gazdar AF. Pathology of small cell carcinoma of the lung and its subtypes: A clinico-pathologic correlation. *In:* Lung Cancer. Vol 1. Livingston RB (Ed). Boston, Martinus Nijhoff, 1981, p. 283.
20. Baker RR, Ettinger DS, Ruckdeschel JD. The role of surgery in the management of selected patients with small-cell carcinoma of the lung. J Clin Oncol 5(5):687, 1987.
21. Lad T. The role of surgery in small cell lung cancer: An intergroup prospective randomized trial (Abstr). Lung Cancer 4:13, 1988.
22. Steel GG. Terminology in the description of drug-radiation interactions. Int J Radiat Oncol Biol Phys 5:1145, 1979.
23. Coleman CN, Turrissi AT. Radiation and chemotherapy sensitizers and protectors. Crit Rev Oncol Hematol 10(3):225, 1990.
24. Turrisi AT, Glatstein E. Principles of combined-modality therapy: Progress, prospects and problems. *In:* Radiation Oncology Rationale, Technique, Results. Moss WT, Cox JD (Eds). St. Louis, Mosby Company, 1988.
25. Carney DN. Recent advances in the biology of small cell lung cancer. Chest 89(Suppl):223S, 1986.
26. Radice PA, Mathews MJ, Ihde DC, et al. The clinical behavior of "mixed" small cell/large cell bronchogenic carcinoma compared to "pure" small cell subtypes. Cancer 50:2894, 1982.
27. Turrisi AT, Glover DJ, Pietra G, Goldwein J. Variant histology limited small cell lung cancer. A poor prognostic indicator. Proc Am Assoc Cancer Res 1989.
28. Aisner SC, Ettinger D, Finkelstein D, et al. The clinical significance of variant morphology small cell carcinoma of the lung. Proc Am Soc Clin Oncol 7:195, 1988.
29. Choi NC, Carey RW. Small cell anaplastic carcinoma of the lung. Reappraisal of current management. Cancer 37:2651, 1976.
30. Looney WB. Special lecture: Alternating chemotherapy and radiotherapy. NCI Monogr 6:85, 1988.
31. Johnson RE, Brereton HD, Kent CH. Small cell carcinoma of the lung: Attempt to remedy causes of past therapeutic failure. Lancet 2:289, 1976.
32. Kent CH, Brereton HD, Johnson RE. "Total" therapy for oat cell carcinoma of the lung. Int J Radiat Oncol Biol Phys 2:427, 1977.
33. Johnson RE, Brereton HD, Kent CH. "Total" therapy for oat cell carcinoma of the lung. Ann Thorac Surg 25:510, 1978.
34. Catane R, Lichter A, Lee YJ, et al. Small cell lung cancer: Analysis of treatment factors contributing to prolonged survival. Cancer 48:1936, 1981.
35. Bleehen NM, Bunn PA, Cox JD, et al. Role of radiation therapy in small cell anaplastic carcinoma of the lung. Cancer Treat Rep 67:11, 1983.
36. Perez CA, Einhorn L, Oldham RK, et al. Preliminary report on a randomized trial of radiotherapy (RT) to the thorax in limited small cell carcinoma of the lung treated with multiagent chemotherapy. Proc Am Soc Clin Oncol 2:190, 1983.
37. Osterlind K, Hansen HH, Hansen HS, et al. Chemotherapy versus chemotherapy plus irradiation in limited small cell lung cancer. Results of a controlled trial with five years follow-up. Br J Cancer 54:7, 1986.
38. Souhami RL, Geddes DM, Spiro SG, et al. Radiotherapy in small cell lung cancer of the lung treated with combination chemotherapy: A controlled trial. Br Med J 288:1643, 1984.
39. Creech R, Richter M, Finkelstein D for the ECOG. Combination chemotherapy with or without consolidation radiation therapy for regional small cell carcinoma of the lung (Abst 756). Proc Am Soc Clin Oncol 7:196, 1988.
40. Perez CA, Einhorn L, Oldham PK, et al. Randomized trial of radiotherapy to the thorax in limited small-cell carcinoma of the lung treated with multi-agent chemotherapy and elective brain irradiation. A preliminary report. J Clin Oncol 2(11):1200, 1984.
41. Bunn PA, Lichter AS, Makuch RW, et al. Chemotherapy alone or chemotherapy with chest radiation therapy in limited stage small cell lung cancer. Ann Intern Med 106(5):655, 1987.
42. Perry MC, Eaton WL, Propert KJ, et al. Chemotherapy with or without radiation therapy

in limited small-cell carcinoma of the lung. N Engl J Med 316:912, 1987.
43. Jackson DV, Zekan PJ, Caldwell RD, et al. VP-16-213 in combination chemotherapy with chest irradiation for small cell lung cancer: A randomized trial of the Piedmont Oncology Association. J Clin Oncol 2:1343, 1984.
44. Goodman GE, Miller TP, Manning MM, et al. Treatment of small cell lung cancer with VP-16, vincristine, doxorubicin (Adriamycin), cyclophsophamide (EVAC), and high-dose chest radiotherapy. J Clin Oncol 1(8):483, 1983.
45. Richmond RC, Powers EL. Radiation sensitization of bacterial spores by cis-diammine dichloroplatinum (II). Radiat Res 88:476, 1981.
46. Douple EB, Richmond DRC. Platinum complexes as radiosensitizers of hypoxic mammalian cells. Br J Cancer 37:98, 1978.
47. Carde P, Leval F. Effect of cis-diammine dichloro-platinum II and x-rays on mammalian cell survival. Int J Radiat Oncol Biol Phys 7:929, 1981.
48. Dewit L. Combined treatment of radiation and cis-diammine dischloro platinum (II): A review of experimental and clinical data. Int J Radiat Oncol Biol Phys 13:403, 1987.
49. Lelieveld P, Scoles MA, Brown JM, Kallman RF. The effect of treatment in fractionated schedules with the combination of x-irradiation and cytotoxic drugs on the RIF-1 tumor and normal mouse strain. Int J Radiat Oncol Biol Phys 11:111, 1985.
50. Shank B, Scher H, Hilaris BS, et al. Increased survival with high-dose multi-field radiotherapy and intensive chemotherapy in limited small cell carcinoma of the lung. Cancer 56:2771, 1985.
51. le Chevalier T, Arriagada R, de Thé H, et al. Combination of chemotherapy and radiotherapy in limited small cell lung carcinoma: Results of alternating schedule in 109 patients. NCI Monogr 6:335, 1988.
52. Arriagada R, Cossett JM, le Chevalier T, Tubiana M. The value of radiotherapy when chemotherapy is the major curative method. Int J Radiat Oncol Biol Phys 19(5):1279, 1990.
53. McCracken JD, Janaki LM, Crowley JJ, et al. Concurrent chemotherapy/radiotherapy for limited small cell carcinoma of the lung. A Southwest Oncology Group Study (Supplemented with personal communication with Dr. McCracken). J Clin Oncol 8:892, 1990.
54. Turrisi AT, Glover DJ, Mason B, Tester W. Concurrent twice-daily multi-field radiotherapy and platinum-etoposide for limited small cell lung cancer (Abst 816). Proc Am Soc Clin Oncol 7:211, 1988.
55. Turrisi A. Personal communication. Eastern Cooperative Oncology Group Data. April 1989.
56. Glatstein E, Johnson B. Personal communication. April 1989.
57. Birch R, Omura GA, Greco FA, Perez CA. Patterns of failure in combined chemotherapy and radiotherapy for limited small cell lung cancer: Southeastern Cancer Study Group experience. NCI Monogr 6:265, 1988.
58. Einhorn L, Greco FA, Cohen H, Birch R. Late consolidation with cisplatin plus VP-16 following induction chemotherapy with cyclophosphamide, Adriamycin, and vincristine in limited small cell lung cancer: A SECSG randomized prospective trial. Proc Am Soc Clin Oncol 6:166, 1987.
59. Woods RL, Levi JA. Chemotherapy for small cell lung cancer: A randomized study of maintenance therapy with cyclophosphamide, adriamycin, and vincristine after remission induction with cisplatinum VP-16-213, and radiotherapy. Proc Am Soc Clin Oncol 3:213, 1984.
60. Splinter TAW. EORTC 08825. Induction vs. induction plus maintenance chemotherapy in small cell lung cancer. Definitive evaluation. Proc Am Soc Clin Oncol 7:202, 1988.
61. Byhardt RW, Cox JD, Libnoch JA, et al. Multiagent chemotherapy, prophylactic neuroaxis irradiation and consolidative irradiation for small cell carcinoma of the lung. Am J Clin Oncol 8:504, 1985.
62. Newman SJ, Hansen HH. Frequency, diagnosis, and treatment of brain metastases in 249 consecutive patients with bronchogenic carcinoma. Cancer 33:492, 1974.
63. Nugent JL, Bunn PA Jr, Mathews MJ, et al. CNS metastases in small cell bronchogenic carcinoma. Cancer 44:1885, 1979.
64. Hansen HH. Should initial treatment of small cell carcinoma include systemic chemotherapy and brain irradiation? Cancer Chemother Rep 4:239, 1973.
65. Bunn PA Jr, Nugent JL, Matthews MJ. Central nervous system metastases in small cell bronchogenic carcinoma. Semin Oncol 5:314, 1978.
66. Lee JS, Benjamin RS, Murphy WK, et al. Successful treatment of brain metastasis with systemic chemotherapy in small cell lung cancer. Proc Am Soc Clin Oncol 7:198, 1988.
67. Lee JS, Benjamin RS, Murphy WK, et al. Successful treatment of brain metastasis with systemic chemotherapy in small cell lung cancer. Lung Cancer 4(Suppl):A103, 1988.
68. Balgan TJ, Marks JE. Comparison of symptomatic and prophylactic irradiation of brain metastases from oat cell carcinoma of the lung. Cancer 47:41, 1981.

69. Jackson DV, Richards F II, Cooper MR, et al. Prophylactic cranial irradiation in small cell carcinoma of the lung. A randomized study. JAMA 237:2730, 1977.
70. Maurer LH, Tulloh M, Weiss RB, et al. A randomized combined modality trial in small cell carcinoma of the lung: Comparison of combination chemotherapy-radiation therapy versus cyclophosphamide-radiation therapy effects of maintenance chemotherapy and prophylactic whole brain irradiation. Cancer 45:30, 1980.
71. Hirsch FR, Paulson OB, Hansen HH, Vraa-Jensen J. Intracranial metastases in small cell carcinoma of the lung: Correlation of clinical and autopsy findings. Cancer 50(11):2433, 1982.
72. Beiler DD, Kane RC, Bernath AM, Cashdollar MR. Low dose elective brain irradiation in small cell carcinoma of the lung. Int J Radiat Oncol Biol Phys 5:941, 1979.
73. Cox JD, Petrovich Z, Paig C, Stanley K. Prophylactic cranial irradiation in patients with inoperable carcinoma of the lung. Cancer 42:1135, 1978.
74. Seydel HG, Creech R, Pagano M, et al. Combined modality treatment of small cell undifferentiated carcinoma of the lung. A cooperative study of the RTOG and the ECOG. Int J Radiat Oncol Biol Phys 9(8):1135, 1983.
75. Johnson DH, Greco FA. Small cell carcinoma of the lung. Crit Rev Oncol Hematol 4:303, 1986.
76. Moss HA, Nannis ED, Poplack DG. The effects of prophylactic treatment of the central nervous system of the intellectual functioning of children with ALL. Am J Med 71:47, 1981.
77. Rowland J, Glidewell O, Sibley R, et al. Effect of cranial radiation (CRT) on neuropsychologic function in children with acute lymphocytic leukemia (ALL). Proc Am Soc Clin Oncol 1:123, 1982.
78. Whitt JK, Wells RJ, McMillan C, et al. Neuropsychological sequelae of cranial irradiation childhood acute lymphocytic leukemia (ALL). Proc Am Soc Clin Oncol 1:50, 1982.
79. Robinson L, Nesbit M, Sather H, et al. Intellectual function in long-term survivors of childhood acute lymphoblastic leukemia (ALL). Proc Am Soc Clin Oncol 1:46, 1982.
80. Meadows AT, Gordon J, Massari DJ, et al. Declines in I.Q. scores and cognitive dysfunctions in children with acute lymphocytic leukaemia treated with cranial irradiation. Lancet 2(8254):1015, 1981.
81. Frytak S, Shaw JN, O'Neill BP, et al. Leukoencephalopathy in small cell lung cancer patients receiving prophylactic cranial irradiation. Am J Clin Oncol 12(1):27, 1989.
82. Ellison N, Bernath A, Kane R, Porter P. Disturbing problems of success: Clinical status of long-term survivors of small cell lung cancer. Proc Am Soc Clin Oncol 1:149, 1982.
83. Catane R, Schwade JG, Yarr I, et al. Follow-up neurological evaluation in patients with small cell lung carcinoma treated with prophylactic cranial irradiation and chemotherapy. Int J Radiat Oncol Biol Phys 7:105, 1981.
84. Scher H, Hilaris B, Wittes R. Long term follow-up of combined modality therapy in small cell carcinoma (SCLC) of the lung. Proc Am Soc Clin Oncol 2:199, 1983.
85. Licciardello J, Bromer R, Karp D, et al. Delayed neurotoxicity (DN) after prophylactic cranial irradiation (PCXRT) of mediastinal irradiation with chemotherapy for patients with small cell lung cancer. Proc Am Soc Clin Oncol 2:199, 1983.
86. Livingston RB. Long-term survivors with small-cell lung cancer (SCLC): A Southwest Oncology Group (SWOG) study. Proc Am Soc Clin Oncol 2:187, 1983.
87. Volk SA, Massour RP, Gandara DR, Redmond J. Morbidity in long-term survivors of small cell carcinoma of the lung. Proc Am Soc Clin Oncol 2:185, 1983.
88. Johnson BE, Inde DC, Bunn PA, et al. Patients with small cell lung cancer treated with combination chemotherapy with or without irradiation. Ann Intern Med 103:430, 1985.
89. Lee JS, Lee YY, Umsawasdi T, et al. Neurotoxicity (NT) in long-term survivors (LTS) of small cell lung cancer (SCLC). Proc Am Soc Clin Oncol 3:330, 1984.
90. Bunn PA. Unpublished observations. Personal communication. April 1989.
91. Feld H. Short course prophylactic cranial irradiation for small cell lung cancer. Am J Clin Oncol 8:371, 1985.
92. Lauer RC, Fleck JF, Antony A, Einhorn L. Is prophylactic cranial irradiation indicated in small cell lung cancer? Proc Am Soc Clin Oncol 7:209, 1988.
93. Rosen ST, Makuch RW, Lichter AS, et al. The role of prophylactic cranial irradiation in preventing central nervous system metastases in small cell lung cancer: Potential benefit restricted to patients in complete response. Am J Med 74:615, 1983.
94. Aroney RS, Aisner J, Wesley MN, et al. Value of prophylactic cranial irradiation given at complete remission in small cell lung carcinoma. Cancer Treat Rep 67:675, 1983.
95. Cox JD, Komaki R, Byhardt RW, Kun LE. Results of whole brain irradiation for metastases from small cell carcinoma of the lung. Cancer Treat Rep 64:957, 1980.
96. Feld R. Complications in the treatment of small cell carcinoma of the lung. Cancer Treat Rev 8:5, 1981.

Chapter 27

NONSMALL-CELL LUNG CARCINOMA

EVERETT E. VOKES, JACOB D. BITRAN, AND SRINIVASAN VIJAYAKUMAR

INTRODUCTION

Lung cancer is a major health care problem globally. The mortality from lung cancer in the United States alone is staggering; 146,000 deaths were reported in 1992 (1). Therapeutic progress in certain histologic types of lung cancer, adenocarcinoma, squamous cell carcinoma, and large-cell carcinoma (otherwise referred to as nonsmall-cell lung cancer [NSCLC]) has occurred slowly. Over the past decade, surgical studies reporting survival statistics of patients with Stage I and II NSCLC have indicated improved results, which reflect improved surgical techniques and better preoperative clinical staging. In contrast, over the same time interval, radiotherapy studies reporting survival statistics of patients with Stage III A and B NSCLC have continued to report limited survival of such patients with a median survival of 8 to 12 months. We believe the current decade offers hope. There have been many Phase II studies employing chemotherapy and radiotherapy and, more recently, randomized trials that ultimately may lead to improved survival statistics for Stage III patients. This chapter will review the current radiotherapeutic approach to NSCLC, review selected chemotherapy and radiotherapy series, and consider future investigations.

RADIOTHERAPY

Clinical investigation of any malignancy requires a uniform patient population, stratification of known prognostic pretreatment factors, and a careful analysis of treatment-related outcome including response duration, sites of treatment failure, and survival. Analyses of the patterns of failure (POF) in patients with locally advanced NSCLC treated with radiotherapy indicate that the majority of patients fail either locally or relapse in systemic visceral sites (2–8). Some generalizations can be made based on the POF for advanced NSCLC.

1. The majority of patients fail within the first 24 months, followed shortly by death.
2. Local failure occurs most frequently in squamous cell carcinoma.
3. In contrast, the majority of patients with large cell or adenocarcinoma fail in systemic sites, particularly the brain.
4. Approximately one-fourth of patients will die without disease progression of intercurrent illness or treatment related toxicity.

Because as many as 40 to 50% of patients with NSCLC will fail locally, it is evident that achieving a greater degree of local control may delay progression of NSCLC, although by itself that may not have much impact on overall survival (8). The importance of local control of NSCLC in improving treatment results must be emphasized (2,9) and is well illustrated by a four-arm randomized study of various radiotherapy dose regimens in patients with locally advanced NSCLC conducted by the Radiation Therapy Oncology Group (RTOG) (10). The objective response rate among the four treatment arms did not alter the POF; however, the patients who achieved an objective response to radiotherapy, regardless of the arm they were randomized to, had an improved survival and a significant delay in the onset of local relapse or systemic metastases, either as a result of radiotherapy itself or of other tumor features correlating with response to radiation. In view of the direct relationship between radiotherapy and local control in NSCLC, three technical facets of dose, treatment volume, and technique in radiotherapy delivery are addressed here in some length.

Dose, Time, and Fractionation

The ideal dose and fractionation scheme for NSCLC is not known. However, fractions of > 300 cGy can lead to significant late normal tissue sequelae when compared to 180- to 200-cGy fractions (11). Thus, 180- to 200-cGy fractionation schemes continue to be recommended. In a recent dose-response analysis for NSCLC, it has been shown that about 8000 cGy may be required for 90% local control (12). The dose that can be delivered in NSCLC is dictated by the surrounding normal tissue tolerance, particularly the tolerance of spinal cord, lung, and heart. The recommended doses are shown in Table 27–1. However, such recommendation should be followed cautiously because the dose requirements in NSCLC continue to be studied carefully and are still evolving. For instance, Cox et al recently showed in a randomized RTOG study that 6960 cGy given in 120-cGy twice-daily fractions resulted in a higher survival than lower doses ($p = 0.02$) (13). In the biologic effects caused by ionizing radiation, a constant fraction of cells is destroyed by a given dose of irradiation. Because the primary site and involved nodes have the highest burden of clonogenic cells, higher doses are required for these sites, compared to sites of subclinical disease, including those areas involved with only microscopic cancer (11,14). For the control of macroscopic disease (> 3 cm), doses exceeding 7000 cGy may be required.

Table 27–1. The Radiotherapeutic Approach in the "Standard" Treatment of Patients with Stage III A/B NSCLC

Volume	Dose (cGy)	Fractionation (cGy)
I. Subclinical Disease—"Large Target Volume" (uninvolved mediastinum and hilar nodes; supraclavicular nodes in selected cases)	4500–5000	180–200
II. Primary and involved nodes with 1- to 2-cm margin—"Target Volume"	6000	180–200
III. Primary and involved nodes "Tumor Volume"	6600–7000	180–200

The necessity of administering more than 6000 cGy to the tumor is well illustrated by the results of studies by Choi and Doucatte (15) and Perez et al (4,5). In a retrospective study, Choi and Doucatte showed that long-term survival improved with increasing doses. With 4000 to 4500 cGy, the 2- and 3-year actuarial survivals were 10% and 3%, respectively. Two- and 3-year actuarial survival rates with 6000 to 6400 cGy, on the other hand, were 36% and 28%, respectively (15). Local tumor control at ≥ 18 months was 76% with 5600 to 6400 cGy, versus 29% with 4000 to 4900 cGy. Similar findings were reported in prospective randomized studies conducted by RTOG (4,5,10). In RTOG study 73-01, patients with unresectable $T_1 N_2$, $T_2 N_2$, $T_3 N_0$, $T_3 N_1$, and $T_3 N_2$ tumors or medically inoperable patients were randomized to 4000-cGy split-course (2000 cGy in 5 fractions in 1 week, followed by 2 weeks rest, and 2000 cGy in 5 fractions in 1 week) or continuous-course radiotherapy with 4000, 5000, or 6000 cGy in 20, 25, or 30 fractions (10). In RTOG 73-02, patients with $T_4 N_{1,2,3} M_0$ and $T_{1,2,3} N_3 M_0$ patients were randomized to 3000-cGy split-course, 6000-cGy split-course, or 4000-cGy continuous-course therapy (4,5). When analyzing the results of both studies, it is clear that the high-dose schedule of 6000 cGy yielded the best results (Table 27–2). The role of hyperfractionated radiotherapy is still being defined (13).

In the mid-1960s and early 1970s, split-course radiotherapy was popular. This entailed an interval of rest between any two cycles of radiotherapy and was primarily developed to improve tolerance. However, this fractionation scheme resulted in inferior cure rates compared to continuous-course radiotherapy. Consequently, such split-course radiotherapy regimens are primarily employed in palliative treatment regimens.

Table 27–2. Importance of Higher Radiation Doses in NSCLC: Summary of Results from RTOG Studies (References 4,5,10)

1. The in-field recurrence was lower with higher doses.
2. A dose response relation was demonstrated in NSCLC and was shown to be statistically significant ($p = 0.017$).
3. The 3-year survival was better with higher radiotherapy doses (15% with 6000 cGy; 10% with 5000 cGy; 6% with 4000 cGy).
4. Supraclavicular nodal failure was 10 to 14% with 3500 cGy vs. 2% with 4500 cGy.
5. The intrathoracic failure was equal (10 to 38%) outside the irradiated volume with different dose categories.

Treatment Volume

A comprehensive volume consisting of the primary tumor, the involved lymph nodes, and the areas at risk for potential microscopic disease should be encompassed by radiotherapy portals. As discussed above, the total radiotherapy dose must be titrated to the extent of involvement. While a dose of 4500 to 5000 cGy should suffice for microscopic disease, 6500 to 7000 cGy or more must be delivered as a boost to areas of bulky tumor involvement. The treatment volume is outlined in Table 27–3 (12,16,17).

Failure to adequately cover the volumes at risk will worsen the results. For instance, in RTOG protocol 73-01, the survival of patients with radiologically negative contralateral hilar nodes was better when these areas were treated in compliance with the protocol (i.e., adequate coverage and dose inhomogeneity ± 5% of prescribed dose) compared to the survival of patients whose treatment included major protocol violations ($p = 0.017$) (4). The median survival was 50 weeks in those with no protocol violations, 43 weeks in patients with minor variations, and 23 weeks with major violations. Choi and Doucatte made similar observations regarding the relationship between radiation treatment volumes and survival in NSCLC (15). When small volumes were irradiated, the 2- and 3-year survivals were 10% and 3%, respectively. With more comprehensive en-bloc volumes, the 2- and 3-year survivals improved to 36% and 28%, respectively (15).

Table 27–3. Volume of Radiation in Patients with Unresectable Nonmetastatic NSCLC

1. Primary tumor with 1- to 2-cm margin.
2. Ipsilateral hilum with 1- to 2-cm margin.
3. Contralateral hilum with 1-cm margin.
4. Entire mediastinum including 6–7 cm inferior to carina.
5. Supraclavicular nodes in selected cases.
6. Shrinking-field technique to be used to titrate the dose to the extent of involvement.

Technique

Attention to technical details of radiotherapy is crucial in improving local control and decreasing normal tissue toxicity. Availability of megavoltage linear accelerators (≥ 4 MeV), simulators, and computerized tomography (CT)-based treatment planning may be essential in the curative radiotherapy approach to NSCLC (12) (Figs. 27–1, 27–2, and 27–3). Optimization of radiotherapy with three-dimensional beam's eye view treatment planning is being investigated currently (12,16,17) and will be implemented by clinical trial cooperative groups in the coming years.

Obtaining a chest CT scan in the treatment position also helps to optimize treatment planning (18). A description of the multiple steps required in the successful planning and execution of a radiotherapy regimen are outside the scope of this chapter.

CHEMORADIATION

Radiotherapy can be applied with curative intent in patients with regionally advanced unresectable NSCLC (4). However, the majority of these patients eventually die of local or distant disease progression (5). Attempts to improve this poor prognosis have focused on the use of chemotherapy. The clinical experience of using chemotherapy in NSCLC as primary treatment for palliation, as adjuvant therapy with surgery and/or radiotherapy, as neoadjuvant therapy prior to radiotherapy or surgery, and with concurrent radiotherapy is reviewed here.

Chemotherapy for Metastatic or Recurrent Disease

As a single-treatment modality, the role of chemotherapy remains strictly palliative. Progress, however, has been made. Several

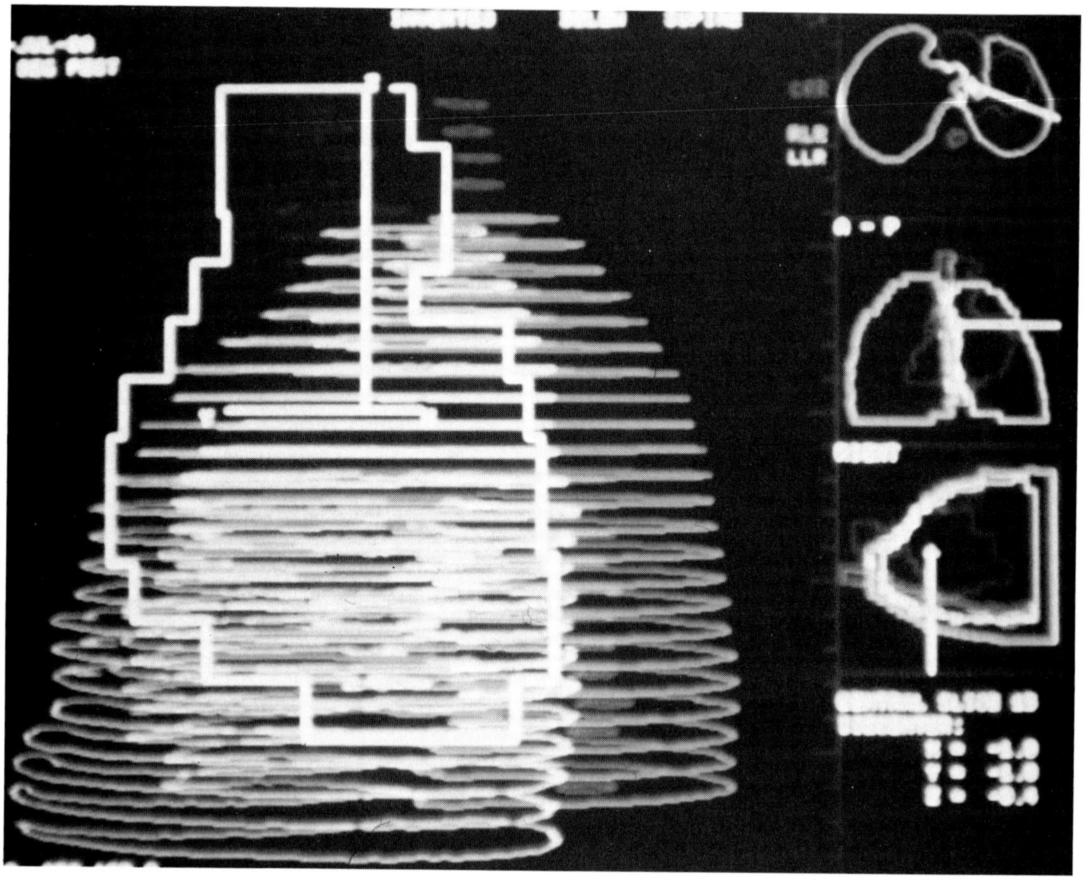

Fig. 27–1. Beam's eye view, from a 20-degree left posterior oblique perspective, of a patient's lungs (blue and purple contours), spinal cord (green contours), and composite target, i.e., tumor plus margin plus regions of possible subclinical disease, such as nodes (red contours). The white outline encompasses the target with an approximately 1-cm margin and thus corresponds to the shape of the appropriate irradiation field from this perspective. Therefore, it can be used as a guide in the delineation of the block. The three icons on the right help the viewer visualize the location of the isocenter and the position of the radiation source. (Figure 27–1 also appears in color in the color section.)

single agents have been shown to produce partial response rates exceeding > 15% in patients with advanced NSCLC; these drugs include cisplatinum, mitomycin-C, vinblastine, vindesine, ifosfamide, and etoposide (19–21).

Combination chemotherapy regimens with reproducible activity in NSCLC have also been defined. Initially, these included regimens based on combinations of drugs such as cyclophosphamide, doxorubicin, and methotrexate. For example, the use of cyclophosphamide, doxorubicin, methotrexate, and procarbazine (CAMP) in 160 patients with metastatic NSCLC resulted in a 26% response rate (22). More recent combination chemotherapy regimens have included the more active single agents mentioned above (23). The combinations of mitomycin-C, cisplatinum, and vinblastine or vindesine (MVP) (24,25) or cisplatinum and etoposide (26,27) have been widely studied. Response rates exceeding 30% have been reported with these regimens.

Despite these advances, the optimal combination of drugs has not been defined to date. The Eastern Cooperative Oncology Group conducted a prospective randomized trial in patients with metastatic NSCLC comparing CAMP to MVP, cisplatinum and etoposide, and a combination of cisplatinum and vindesine (24). While MVP produced the

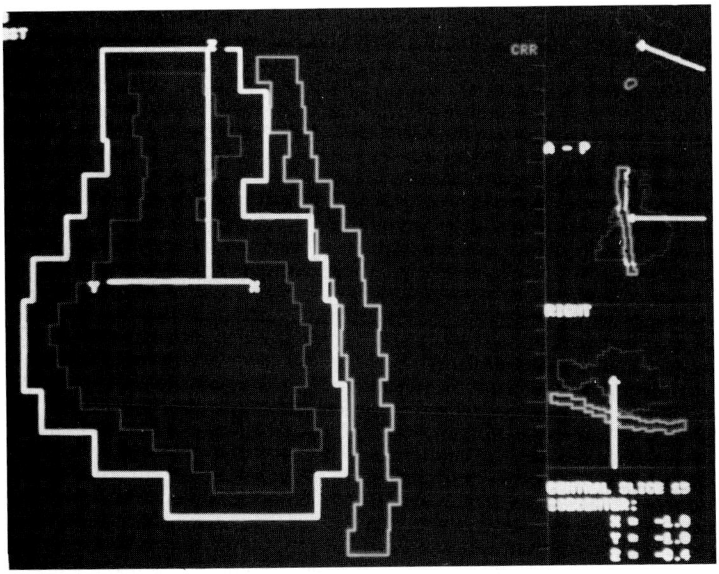

Fig. 27–2. Beam's eye view of the target (red) and spinal cord (blue) of the same patient from the same perspective as in Figure 27–1. The outlines indicate the largest extent of the projection, laterally, of the corresponding contour at each CT slice level, joined in a stepwise manner. The white outline is the same as in Figure 27–1 and it clearly avoids the cord. (Figure 27–2 also appears in color in the color section.)

highest response rate (31%), the median survival for patients treated with MVP was not longer than that in the other treatment groups. The response rate to CAMP was only 17%; however, toxicity was also significantly lower in patients receiving CAMP. More recently, ECOG compared MVP to single-agent chemotherapy followed by MVP at first progression. Patients treated with single-agent carboplatin followed by MVP had a significantly prolonged survival (despite a low initial response rate to carboplatin) compared to other treatment arms (28).

While response rates exceeding 30% can be achieved with the more recent combination regimens, responses are usually partial and of limited duration. At the same time, patients are exposed to considerable toxicities. The use of chemotherapy outside an investigational setting could therefore be recommended only if prolongation of survival as a direct consequence of the use of chemotherapy could be demonstrated. This question has been addressed in several randomized studies (29).

Cormier et al compared a regimen consisting of methotrexate, doxorubicin, cyclophosphamide, and CCNU to placebo in 39 patients with NSCLC (30). A 35% response rate was seen in the chemotherapy arm, while no patient responded in the control group. The median survival was also superior in the chemotherapy arm (31 weeks vs. 9 weeks). Rapp et al compared two chemotherapy regimens (cyclophosphamide, doxorubicin, cisplatinum and cisplatinum plus etoposide) to best supportive care (31). A significant prolongation of survival was found for both chemotherapy arms compared to best supportive care on the control arm. Woods et al reported a trial comparing a combination of cisplatinum and vindesine to no treatment; the difference in median survival (17 vs. 27 weeks) favored chemotherapy treated patients but was not statistically significant (32). Ganz et al reported a similar trend in survival favoring the chemotherapy group that was not statistically significant (33). More recently, Cellerino et al (34) reported a trial that demonstrated a median survival of 34 vs. 21 weeks favoring patients treated with chemotherapy but that also failed to achieve statistical significance ($p = 0.1$). In summary, these trials indicate a consistent trend for a small improvement in survival rates in patients receiving chemotherapy (35), although statistical significance is not always achieved. They also support the continued investigation of chemotherapy in NSCLC to identify more active regimens and may support the use of chemotherapy as standard therapy in this group of patients.

In addition, they raise the question of whether chemotherapy can be used more successfully earlier in the natural history of NSCLC, i.e., as adjuvant chemotherapy in resectable patients, as neoadjuvant chemotherapy, or concomitantly with radiotherapy in

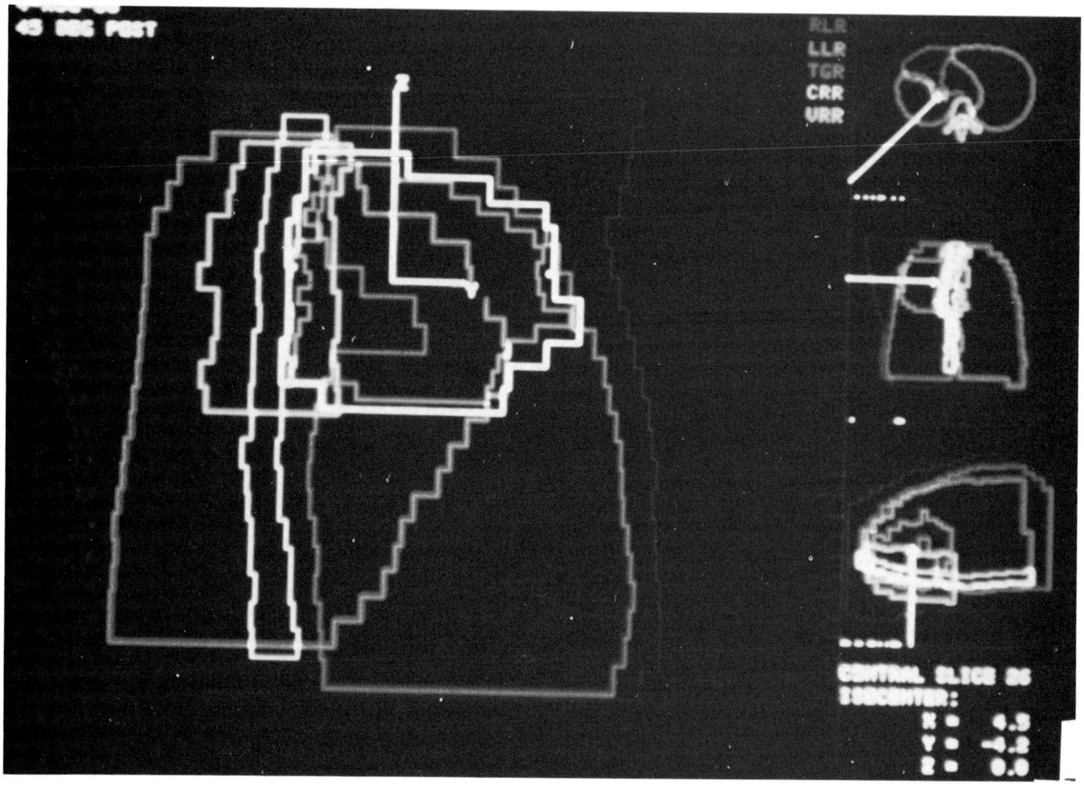

Fig. 27–3. Beam's eye view, from a 45-degree right posterior oblique perspective, of a patient with adenocarcinoma in the posterior aspect of the superior lobe of the right lung, with extension into the pleura. Shown are outlines of the external contours (red), right lung (green), left lung (yellow), target (dark blue), spinal cord (purple), and vertebrae (light blue). The white outline frames the target with an 0.5-cm margin, yet it barely clears the cord. (Figure 27–3 also appears in color in the color section.)

patients with regionally advanced, unresectable NSCLC.

Adjuvant Chemotherapy

Adjuvant chemotherapy targets fewer tumor cells than those present in the large tumor masses in patients with unresectable or metastatic disease. Therefore, a positive impact on survival might be easier to achieve. This question has been addressed in several studies (36).

Several earlier studies evaluating adjuvant chemotherapy in a randomized fashion showed either no benefit or decreased survival in patients treated with adjuvant chemotherapy (37–39). It has been pointed out that specific chemotherapy drugs or doses used in these trials were suboptimal and that the randomization process was not stratified for important prognostic factors (36).

The Lung Cancer Study Group has published two randomized studies investigating postsurgical chemotherapy using an active combination of drugs and proper stratification (Table 27–4) (40–42). Completely resected patients with Stage II and III adenocarcinoma or large-cell undifferentiated carcinoma (patients with disease in the most proximal mediastinal lymph node were ineligible) were stratified according to clinical center, stage of disease, prior weight loss of greater or less than 10%, and presence or absence of cardiac arrhythmias. Patients were then randomized to receive either adjuvant chemotherapy with cyclophosphamide, doxorubicin, and cisplatinum (CAP) monthly for six cycles or immunotherapy with intrapleural BCG (Bacillus Calmette-Guerin vaccine) daily doses of isoniazid for 12 weeks, and levamisole administered

Table 27–4. Randomized Studies of Adjuvant Postsurgical CAP Chemotherapy by the Lung Cancer Study Group

Study	No. of Patients	Control Arm Treatment	Med-Survival (mos) CAP/Control	Recurrence-Free Survival (%) or Overall Survival CAP/Control
1. Holmes et al (40)	130	BCG, Isoniazid, Levamisole	$p = 0.078$	$p = 0.146$
2. Lad et al (41) Sadeghi et al (42)	164	Radiation Therapy, 4000 cGy in 5 weeks	$p = 0.08$	$p = 0.006$

CAP = cyclophosphamide, Adriamycin, cisplatinum; BCG = Bacillus Calmette-Guerin vaccine.

orally for 3 consecutive days every other week for 18 months (40). Of 141 randomized patients, 130 were eligible and included in the analysis. The estimated median time to recurrence was 7 months longer in the chemotherapy group, as was the estimated median survival, although statistical significance was not achieved. Systemic disease recurrence was most commonly observed, and the brain was the single most common site involved. As the survival of the control group receiving immunotherapy was similar to earlier survival data reported for similar cohorts of patients treated with surgery alone, the authors considered a negative effect of the immunotherapy on patient survival in this study unlikely and attributed the trend in improved survival to the effect of chemotherapy.

Another study investigated the use of postoperative thoracic radiotherapy with or without CAP chemotherapy in patients with incompletely resected NSCLC (41,42). These included patients with ipsilateral microscopic or macroscopic residual disease or disease in the highest paratracheal lymph node. All patients received radiotherapy with 2000 cGy in five fractions over 5 days followed by a 3-week rest period and a second identical treatment. Patients randomized to the chemotherapy arm also received six monthly cycles of CAP, the first two cycles of which were administered on the first day of each radiotherapy cycle; 164 eligible patients were analyzed. Patients receiving chemotherapy had a significantly longer recurrence-free survival than the radiotherapy-only patients ($p = 0.006$). Survival was not significantly different ($p = 0.146$); the median survival for all patients was 15 months, and 34% of patients were alive 2 years following initial resection. Of documented disease recurrences, 82% were systemic; brain metastases were most frequently observed.

These two studies by the Lung Cancer Study Group indicate a possible positive effect of CAP chemotherapy on survival if administered as adjuvant chemotherapy to patients with NSCLC. However, in both trials, statistical significance for survival was not achieved and the incidence of systemic disease recurrence remained high. This indicated the need to pursue more effective adjuvant chemotherapy regimens in future trials.

Neoadjuvant Chemotherapy

Neoadjuvant chemotherapy is under investigation in a number of solid tumors. It is hoped that the initial administration of chemotherapy will lower the locoregional tumor burden and allow subsequent curative local therapy and/or the use of less radical surgical procedures. In addition, the early use of systemic therapy might eradicate micrometastases and prevent distant failure, a highly prevalent problem in NSCLC (43). A large number of studies have been published investigating this concept in the Phase II setting. Most of these investigate the use of two to three cycles of cisplatinum-based chemotherapy prior to surgery and/or radiotherapy.

Fram et al administered a combination of cyclophosphamide, doxorubicin, and cisplatinum for two cycles prior to radiotherapy to 30 patients with regionally advanced NSCLC (44). A response rate of 47% was documented and, following radiotherapy, 66% of the patients had objective disease regression.

The median survival for all patients was 9 months. Locoregional recurrence was observed less frequently in patients having PR or CR (5 of 19) after radiotherapy compared to those patients who had less than PR (8 of 10). Skarin et al investigated the same chemotherapy prior to surgery in 41 patients with resectable disease (45). The response rate to chemotherapy was 53%. The median survival was 32 months.

Eagan et al reported on 39 patients with regionally advanced NSCLC (46). Although 20 patients (51%) had an initial response to chemotherapy, the median survival for all patients was 11 months only. For 19 patients who underwent subsequent thoracotomy (all 19 had responded to neoadjuvant chemotherapy), the median survival was 15 months and the 2-year survival rate was 10%. The patients who underwent thoracotomy were noted to have a low local recurrence rate; however, there was a high distant failure rate.

Spain et al treated 22 inoperable patients with three to four cycles of mitomycin-C, cisplatinum, and vinblastine (47); 73% of patients responded. At a median follow-up in excess of 4 years, the median survival was 19 months. Osoba et al treated 30 patients with unresectable Stage II or III disease with two cycles of bleomycin, etoposide, and cisplatinum prior to split-course radiotherapy (48). Of 25 patients evaluable for response to chemotherapy, one had a complete response and 10 had a partial response. The median survival had not been reached at 52 weeks of follow-up time.

At the University of Chicago, we treated 27 patients with regionally advanced NSCLC with two cycles of neoadjuvant etoposide, vinblastine, and cisplatinum (49). Twenty-three patients were evaluable for response; 13 patients had a partial response, while 10 patients had stable disease or disease progression. Subsequent local therapy consisted of surgery followed by radiotherapy in four patients and radiotherapy alone in 14 patients. Five patients did not receive local therapy. The median time to disease progression for the 13 patients who had a partial response to neoadjuvant chemotherapy was 8 months. The median survival for all patients was 8 months.

Martini et al published their pilot data on the use of neoadjuvant MVP in patients with clinical N_2 disease (50); 30 of 41 patients responded to the chemotherapy and 28 underwent resection. The 3-year actuarial survival was 34%, and the median survival for resected patients was not reached.

Finally, Johnson et al administered cisplatinum and vinblastine to 28 patients with unresectable disease followed by radiation therapy (51). The response rate to chemotherapy was 54%; the median survival was 12 months.

In summary, these Phase II trials show that response rates to cisplatinum-based chemotherapy in the neoadjuvant setting consistently exceed those obtained for patients with metastatic or recurrent disease. They also demonstrate that patients who achieve partial or complete response have a prolonged survival compared to nonresponding patients. The toxicities are usually acceptable, and the administration of neoadjuvant chemotherapy to patients with NSCLC does not preclude administration of subsequent standard local therapy.

However, does neoadjuvant chemotherapy improve local and distant control rates in NSCLC? The survival data from these pilot trials are conflicting and certainly do not allow one to conclusively answer this question.

To answer this question, randomized trials are necessary. Four such trials have been reported (52–58). Dillman et al compared the administration of two cycles of cisplatinum and vinblastine followed by radiotherapy to radiotherapy alone in 155 patients with unresectable disease (52). The median survival was 14 months for the group receiving chemotherapy, compared to 10 months for patients treated with radiotherapy only ($p = 0.0066$); in addition, the 3-year survival was 24% vs. 11% in favor of the chemotherapy group.

A similar trial by Arriagada et al included 53 patients with unresectable disease (53–55). The chemotherapy investigated included vindesine, cyclophosphamide, cisplatinum, and lomustine. Initially, a statistically significant decrease in the incidence of distant metastases was reported (53,54); with longer follow-up, an initial trend in survival also became statistically significant (2-year survival was 21% vs. 14% in favor of the chemotherapy group) (55).

Mortin et al reported no significant difference in time to progression or survival using a combination of methotrexate, doxorubicin, cyclophosphamide, and lomustine (MACC) in unresectable patients (56). It has been pointed out, however, that this trial may have included too few patients to identify a smaller difference in survival and that the chemotherapy used did not include the most active agents in this disease (57). A fourth trial involving 238 patients was reported by Mattson et al, who used a three-drug regimen of cyclophosphamide, doxorubicin, and cisplatinum administered at low-dose intensity and also failed to show a beneficial effect on survival by the chemotherapy (58).

Concomitant Chemoradiation

An alternative approach to neoadjuvant chemotherapy has been the integration of chemotherapy into multimodality treatment plans through the use of concomitant chemoradiation. In these regimens, chemotherapeutic agents are used as radioenhancers in an effort to increase the local antitumor efficacy of radiotherapy (59–61). In addition to local radiation enhancement, the systemic activity of the chemotherapy may eradicate microscopic disease outside of the field being irradiated (spatial cooperation of chemotherapy and radiotherapy). This concept is particularly attractive in the therapy of regionally advanced NSCLC, in which improvement in the control rates of the frequently bulky regional disease is needed, along with an improvement of distant control rates through early eradication of distant micrometastases.

A large number of clinical trials have been conducted (59–62), employing either single-agent or combination chemotherapy and utilizing a variety of radiotherapy schedules. Three randomized trials have been conducted comparing radiation alone to concomitant chemoradiation. No significant prolongation was reported with single-agent hydroxyurea (63) or low doses of single-agent cisplatinum (15 mg/m^2/week) (64). The Japan Radiation-ACNU study group tested this single agent at 30 mg/m^2/week during radiation (65). A significant increase in CR rate was reported (55% vs. 14%). There was no significant impact on survival, although the 2-year survival was 19% for the concomitant study arm vs. 6% for the radiation-alone study arm.

Schaake-Koning et al reported an interesting randomized Phase II trial (66). Patients either received radiotherapy only (5500 cGy, split course) or the same radiation with weekly cisplatinum (30 mg/m^2) or daily cisplatinum (6 mg/m^2) for an identical total cisplatinum dose in the latter two arms. While overall response rates were similar in all three study groups, the 2-year survival rates were 14% (radiotherapy alone), 17% (radiotherapy with weekly cisplatinum), and 34% (radiotherapy with daily cisplatinum). These data suggest the latter to be the most promising schedule, which is now undergoing further investigation in a Phase III comparison to radiotherapy alone.

Additional pilot trials have been published (67–76). Several of these utilize 5-fluorouracil (5-FU) with concomitant-chemotherapy-based split-course radiotherapy as initially reported by Byfield et al. These chemoradiation schedules are in design analogous to the customary administration of combination chemotherapy in cycles. It is hoped that the treatment interruptions will render concomitant therapy not only more tolerable for the patient but also will allow for the administration of more effective chemotherapy in regard to the dose and the number of drugs. Byfield et al used a 120-hour continuous infusion of 5-FU with simultaneous radiotherapy (72). A 5-day course of therapy was followed by a 3-week rest period followed by additional therapy to a total of 5000 cGy to the tumor. In this study, both the 5-FU dose (20 to 35 mg/kg/day) and the daily fractions of radiotherapy (200 to 400 cGy per fraction) were escalated in cohorts of patients; 35 mg/kg/day of 5-FU was found to be the maximally tolerated dose with mucositis being dose-limiting. No recommendations on the radiotherapy fraction size were made. Overall, 10 of 28 evaluable patients in this Phase I study achieved a CR and the median survival for all patients was 290 days.

Taylor et al expanded on this observation by adding cisplatinum to the combination (74); 64 patients with NSCLC were treated with four cycles of cisplatinum, 5-FU, and radiotherapy, all administered every other week to a total dose of 4000 cGy, followed by reevaluation for surgery and two additional cycles of this regimen planned for patients with incomplete resections. Eight percent of patients had a clinical CR and 48% had a PR; 39 of 68 patients (61%) underwent surgery, nine of these had no evidence of disease on histologic examination of the specimen, eight had microscopic tumor only, and 22 had gross residual disease (74). Thus, clinical and pathologic response were shown to correlate poorly. The median time to failure was 6.5 and at a mean follow-up of 17 months, estimated 12- and 18-month survival figures were 61% and 47%, respectively.

A follow-up trial added etoposide to this combination and increased the cycle duration from 14 to 21 days (2 weeks of treatment interruption) (75). The median survival was 13 months, and 3-year actuarial survival and disease-free survival rates were 30% and 23%, respectively. It is not clearly apparent that this regimen is superior to the previously studied regimen, which did not include etoposide.

Experience with concomitant chemoradiation at our institution has focused on the combination of 5-FU, leucovorin, hydroxyurea (HU), and radiotherapy (73) because both drugs have been shown to enhance the efficacy of radiation in randomized studies (59). In a Phase II study, we administered 5-FU, leucovorin, and HU with concomitant radiotherapy to 23 patients with Stage III NSCLC. The treatment schedule called for concomitant administration of all therapy every other week. In 23 patients, we saw one complete response and 13 partial responses for an overall response rate of 61%. Twelve patients progressed outside the irradiated field, while only three patients progressed in the chest. This suggested activity of this regimen within the irradiated field but insufficient systemic activity. The addition of increased systemic therapy is currently being investigated.

It is not possible presently to assess the late toxic effects of concomitant chemoradiation. The acute toxicities of nausea and vomiting and myelosuppression are usually not severe and are readily managed. The cardiotoxic events of 5-FU when combined with radiotherapy are of concern and it is obvious that patients must be watched closely in any experimental trial that utilizes 5-FU and radiotherapy simultaneously (77). Late toxic effects related to the lung, esophagus, myocardium, and pericardium are obvious areas of concern.

Clearly, some of the trials using concomitant chemoradiation have promising early results, especially where protracted chemoradiation schedules are involved. However, most patients eventually experience disease recurrence, either inside or outside the irradiated field. Many other questions must be addressed in additional trials. What are the optimal radiotherapy fraction sizes? Should protracted radiotherapy schedules be used? Is surgery a necessary component in this treatment? What, if any, late sequelae that are as yet undescribed can result from concomitant chemoradiation? After some of these questions have been considered, randomized studies will be needed to directly compare these regimens to standard therapy.

Future Prospects

Phase III trials that are currently under way may validate the superiority of neoadjuvant chemotherapy followed by radiotherapy with or without surgery compared to radiotherapy alone or of concomitant chemoradiation compared to radiotherapy alone. The areas that will be addressed in future trials will include newer and possibly more effective radiotherapy fractionations, monoclonal antibodies as a way of targeting radiotherapy or drugs to small volumes of tumor, Biologic Response Modifiers (BMR) as cytostatic agents or modulators of chemotherapy or radiation, and the discovery of better chemotherapeutic agents. Several promising new agents are currently being investigated, including navelbine, taxol, edatrexate, gemcitabine, and the camphothecin analogs.

While advances in the treatment of NSCLC have been slow, some important steps have been undertaken in the past 10 years. Therapeutic progress will continue, and we hope it will result in increasing numbers of patients with NSCLC achieving complete response and ultimately cures. In the meantime, a renewed focus on primary (smoking cessation) and secondary prevention (chemoprevention) will be important additional activities in reducing the death rates from this disease.

Acknowledgement

The authors wish to thank Mrs. Susan Jarman for her assistance in the preparation of this manuscript.

REFERENCES

1. Boring TC, Squires TS, Tong T. Cancer Statistics 1992. CA 42(1):19, 1992.
2. Eisert DR, Cox JD, Komaki R. Irradiation for bronchial carcinoma: Reasons for failure, I. Analysis of local control as a function of dose, time and fractionation. Cancer 37:2665, 1976.
3. Stanley K, Cox JD, Petrovich Z, Paig C. Patterns of failure in patients with inoperable carcinoma of the lung. Cancer 47:2725, 1981.
4. Perez CA, Stanley K, Grundy G, et al. Impact of irradiation technique and tumor extent in tumor control and survival of patients with unresectable non-oat cell carcinoma of the lung. Cancer 50:1091, 1982.
5. Perez CA, Pajak TF, Rubin P, et al. Long-term observations of the patterns of failure in patients with unresectable non-oat cell carcinoma of the lung treated with definitive radiotherapy. Cancer 59:1874, 1987.
6. Shields TW. Treatment failures after surgical resection of thoracic tumors. Cancer Treat Symp 2:69, 1983.
7. Aisner J, Forastiere A, Aroney R. Patterns of recurrence for cancer of the lung and esophagus. Cancer Treat Symp. 2:87, 1983.
8. Johnson DH, Einhorn LH, Barolucci, et al. Thoracic radiotherapy does not prolong survival in patients with locally advanced, unresectable non-small cell lung cancer. Ann Intern Med 113:33, 1990.
9. Suite HD. The scope of the problem of primary tumor control. Cancer 61:2141, 1988.
10. Perez CA, Stanley K, Rubin P, et al. A prospective randomized study of various doses and fractionation schedule in the treatment of inoperable non-oat cell carcinomas of the lung. Cancer 45:2744, 1980.
11. Fletcher GH. Textbook of radiotherapy. 3rd ed. Philadelphia, Lea & Febiger, 1980.
12. Vijayakumar S, Myrinathopoulos LC, Rosenberg I, et al. Optimization of radical radiotherapy with beam's eye view techniques for non-small cell lung cancer. Int J Radiat Oncol Biol Phys 21:779, 1991.
13. Cox JD, Azarnia N, Byhardt RW, et al. A randomized Phase II/II trial of hyperfractionated radiation therapy with total doses of 60.0 Gy to 79.2 Gy. Possible survival benefit with ≥ 69.6 Gy in favorable patients with Radiation Therapy Oncology Group Stage III non-small cell lung carcinoma. Report of Radiation Therapy Oncology Group 83–11. J Clin Oncol 8:1543, 1990.
14. Perez CA, Brady LW. Principles and Practice of Radiation Oncology. Philadelphia, JB Lippincott Co., 1987, p. 1.
15. Choi NCH, Doucatte JA. Improved survival of patients with resectable non-small cell bronchogenic carcinoma by an innovative high dose en bloc radiotherapeutic approach. Cancer 48:101, 1981.
16. Vijayakumar S, Low N, Chen GTY, et al. Beam's eye view-based photon radiotherapy I. Int J Radiat Oncol Biol Phys 21:1575, 1991.
17. Vijayakumar S, Rubin S, Myrianthopoulos L, et al. Beam's eye view based photon radiotherapy-practical aspects. Applied Radiology 21(11):82, 1992.
18. Kline RW, Foley WD, Gillin MT. Computed tomography and radiation therapy treatment planning. *In:* Oncologic Imaging. Bragg DG, Rubin P, Youker JE (Eds). Amsterdam, Pergamon Press, 1985, p. 573.
19. Kris MG, Gralla RJ, Wertheim MS, et al. Trial of the combination of mitomycin, vindesine, and cisplatin in patients with advanced non-small cell lung cancer. Cancer Treat Rep 70:1091, 1986.
20. Kalstersky J. Therapy with cisplatin and etoposide for non-small-cell lung cancer. Semin Oncol 13(Suppl 3):104, 1986.
21. Joss RA, Cavalli F, Goldhirsch A, et al. New agents in non-small cell lung cancer. Cancer Treat Rev 11:205, 1984.
22. Shepard KV, Golumb HM, Bitran JD, et al. CAMP chemotherapy for metastatic non-oat cell bronchogenic carcinoma. Cancer 56:2385, 1985.
23. Bonomi P. Brief overview of combination chemotherapy in non-small-cell lung cancer. Semin Oncol 13(Suppl 3):89, 1986.
24. Ruckdeschel JC, Finkelstein DM, Etting DS, et al. A randomized trial of the four most active regimens for metastatic non-small-cell lung cancer. J Clin Oncol 4:14, 1986.
25. Schulman P, Budman DR, Weiselberg L, et al. Phase II trial of mitomycin, vinblastine, and cisplatin (MVP) in non-small cell bronchogenic carcinoma. Cancer Treat Rep 67:943, 1983.
26. Splinter T, Kok T, Kho S, et al. A multicenter phase II trial of cisplatin and oral etoposide (VP-16) in inoperable non-small-cell lung cancer. Semin Oncol 13(Suppl 3):97, 1986.
27. Longeval E, Klastersky J. Combination chemotherapy with cisplatin and etoposide in bronchogenic squamous cell carcinoma and adenocarcinoma. Cancer 50:2751, 1982.
28. Bonomi PH, Finkelstein DM, Ruckdeschel JD, et al. Combination chemotherapy versus single agents followed by combination chemo-

therapy in stage IV non-small-cell lung cancer. A study of the Eastern Cooperative Oncology Group. J Clin Oncol 7:1602, 1989.

29. Vokes EE, Vijayakumar S, Bitran JD, et al. Role of systemic therapy in advanced non-small cell lung cancer. Am J Med 89:777, 1990.
30. Cormier Y, Bergeron D, La Forge J, et al. Benefits of polychemotherapy in advanced non-small-cell bronchogenic carcinoma. Cancer 50:845, 1982.
31. Rapp E, Pater JL, Willan A, et al. Chemotherapy can prolong survival in patients with advanced non-small-cell lung cancer—Report of a Canadian multicenter randomized trial. J Clin Oncol 6:663, 1988.
32. Woods RL, Williams CJ, Levi J, et al. A randomized trial of cisplatin and vindesine versus supportive care only in advanced non-small cell lung cancer. Br J Cancer 61:608, 1990.
33. Ganz PA, Figlin RA, Haskell CM, et al. Supportive care versus supportive care and combination chemotherapy in metastatic non-small cell lung. Does chemotherapy make a difference? Cancer 63:1271, 1989.
34. Cellerino R, Tummarello D, Guidi F, et al. A randomized trial of alternating chemotherapy versus best supportive care in advanced non-small cell lung cancer. J Clin Oncol 9:1453, 1991.
35. Vokes EE, Bitran JD, Vogelzang NV. Chemotherapy for non-small cell lung cancer. The continuing challenge. Chest 99:1326, 1991.
36. Holmes EC. Surgical adjuvant chemotherapy in non-small cell lung cancer. Semin Oncol 15:255, 1988.
37. Slack NH. Bronchogenic carcinoma. Nitrogen mustard as a surgical adjuvant and factors influencing survival. Cancer 25:987, 1970.
38. Shields TW, Higgins GA, Humphrey EW, et al. Prolonged intermittent adjuvant chemotherapy and hydroxyurea after resection of carcinoma. Cancer 50:1713, 1982.
39. Brunner KW, Marthaler T, Muller W. Effects of long-term adjuvant chemotherapy with cyclophosphamide (NSC-26271) for radically resected bronchogenic carcinoma. Cancer Chemother Rep 4:125, 1973.
40. Holmes EC, Gail M. Surgical adjuvant therapy for stage II and stage III adenocarcinoma and large-cell undifferentiated carcinoma. J Clin Oncol 4:710, 1986.
41. Lad T, Rubinstein L, Sadeghi A. The benefit of adjuvant treatment for resected locally advanced non-small cell lung cancer. J Clin Oncol 6:9, 1988.
42. Sadeghi A, Payne D, Rubinstein L, et al. Combined modality treatment for resected advanced non-small cell lung cancer. Local control and local recurrence. Int J Radiat Oncol Biol Phys 15:89, 1988.
43. Vokes EE. Sequential combined modality therapy for stage III non-small cell lung cancer. Hematol Oncol Clin North Am 4:1133, 1990.
44. Fram R, Skarin A, Balikian J, et al. Combination chemotherapy followed by radiation therapy in patients with regional stage III unresectable non-small cell lung cancer. Cancer Treat Rep 69:587, 1985.
45. Skarin A, Jochelson M, Shelton T, et al. Neoadjuvant chemotherapy in marginally resectable stage III-M_0 non-small cell lung cancer; Long-term follow-up in 41 patients. J Surg Oncol 40:266, 1989.
46. Eagan RT, Ruud C, Lee RE, et al. Pilot study of induction therapy with cyclophosphamide, doxorubicin, and cisplatin and chest irradiation prior to thoracotomy in initially inoperable stage III M_0 non-small cell lung cancer. Cancer Treat Rep 71:895, 1987.
47. Spain RC. Neoadjuvant mitomycin-C, cisplatin, and infusion vinblastine in locally and regionally advanced non-small cell lung cancer. Problems and progress from the perspective of long term follow-up. Semin Oncol 15:6, 1988.
48. Osoba D, Rusthoven JJ, Evans WK, Turnbull KA. Combined chemotherapy and radiation therapy for non-small-cell lung cancer. Semin Oncol 13(Suppl 3):121, 1986.
49. Vokes EE, Bitran JD, Hoffman PC, et al. Neoadjuvant vindesine, etoposide, and cisplatin for locally advanced non-small-cell lung cancer. Final report of a phase II study. Chest 96:110, 1989.
50. Martini N, Kris MG, Gralla RJ, et al. The effects of preoperative chemotherapy in the resectability of non-small cell lung carcinoma with mediastinal lymph node metastases (N_2 M_0). Ann Thorac Surg 45:370, 1988.
51. Johnson DH, Strupp J, Grego AF, et al. Neoadjuvant cisplatin plus vinblastine chemotherapy in locally advanced non-small cell lung cancer. Cancer 68:1216, 1991.
52. Dillman RO, Seagren SL, Propert K, et al. A randomized trial of induction chemotherapy plus high-dose radiation versus radiation alone in stage III non-small cell lung cancer. N Engl J Med 323:940, 1990.
53. Arriagada R, le Chevalier T, Quoix E, et al. ASTRO plenary. Effect of chemotherapy on locally advanced non-small cell lung carcinoma. A randomized study of 353 patients. Int J Radiat Oncol Biol Phys 20:1183, 1991.
54. Le Chevalier T, Arriagada R, Quoix E, et al. Radiotherapy alone versus combined chemotherapy and radiotherapy in nonresectable

non-small cell lung cancer. First analysis of a randomized trial in 353 patients. J Natl Cancer Inst 83:417, 1991.

55. Le Chevalier T, Arriagada R, Tarayre M, et al. Significant effect of adjuvant chemotherapy on survival in locally advanced non-small-cell lung carcinoma. J Natl Cancer Inst 84:58, 1992.
56. Morton RF, Jett JR, McGinnis WL, et al. Thoracic radiation therapy alone compared with combined chemoradiotherapy for locally unresectable non-small cell lung cancer. A randomized phase III trial. Ann Intern Med 115:681, 1991.
57. Ihde DC. Chemotherapy combined with chest irradiation for locally advanced nonsmall cell lung cancer. Editorial. Ann Intern Med 115:736, 1991.
58. Mattson K, Holsti LR, Holsti P, et al. Inoperable non-small cell lung cancer. Radiation with or without chemotherapy. Eur J Cancer Clin Oncol 24:477, 1988.
59. Vokes EE, Weichselbaum RR. Concomitant chemoradiotherapy. Rationale and clinical experience in patients with solid tumors. J Clin Oncol 8:911, 1990.
60. Tannock IF, Rotin D. Keynote address. Mechanisms of interaction between radiation and drugs with potential for improvements in therapy. NCI Monogr 6:77, 1988.
61. Fu KK, Phillips TL. Biologic rationale of combined radiotherapy and chemotherapy. Hematol Oncol Clin North Am 5:737, 1991.
62. Belani CP. Sequential and concurrent chemotherapy and thoracic radiation therapy for locally advanced non-small cell lung cancer. J Infus Chemother 2:27, 1992.
63. Landgren RC, Hussey DH, Barkley HT, et al. Split course irradiation compared to split course irradiation plus hydroxyurea in inoperable bronchogenic carcinoma. A randomized study of 53 patients. Cancer 34:1598, 1974.
64. Soresi E, Clerici M, Grilli R, et al. A randomized clinical trial comparing radiation therapy vs. radiation therapy plus cis-dichlorodiamine platinum (II) in the treatment of locally advanced non-small cell lung cancer. Semin Oncol 15(Suppl 7):20, 1988.
65. Japan Radiation-ACNU Study Group. A randomized prospective study of radiation versus radiation plus ACNU in inoperable nonsmall cell carcinoma of the lung. Cancer 63:249, 1989.
66. Schaake-Koning C, Maat B, van Houtte P, et al. Radiotherapy combined with low-dose cis-dichloroplatinum (II) (CDDP) in inoperable nonmetastatic non-small cell lung cancer (NSCLC). A randomized three arm phase II study of the EORTC lung cancer and radiotherapy cooperative groups. Int J Radiat Oncol Biol Phys 19:967, 1990.
67. Eagan RT, Lee RE, Frytak S, et al. Randomized trial of thoracic irradiation plus combination chemotherapy for unresectable adenocarcinoma and large cell carcinoma of the lung. Int J Radiat Oncol Biol Phys 5:1401, 1979.
68. Robinow JS, Shaw EG, Eagan RT, et al. Results of combination chemotherapy and thoracic radiation therapy for unresectable non-small cell carcinoma of the lung. Int J Radiat Oncol Biol Phys 17:1203, 1989.
69. Boven E, Tierie TJ, Pinedo HM. Combined radiation and daily low-dose cisplatin for inoperable, locally advanced non-small cell lung cancer. Results of a phase II trial. Semin Oncol 15(Suppl 7):18, 1988.
70. Mira JG, Taylor SL, Stephens RL, Chen T. Simultaneous chemotherapy—Radiotherapy with prophylactic cranial radiation for inoperable adeno and large cell lung carcinoma. A Southwest Oncology Group study. Int J Radiat Oncol Biol Phys 15:757, 1988.
71. Friess GG, Balkadi M, Harvey WH. Concurrent cisplatin and etoposide with radiotherapy in locally advanced non-small cell lung cancer. Cancer Treat Rep 71:681, 1987.
72. Byfield JE, Stanton W, Sharp TR, et al. Phase I-II study of 1230 hour infused 5-FU and split course radiation therapy in localized nonsmall cell cancer. Cancer Treat Rep 67:933, 1983.
73. Vokes EE, Vijayakumar S, Hoffman PC, et al. 5-fluorouracil with oral leucovorin and hydroxyurea and concomitant radiotherapy for stage III non-small cell lung cancer. Cancer 66:437, 1990.
74. Taylor SG, Trybula M, Bonomi PD, et al. Simultaneous cisplatin fluorouracil infusion and radiation followed by resection in regionally localized stage III, non-small cell lung cancer. Ann Thorac Surg 43:87, 1987.
75. Recine D, Rowland K, Reddy S, et al. Combined modality therapy for locally advanced non-small cell lung carcinoma. Cancer 66:2270, 1990.
76. Lokich J, Chaffey J, Neptune W. Concomitant 5-fluorouracil infusion and high-dose radiation for stage III non-small cell lung cancer. Cancer 64:1021, 1989.
77. Gradishar WJ, Vokes EE. 5-Fluorouracil cardiotoxicity. A critical review. Ann Oncol 1:409, 1990.

Chapter 28

GYNECOLOGIC SYSTEM

MADHU J. JOHN AND MARSHALL S. FLAM

INTRODUCTION

Even though the number of deaths due to cervical cancer (CC) in developed countries is comparatively small, there are several compelling reasons for developing newer strategies in the management of this cancer. First, CC is the single most prevalent and lethal female cancer in several developing countries of South America, Africa and Asia (1,2). Indeed, in several of these countries, where tobacco consumption is not a deeply entrenched habit yet, and where lung cancer is not nearly the health problem it is in the USA or Europe, CC may be the most prevalent and lethal of all cancers, male or female. It is common to see 40 to 60% of patients in cancer wards in several countries with CC; in addition, the vast majority of these women have advanced disease (2).

Second, several reports from various countries suggest an increasing incidence of CC in younger women (2–6). These cancers appear to be more aggressive in their natural history and more resistant to conventional therapies than cancers seen in older women (3,7–10). Also, increasing incidences of human papilloma virus (HPV) infections have correlated to increasing incidence of invasive carcinoma of the cervix (11,12).

Finally, the last major advance in the development of therapy for cervical carcinoma took place three decades ago with the introduction of the megavoltage radiotherapy machines. There is some indication that refinements of surgical and radiotherapeutic technique might have a marginal effect on improving survival statistics in CC since then. Also, the introduction of several chemotherapeutic drugs in the last decade had little impact on the treatment of this primary disease.

Thus, despite the fact that the incidence of cervical carcinoma may be actually declining in this country (13,500 new cases, 4400 deaths per year) (13), newer therapeutic approaches are needed in an increasingly global society where most women present with advanced disease and younger women face an imminent epidemic of a virulent variant of CC.

TRADITIONAL TREATMENT APPROACHES

The preferred management for most cervical cancers is a combination of external megavoltage radiotherapy (RT) and intracavitary radioisotopic treatment. All stages of cervical cancer may be treated with this combination with fairly good results. Earlier stages (FIGO IB, IIA) require less external radiotherapy; intracavitary treatment is the mainstay of treatment for women with such early disease. External radiotherapy becomes increasingly important with advanced disease in the parametrium and vagina. Surgical management is a feasible and sometimes preferred alternative to radiotherapy in earlier invasive cervical carcinoma (FIGO Stages IA, IB, IIA), providing equally good chances of survival.

Survival statistics vary from country to country (2). Even within the United States, there appears to be a wide range in probability of survival in several institutions (3). Five-year survival rates for Stages IIA and IIB range from 30 to 75%, for Stages IIIA and IIIB between 10% and 60%, and for Stage IVA between 0 and 25%. More realistic figures may be obtained from two comprehensive studies which indicate 5-year survival rates of 50% for FIGO Stage IIB, 28% for FIGO Stage IIIB, and 10% for FIGO Stage IVA (2,14). Because these figures reflect cure rates in developed countries with access to state-of-the-art armamentarium and skill, it can be deduced with impunity that the number of women who develop this disease and die from it in less developed nations, where CC is endemic, is substantial. The patterns of care study in cancers of the cervix conducted in the United States suggest several reasons for these vast discrepancies in survival statistics, including improper pretreatment evaluation and nonconformity in treatment technique (14). Nevertheless, the fact remains that, after three decades of megavoltage radiotherapy, no significant improvements in survival have resulted despite improved treatment techniques such as interstitial brachytherapy; newer isotopes; high LET radiotherapy; more sophisticated treatment planning support; and the addition of other modalities such as hyperbaric oxygen, hypoxic cell sensitizers, and hyperthermia. The major problems with these newer techniques have been their unavailability for general use and a lack of evidence suggesting definitive improvement over standard therapy with acceptable morbidity.

Thus, several recognizable subsets of the population with invasive cervical cancer exist and require more than conventional surgery or radiotherapy. Patients may include women with the Stage IB barrel-shaped cervical cancer, younger women under age 35; patients with para-aortic nodal metastases, and patients with advanced stages of the disease (certain FIGO Stages IIBs, III, and IVA).

CHEMORADIATION FOR CERVICAL CANCER

Rationale

The rationales for the use of chemoradiation in cervical cancer are the lack of improvement in survival rates in advanced cervical cancer, the possibility of an increase in a clinically aggressive variant of the tumor in younger women, the increasing realization of the importance of distant metastases as local control improves, and the accumulating evidence of the effectiveness of chemoradiation in other epithelial tumors.

Stagnant Survival Rates

Table 28–1 shows the survival rates and patterns of failure for advanced cervical cancers from two major institutions (15,16). Table 28–2 shows 5-year survival figures for Stage III cervical cancer in the United States as well as other industrialized nations (14–20). In one of the few reports from the African continent, the 2-year survival for Stage III patients was 22% (21). Table 28–1 shows that, in Stages III and IV cervical carcinoma, treatment failure is primarily related to local control, but that distant metastases constitute a sizable proportion of failures with increasing disease. Considering the fact that both the major institutions quoted here use the highest doses known to the central and lateral pelvic points, it is clear that the biologic effect at these points has to be augmented—by higher doses through altered fractionation, radioenhancers or drugs—in order to increase local control and survival. If, indeed, the distant failure rate is distinct from the local failure rate, the use of systemic therapy or drugs becomes mandatory in such advanced disease. Applying the concept of potential for increased cure as a function of perfect local control as developed by Suit to their experience with 183 patients with CC, Potish and associates have predicted that the next major advance in the cure of CC will come with improvements in the management of distant rather than local disease (22). Table 28–2 shows that considerable differences exist in survival among nations and even among major and minor institutions within the USA. The situation is probably worse in developing countries, where statistics and treatment modalities are hard to come by, where the incidence of CC is higher, and where most patients present with advanced disease.

The yWACC Syndrome

The overall incidence of CC is declining, but there is a definite shift in its occurrence to younger age groups (3–6,23). Some debate exists as to whether the occurrence of CC in women under 35 years is associated with a worse prognosis. However, the reports that suggest that this is so (3–10,23) outnumber by far those that suggest that age alone is a poor indicator of prognosis (24–26). Most

Table 28–1. Patterns of Failure and Survival in Advanced Cervical Cancer in Two Major Institutions in the Megavoltage Era

Institution	Stage	Local Recurrence (%)	Distant Metastases (%)	5-Year Survival (%)
MD Anderson (15)	III	37	20	45
	IV	71	50	21
Mallinckrodt (16)	III	37	32	45
	IV	78	39	18

clinical oncologists are now familiar with the clinical entity of the *y*ounger *w*oman with *a*ggressive *c*ervical *c*ancer, which for facile use may be termed the **yWACC Syndrome.**

Several reports indicate an increasing prevalence of adenocarcinoma and adenosquamous carcinoma of the cervix (27–31). Peters et al show a 8% rise per year in the incidence of adenocarcinoma of the cervix in women below 35 years between 1972 and 1982 in Los Angeles County (30). Angel et al, in their study of 89 patients with Stage I cervical adenocarcinoma over 25 years, note a sevenfold increase in its incidence in the last decade and that treatment results with radiation, surgery or its combination did not improve results (32). The roles of oral contraceptives (30), the herpesvirus type II (33), and the HPV virus (11,12) have been hypothesized as promoting agents for this syndrome, but no direct etiologic link have been made.

Whatever the etiologic factors, there are plausible reasons to believe that these variants of CC in younger women are biologically different and require more aggressive treatment than standard radiotherapy, surgery, or a combination of the two.

Other Poor-Prognostic Subpopulations

Besides patients with advanced Stages III and IV cervical cancer, several subpopulations may inherently carry a poor prognosis. Analysis of the national survey conducted by the Patterns of Care Study (PCS) by Lanciano and colleagues have determined that pretreatment factors associated with poor prognosis include lower performance status, younger age, and bilateral parametrial and bilateral pelvic wall involvement (34,35).

Several authors have noted correlations between poorly differentiated histology, lymphatic permeation, pathologic variants such as adenosquamous glassy-cell carcinoma, clear-cell carcinoma, and small-cell carcinomas with poor survival (36). Other factors related to tumor bulk include barrel-shaped Stage I and II tumors and endometrial extension, which are associated with greater incidence of distant metastases and reduced survival (36–38).

Thus, several subpopulations of patients besides those with advanced-stage CC have been identified as having reduced survival rates with conventional radiotherapy, surgery, or their combinations. The concept of chemoradiation, whether sequential, concurrent, or alternating, offers an attractive option that has already caught the imagination of several investigators but requires considerable research still.

CHEMOTHERAPY USE IN CC

Palliative

Inasmuch as the advent of chemotherapeutic agents had spectacular results in the

Table 28–2. Selected Worldwide Survival Statistics for Stage III Cervical Cancer

Institution/Location	5-Year Survival (%)	Institution/Location (No. of Patients)	5-Year Survival (%)
MD Anderson/USA (15)	45	Germany (20)	31
Mallinckrodt/USA (16)	45	Krakow/Poland (2)	21
Christie/UK (17)	45	Nigeria/Africa (20)	22*
Paris/France (18)	43	163 sites/USA (14)	28†
Yugoslavia (19)	34	World average/Kottmeier (2)	28

*2-year survival
†4-year survival - PCS series

management of other tumors, notably in testicular cancer, their effect on cervical cancer was marginal or transient or both at best. Even so, the individual drugs that appear most effective in the disease are cisplatinum, mitomycin-C, high-dose methotrexate, Adriamycin, ifosfamide, and 5-fluorouracil (5-FU), with response rates between 15 and 38% (39). Combinations of drugs, usually CDDP- or bleomycin-based, were used primarily in patients with recurrent disease following conventional treatment with RT and surgery. In short, these drugs in various combinations appeared most suited either for palliative treatment or as agents for induction or consolidation therapy in a definitive treatment regimen.

Definitive

Neoadjuvant Chemotherapy

For primary management of CC, chemotherapy (CT) has been used in neoadjuvant fashion prior to radiotherapy or in concurrent fashion. Most of the experience in neoadjuvant therapy has been in the use of intra-arterial chemotherapy prior to pelvic radiotherapy. The rationale for using intra-arterial chemotherapy in CC was to decrease the size of bulky tumors so that conventional radiotherapy (or surgery in a few cases) would be used successfully with lesser morbidity (decreased treatment volume). The intra-arterial route was used by investigators in the belief that, by infusing the artery feeding the tumor, a greater intratumor drug concentration would result and toxicity would be reduced.

A select number of reports of neoadjuvant intra-arterial chemotherapy is included in Table 28–3 (40–43). Most such reports describe difficulties with consistent intratumoral distribution of drugs, moderate to severe toxicities (renal failure being most prominent), and mostly transient responses. On the other hand, there was often a dramatic improvement in pelvic pain. It appears that intra-arterial chemotherapy requires further clinical investigation, and may be particularly useful in women with intractable pelvic pain and those who are unlikely to respond to surgical and radiotherapeutic intervention.

Several studies using various combinations of drugs prior to radiotherapy have been reported (44–49). Most of them concluded that their particular combination of drugs caused marked tumor shrinkage, making radiotherapy easier to deliver. No overall superiority over radiotherapy alone was claimed. The only randomized prospective study in this group showed that BOMP chemotherapy was associated with unacceptable toxicity and adversely affected survival in Stage IIIB patients (49).

Concurrent Chemoradiation

Most of the experience in combining drugs and RT in CC has been in concurrent fashion (50–77). Here too, as in other epithelial cancers of the esophagus and anal canal, the vast majority of reports involve one of 2 combinations, e.g., 5-FU + mitomycin-C or 5-FU + CDDP. With few exceptions, notably the reports of Piver and co-workers, who have reported on mainly Stage IIB patients treated with hydroxyurea and RT, (54,55) most reports concern advanced disease such as poor prognostic Stage IIB disease or Stages III and IVA.

In order to begin to understand these vast data, it is best that the experience in concur-

Table 28–3. Intra-arterial Chemotherapy as Induction Prior to Radiotherapy in Cervical Cancer

Series (Reference)	No. of Patients	Drugs	Response Rate (%)	Overall Survival (%)
1. Fallappa (40)	25	MTX, ADR	80	—
2. Rettenmaier et al. (41)	9	CDDP	56	—
3. Iglesias (42)	19	Mito-C, BLM, CDDP	53	18
4. Patton et al. (43)	46	Mito-C, BLM, CDDP, VCR given I.V.	76	30

MTX = methotrexate; ADR = Adriamycin/doxorubicin; CDDP = cisplatinum; Mito-C = mitomycin-C; BLM = bleomycin; VCR = vincristine.

rent chemoradiation in CC be divided into 4 categories: the NCOG/RTOG research group experience, the hydroxyurea experience of Piver et al, the Princess Margaret experience with 5-FU and mitomycin-C, and a miscellaneous group where mostly the combination of 5-FU and cisplatinum is used.

THE NCOG/RTOG EXPERIENCE

Based on some of the rationale described above, a pilot project using empiric combinations of 5-FU, mitomycin-C (mito-C) and cisplatinum (CDDP) and external and intracavitary radiotherapy was initiated at UCSF-Fresno in 1983 for advanced CC. The published results showed a 90% survival for 10 patients followed for 14 to 45 months (median 28 months) (50). Acute toxicity was tolerable and long-term toxicity was seen in two patients with transient rectal ulcers.

This result provided the framework for an intergroup Northern California Oncology Group (NCOG) and Radiation Therapy Oncology Group (RTOG) study (51). Thirty-eight patients were treated on a protocol identical to the pilot as described in Table 28–4. Seventy-one percent of these patients had Stage III disease. The complete response rate and actuarial 2-year survival rate was 63%. Of 36 patients evaluable for toxicity, 11% had Grade 3 nonhematologic toxicity and 11% had reversible grade 4 hematologic toxicity.

Building on the above study, RTOG conducted a second-generation chemoradiation protocol on 60 patients with advanced cervical cancer (52). The protocol described in Table 28–4 was altered by increasing the RT dose to the lateral pelvic wall by 10% and reducing the mitomycin-C dose by 25%. Compared to the results of the previous protocol, both Grade 4 hematologic (2%) and Grade 3 nonhematologic (8%) toxicity were decreased. Complete response rates were improved from 63% to 77%. Early (1-year) actuarial survival rates were also improved from 71 to 81%. RTOG has presently undertaken a Phase III comparison study between chemoradiation and extended-field RT for cervical cancer.

Table 28–4. Schema of Intergroup NCOG/RTOG Phase I-II Protocol for Patients with Stages IIB-IVA Carcinoma of the Cervix

Radiotherapy:	180 cGy/day, 5 times/week to pelvis, total 3600 cGy. Parametrial boost 900 cGy followed by 2 intracavitary cesium applications for a total of 4000 mg hrs of Ra equivalent.
Chemotherapy:	1. 5-FU 1g/m^2/day × 4 days by infusion during week 2 of external RT and first cesium application. 2. Mitomycin-C: 10 mg/m^2 I.V. bolus on day 1 of first 5-FU infusion. 3. CDDP: 75 mg/m^2 I.V. during day 1 of second 5-FU infusion.

THE HYDREA TRIAL

Since 1968, when Hreshcyshyn first introduced the combination of hydroxyurea (hydrea, HU) and irradiation for CC, several reports of randomized trials using HU have emerged from Roswell Park Memorial Institute (Piver et al) and the Gynecology Oncology Group (GOG) (53–61).

Hydroxyurea appears to exert its radioenhancement by means of inhibiting repair of sublethal radiation injury, killing cells in the relatively radioresistant S phase of the cell cycle, and consequently synchronizing and accumulating cells in the G_1 phase, which is radiosensitive. Its primary toxicity in these studies was leukopenia; small-bowel toxicity was minimal.

The 1974 study of Piver et al (54) showed statistically improved survival ($p < 0.002$) for patients with Stages IIB and IIIB treated with RT + HU compared to RT + placebo (67% vs. 32%). This was confirmed by a GOG study (56) with a p value < 0.05 between the two groups. However, its validity was considered suspect because of large numbers of inevaluable patients. Subsequent studies have confirmed the superiority of the RT + HU combination for Stage IIB patients (55,57) but not for Stage IIIB or IVA patients (55,59). The GOG is presently conducting a randomized trial comparing RT + HU versus RT + 5-FU and CDDP.

THE PRINCESS MARGARET SERIES

Thomas and co-workers have conducted a series of Phase I-II studies at the Princess Margaret Hospital (PMH) with 5-FU ± mitomycin-C and concurrently with radiotherapy

Table 28–5. Results of Chemoradiation (5-FU ± Mitomycin-C) for Advanced Cervical Cancer at the Princess Margaret Hospital

FIGO Stage	No. of Patients	3-Year Pelvic Control (%)	3-Year Survival (%)
IB	38	84	71
II	63	86	69
III	89	52	43
IV	10	36	40
TOTAL	200	67(58*)	54

*Radiation controls

on women with advanced cervical cancer, including those with periaortic nodal involvement. The results for each stage of disease are summarized in Table 28–5.

The major finding from these series was the increased incidence of bowel toxicity in patients receiving mitomycin-C + 5-FU (22%) compared to those receiving 5-FU alone (7%) ($p < 0.005$) (62). This conclusion was derived from a multivariate analysis despite a marked variation in RT dose, fractionation, and field sizes. As a result, further trials at that institution are being conducted without the use of mitomycin-C.

These investigators at PMH also reported on their experiences with treating 17 patients with similar chemoradiation for recurrent disease following surgery for carcinoma of the cervix (63). Eight of seventeen (47%) were alive and disease-free 21 to 58 months after therapy. This outstanding result was achieved despite overwhelming poor-prognostic features such as pelvic side wall disease, and with acceptable morbidity.

MISCELLANEOUS STUDIES

Table 28–6 illustrates select trials of concurrent radiotherapy and various chemotherapeutic agents (64–76). The combinations most commonly used are 5-FU + CDDP and 5-FU + mitomycin-C; these are tabulated separately. A few single-drug or unusual-drug-combination studies are listed together.

Most studies have few patients as primarily single institution pilots. Generally, concurrent chemoradiation appears to be tolerated well in these reports. Whether they are effective and require further examination in prospective studies cannot be determined on the base of the data available. As seen above, it appears that most research organizations have opted for the 5-FU + CDDP

Table 28–6. Select Trials of Concurrent Chemoradiation in Advanced Cervical Cancer

Series (Reference)	No. of Patients	Drugs	Disease-free Survival (%)	Follow up (months) Range/Median
1. Kuske et al. (64)	15	5-FU, CDDP	53	12–36/-
2. Grigsby et al. (65)	18	5-FU, CDDP	66	6–20/-
3. Roberts et al. (66)	18	5-FU, CDDP	50	-/17
4. Runowicz et al. (67)	16	5-FU, CDDP	81	-/12
5. Heaton et al. (68)	29	5-FU, CDDP	65	12–76/29
6. Thomas et al. (69)	27	5-FU, Mito-C	59	4–26/6
7. Evans et al. (70)	10	5-FU, Mito-C	70	7–38/18
8. Ludgate et al. (71)	38	5-FU, Mito-C	71	5–36/20
9. Kalra et al. (72)	6	5-FU, Mito-C	66	0–45/24
10. Drescher et al. (73)	10	5-FU	10	3–24/8
11. Potish et al. (74)	22	CDDP	81	-/12
12. Monyak et al. (75)	38	CDDP	52	-/36
13. Malviya et al. (76)	19	CDDP, Mito-C	73	9–22/-
14. John et al. (50)	10	5-FU, CDDP, Mito-C	80	14–45/28

- = not stated

combination (with radiotherapy) for future studies. However, on account of mitomycin-C's effectiveness against hypoxic cells which are inherently radioresistant, it may be worthwhile to incorporate this drug in some limited role to the 5-FU + CDDP + RT combination in future protocols.

OTHER GYNECOLOGICAL MALIGNANCIES

The use of chemoradiation in the management of carcinoma of the vagina, vulva, endometrium, and ovary has been sparsely reported in the literature to date. Thomas et al reported on a series of 33 patients with vulvar carcinoma treated with chemoradiation, as adjuvant treatment postsurgery (9 patients), for postsurgical recurrence (15 patients) and as definitive treatment (9 patients) (77). Seven of the 9 patients treated definitively were rendered disease-free after chemoradiation alone or (in 3 cases) with the addition of minimal surgery. They concluded that chemoradiation increased locoregional control and may help preserve normal anatomy. They also noted a relative lack of associated morbidity in these patients.

Evans et al reported on 11 patients with advanced carcinoma of the vagina (7) and vulva (4). Survival by site was 100% in the vulva and 66% in the vagina with a mean follow-up of 26 months (70).

The experience in treating primary tumors of the endometrium and ovary with chemoradiation is minimal at the present time.

CONCLUSIONS

Stagnant survival rates in advanced cervical cancer since the megavoltage era was introduced to radiotherapy have spurred the addition of various chemotherapeutic agents in its management. The identification of several subpopulations of cervical cancers that appear to be particularly resistant to conventional treatment is another compelling reason to develop more aggressive treatment approaches such as chemoradiation.

The experience with sequential chemoradiation is primarily with intra-arterial chemotherapy, results of which are erratic and often marred by toxicity.

The concurrent use of chemotherapy and radiotherapy has primarily involved the drug hydroxyurea (hydrea) and the combinations of 5-FU + CDDP and 5-FU + mitomycin-C. The latter two combinations have been primarily used in pilot studies and are only now being tested in prospective multi-institutional studies. The addition of hydroxyurea to RT appears to have had a definite positive effect on the cure rate of Stage IIB carcinoma of the cervix.

Just as with anal and esophageal cancers, the composition of the optimal chemoradiation regimen is undefined at this time. Unlike the results of chemoradiation in those two GI tract tumors, the results of chemoradiation in cervical cancer is less striking. Therefore, prospective randomized studies comparing radiotherapy alone with chemoradiation are definitely in order.

REFERENCES

1. Day NE. A new measure of age standardized incidence. The cumulative rate. *In:* Cancer incidence in five continents. Vol III. Waterhouse J, Muir C, Correa P (Eds). Lyon, International Agency for Research in Cancer. 1976.
2. Annual Report on the Results of Treatment in Gynecological Cancer. Vol. 18. Kottmeier HL, Kolstad P, McGarrity KA, Peterson F, and Ulfelder H (Eds). Stockholm, International Federation of Obstetrics and Gynecology, 1982.
3. Stuart GCE, Robertson DI, Fedorkow DM, et al. Recurrent and persistent squamous cell cervical cancer in women under age 35. Gynecol Oncol 30:163, 1988.
4. Carmichael JA, Clark DH, Moher D, et al. Cervical cancer in women aged 34 and younger. Am J Obstet Gynecol 154:264, 1986.
5. Green GH. Cervical cancer and cytology in New Zealand. Brit J Obstet Gynaecol 85:881, 1978.
6. Beral V, Booth M. Predictions of cervical cancer incidence and mortality in England and Wales. Lancet 1:495, 1986.
7. Stanhope CR, Smith JP, Wharton JT, et al. Carcinoma of the cervix: The effect of age on survival. Gynecol Oncol 10:188, 1980.
8. Gynning I, Johnsson JE, Alm P, Trope C. Age and prognosis in Stage IB squamous cell carcinoma of the uterine cervix. Gynecol Oncol 15:18, 1983.
9. LaVecchia C, Franceschi S, Decarli A, et al. Invasive cervical cancer in young women. Brit J Obstet Gynaecol 91:1149, 1984.

10. Prempree T, Patanphan V, Sewchand W, Scott RR. The influence of patient's age and tumor grade on the prognosis of carcinoma of the cervix. Cancer 51:1764, 1983.
11. Crum CP, Levine RU. Human papillomavirus infection and cervical neoplasia. New perspectives. Int J Gynecol Pathol 3:376, 1984.
12. Reid R, Crum CP, Herschman BR, et al. Genital warts and cervical cancer III. Subclinical papillomarviral infection and cervical neoplasia are linked by a spectrum of continuous morphologic and biologic change. Cancer 53:943, 1984.
13. Boring CC, Squires TS, Tong T. Cancer Statistics 1992. 42(1):19, 1992.
14. Hanks GE, Herring DF, Kramer S. Patterns of care outcome studies. Results of the national practice in cancer of the cervix. Cancer 51:959, 1983.
15. Jampolis S, Andras EJ, Fletcher GH. Analysis of sites of causes of failures of irradiation in invasive squamous cell carcinoma of the intact uterine cervix. Radiology 115:681, 1975.
16. Perez CA, Camel HM, Walz BJ, et al. Radiation therapy alone in the treatment of carcinoma of the uterine cervix. A 20 year experience. Gynecol Oncol 23:127, 1986.
17. Hunter RD, Cowie VJ, Blair V, Cole MP. A clinical trial of two conceptually different radical radiotherapy treatments in Stage III carcinoma of the cervix. Clin Radiol 37:23, 1986.
18. Fenton J, Decroix Y. Exclusive radiotherapy of late stage II and stage III carcinoma of the uterine cervix. Bull du Cancer 66:542, 1979.
19. Kovacic J, Cavic M, Omahen A, et al. The treatment of invasive carcinoma of the cervix at the Department of Gynecology and Obstetrics in Ljubljana. Eur J Gynecol Oncol 1:65, 1980.
20. Prignitz R, Hess F, Kleinsorge F, et al. Radiotherapy of cervix and uterus carcinomas (Marburg results of 1960 to 1975). Strahlentherapie 159:326, 1983.
21. Nnatu SNN, Durosinmi-Etti FA. The problems with the management of carcinoma of the cervix in Nigeria-Lagos experience. East Afr Med J 62(5):347, 1985.
22. Potish RA, Farniok KE, Twiggs LB. The interplay of local and distant control in the cure of cervical cancer. Cancer 66:2514, 1990.
23. Yule R. Mortality from carcinoma of the cervix. Lancet 1:1031, 1978.
24. Russell JH, Blair V, Hunter RD. Cervical carcinoma: Prognosis in patients. Brit Med J 295:300, 1987.
25. Meanwell CA, Kelly KA, Wilson S, et al. Young age as a prognostic factor in cervical cancer: Analysis of population based data from 10,022 cases. Brit Med J 296:386, 1988.
26. Chu J, White E. Decreasing incidence of invasive cervical cancer in young women. Am J Obstet Gynecol 157:1105, 1987.
27. Tasker JT, Collins JA. Adenocarcinoma of the uterine cervix. Am J Obstet Gynecol 118:344, 1974.
28. Gallup DG, Abell MR. Invasive adenocarcinoma of the uterine cervix. Obstet Gynecol 49:596, 1977.
29. Fu YS, Reagan JW, Hsu JG, et al. Adenocarcinoma and mixed carcinoma of the uterine cervix. I. Clinicopathologic study. Cancer 49:2560, 1982.
30. Peters RK, Chao A, Mack TM, et al. Increased frequency of adenocarcinoma of the uterine cervix in young women in Los Angeles County. J Natl Cancer Inst 76(3):423, 1986.
31. Leminen A, Pavonen J, Forss M, et al. Adenocarcinoma of the uterine cervix. Cancer 65:53, 1990.
32. Angel C, DuBeshter B, Lin JY. Clinical presentation and management of Stage I cervical adenocarcinoma: A 25 year experience. Gynecol Oncol 44:71, 1992.
33. Kessler II. Human cervical cancer as a venereal disease. Cancer Res 36:783, 1976.
34. Lanciano RM, Won M, Coia LR, Hanks GE. Pretreatment and treatment factors associated with improved outcome in squamous cell carcinoma of the uterine cervix. A final report of the 1973 and 1978 Patterns of Care studies. Int J Radiat Oncol Biol Phys 20:667, 1991.
35. Lanciano RM, Won M, Hanks GE. A reappraisal of the International Federation of Gynecology and Obstetrics staging system for cervical cancer. Cancer 69:482, 1992.
36. Perez CA. Uterine cervix. *In:* Principles and Practice of Radiation Oncology. 2nd ed. Perez CA, Brady LW (Eds). Philadelphia, JB Lippincott, 1992, p. 1143.
37. Fletcher GH. Uterine cervix. *In:* Textbook of Radiotherapy. 3rd ed. Fletcher GH (Ed). Philadelphia, Lea & Febiger, 1980, p. 720.
38. Grimard L, Genest P, Girard A, et al. Prognostic significance of endometrial extension in carcinoma of the cervix. Gynecol Oncol 31:301, 1988.
39. Muscato MS, Perry MC, Yarbro JW. Chemotherapy of cervical carcinoma. Semin Oncol 9:373, 1982.
40. Falappa P, Trodella L, Controneo AR, et al. Advanced carcinoma of the cervix treated by continuous pelvic arterial infusion with cytostatics and radiation therapy. Eur J Radiol 2:307, 1982.

41. Rettenmaier MA, Moran MF, Ramsinghani NF. Treatment of advanced and recurrent squamous carcinoma of the uterine cervix with constant intra-arterial infusion of cisplatin. Cancer 61:1301, 1988.
42. Iglesias X. Intraarterial infusion of chemo beneficial in treating cervical ca. Oncol Times 10:15, 1988.
43. Patton TJ Jr, Kavanagh JJ, Delclos L, et al. Five year survival in patients given intra-arterial chemotherapy prior to radiotherapy for advanced squamous carcinoma of the cervix and vagina. Gynecol Oncol 42:54, 1991.
44. Hakes T, Wertheim M, Daghestam A, et al. Adjuvant chemotherapy for poor-risk Stage 1B/2A cervix carcinoma patients—a pilot study with cisplatin/bleomycin. Proc Am Soc Clin Oncol 3:171, 1984.
45. Kirsten F, Atkinson KH, Coppleson JV, et al. Combination chemotherapy followed by surgery or radiotherapy in patients with locally advanced cervical cancer. Br J Obstet Gynaecol 94:583, 1987.
46. Symonds RP, Habeshaw T, Watson ER, Kaye SB. Combination chemotherapy prior to radical radiotherapy for stage III and IV carcinoma of the cervix. Clin Radiol 38:273, 1987.
47. Soeters R, Bloch B, Levin W, et al. Combined chemotherapy and radiotherapy in patients with advanced squamous carcinoma of the cervix (cis-platinum-bleomycin-vinblastine). Gynecol Oncol 33:44, 1989.
48. Rabinovich MG, Focaccia G, Ferreyra R, et al. Neoadjuvant chemotherapy for cervical carcinoma. Obstet Gynecol 78:685, 1991.
49. Souhami L, Gil RA, Allan SE, et al. A randomized trial of chemotherapy followed by pelvic radiation therapy in stage IIIB carcinoma of the cervix. J Clin Oncol 9:970, 1991.
50. John M, Cooke K, Flam M, et al. Preliminary results of concomitant radiotherapy and chemotherapy in advanced cervical carcinoma. Gynecol Oncol 28:101, 1987.
51. John M, Flam M, Sikic B, et al. Preliminary results of concurrent radiotherapy and chemotherapy in advanced cervical carcinoma: A phase I-II prospective intergroup NCOG-RTOG study. Gynecol Oncol 37:1, 1990.
52. John M, Flam M, Marcus S, et al. RTOG-85-15: A second generation phase II chemoradiation protocol for advanced cervical cancer. Proc Am Soc Clin Oncol 10:190, 1991.
53. Hreschyshyn MM. Hydroxyurea with irradiation for cervical carcinoma—a preliminary report. Cancer Chemother Rep 52:601, 1968.
54. Piver MS, Barlow JJ, Vongtama V, Webster J. Hydroxyurea and radiation therapy in advanced cervical cancer. Am J Obstet Gynecol 120:969, 1974.
55. Piver MS, Barlow JJ, Vongtama V, Blumenson L. Hydroxyurea as a radiation sensitizer in women with carcinoma of the uterine cervix. Am J Obstet Gynecol 129:379, 1977.
56. Hreschyshyn MM, Aron BS, Boronow RC, et al. Hydroxyurea or placebo combined with radiation to treat Stages IIIB and IV cervical cancer confined to the pelvis. Int J Radiat Oncol Biol Phys 5:317, 1979.
57. Piver MS, Barlow JJ, Vongtama V, Blumenson L. Hydroxyurea: A radiation potentiator in carcinoma of the uterine cervix. Am J Obstet Gynecol 147:803, 1983.
58. Piver MS, Krishnamsetty RM, Emrich LJ. Survival of nonsurgically staged patients with negative lymphangiograms who had stage IIB carcinoma of the cervix treated by pelvic radiation plus hydroxyurea. Am J Obstet Gynecol 151:1006, 1985.
59. Piver MS, Vongtama V, Emrich LJ. Hydroxyurea plus pelvic radiation versus placebo plus pelvic radiation in surgically staged stage IIIB cervical cancer. J Surg Oncol 35:129, 1987.
60. Stehman FB, Bundy BN, Keys H, et al. A randomized trial of hydroxyurea versus misonidazole adjunct to radiation therapy in carcinoma of the cervix: A preliminary report of a Gynecology Oncology Group study. Am J Obstet Gynecol 159:87, 1988.
61. Piver M, Khalil M, Emrich LJ. Hydroxyurea plus pelvic irradiation versus placebo plus pelvic irradiation in nonsurgically staged stage IIIB cervical cancer. J Surg Oncol 42:120, 1989.
62. Thomas G, Dembo A, Fyles A, et al. Concurrent chemoradiation in advanced cervical cancer. Gynecol Oncol 38:446, 1990.
63. Thomas GM, Dembo AJ, Black B, et al. Concurrent radiation and chemotherapy for carcinoma of the cervix recurrent after radical surgery. Gynecol Oncol 27:254, 1987.
64. Kuske R, Perez C, Grigsby P, et al. Phase I/II study of definitive radiotherapy and chemotherapy (cisplatin and 5-fluorouracil) for advanced or recurrent gynecological malignancies: A preliminary report. Am J Clin Oncol 12:467, 1989.
65. Grigsby PW, Perez CA. Efficacy of 5-fluorouracil by continuous infusion and other agents as radiopotentiators for gynecologic malignancies. *In:* Concomitant continuous infusion chemotherapy and radiation. Rotman M, Rosenthal CJ (eds), Berlin, Springer-Verlag, 1991, p. 259.
66. Robert WS, Kavanagh JJ, Greenberg H, et al. Concomitant radiation therapy and chemo-

therapy in the treatment of advanced squamous carcinoma of the lower female genital tract. Gynecol Oncol 34:183, 1989.
67. Runowicz CD, Wadler S, Rodriguez-Rodriguez L, et al. Concomitant cisplatin and radiotherapy in locally advanced cervical carcinoma. Gynecol Oncol 34(3):395, 1989.
68. Heaton D, Yordan E, Reddy S, et al. Treatment of 29 patients with bulky squamous cell carcinoma of the cervix with simultaneous cisplatin, 5-fluorouracil and split-course hyperfractionated radiation therapy. Gynecol Oncol 38:323, 1990.
69. Thomas G, Dembo A, Beale F, et al. Concurrent radiation, mitomycin-C and 5-fluorouracil in poor prognosis carcinoma of cervix. Preliminary result of phase I, II study. Int J Radiat Oncol Biol Phys 10:1785, 1984.
70. Evans LS, Kersh CR, Constable WC, Taylor PT. Concomitant 5-fluorouracil, mitomycin-C and radiotherapy for advanced gynecological malignancies. Int J Radiat Oncol Biol Phys 15:901, 1988.
71. Ludgate SM, Crandon AJ, Hudson CN, et al. Synchronous 5-fluorouracil, mitomycin-C and radiation therapy in the treatment of locally advanced carcinoma of the cervix. Int J Radiat Oncol Biol Phys 15:893, 1988.
72. Kalra J, Cortes E, Chen S, et al. Effective multimodality treatment for advanced epidermoid carcinoma of the female genital tract. J Clin Oncol 3:917, 1985.
73. Drescher CW, Reid GC, Terada K, et al. Continuous infusion of low-dose 5-fluorouracil and radiation therapy for poor prognosis squamous cell carcinoma of the uterine cervix. Gynecol Oncol 44(3):227, 1992.
74. Potish RA, Twiggs LB, Adcock LL, et al. Effect of cisplatinum on tolerance to radiation therapy in advanced cervical cancer. Am J Clin Oncol 9:387, 1986.
75. Monyak DJ, Twiggs LB, Potish RA, et al. Tolerance and preliminary results of simultaneous therapy with radiation and cisplatin for advanced cervical cancer. NCI Monogr 6:369, 1988.
76. Malviya VK, Deppe G, Kim Y, Gove N. Concurrent radiation therapy, cis-platinum and mitomycin-C in patients with poor prognosis cancer of the cervix. A pilot study. Am J Clin Oncol 12:434, 1989.
77. Thomas G, Dembo A, DePetrillo A, et al. Concurrent radiation and chemotherapy in vulvar carcinoma. Gynecol Oncol 34:263, 1989.

Chapter 29

BLADDER

ROBERT S. MILLER, FRANK M. TORTI, AND WILLIAM U. SHIPLEY

CONVENTIONAL TREATMENT RESULTS

Unfortunately, past treatment of patients with muscle-invading bladder carcinoma by either radical surgery or radical radiotherapy has been, for the majority of patients, unsuccessful. Fewer than 50% of the patients have lived 5 or more years. Among the treated population, both cured and not cured, these treatments have often been associated with significant morbidity and with a decrease in the patient's quality of life. The comparisons of treatment results have often been made more confusing by authors comparing their own recent results with those of others or with "historical controls" from their institution. In most instances, these control groups of patients were staged and treated by different techniques. Such a comparison is always hazardous in the analysis of results and often results in incorrect data because of "stage migration" (the changes in the techniques of staging over a period of time) and because of known and unknown types of patient selection (1). Staging by clinical criteria (depth of tumor invasion on material recovered from the transurethral resection and the results of the bimanual examination under anesthesia) has an error rate as high as 50% between the clinical and pathologic (based on this histologic review of the tumor in the cystectomy specimen) stages for patients with muscle-invading tumors (2,3). Nevertheless, it is necessary to use clinical staging to compare "accurately" the results from different treatments to ensure that, on average, patients had similar potential curability at the initiation of treatments.

For two decades, radical megavoltage radiotherapy has offered the opportunity and hope of local control of the cancer without the loss of bladder function that results from cystectomy. However, numerous reported series over the last two decades show that the risk of local recurrence following radical radiotherapy is 50 to 70% (4–8) as compared to a 10 to 25% pelvic recurrence rate recurrence rate (2,4,9,10) following treatment by adjunctive preoperative radiation therapy and radical cystectomy (Table 29–1). Quite clearly, radical cystectomy can lower the pelvic recurrence rate (relative to radical radiotherapy), but there is little, possibly 10%, improvement in overall patient survival when these treatments are compared at 5 years or more (Table 29–1). Mainly, this occurs because patients presenting with invasive, apparently localized tu-

Table 29–1. Invasive Bladder Tumors: Treatment Results

Initial Treatment	Clinical Stages	Pelvis Remaining Tumor-Free	5-year Survival	References
Cystectomy	T2-T3	?	26–40%	97–99
Radiotherapy	T2-T3	24–56%	22–39%	4–8
Preoperative radiotherapy and cystectomy	T2-T3	88–100%	40–54%	2,6,9–11,97

mors have a significant probability (40 to 65%) of subsequently developing distant metastases, whether they are treated by radical cystectomy (4,9–11) or radical radiotherapy (4,7).

In the decade of the 1970s, there was considerable interest in exploring the relative efficacy of neutron irradiation to that of high energy photons. At that time, only moderate energy (up to 15 MeV) neutron beams were available. Several studies including two randomized Phase III trials were done in patients with clinically localized bladder carcinoma and reviewed by Russell et al (12). These indicated no therapeutic gain from moderate energy neutrons. In fact, the dose of neutrons selected caused a higher incidence of radiation injury (relative to photons). However, it still resulted in no additional benefit in overall survival or in local tumor control. Over the next decade, when high-energy neutron beams are available in some centers, further trials should be carried out.

PROGNOSTIC FACTORS FOR RADIOCURABILITY

For patients to be treated well by radiation therapy, close coordination and cooperation between the urologic surgeon and the radiation therapist is necessary. The urologist does the initial thorough evaluation of the patient and plays the major role in the selection of treatment. Because the local tumor recurrence rate for all patients undergoing radical radiotherapy is 50% or more, it is clearly desirable to identify, if possible, subgroups that will be relatively more likely to have external beam radiation therapy succeed. Blandy and colleagues were the first to report a favorable and significant correlation between achieving a complete tumor response and survival (5). Other prognostic factors are reported to be significant for local curability in patients treated with radical radiotherapy for clinical Stage T_2 and T_3 disease.

1. The absence of ureteral obstruction on excretory urography (7,13).
2. The presence of papillary histologic characteristics (7).
3. That a visibly "complete" resection of tumor (usually by transurethral resection) prior to radiation therapy was accomplished (4,7).

SYSTEMIC CHEMOTHERAPY

Major progress has been made in recent years in the development of chemotherapeutic regimens for the treatment of muscle-invasive transitional cell carcinoma of the bladder, once regarded as a tumor that was largely resistant to chemotherapy. The identification of drugs that are active in this disease has evolved from studies ranging from predominantly drug-oriented Phase I and II trials of single agents, which often included few patients with bladder cancer, to cooperative group trials of drug combinations (14). Objective response rates have exceeded 60% in some series (15), with a significant number of complete responses reported. Despite these encouraging results, there have still been few prospective randomized Phase III trials comparing one combination regimen to another or to single agents (16), and an advantage in terms of improving overall survival has not clearly been demonstrated. Nevertheless, the fact that the majority of patients with muscle-invasive transitional cell carcinoma (TCC) of the bladder will die of their disease within 2 years of diagnosis despite primary surgery and/or radiotherapy underscores the need for effective chemotherapy for both micrometastatic and clinically apparent disease.

Single Agents

Various individual agents have shown activity in TCC of the bladder, with response rates varying from 15 to 50% (Table 29–2) (17,18). Reported response rates for any given agent vary widely, and this may be due partly to the heterogeneity of the patients studied, inaccuracies in staging (especially clinical vs. pathologic staging), and variability in response criteria utilized (14). Cisplatinum and methotrexate are the most active drugs, with doxorubicin and vinblastine possessing important activity (15). Other conventional cytotoxic agents have shown minimal single agent activity but appear to have enhanced efficacy in combination.

Cisplatinum

In 1976, Yagoda et al first reported an overall response rate of 35% in 23 evaluable

Table 29–2. Single Agent Activity in Advanced Bladder Cancer

Drug	No. Evaluable Patients	% Response (CR + PR)	References
Hexamethylmelamine	26 (bilharzial)	38	43
Cisplatinum	257*	34	20,21,61,100–104
Cyclophosphamide	98*	31(?)	14
Methotrexate	134*	29	22,23,105
Gallium nitrate	26	27	24
Mitomycin C	48*	21	17
5-Fluorouracil	72*	19	27,28,33
Vinblastine	28	18	31
Amsacrine	25	16	107
Doxorubicin	114*	15	27–30
Carboplatin	149*	15	40
VM-26	40	5	36
Neocarcinostatin	19	5	24
Vincristine	23	4	32
VP-16	49*	2	34,35,106

*Represents data pooled from several studies

patients with advanced measurable bladder cancer treated with cisplatinum at a dose of 1.25 to 1.6 mg/kg every 3 or 4 weeks, including eight responses, all partial, in 14 patients who had no prior chemotherapy (19). Subsequent Phase II trials at Memorial Sloan-Kettering Cancer Center confirmed an overall response rate of 36% (20); however, the median duration of response was only 5 months. Pooled data from eight separate studies, some of which were randomized, are shown in Table 29–2. With a range of dosages from 50 to 100 mg/m^2, cisplatinum as a single agent has an overall response rate of 34%, with rare complete responses. In the most recent study cited (21), Hillcoat showed essentially the same response rate (31%) and time to disease progression (6.6 months) as did Yagoda in the 1970s. Cisplatinum remains the single most active drug for the treatment of advanced TCC. However, the optimum dose is not known, and it is not clear whether a dose-response relationship exists for the drug, as is the case with some other solid tumors such as testicular or ovarian carcinomas.

Methotrexate

This drug has been used in a variety of dosage schedules and routes in a large number of studies, but many, especially those prior to 1980, do not adequately define patient selection and response criteria. Turner treated 64 patients with 50 mg IV, 100 mg IV, and 200 mg IM with folinic acid rescue and found objective clinical responses (complete and partial) in 3 of 25, 12 of 23, and 8 of 16 patients, respectively (22). Natale et al reported one objective response in evaluable patients with measurable, bidimensional lesions who received 250 mg/m^2 with folinic acid rescue, and 10 responses in 33 similar patients receiving 0.5 to 1.0 mg/kg (23). The overall response rate for methotrexate used as a single agent ranges from 18 to 38%, with a median of approximately 30% (15). There have been no randomized studies comparing low- vs. high-dose methotrexate, although in a small number of patients treated at higher doses, responses as high as 45% are reported (24).

Doxorubicin

Early trials with Adriamycin at a dose of 60 to 75 mg/m^2 every 3 weeks showed objective remissions in 36% of 39 patients (25), and a dose-response relationship was suggested (26). Subsequent studies have failed to reproduce this initial response rate, and as a single agent, the drug is considered to produce responses in about 15% of patients treated (27–30). Median duration of response is 3 to 5 months (14).

Vinca Alkaloids

A limited number of patients have been treated with vinblastine as a single agent.

Blumenreich et al obtained responses in 5 of 28 patients (18%), three of whom had received prior chemotherapy, with doses of 0.10 to 0.15 mg/kg each week (31). Vincristine showed little antitumor efficacy and prohibitive toxicity as a single agent (32).

5-Fluorouracil

Older trials with 5-fluorouracil (5-FU) showed a wide range of response rates, and this may be the result of heterogeneous patient populations, different administration schedules, and inadequately defined response criteria. Three more recent trials employing the drug as a weekly bolus found responses in 3 of 11, 7 of 36, and 4 of 15 patients (27,28,33).

Other Drugs

Occasional responses have been seen with the podophyllotoxin derivatives VM-26 and VP-16, but their activity as single agents is limited (34–36). Cyclophosphamide has been studied in several older trials, but its single-agent efficacy using modern response criteria is not known (17). Mitomycin C has been reported to have an overall response rate of 21% in trials completed before 1975 (17). Hexamethylmelamine has been studied in bilharzial bladder cancer, usually of squamous histology, in which it appears to have some activity (37). However, when this drug was compared to 5-FU, Adriamycin, and cyclophosphamide in a randomized SWOG study, no activity could be demonstrated in TCC (38).

New and Investigational Agents

In an attempt to circumvent the nephro- and neurotoxicity associated with cisplatinum, carboplatin has been studied in several tumor types. In TCC of the bladder, carboplatin appears to have less activity as a single agent than cisplatinum. In a report by the Medical Research Council in Great Britain, carboplatin given by monthly injection produced only three partial responses (PRs) and no complete responses (CRs) in 48 patients (39). Pooled data from Phase II trials show only a 15% response rate in 149 patients (40). Studies in drug scheduling using human urothelial tumors grown in nude mice showed that carboplatin was more efficacious with more frequent doses (41), and a pilot study utilizing 24-hour infusions of the drug showed a higher objective response rate (42).

Ifosfamide is active in bilharzial bladder cancer (43), but it is largely untested in TCC. Other drugs with some activity in TCC are listed in Table 29–2. Few studies have used lymphokines or other biologic agents in muscle-invasive disease. Alpha-interferon can produce complete remissions in carcinoma in situ when used intravesically (44), and interleukin-2 produced three local complete responses in six patients treated with intralesional injection of primary bladder tumors (45), but the systemic activity of such agents is not known.

Combination Regimens

The highest rates for complete and partial responses in TCC have been seen with multidrug combinations. The most efficacious regimens combine cisplatinum and methotrexate, the two most active drugs, in various doses and schedules. However, multiple other regimens have been tested and shown to have at least modest antitumor activity. Further Phase III studies are needed to confirm the superiority of multidrug regimens, especially considering the increased toxicity of many combinations.

Non-Cisplatinum-Containing Regimens

Although several different combinations lacking cisplatinum have been studied, most are less effective for advanced TCC than those containing cisplatinum. The elimination of cisplatinum may attenuate neurologic and renal toxicity, but many of these regimens are based on doxorubicin (Adriamycin, ADR), and cardiac toxicity may limit the dose (18). Merrin et al (46) reported a 50% response rate in 18 patients treated with cyclophosphamide and ADR, but subsequent investigators have been unable to reproduce these results, even with higher doses of cyclophosphamide (47). Tannock et al combined methotrexate with ADR and cyclophosphamide (MAC) and showed objective responses in 15 of 38 patients with measurable disease and 4 of 14 patients with nonmeasurable, evaluable lesions (48). Adriamycin has been combined with 5-FU by several investigators. Cross found three CRs and four

PRs in 20 patients using 5-FU 500 mg/m^2 and ADR 50 mg/m^2 every 3 weeks (49). Using similar doses, Martino found 8 objective responses in 21 patients, but 12 patients had severe leukopenia, and there was one septic death (50). The combination of ADR, cyclophosphamide, and 5-FU has not shown greater efficacy than single agents alone, and chemotherapy-related deaths have been reported (33,38,51).

Other combinations studied include VM-26 and ADR, which together appear to be less effective than ADR alone (52). The combination of vinblastine 4 mg/m^2 and methotrexate 40 mg/m^2 given as weekly outpatient doses induced 19 complete or partial responses in 47 evaluable patients without significant toxicity (53). Although the 95% confidence limits for this combination overlapped those for methotrexate as a single agent, the duration of response was longer, and this combination might play some role as a salvage for patients failing single-agent cisplatinum.

Cisplatinum-containing Combinations

Cisplatinum-based regimens for advanced TCC can be divided into those with methotrexate and those without methotrexate. In the latter group, cisplatinum has been combined with ADR, cyclophosphamide, 5-FU, and VM-26 (54–61). Table 29–3 summarizes the most active combinations. The combination of cisplatinum, ADR, and cyclophosphamide (CISCA or CAP) has been the most extensively studied. It was first reported in 1977 to produce CR + PR in 9 of 10 patients with metastatic TCC (54), but subsequent results have been more modest. The Memorial group used cisplatinum 70 mg/m^2 on day 1, cyclophosphamide 250 mg/m^2 on day 2, and Adriamycin 45 mg/m^2 on day 3, and reported 13 complete or partial remission in 28 evaluable patients, with a median duration of response of eight months (55). Sites of response included lung lesions and lymph nodes, and usually occurred within the first three cycles. Pooled data from four reports (56–59) using these drugs are shown in Table 29–3. Two of these studies randomized patients between single agent cisplatinum and the combination (58,59). No statistical difference in overall response, duration of response, or survival could be found, but the multidrug combination showed significantly more life-threatening toxicity (58).

Results of randomization between cisplatinum and cisplatinum plus Adriamycin in a SWOG trial also showed no differences in response or survival (60). A National Bladder Cancer Group study comparing single agent cisplatinum and cyclophosphamide again demonstrated no advantage to the combination (61). Representative reports from cisplatinum combinations with adriamycin ± 5-FU ± VM-26 are shown in Table 29–3. Two recent reports (62,63) have shown promising results using cisplatinum combined with 4- or 5-day continuous infusions of 5-FU, perhaps taking advantage of the theoretical synergy between these two drugs. Mucositis and myelosuppression were significant, however.

Cisplatinum plus Methotrexate-based Regimens

Combination regimens containing both cisplatinum and methotrexate have shown

Table 29–3. Cisplatinum Regimens for Advanced Bladder Cancer (Non-MTX-Containing)

Regimen	No. evaluable patients	% response (CR + PR)	References
CDDP 50 mg/m^2 + DOX 50 mg/m^2 + 5-FU 500 mg/m^2 + VM-26 100 mg/m^2	14	72	110
CDDP 20 mg/m^2 × 5 + DOX 50 mg/m^2 + 5-FU 500 mg/m^2	17	65	109
CDDP 60 mg/m^2 + DOX 60 mg/m^2 (12 hrs later)	35	57	18
CDDP 70 mg/m^2 + VM-26 100 mg/m^2	41	51	111
CDDP 50 mg/m^2 (day 2) + DOX 50 mg/m^2 (day 1)	37	43	60
CDDP 40-60 mg/m^2 + CTX 400 mg/m^2 + DOX 40 mg/m^2	152*	39	56–59
CDDP 50 mg/m^2 + CTX 650 mg/m^2	17	35	108

*Represents data pooled from several studies
CDDP = cisplatinum, DOX = doxorubicin (Adriamycin), CTX = cyclophosphamide (cytoxan), 5-FU = 5-fluorouracil

the highest reproducible overall response rates, the most CRs, and the longest durations of response compared with other multidrug combinations (14). Toxicity has been significant and prohibitive in some patients, especially the elderly and those with diminished creatinine clearance prior to chemotherapy. The renal dysfunction caused by cisplatinum has been potentiated by methotrexate toxicity in some cases, although a pharmacokinetic study in 1984 at the University of Glasgow failed to show a diminution of methotrexate clearance by concomitant administration of cisplatinum at 50 mg/m^2 (64). Several groups have reported on two-drug combinations of cisplatinum and methotrexate, using cisplatinum 70 to 100 mg/m^2 and methotrexate 40 to 200 mg/m^2 (with or without folinic acid rescue) on a variety of schedules (21,65–67). The response rates ranged from 45 to 68%, using pooled data from these four studies, an overall response rate of 49% was seen, with 22 of 135 (16%) achieving a CR. One of these reports (21) randomized patients to cisplatinum vs. cisplatinum + methotrexate. Although the response rate and median survival for the combination were higher, the values did not achieve statistical significance in the 53 patients studied. The combination caused significantly more hematologic toxicity and mucositis.

The two most efficacious regimens to date in the treatment of advanced TCC of the bladder are CMV (*c*isplatinum, *m*ethotrexate, and *v*inblastine), developed at Stanford University Medical Center and investigated by the Northern California Oncology Group, and MVAC (*m*ethotrexate, *v*inblastine, *A*driamycin, and *c*isplatinum), developed at Memorial Sloan-Kettering Cancer Center. The CMV regimen (Table 29–4) uses methotrexate 30 mg/m^2 and vinblastine 4 mg/m^2 on day 1, followed in 12 to 24 hours by cisplatinum 100 mg/m^2 (68,69). Methotrexate and vinblastine are repeated at day 8, and the whole cycle is repeated on day 22. The doses of methotrexate and vinblastine are modified for hematologic toxicity. The doses of cisplatinum and methotrexate are adjusted for creatinine clearance. Of 50 evaluable patients with measurable disease by physical examination, chest x-ray, or CT scan, 14 achieved a complete response to CMV and 14 others achieved a partial response for an overall response rate of 56% (68). Complete responses were noted in all sites including retroperitoneal nodes, liver, lung, bladder, and bone. The median time of survival was 8 months, with responders surviving significantly longer than nonresponders. Toxicities in the 50 patients included moderate to severe mucositis in 13, fever and neutropenia in 14, and transient elevation of serum creatinine > 2.0 mg/dL in 15. Two patients died

Table 29–4. CMV Regimen (Stanford) for Advanced TCC

Drugs	Day 1	Day 2	Day 8
Cisplatinum		100	
Methotrexate	30		30
Vinblastine	4		4

All doses in mg/m^2. Cycles are repeated every 21 days.

Dose Modification of Methotrexate and Vinblastine for Myelosuppression
(% of initial calculated dose)*:

	Platelet Count			
WBC	≥150K	100–149K	75–99K	<75K
≥3.5	100	100	50	0
3.0–3.4	75†	75†	50	0
2.5–2.9	50	50	0‡	0
<2.5	0	0	0	0

*If day 1 dose of subsequent cycles (day 22) falls into the 0 to 50% range, delay the initiation of cycles up to 2 weeks.
†100% of calculated dose to be given for platelet and WBC counts at this level on day 8.
‡50% of calculated dose to be given for platelet and WBC counts at this level on day 8.

Dose Modification of Cisplatin for Nephrotoxicity
(% of initial calculated dose):

Creatinine Clearance (mL/min)	% Calculated Cisplatinum Dose
>60	100
45–60	50
<45	0

Dose Modification of Methotrexate for Nephrotoxicity

NO methotrexate is given if any of the following occur:
1. Creatinine clearance decreases by greater than 30 mL/min.
2. Creatinine clearance decreases to < 45 mL/min.
3. Serum creatinine ≧ 2.0 mg/dL, regardless of creatinine clearance.

septic deaths, but both had been treated at the higher doses of methotrexate and vinblastine (40 mg/m^2 and 5 mg/m^2, respectively) specified by the original protocol. Two additional reports confirm these results. Rosenberg and Williams employed the same doses and schedule as NCOG and found a 47% CR rate and a 12% PR rate in 17 evaluable patients (70). Using a 1-monthly 3-day regimen, with cisplatinum divided into two doses of 45 mg/m^2, Walther and Walker achieved 6 of 19 CRs and 8 of 19 PRs with acceptable toxicity (71). It remains to be seen whether these responses will be durable.

The MVAC regimen developed by the Memorial group differs from CMV in both schedule (drugs are given on days 1, 2, 15, 22, and the cycle is repeated every 28 days) and dose (cisplatinum and vinblastine are decreased to 70 mg/m^2 and 3 mg/m^2, respectively), as well as by the addition of Adriamycin. In the initial report of 24 evaluable patients with bidimensionally measurable disease, 12 achieved a CR and five achieved a PR for an overall response rate of 71% (72). All sites of metastatic disease responded, including peripheral lymph nodes or subcutaneous masses in 100% of responding patients with these indicator lesions. Hematologic toxicity was significant, with 24% of patients having a WBC at nadir of 1000/mm^3 or less, four episodes of fever and neutropenia, and one septic death in a patient with an initial Karnofsky performance score of 40. Only three patients had a creatinine $\geq$ 2.1 mg/dL. A follow-up report of 92 patients showed CR in 37% $\pm$ 10% ($\pm$ percent confidence limits) and PR in 31% $\pm$ 10%, with 17 of 31 completely responding patients surviving 26+ to 49+ months (73). Relapses in the brain occurred in 18% of responders, half of whom did not have a systemic relapse, suggesting that the CNS may be a sanctuary site in patients who achieve a remission elsewhere.

Using the same doses as MVAC but modifying the schedule, Simon and Srougi reported 4 of 12 CRs and 5 of 12 PRs in evaluable patients (74). Tannock et al treated 41 patients with the Memorial MVAC schedule and noted an overall response rate of only 40% in 30 evaluable patients (75). Toxicity was formidable, with 90% of patients having a WBC $<$ 500/mm^3 and one dying of sepsis. The authors caution against the "widespread use" of MVAC, especially considering the lack of statistically significant benefit in terms of response or survival shown in previously reported randomized trials of cisplatinum vs. cisplatinum-containing combinations (21,58–60). Additionally, a preliminary report in which 69 patients were randomized to CISCA (cyclophosphamide, adriamycin, cisplatinum) or MVAC also showed no statistically significant difference in response rates, although a trend toward higher response rates with MVAC was noted [68% vs. 44%, $p > 0.07$] (76).

Other variant combinations of methotrexate and cisplatinum have been reported. Weekly M-VAC-L (*c*isplatinum 25 mg/m^2, *A*driamycin 15 mg/m^2, *v*inblastine 4 mg/m^2, *m*ethotrexate 15 mg/m^2, and *l*eucovorin 20 mg po for 3 days) produced pathologic CRs in 10/19 patients with resectable tumors (77). In another report, the substitution of epirubicin for Adriamycin in the Memorial schedule did not alter the efficacy of the regimen in 30 patients receiving it (78). It remains to be seen whether epirubicin in this regimen (MVEC) truly results in decreased cardiac toxicity when compared with MVAC. An interesting report from the United Kingdom using a combination of carboplatin, methotrexate, mitoxantrone, and vinblastine in 40 patients showed complete responses in 27% and partial responses in 36% (79). Despite the greater myelosuppressive effects of carboplatin vs. cisplatinum, hematologic toxicity was relatively mild, although nine patients were admitted with fever and neutropenia. Combinations of carboplatin with methotrexate and other active agents deserve further study. The increasing availability of hematopoietic growth factors in clinical practice may enable investigators to use higher doses of myelosuppressive drugs such as carboplatin in combination with other agents for advanced bladder cancer (80).

Neoadjuvant Chemotherapy

The impressive results of combination chemotherapy based on cisplatinum and methotrexate have led many investigators to use the drugs in a neoadjuvant fashion, prior to definitive therapy for the primary bladder lesion. The theoretical benefits of this approach include reducing the size of the original tumor, to make marginally resectable lesions prior to chemotherapy operable; identifying which tumors are "sensitive" to chemotherapy for purposes of postoperative adjuvant chemotherapy; treating micrometastatic disease at a time when the tumor burden is the smallest and most kinetically active; and sterilizing the primary bladder tumor to prevent dissemination of malignant cells in the operative field at cystectomy (81).

There has been a proliferation of trials of neoadjuvant chemotherapy prior to cystectomy, most using the CMV or MVAC regimens. There is considerable variability in these trials, because of differences in patient selection, the inclusion of some patients with T_1 and T_2 lesions, the extent of restaging, and criteria for response (24). In 1988, the Memorial group reported on 50 patients with T_{2-4} N_0 M_0 who received one to five cycles of MVAC in an attempt to "downstage" the primary bladder lesion (82). A significant decrease in the T stage as assessed by transurethral resection was observed, with 57% of 44 evaluable patients achieving T_0 and 11% Tis. Of the 32 patients who underwent surgical staging (cystectomy or laparotomy with lymph node biopsy), stage P_O (no evidence of disease in adequate biopsy specimens) was achieved in 39% of 23 patients originally with T_3 lesions and in 14% of patients with T_4 lesions. The study also demonstrated the limitations of clinical restaging, with an error rate of 38% when clinical staging was compared with pathologic staging (82).

Other groups report similar results in small numbers of patients, with two to four cycles of MVAC preoperatively producing downstaging in the primary tumor in the majority of patients (83,84). The Stanford group used four cycles of neoadjuvant CMV chemotherapy and found 12 clinical CRs in 24 evaluable patients, although 8 of these were found to have residual tumor at the time of surgery (85). Eleven of the 12 patients were alive without disease at 15 to 46 months.

Although it is clear that dramatic downstaging of bulky bladder lesions does occur often, the exact role of neoadjuvant chemotherapy remains uncertain. Most data from neoadjuvant trials are not mature enough and patient numbers not great enough to determine whether initial chemotherapy confers a significant survival advantage. The Massachusetts General Hospital and the Radiation Therapy Oncology Group have a randomized trial underway with and without neoadjuvant methotrexate, cisplatinum, and vinblastine in patients with muscle-invasive tumors who are being treated on a selective bladder-sparing regimen of pelvic irradiation (to 4000 cGy) plus cisplatinum. Complete responders (negative biopsy of the original tumor site on cystoscopic reevaluation) have consolidation radiotherapy to 6480 cGy plus additional cisplatinum; incomplete responders undergo immediate radical cystectomy.

ECOG and SWOG have initiated a randomized trial with and without MVAC prior to radical cystectomy for patients with muscle-invading tumors. The EORTC have also recently initiated a randomized trial testing the addition of neoadjuvant CMV chemotherapy to definitive local treatment of invasive bladder cancer. We will need to await the results from such trials to determine whether initial chemotherapy will improve upon the outcomes achieved by the definitive local treatment: either radical cystectomy, radical radiotherapy, or chemoradiation.

CHEMORADIATION: OPPORTUNITIES FOR SUCCESSFUL BLADDER-SPARING APPROACHES

Following the demonstration by Yagoda (13) of significant objective response rates with cisplatinum against metastatic tumors, trials combining systemic cisplatinum with radical radiotherapy were initiated (86–89). The National Bladder Cancer Group treated 70 patients with stage T_2–T_{4b} cancer who were not candidates for cystectomy with combined cisplatinum (70 mg/m^2) plus radiotherapy (6480 cGy) (88). The actuarial 4-year survival rate for all entered patients was significantly better for patients with clinical stage T_2 tumors (64%) than for those with clinical stages T_3 or T_4 tumors (24%). Jakse and colleagues from Innsbruck treated patients with Stage T_3 and T_4 tumors with cisplatinum plus 6000 cGy radiation and, in some instances, Adriamycin (87). They found a 46% overall survival and a 66% survival for the completely responding patients. A similar excellent result is reported by

Sauer and colleagues from Erlangen (90). They report a complete response rate of 85% for 33 patients with stage T_2–T_4 tumors treated with infusion cisplatinum plus 5000 to 5600 cGy.

The randomized Phase III trial by Richards and colleagues (91) failed to show an improvement in the patient survival or local control when conventional external beam was combined with 5-FU, and Adriamycin was given after radical radiotherapy. However, Rotman and colleagues reported a 61% complete response rate using concomitant 5-FU infusion with external beam radiation and occasionally mitomycin C for 18 patients with advanced bladder carcinoma (89). To date, the "indications" for increased efficacy of chemotherapy plus radiation (relative to radiation alone) is based on the above reports of higher complete response rates with a combined approach. The complete response rates for definitive radiation alone range from 40 to 51% (5,6,8,91); the complete response rates using cisplatinum or infusional 5-FU plus full-dose radiation range from 75 to 85% (87–90). The local tumor complete response rate following single or multiple agent chemotherapy without radiation therapy ranges from 9 to 52% (63,69,73,92,93).

A recent approach is to use the response of the primary tumor to single- or multiple-agent chemotherapy plus radiotherapy, when given as neoadjuvant treatment, as a way to select patients for bladder preservation (94–96). The goal is to select *only* those patients who have a very high likelihood of having a permanent local cure of their bladder cancer. Only patients who have had a complete response to up-front chemotherapy plus radiotherapy to an intermediate dose of 4000 to 4500 cGy are selected for definitive radiation therapy. By using these criteria at the Massachusetts General Hospital, we have been able to select approximately two thirds of our patients for bladder preservation while one third of the patients with stage T_2–T_4 tumors have gone on to immediate cystectomy (94,96). We have used the schema outlined in Figure 29–1. Forty-four consecutive patients with biopsy-proven muscle invasive stage T_2–T_4 bladder tumors underwent a debulking transurethral resection followed by MCV chemotherapy (methotrexate 30 mg/m^2 given on days 1, 15, and 22; cisplatinum 70 mg/m^2 given on day 2; and vinblastine 3 mg/m^2 given on days 2, 15, and 22 of a 28-day cycle). After two cycles, the patients had a repeat cystoscopic biopsy, bimanual evaluation, and saline barbotage for cytologic examination. The patients then received 4000 cGy to the bladder and pelvic lymphatics using a 4-field box technique with high energy photons (usually

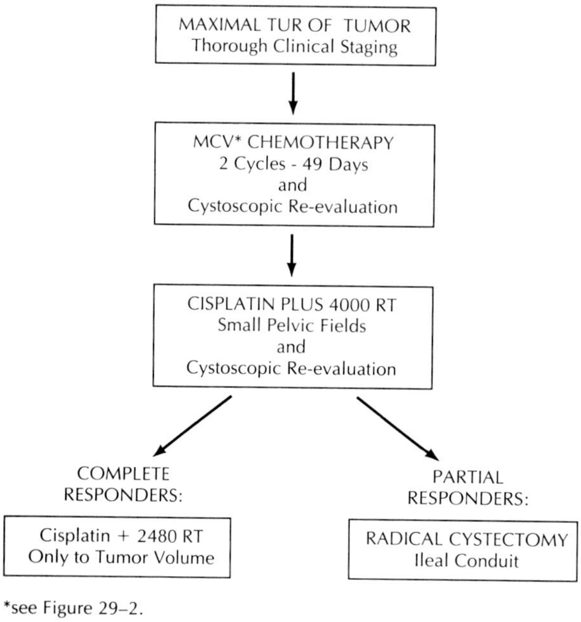

Fig. 29–1. The Massachusetts General Hospital protocol (Invasive bladder carcinoma protocol 180) of neoadjuvant chemoradiation as a means of bladder preservation in invasive bladder carcinoma.

25 MV). Cisplatinum (70 mg/m^2) was given a day prior to the start of the radiation and again on day 22. Repeat evaluation included cystoscopic biopsy, and a repeat pelvic CT scan. If the patient had a complete response (CR), additional radiotherapy to the tumor-bearing column was delivered to bring the total dose to 6480 cGy with an additional dose of cisplatinum given on day 43 of the radiation. Patients who had residual tumor following the 4000 cGy plus cisplatinum were advised to undergo cystectomy.

Thirty-six of the first 44 patients completed the full protocol (i.e., either full radiation therapy of 6480 cGy or radical cystectomy after MCV and 4000 cGy plus cisplatinum). Forty-three percent of patients achieved a CR after MCV and 65% after 4000 cGy plus cisplatinum. To be a CR, or a cT_0, the patient had to have a negative tumor-site biopsy and a negative bladder-washing cytologic examination. A PR required a negative tumor-site biopsy but a positive cytologic examination. Five additional patients achieved a PR following MCV and three patients were in PR following 4000 cGy and cisplatinum. Only 43% of the patients had a persistently positive tumor-site biopsy following MCV and only 26% had a positive tumor-site biopsy following 4000 cGy and cisplatinum. To date, 25 patients have completed the consolidation radiation therapy and cisplatinum to 6480 cGy, with 22 (88%) being complete responders 3 months following completion of the radiation and 19 (76%) remaining without evidence of tumor in the bladder—in *maintained* CR or cTO status. Six of the 25 patients have had recurrent or persistent tumor in the bladder to date. Two have had recurrence of invasive tumors and have undergone radical cystectomy without undue difficulty. Four have developed Tis (carcinoma in situ) and have undergone intravesical therapy. Two of these four patients are disease-free and two have a persistent positive urine cytology. Thus, of the 25 patients treated with planned bladder preservation, 21 or 84% have tumor-free bladders, although the follow-up is still short, ranging from 6 to 28 months.

In addition to 8 patients who did not complete the protocol as planned due to toxicity, dosage modifications of the drug were required in 59% of the patients for either low blood counts, stomatitis, or renal toxicity. Further, we observed a level of treatment toxicity that these aging patients would not tolerate. While not life-threatening, this regimen resulted in discomforture of a degree that 12 of the 25 patients who received the full radiation dose failed to receive the last dose of cisplatinum. The patients' knowledge of their local tumor status (i.e., being a CR) may have influenced this event.

Because, to date, it is still uncertain whether neoadjuvant chemotherapy will add improved efficacy in bladder preservation or increase patient survival by sterilizing initially undetected micrometastatic disease, we initiated (in May 1988) a randomized Phase III trial at Massachusetts General Hospital to study this important question (Fig. 29–2). To date, this trial has proved acceptable to patients and physicians and has accrued 55 patients in the first 18 months, an accrual rate from our single institution of 3 patients per month.

Response Durability with Bladder Preservation Treatments

For a bladder-preserving treatment to be a success, a complete response must be achieved *and* maintained. This requires complete tumor cell sterilization and that the retained bladder not develop a tumor recurrence. Table 29–5 reviews the published information on the durability of a complete response following radiation therapy and/or chemotherapy. Although all listed series include patients with follow-up well under 5 years, the data in this table suggest that significant levels of durable complete responses are being achieved by combined chemotherapy and radiation. Such criteria of tumor sterilization by follow-up reevaluation of treated bladders in vivo is a more meaningful way to document cure than is a "pathologic complete response." Interpretation of this information is hazardous because pathologic staging can give false positive information (when only nonviable or nonclonogenic tumor cells are seen microscopically) or false negative (when sectioning has missed viable tumor cells that would ultimately lead to a recurrence). The available results with chemotherapy alone (Table 29–5) suggest that the durability of a complete response in the primary bladder tumor

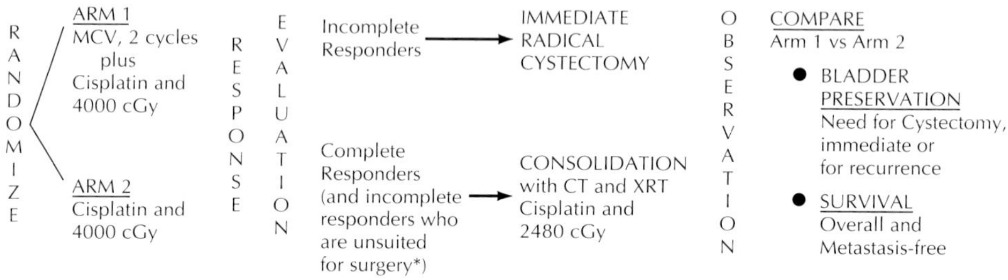

STRATIFY: 1. Clinical T stage (T2, T3 or T4).
2. Known bladder tumor remaining after entry TURB (yes or no).
3. Cystectomy candidate (yes or no *—per clinician or patient).

MCV: Methotrexate, 30mg/M^2; Cisplatin, 70mg/M^2; Vinblastine, 3mg/M^2
TURB: Transurethral Resection of Bladder tumor by institutional urologist.

Fig. 29–2. A Massachusetts General Hospital randomized trial (invasive bladder carcinoma protocol 880) with and without neoadjuvant MCV chemotherapy in addition to transurethral surgery, cisplatinum with radiation therapy for selective bladder preservation in patients with muscle-invading bladder cancer.

may not be satisfactory with this approach (4,63,93). Patients with an excellent clinical response to chemotherapy are relatively uncommonly found to be pathologic complete responders (93). The true success of bladder-preserving treatment by chemotherapy and/or radiotherapy requires a 3- to 5-year follow-up for investigators to be confident that such treatment has sterilized the bladder of cancer.

Note

This text is partly based on a recent review prepared for the National Conference on Advances in Cancer Management of the American Cancer Society, December 7–9, 1988 in Los Angeles. (This review has been published as: Shipley WU, Prout FR Jr, Kaufman DS. Bladder cancer: Advances in laboratory

Table 29–5. Durability of a Complete Response with Bladder Preservation Following Radiation and/or Chemotherapy

Treatment	Series	Number of Patients	Clinical Stage	% Complete Response	% Maintained Complete Response
RT Alone:					
6400 cGy	London (8)	138	T2–3	47	39
RT + CT:					
CDDP and 6480 cGy	NBCG #8 (88)	57	T2–4	79	58
CDDP and 6000 cGy ± ADR	Innsbruck (87)	44	T3–4	75	65
5-FU and 6000–6500 cGy ± MMC	SUNY, Brooklyn (89)	18	T1–4	61	61†
CDDP and 5000–5600 cGy	Erlangen (90)	33	T2–4	85	70
MCV plus CDDP and 6480 cGy	MGH #180 (94)	25*	T2–4	88	76†
CT Alone:					
CDDP and 5-FU	Nice (63)	19	T2–4a	47	20
M-VAC	MSKCC (93)	23	T2–4	52	30‡

*Selected for, and completed, 6480 cGy and CDDP from initial group of 42
†Not including 2 patients back into maintained CR by intravesical therapy for Tis.
‡Not including 5 patients back into maintained CR by intravesical therapy for Tis.
Chemotherapy (CT): CDDP = cisplatinum, ADR = adriamycin (doxorubicin), 5-FU = 5-fluorouracil, MMC = mitomycin C, MCV = methotrexate, cisplatinum, vinblastine, M-VAC = methotrexate, vinblastine, adriamycin, cisplatinum, RT = Radiotherapy (dose in centigray)

innovations and clinical management. Cancer 65:675, 1990.)

REFERENCES

1. Tomkin K, Tannock I. Evaluation of response and morbidity following treatment of bladder cancer. *In:* The Management of Bladder Cancer. Raghavan D (Ed). London, Edward Arnold, 1988, p. 228.
2. Batata NA, Chu FCH, Hilaris BS, et al. Preoperative whole pelvis versus true pelvis irradiation and/or cystectomy for bladder cancer. Int J Radiat Oncol Biol Phys 7:1349, 1981.
3. Skinner DG, Tift JP, Kaufman JJ. High-dose, short-course preoperative radiation therapy and immediate single stage radical cystectomy with pelvic node dissection in the management of patients with bladder cancer. J Urol 127:671, 1982.
4. Miller LS, Johnson DE. Megavoltage radiation for bladder carcinoma. Alone, postoperative, or preoperative. Seventh National Cancer Conference Proceedings, 1973, p. 771.
5. Blandy JT, England HR, Evans SJW, et al. T3 bladder cancer—the case for salvage cystectomy. Br J Urol 52:506, 1980.
6. Bloom HJG, Hendry WF, Wallace DM, Skeet RG. Treatment of T_3 bladder cancer: Controlled trial of preoperative radiotherapy and radical cystectomy versus radical radiotherapy. Second report and review. Br J Urol 54:136, 1982.
7. Shipley WU, Rose MA, Perrone TL, et al. Full-dose irradiation for patients with invasive bladder carcinoma: Clinical and histological factors prognostic of improved survival. J Urol 134:679, 1985.
8. Blandy JP, Jenkins BJ, Fowler CG, et al. Radical radiotherapy and salvage cystectomy for T2 and T3 cancer of the bladder. *In:* The Management of Advanced Cancer of Prostate and Bladder. Smith P, Pavone-Macaluso N (Eds). New York, A. R. Liss, Inc., 1988, p. 447.
9. van der Werf-Messing B. Carcinoma of the urinary bladder T3 Nx M0 treated by preoperative radiation followed by simple cystectomy. Int J Radiat Oncol Biol Phys 8:1849, 1982.
10. Shipley WU, Coombs LJ, Prout, Jr., GR, et al. Preoperative irradiation and radical cystectomy for invasive bladder cancer—patterns of failure and prognostic factors associated with patient survival and disease progression. J Urol 135(4,pt.2):222A (Abs 473), 1986.
11. Boileau MA, Johnson ED, Chan RC, Bonsalez MO. Bladder carcinoma. Results with preoperative radiation therapy and radical cystectomy. Urology 16:569, 1980.
12. Russell KJ, Laramore GE, Griffin TW, et al. Fast neutron radiotherapy for the treatment of carcinoma of the urinary bladder. Am J Clin Oncol (CCT) 12(4):301, 1989.
13. Greiner R, Skaleric KC, Veraguth P. The prognostic significance of ureteral obstruction in carcinoma of the bladder. Int J Radiat Oncol Biol Phys V2:1095, 1979.
14. Yagoda A. Chemotherapy of metastatic bladder cancer. Cancer 45:1879, 1980.
15. Chun HG, Dorr FA. Systemic chemotherapy of transitional cell carcinoma of the urothelium. *In:* Cancer Chemotherapy: Investigations and Therapeutic Advances. Muggia F (Ed). Boston, Kluwer Academic Publishers, 1988, p. 151.
16. Yagoda A. Neoadjuvant chemotherapy in bladder cancer. Urology 31:9, 1988.
17. Torti FM, Harker WG. Chemotherapy of advanced transitional cell carcinoma of the uroepithelium. Cancer Chemother Pharmacol 11(Suppl):S1–S4, 1983.
18. Roemeling RV, Hrushesky WJM. Advanced transitional cell bladder cancer: A treatable disease. Semin Surg Oncol 2:76, 1986.
19. Yagoda A, Watson RC, Gonzalez-Vitale JC, et al. Cis-dichlorodiammineplatinum (II) in advanced bladder cancer. Cancer Treat Rep 60:917, 1976.
20. Yagoda A. Phase II trials with cis-dichlorodiammineplatinum (II) in the treatment of urothelial cancer. Cancer Treat Rep 63:1565, 1979.
21. Hillcoat BL, Raghavan D, Matthews J, et al. A randomized trial of cisplatin versus cisplatin plus methotrexate in advanced cancer of the urothelial tract. J Clin Oncol 7:706, 1989.
22. Turner AG. Methotrexate in advanced bladder cancer. Cancer Treat Rep 65 (Suppl 1):183, 1981.
23. Natale RB, Yagoda A, Watson RC, et al. Methotrexate. An active drug in bladder cancer. Cancer 47:1246, 1981.
24. Yagoda A. Chemotherapy of urothelial tract tumors. Cancer 60:574, 1987.
25. O'Bryan RM, Luce JK, Talley RW, et al. Phase II evaluation of adriamycin in human neoplasia. Cancer 32:18, 1973.
26. O'Bryan RM, Baker LH, Gottlieb JE, et al. Dose response evaluation of adriamycin in human neoplasia. Cancer 39:1940, 1977.
27. Fossa SD, Gudmundsen TE. Single-drug chemotherapy with 5-FU and adriamycin in metastatic bladder carcinoma. Br J Urol 53:320, 1981.
28. Knight EW, Pagand M, Hahn RG, et al. Com-

parison of 5-FU and doxorubicin in the treatment of carcinoma of the bladder. Cancer Treat Rep 67:514, 1983.

29. Weinstein SH, Schmidt JD. Doxorubicin chemotherapy in advanced transitional cell carcinoma. Urology 8:336, 1976.
30. Yagoda A, Watson RC, Whitmore WF, et al. Adriamycin in advanced urinary tract cancer. Cancer 39:279, 1977.
31. Blumenreich MS, Yagoda A, Natale RB, et al. Phase II trial of vinblastine sulfate for metastatic urothelial tract tumors. Cancer 50:435, 1982.
32. Richards B, Newling D, Fossa S, et al. Vincristine in advanced bladder cancer. A European organization for research on treatment of cancer (EORTC) phase II study. Cancer Treat Rep 67:575, 1983.
33. Smalley RV, Bartolucci AA, Hemstreet G, et al. A phase II evaluation of a 3-drug combination of cyclophosphamide, doxorubicin and 5-fluorouracil in patients with advanced bladder carcinoma or stage D prostatic carcinoma. J Urol 125:191, 1981.
34. Nissen NI, Pajak TF, Leone LA, et al. Clinical trial of VP 16-213 (NSC 141540) I.V. twice weekly in advanced neoplastic disease. Cancer 45:232, 1980.
35. Panduro J, Hansen H. Oral VP-16-213 in transitional cell carcinoma of the bladder: A phase II study. Cancer Treat Rep 65:703, 1981.
36. Qazi R, Elson P, Khandekar JD. Phase II evaluation of VM-26 in patients with metastatic transitional cell carcinoma of the urinary tract: Eastern Cooperative Oncology Group Study. Cancer Treat Rep 66:405, 1982.
37. Gad-El-Mawla N, Hamza MR, Zikri ZK, et al. Chemotherapy in invasive carcinoma of the bladder: A review of phase II trials in Egypt. Acta Oncol 28:73, 1989.
38. Gagliano RG, Stephens RL, Costanzi JJ, et al. Randomized trial of hexamethylmelamine versus 5-FU, doxorubicin, and cyclophosphamide (FAC) in advanced transitional cell bladder carcinoma: A Southwest Oncology Group Study. Cancer Treat Rep 68:1025, 1984.
39. Medical Research Council Working Party on Urological Cancer, Subgroup in Advanced Bladder Cancer. A phase II study of carboplatin in metastatic transitional cell carcinoma of the bladder. Eur J Cancer Clin Oncol 23:375, 1987.
40. Canetta R, Bragman K, Smaldone L, et al. Carboplatin: Current status and future prospects. Cancer Treat Rev 15 (Suppl B):17, 1988.
41. Kyriazis AP, Yagoda A, Kyriazis AA, et al. Response of nude mouse-grown human urothelial cancer to cis-diamminedichloroplatinum (II), diammine [1,1-cyclobutanedicarboxylato(2)-0,0'-platinum], and mitoguazone dihydrochloride. Cancer Res 45:2012, 1985.
42. Creekmore SP, Waters WB, Vogelzang NJ, et al. Antitumor activity of 24-hour CBDCA infusions in metastatic transitional cell carcinoma (meeting abstract). Proc Am Soc Clin Oncol 5:A393, 1986.
43. Gad-El-Mawla N, Hamza MR, Zikri Z, et al. Chemotherapy of advanced bladder cancer: Further phase II studies (Meeting abstract). Proc Am Soc Clin Oncol 4:109, 1985.
44. Torti FM, Shortliffe LD, Williams RD, et al. Alpha-interferon in superficial bladder cancer: A Northern California Oncology Group Study. J Clin Oncol 6:476, 1988.
45. Pizza G, Severini G, Menniti D, et al. Tumour regression after intralesional injection of interleukin 2 (IL-2) in bladder cancer. Preliminary report. Int J Cancer 34:359, 1984.
46. Merrin C, Cartagena R, Wajsman Z, et al. Chemotherapy of bladder carcinoma with cyclophosphamide and adriamycin. J Urol 114:884, 1975.
47. Yagoda A, Watson RC, Grabstald H, et al. Adriamycin and cyclophosphamide in advanced bladder cancer. Cancer Treat Rep 61:97, 1977.
48. Tannock IF, Gospodarowicz M, Evans WK. Chemotherapy for metastatic transitional carcinoma of the urinary tract: A prospective trial of methotrexate, adriamycin, and cyclophosphamide (MAC) with cis-platinum for failure. Cancer 51:216, 1983.
49. Cross RJ, Glashan RW, Humphrey CS, et al. Treatment of advanced bladder cancer with adriamycin and 5-fluorouracil. Br J Urol 48:609, 1976.
50. Martino S, Samal B, Al-Sarraf M. Phase II study of 5-fluorouracil and adriamycin in transitional cell carcinoma of the urinary tract. Cancer Treat Rep 64:161, 1980.
51. McGeorge A, Hart AJL, Rundle JSH, et al. The treatment of advanced carcinoma of the bladder with combination chemotherapy. Br J Urol 54:366, 1982.
52. Rodriguez LH, Johnson DE, Holoye PY, et al. Combination VM-26 and adriamycin for metastatic transitional cell carcinoma. Cancer Treat Rep 61:87, 1977.
53. Ahmed T, Yagoda A, Needles B, et al. Vinblastine and methotrexate for advanced bladder cancer. J Urol 133:602, 1985.
54. Sternberg JJ, Bracken RB, Handel PB, et al. Combination chemotherapy (CISCA) for ad-

vanced urinary tract carcinoma. JAMA 238:2282, 1977.
55. Schwartz S, Yagoda A, Natale RB, et al. Phase II trial of sequentially administered cisplatin, cyclophosphamide and doxorubicin for urothelial tract tumors. J Urol 130:681, 1983.
56. Kedia KR, Gibbons C, Persky L. The management of advanced bladder carcinoma. J Urol 125:655, 1981.
57. Mulder JH, Fossa SD, De Pauw M, et al. Cyclophosphamide, adriamycin and cisplatin combination chemotherapy in advanced bladder carcinoma: An EORTC phase II study. Eur J Cancer Clin Oncol 18:111, 1982.
58. Khandekar JD, Elson PJ, DeWys WD, et al. Comparative activity and toxicity of cis-diamminedichloroplatinum (DDP) and a combination of doxorubicin, cyclophosphamide, and DDP in disseminated transitional cell carcinomas of the urinary tract. J Clin Oncol 3:539, 1985.
59. Troner M, Birch R, Omura GA, et al. Phase III comparison of cisplatin alone versus cisplatin, doxorubicin and cyclophosphamide in the treatment of bladder (urothelial) cancer: A Southeastern Cancer Study Group trial. J Urol 137:660, 1987.
60. Gagliano R, Levin H, El-Bolkainy MN, et al. Adriamycin versus adriamycin plus cis-diamminedichloroplatinum (DDP) in advanced transitional cell bladder carcinoma. A Southwest Oncology Group study. Am J Clin Oncol 6:215, 1983.
61. Soloway MS, Einstein A, Corder MP, et al. A comparison of cisplatin and the combination of cisplatin and cyclophosphamide in advanced urothelial cancer. Cancer 52:767, 1983.
62. Kish JA, Ensley JF, Tapazoglou E, et al. Cisplatinum and 5-fluorouracil infusion for advanced bladder cancer (meeting abstract). Proc Annual Meeting, Am Soc Clin Oncol 7:A486, 1988.
63. Amiel J, Quintens H, Thyss A, et al. Transurethral resection (TUR) and neoadjuvant chemotherapy as primary treatment for pT2–pT4, Nx, M0 bladder cancer (meeting abstract). J Urol 139(4, part 2):269A, 1988.
64. Kaye SB, McWhinnie D, Hart A, et al. The treatment of advanced bladder cancer with methotrexate and cis-platinum—a pharmacokinetic study. Eur J Cancer Clin Oncol 20:249, 1984.
65. Carmichael J, Cornbleet MA, MacDougall RH, et al. Cis-platin and methotrexate in the treatment of transitional cell carcinoma of the urinary tract. Br J Urol 57:299, 1985.
66. Oliver RTD, Kwok HK, Highman WJ, et al. Methotrexate, cisplatin and carboplatin as single agents and in combination for metastatic bladder cancer. Br J Urol 58:31, 1986.
67. Stoter G, Splinter AW, Child JA, et al. Combination chemotherapy with cisplatin and methotrexate in advanced transitional cell cancer of the bladder. J Urol 137:663, 1987.
68. Harker WG, Meyers FJ, Freiha FS, et al. Cisplatin, methotrexate, and vinblastine (CMV): An effective chemotherapy regimen for metastatic transitional cell carcinoma of the urinary tract. A Northern California Oncology Group study. J Clin Oncol 3:1463, 1985.
69. Meyers FJ, Palmer JM, Freiha FS, et al. The fate of the bladder in patients with metastatic bladder cancer treated with cisplatin, methotrexate and vinblastine: A Northern California Oncology Group study. J Urol 134, 1118, 1985.
70. Rosenberg SJ, Williams RD. Cis-platinum, methotrexate, and vinblastine combination chemotherapy (CMV) for advanced carcinoma of the bladder and upper urinary tract. J Urol 137 (4, Part 2):157A(Abs. 216), 1987.
71. Walther PJ, Walker RA. Treatment of advanced bladder carcinoma with once-monthly methotrexate, vinblastine, and cisplatin (meeting abstract). J Urol 137 (4, Part 2):157A (Abs. 215), 1987.
72. Sternberg CN, Yagoda A, Scher HI, et al. Preliminary results of M-VAC (methotrexate, vinblastine, doxorubicin and cisplatin) for transitional cell carcinoma of the urothelium. J Urol 133:403, 1985.
73. Sternberg CN, Yagoda A, Scher HI, et al. M-VAC (methotrexate, vinblastine, doxorubicin and cisplatin) for advanced transitional cell carcinoma of the urothelium. J Urol 139:461, 1988.
74. Simon SD, Srougi M. Systemic MVAC chemotherapy for primary treatment of locally invasive transitional cell carcinoma of the bladder (TCCB): A pilot study (meeting abstract). Proc Am Soc Clin Oncol 5:111, 1986.
75. Tannock I, Gospodarowicz M, Connolly J, et al. M-VAC (methotrexate, vinblastine, doxorubicin and cisplatin) chemotherapy for transitional cell carcinoma: The Princess Margaret Hospital experience. J Urol 142:289, 1989.
76. Logothetis C, Chong C, Dexeus F, et al. Preliminary results of a prospective randomized trial comparing CISCA to MVAC chemotherapy for patients (pts) with advanced transitional cell carcinomas (TCC) of the urothe-

lium (meeting abstract). Proc Am Soc Clin Oncol 7:A517, 1988.
77. Ervin TJ, Hayes DM, Dorsk BM, et al. A pilot trial of outpatient weekly methotrexate with leucovorin, vinblastine, doxorubicin (adriamycin) and cisplatin (M-VAC-L) in stages II, III, and IV transitional cell carcinoma of the urothelium (TCC-U) (meeting abstract). Proc Annual Meeting, Am Soc Clin Oncol 8:A540, 1989.
78. Ruther U, Bauerle K, Rassweiler J, et al. Chemotherapy with MVEC in advanced carcinoma of the bladder and upper urinary tract (meeting abstract). ECCO-4. Fourth European Conference on Clinical Oncology and Cancer Nursing. Acta Oncol 27(5):465, 1988.
79. Waxman J, Abel P, James N, et al. New combination chemotherapy programme for bladder cancer. Br J Urol 63:68, 1989.
80. Gabrilove JL, Jakubowski A, Scher H, et al. Effect of granulocyte colony-stimulating factor on neutropenia and associated morbidity due to chemotherapy for transitional-cell carcinoma of the urothelium. N Engl J Med 318:1414, 1988.
81. Herr HW. Neoadjuvant chemotherapy for invasive bladder cancer. Semin Surg Oncol 5:266, 1989.
82. Scher HI, Yagoda A, Herr HW, et al. Neoadjuvant M-VAC (methotrexate, vinblastine, doxorubicin and cisplatin) effect on the primary bladder lesion. J Urol 139:470, 1988.
83. Vogelzang NJ, Chodak GW, Awan AM, et al. Neoadjuvant chemotherapy for locally invasive transitional cell carcinoma of the bladder (TCCB) (meeting abstract). Proc Am Assoc Cancer Res 28:204, 1987.
84. Miller RJ, Bahnson RR, Banner B, et al. Neoadjuvant methotrexate, vinblastine, doxorubicin, and cisplatin for locally advanced transitional cell carcinoma of the bladder. Cancer 65:207, 1990.
85. DeVries CR, Greiha FS, Torti FM. Combination CMV chemotherapy plus surgery for advanced urothelial carcinoma (meeting abstract). Proc Am Soc Clin Oncol 7:A481, 1988.
86. Raghavan D. First-line intravenous chemotherapy for invasive bladder cancer. *In:* The Management of Bladder Cancer. Raghavan D (Ed). London, Edward Arnold, 1988, p. 285.
87. Jakse G, Frommhold H. Treatment of locally advanced bladder cancer by radiotherapy and chemotherapy. *In:* Management of advanced cancer of the prostate and bladder. Smith P, Pavone-Macaluso M (Eds). New York, A. R. Liss, Inc., 1988, p. 431.
88. Shipley WU, Prout, Jr. GR, Einstein AB, et al. Treatment of invasive bladder cancer by cisplatin and irradiation in patients unsuited for surgery: A high success rate in clinical stage T2 tumours in a National Bladder Cancer Group trial. JAMA 258:931, 1987.
89. Rotman M, Macchia R, Silverstein R, et al. Treatment of advanced bladder carcinoma with irradiation and concomitant 5-fluorouracil infusion. Cancer 59:710, 1987.
90. Sauer R, Schrott KM, Dunst J, et al. Preliminary results of treatment of invasive bladder carcinoma with radiotherapy and cisplatin. Int J Radiat Oncol Biol Phys 15:871, 1988.
91. Richards B, Bastable JR, Freedman L, et al. Adjuvant chemotherapy with adriamycin and 5-fluorouracil in T_3, N_x, M_0 bladder cancer treated with radiotherapy. Brit J Urol 55:386, 1983.
92. Oliver RTD, England HR, Risdon RA, et al. Methotrexate in the treatment of metastatic and recurrent primary transitional cell carcinoma. J Urol 131:483, 1984.
93. Scher HI, Herr HW, Sternberg C, et al. Neoadjuvant chemotherapy for invasive bladder cancer: Experience with the M-VAC regimen. Br J Urol 64:250, 1990.
94. Kaufman DS, Prout, Jr. GR, Shipley WU, et al. Upfront MCV chemotherapy plus cisplatin and radiotherapy: Its efficacy in successful bladder preservation in 50 patients with invasive bladder cancer (meeting abstract). Proc Am Soc Clin Oncol 8:129, 1989.
95. Porter AT, Tester W, Pilepich M, et al. Preliminary results of the RTOG Protocol 85-12 evaluating the study of the use of combined modality therapy with organ preservation in muscle invasive carcinoma of the bladder. Int J Radiat Oncol Biol Phys 15(Suppl):212, 1988.
96. Marks LB, Kaufman DS, Prout GR Jr et al. Invasive bladder carcinoma. Preliminary report of selective bladder conservation by transurethral surgery, chemotherapy, and radiation. Int J Radiat Oncol Biol Phys 15:887, 1988.
97. Prout GR Jr. The surgical management of bladder cancer. Urol Clin North Am 3:149, 1976.
98. Marshall VF, McCarron, Jr. JP. The curability of vesical cancer: Greater now or then? Cancer Res 37:2753, 1977.
99. Montie JE, Straffon RA, Stewart BH. Radical cystectomy without radiation therapy for carcinoma of the bladder. Eur Urol 131:477, 1984.
100. Fagg SL, Dawson-Edwards P, Hughes MA, et al. Cis-diamminedichloroplatinum (DDP) as

initial treatment of invasive bladder cancer. Br J Urol 56:296, 1984.
101. Herr HW. Cis-diamminedichloride platinum II in the treatment of advanced bladder cancer. J Urol 123:853, 1980.
102. Merrin CE. Treatment of genitourinary tumors with cis-dichlorodiammineplatinum (II): Experience in 250 patients. Cancer Treat Rep. 63:9, 1979.
103. Oliver RTD, Newlands ES, Wiltshaw E, et al. A phase 2 study of cis-platinum in patients with recurrent bladder carcinoma. Br J Urol 53:444, 1981.
104. Peters PC, O'Neill MR. Cis-diamminedichloroplatinum as a therapeutic agent in metastatic transitional cell carcinoma. J Urol 123:375, 1980.
105. Oliver RTD. Methotrexate as salvage or adjunctive therapy for primary invasive carcinoma of the bladder. Cancer Treat Rep 65(Suppl 1):179, 1981.
106. Walther PJ, Williams SD, Troner M, et al. Phase II study of etoposide for carcinoma of the bladder: The Southeastern Cancer Study Group experience. Cancer Treat Rep 70:1337, 1986.
107. Al-Sarraf M, Frank J, Smith JA, et al. Phase II trial of cyclophosphamide, doxorubicin, and cisplatin (CAP) versus amsacrine in patients with transitional cell carcinoma of the urinary bladder: A Southwest Oncology Group study. Cancer Treat Rep 69:189, 1985.
108. Dexeus F, Logothetis C, Samuels M, et al. Cyclophosphamide and weekly cisplatin therapy for metastatic urothelial malignancies (Meeting abstract). Proc Am Assoc Cancer Res 27:181, 1986.
109. Williams SD, Donohue JP, Einhorn LH. Advanced bladder cancer: Therapy with cis-dichlorodiammineplatinum (II), adriamycin, and 5-fluorouracil. Cancer Treat Rep 63:1573, 1979.
110. Francini M, Veronesi A, Dal Bo V, et al. Pre-surgery chemotherapy in bladder cancer. Prog Clin Biol Res 260:585, 1988.
111. Stoter G, van Oosterom AT, Mulder JH, et al. Combination chemotherapy with cisplatin and VM-26 in advanced transitional cell carcinoma of the bladder. Eur J Cancer Clin Oncol 20:315, 1984.

Chapter 30

PROSTATE

PHILIP J. STELLA AND MILJENKO V. PILEPICH

BACKGROUND

Cancer of the prostate is the second leading cause of death from cancer in men in the United States, the first being lung cancer. Its incidence has been increasing steadily. It is not clear whether the observed rapid increase in the reported cases is related to an improvement in detection or an actual increase in the affliction rate. It is estimated that approximately 132,000 new cases occur annually and that approximately 34,000 deaths are attributed to prostate cancer (1). When observed over time, the incidence and mortality rates diverge, the mortality rate showing only a modest increase and the incidence rate increasing more rapidly (2). Analysis of the incidence of prostate cancer by stage indicates a minimal increase of cases with distant and regional disease and a steady increase of cases with localized disease. This phenomenon may be a reflection of earlier detection.

The natural history of prostate carcinoma is highly variable and unpredictable. Although, in many patients, prostate cancer can remain indolent for a number of years without significantly impacting the patient's quality of life and survival, some forms disseminate rapidly and result in early death. Therapeutic interventions are unlikely to produce significant impact in either of these two extremes of the biologic spectrum. Because carcinoma of the prostate seems to be an indolent disease in a significant proportion of patients, one of the major challenges in the management of this tumor is the identification of patients in whom the cancer is likely to exert a detrimental effect on the quality of life and survival if left untreated.

Most prostate cancers arise in the periphery of the gland, usually extending toward the center of the gland first before penetrating the prostatic capsule. Lymphatic invasion occurs commonly and usually entails involvement of the obturator nodes as the most common site, followed by the hypogastric, external iliac and presacral lymph nodes. The incidences of lymphatic invasion as well as hematogeneous metastases correlate with the degree of histologic differentiation and extent of the primary tumor (3).

CURRENT TREATMENT APPROACHES

Although less than one third of men afflicted by prostate cancer die of the disease, the disparity of the incidence and mortality rate may reflect primarily the natural history of the disease and other factors rather than the effect of treatment. Although undoubtedly the definitive modes of treatment (surgical resection and radiotherapy) do cure a proportion of patients with carcinoma of the prostate, the impact of these modalities on the mortality rate is difficult to quantify. In a proportion of patients, the disease is indolent and would not result in death even if left untreated. In others, the disease is so virulent that patients die rapidly regardless of treatment. The matter is complicated further by the advanced age of most patients with a multitude of competing and potential causes for mortality.

Localized Disease

The accepted curative (definitive) modalities in the treatments of patients with disease localized to the prostate (Stages A_2 and B) include **radical prostatectomy** and **de-**

finitive radiotherapy. Historically, the overall results in terms of disease-free survival and survival associated with these two modalities appear comparable. In a randomized VA study comparing radiotherapy versus prostatectomy, the results were suggestive of a superior outcome in surgically treated patients (4). Suboptimal design of the study and the striking difference in outcome compared to a number of other studies provoked serious doubts as to the validity of the VA study (5). As reflected in the consensus statement of the NIH conference of 1987, the available data indicate comparable outcome in patients with localized disease treated either surgically or with definitive radiotherapy (6).

Regional Disease

Patients with regional disease, with tumor penetrating through the capsule, into the seminal vesicles, and/or involving pelvic lymphatics, are generally treated with **radiotherapy.** Considerable experience has been accumulated with the use of radiotherapy in Stage C and D-1 disease. The data from Stanford indicate that approximately 60% of the patients with Stage C disease remain alive at 5 years (7). This percentage decreases to approximately 35% at 10 years and 18 percent at 15 years. These results are similar to those in the RTOG studies, although the follow-up is shorter (8).

Patients who undergo prostatectomy for apparently localized disease and are found to have transcapsular extension and involvement of the resection margins are often treated with postoperative radiotherapy. Although the impact of postoperative radiotherapy on survival remains unquantified, the incidence of local recurrence is reduced dramatically (9,10).

Metastatic Disease

Metastatic disease has traditionally been the domain of **hormonal management.** Hormonal management in carcinoma of the prostate is based on the dependency of cancer cells on androgen. Androgen deprivation may be achieved by ablation of the endocrine glands, suppression of LH release, inhibition of androgen synthesis, or inhibition of androgen action (receptors). Traditionally, **orchiectomy** and **estrogen administration** were the principal forms of hormonal manipulation; currently, there is much interest in the use of luteinizing hormone-releasing hormone (LH-RH) agonists. They seem to be as effective as estrogen and are associated with less toxicity (11).

Although hormonal manipulation produces a response in the majority of patients and some of the responses are dramatic and complete, the overwhelming majority of patients do eventually progress while on hormonal therapy. This is explained by the recognized heterogeneity of cancer cell populations, which differ in their requirements for androgen. Some are androgen dependent, some are dependent only to a limited extent, and some are independent and the source of relapse.

The treatment of hormone-refractory prostate cancer presents a major challenge to those involved in the care of these patients. Despite the fact that approximately 80% of patients with metastatic prostate cancer enjoy an objective and subjective response to first-line hormonal therapy, those who fail have an extremely poor prognosis (12).

Stimulation of androgen response in cells by adrenal androgens and/or their derivatives has been considered a potential source of failure (13). There is evidence that the androgens of adrenal origin can be converted to dehydrotestosterone and are of clinical significance. Nevertheless, it is clear that most patients will eventually progress even if their adrenal androgens are blocked, presumably because of the hormone-resistant cells rather than the adrenal androgen stimulation.

Evaluation of the various treatment options in relapsing patients is made difficult by a lack of consensus as to what represents a response, which is subject to a great divergence of opinion (14). The Memorial Sloan-Kettering criteria (at least 50% reduction in the measurable lesion) are fairly standard for solid tumors, but unfortunately exclude patients with bone only disease. The National Prostate Cancer Project (NPCP) criteria are probably the most commonly accepted; these are listed in Table 30–1 (15). In the NPCP studies, stable disease is considered a response because patients had to have evidence of progressive disease prior to going on the study. Support of this is provided by

Table 30–1. NPCP Criteria for Determination of Response to Therapy

Complete response—all of the following criteria:
1. Masses, if present, totally disappeared and no new lesions appeared.
2. Elevated acid phosphatase, if present, returned to normal.
3. Osteolytic lesions, if present, recalcified.
4. Osteoblastic lesions, if present, disappeared, with a negative bone scan.
5. If hepatomegaly is a significant indicator, there must be a complete return in liver size to normal, that is no distension below both costal margins at the xiphoid process during quiet respiration without liver movement, and normalization of all pretreatment abnormalities of liver function, including bilirubin mg % and serum glutamic oxaloacetic transaminase.
6. No significant cancer-related deterioration in weight (>10%), symptoms or performance status.
7. All complete regressions will be reviewed by a committee of 3 investigators: the protocol chairman and 2 investigators appointed by the central office. If the patient is from the protocol chairman's institution, a substitute reviewer will be appointed.

Partial response—any of criteria 1 to 4 and criteria 5 to 7:
1. Recalcification of ≥ 1 of any osteolytic lesions.
2. A reduction by 50% in the number of increased uptake areas on the bone scan.
3. Decrease of ≥ 50% in cross-sectional area of any measurable lesions.
4. If hepatomegaly is a significant indicator there must be at least a 30% reduction in liver size indicated by a change in the measurements and at least a 30% improvement of all pre-treated abnormalities of liver function, including bilirubin mg/dL and serum glutamic oxaloacetic transaminase.
5. No new sites of disease.
6. Acid phosphatase returned to normal.
7. No deterioration in weight (>10%), symptoms, or performance status.

Stable—all of the following criteria:
1. No new lesions occurred and no measurable lesions increased >25% in cross-sectional area.
2. Elevated acid phosphatase, if present, decreased, although it need not have returned to normal.
3. Osteolytic lesions, if present, did not appear to worsen.
4. Osteoblastic lesions, if present, remained stable on the bone scan.
5. Hepatomegaly, if present, did not appear to worsen >30% increase in the measurements and symptoms of hepatic abnormalities did not worsen, including bilirubin mg % and serum glutamic oxaloacetic transaminase.
6. No significant cancer-related deterioration in weight (>10%), symptoms or performance status.

Progression—any of the following criteria:
1. Significant cancer-related deterioration in weight (>10%), symptoms or performance status.
2. Appearance of new areas of malignant disease by bone scan or x-ray or in soft tissue by other appropriate techniques.
3. Increase in any previously measurable lesion by >25% in cross-sectional area.
4. Development of recurrent anemia, secondary to prostatic cancer (not chemotherapy).
5. Development of ureteral obstruction.

Note: an increase in acid or alkaline phosphatase alone is not to be considered an indication of progression. These should be used in conjunction with other criteria.

Slack et al, who reviewed the NPCP data as to the survival and found similar survival curves for both partial and stable disease patients (16). Compilation of data from a number of series indicate that a response rate of 20 to 30% can be achieved with second-line hormonal management (14). Aminoglutethimide and Estramustine have been extensively studied resulting in a response in about a quarter of the patients treated.

Recently Labrie et al championed the concept of **total androgen blockade** using LH-RH agonists (or bilateral orchiectomy) in combination with androgen-blocking agent Flutamide (17). In a Phase II study of 209 previously treated patients showing progression after orchiectomy, the addition of Flutamide to either orchiectomy or an LH-RH agonist resulted in a 6.2% complete response, 9.6% partial response, and 18.6% stable disease for a total response rate of 34.5% by NPCP standards. This figure is not substantially different from response rates noted in other studies (14). The concept of total androgen blockage (at least as first-line therapy) is supported by the recently published data by Crawford et al (18). A total of 603 patients were randomized in a double-blinded fashion to Leuprolide with or without Flutamide. On progression, patients receiving the placebo were crossed over and given Flutamide. Patients who were initially assigned to the combination and found to have progressive disease were removed from the study and treated at the discretion of the investigator. In essence, this study was testing the early versus late application of Flutamide. The response rate by NPCP criteria was similar with an overall response of 92% with the combination and 89% with Leuprolide alone. There was also no difference in complete response at 7.9 and 7.1%, respectively. The progression-free and overall survival, however, favored the combination arm. There was an advantage in progression free survival with the combination arm, (16.5 vs. 13.9 months) and also an advantage in overall survival (35.6 vs. 28.3 months; p = 0.035). These differences were particularly evident in men with minimal disease and with a good performance status. Randomized controlled studies are needed to test the use of total androgen blockade in relapse after initial hormonal therapy.

Traditionally, **chemotherapy** has been applied to patients relapsing on hormonal management. There have also been several attempts to use chemotherapy in an adjuvant fashion in patients with limited disease. Response rates for the available single agent Phase II trials in hormone-resistant prostate cancer are shown in Table 30–2. These are made up of a small number of patients in whom the response criteria are sometimes unspecified or variable. The more active agents include doxorubicin, cyclophosphamide, cisplatinum, 5-fluorouracil (5-FU), estramustine, and prednimustine. New agents such as mitoxantrone, vindesine, and VP-16 may hold some promise as well.

NPCP performed a series of studies of chemotherapy regimens in hormone resistant disease. The first two studies included a standard-treatment control arm comprised of patients treated with various palliative measures including radiation and further hormonal therapy (19,20). These two studies are important, in that patients on the standard-treatment arm did not get crossed over, thus allowing comparison of survival. Patients on Study 200 received more than 2000 cGy to the pelvis, and therefore relatively nonmyelosuppressive regimens were used. Chemotherapy was modestly better than standard care. Of the 79 responders, however, only 11 or 14% could be classified as partial or complete. Unfortunately, response did not translate into significant survival advantage over the standard treatment control arm. Other studies testing a variety of chemotherapeutic regimens failed to confirm the superiority of tested combination regimens or single agents (14,21–27).

Table 30–2. Single-agent Phase II Trials in Hormone-resistant Prostate Cancer

Drug	Eligible Patients/Responders	Response CR&PR	Stable	Improved
Doxorubicin (Adriamycin)	139/35	13	18	3
Carmustine	15/2	*	*	*
Lomustine	19/2	*	*	*
Cyclophosphamide	57/8	*	*	*
Cisplatinum	146/35	24	8	3
Estramustine	398/122	15	17	42
5-Fluorouracil	24/12	4	3	0
Hydroxyurea	130/19	15	4	0
Mithramycin	42/4	*	*	*
Mitomycin C	4/0	0	0	0
Melphalan	15/1	0	0	1
Mitoxantrone	87/32	2	30	*
Nitrogen mustard	34/12	0	0	2
Prednimustine	23/5	0	0	5
Vincristine	22/2	*	*	*
m-Amsacrine	40/10	0	10	0
Asziridinyl-Benzoquinone	36/16	*	13	3
Dihydroxy-anthracenedione	35/7	*	5	0
Hexamethylmelamine	14/0	0	0	0
Mitoguazone	48/6	6	0	0
Neocarzinostatin	14/0	0	0	0
Vindesine	27/16	5	11	0
VP-16	28/7	2	4	1

*Not stated.

The NPCP also conducted trials using **chemotherapy combined with hormonal agents** in newly diagnosed prostate cancer patients with metastatic disease (28–30). These studies had a DES/orchiectomy control arm. There was no difference in the number of responses, complete responses, or survival over orchiectomy/DES alone. Seifter and colleagues conducted a study of combination chemotherapy with cytoxan, Adriamycin, and cisplatinum before any hormonal manipulation (31). Using criteria standard for solid tumors, 7 of 21 evaluated patients enjoyed a partial remission and another 6 had stable disease. Importantly, upfront chemotherapy did not adversely affect subsequent response to hormonal therapy, with 13 of 19 (68%) responding and an additional four patients enjoying stable disease.

Androgen priming has been tested in a randomized study by Manni in which 85 patients with progressive prostate cancer refractory to orchiectomy were treated continuously with aminoglutethimide and hydrocortisone and cytoxan, Adriamycin, and 5-FU every 3 weeks and randomized to receive the synthetic androgen, fluoxymesterone, 5 mg. b.i.d. 3 days before and on the day of chemotherapy (32). There was no significant difference in response or duration of response between control and stimulation arms. Overall survival, however, favored the control arm over the stimulation arm with median survivals of 15 months versus 10 months respectively. The toxicity of the stimulation arm was significant, accounting for a high dropout rate on that particular arm.

ADJUVANT THERAPY

Adjuvant therapy has not been adequately tested in prostate cancer. In the initial Veteran's Administration Study, no survival benefit could be detected in patients with Stage I and II disease treated with 5 mg of DES after prostatectomy (33). There was, as is well known, an appreciable cardiovascular mortality associated with administration of DES, which in all likelihood counteracted the potential beneficial effects of androgen deprivation.

The Mayo Clinic experience with adjuvant hormonal manipulation in patients with Stage D-1 prostate cancer has attracted considerable interest. In a nonrandomized study, patients undergoing adjuvant bilateral orchiectomy at the time of radical prostatectomy and pelvic lymphadenoectomy enjoyed a longer freedom from progression and survival over those undergoing orchiectomy at the time of progression (34). Meyers and co-workers were able to show that ploidy status and immediate adjuvant endocrine therapy were a powerful prognostic determinator in Stage D-1 patients. Diploid patients appeared to have a significant advantage in terms of disease-free survival with the immediate endocrine treatment, whereas nondiploid patients did not fare as well.

Radiation-Hormonal Combinations

A potentially promising area of adjuvant hormonal manipulation is in patients with bulky primary tumors who are treated with definitive radiotherapy. Primary tumor size (bulk) is a powerful predictor of tumor control indefinitively irradiated patients. The use of hormonal manipulation as a means of cytoreduction in combination with radiotherapy has been under investigation over the last several years. Green tested the use of estrogen for 2 months prior to and concurrent with radiotherapy in 25 patients with bulky primary disease (35). These patients were then compared with those treated with radiotherapy alone and those who were treated after failing on estrogen. The complete response rate was recorded in 72% of the patients treated with estrogen followed by radiotherapy and 55% of those treated with radiotherapy alone.

The Radiation Therapy Oncology Group (RTOG) started testing the concept of hormonal cytoreduction as an adjuvant to definitive radiotherapy in the early 1980s. In a Phase II randomized study, megestrol was compared to the diethylstilbestrol (DES) as cytoreductive agents prior to initiation of radiotherapy and continued throughout the radiotherapy course (36). A total of 203 patients were accessioned; 197 were analyzable. Although the incidence of drug-related toxicity was significantly higher in the DES arm, there was no significant difference in the rate of tumor regression and the incidence of complete response. At 3 years, only 6.5% of evaluable patients manifested evidence of local failure.

In a subsequent Phase I-II study, a "total androgen blockage regimen" was tested as a means of cytoreduction (37). The study was conducted in 1986. Thirty-one cases were entered and 30 were analyzable. The patients had locally advanced tumors, either Stage B-2 or C. Cytoreductive regimen consisted of Zoladex (a Depot-LH-RH agonist) and Flutamide. The drugs were administered for 2 months prior to initiation of radiotherpy and during the radiotherapy course for a total duration of approximately 4 months. With a minimum follow-up of 2 years, clearance of the primary lesions (by clinical examination) was documented in 28 of 30 patients. The remaining two patients died during the first post-treatment year (of unrelated causes).

The observed primary tumor clearance rates on both RTOG cytoreduction studies appear superior to those of historical controls. A Phase III study testing the concept of hormonal cytoreduction using total androgen blockage with Zoladex and Flutamide comparing it with radiotherapy alone has recently been completed (RTOG 86-10). The data are not yet available.

Chemoradiation

Experience with the use of concomitant radiotherapy and chemotherapy with cytotoxic agents is virtually nonexistent. Some investigation has been going on in the area of hypoxic sensitizers. A pilot study using SR-2508 is being carried on at The Joint Center for Radiation Therapy in Boston. Twenty-five patients with locally advanced disease received definitive radiotherapy in conjunction with SR-2508. At 3 months, 70% of patients showed no evidence of disease clinically (Coleman, verbal communication). RTOG has recently completed a Phase II pilot trial of external beam radiation and SR-2508 in locally advanced prostate carcinomas. The results are not yet available. The regimen remains to be tested in a Phase III trial.

FUTURE DIRECTIONS

The use of chemoradiation on prostatic cancer remains untested. Drugs such as methotrexate, 5-FU and cisplatinum have been used concomitantly with radiotherapy in the treatment of bladder cancer and GI malignancies, providing data about normal (pelvic) tissue tolerance for the concommitant use of these drugs and radiotherapy. Studies testing the potential benefit of such a combined approach on tumor control and survival remain to be carried out.

REFERENCES

1. Boring CC, Squires TS, Tong T. Cancer Statistics, 1992 CA: 42:19, 1992.
2. Sondik E. Incidence, survival and mortality trends in prostate cancer. *In:* A Multidisciplinary Analysis of Controversies in the Management of Prostate Cancer. Coffey DS, Resnick MI, Dorr FA, Karr JP (Eds). New York, Plenum Press, 1988, p. 9.
3. Barzell W, Beau MA, Hilaris BS, Whitmore WF Jr. Prostatic adenocarcinoma, relationship of grade and local extent to the pattern of metastases. J Urol 118:278, 1977.
4. Paulson DF, Lin GH, Hinshow W, Stephani S, Uro-Oncology Research Group. Radical surgery versus radiotherapy for adenocarcinoma of the prostate. J Urol 128:502, 1982.
5. Pilepich MV, Bagshaw MA, Asbell SO, et al. Definitive radiotherapy in resectable (stage A_2 and B) carcinoma of the prostate—results of a national overview. Int J Radiat Oncol Biol Phys 13:659, 1987.
6. Consensus Conference. The management of clinically localized prostate cancer. JAMA 258:2727, 1987.
7. Bagshaw MA. Radiation therapy in carcinoma of the prostate: Pathology, staging and treatment. Curr Prob Cancer 12:347, 1988.
8. Pilepich MV, Krall JM, Sause WT, et al. Prognostic factors in carcinoma of the prostate—analysis of RTOG study 75-06. Int J Radiat Oncol Biol Phys 13:339, 1987.
9. Lange PH, Narayan P. Understaging and undergrading of prostate cancer: Argument for post-operative radiation as adjuvant therapy. Urology 21:113, 1983.
10. Pilepich MV, Walz BJ, Baglan RJ. Postoperative irradiation in carcinoma of the prostate. Int J Radiat Oncol Biol Phys 10:1869, 1984.
11. The Leuprolide Study Group. Leuprolide versus Diethylstilbestrol for metastatic prostate cancer. N Engl J Med 31:1281, 1984.
12. Resnick MI and Grayhack JT. Treatment of stage IV carcinoma of the prostate. Urol Clin North Am 2:141, 1975.
13. Labrie F, Dupont A, Giguère M, et al. Combination therapy with Flutamide and castration (orchiectomy or LHRH agonist): The minimal endocrine therapy in both untreated and previously treated patients. J Steroid Biochem 27:525, 1987.
14. Raghavan D. Non-hormone chemotherapy for prostate cancer: Principles of treatment and application to the testing of new drugs. Semin Oncol 15:371, 1988.

15. Loening SA, Beckley S, Brady MF, et al. Comparison of estramustine phosphate, methotrexate and cisplatinum in patients with advanced, hormone refractory prostate cancer. J Urol 129:1001, 1983.
16. Slack NH, Mittelman A, Brady MF, et al. The importance of the stable category for chemotherapy treated patients with advanced and relapsing prostate cancer. Cancer 46:2393, 1980.
17. Labrie F, Dupont A, Giguère M, et al. Benefits of combination therapy with flutamide in patients relapsing after castration. Br J Urol 61:341, 1988.
18. Crawford ED, Eisenberger MA, McLeod DG, et al. A controlled trial of leuprolide with and without flutamide in prostatic carcinoma. N Engl J Med 321:419, 1989.
19. Murphy GP, Gibbons RP, Johnson DE, et al. A comparison of estramustine phosphate and streptozotocin in patients with advanced prostatic carcinoma who have had extensive irradiation. J Urol 118:288, 1977.
20. Scott WW, Gibbons RP, Johnson DE, et al. The continued evaluation of the effects of chemotherapy in patients with advanced carcinoma of the prostate. J Urol 116:211, 1976.
21. Eisenberger MA. Chemotherapy for prostate carcinoma. NCI Monogr 7:151, 1988.
22. Loening SA, Scott WW, DeKernion J, et al. A comparison of hydroxyurea, Methyl-chloroethyl-cyclohexy-nitrosourea and cyclophsophamide in patients with advanced carcinoma of the prostate. J Urol 125:812, 1981.
23. McLeod DG, Murphy GP, Priore R. Comparison of megace, stilphostrol, megace plus DES, or streptozotocin in metastatic prostatic cancer in patients with hormonal failure and prior radiotherapy. Urology 32:431, 1988.
24. Murphy GP, Gibbons RP, Johnson DE, et al. The use of estramustine and prednimustine versus prednimustine alone in advanced metastatic prostatic cancer patients who have received prior irradiation. J Urol 121:763, 1979.
25. Schmidt JD, Scott WW, Gibbons RP, et al. Comparison of procarbazine, imidazole-carboxamide and cyclophosphamide in relapsing patients with advanced carcinoma of the prostate. J Urol 121:185, 1979.
26. Soloway MS, Beckley S, Brady MF, et al. A comparison of estramustine phosphate versus cisplatinum alone versus estramustine phosphate plus cisplatinum in patients with advanced hormone refractory prostate cancer who had had extensive irradiation to the pelvis or lumbosacral area. J Urol 129:56, 1983.
27. Soloway MS, deKernion JB, Gibbons RP, et al. Comparison of estramustine phosphate and vincristine alone or in combination for patients with advanced, hormone refractory, previously irradiated carcinoma of the prostate. J Urol 125:664, 1981.
28. Huben RP, Murphy GP. A comparison of diethylstilbestrol or orchiectomy with buserelin and with methotrexate plus diethylstilbestrol or orchiectomy in newly diagnosed patients with clinical stage D_2 cancer of the prostate. Cancer 62:1881, 1988.
29. Murphy GP, Beckley S, Brady MF, et al. Treatment of newly diagnosed metastatic prostate cancer patients with chemotherapy agents in combination with hormones versus hormones alone. Cancer 51:1264, 1983.
30. Murphy GP, Huben RP, Priore R. Results of another trial of chemotherapy with and without hormones in patients with newly diagnosed metastatic prostate cancer. Urology 28:36, 1986.
31. Seifter EJ, Bunn PA, Cohen MH, et al. A trial of combination chemotherapy followed by hormonal therapy for previously untreated metastatic carcinoma of the prostate. J Clin Oncol 4:1365, 1986.
32. Manni A, Bartholomew M, Caplan R, et al. Androgen priming and chemotherapy in advanced prostate cancer: Evaluation of determinants of clinical outcome. J Clin Oncol 6:1456, 1988.
33. Byar DP, Corle DK. Hormone therapy for prostate cancer: Results of the Veterans Administration Cooperative Urological Research Group Studies. NCI Monogr 7:165, 1988.
34. Myers RP, Therneau TM, Zincke H, Utz DC. Radical prostatectomy and the influence of early endocrine therapy for stage D, prostate cancer. Long-term follow up study. *In:* A multidisciplinary analysis of controversies in the management of prostate cancer. Coffey DS, Resnick FA, Dorr FA, Karr JR (Eds). New York, Plenum Press, 1988, p. 16.
35. Green N, Boder H, Broth E, et al. Improved control of bulky prostate carcinoma with sequential estrogen and radiation therapy. Int J Radiat Oncol Biol Phys 10:971, 1984.
36. Pilepich MV, Krall JM, John MJ, et al. Hormonal cytoreduction in locally advanced carcinoma of the prostate treated with definitive radiotherapy: Preliminary results of RTOG 83-07. Int J Radiat Oncol Biol Phys 16:813, 1989.
37. Pilepich MV, Al-Sarraf J, John MJ, et al. Phase II RTOG study of hormonal cytoreduction with flutamide and zoladex in locally advanced carcinoma of the prostate treated with definitive radiotherapy. Am J Clin Oncol 13:461, 1990.

Part IV

TOXICITY

Section A

ORGAN-SPECIFIC TOXICITY

Chapter 31

BONE MARROW TOXICITY

LOUIS S. CONSTINE III AND PHILIP RUBIN

Tumor cell killing by radiation and chemotherapy, individually and in tandem, is dose-dependent. Coincidental bone marrow injury, as reflected by a depression in peripheral blood counts, is frequently the dose-limiting toxicity because the risks for infection and bleeding increase accordingly. Strategies to protect hematopoietic progenitor cells or bone marrow stroma from therapy-induced death, or to accelerate hematopoiesis following therapy, would ideally permit more intensive treatment without the associated risks. To understand the impact of radiation and chemotherapy on the bone marrow organ, its organization and function must be considered. New insights into the complexity of this critical organ offer the potential to modulate and modify its response to cancer therapy.

STRUCTURE AND FUNCTION

The pluripotent stem cell replicates and differentiates along lymphoid or myeloid lineages through a complicated process regulated by a network of hematopoietic growth factors and cellular interactions (1,2). The cascade through myeloid differentiation leads to erythrocytes, platelets, granulocytes, and macrophages, and the lymphoid cascade to T and B cells (Fig. 31–1). Families of growth factors (or cytokines) that control these processes of replication and differentiation have been identified. The hematopoietic progenitor cells and their offspring are cradled on a stroma of endothelial cells, adventitial cells, fibroblasts, macrophages, and fat cells within the bone marrow. This microenvironment (ME) is both supportive

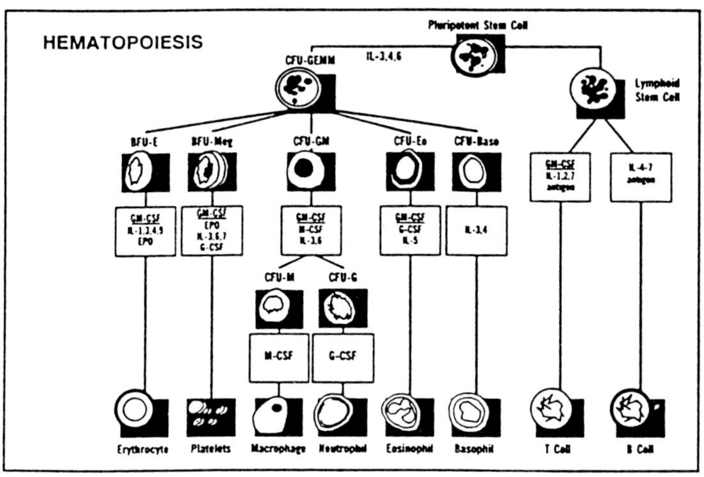

Fig. 31–1. Hematopoiesis and its regulation by growth factors. CFU-GEMM = colony-forming units for granulocytes, erythrocytes, macrophages, megakaryocytes; BFU = burst-forming units; CSF = colony-stimulating factor; IL = interleukin; EO = eosinophil; Meg = megakaryocytes; EPO = erythropoietin; Baso = basophil.

and directive in the developmental and replicative processes. Not only do the stromal elements respond to and secrete growth factors, but the geometric niches formed by the stroma maintain cell-to-cell contact of progenitors and their offspring. It is likely that lineage-specific differentiation occurs in these niches as a consequence of the biochemical milieu defined by specific extracellular matrix proteins (3).

The geographic distribution of the bone marrow is particularly relevant to understanding radiation effects. Although variations occur, the major functional sites are the pelvis and vertebrae, as depicted in a skeletal portrayal based upon semiquantitative histopathologic studies (Fig. 31–2). In addition to the pelvis and vertebrae, the ribs, sternum, skull, scapulae, and proximal portions of the femur and humerus contain virtually all of the functioning marrow (4). In children, the humerus, femur and other long bones are active, but marrow retraction from the peripheral (appendicular) toward central (axial) skeleton, and from diaphyseal to metaphyseal in individual long bones occurs (Fig. 31–3). By age 20 years, the mature adult distribution pattern is present (5).

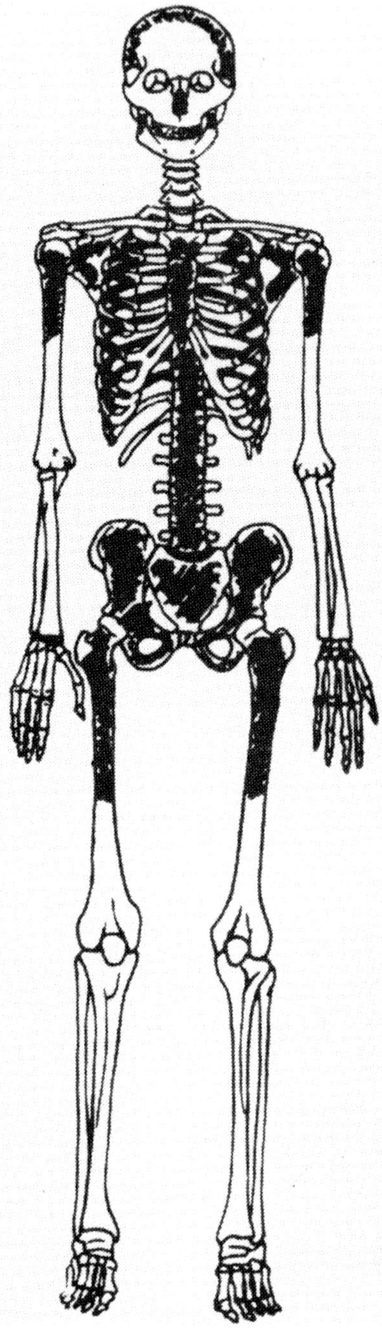

Fig. 31–2. Bone marrow distribution in adult humans as determined by autopsy findings: active regions are shaded. (From Hashimoto M. Kyushu J Med Sci 11:103, 1960.)

MECHANISMS AND ASSESSMENT OF DAMAGE

Bone marrow dysfunction in the setting of cancer therapy has several possible etiologies (6).

1. Direct injury to hematopoietic stem cells or their depletion.
2. Structural or functional damage to the stroma or microcirculation.
3. Injury to other accessory cells which have regulatory (CSF-secreting) functions.
4. Perturbation of bone marrow function by the underlying disease (e.g., leukemia).
5. An inherent defect in bone marrow stem cells associated with the underlying disease.

These various injuries translate into a disturbance in the production and release of growth factors, and in the finely tuned cell-to-cell interactions important for marrow functioning. Thus, the regulation or process of hematopoiesis is disrupted.

The acute and chronic consequences of bone marrow injury by cytotoxic therapy

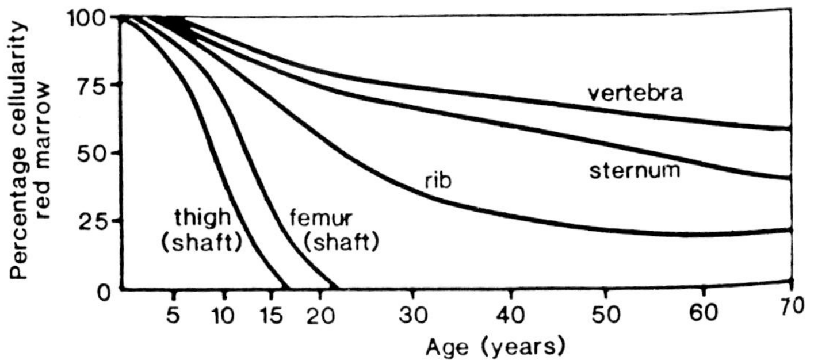

Fig. 31–3. The relative amount of red and yellow bone marrow in different anatomic sites as a function of age. (From Kricun ME. Skeletal Radiol 14:10, 1985. Modified from Custer RP, Anefedt FE. J Lab Clin Med 17:960, 1932.)

can be considered in the context of these mechanisms. However, dissecting out the most relevant variables can be difficult due to limitations in the assessment of structure and function. **Peripheral blood counts** fail to demonstrate the true extent of marrow suppression or its likelihood of tolerating additional cytotoxic therapy because of the ability for the bone marrow to transiently compensate for injury. Figure 31–4 illustrates this in children treated with chemotherapy for acute lymphoblastic leukemia. **Progenitor cell cultures** such as colony-forming units for granulocytes, macrophages (CFU-GM), burst-forming units for erythrocytes (BFU-E), colony-forming units for granulocytes, erythrocytes, macrophages, megakaryocytes (CFU-GEMM); **histopathology** (bone marrow aspirate and biopsy), **radioisotopic scanning** (^{111}In ^{52}Fe, ^{99m}Tc-sulfur colloid reflecting the myeloid, erythroid and reticuloendothelial compartments respectively); and **stromal cell cultures** such as colony-forming units for fibroblasts (CFU-F), are all used to evaluate various quantitative or functional aspects of the bone marrow but are all limited in scope. Their ability to demonstrate irradiation effects is particularly marginal because of volume and dose considerations. Small segments or large compartments of previously active marrow may become aplastic, hypoplastic, or hyperplastic, and previously quiescent areas may become active (7). Finally, chronic marrow damage from cytotoxic therapy depends on stromal or stem cell defects resulting from the underlying malignancy (e.g., leukemia) or the specific cytotoxic agents used. Normal numbers of mature hematopoietic cells probably result from an increase in stem cell cycling with amplification, and the longterm capacity for normal marrow to function or to respond to stress is not immediately apparent (8). Nevertheless, our current under-

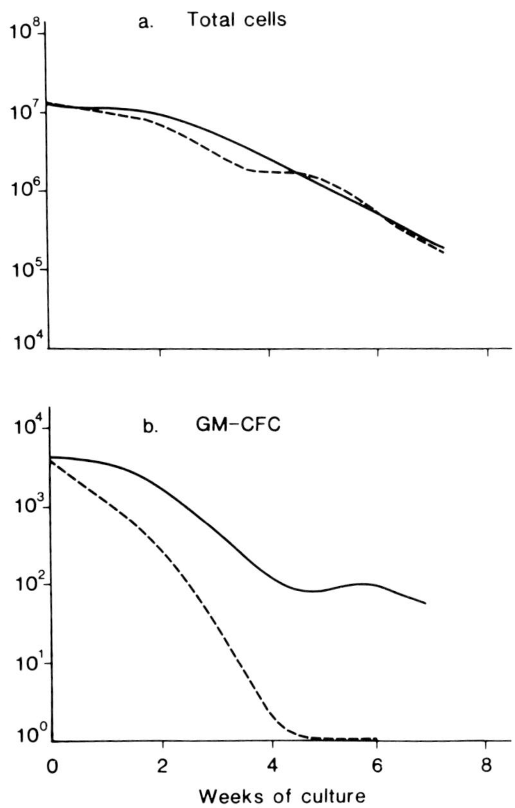

Fig. 31–4. Production of nucleated cells and of GM-CFCs in longterm bone marrow cultures from 20 children in hematological remission after treatment for ALL (dashed line) compared to nine matched controls (full line). Ordinate shows the numbers measured in suspension at the times indicated. (From Testa N, et al. Long-term bone marrow damage after treatment for acute lymphoblastic leukemia. *In:* Hematopoiesis: Long-Term Effects of Chemotherapy and Radiotherapy. Testa N, Gale R (Eds). New York, Marcel Dekker, 1988, p. 279.)

standing of bone marrow damage following cytotoxic therapy is based on the aforementioned evaluations.

MANIFESTATIONS OF TOXICITY

The acute sequelae of marrow toxicity are well known to the clinician and are only briefly noted in this chapter. Depression of each hematopoietic cell lineage translates into potential or observed difficulties for the patient. The definitions of granulocytopenia, thrombocytopenia, and anemia are all somewhat arbitrary and appropriately operational in nature.

1. **Severely granulocytopenic** (or neutropenic) patients are generally considered to be those with an absolute granulocyte count (consisting of polymorphonuclear cells and band forms) of 500/µL or less. These patients are at substantial risk for infection (9). Counts between 500/µL and 1000/µL and declining due to antineoplastic therapy are considered by most oncologists to represent moderately severe neutropenia. Most patients clinically tolerate granulocyte counts between 1000 and 1500/µL.
2. **Thrombocytopenia** has been strictly defined as a platelet count below 140,000/µL, but the manifestations of bruising, petechiae, and mucosal bleeding rarely occur with counts of 100,000/µL or above, and in fact are infrequent unless counts fall below 20,000/µL (10). Intracranial hemorrhage is particularly rare, and most episodes occur at counts less than 10,000/µL.
3. **Anemia** prompting red blood cell transfusion is even more difficult to define because various clinical judgments are used. In practice, hematocrits as low as 23 to 25% are tolerated by most patients.

Chronic marrow injury following cytotoxic therapy is poorly understood. The hematopoietic system appears to recover promptly after doses of chemotherapy and radiotherapy, as seen in Figure 31–5. However, heavily treated patients are known to have a reduced tolerance to additional therapy, showing lower nadirs of peripheral counts, particularly platelets. Although this subject is further discussed elsewhere in this chapter, decreased marrow functioning as reflected by marrow scanning after radiotherapy (11), or the CFU-GM pool after chemotherapy (12) has been demonstrated up to 5 years following therapy. Hypoplastic and myelodysplastic syndromes have been observed at late intervals, but may represent a mutagenic or carcinogenic event.

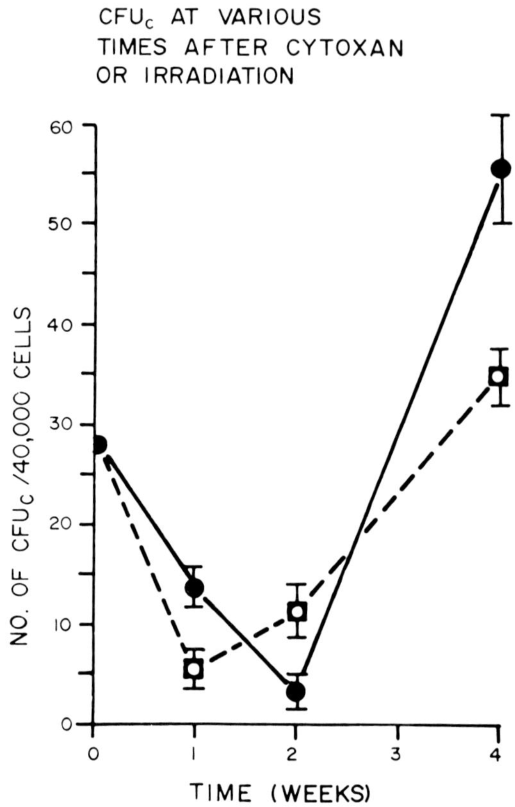

Fig. 31–5. Colony-forming units for granulocytes-macrophages at various times after radiation (open squares) or cytoxan (closed circles). (From Rubin P, Scarantino C. Int J Radiat Oncol Biol Phys 4:3, 1978, Pergamon Press Ltd.)

ACUTE TOXICITY FROM CHEMOTHERAPY

Antineoplastic drugs are selected for their toxicity to malignant cells, and concomitant bone marrow suppression is an expected side effect of most of these agents. The degree of toxicity varies according to drug type and dose (13). Table 31–1 categorizes several drugs according to their relative degrees of myelosuppression. The rate at which this marrow suppression occurs also varies. An immediate decrease in granulocytes within 48 hours can be seen after hydroxyurea. However, the depression in peripheral blood counts caused by most chemotherapeutic agents, including the alkylators and anthracyclines, is not apparent for 1 to 3 weeks due to their effect on relatively immature cells. This time course is best explained by the kinetics of cell maturation and egress from the marrow, the life span of the mature peripheral blood cells (6 hours for granulocytes, 10 to 12 days for platelets, and 120 days for erythrocytes) and the bone marrow reserve. Granulocyte counts decline prior to the platelets and anemia can take several weeks to develop. A few drugs, such as the nitrosoureas and mitomycin C, cause a count depression, which is not observed for 3 to 5 weeks. The observed thrombocytopenia is often more severe and precedes leukopenia. This rate of change also varies according to several other parameters, including the drug dose, schedule and route of administration, and concomitant or previous treatment with other drugs or irradiation (13).

Although the mechanisms by which suppression occurs are those previously listed under "Mechanisms of damage," the precise explanation for this action by each particular drug is poorly defined and not necessarily identical to its antineoplastic action. As suggested in the previous paragraph, the level of cell maturation appears to be relevant. It should be noted that much of the information available to us is derived from studies in mice. Using this model, the spleen colony-forming unit (CFU-S) is considered a stem cell, whereas the CFU-GM is a progenitor cell more committed to differentiation (granulocytes and macrophages). Alkylating agents affect both, but sublethal doses allow preservation of sufficient CFU-S for recovery (Table 31–2). Additional examples include the relative sparing of the CFU-S by 5-FU and cyclophosphamide, which thus preferen-

Table 31–1. Antineoplastic Drug Category/Agent with Relative Degree and Duration of Myelosuppression

		Myelosuppression	
Drug or Drug Class	Degree of Suppression*	Nadir (days)	Duration of Marrow Recovery (days)
Anthracycline	III	6–13	21–24
Vinca alkaloids	I–II	4–9	7–21
Mustard alkylator			
nitrogen mustard	III	7–14	28
Antifolates	III	7–14	14–21
Antipyrimidines	III	7–14	22–24
Antipurines	II	7–14	14–21
Podophyllotoxins	II	5–14	22–28
Alkylators	II	10–21	18–40
Nitrosoureas	III	26–60	35–85
Miscellaneous†			
Busulphan	III	11–30	24–54
Cisplatin	I	14	21
Dacarbazine	III	21–28	28–35
Hydroxyurea	II	7	14–21
Mithramycin	I	5–10	10–18
Mitomycin C	II	28–42	42–56
Procarbazine	II	25–36	35–50
Razoxane (ICRF)	II	11–16	12–25

*I = mild, II = moderate, III = severe (based on common dose schedules).
†Agents differing from their class of compounds.
Reprinted with permission from Hoagland HC. Semin Oncol IX(1):95, 1982.

Table 31–2. Differing Effects of Chemotherapeutic Agents on the Spleen Colony-Forming Units (CFU-S) of Mouse Bone Marrow

Drug	Self-Reproduction Capacity Immediately After Treatment (% Control)	Longterm CFU-S Numbers (% Control)
Hydroxyurea (HU)	—	100
5-Fluorouracil (5-FU)	75	100
Methotrexate (MTX)	100	100
6-Mercaptopurine (6-MP)	95	100
Cyclophosphamide (CTX)	776	96
Vinblastine (VBL)	100	85
L-Phenylalanine mustard (L-PAM)	—	65
Busulfan (BUS)	11–38	30–60
Bischlorethylnitrosourea (BCNU)	24–25	30–60

Modified from Testa N, et al. Long term bone marrow damage after cytotoxic treatment. *In:* Hematopoiesis: Long-Term Effects of Chemotherapy and Radiation. Testa N, Gale R (Eds). New York, Marcel Dekker, 1988, p. 75.

tially affect more mature cells, particularly neutrophils (14,15). Conversely, the nitrosoureas appear to damage a precursor whose maturation period is 3 to 4 weeks, and busulfan damages stem cells only when administered in high doses (16) (Table 31–2).

Other explanations including effects on regulatory cells (and thus growth factor secretion) or cell-to-cell interactions are also possible (16). For example, recent data suggest that chemotherapy may affect the erythropoietin response to anemia, causing a deregulation in the normal control of red blood cell production (17). The acute effects of drugs on hematopoietic cells may also involve mechanisms referable to cell cycling characteristics. Some agents, such as many **antimetabolites** (e.g., Ara-C, 5-FU, 5-azacytadine), are cycle phase-specific for hematopoietic progenitors, and have plateaus in their dose survival curves that differ for each agent; fractional survival after single doses ranges from 5 to 80%. The length of drug exposure also influences survival characteristics. Other drugs, including some **alkylating** agents, **antibiotics,** and m-AMSA, kill cells in all phases of the cell cycle and noncycling cells, and have exponential survival curves (18–20). Hydroxyurea directly inhibits DNA synthesis in the bone marrow (21). The importance of understanding these issues relates to the potential for reversibility of toxicity because drugs that have direct effects on blood cells but spare the microenvironment are associated with marrow recovery.

CHRONIC TOXICITY FROM CHEMOTHERAPY

Chronic marrow damage following cytotoxic therapy may be subclinical and thus not apparent until the marrow is stressed by additional therapy, or exposed to otherwise tolerable external factors. Through an increase in cycling and amplification of precursor cells, normal peripheral counts persist, thereby "hiding" such damage until depletion of stem cells occurs. However, injury to the hematopoietic progenitors can only partially explain the occurrence of chronic marrow injury. It is the interplay between these cells and the microenvironment, with its supportive and regulatory functions, that must be considered to understand potential longterm sequelae.

Damage to the stem cell compartment can be conceptualized as resulting from a permanent reduction in stem cell numbers or their intrinsic proliferative potential (12). A long-lasting depletion of cells is a characteristic effect of some chemotherapeutic agents, such as busulfan and the nitrosoureas, but not of others such as the antimetabolites and many alkylating agents. A loss of the proliferative potential of individual stem cells may be conceived of as premature senescence or aging, which impairs the stem cell compartment from endlessly repopulating the marrow. Evidence of this defect was provided by Botnick using serial transplantation experiments in a murine model; certain chemotherapeutic agents decreased the repopulating capability of the stem cells (22). This effect appears to be substantial following the use of BCNU and busulfan, but not after the use of antimetabolites. This is consistent with the preferential effect of the former drugs on the pluripotent subpopulation of stem cells that are less actively cycling, and of the latter drugs on the more mature (committed) actively proliferating subpopulation. In vivo correlates in the murine model are demonstrable, such as the development of late marrow hypoplasia after busulfan and the nitrosoureas (23).

Damage to the marrow microenvironment (ME), including its vasculature, is a critical component of chronic bone marrow injury. Conceptually, this target may be easily disrupted due to the necessity for several cell populations to appropriately interact in order to maintain the integrity of both the supportive and regulatory functions (16). The complexity and importance of such cellular interactions make the study of the ME difficult. Assays of individual cell populations, such as the CFU-F (fibroblastic-reticular precursors), are inadequate reflections of ME integrity. Other assays, such as longterm bone marrow culture systems, or ectopic hematopoiesis in implanted femora, provide additional insight. Using these systems, select drugs can be shown to cause injury, such as cyclophosphamide to the CFU-F (24), or busulfan to subcutaneously implanted femora (25). Studies in progress on the longterm effects of therapy on the stroma in allogeneic bone marrow transplant recipients should provide additional information.

Studies to date on populations of patients treated for various cancers confirm the existence of longterm injury after cytotoxic therapy (Table 31–3). For some diseases, such as acute lymphoblastic leukemia, information exists on the presence of stem cell and ME injury. In this setting, peripheral blood counts and CFU-F numbers are normal, but CFU-GMs are reduced in number although accelerated in their cycling, and the capacity of the marrow stroma to support hematopoiesis in longterm bone marrow cultures is low (26). In most other studies, only generalizations can be made (Table 31–3).

ACUTE TOXICITY FROM RADIATION THERAPY

The bone marrow is extremely radiosensitive to the degree that some injury is produced by any fractional dose. Peripheral blood cell counts acutely and progressively decrease in number due to the destruction of both mature and progenitor cells. The sequence and rate of decline (Fig. 31–6) are similar to those caused by the majority of chemotherapeutic agents, which again reflects the kinetics of bone marrow cell production, maturation, egress, and longevity, as well as the bone marrow reserve. *Lymphopenia* occurs almost immediately after even modest radiation doses because these cells are exquisitely sensitive and die in interphase. After 3000 to 4000 cGy to large bone marrow volumes, neutropenia occurs in the first week, followed by thrombocytopenia in 2 to 3 weeks and anemia in 2 to 3 months. Early recognition of this sensitivity prompted investigations to characterize the morphologic and functional consequences of marrow irradiation. Knopse et al performed animal studies with single irradiation doses and demonstrated a rapid loss of cellularity with sinusoidal dilatation (1 to 4 days), immediately followed by an increasing deposition of fat and collagen (by 14 days). By 3 months, fibrosis and fatty replacement obliterated the marrow cavity. Hematopoietic and sinusoidal regeneration occurred between 6 and 12 months only at the lower doses (27). Rubin demonstrated that, within 2 weeks following irradiation of rabbit marrow, there is a dose-related depletion of bone marrow cells (28). Studies in humans performed by Sykes et al.* actually preceded much of the animal experimentation, and revealed consistent data (29). A sequence of histologic alterations occurred due to the accumulation of radiation doses administered in successive fractions:

1. At 3 days (400 cGy*), there was a moderate decrease in nucleated cells, especially red cell and granulocyte precursors.
2. At 8 days (1000 cGy), there was dilatation of sinusoids with hemorrhage, and an absence of young hematopoietic precursors.
3. At 16 days (2000 cGy), the cellularity (nucleated) had decreased to 20%.

---

*Sykes data were obtained and presented using the original irradiation unit of R or roentgen, and not in centigray (cGy) as indicated.

Table 31–3. Observations Indicating Long-Lasting Damage to the Hematopoietic System Due to Chemotherapy

Malignancy	Drugs (Dose, Schedule)	Parameter	Type of Damage	Permanence of Damage
Gastric	Mitomycin-C	Blood count	Thrombocytopenia	Long-lasting, reversible
	Nitrosoureas BCNU or Me-CCNU	Blood count	Neutropenia, thrombocytopenia	Long-lasting
		GM-CFC in peripheral blood	Almost complete disappearance	Long-lasting
		GM-CFC in bone marrow	Reduction, severe	Long-lasting after regeneration of peripheral blood granulocytes
Brain	Me-CCNU (120 mg/m^2 q 3 wk)	Blood count	Severe myelosuppression	Long-lasting
Breast	L-Phenylalanine mustard	Bone marrow granulocyte reserve	Hypocellular marrow with reduced PMN reserve	8–21 months after cessation of chemotherapy
	Adriamycin (50 mg/m^2)+	Peripheral blood granulocytes	Decrease	6–8 months after chemotherapy
	Cyclophosphamide (500 mg/m^2) × 6 q 4 wk	GM-CFC in bone marrow	Delayed regeneration and reduced numbers	55 days after chemotherapy
		GM-CFC in peripheral blood	Reduced	For at least 5 years after chemotherapy
	Cyclophosphamide + Methotrexate + 5-Fluorouracil	GM-CFC in peripheral blood	Reduced	More than 1 year
Small-cell lung	Adriamycin + Cyclophosphamide + Vincristine q 3 wk	GM-CFC in bone marrow	Delayed regeneration	No longterm follow-up

Modified from Lohrmann H, Schremi W. Long term hematopoietic after cytotoxic drug therapy for solid tumors. *In:* Hematopoiesis: Long-term Effects of Chemotherapy and Radiation. Testa N, Gale R (Eds). New York, Marcel Dekker, 1988, p. 325.

4. At 35 days (5000 cGy—end of therapy), hypoplasia is extreme and fat has accumulated, but sinusoids are less dilated.
5. At 3 months, 50% of patients show a reappearance of the young hematopoietic cells but cellularity is still reduced.
6. At 5 to 12 months, recovery continues in some patients, but others show a second irreversible picture of marrow depression.

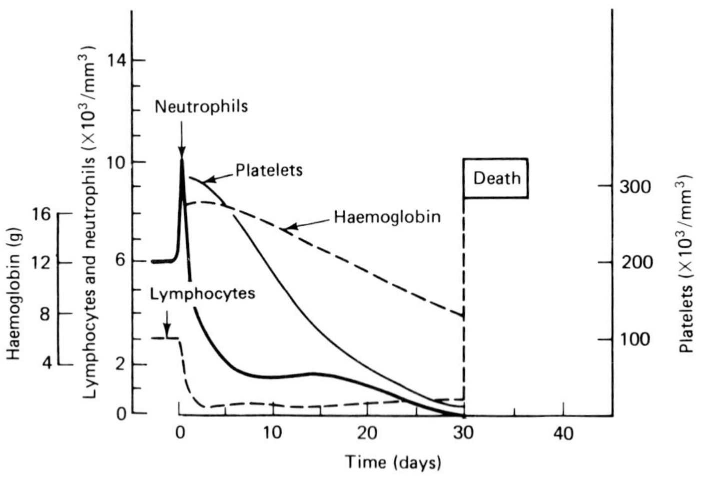

Fig. 31–6. Temporal sequence of changes in numbers of neutrophils, platelets, and lymphocytes and hemoglobin concentration, after lethal total body irradiation. (From Andrew GA. Radiat Res 7:390, 1967.)

The acute response of the marrow organ to single total body exposures provides additional insight and relevance in this era when bone marrow transplantation (BMT) is commonplace. Following total body doses of 150 to 750 cGy, a rapid depletion of vital stem cells occurs within one week (30). Death usually results from granulocytopenia and thrombocytopenia. Doses of 300 to 500 cGy result in a lethal dose (LD) of 50/100 (50% of patients dying within 100 days). Doses of 750 to 1050 cGy are associated with more frequent death rates and shorter intervals to death (31). However, these doses are well tolerated if healthy compatible marrow is infused. The microvasculature survives these doses and allows implantation and proliferation of transferred stem cells (32). Fractionated total body irradiation (TBI) doses are rarely used except in the setting of BMT when combined with chemotherapy, which precludes identification of the rate of marrow ablation due to TBI. Other clinical applications have included non-Hodgkin's lymphoma, in which 10 to 15 cGy were given two or three times weekly to total doses as high as 300 to 450 cGy and well tolerated (33). In multiple myeloma and chronic lymphocytic leukemia, similar schedules to total doses of 150 cGy caused severe thrombocytopenia, presumably due to marrow defects associated with these diseases (34,35). This assumption is supported by the data of Rubin et al. using a rabbit model in which small daily doses of 5 to 25 cGy given repeatedly to very high total doses are well tolerated, greatly exceeding the single dose of LD 50/30 (dose resulting in death of 50% of animals within 30 days) (36).

The radiation dose, dose rate, and treatment volume all affect the acute response of the bone marrow to therapy. Although the complex compensatory mechanisms of the marrow are primarily relevant to understanding chronic radiation effects (discussed in the next section), some come into play acutely. When small fields comprising only 10 to 15% of the bone marrow are irradiated, the unexposed bone marrow responds by increasing its population of progenitor cells (7,37). Often the bone marrow organ fails to regenerate the small irradiated portion of marrow because the compensatory process is able to meet the demands for hematopoiesis. Thus, acute effects are not seen. Conversely, exposures to larger but less than total body fields are associated with peripheral blood count depressions in the sequence previously noted.

Greater understanding of these phenomena is provided by studies of the effects of irradiation on the release of growth factors from the marrow stroma. In mice, the CFU-Ss decrease in the shielded areas of bone marrow soon after irradiation, probably due to stem cell differentiation and cell migration to other regions of the body. Within a few more hours, the unirradiated stem cells are triggered into proliferation. Humoral (growth) factors probably mediate these events (37,38). Bierkens et al. have reviewed the effect of in vitro irradiation on growth factor production in plateau-level stromal cultures (primarily cloned cell lines and longterm culture systems) (39). As shown in Table 31–4 irradiation can induce the appearance of locally synthesized factors, creating the appropriate biochemical milieu for replication and maturation of hematopoietic precursors (40–48). Most frequently, the measurable growth factor concentration is positively correlated with radiation dose and negatively correlated with the relative number of mature hematopoietic cells. Other explanations for the appearance of these factors include radiation-induced elimination of an inhibitory cell population of hematopoietic cells that would otherwise internalize such factors. Conflicting data on the identification of such growth factors induced by irradiation probably relate to the different cell targets and assay systems tested. The autocrine, paracrine, and endocrine effects of the release of growth factors are currently under investigation, but an endocrine effect might explain the resiliency of the bone marrow to irradiation of small or larger segments.

CHRONIC TOXICITY FROM RADIATION THERAPY

The traditional orientation of the radiation oncologist toward identifying the chronic sequelae of therapy has provided a wealth of information on these effects in the bone marrow (7,49,50). If the appropriate assay is used, residual effects of all but the lowest doses of radiation therapy can be detected; their clinical importance, however, varies according to the fascinating capacity of the

Table 31–4. Effect in Vitro Irradiation on Growth Factor Production in Plateau-Level Stromal Cultures

Culture System	Assay	Target Cell Pop* in Bioassays	Growth Factor Production* M-CSF	GM-CSF	IL-3	Meg-CSF	Novel Growth Factor	Ref
Murine LTBMCs	Agar overlay CM[a] Anti-CSF blocking RIA[b]	FBM[d]	–	+	–	+	–	40
Murine LTBMCs	Agar overlay CM[a]	FBM[d]	–	+[1]	–	–	–	41
Murine LTBMCs	Agar overlay CM[a]	FBM[d]	–	+[2]	–	–	–	42
Murine LTBMCs	Agar overlay CM[a] Anti-CSF blocking	FDC[e]	±	+	N.D.	–	–	43
Murine LTBMCs	Agar overlay CM[a]	FBM[d] FDC[e]	+	+[3]	–	–	–	44
Murine nude LTBMCs	Agar overlay	FBM[d]	–	–	–	–	–	45
Cloned SCL[c]	RIA[b]	FDC[e]	–	–	–	–	–	–
Cloned SCL[c]	Agar overlay CM[a] RIA[b]	FBM[d]	–	N.D.	N.D.	–	–	46
Cloned SCL[c]	Agar overlay CM[b] RIA[b] Northern blot hybridization	FBM[d] FDC[e]	–	N.D.	N.D.	–	+[4]	47
Cloned SCL Murine LTBMC	Agar overlay CM [a] Northern blot hybridization	FMB[d] FDC[e]	–	±[5]	N.D.	–	+[4]	48

[a]CM: condition median; [b]RIA: radioimmunoassay; [c]SCL: stromal cell line; [d]FBM: fresh bone marrow; [e]FDC: factor-dependent cell line. *No report on G-CSF.
[1]Colony morphology is described as 8% granulocytic; 80% macrophage and 12% mixed.
[2]Exact nature of CSF is not determined; relative increase of GM-colonies in agar-overlay suggest production of GM-CSF.
[3]The stimulation of GM-CSF/IL-3 dependent cell-line FDC-P1 is an indication for the presence of multi-CSF; this may be GM-CSF or IL-3.
[4]The production of a growth factor is suggested: Transforming growth factor (TGF).
[5]In D2xRII stromal clone, mRNA for GM-CFC is detected but no evidence is seen for increase after irradiation.
LTBMC = Long-term bone marrow cultures
N.D. = no data
Modified with permission from Bierkens J, et al. Eur J Haematol 43:95.

bone marrow to sense and compensate for such injury. An appreciation of the extensive communication network that apparently exists in this organ is necessary to understand the patterns of bone marrow function following radiation therapy:

1. **Regeneration** within the irradiated field
2. **Hyperactivity** in unirradiated regions
3. **Extension of function** into previously quiescent regions
4. **Extramedullary hematopoiesis**

The contrasting radiosensitivities of the bone marrow stroma and hematopoietic stem cells, and the elaboration of growth factors following irradiation, underlie the mechanisms for compensation of damage. Early investigations in mice by Fried et al demonstrated that the stromal cells supporting hematopoietic regeneration were more radioresistant than the CFU-S; single whole-body doses of 500 cGy or less did not consistently affect the ME but destroyed more than 99% of CFU-S (51). The stroma both proliferates and supports hematopoiesis, and these capacities are diverse in their radiosensitivity. Low single doses of less than 600 cGy can prevent the establishment of a stromal layer in longterm culture systems (52) and prevent stromal cell proliferation (53).

Conversely, greater than 10,000 cGy to the stroma are tolerated in terms of the ability of hematopoietic cells to adhere and produce growth factors (53,54), or support progenitor cell proliferation (53). The influence of dose fractionation and rate are also relevant because of the contrasting ability of the stromal and hematopoietic precursors to repair damage. In vitro studies by Laver provide D_0 values of 130 cGy and 115 cGy for CFU-F and CFU-GM respectively; however, the CFU-F survival curve exhibits a shoulder (n = 1.3), whereas the CFU-GM curve does not (n = 1.0) (52).* Similar D_0 values for CFU-S and other progenitors have been demonstrated by Hendry (Fig. 31–7) (55). Various survival curves have been demonstrated for the stroma, apparently dependent on the assay used (Fig. 31–8) (39). Greenberger et al. have shown the relevance of low (5 cGy/min) and high (120 cGy/min) dose rates to several parameters of marrow stromal cell support for engrafted hematopoietic stem cells (56). Conversely, the radiosensitivity of multipotential stem cells is independent of dose rate (55). The understanding of these data must await further investigation because of the demonstrated differences between the ability for marrow stroma to regenerate and repair damage when assayed in vitro versus in vivo (57,58).

A cascade of direct and indirect responses of both irradiated and unirradiated bone marrow regions underlies the patterns of marrow activity observed after therapy. On the most basic level, the individual radiosensitivities of the ME and hematopoietic stem cells determine the potential for any locally irradiated region to maintain function. On a higher level, the interactive capabilities of

*Please refer to Chapter 6 for explanation of these parameters of radiation injury.

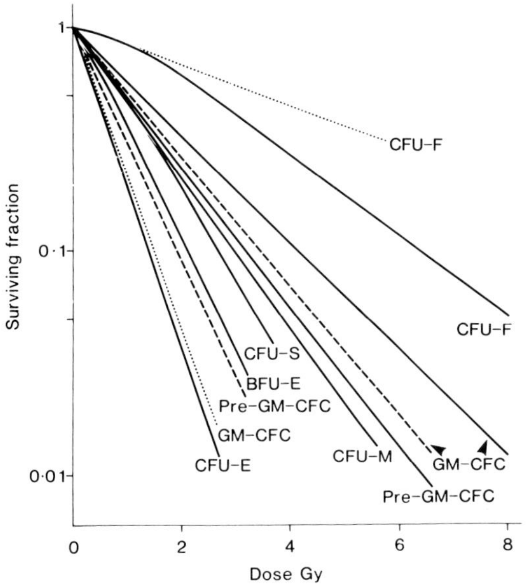

Fig. 31–7. Survival of hematopoietic and stromal progenitor cells after doses of low LET radiation (usually gamma-rays): (——) mouse; (– – –) human; (. . .) dog. CFU-F = colony-forming units for fibroblasts; GM-CFC = colony-forming units for granulocytes-macrophages; CFU-S = spleen colony forming units; BFU-E = burst-forming units for erythrocytes; CFU-M = colony-forming units for macrophages; CFU-E = colony-forming units for erythrocytes. (From Hendry J. Radiother Oncol 3:331, 1985.)

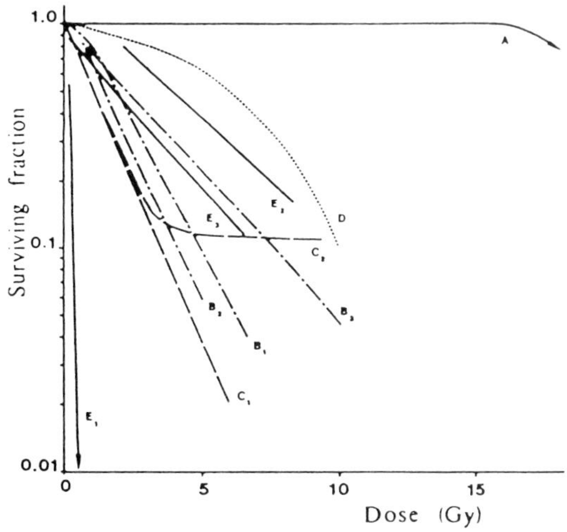

Fig. 31–8. Radiosensitivity of the marrow stroma using different assays. A: loss of sinusoids at 1 year; B1: CFU-F after in vivo irradiation (420 cGy/min.); B2: CFU-F after in vitro irradiation, B3: CFU-F after in vivo low-dose rate (1.4 cGy/min.) irradiation, C1 and C2: CFU-S in kidney implants using 400 cGy/min. and 160 cGy/min., respectively; D: CFU-S and GM-CFC and CFU-F content in subcutaneous femur implants; E1: nonadherent CFU-S in type I longterm bone marrow cultures after 7 weeks; E2 and E3: nonadherent and adherent CFU-S in type II longterm bone marrow cultures after 5 weeks. (From Bierkens J, et al. Eur J Haematol 43:95, 1989, Pergamon Press Ltd.)

treated and untreated bone marrow volumes determine the potential for the organism to sustain radiation injury. Table 31–5 is an attempt to categorize what must be a continuum of events in this regard.

1. When a small field with less than 10 to 15% of the bone marrow organ is irradiated beyond (fractionated) total doses of 3000 cGy or single doses of 2000 cGy, permanent ablation or hypoplasia occurs (24,59–61). The capacity of the unexposed bone marrow to compensate by accelerating its rate of hematopoiesis is sufficient, obviating the need for in-field regeneration.
2. When large fields of 25 to 50% of the bone marrow are irradiated, permanent ablation or hypoplasia occurs at similar dose levels as for small fields. However, the unirradiated marrow becomes hyperactive in order to meet the demands for hematopoiesis. This is best demonstrated by the failure of bone marrow to regenerate in-field after 3000 to 4000 cGy mantle irradiation for Hodgkin's disease (62–64).
3. When subtotal body volumes including 50 to 70% of the bone marrow organ are irradiated, a mosaic of events occurs to compensate for the ensuing large volume of bone marrow suppression (see Fig. 31–5). Hematopoietic activity increases in the unexposed marrow segments, followed by extension of functioning marrow into previously quiescent areas, such as the femora and humeri (11,37). Parmentier et al have shown hyperactivity in the nonirradiated bone marrow 8 to 13 years after exposure (62). Paradoxically, in-field marrow regeneration also occurs between doses of 3500 to 4000 cGy (7,11,62,64). This suggests both a capacity for the stroma to sustain high fractionated radiation doses, and for disparate bone marrow regions to respond to each other.

PATTERNS OF REGENERATION

The temporal pattern of bone marrow regeneration is variable in patient studies, and for previously noted reasons, lags behind the recovery in peripheral blood counts. Rubin studied patients treated for Hodgkin's disease with 4000 to 4500 cGy total nodal irradiation (encompassing 60 to 70% of the bone marrow) and noted depression of the WBC to 2500/μL or less in 63% of patients, and of the platelets to 50,000/μL or less in 41%. Although count recovery occurred in 1 to 2 months after completion of therapy in 90% of patients, bone marrow regeneration and recovery required a much longer time. using ^{99m}Tc-S colloid (phagocytosed by reticuloendothelial cells) as a tracer for active marrow, the sequence of alterations was as follows: full suppression of uptake in the cervicothoracic spine after mantle irradiation; then lumbar and sacroiliac suppression following completion of para-aortic and pelvic irradiation. At 6 to 12 months there was no evidence of in-field bone marrow regeneration (Fig. 31–9). At 1 to 2 years there was a gradual return of in-field bone marrow activity with 54% of the patients showing partial or complete regeneration. At 2 to 3 years

Table 31–5. Bone Marrow Regeneration (BMR) Patterns and Compensatory Mechanisms

	Regeneration			Doses (cGy)	
Techniques (Irradiation)	Exposed Bone Marrow	Unexposed Bone Marrow	Extension	Daily	Total
Small field	N	Local-regional ↑ BMR	N	200	> 4000
Large field	N	Generalized ↑ ↑ BMR	N	200	> 3000
Subtotal body	Suppressed BMR which then recovers	Generalized ↑ ↑ BMR	↑ ↑	200	4000
Total body	Active	—	N	5–10	> 100

N: None; ↑: increased activity; ↑ ↑: greatly increased activity.
Modified with permission from Rubin P. Int J Radiat Oncol Biol Phys 10:5, 1989.

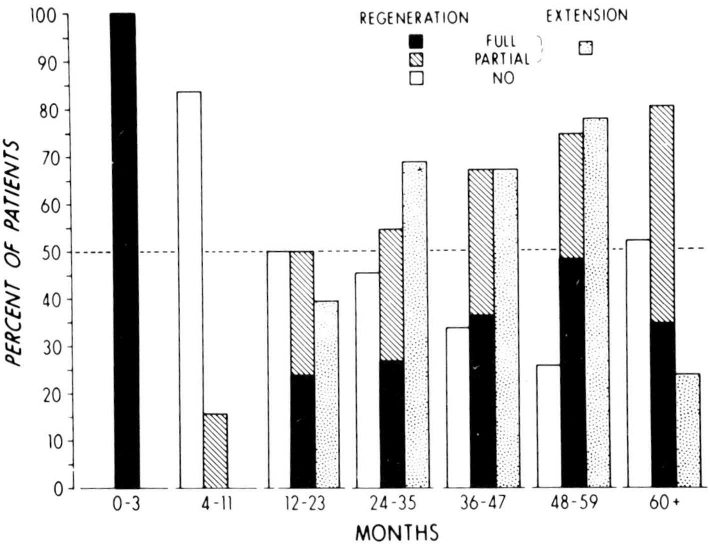

Fig. 31–9. Pattern of bone marrow regeneration and extension in Hodgkin's disease patients (after total nodal irradiation) as determined by ^{99m}Tc-S colloid. (From Rubin P, Scarantino C. Int J Radiat Oncol Biol Phys 4:3, 1978, Pergamon Press Ltd.)

66% of the irradiated sites showed regenerative activity, equally divided between partial and complete. At 4 to 5 years the rate had increased to 75%, the level at which it appeared to remain. Extension of bone marrow activity into previously quiescent regions of the femora was not seen until after 1 year. Extension was apparent in 37% of patients by 2 years, 68% by 3 years, and 77% by 5 years (7,11). Subsequently, this marrow activity appeared to decrease gradually, suggesting that the drive mechanism had abated. Presumably, endocrine effects of growth factors are involved in this scenario.

The scanning studies of Knopse et al using ^{52}Fe to trace recovery of erythropoietic marrow in irradiated lymphoma patients provide consistent findings. Regeneration was evident 2 years after 4000 to 5000 cGy in 7 of 8 patients, though 6 of 8 also showed persistent suppression in at least one irradiated field. Forty percent of patients showed extension of bone marrow into the peripheral skeleton by 12 months, whereas less extension was seen at more than 24 months (65). Although other reports attest to patient variability in the time course and degree of bone marrow regeneration and extension following irradiation, the above general patterns of regeneration hold true.

Data from animal models are consistent with the slow regenerative pattern seen in patients. Following TBI or partial body irradiation in mice, the stem cell (CFU-S) pool is reduced at 6 to 18 months, whether bone marrow samples are taken from within or at distances from the irradiated field (66). Rubin irradiated rabbits with 2000 to 3000 cGy in 200 cGy fractions and observed cortical regeneration beginning at 3 months, but not until 6 months following 4000 to 5000 cGy. Bone marrow regeneration was first seen in the cortex and along endosteum with the central marrow cavity being repopulated in a centrifugal fashion, and not randomly throughout the marrow cavity as seen after BMT (28). Data from Maloney et al. suggest that the stromal stem cell domains within the irradiated marrow cavity are reduced at these time intervals, probably reflecting damage to the microenvironment (67). Knopse et al recently performed experiments using cellulose ester membranes coated with stromal cells from bone marrow or bone and implanted intraperitoneally in mice (68). These studies show that stromal cells produce substances that can induce differentiation of early mesenchymal, prestromal cells into stromal cells that are capable of providing a ME supportive of hematopoiesis. This is consistent with the data in rabbits from Rubin and emphasizes the importance of growth factors in bone marrow regeneration.

In summary, although hematopoietic stem cells are exquisitely radiosensitive, damage to the bone marrow stroma primarily accounts for chronic radiation injury. Although such injury can be detected in vitro after less than 500 cGy, the capacity for repair in vivo appears to be great, particularly after fractionated irradiation. Marrow recovery can occur over extended periods, but this depends on the volume irradiated. Irreversible injury after doses greater than 5000 cGy is a consequence of irreparable damage to the microvasculature manifested by irrevocable bone marrow fibrosis.

TOXICITY FROM CHEMORADIATION

Therapeutic strategies for combining these modalities are based on the goal of tumor eradication, but must also take into account dose-limiting toxicities, notably marrow suppression. The observed interactions are founded on the previously discussed mechanisms for acute and chronic toxicity, but nevertheless are not entirely understood. The complexity of the interactions is nicely illustrated by the studies of Kovacs et al on the alteration in hematopoietic reserve that follows radiotherapy and different chemotherapeutic agents (69). CFU-S and CFU-GM recovery kinetics were assessed in mice in the setting of drug treatment followed by 450 cGy TBI. Treatment with Adriamycin, which affects the more primitive hematopoietic precursor cells, caused an increased radiosensitivity of the bone marrow both immediately and progressively over prolonged (and perhaps permanent) intervals. The radioenhancing effects of cyclophosphamide and 5-FU, which are more selectively harmful to relatively mature, hematopoietic cells, are seen shortly after treatment (Fig. 31–10) Cyclophosphamide, in addition, produced a prolonged stromal effect, resulting in a second, though transient, interval of increased radioenhancement.

Taken together, the data showed that the selectivity of drugs for different hematopoietic cell subpopulations determined the temporal consequences of radiation tolerance of the marrow after chemotherapy. The drugs that diminish radiation tolerance at prolonged intervals do so in a dose-dependent manner and affect the more primitive stem cells. Thus, the initial drug-induced lesion in the stem cell compartment, resulting in long-term sensitization to radiation damage, involves a major restriction (in either cell number or intrinsic proliferative potential) of the capacity for recovery from subsequent radiation insult. Hellman and Hannon also studied the effects of Adriamycin on the radiation response of murine hematopoietic stem cells (70). Although small Adriamycin doses did not alter the single dose radiation survival curve, larger doses resulted in a

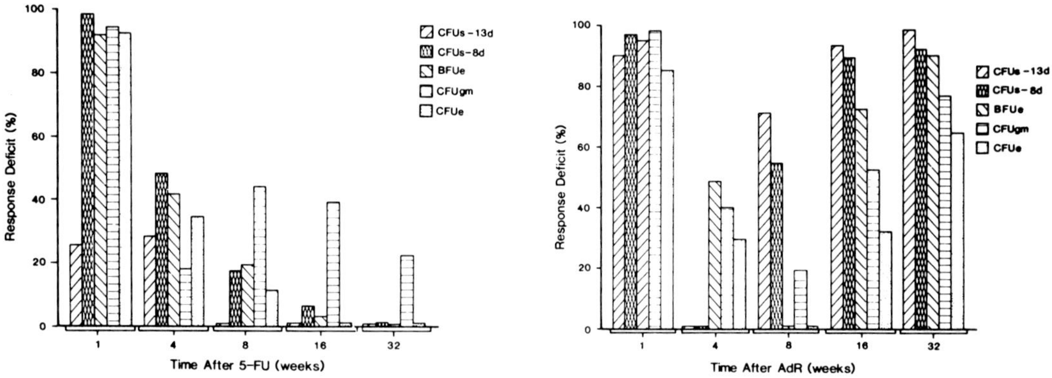

Fig. 31–10. A. Effect of a single maximum tolerated dose of 250 mg/kg 5-FU on the subsequent radiation response deficit of the hematopoietic compartments. Significance of difference between the treated and control data at each time point (0 to 28 days) used to generate the response curves was established by a Student's t-test. Each control and treated time point following 450 cGy of total body irradiation was obtained from analysis of the marrow of 5 to 10 animals. Irradiation occurred at either 1, 4, 8, 16, or 32 weeks after drug treatment. B. Effect of a single maximum tolerated dose of 10 mg/kg adriamycin on the subsequent response deficit of the hematopoietic compartments. Experimental conditions are identical to those described in (A). (From Kovacs C, et al. NCI Monogr 6:45, 1988.)

modification of the curve with disappearance of the shoulder, indicating repair inhibition. However, when fractionated radiation doses followed Adriamycin, repair was not inhibited. It was hypothesized that Adriamycin prevented the cells from entering a radiosensitive phase of the cell cycle and thus permitted the cell to benefit from sublethal damage repair. Further experiments are necessary to clarify these points.

From the standpoint of hematologic toxicity, the optimal sequencing of radiotherapy and chemotherapy would maximize the likelihood of delivering both in full doses. The cytotoxic agent that is most often associated with injury to hematopoietic stem cells or stroma would conceptually be better tolerated at the end rather than the beginning of therapy. From the previous discussions, it would appear that, depending on the chemotherapeutic agents employed, the ideal sequencing would most often be chemotherapy followed by irradiation. This is a consequence of the relatively increased radiosensitivity of less committed hematopoietic cells and stroma to irradiation. Conversely, when chemotherapeutic agents, which also preferentially damage stem cells, are used, sequencing may be less critical.

Additional considerations in this regard relate to the kinetics of cell turnover following cytotoxic therapy. Most commonly, chemotherapy is associated with a 2-to-3-week period of myelosuppression followed by a stimulation of early and more committed cells, so that the bone marrow is "turned on." Irradiation of limited volumes after chemotherapy should be well tolerated since unirradiated areas are compensating with increased cell replication. However, it might also be expected that local field irradiation followed by chemotherapy would be well tolerated. Conversely, when large field irradiation precedes chemotherapy, tolerance might be expected to be poor. This could result not only from the ablation or suppression of bone marrow segments, but the increased sensitivity of the unexposed marrow which has become hyperactive. With a greater proportion of progenitor cells cycling in the unirradiated segments as a compensatory mechanism, increased chemosensitivity is likely.

Experimental data available on this subject are sparse. Rubin and Scarantino studied rabbits treated with 1 g/m^2 cyclophosphamide preceded or followed by 1000 cGy hemibody irradiation (7). Bone marrow regeneration occurred at a slower rate than in animals treated with either modality alone, and no significant difference in CFU-GM numbers was seen at one month followed the combination in either sequence.

Clinical data are also sparse. Hreschchyshyn studied patients with ovarian cancer given melphalan before or after irradiation; preirradiation chemotherapy was marginally less toxic (Table 31–6) (71). In patients treated for Hodgkin's disease, MOPP chemotherapy is better tolerated preceding rather than following total nodal irradiation, although regimens that alternate cycles of chemotherapy and irradiation appear optimal in this regard (72). Studies of patients treated with combined irradiation and chemotherapy for bowel or small cell lung cancer simply attest to the increase in myelosuppression compared to chemotherapy alone (73–75).

The chronic toxicities that follow the combined modes would be expected to be at least additive in terms of reduction or premature senescence of the hematopoietic stem cell compartment or injury to the stroma. Data from bone marrow transplant patients treated with TBI and chemotherapy indicate progressive stem cell depletion over time, presumably resulting from an increased demand on stem cells for differentiation that takes precedence over self-renewal (49,76).

FUTURE DIRECTIONS IN MINIMIZING BONE MARROW TOXICITY

Strategies to minimize the hematologic sequelae of irradiation and chemotherapy, alone or in combination, will be built on our understanding of the mechanisms for normal marrow functioning and toxicity. A variety of avenues are possible and being tested. Some are described in greater detail in Chapter 45.

1. **Chemical agents** that protect bone marrow from cytotoxic therapy, such as WR-2721, have not shown impressive efficacy to date but continue to be explored (77,78). Biologic agents such as interleukin-1 are also under investigation in this regard (79,80).

Table 31–6. Results of Postoperative Treatment of Women with Stage III Ovarian Cancer, by Radiotherapy or Melphalan Either Alone or in Both Sequences

Regimen	No. of Patients Evaluated	Chemotherapy: WBC< 3000 or Platelets <75,000 (%)	Radiotherapy: WBC < 3000 or Platelets <75,000 (%)	Other Toxicity (%)
I	37	0 (0.0)	7 (18.9)	17
II	30	13 (43.3)	7 (23.2)	15
III	37	11 (29.7)	0 (0.0)	6
IV	38	7 (18.4)	7 (18.4)	9

Key: Regimen I = Radiation alone: Regimen II = Radiation followed by melphalan; Regimen III = Melphalan alone; Regimen IV = Melphalan followed by radiation.
Radiation dose: 2500–3000 cGy (5x/week, 4–6 weeks) to pelvis and abdomen. Supplement 2000 cGy to tumor out of pelvis and 3000 cGy to tumor in pelvis. Following chemotherapy, radiation is started 4–8 weeks after last drug treatment.
Chemotherapy: Melphalan 0.2 mg/kg/day for 5 days q. 4 weeks (x3 months).
Modified with permission from Hreschchyshyn M. NCI Monogr 42:155, 1976.

2. **Expanding the hematopoietic system** before or after therapy through the use of growth factors (e.g., IL-1, IL-3, GM-CSF) is an important approach. The stem cell reserve could be increased, or more cells could be recruited into the maturing cell compartments (81,82).
3. **Correcting stromal cell or microenvironmental damage** is likely to be the most difficult problem. Approaches that include the use of stromal growth factors or methods to effectively replace or replenish the stroma are possible avenues (83).

The bone marrow organ continues to be a fascinating and important organ for study. The possibilities of manipulating its response to therapy increase in tandem with our understanding of its behavior.

REFERENCES

1. Clark SC, Kamen R. The human hematopoietic colony-stimulating factors. Science 236:1229, 1987.
2. Sieff C. Hematopoietic growth factors. J Clin Invest 79:1549, 1987.
3. Vuillet MH, Leroy C, Parmentier C, et al. Lineage and stage-specific adhesion of human hematopoietic precursor cells (HPC) to extracellular matrices (ECM). Blood 68(Suppl):500, 1986.
4. Atkinson H. Bone marrow distribution as a factor in estimating radiation to the blood forming organs: A survey of present knowledge. J Coll Radiol Austr 6:149, 1962.
5. Custer RP, Ahlfedt FE. Studies on the structure and function of bone marrow II. Variations in cellularity in various bones with advancing years of life and their relative response to stimuli. J Lab Clin Med 17:960, 1932.
6. Gale RP. Antineoplastic chemotherapy myelosuppression: Mechanisms and new approaches (Keynote address). Exp Hematol 13:3, 1985.
7. Rubin P, Scarantino C. The bone marrow organ: The critical structure in radiation-drug interaction. Int J Radiat Oncol Biol Phys 4:3, 1978.
8. Testa N, Henry J, Molineux G. Long-term bone marrow damage in experimental systems and in patients after radiation or chemotherapy. Anticancer Res 5:101, 1985.
9. Rubin M, Hathorn J, Pizzo P. Controversies in the management of febrile neutropenic cancer patients. Cancer Invest 6:167, 1988.
10. Buchanan G. Hematologic supportive care. *In:* Principles and Practice of Pediatric Oncology. Pizzo P, Poplack D (Eds). Philadelphia, JB Lippincott, 1989, p. 823.
11. Rubin P, Landman S, Mayer E, et al. Bone marrow regeneration and extension after extended field irradiation in Hodgkin's disease. Cancer 32:699, 1973.
12. Lohrmann H, Schremi W. Long-term hemopoietic damage after cytotoxic drug therapy for solid tumors. *In:* Hematopoiesis: Long-Term Effects of Chemotherapy and Radiation. Testa N, Gale R (Eds). New York, Marcel Dekker, 1988, p. 325.
13. Gale R. Myelosuppressive effects of antineoplastic chemotherapy. *In:* Hematopoiesis: Long-Term Effects of Chemotherapy and Radiation. Testa N, Gale R (Eds). New York, Marcel Dekker, 1988, p. 63.

14. Schremi W, Lohrmann H, Anger B. Stem cell defects after cytoreductive therapy in man. Exp Hematol 13(suppl 16):31, 1985.
15. Hodgson G, Bradley T. Properties of stem cells surviving 5-fluorouracil treatment: Evidence for a pre-CFU-S cell? Nature 281:381, 1979.
16. Testa N, Hendry J, Molineux, G. Long-term bone marrow damage after cytotoxic treatment. *In:* Hematopoiesis: Long-Term Effects of Chemotherapy and Radiation. Testa N, Gale R (Eds). New York, Marcel Dekker, 1988, p. 75.
17. Miller C, Jones R, Piantadosi S, et al. Decreased erythropoietin response in patients with the anemia of cancer. N Engl J Med 322:1689, 1990.
18. Miller A, Weiner R. Long-term bone marrow damage after acute nonlymphocytic leukemia. *In:* Hematopoiesis: Long-Term Effect of Chemotherapy and Radiation. Testa N, Gale R (Eds). New York, Marcel Dekker, 1988, p. 289.
19. Marsh JC. The effects of cancer chemotherapeutic agents on normal hematopoietic precursor cells: A review. Cancer Res 36:1853, 1976.
20. Marsh JC. Correlation of hematologic toxicity of antineoplastic agents with their effects on bone marrow stem cells: Interspecies studies using an in vivo assay. Exp Hematol 13(Suppl 16):16, 1985.
21. Kennedy B, Yarbro J. Metabolic and therapeutic effects of hydroxyurea in chronic myelogenous leukemia. JAMA 195:1038, 1966.
22. Botnik LE, Hannon EC, Hellman S. Late effects of cytotoxic agents on the normal tissue of mice. Front Radiat Ther Oncol 13:36, 1979.
23. Morley A, Trainor K, Seshadri R. Chronic hypoplastic marrow failure and residual injury. Blood Cells 4:253, 1978.
24. Molineux G, Xu C, Hendry J, Testa N. A cellular analysis of long-term hematopoietic damage in mice after repeated treatment with cyclophosphamide. Cancer Chemother Pharmacol 18:11, 1986.
25. Fried N, Musseini S, Knopse W, Trobaugh F. Studies on the source of hematopoietic tissue in the marrow of subcutaneously implanted femurs. Exp Hematol 1:29, 1973.
26. Testa N, Bhavnani M, Will A, Morris-Jones P. Long-term bone marrow damage after treatment for acute lymphoblastic leukemia. *In:* Hematopoiesis: Long-term Effects of Chemotherapy and Radiation. Testa N, Gale R (Eds). New York, Marcel Dekker, 1988, p. 279.
27. Knopse W, Blom J, Crosby W. Regeneration of locally irradiated bone marrow. I. Dose dependent long-term changes in the rat, with particular emphasis upon vascular and stromal reaction. Blood 28:398, 1966.
28. Rubin P. Regeneration of bone marrow in rabbits following local, fractionated irradiation. Cancer 32:847, 1973.
29. Sykes M, Chu F, Savel H, et al. The effects of varying dosages of irradiation upon sternal marrow regeneration. Radiology 83:1084, 1964.
30. Tubiana M, Frindel E, Croizat H. Effects of radiation on bone marrow. Pathol Biol (Paris) 27:326, 1979.
31. Reactor safety study. Appendix VI. USNRC, Washington 1400 (NUREG 75/014), 1975.
32. Kim T, Khan F, Galvin J. A report of the working party: Comparison of total body irradiation techniques for bone marrow transplantation. Int J Radiat Oncol Biol Phys 6:775, 1980.
33. Carbell S, Chaffey J, Rosenthal D, et al. Results of total body irradiation in the treatment of advanced non-Hodgkin's lymphoma. Cancer 43:994, 1979.
34. Rubin P, Bennet J, Begg C, et al. The comparison of total body irradiation versus chlorambucil and prednisone for remission induction of active chronic lymphocytic leukemia: An ECOG Study. I. Total body irradiation, response and toxicity. Int J Radiat Oncol Biol Phys 7:1623, 1981.
35. Bergsagel D. Total body irradiation for myelomatosis. Br Med J ii:325, 1971.
36. Rubin P, Constine L, Scarantino C. The paradoxes in patterns of mechanisms of bone marrow regeneration after irradiation. II. Total body irradiation. Radiother Oncol 2:227, 1984.
37. Scarantino C, Rubin P, Constine L. The paradoxes in patterns and mechanism of bone marrow regeneration after irradiation. I. Different volumes and doses. Radiother Oncol 2:215, 1984.
38. Croizat H, Frindel E, Tubiana M. Abscopal effect of irradiation on hematopoietic stem cells of shielded bone marrow. Role of migration. Int J Radiat Oncol Biol Phys 30:347, 1976.
39. Bierkens J, Hendry J, Testa N. The radiation response and recovery of bone marrow stroma with particular reference to long-term bone marrow cultures. Eur J Haematol 43:95, 1989.
40. Gualtieri R, Shadduck R, Baker D, Quesenberry P. Hematopoietic regulator factors produced in long-term murine bone marrow cultures and the effect of in vitro irradiation. Blood 64:516, 1984.
41. Song Z, Quesenberry P. Radioresistant murine marrow stromal cells: A morphologic and functional characterization. Exp Hematol 12:523, 1984.

42. Naparstek E, Donnelly T, Kase K, Greenberger J. Biologic effects of in vitro X-irradiation of murine long-term bone marrow cultures on the production of granulocyte-macrophage colony-stimulating factors. Exp Hematol 13:701, 1985.
43. Alberico T, Ihle J, Liang C, et al. Stromal growth factor production in irradiated lectin exposed long-term murine bone marrow cultures. Blood 69:1120, 1987.
44. Gualtieri R. Consequences of extremely high doses of irradiation on bone marrow stromal cells and the release of hematopoietic growth factors. Exp Hematol 15:952, 1987.
45. Greenberger J, Klassen V, Kase K, et al. Effects of low dose rate irradiation on plateau phase bone marrow stromal cells in vitro: Demonstration of a new form of non-lethal, physiologic damage to support hematopoietic stem cells. Int J Radiat Oncol Biol Phys 10:1027, 1984.
46. Neparstek E, Donnelly T, Shadduk R, et al. Persistent production of colony-stimulating factor (CSF-1) by cloned bone marrow stromal cell line D2XR11 after X-irradiation. J Cell Physiol 126:407, 1986.
47. Naparstek E, Pierce J, Metcalf D, et al. Induction of growth alteration in factor-dependent hematopoietic progenitor cell lines by cocultivation with irradiated bone marrow stromal cell lines. Blood 67:1395, 1986.
48. Naparstek E, Fitzgerald T, Sakakeeny M, et al. Induction of malignant transformation of cocultivated hematopoietic stem cells by X-irradiation of murine bone marrow stromal cells in vitro. Cancer Res 46:4677, 1986.
49. Knopse W. Long-term bone marrow damage after irradiation. *In:* Hematopoiesis: Long-term Effects of Chemotherapy and Radiation. Testa N, Gale R (Eds). New York, Marcel Dekker, 1988, p. 93.
50. Parmentier C, Morardet N, Tubiana M. Long-term bone marrow damage after treatment for lymphomas. *In:* Hematopoiesis: Long-term Effects of Chemotherapy and Radiation. Testa N, Gale R (Eds). New York, Marcel Dekker, 1988, p. 301.
51. Fried W, Chamberlin W, Kedo A, Varone J. Effects of radiation on hematopoietic stroma. Exp Hematol 4:310, 1976.
52. Laver J, Ebell W, Castro-Malaspina H. Radiobiological properties of the human hematopoietic microenvironment: Contrasting sensitivities of proliferative capacity and hematopoietic function to in vitro irradiation. Blood 67:1090, 1986.
53. Zuckerman K, Rhodes R, Sparks B, Chenier B. Radioresistance of stromal cells supportive of hematopoiesis in murine long-term bone marrow cell cultures. Exp Hematol 13:372, 1985.
54. Gualtieri R, McGraw J. Bone marrow stromal cells survive mega-dose irradiation and continue to produce hematopoietic growth factor(s). Blood 66 (Suppl 1):152, 1985.
55. Hendry J. The cellular basis of long-term marrow injury after irradiation. Radiother Oncol 3:331, 1985.
56. Greenberger J, Fitzgerald T, Klassen V, et al. Alteration in hematopoietic stem cell seeding and proliferation by both high and low dose rate irradiation of bone marrow stromal cells in vitro. Int J Radiat Oncol Biol Phys 14:85, 1988.
57. Chertkov J, Drize N, Gurevitch O. Hemopoietic stromal precursors in long-term culture of bone marrow. II. Significance of initial packing for creating a hemopoietic microenvironment and maintaining stromal precursors in the culture. Exp Hematol 11:243, 1983.
58. Knopse W, Husseini S. Hematopoiesis on cellulose ester membranes (CEM). X. Effects of in vivo irradiation of stromal cells prior to application on CEM. Exp Hematol 14:975, 1986.
59. Slanina J, Musshoff K, Rahner T, Stiasny R. Long-term side effects in irradiated patients with Hodgkin's disease. Int J Radiat Oncol Biol Phys 2:1, 1977.
60. Croizat H, Frindel E, Tubiana M. Proliferative activity of stem cells in the bone marrow of mice after single and multiple irradiations (total and partial body) Int J Radiat Oncol Biol Phys 18:347, 1970.
61. Rubin P. The Franz Buschke Lecture: Late effect of chemotherapy and radiation therapy: A new hypothesis. Int J Radiat Oncol Biol Phys 10:5, 1984.
62. Parmentier C, Morardet N, Tubiana M. Late effects on human bone marrow after extended field radiotherapy. Int J Radiat Oncol Biol Phys 9:1303, 1983.
63. Morardet N, Parmentier C, Flamant R. Etude par le fer 59 des effets de la radiothérapie´ etendue des hématosarcomes sur l'érythropoièse. Biomedicine 18:228, 1973.
64. Sacks E, Goris M, Glatstein E, et al. Bone marrow regeneration following large field radiation. Influence of volume, age, dose and time. Cancer 42:1057, 1978.
65. Knopse W, Rayudu V, Cardello M, et al. Bone marrow scanning with 52 iron (^{52}Fe). Regeneration and extension of marrow after ablative doses of radiotherapy. Cancer 37:1432, 1976.
66. Croizat H, Frindel E, Tubiana M. Long term radiation effects on the bone marrow stem

cells of C3H mice. Int J Radiat Oncol Biol Phys 36:91, 1979.

67. Maloney M, Lamela R, Patt H. Decrease in hematopoietic stem cell domains as a delayed effect of x-irradiation. Int J Cell Cloning 1:206, 1983.
68. Knopse W, Husseini S, Fried W. Hematopoiesis on cellulose ester membranes. XI. Induction of new bone and a hematopoietic microenvironment by matrix factors secreted by marrow stromal cells. Blood 74:66, 1989.
69. Kovacs C, Evans M, Hooker J, Johnke R. Long-term consequences of chemotherapeutic agents on hematopoiesis: Development of altered radiation tolerance. NCI Monogr 6:45, 1988.
70. Hellman S, Hannon E. Effects of adriamycin on the radiation response of murine hematopoietic stem cells. Rad Res 67:162, 1976.
71. Hreschchyshyn M. Results of the Gynecologic Oncology Group trials on ovarian cancer: A preliminary report. *In:* Symposium on Ovarian Carcinoma. NCI Monogr 42:155, 1976.
72. Hoppe R, Portlock C, Glatstein E, et al. Alternating chemotherapy and irradiation in the treatment of advanced Hodgkin's disease. Cancer 43:472, 1979.
73. Sugarbaker P, Gianola F, Barofsky I, et al. 5-Fluorouracil chemotherapy and pelvic radiation in the treatment of large bowel cancer. Cancer 58:826, 1986.
74. Abrams R, Lichter A, Bromer R, et al. The hematopoietic toxicity of regional radiation therapy. Correlations for combined modality therapy with systemic chemotherapy. Cancer 55:1429, 1985.
75. Lee J, Umsawasdi T, Dhingra H, et al. Effects of brain irradiation and chemotherapy on myelosuppression in small-cell lung cancer. J Clin Oncol 4:1615, 1986.
76. Siminovitch L, Till J, McCulloch E. Decline in colony-forming ability of marrow cells subjected to serial transplantation into irradiated mice. J Cell Comp Physiol 64:23, 1964.
77. Constine L, Zagars G, Rubin P, Kligerman M. Protection by WR-2721 of human bone marrow function following irradiation. Int J Radiat Oncol Biol Phys 12:1505, 1986.
78. Glover D, Glick J, Weiler C, et al. Phase I/II trials of WR2721 and Cis-platinum. Int J Radiat Oncol Biol Phys 12:1509, 1986.
79. Neta R, Douches S, Oppenheim J. Interleukin-1 is a radioprotector. J Immunol 136:2483, 1986.
80. Constine LS, Harwell S, Kong P, et al. Interleukin 1 alpha stimulates hemopoiesis but not tumor cell proliferation and protects mice from lethal total body irradiation. Int J Radiat Oncol Biol Phys 20:447, 1991.
81. Appelbaum F. The clinical use of hematopoietic growth factors. Semin Hematol 26(Suppl):7, 1989.
82. Metcalf D. The colony stimulating factors. Discovery development and clinical applications. Cancer 65:2185, 1990.
83. Dexter T. Recent advances in the knowledge of the hemopoietic system. Possible ways of correcting long-term damage. *In:* Hematopoiesis: Long-term Effects of Chemotherapy and Radiation. Testa N, Gale R (Eds). New York, Marcel Dekker, 1988, p. 389, 1988.
84. Hoagland HC. Hematologic complications of cancer chemotherapy. Semin Oncol IX(1):95, 1982.
85. Hashimoto M. The distribution of active marrow in the bones of the normal adult. Kyushu J Med Sci 11:103, 1960.
86. Andrew GA. Radiation accidents and their management. Radiat Res 7(Suppl):390, 1967.

Chapter 32

GASTROINTESTINAL TOXICITY

LEONARD L. GUNDERSON, JAMES A. MARTENSON, JR. AND STEPHEN R. SMALLEY

The intent of this chapter is to evaluate acute and chronic gastrointestinal (GI) tolerance as a function of treatment with irradiation alone or in combination with chemotherapy. During the past two decades, the use of aggressive combinations of radiation and chemotherapy has increased for both thoracic and abdominal malignancies. For many abdominal malignancies, the stomach and small intestine are the dose-limiting structures in such treatment combinations. When an organ is involved by malignancy, the exact influence of treatment on tolerance is difficult to define. If a locally advanced tumor has altered the structural integrity of its host organ, subsequent control of tumor by aggressive treatment combinations may result in a dysfunctional organ. Also, recurrent tumor can cause the same signs and symptoms as treatment-related complications. As we attempt to place organ tolerance into perspective, it should be noted that a higher incidence of complications is usually acceptable in cases in which an organ is involved by tumor than with cases where it is not involved by disease. Similarly, more complications are acceptable when unresectable disease is present than when all known disease has been resected.

ESOPHAGUS

The tolerance of the esophagus to irradiation alone or in combination with chemotherapy is often difficult to interpret from available human and animal data (1). Most relevant data are found in patients irradiated for lung cancer (organ uninvolved) or esophageal cancer (organ involved). Survival is limited in both of these patient populations, and therefore the number of patients at risk for late complications is small. Because reported complication rates often use the original patient population as the denominator, the risk of serious toxicity is often underestimated for a given point in time. With esophageal cancers, treatment-related toxicity may be difficult to distinguish from effects of the primary tumor (2,3). For example, 67% of patients in a Princess Margaret Hospital (PMH) series developed a stricture following irradiation (3). Persistent or recurrent tumor was clinically considered to be the cause of stricture in 73%, and the remaining 27% were felt to be due to benign causes. Autopsies were subsequently performed in five patients assumed to have benign stricture by clinical criterion (including negative endoscopic biopsy). Recurrent tumor was found at the site of stricture in four of the five patients. The authors estimated that postradiation esophageal stricture is due to persistent or recurrent tumor in 95% of irradiated patients.

The incidence of severe acute esophagitis in patients irradiated for esophageal cancer is generally less than 10% (4–6) (Table 32–1). The addition of a variety of chemotherapeutic agents has *not* resulted in an obvious increase in severe acute or late complications (6–12), with the possible exception of the Harvard-New England Deaconess experience with continuous infusion 5-fluorouracil (5-FU) (11) (Table 32–1). However, as noted above, the rate of esophageal complication rates reported in esophageal cancer

Table 32–1. Acute And Late Toxicity In Esophageal Cancer Patients Treated By Radiation Therapy ± Chemotherapy

Author (No.)	Institution	Number of Patients	Radiation Dose (Gy)	Fraction Size (Gy)	Chemotherapy	Number With Acute Esophagitis* (%)	Late Esophageal Complication** (#, %)
Elkon, et al (4)	Rush Presbyterian–St. Luke's Hospital	55[§§]	Variable	Not stated	None	None noted	3 (5)
Langer, et al (5)	Massachusetts General Hospital	46	50–69	1.8	None	4 (9)	9 (20)
Richmond, et al (6)	Henry Ford Hospital	17	40–60	2–2.5	None	None noted	2 (12)
		25	56–60	2–2.5	5-FU, CDDP	None noted	1 (4)
Keane, et al (7)	Princess Margaret Hospital	35	25–50	2.5	5-FU, Mito-C	None noted	8 (23)
Marcial, et al (8)	Radiation Therapy Oncology Group	25[†]	50	2.5	VCR BLEO MTX 5-FU FA	2 (8)	None noted
John, et al (9)	UCSF-Fresno	30	50.4	1.80	5-FU, CDDP, Mito-C MTX, FA	2 (7)	2 (7)
Byfield, et al (10)	University of California, San Diego	6	50–60	2.5	5-FU	0 (0)[††]	None noted
Lokich, et al (11)	Harvard New England Deaconess	12	44–69	1.8–2.0	5-FU	2 (17)	4 (57)[§]

Abbreviations: 5-FU, 5-fluorouracil; Mito-C, mitomycin-C; CDDP, cisplatinum; VCR, vincristine; BLEO, bleomycin; MTX, methotrexate; FA, folinic acid.
*Includes esophagitis described as "severe" or of sufficient intensity to require treatment interruption.
**Includes stenosis, fistula, perforation, bleeding.
§Only 7 patients at risk for late esophageal complications.
§§Number of patients treated for cure.
†Number of patients evaluable for toxicity.
††One patient complained of esophageal pain.
Modified from Gunderson LL, Martenson JA. Front Radiat Ther Oncol 23:277, 1989.

literature must be interpreted with caution because it is not always possible to distinguish between tumor and treatment-related toxicity.

Incidental Esophageal Toxicity

The normal esophagus is usually within the irradiation field of lung cancer patients. When conventional treatment fractions are used, acute esophagitis is almost always observed after 2000 to 4000 cGy (13). When total doses do not exceed 4500 cGy, severe esophagitis is rare, and symptoms usually resolve in 7 to 10 days (13,14) (Table 32–2).

Chronic injury resulting in esophageal stricture is rare following doses ≤ 4500 cGy in the treatment of lung cancer (14) (Table 32–2). In a Mallinkrodt series, the risk of clinically significant chronic esophageal damage is appreciably increased above doses of 6000 cGy (13) (Fig. 32–1) The only long-term chronic problem that occurred at < 6000 cGy was due to a short time-dose fractionation scheme.

Chemotherapeutic agents can significantly alter the tolerance of irradiated normal esophagus (15–17). The incidence of severe esophagitis was 20 to 50% in a series of lung cancer patients treated at the Mayo Clinic

Table 32–2. Incidence of Severe Acute and Chronic Esophageal Complications in Lung Cancer Patients Treated on RTOG 73-01

Esophageal Dose* (cGy)	Number of Patients	Incidence of Severe Acute Esophagitis (%)	Incidence of Esophageal Stricture (%)
2500	93	1	0
4000–4500	272	1–3	0–1

*Estimate, based on upper limit of dose to spinal cord.
Adapted with permission from Perez C, et al. Cancer 45:2744, 1980.

with a combination of irradiation, cyclophosphamide, Adriamycin, cisplatinum, and bleomycin. The dose of bleomycin had a direct relationship to the risk of esophagitis (17) (Table 32–3). Other agents that appear to increase acute radiation esophagitis include actinomycin D, and vinblastine (15,16) (Table 32–3).

Summary

In summary, doses of 4500 to 6000 cGy in standard fractionation, alone or in combination with chemotherapy, usually result in acceptable chronic tolerance of the normal esophagus. When chemotherapy is combined with irradiation, the incidence of acute esophagitis may increase. Bleomycin, Actinomycin D, vinblastine, and infusion 5-FU have each been implicated in this regard.

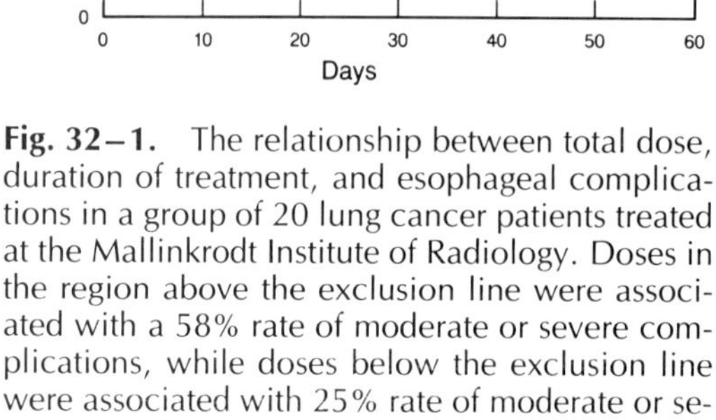

Fig. 32–1. The relationship between total dose, duration of treatment, and esophageal complications in a group of 20 lung cancer patients treated at the Mallinkrodt Institute of Radiology. Doses in the region above the exclusion line were associated with a 58% rate of moderate or severe complications, while doses below the exclusion line were associated with 25% rate of moderate or severe complications. (Adapted from Seaman WB, Ackerman LV. Radiology 68:534, 1957. The ordinate was modified to account for a conversion from roentgens, in the original figure, to cGy in the above figure. The exclusion line was not present in the original figure.)

STOMACH

In a Massachusetts General Hospital (MGH) series, a group of 46 patients with gastric cancer were irradiated (18). In most patients, the irradiated stomach was uninvolved by gross malignancy after the gastric lesion had been resected, but in 13, the lesion was not resected. The entire stomach or remaining stomach was usually included to a minimum dose of 4500 cGy in 25 fractions over 5 weeks, and portions of the stomach were sometimes included within a reduced field to 5040 to 5220 cGy. Most patients were treated with 10 MV photons with parallel-opposed fields. Forty of 46 patients received chemotherapy in conjunction with their irradiation. From a chronic toxicity standpoint, 34 patients were at risk ≧ 12 months and 25 at risk ≧ 18 months. There was no evidence of chronic injury to either stomach or liver in this series of patients.

In a Mayo Clinic phase I/II tolerance study of multiple daily fractions ± 5-FU for gastric carcinoma, an attempt was made to combine two fractions of irradiation per day with 5-FU (19). Both 165 cGy per fraction and 150 cGy per fraction were intolerable from an acute GI endpoint. Patients had prolongation of acute symptoms persisting for as long as 2 to 4 weeks after completion of combined modality treatment. Normally, with 1 fraction of 180 cGy per day plus 3 days of 5-FU (500 $mg/m^2/d$) during weeks 1 ± 5, most acute GI symptoms ameliorate within several days to a week of completion of treatment. In an occasional patient, the second sequence of

Table 32–3. Incidence of Radiation Esophagitis in Lung Cancer Patients Treatment with and without Chemotherapy

Institution (Ref. No.)	Number of Pts.	Radiation Dose*	Fraction Size*	Chemotherapy	Esophagitis (%)	Comments
Eastern Solid	115	5000 R	200 R	None	17 (15)	3-arm randomized prospective study
Tumor Group (15)	113	5000 R	200 R	5-FU	15 (13)	
	114	5000 R	200 R	Actinomycin-D	24 (21)	
British Columbia	93	4000 cGy	500 cGy	None	13 (14)	Choice of treatment made by date of birth
Cancer Institute (16)	101	4000 cGy	500 cGy	Vinblastine	30 (30)	
Mayo Clinic (17)	12	4000 cGy	400 cGy	CAP-BLEO	8† (67)	Bleomycin dose 10 units twice weekly
	10	4000 cGy	400 cGy	CAP-BLEO	6† (60)	Bleomycin dose 5 units twice weekly

Abbreviations: R, Roentgens; cGy, centigray; 5-FU, 5-fluorouracil; CAP-BLEO, cyclophosphamide, Adriamycin, platinum, bleomycin
*R, Roentgen is the original unit of radiation; 1 R ≈ 0.9 rad ≈ 0.9 centigray
†Severe or life-threatening toxicity was observed in 6/12 (50%) patients with bleomycin dose of 10 units twice weekly and only 2/10 (20%) patients with a bleomycin dose of 5 units twice weekly.
Modified with permission from Gunderson LL and Martenson JA. Front Rad Ther Oncol 23:277, 1989.

5-FU during the last week of irradiation can increase the severity as well as duration of GI toxicity. When two fractions of 150 cGy per day were given without 5-FU, tolerance was improved and was more comparable to one fraction of 180 cGy plus 5-FU.

Incidental Gastric Toxicity

The classic data on gastric injury were reported in the Walter Reed testicular cancer experience (20) (Table 32–4). The treatment technique was usually one field per day with doses delivered over 3 to 4 weeks with 1 MV supervoltage machine. In view of the use of low kilovoltage, short time dose fractionation schemas, and one field per day treatments, tolerance data generated from that series is not very applicable to modern treatment techniques.

With higher energy supervoltage machines and standard fractionation of 180 to 200 cGy per fraction five days per week, most data suggest that the TD 5/5 * for stomach is probably 4500 to 5000 cGy. A small segment of the stomach is invariably included within a para-aortic irradiation field in hundreds of patients treated for cervical and testicular cancers. The chronic risk of gastric toxicity varied from 0 to 8% with total doses varying from 4000 to 5500 cGy at 180 to 200 cGy per fraction (21,22). In

*TD 5/5 = tolerance dose of irradiation that will result in ≤ 5% risk of severe toxicity at 5 years [based on standard daily fraction size of 180 to 200 cGy]

Table 32–4. Radiation-Induced Gastric Injury, Walter Reed data*

	2500–3400 R	3500–4400 R	4500–5400 R	5500–6400 R
Total Cases	15	32	61	22
% with problems	20	25	50	63
% Dyspepsia	13	3	2	—
% Gastritis	—	21	21	32
% Ulcer	7	—	15	14
% Ulcer & perforation or obstruction	—	—	11	18

*Radiation usually given over 3–4 weeks (short fractionation schemes) with low kv (≤ 1 MeV); treatment of 1 field/day.
R, Roentgen; former unit of radiation dose; 1 R ≈ 0.9 rad ≈ 0.9 cGy
Modified with permission from Roswit B, et al. Front Radiat Oncol 6:160, 1972.

series with doses ≤ 5000 cGy, the incidence of reported gastric problems has been 0 to 2% (22).

A good analysis of gastric and duodenal tolerance exists in biliary duct data from Buskirk and others from the Mayo Clinic (23,24). For locally unresectable or residual biliary cancer, three aggressive treatment regimens were utilized: (1) external irradiation alone or combined with 5-FU, 4500 cGy/25 fractions in 5 weeks to a tumor/nodal field with a reduced field boost for 1000 to 2000 cGy fractions; (2) and (3) Similar external beam irradiation to a tumor nodal field combined with a boost with intraoperative radiotherapy (IORT), either with electrons or brachytherapy. Distal stomach and the duodenal C-loop are usually included to 4500 cGy (23). With brachytherapy, patients received a dose of 1500 to 2500 cGy which was usually calculated at a 1 cm radius from the transcatheter iridium. A dose versus complications analysis was performed in patients who received external alone or external combined with IORT electrons (with IORT, one could exclude the duodenum and stomach). With external doses ≤ 5500 cGy to the duodenum and/or stomach, the risk of severe GI complications varied from 5 to 10%, depending on what parameter was evaluated. At ≥ 5500 cGy, 180 cGy fractions/5 days a week, 33% of patients developed severe problems. In patients who received external irradiation plus iridium, the dose to the external field was limited to 5040 cGy, but most received an additional radiation dose to the duodenum and/or stomach from the iridium boost (higher doses with distal lesions). There was a 30 to 40% incidence of severe complications in the duodenum or stomach in this group of patients.

Summary

With 180 cGy fractions and 6 to 10+ MV photons, one can safely treat all or most of the stomach to a dose of 4500 to 5000 cGy with a 5 to 10% risk of severe radiation damage. If doses exceed 5500 cGy, the incidence of severe complications rises sharply to 30 to 40%, suggesting a steep dose response tolerance curve for stomach with or without the duodenum. While patients usually have acceptable acute tolerance with 5-FU and one daily fraction of irradiation, an occasional patient has prolongation of acute symptoms when a second 3-day sequence of 5-FU is given during the last week of irradiation. When bolus 5-FU is combined with twice-daily fractions of 150 to 165 cGy, tolerance is unacceptable.

SMALL INTESTINE

Data regarding the effect of irradiation, chemotherapy, or chemoradiation on small bowel involved by carcinoma are unavailable in view of the rarity of such tumors. Therefore, in this section, discussion is related to the incidental effects of irradiation alone and chemoradiation on normal small bowel.

Radiation Alone

When parallel opposed fields are used for postoperative irradiation of rectal cancer instead of four-field techniques, the incidence of small bowel obstruction requiring reoperation nearly doubles when compared with surgery alone (25) (Table 32–5). With multiple field techniques, the risk of small bowel obstruction is equivalent to surgery alone, although reoperation in the irradiated group

Table 32–5. Incidence of Small Bowel Obstruction in Relation to Radiation Field Design in Postoperative Pelvic Irradiation for Rectal Cancer

	M.D. Anderson* %	LDS Hospital* %	Massachusetts General† %
Operation alone	5	—	5
Operation + postoperative RT	10–12**	10	4

RT Technique: *AP:PA; †AP:PA and laterals.
**Original incidence of 17.5% was reduced to 10–12% by reduction of superior field extent
(From Gunderson LL, et al. Int J Radiat Oncol Biol Phys 11:1379, 1985, Pergamon Press Ltd.)

will predictably be more difficult. When small bowel series are obtained with cross-table lateral views, a moderate amount of anteriorly located small intestine may be observed, and much of it can be excluded if lateral fields are used as a component of treatment (25,26). Because complications from radiation have a volume/dose relationship for most tissues and organs, multiple field treatment techniques to decrease the volume of irradiated small bowel should be used whenever feasible.

If postoperative irradiation is used in an adjuvant setting for colon cancer, multiple field techniques can rarely be used to decrease the volume of irradiated small bowel. Commonly obtained preoperative diagnostic studies do not allow adequate reconstruction of the target volume, which could result in a more limited treatment field (barium enema plus pathologic findings reconstruct only cephalocaudal tumor extent; routine use of preoperative CT would not be cost-effective). In the publication by Duttenhaver et al (27), 80 patients with colon cancer were treated in an adjuvant setting at MGH with the same dose criteria that were used as in the MGH rectal series (4500 cGy/25 fractions/5 weeks to a tumor ± nodal field, 5040 cGy within boost volume). By using the specialized technique of decubitus position during a portion of the treatment course, they often obtained a shift of small bowel and decreased volume within irradiation fields when compared with a more standard supine treatment position. In that series, morbidity was analyzed as a function of the degree of shift of small bowel. Five of 80 patients developed severe morbidity, but only two (2.5%) required operative intervention.

An excellent analysis of dose-volume relationship regarding small bowel complications was performed by Gallagher et al (26). The volume of small bowel within radiation fields was reconstructed for a variety of irradiated sites. Patients who had no prior surgery or a pelvic operation other than abdominoperineal resection, had substantially less volume of small bowel within irradiated fields than those who had abdominoperineal resection. Moderate to marked differences occurred with AP:PA versus four field techniques and some advantage was found to treating patients in a prone position with external compression and bladder distention. Dose and volume had a relationship to both acute and chronic effects. Five patients subsequently developed small bowel obstruction (none of 75 with no previous pelvic surgery, 3 of 25 (12%) with abdominoperineal resection, and 2 of 50 (4%) with other pelvic operations).

Chemoradiation

Because standard treatment for rectal cancer has evolved to postoperative irradiation plus chemotherapy in most centers on the basis of randomized GTSG* (28,29) and Mayo/NCCTG† trials (30), the tolerance of small bowel with combined modality regimens needs to be reviewed. In the initial GTSG trial parallel, opposed irradiation fields were used. The incidence of severe small bowel complications appeared excessive with the combined treatment arm of irradiation plus chemotherapy with two treatment-related deaths (2 of 46 patients at risk or 4% mortality rate). Patients received bolus 5-FU during weeks 1 and 5 of irradiation followed by maintenance 5-FU plus MeCCNU. The Mayo/NCCTG trial was the first combined modality adjuvant rectal trial that mandated multiple-field irradiation techniques. This was a two-arm trial of postoperative irradiation ± chemotherapy (approximately 100 patients/arm). In the combined modality arm, 5-FU was given during weeks 1 and 5 of irradiation, and a course of 5-FU plus MeCCNU was given before and after irradiation. In the published 1991 analysis with minimum five-year follow-up, the incidence of severe small bowel complications was < 5% in both groups. As seen in Table 32–5, this risk is essentially the same as the incidence of small bowel problems requiring reoperation with surgery alone.

Summary

Small bowel toxicity is often the most serious (and occasionally dose-limiting) toxicity of radiotherapy for abdominal and pelvic malignancies. Several treatment modification techniques have been shown to drastically reduce the incidence of such complications.

*GTSG = Gastrointestinal Tumor Study Group
†NCCTG = North Central Cancer Treatment Group

There is some evidence that these techniques may be beneficial in ameliorating the potentially increased complication rate associated with previous surgery and concomitant adjuvant chemotherapy.

LARGE BOWEL

With large bowel cancers, irradiation is usually combined with surgical resection, except for select early lesions for which endocavitary irradiation alone is a suitable treatment alternative. Most information regarding large-bowel radiation tolerance has been obtained in the setting of an uninvolved organ being included in the radiation field of another malignancy (i.e., rectum ± sigmoid included in AP:PA and lateral fields for prostate, bladder, and gynecologic malignancies). In such a situation, severe chronic complication rates greater than 5% would usually be unacceptable for primary irradiation of early stage disease or for adjuvant irradiation combined with resection (the circumference of the rectum can be irradiated to a dose of 5500 to 6000 in 180 to 200 cGy fractions with a chronic severe risk ≤ 5%). For locally advanced or unresectable lesions, a toxicity risk of 10 to 25% may be accepted by patient and physician. The mid and lower rectum are often carried to higher radiation doses than other sites in the large bowel because dose limiting small bowel and stomach can be excluded.

Little data have been generated on large-bowel tolerance when involved by malignancy. In a PMH trial of primary irradiation for rectal cancer, Cummings noted that severe rectal or sigmoid problems were infrequent when using doses of 4500 to 5000 cGy in 250 cGy fractions (31). Of 27 patients in whom the primary lesion was controlled by irradiation alone, 1 developed sigmoid and small bowel necrosis requiring resection and 1 developed rectal bleeding and pelvic fibrosis responding to medical management only. Although various irradiation techniques were used, an attempt was often made to limit the treatment field to the posterior pelvis with multiple field or arc techniques for the last 8 fractions. When preoperative irradiation is delivered prior to resection of rectal cancers, the risk of anastomotic leaks is < 5% if unirradiated bowel is used for the proximal limb of the anastomosis (32).

Incidental Large Bowel Toxicity

In this section, the discussion of large bowel tolerance is based on rectal tolerance generated in prostate and anal canal cancer series, where external beam radiotherapy was used exclusively. Although rectal tolerance information exists in the gynecologic literature, it is obfuscated because external irradiation is usually combined with brachytherapy. Some animal data are presented that discuss the influence of diet and medications on rectal healing after radiation injury.

The majority of prostate radiation series use multiple field techniques, with boost field doses to 6500 to 7000 cGy, that spare the posterior wall of the rectum. Analyses have shown that the incidence of bowel complications increases with doses in excess of 7000 cGy (33–36). Although the colostomy incidence is at or below 1% in most series (Table 32–6), an exception to this was a 6% incidence in an M.D. Anderson Hospital (MDAH) series (37). Table 32–7 evaluates local control and complications in the MDAH series as a function of stage and dose. The only severe complication seen at the 6500 cGy level at MDAH was in a patient treated with large field rotation cobalt-60. Most of the severe problems were at the 7000 cGy dose level. Prior to 1976, although

Table 32–6. Rectal Tolerance with External Irradiation of Prostate Cancer

Institution (Ref No.) Author	Stage	Dose to Prostate (cGy)	No. Patients	Colostomy Incidence	Radiation Ulcer
Mallinkrodt (36) (Pilepich et al.)	B&C	6500–7000 cGy (1000 cGy/wk, AP-PA)	267	0.37%	—
M.D. Anderson (37) (Hussey and Chan)	C	6500–7000 cGy (1000 cGy/wk, 4-field)	165	6%	—

Table 32–7. Local Control and Complication Rates for Prostate Cancer by Tumor Dose (M.D. Anderson Data)

	Local Control%		Complications*%	
Stage	~6500 cGy	~7000 cGy	~6500 cGy	~7000 cGy
C_1	94 (16/17)	92 (68/74)	6 (1/17)	11 (8/74)
C_2	62 (8/13)	79 (27/34)	0 (0/13)	12 (4/34)
Total	80 (24/30)	88 (95/108)	3 (1/30)	11 (12/108)

*Only complication in group receiving ~6500 cGy was in patient treated with large fields using a rotation technique with ^{60}Co.
Modified with permission from Hussey D, Chan R. Cancer Treat Symp 2:51, 1983.

four field techniques were utilized, most patients had only one field per day treated. Since 1976, there have been no colostomies in the MDAH prostate series with the dose limited to 6500 cGy in most patients (personal communication, D. Hussey 3/88).

In the treatment of anal cancer, the entire circumference of the lower rectum is included to doses of 6000 to 7000 cGy in 180 to 200 cGy fractions with external irradiation alone (38–41) or 4000 to 5500 cGy plus chemotherapy (41–43). The incidence of severe rectal complications is ≤ 5%.

Animal Data

As noted in an animal model by Trott et al, several factors can alter the severity of chronic large-bowel damage (44). In that trial, a 24 mm. segment of Wistar rat large bowel was irradiated with 2300 cGy in a single fraction, and 90% developed a chronic radiation ulcer. Modification of the ulcer healing process in control animals that were irradiated and did not receive any special treatment was compared with that found in animals treated with cortisone, Neomycin, Metamucil (laxative), or combinations thereof. Some animals were fed a standard rodent diet, others a residue-free synthetic diet, and some received both in sequence. Survival was increased in animals that received daily cortisone enemas plus Neomycin in the drinking water after irradiation, or in those who had Metamucil added to their diet. Animals that received the synthetic diet after irradiation survived as long as the diet was continued, but over 90% developed progressive large-bowel obstruction when the synthetic diet was stopped and the subject placed on a normal diet (the hard pellet-like stools that were produced abraded the surface of the bowel and did not allow the radiation-induced ulcer to heal).

Summary

The animal model reflects what can be seen in the clinical setting in which radiation damage can be modified by steroids, stool softener or Metamucil, and diet. When radiation ulcers do not heal with conservative management, diversion with a temporary colostomy can be successful. Biopsies of heavily irradiated rectal wall could cause ulceration if performed repetitively. In summary, the damage caused by radiation can be modified for better or worse by later diagnostic and treatment choices.

ANUS

In most clinical situations, including lower pelvic irradiation, if multiple field techniques are used, the full circumference of the anus is often spared. Therefore, most information regarding anal tolerance is derived from series in which the anus is involved with malignancy. Tolerance is evaluated with different modalities including external beam irradiation alone or in combination with chemotherapy, or brachytherapy with or without external irradiation.

Acute Toxicity

Radiation Alone

Nearly all patients who receive irradiation to the anus experience an acute, self-limited perineal skin reaction, which can range from mild, nearly asymptomatic tanning of the skin to intense erythema and moist desquamation. The frequency and severity of reported significant acute toxicity varies widely in the medical literature (38,39,41). Cantril et al, for example, evaluated acute toxicity in a series of 39 patients treated with radiation therapy for anal cancer (92% by external beam radiation therapy alone) with daily fraction sizes of 180 to 225 cGy to total doses of 4400 to 8050 cGy (38). Eighteen percent experienced a "moderate" acute perineal skin reaction, 20% experienced a "severe" acute perineal skin reaction, and 62% experienced a "mild" reaction or no reaction. In contrast, in a PMH series using a larger fraction size of 250 cGy, "virtually all" patients developed moist desquamation, even after doses as low as 2500 cGy in ten fractions (41).

Chemoradiation

The use of combined chemotherapy and radiation therapy does not appear to result in a large increase in acute perineal toxicity when compared to use of radiation therapy alone (41–43). In the PMH experience, for example, moist desquamation was common, regardless of whether patients were treated by radiation therapy alone or radiation therapy combined with infusion 5-FU and mitomycin-C (41). In their series, a treatment break had to be introduced in order to achieve acceptable acute tolerance. Byfield et al reported most desquamation in 6 of 11 patients treated by 3 to 5 cycles of 5-FU 25 mg/kg per 24 hours over 5 days in combination with 1000 cGy of RT per week, given in 250 cGy fractions with a minimum of 9 days of rest between cycles (42).

Chronic Toxicity

Significant late complications following radiation therapy for anal cancer include anal necrosis, ulceration, stricture, and chronic bleeding. In patients with large, extensively infiltrating or circumferential tumors, late complications may occur in a setting where the neoplastic process itself has significantly damaged normal anatomy. Even when tumors totally regress as a function of treatment, late anal complications may occur because the normal tissues are unable to totally repair themselves because of pre-existent neoplastic destruction. In the Institut Gustave-Roussy (IGR) series, for example, severe grade 3 complications were "often associated with rectovaginal fistulae and destruction of the anal canal by extensive tumors" (39). The frequency of severe, grade 3 complications was directly related to the size of the tumor. Among patients with T_1 and T_2 tumors, only 2 of 33 (6%) developed severe complications. In contrast, 3 of 25 (12%) with T_3 tumors and 4/6 (67%) with T_4 tumors developed severe complications.

The overall rate of serious anal complications following external irradiation for anal cancer ranges from 0 to 22% with 0 to 13% requiring a colostomy as a result of anal complications (38,39,41,43) (Table 32–8). No obvious differences exist in late severe complication rates for patients treated by irradiation alone compared to those treated by chemoradiation (Table 32–8).

Summary

In summary, significant self-limited acute toxicity is seen in the vast majority of patients treated for anal cancer. Long-term complications of anal necrosis, stricture, and/or bleeding are seen in up to 25% of patients (range 0 to 25%) treated by external and/or interstitial irradiation with or without chemotherapy (45,46). The incidence of colostomy for complications is 4 to 5% in most series. In many cases, these complications result from destruction of normal anatomy by the neoplastic process itself rather than radiation-induced damage. Although the precise tolerance of the anus remains unknown, doses in the range typically used for treating anal cancer leave the majority of patients with functional anal anatomy.

The incidence of both acute and chronic complications due to the nonsurgical treatment approaches discussed in this section must be kept in perspective by considering alternative treatment. A decade ago, the treatment of choice for most anal cancers was abdominoperineal resection. In the current irradiation or chemoradiation series, colostomy-free survival ranges from 70 to 90+% (including colostomies performed for

Table 32–8. Severe Late Anal Complications Following Irradiation ± Chemotherapy

Author (Ref. No.)	Total Tumor Dose (cGy)	Daily Fraction Size (cGy)	Duration of RT* (wks)	Chemotherapy	No. of Patients	No. of Patients with Severe Late Complications (%)	No. of Patients with Colostomy Resulting from Complication (%)
Cantril et al. (38)	4410–8050	180–225	NS	None	32†	7(22)	2‡(6)
Eschwedge et al. (39)	6000–6500	Usually 200	6–6 ½	None	64	9(14)	NS
Cummings et al. (41)	4500–6000	Usually 250	4–6	None	25	3(12)	1(4)
	5000	250	4	5–FU Mito C	30	4(13)	4(13)
Flam et al. (43)	4140–5040	180	4–6	5–FU Mito C	30	0(0)	0(0)

*Duration of RT is given exclusive of treatment breaks.
†Includes one patient treated preoperatively who subsequently refused surgery. Excludes patients who underwent radioactive implantation.
‡One case was treated via an external Cesium-137 source to 11,000 cGy (maximum dose). The other case was a patient with an 8 cm tumor treated to a total of 6900 cGy.
Abbreviations: NS = not stated; 5-FU = 5-fluorouracil; Mito C = mitomycin C; RT = radiation therapy

disease persistence as well as for complication).

MANAGEMENT OF GI TOXICITY

Acute Toxicity

Acute GI toxicity secondary to radiotherapy, chemotherapy, or a combination of the two modalities can interrupt and delay a treatment course or may jeopardize the administration of optimal doses of either modality. In either instance, a decrease in cure rates may be the possible consequence. With radiotherapy, such toxicity is related to the method of radiation, radiation fraction size, total dose, field size, and volume and specific parts of GI tract included in the irradiation field. With chemotherapy, the relationship is less obvious except for being dose-related. Some toxicities may be explained on the basis of proclivities of drug metabolites to accumulate at specific sites (5-FU metabolites on mucous membranes causing stomatitis and diarrhea). Others, such as nausea and vomiting, may be due to a secondary increase in neurotransmittors or a direct central nervous system effect.

Emesis

Both peripheral (GI tract) and central (chemoreceptor trigger zone) effects may be responsible for the nausea and vomiting caused by radiotherapy and chemotherapy. Several groups of drugs, individually or in combination, have been found effective in combating chemoradiation-induced nausea and vomiting (47). They include phenothiazines, metoclopramide, corticosteroids, benzodiazapines, antihistamines, and anticholinergics. Cannabinoids were the focus of transient interest and research and were found to be fairly ineffective in tolerable doses. The new family of serotonin antagonists have been found to be effective and relatively safe and may replace some of the antiemetics described above.

Enterocolitis

Acute damage to small and large bowel by chemoradiation is manifest by nausea, vomiting, diarrhea, and occasionally rectal bleeding. Histopathologically, such damage is due to denudation of intestinal lining leading to hyperemia and mucosal ulceration. The antibiotics mitomycin C and antinomycin D, methotrexate, and 5-FU are the chemotherapeutic agents most frequently associated with acute diarrhea.

Management of acute enterocolitis may include modification of radiation fields, as discussed earlier, or temporary cessation of such treatment. Dietary changes may include an initial fluid diet, followed by the institution of a low residue lactose-free diet, the administration of antiperistaltics such as diphenoxylate (Lomotil) or loperamide (Imodium), and occasionally broad-spectrum antibiotics to control altered intestinal flora. Acute proctitis may be managed with some of the above methods and the addition of intrarectal steroids and sitz baths. Perineal dermatitis may also be managed with sitz baths and topical steroids. Some institutions use liberal applications of broad spectrum sulfa cream (sulfadiazine 1%, Silvadene).

Chronic Toxicity

Chronic enterocolitis usually manifests itself a few months to several years after chemoradiation. Histopathologically, this is due to the phenomenon of endarteritis obliterans of intestinal capillaries manifesting clinically as telangiectasia, fibrosis, and strictures. Painless rectal ulceration and bleeding are characteristic longterm effects of damage from radiation in pelvic malignancies such as cervical and prostate cancers. These are usually managed conservatively by converting to a nonabrasive diet and using stool softeners. Occasionally, laser treatment to obliterate telangiectic blood vessels at the ulcer base may be required for hemostasis. In a few cases that have been nonresponsive to such measures, a temporary colostomy may be necessary. For esophagal and rectal strictures, graded attempts at dilatation are generally satisfactory.

It is radiobiologically predicted that hyperfractionated radiotherapy (multiple small fractions daily) will decrease the incidence of severe chronic side effects. Contrarily, there exists a potential for an increase in long-term effects from chemoradiation. As hyperfractionation and chemoradiation become increasingly used in head and neck, gynecologic, and certain gastrointestinal cancers, one can only hope that the two theoretically offsetting outcomes will become a practical reality. At the present time, with long-term follow-up of anal cancer patients treated with chemoradiation, there is no evidence of any significant increase in chronic effects (Table 32–8) (38,39,41,43).

Modification of Radiotherapy and Chemotherapy Administration

Multiple radiotherapeutic techniques to minimize both acute and chronic side effects have been attempted and shown to be clinically successful. Basically, they involve the minimization of radiation dose to normal tissues surrounding the areas of gross or occult tumor. They include the following.

1. The use of custom-made blocks and shaped radiation fields to decrease the volume of irradiated stomach and small intestine.
2. Patients with pelvic malignancies treated in prone position with a full bladder to reduce the volume of small bowel in the field (this is contraindicated if the bladder is involved by tumor).
3. The possibility of reducing doses to extended fields for chemoradiation regimens when compared to doses used for radiotherapy alone. Standard radiation fields encompass not only gross malignancy but areas of potential involvement by microscopic disease. When combined with effective chemotherapy, radiotherapy fields could possibly be reduced with the tacit understanding that the systemic agent(s) may be capable of killing microscopic foci of tumor far removed from the primary tumor bulk. This concept will have to be evaluated carefully to achieve the proper balance between local control and toxicity.
4. Use of multiple fields with at least two fields being treated daily.
5. Use of high energy (4 to 10 MeV photons) supervoltage radiotherapy equipment.

Chemotherapy-induced gastrointestinal toxicity can best be reduced or prevented by prophylactic use of antiemetics, sedatives, and tranquilizers (48). Some of the effective antiemetic agents used have been outlined above. The phenomenon of delayed emesis occurring on days 1 to 4 following cisplatinum administration can be palliated with a regimen combining dexamethasone and metoclopramide. Anticipatory emesis associated with both radiotherapy and chemotherapy may not respond to conventional antiemetics and often requires desensitization with behavior therapy.

The toxicity of certain drugs can be manipulated by altering their route of administration. For example, the incidence of stomatitis secondary to infusional 5-FU may be decreased by administering the drug by bolus injection.

The diarrhea and dehydration associated with long-term infusion of 4-fluoro-2-doxyuridine (FUdR) or 5-FU plus high-dose leucovorin (200 mg/m^2) can be life-threatening. Circadian-based infusion of FUdR delivering most of the daily dose during the late hours of the day can markedly reduce this gastrointestinal toxicity (49).

Chen et al have reported that the addition of aclarubicin (ACR) to a continuous infusion schedule of cisplatinum for recurrent gynecologic adenocarcinomas resulted in *no* gastrointestinal toxicity. They explained this lack of toxicity as being due to a low-level consistent plasma concentration of platinum secondary to ACR (50).

Animal data suggest that pretreatment with heavy meals such as bismuth salts decreases the lethality and gastrointestinal toxicity associated with cisplatinum and alkylating agents (51).

CONCLUSIONS

An updated interpretation of radiation tolerance doses for gastrointestinal tract organs is shown in Table 32–9. In an earlier evaluation of GI tolerance, data presented by Rubin and Casarett were based on daily fractions of 200 cGy and lower-energy supervoltage equipment (52). The upper estimates of tolerance in the TD 5/5 column in the current table are based on the availability of higher-energy supervoltage machines in most institutions and the use of 180 cGy fractions 5 days per week. For those who deliver 1000 cGy/week in 5 fractions, the lower estimates of tolerance are recommended. As was the case in Rubin and Casarett's original tolerance estimates, the current recommendations are based on our interpretation of the literature combined with our personal experience.

Since the mid-1970s, the use of combined modality treatment has markedly increased in an attempt to achieve radiation sensitization with chemotherapy or radiation dose modifiers and to decrease the high incidence of systemic metastases. For most GI malignancies, combinations of radiation and chemotherapy have become increasingly common, if not the accepted standard, as either primary treatment (anus and esophageal; unresectable pancreas, large bowel ± gastric) or adjuvant treatment after resection (rectum, pancreas ± other). Because optimal treatment regimens do not yet exist for most locally advanced malignancies, an ongoing evaluation of normal tissue tolerance by modality will be necessary.

Acknowledgements

The authors appreciate the efforts of Julie Chambers and the Mayo Clinic Typing Service for assistance in the preparation of the manuscript. We are indebted to our wives and families for the support received in personal and professional endeavors.

Table 32–9. Radiation Tolerance Doses* (in cGy), Gastrointestinal Tract

Organ	Injury at 5 years	1%–5% $TD_{5/5}$	25%–50% $TD_{50/5}$	Volume or Length
Esophagus	Ulcer, stricture	6000–6500	7500	75 cm^3
Stomach	Ulcer, perforation	4500–5000	5500	100 cm^3
Intestine (small)	Ulcer, stricture	4500–5000	5500	100 cm^3
Colon	Ulcer, stricture	5500–6000	7500	100 cm^3
Rectum	Ulcer, stricture	5500–6000	7500	100 cm^3
Anus	Ulcer, stricture	6000–6500	≥ 7500	Whole

*Compiled by Gunderson and Martenson, 1988 (literature interpretation, personal experience). Based on supervoltage 4–10 MV, 900 cGy/week (5 × 180 cGy).

This chapter is supported in part by NCI GI Program Project Grant CA 31224.

REFERENCES

1. Phillips TL, Margolis L. Radiation pathology and the clinical response of lung and esophagus. Front Radiat Ther Oncol 6:254, 1972.
2. Cederqvist C, Nielson J, Bertelsen A, Hansen HS. Cancer of the oesophagus. II. Therapy and outcome. Acta Chir Scand 144:233, 1978.
3. Beatty JD, DeBoer G, Rider WD. Carcinoma of the esophagus: pretreatment assessment, correlation of radiation treatment parameters with survival, and identification and management of radiation treatment failure. Cancer 43:2254, 1979.
4. Elkon D, Lee MS, Hendrickson FR. Carcinoma of the esophagus: Sites of recurrence and palliative benefits after definitive radiotherapy. Int J Radiat Oncol Biol Phys 4:615, 1978.
5. Langer M, Choi NC, Orlow E. Radiation therapy alone or in combination with surgery in the treatment of carcinoma of the esophagus. Cancer 58:1208, 1986.
6. Richmond J, Seydel HG, Bae Y, et al. Comparison of three treatment strategies for esophageal cancer within a single institution. Int J Radiat Oncol Biol Phys 13:1617, 1987.
7. Keane TJ, Harwood AR, Elhakim T, et al. Radical radiation therapy with 5-fluorouracil infusion and mitomycin C for oesophageal squamous carcinoma. Radiother Oncol 4:205, 1985.
8. Marcial VA, Valez-Garcia E, Cintron J, Ydrach AA. Radiotherapy preceded by multidrug chemotherapy in carcinoma of the esophagus: A pilot study of the Radiation Therapy Oncology Group. Cancer Clin Trials 3:127, 1980.
9. John MJ, Flam MS, Mowry PA, et al. Radiotherapy and chemoradiation for nonmetastatic esophageal carcinoma. A critical review of chemoradiation. Cancer 63:2397, 1989.
10. Byfield JE, Barone R, Mendelsohn J, et al. Infusional 5-fluorouracil and x-ray therapy for non-resectable esophageal cancer. Cancer 45:703, 1980.
11. Lokich JJ, Shea M, Chaffey J. Sequential infusional 5-fluorouracil followed by concomitant radiation for tumors of the esophagus and gastroesophageal junction. Cancer 60:275, 1987.
12. Gunderson LL, Martenson JA. Gastrointestinal tract radiation tolerance. *In:* Radiation Tolerance of Normal Tissues. Vaeth J (Ed). Karger, Basel, 23:277, 1989.
13. Seaman WB, Ackerman LV. The effect of radiation on the esophagus: Clinical and histologic study of the effects produced by the betatron. Radiology 68:534, 1957.
14. Perez CA, Stanley K, Rubin P, et al. A prospective randomized study of various irradiation doses and fractionation schedules in the treatment of inoperable non-oat-cell carcinoma of the lung. Cancer 45:2744, 1980.
15. Hall TC, Dederick MM, Chalmers TC, et al. A clinical pharmacologic study of chemotherapy and x-ray therapy in lung cancer. Am J Med 43:186, 1967.
16. Coy P. A randomized study of irradiation and vinblastine in lung cancer. Cancer 26:803, 1970.
17. Eagan RT, Fleming TR, Lee RE, et al. Chemotherapy response as a prognosticator for survival in patients with limited squamous cell lung cancer treated with combined chemotherapy and radiotherapy. Int J Radiat Oncol Biol Phys 6:879, 1980.
18. Gunderson LL, Hoskins RB, Cohen AC, et al. Combined modality treatment of gastric cancer. Int J Radiat Oncol Biol Phys 9:965, 1983.
19. O'Connell MJ, Gunderson LL, Moertel CG, Kvols LK. A pilot study to determine clinical tolerability of intensive combined modality therapy for locally unresectable gastric cancer. Int J Radiat Oncol Biol Phys 11:1827, 1985.
20. Roswit B, Malsky SJ, Reid CB. Radiation tolerance of the gastrointestinal tract. Front Radiat Ther Oncol 6:160, 1972.
21. Goldstein HM, Rogers LF, Fletcher GH, Dodd GD. Radiological manifestations of radiation induced injury to the normal upper gastrointestinal tract. Radiology 117:135, 1975.
22. Smalley SR, Gunderson LL. Tumors of the stomach. *In:* Principles and Practice of Radiation Oncology. 2nd Ed. Perez C and Brady L (Eds). Philadelphia, J B Lippincott, 1992, p. 985.
23. Buskirk SJ, Gunderson LL, Adson MA, et al. Analysis of failure following curative irradiation of gallbladder and extrahepatic bile duct carcinoma. Int J Radiat Oncol Biol Phys 10:2013, 1984.
24. Buskirk SJ, Gunderson LL, Schild SE, et al. Analysis of failure following curative irradiation of extrahepatic bile duct carcinoma. Ann Surg 215:125, 1992.
25. Gunderson LL, Russell AH, Llewellyn HJ, et al. Treatment planning for colorectal cancer: Radiation and surgical techniques and value of small bowel films. Int J Radiat Oncol Biol Phys 11:1379, 1985.
26. Gallagher MJ, Brereton HD, Rostock RA, et al. A prospective study of treatment techniques to minimize the volume of pelvic small bowel with reduction of acute and late effects associated with pelvic irradiation. Int J Radiat Oncol Biol Phys 12:1565, 1986.

27. Duttenhaver JR, Hoskins RB, Gunderson LL, Tepper JE. Adjuvant postoperative radiation therapy in cancer of the colon. Cancer 57:955, 1986.
28. Gastrointestinal Tumor Study Group. Prolongation of the disease-free interval in surgically resected rectal cancer. N Engl J Med 312:1465, 1985.
29. Gastrointestinal Tumor Study Group. Survival after postoperative combination treatment of rectal cancer. N Engl J Med 315:1294, 1986.
30. Krook JE, Moertel CG, Gunderson LL, et al. Effective surgical adjuvant therapy for high-risk rectal cancer. N Engl J Med 324:709, 1991.
31. Cummings BJ, Rider WD, Harwood HR, et al. Radical external beam radiation therapy for adenocarcinoma of the rectum. Dis Col Rectum 26:30, 1983.
32. Roberson SH, Heron HC, Kerman HD, Bloom TS. Is anterior resection of the rectosigmoid safe after preoperative radiation? Dis Colon Rectum 28:254, 1985.
33. Leibel SA, Hanks GA, Kramer S. Patterns of care outcome studies: Results of the national practice in adenocarcinoma of the prostate. Int J Radiat Oncol Biol Phys 10:401, 1984.
34. Pilepich MV, Asbell SO, Krall JM, et al. Correlation of radiotherapeutic parameters and treatment morbidity—analysis of RTOG study 77-06. Int J Radiat Oncol Biol Phys 13:1007, 1987.
35. Pilepich MV, Krall JM, Sause WT, et al. Correlation of radiotherapeutic parameters and treatment related morbidity in carcinoma of the prostate—analysis of RTOG study 75-06. Int J Radiat Oncol Biol Phys 13:351, 1987.
36. Pilepich MV, Perez CA, Walz BJ, Zivuska FR. Complications of definitive radiotherapy for carcinoma of the prostate. Int J Radiat Oncol Biol Phys 7:1341, 1981.
37. Hussey DH, Chan RC. Patterns of failure in patients treated by radiotherapy for genitourinary tumors. Cancer Treatment Symposia 2:51, 1983.
38. Cantril ST, Green JP, Schall GL, Schaupp WC. Primary radiation therapy in the treatment of anal carcinoma. Int J Radiat Oncol Biol Phys 9:1271, 1983.
39. Eschwege F, Lasser P, Chavy A, et al. Squamous cell carcinoma of the anal canal: Treatment by external beam irradiation. Radiother Oncol 3:145, 1985.
40. Papillon J. Radiation therapy in the management of epidermoid carcinoma of the anal region. Dis Colon Rectum 17:181, 1974.
41. Cummings B, Keane T, Thomas G, et al. Results and toxicity of the treatment of anal canal carcinoma by radiation therapy or radiation therapy and chemotherapy. Cancer 54:2062, 1984.
42. Byfield JE, Barone RM, Sharp TR, Frankel SS. Conservative management without alkylating agents of squamous cell anal cancer using cyclical 5-FU alone and x-ray therapy. Cancer Treat Rep 67:709, 1983.
43. Flam MS, John MJ, Mowry PA, et al. Definitive combined modality treatment of carcinoma of the anus. A report of 30 cases including results of salvage therapy in patients with residual disease. Dis Colon Rectum 30:495, 1987.
44. Trott SR, Breiter N, Spiethoff A. Experimental studies on the pathogenesis of the chronic radiation ulcer of the large bowel in rats. Int J Radiat Oncol Biol Phys 12:1637, 1986.
45. Ramming KP, Juilard G, Parker R, Eilber F. Management of carcinoma of the rectum and anus without abdominoperineal resection. Am J Surg 152:16, 1986.
46. Hintz BL, Charyulu KN, Sudarsanam A. Anal carcinoma: basic concepts and management. J Surg Onc 10:141, 1978.
47. Stewart DJ. Cancer therapy, vomiting, and antiemetics. Can J Physiol Pharmacol 68:304, 1990.
48. Gralla RJ. Treatment of emesis. *In:* Manual of Oncologic Therapeutics 1989–1990. Wittes RE (Ed). Philadelphia, J B Lippincott, 1989, p. 490.
49. Lanning RM, von Roemeling R, Hrushesky WJ. Circadian-based infusional FUDR therapy. Oncol Nurs Forum, 17:49, 1990.
50. Chen JT, Hirai Y, Shimizu Y, et al. New cisplatin schedule in combination with aclarubicin (ACR) with high response rate in recurrent gynecological adenocarcinomas. Gynecol Oncol 38:1, 1990.
51. Basu A, and Lazo JS. A hypothesis regarding the protective role of metallothioneins against the toxicity of DNA interactive anticancer drugs. Toxicol Lett 50:123, 1990.
52. Rubin P, Casarett G. A direction for clinical radiation pathology—the tolerance dose. Front Radiat Ther Oncol 6:1, 1972.

Chapter 33

PULMONARY TOXICITY

MACK ROACH III AND THEODORE L. PHILLIPS

As the benefits of combining chemotherapy and radiation therapy have become more apparent, so too have the complications associated with this approach (1–5). For the thorax, more than any other anatomic region, locally excessive toxicity due to radiation-drug interactions may result in total disability or even death. The merits and the morbidity associated with combined modality therapy have been well documented. Randomized trials, pilot studies, retrospective reviews, and anecdotal reports suggest either an improvement in survival or local control associated with the use of thoracic combined modality therapy (CMT) (3–10). The purpose of this chapter is to summarize some of the available data that allow us to assess the risk-benefit ratio of CMT in relation to pulmonary morbidity and mortality.

Thoracic CMT is commonly used in the management of lung cancer, breast cancer, and esophageal cancer (1–10). Based on these sites alone, more than 155,000 patients per year may be candidates for CMT (11). Other relatively common indications for thoracic CMT include its use in the management of Hodgkin's and non-Hodgkin's lymphomas and in conjunction with total body irradiation (TBI) during preparation for bone marrow transplantation (BMT) (12–14).

Unfortunately, the normal tissue tolerance of lung imposes restraints on the use of CMT, such that the delivery of tumorcidal doses is frequently compromised. In addition to limiting the volume of lung irradiated, our ability to use combined modality therapy safely is dependent on dose, time, and tolerance factors (15,16). Because both radiation and chemotherapy are potentially toxic to the lung, it is not surprising that pulmonary toxicity increases when the two modalities are combined. However, considerable variation exists for the risk and severity of toxicity, depending on the specific drug and how and when the radiation and drugs are combined. In order to evaluate the impact of the combined use of these modalities, it is instructive to first briefly review the pulmonary toxicity associated with each modality independently. Drugs that have been reported to be intrinsically toxic to the lung will be discussed separately from those drugs not known to be intrinsically pulmonary toxic in an attempt to clarify the nature of the expected differences in drug-radiation interactions (if such a difference does in fact exist).

RADIATION-INDUCED PULMONARY TOXICITY

Mechanisms

The effects on the lung of radiation, whether administered by Cobalt-60 (gamma rays) or by means of the conventional linear accelerator (x-rays) are thought to be mediated through damaged DNA. Both forms of radiation are indirectly ionizing and produce fast recoil electrons. Their biologic effects may be due to direct action (the recoil electron interacts with the target molecule) or to indirect action (the recoil electron interacts with water to produce an OH radical, which diffuses to the target molecule) (17). It is believed that approximately two thirds of the biologic effects are due to indirect action and that this may be modified by chemical sensitizers or protectors. These organic peroxides fix chemical lesions, which result in the generation of both repairable and nonrepairable DNA damage. High linear energy transfer (HiLET) radiation, which includes neutrons and heavy charged particles, can induce DNA damage by direct action with much less dependence on the intermediate presence of oxygen and is associated with less repairable damage. In either case, the expression of radiation damage is generally not seen until the target cell enters mitosis. Differentiated normal tissues with low mitotic activity, such as the heart and spinal cord, tend to express the effects of radiation much later than cells from more kinetically active cells such as the bronchial epithelium.

Histopathology

The phases of pulmonary toxicity have been classified as exudative, proliferative, and fibrotic by some investigators, as early, intermediate, and late by others; and simply as early and late by others (18–20). To confuse matters further, some investigators have suggested that even the initial pneumonitis (classically called an acute event) is actually a late event, as is the fibrosis (21). These descriptive classification schemes depend on whether the emphasis is placed on the histopathologic changes, the timing with which changes are observed, or the presence of a recognized clinical syndrome.

The cells thought to be primarily involved in the expression of this injury include the Type I epithelial cells (flat alveolar cells), the Type II epithelial cells (surfactant producing alveolar cells), interstitial cells, and endothelial cells (22). This description is somewhat simplistic because more than 40 different cell types have been reported to demonstrate detectable changes by light or electron microscopy (23,24). The fact that the alveolar cells are the most actively dividing cellular component in the lung (excluding lymphoid cells) and the fact that the type I alveolar cells turn over three times faster than the type II cells, one might expect them to be the dose-limiting cell line (25). However, histologically, they seem to be relatively spared following radiation (23).

The critical role of the surfactant producing type II cells and the histopathologic similarity between radiation damage and other surfactant deficient states have prompted a number of investigators to argue that they might well be the primary target (19,25,26). Rubin et al correlated surfactant levels measured by bronchial lavage with lethality following fractionated and single dose radiation in mice and rabbits and attempted to use it as a marker for late effects (26). Although they reported a strong correlation between rising surfactant levels and lethality, the variation in the interval between rising levels and the lack of correlation of the threshold dose for the surfactant release response or the LD_{50} (dose associated with a 50% chance of a lethal outcome) cast doubts on the specificity of this marker. Furthermore, in a previous study, they found no dose-response relationship following single fractions with the loss of lamellar bodies (a marker for type II cells) and found greater lamellar body loss with fractionated radiotherapy than with single fraction treatment (the opposite of what might be expected if the loss of these cells correlated with long-term toxicity).

Vascular changes might play a critical role in the expression of late toxicity in the postirradiated lung (18,22,27). Studies of the effects of radiation on the microvasculature, using several animal models, revealed two distinct dose-related phases of toxicity, which bring to mind the phases of pulmonary toxicity (27). However, this pattern of injury response has been shown to be common to a number of organs (22). Further, support for the possible critical role for vascular injuries is the finding that drugs, such as captopril (an angiotensin-converting enzyme inhibitor which is thought to be a marker of endothelial function), have been shown to reduce radiation-induced damage (21).

Radiation Pneumonitis and Fibrosis

Radiation pneumonitis is the second most common potentially life-threatening complication of thoracic irradiation. Several excellent reviews have been published describing this syndrome in some detail (18–21,28). For the sake of this review, the term "radiation pneumonitis" is used to refer to the symptomatic syndrome as opposed to the radiographic diagnosis, as has been suggested by some authors (29–31). This syndrome is characterized by cough, dyspnea, occasionally fever, and less frequently, chest pain. The onset is usually between 2 and 3 months following radiation, but it may occur earlier or as late as 6 months. The syndrome may last as little as a week or for months, and is rarely progressive and fatal. Findings on examination may include a pleural friction rub and/or tachycardia. Laboratory findings typically reveal leukocytosis, an elevated sedimentation rate, and radiographic findings which reflect the portion of the lung irradiated.

In order to weigh the risks and benefits of CMT, it is useful to quantitate the severity of radiation pneumonitis. The failure of most published series to use uniform criteria for defining radiation pneumonitis precludes precise estimation of the incidence and severity of radiation pneumonitis (29–31). Table 33–1 summarizes the late radiation morbidity scoring scheme used by the Radiation Therapy Oncology Group (RTOG) and EORTC (European Oncology Research Therapy Cooperative). Using these well-defined criteria and data gathered from prospective randomized trials using conventional fractionation for a total of 6000 cGy in the treatment of inoperable lung cancer, the incidence of Grade 3 or 4 radiation pneumonitis is approximately 10%. Grade 4 and 5 severity pneumonitis is much less common, occurring in approximately 1% of patients (32,33). The incidence of pneumonitis due to treatment of other sites (e.g., breast) is likely to be lower, but varies depending on the irradiated lung volume and technique used. The observed incidence of pneumonitis is likely to be higher in a patient population that has a higher incidence of COPD (chronic obstructive pulmonary disease) and which is older.

Generalized radiation pneumonitis, perhaps mediated by a hypersensitivity reaction, has been reported as an unusual complication of radiation (28,29,34–36). Because most of the case reports fail to exclude other possible causes of diffuse infiltrates such as viral pneumonia, Legionella pneumophila, Pneumocystis carinii, or the presence of a drug-induced syndrome, it is difficult to estimate the incidence of this syndrome. It does appear to be rare and may be associated with the treatment of relatively small volumes (36).

Whether or not pneumonitis occurs, some degree of fibrosis usually does. The independence between early and late pulmonary toxicity is supported by animal work by Moss and Haddy and later by van den Brenk (19,37). These authors demonstrated that *early toxicity can be reduced and late effects exacerbated by high pressure oxygen.* These data suggest the possibility that different cellular targets and different mechanisms are involved in acute radiation pneumonitis and late fibrosis.

Whether the late end-point is pneumonitis or fibrosis, small differences in dose per fraction can dramatically alter lung tolerance. McDonald et al reported late deaths due to pulmonary fibrosis in laboratory animals with differences in doses as small as 120 to 260 cGy between those animals demonstrating a recognized clinical event and a lethal event (21). These data and others emphasize the very steep dose response curve for pulmonary damage following single fractions in the dose range of 1000 cGy to 1200 cGy (Fig. 33–1) (21,31,38,39). In addition to radiation pneumonitis and fibrosis, occasionally pleural effusions have been reported. These effusions are generally small and frequently disappear spontaneously, but may last more than 3 years (28). Much less commonly, spontaneous pneumothoraces and rib fractures have been reported. These complications are expected to be less common

Table 33–1. Pulmonary Toxicity Grading Scale: RTOG/EORTC

Grade 0	Grade 1	Grade 2	Grade 3	Grade 4	Grade 5
None	Asymptomatic or mild symptoms (dry cough), slight radiographic appearances	Moderate symptomatic, fibrosis or pneumonitis (severe cough), fever, patchy radiographic appearances	Severe symptomatic fibrosis or pneumonitis, dense radiographic changes	Severe respiratory insufficiency/ continuous O_2/ assisted ventilation	Death directly related to radiation late effects

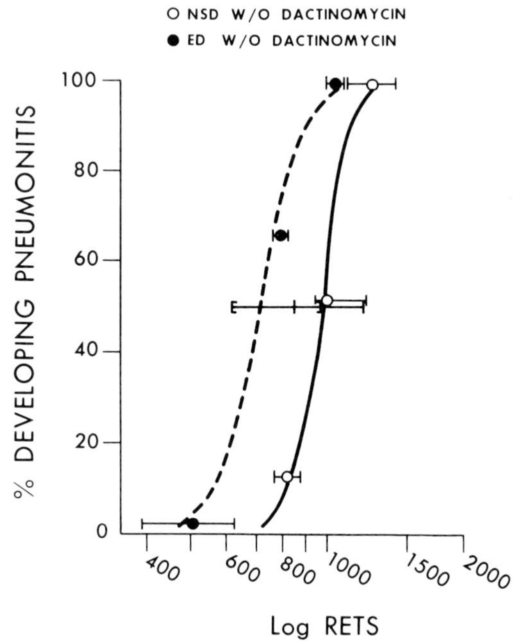

Fig. 33–1. Comparison of the ED equation of Wara et al, and the NSD equation of Ellis et al. Note the steep dose-response curve in the range of 1000 to 1200 cGy. (From Wara WM, et al. Cancer 32:547, 1973.)

these days with the widespread use of higher energy radiation and the use of standard fractionation.

Finally, perhaps the most serious complication of radiation therapy is local failure. Any analysis that fails to take this into account neglects the reality that only patients with life-threatening diseases requiring aggressive treatment are offered this approach in the first place! Fear of complications such as radiation pneumonitis should not be an excuse for inadequate treatment.

Treatment Volume and Pulmonary Functions

The physiologic changes associated with radiation of the lung have been studied extensively. Studies published in the 1960s emphasized the progressive decline of lung volumes, an impairment of the diffusing capacity, and an increase in the work of breathing (40–43). The severity of these effects was noted to be related to the volume of lung irradiated. For example, patients treated following mastectomy were noted to have recovered normal function by 18 months (43). Other studies associated with the treatment of large volumes showed little to no recovery from radiation-induced damage. Although considerable variation was noted from person to person, the early postradiation effects were not deemed sufficient to omit radiation even in patients with severely compromised pulmonary function (41).

More recent studies have attempted to correlate standard pulmonary function studies with the status of the postirradiated lung and pretreatment features (44–45). Choi et al found that in patients with a relatively high initial FEV-1 there was a significant decrease in FEV-1, FVC, MBC, PEFR*, and diffusion capacity, as well as an increase in airway resistance. In contrast, most patients with low initial values or obstructive lesions actually demonstrated improvement in pulmonary functions (44). Curran et al evaluated the influence of elective nodal irradiation on postirradiation pulmonary functions. They compared five different treatment volumes ranging from tumor only plus a 2-cm margin to tumor plus mediastinal, bilateral supraclavicular fossae, as well as hilar irradiation. Although larger treatment volumes tended to correlate with larger declines in the pretreatment FEV-1, there was a considerable range of effects observed so that accurate predictions of postirradiation pulmonary function were not possible (45). These data suggest that the highly variable size and location of lung tumors, as well as the variation in the degree of obstruction, the level of baseline pulmonary dysfunction, and the regeneration capacity, preclude precise prediction of postirradiated pulmonary function. Larger treatment volumes are associated with large decrements in pulmonary function, but in the vast majority of cases, the changes observed are mild to moderate.

Dose Per Fraction Considerations

The impact of dose per fraction on pulmonary toxicity is even more critical than total dose, volume or time (31,38,46). The Ellis equation attempted to provide us with practical guidelines for adjusting total dose for time, dose per fraction and normal tissue

*FEV-1 = forced expiratory volume in one second, FVC = forced vital capacity, MBC = maximum breathing capacity, PEFR = peak expiratory flow rate.

tolerance (46). Wara and coworkers modified Ellis' nominal standard dose (NSD) formula and proposed the estimated dose (ED) equation shown below (38):

$$\text{Total Dose} = \text{ED} \times N^{0.377} \times T^{0.058}$$

When N = number of fraction and T = time

This equation was developed specifically to estimate pulmonary damage and is based on experimental radiation pneumonitis in LAF-1 mice and verified by application to 51 patients treated with 92 separate lung fields. The ED formula was found to be a more accurate predictor of radiation pneumonitis than the NSD formula. Based on this data, the authors cautiously concluded that 2500 cGy in 20 fractions represented a relatively safe estimate for whole lung tolerance (see Fig. 33–1). Mah et al, using the same model, reported a similar dose for an associated risk of 5% toxicity but with a somewhat higher lung tolerance for a 50% risk of toxicity (31).

More recently, the so-called linear quadratic equation (L-Q equation) has been adopted by many clinical investigators as the most useful model for comparing various dose and fractionation schemes (47). This equation can be written as follows:

$$\text{Effect} = E = n(\alpha d + \beta d_2)$$

where d = dose per fraction
α = non repairable effects
β = repairable effects
n = number of identical fractions

For comparing two different fractionation schemes, assuming a similar overall treatment time, the L-Q equation can be written as follows:

$$D_2/D_1 = (1 + d_1\,\beta/\alpha)/(1 + d_2\,\beta/\alpha)$$

where D_1 or D_2 = Total dose,
d_1 or d_2 = dose/fraction,
n_1 or n_2 = number of fractions
$D_1 = n, d_1$ and
$D_2 = n_2\, d_2$

Assuming an α/β ratio of 3 for lung and 10 for tumor, the late effects of radiation delivered (120 cGy fractions given b.i.d., separated by 6 hours) to 6960 cGy would be expected to be equivalent to the late effects using conventional fractionation to a total of 5800 cGy. The early responding tissue such as tumor and the epithelium of the esophagus would be expected to respond as though they had been treated with a dose of 6500 cGy using conventional fractionation. This model predicts an increase in acute effects including tumor response but a decrease in late effects such as pulmonary fibrosis. In contrast, a fractionation scheme using 300 cGy fractions delivered every other day over a similar period of 6 weeks would require a dose reduction to 5100 cGy to yield similar late effects. This would result in an effect on early responding tissues and tumor equivalent to 5500 cGy by conventional fractionation. This would correspond to nearly a 10% reduction in the effective dose to the tumor without sparing late complications despite decreasing the number of treatments from 30 to 17.

Conclusions

In summary, using radiation alone (e.g., for lung cancer) delivered by conventional fractionation to 6000 cGy or hyperfractionated 120 cGy b.i.d. (separated by 6 hours) to 6960 cGy, the incidence of Grade 3 or 4 radiation pneumonitis is on the order of 10%. Somewhat higher incidences may be expected with unusually large volumes and a lower incidence with smaller volumes (e.g., breast cancer). Grade 4 and 5 severity pneumonitis is much less common. The use of larger doses per fraction or the addition of chemotherapy (as will be discussed) is associated with a markedly higher risk. Single-dose whole lung tolerance is much lower than the tolerance for fractionated radiotherapy. For example, 750 cGy and 1000 cGy in single fractions have been associated with risk for radiation pneumonitis, perhaps as high as 5% and 50% respectively (39).

CHEMOTHERAPY-INDUCED PULMONARY TOXICITY

In this section, we briefly review common cytotoxic drugs which have been reported to be intrinsically pulmonary toxic. For a more detailed discussion, the reader is referred to a number of more comprehensive reviews (48–52). The cytotoxic drugs classically associated with intrinsic pulmonary toxicity are summarized in Table 33–2 (48–66). Numerous other cytotoxic drugs have been implicated as being pulmonary toxic (e.g., nitrogen mustard, chlorambucil, melphalan, mercaptopurine, vinblastine), but these drugs are less well described in the literature and are excluded (48–53,67). Also excluded from this discussion are pulmonary toxic drugs that are not cytotoxic to tumor but are frequently given to cancer patients, such as tetracycline, methadone, dilantin, and penicillin (51). To what extent these drugs may contribute to the pulmonary toxicity observed in patients treated with combined modality therapy is unknown. Clinically, the features of drug-induced pneumonitis are similar to those noted with radiation pneumonitis including symptoms such as cough, dyspnea, and fever. As with the radiation syndrome, pulmonary function tests are usually remarkable for a reduction in the diffusion capacity and demonstrate a restrictive defect. No consistent criteria have been used in the various reports. Consequently, the precise incidence and/or severity of toxicity from any particular drug is difficult to state with certainty. Histologic changes are most sensitive and are present when clinical signs and symptoms are absent.

When more than a single pulmonary toxic drug is included as part of a multi-drug regimen, the result may be enhanced toxicity contributing to the uncertainty of the nature and incidence of individual drug-induced toxicity (53). Furthermore, the route of delivery and the dose of drug received vary considerably from one series to the next and may confound estimates of risk and the identification of a possible dose-response relationship. For example, treatment with 100 to 500 units of Bleomycin is associated with a low and relatively constant risk of pulmonary toxicity. However, with a cumulative dose above 500 units, there is a rapid rise in the risk for clinically significant toxicity. Bleomycin toxicity may be reduced if the drug is administered by intramuscular injection or by continuous intravenous (I.V.) infusion, compared to I.V. bolus (54,55).

In general, the similarities overshadow the differences in the drug-induced pulmonary toxic syndromes. However, some characteristic differences are associated with pulmonary toxicity from the various drugs (Table 33–2). For example, there is a clear dose response relationship for Bleomycin and BCNU. For other drugs, duration of treatment more than 8 months (Busulphan) or frequency of treatment (methotrexate; MTX) may be risk factors. Bleomycin- and mitomycin C-induced pulmonary toxicity have been noted to be exacerbated by oxygen therapy (50,52,65). Characteristic differences in the radiographic appearance have also been reported with these drugs (51). For example, although pleural effusions are uncommon in drug-induced pneumonitis, they have been described in association with bleomycin, busulfan, and methotrexate (48,49).

Table 33–2. Chemotherapeutic Agents Intrinsically Toxic to Pulmonary Tissues

Drug (References)	Frequency (%)	Reversible	Dose Response	Miscellaneous Risk Factors
Bleomycin (48–58)	4.0–46	±	2+	Age, oxygen, I.V. bolus
BCNU (48–52,59–62)	20–30	–	2+	Cytoxan?, lung disease
CTX* (48–52,63)	Rare	+	–	—
Busulfan (48–52)	2.5–11.5	±	+	> 8 months duration of treatment
MTX* (48–52,64)	2.5–8	3+	–	Oxygen, frequency of administration
Mitomycin C (48,52,65,66)	8	2+	–	Oxygen therapy
PCZ* (48–52)	Rare	3+	–	—

*MTX = Methotrexate, PCZ = Procarbazine, CTX = Cytoxan

In addition to differences in risk factors for manifesting toxicity, there are differences in the likelihood that the syndromes will be reversible. The toxic pulmonary reactions associated with hypersensitivity-type reactions are reversible and often steroid-responsive. In contrast, the toxic events associated with high-dose bleomycin and Bischloroethylnitrosourea (BCNU) tend to be less reversible and less responsive to steroids. Bleomycin may be associated with both hypersensitivity and dose-related reactions, with the former being more reversible. To what extent other drugs might also be capable of causing more than one type of reaction is unclear. In the next section, we review experimental data pertinent to the pulmonary toxicity associated with combining intrinsically and non-intrinsically pulmonary toxic drugs.

CHEMORADIATION AND PULMONARY TOXICITY—EXPERIMENTAL RESULTS

Quantification and Schedule Dependence

In an effort to quantify the interactions between radiation and chemotherapy in the lung, several investigators have used animal models and calculated the dose-effect factor (DEF) (68–72). DEF is defined as follows:

$$\text{DEF} = \frac{\text{dose to achieve a specific effect without drug}}{\text{dose to achieve a specific effect with the drug present.}}$$

Therefore, if for example, a specific drug interacted with radiation so that the dose required to cause pneumonitis could be reduced by half, the DEF would be 2. Table 33–3 summarizes the dose effect factors relevant to the lung from a number of selected studies available (68,69,71–78). Of note, the lung DEF values vary somewhat from one study to the next depending upon the drug, the animal model used, and the end-point used. Most of the studies included in Table 33–3 used LD_{50} or fibrosis as end-points, whereas others used breathing rates per minute. Surprisingly, no clear relationship is apparent when comparing the drugs that are intrinsically pulmonary toxic and the DEFs reported in animal models (comparing Tables 33–2 and 33–3).

The critical dependence of drug/radiation interactions on the interval between delivery of each has been a consistent theme among these studies. von der Maase et al (data shown in Table 33–3) evaluated the effects of single-drug doses administered 15 minutes before graded single doses of radiation and at different intervals from 28 days before to 28 days after a fixed radiation dose (71). The largest DEF values were found when the drug was given 15 minutes before radiation for Adriamycin, bleomycin, cyclophosphamide, and mitomycin C.

An effect was seen when Adriamycin was administered 7 days before or 7 days after radiation, whereas bleomycin and cyclophosphamide-enhanced responses were noted if they were administered from 24 hours to 3 days after radiation. The effect of mitomycin C was observed when the drug was given 24 hours before to 24 hours after

Table 33–3. Dose-effect Factors for Lung from Selected Series

DRUGS	Phillips (68,69)	von der Maase (71)	Others (72–78)
Actinomycin D	1.3–1.6	—	1.53
Adriamycin	1.31	1.6	1.57 1.67
BCNU	0.78	—	—
Bleomycin	1.16	1.41	1.02–1.22
Cisplatinum	1.22	0.94	0.97–1.38
Cytoxan	2.05	2.05	1.07–1.3
5-FU	0.98	1.00	—
Melphalan	1.05	—	—
Methotrexate	1.61	1.03	—
Mitomycin C	—	1.73	—
Nitrogen mustard	0.97	—	—
Vincristine	0.91	—	—

radiation, but 5-FU, MTX, and cisplatinum (CDDP) had no effect on the radiation response at any of the investigated intervals. These studies used large single doses per fraction (range 1000 to 2200 cGy), and therefore may not be applicable to clinical practice in humans.

Tanabe and coworkers studied the effects of fractionated irradiation combined with CDDP on SCCVII/St tumors and the lung of the C3H/KM mouse (76). In contrast to the findings of von der Maase, schedule-dependent enhancement was noted as summarized in Table 33–4. In addition to measuring DEF by tumor response, these investigators measured the so-called therapeutic gain factor (TGF). TGF is defined as follows:

$$TGF = \frac{\text{DEF tumor}}{\text{DEF normal tissue (lung)}}$$

Using this experimental animal model, they found that either concurrent daily CDDP and radiation or a large single dose of CDDP administered 24 hours before or after 5 days of radiation yielded the highest TGF values (Table 33–4). Figure 33–2 demonstrates the critical dependence of DEF on the time of drug delivery and radiation. More recently, this same group of investigators reported even higher schedule dependent TGFs with the addition of other drugs (78). This work brings focus to the fact that knowing the DEF is not likely to be as important as knowing the TGF when predicting the risk of pulmonary toxicity. Unfortunately, very little literature is available to provide clinically useful information in this regard.

Clinical Relevance

Several important conclusions can be reached from this data regarding its relevance to clinical applicability in humans. First, drugs which are not intrinsically pulmonary-toxic may enhance the effects of fractionated radiation on the lung as much as or more than intrinsically toxic drugs. This suggests that drug enhancement of radiation effects in the lung is probably mediated

Table 33–4. DEF and TGF 5 Months after Cisplatinum (CDDP) and Radiation (SCC VII/St. Tumor and Lung)

5-Day Treatment Scheme	Drug (c or C), Time Interval (hr), Irradiation (X)	DEF	TGF (Max)
1	c c c c c 0 0 0 0 0 X X X X X	1.02	1.78
2	c c c c c 2 2 2 2 2 X X X X X	1.12	1.45
3	X X X X X 6 6 6 6 6 c c c c c	1.27	1.31
4	C 24 X X X X X	0.94	1.86
5	X X X X X 24 C	0.98	1.68
6	X X X X X 72 c c c c c	1.25	1.23
7	c c c c c 72 X X X X X	1.28	1.24

C = 12 mg/kg CDDP, c = 2.4 mg/kg CDDP, X = radiation 400 cGy per fraction
Modified with permission from Tanabe M, et al, Int J Radiat Oncol Biol Phys 13:1523, 1987 (76).

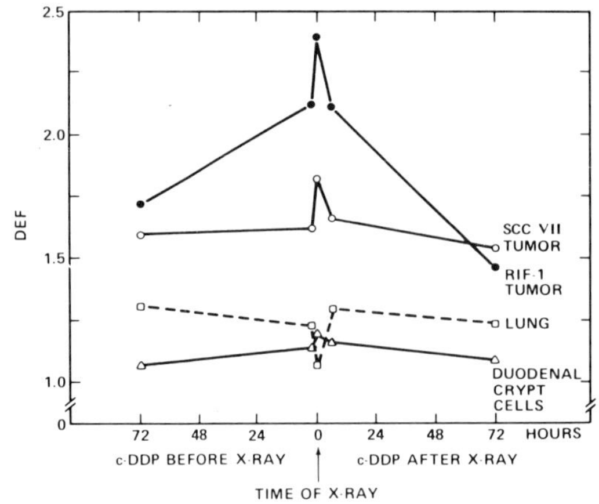

Fig. 33–2. Mean DEF for tumor cell growth inhibition, late lung injury, and crypt cell kill as a function of the scheduling of C-DDP and irradiation. The peak DEF corresponds to drug administration immediately prior to each x-ray dose. (From Tanabe M, et al. Int J Radiat Oncol Biol Phys 13:1523, 1987.)

through different mechanisms than the mechanisms associated with intrinsic pulmonary toxicity. This hypothesis is supported by the lack of correlation between DEF measurements and the intrinsic pulmonary toxicity capacity of the drugs studied, and furthermore by critical schedule dependence of the measured DEF but not the intrinsic toxicity. This hypothesis does not exclude the possibility that clinically significant pulmonary toxicity could occur due to the mechanisms of intrinsic pulmonary toxicity and radiation-mediated mechanisms, but because the end-point for most of these animal models is usually a lethal event, this would result in literal "overkill." That is, if you give enough drug to result in a lethal event, adding it to any amount of radiation is not likely to yield meaningful information.

Secondly, experimental models using large single doses of radiation are not likely to give us useful information on how best to combine radiation and chemotherapy. This is because late-responding tissue, such as lung, tolerates large fractions poorly, and normal tissue tolerance is the main dose-limiting problem.

Thirdly, the time interval between the administration of a drug and radiation may be more critical than generally appreciated. All combined modality treatment schedules designed to answer clinical questions about the optimal way to treat cancer should include details about the time interval between modalities designed explicitly into the protocol.

CHEMORADIATION AND PULMONARY TOXICITY—CLINICAL RESULTS

We have reviewed the toxic effects of radiation alone, of intrinsically pulmonary toxic drugs, and experimental data which predict enhancement of the effects of radiation by specific drugs. How does this compare with clinical experience? Inasfar as there have been many thousands of patients treated with CMT who are at risk for pulmonary toxicity, it is not surprising that it did not take long for the literature to explode with reports of enhanced toxicity (1–3,5). Also not surprising is the fact that the most dramatic reports have been associated with the use of large dose-per-fraction radio-therapy.

The most impressive body of literature (relative to the number of patients undergoing this treatment) emphasizing the toxic effects of radiation on the lung is in association with BMT using large single fractions (79,80). Typically, patients in these series were treated with single doses on the order of 900 cGy to 1300 cGy and were found to have an incidence of interstitial pneumonitis of 40 to 80%. Many of these idiopathic cases are attributable to radiation toxicity. These results are surprisingly similar to the experimental findings of Wara and coworkers in 1973 (38).

The excessive toxicity associated with the use of large dose-per-fraction has resulted in the adoption of fractionated radiotherapy schedules for patients undergoing TBI at BMT centers around the world. Radiobiologic considerations have brought further attention to and support for the use of fractionated radiation schedules (81–83). Unfortunately, the adoption of some of these fractionation schedules may have been overly conservative. A recent retrospective review by Socie et al involving 180 patients undergoing BMT for chronic myelogenous leukemia revealed that, although fractionated TBI (200 cGy b.i.d. for 3 days) reduced pulmonary toxicity compared to single fraction therapy (1000 cGy), there was a higher relapse rate resulting in similar overall survivals in both groups (84). These findings are consistent with what one might predict based on the linear quadratic equation discussed earlier. Using this equation, a significantly larger fractionated total dose would be required to yield a similar biologic effect on early responding tissues (including leukemia cells).

The most common site for which CMT plays a role is in the management of lung cancer. Because the lung is included in the target of interest, only limited sparing is possible. The chemotherapy regimes most commonly used include drugs that are either intrinsically pulmonary toxic or at least have been demonstrated to enhance the effects of radiation (see Tables 33–2 and 33–3). Tables 33–5 and 33–6 (85–103) summarize some of the series available in the literature utilizing CMT for nonsmall-cell and small-cell lung cancer (see Chapters 26 and 27 for further details).

Of interest, in those series which delivered all of the radiation using fraction sizes greater than 250 cGy, 6 of 10 (60%) reported an incidence of radiation pneumonitis of 20% or more. Included in four of the series not reporting such an incidence is one that used 267 cGy fractions, one using less intensive chemotherapy than is commonly used now, one with an incidence of pneumonitis of 17% and one series with only 29 patients and a reduction of chemotherapy during radiation.

In contrast, among the series using fraction sizes < 250 cGy only 1 of 11 (9%) reported an incidence of radiation pneumonitis > 20%. This one series used high-dose cisplatinum, 200 cGy fractions, large fields, and no correction for lung inhomogeneity. In this series, we noted pneumonitis in 3 of the first 11 patients (27%) and modified our radiation technique to treat smaller volumes. Two additional episodes of less severe pneumonitis occurred in the next 11 patients (18%) (6).

These data again emphasize the importance of the dose per fraction. The radiation pneumonitis seen in patients treated with combined modality therapy appears to have more to do with fraction size than the drugs. This is not to say that the radiation effects are not enhanced, but rather that large doses are enhanced more than smaller ones. If, for example, 400 cGy fractions are used in combination with drugs and result in a DEF of 1.5, at least some of the fractions may be

Table 33–5. Pulmonary Toxicity and CMT in Limited Small-cell Lung Cancer

First Author (Ref.), Year	No. Patients	RT Dose per Fraction (cGy)	Total Dose (cGy)	Drug Schedule	Radiation Pneumonitis %/ Deaths (%)
Goodman (85) 1991	56	180	4500	CDDP, E, + CAV concurrent	0/0
Mornex (86) 1990	77	150–180 (BID)	5100*	A, E, Ifos alternating	21/1
McCracken (87) 1990	138	180	4500	CDDP, E, V concurrent	9/0
Turrisi (15) 1990	40	150 (BID)	4500	CDDP, E + CAV concurrent	NA/5
Coy (89) 1988	168	250	2500–3750	CAV + CDDP, E alternating	2/0
Pater (88) 1989	233	267	4000	CAV + CDDP, E concurrent	2/<1
Perry (3) 1987	125	200	5000	CEV + CAV concurrent	9/0
Perry (3) 1987	145	200	5000	CEV+ CAV alternating	6/0
Brooks (5) 1986	40	267	4000	CM, CU concurrent	28/15
Perez (90) 1984	104	300 × 10+ 250 × 4	4000*	CAV alternating	1/NA
Shanks (91) 1980	24	250	4500	CAV + CDDP, E alternating	13/8
Maurer (92) 1980	258	320	3200	CM/CMV/C/MV alternating	0/0
Hornback (93) 1976	29†	300	3600*	CAV‡ concurrent	0/0
Einhorn (1) 1976	13†	400	4000*	B, CAV‡ concurrent	38/23

A = Adriamycin, B = Bleomycin, C = Cytoxan, CDDP = Cisplatinum, CU = CCNU, E = VP16, Ifos = Ifosfamide, M = Methotrexate, V = Vincristine

*Split course schedule

†Includes some patients with extensive disease

‡chemotherapy dose reduced during radiation

Table 33–6. Pulmonary Toxicity and CMT in Nonsmall-Cell Lung Cancer

First Author (Ref) Year	No. Patients	RT Dose per Fraction (cGy)	Total Dose (cGy)	Drugs Schedule	Radiation Pneumonitis %/ Deaths (%)
Gandara (6) 1991	22	200	6000*	CDDP alternating	23/0
Recine (94) 1990	60	200	4000–6000*(+)	CDDP, E, 5-FU alternating	8/0
Dillman (4) 1990	78	200	6000	CDDP, VLB alternating	1/0
Weitberg (95) 1990	44	NA	5600–5900	CDDP, E	0/0
Mirimanoff (96) 1990	50	150 (BID)	6300	CDDP, MC, Vd	10/NA
Pincus (97) 1988	31	200	4000–6000*(+)	5-FU, CDDP, E concurrent	13/0
Sadeghi (98) 1988	82	400	4000	C, A, CDDP concurrent	17/0
Friess (99) 1988	20	180	5500–6100	CDDP, E concurrent	0/0
Verschoore (2) 1987	27	400	4000*	A	54/15
van Harskamp (100) 1987	37	300	4800*	CDDP concurrent	22/0
Crowley (101) 1985	14	300	5100*	CDDP, VLB, MC alternating	21/NA
Madej (102) 1984	101	300	3000–4200	C, A, M, P± CDDP alternating	NA/4
Chan (103) 1976	13	400	4000*	B concurrent	23/0

(+) = Inoperable patients taken to the higher dose, NA = Not available
A = Adriamycin, B = Bleomycin, C = Cytoxan, CDDP = Cisplatinum, CU = CCNU, E = VP16 and Ifos = Ifosfamide, M = Methotrexate, MC = Mitomycin C, P = Procarbazine, V = Vincristine, VLB = Vinblastine, Vd = Vindesine, 5-FU = 5-Fluorouracil
*Split course schedule.

radiobiologically equivalent to 600 cGy. If lung inhomogeneity correction factors are excluded, even a single treatment could be associated with a risk of radiation pneumonitis approaching 5%.

This does not mean that drug effects are not also important. It is clear that certain specific drugs should be used cautiously. For example, according to a review by Catane et al, patients treated with combined bleomycin and radiation experienced a doubling of their risk of pneumonitis, and their mortality increased from 2.2% to 10% (56). Several investigators have reported their experience using bleomycin in combination with other agents and radiation for Hodgkin's disease. Two prospective randomized trials comparing MOPP and ABVD combined with irradiation demonstrated a higher incidence of radiation pneumonitis in the ABVD arm (104,105). In the report by Santoro et al, the toxicity was mild, however, and a survival advantage was seen in the ABVD arm (104). In the trial reported by Cosset et al, toxicity was again noted to be mild and correlated with fraction size greater than 200 cGy and dose greater than 3500 cGy (105). Several other series have confirmed these findings, noting an excellent outcome and tolerable toxicity for patients treated with a bleomycin-containing regimen and radiation for Hodgkin's disease (106–108).

SUMMARY

By far the most common and serious complication of combined modality therapy is local failure. For most solid tumors, the probability of tumor-related morbidity and mortality exceeds the probability of serious complications by a factor of at least 3 and treatment-related mortality by a factor of 10. Using the doses required to obtain local control of gross disease, some degree of measurable damage to the lung is inevitable. Although numerous factors contribute to the risk of clinically significant pulmonary toxicity (e.g., treatment volume, total dose, extent of underlying pulmonary dysfunction, the use of chemotherapy), the fraction size is probably the most critical. The incorporation of information regarding the TGF associated with specific radiation/drug combinations derived by using the appropriate site-specific experimental model should allow us to decrease toxicity and improve our treatment results. The development of radioprotective agents should add to the tolerance of normal tissues, further extending our ability to heal and yet "do no harm."

REFERENCES

1. Einhorn L, Krause M, Hornback N, Furnas B. Enhanced pulmonary toxicity with bleomycin and radiotherapy in oat cell lung cancer. Cancer 37:2414, 1976.
2. Verschoore J, Lagrange J, Boublil J, et al. Pulmonary toxicity of a combination of low-dose doxorubicin and irradiation for inoperable lung cancer. Radiother Oncol 9:281, 1987.
3. Perry MC, Eaton WL, Propert KJ, et al. Chemotherapy with or without radiation therapy in limited small-cell carcinoma of the lung. N Engl J Med 316:912, 1987.
4. Dillman RO, Seagren SL, Propert KJ, et al. A randomized trial of induction chemotherapy plus high-dose radiation versus radiation alone in stage III non-small-cell lung cancer. N Engl J Med 323:940, 1990.
5. Brooks BJ, Seifter EJ, Walsh TE, et al. Pulmonary toxicity with combined modality therapy for limited stage small-cell lung cancer. J Clin Oncol 4:200, 1986.
6. Gandara DR, Valone F, Perez EA, et al. Rapidly alternating radiotherapy and high dose cisplatin chemotherapy in stage IIIB non-small cell lung cancer: Results of a phase I-II study. Int J Radiat Oncol Biol Phys 20:1047, 1991.
7. McCracken JD, Janaki LM, Taylor SB, et al. Concurrent chemotherapy and radiotherapy for limited small-cell carcinoma of the lung: A Southwest Oncology Group Study. Semin Oncol 13(Suppl 3):31, 1986.
8. Thomas WW, McNeese MD, Fletcher GH, et al. Multimodal treatment for inflammatory breast cancer. Int J Radiat Oncol Biol Phys 17:739, 1989.
9. John MJ, Flam MS, Mowry PA, et al. Radiotherapy alone and chemoradiation for non-metastatic esophageal carcinoma. Cancer 63:2397, 1989.
10. Herskovic A, Martz K, Al-Sarraf M, et al. Intergroup Esophageal Study: Comparison of radiotherapy (RT) to radio-chemotherapy combination: A phase III trial. Proceedings of ASCO, 1991, p. 401.
11. Boring CC, Squires TS, Tong T. Cancer Statistics, 1991. Ca—A Cancer Journal for Clinicians; 41(1), 1991.
12. Hoppe RT. Combined modality studies in the treatment of Hodgkin's Disease. *In:* Bleomycin Chemotherapy. Sikic BI, Rosencweig M, Carter SK (Eds). New York, Academic Press, Inc, 1985, p. 155.
13. Hoppe RT. The role of radiation therapy in the management of the non-Hodgkin's lymphomas. Cancer 55:2176, 1985.
14. Antman K, Gale RP. Advanced breast cancer: High-dose chemotherapy and bone marrow autotransplants. Ann Intern Med 108:570, 1988.
15. Turrisi A, Wagner H, Glover D, et al. Limited small cell lung cancer (LSCLC): Concurrent BID thoracic radiotherapy (TRT) with Platinum-Etoposide (PE): An ECOG study. Proceedings of ASCO (Abstract 887), vol 9, 1990.
16. Thames HD, Peters LJ, Ang KK. Time-dose considerations for normal tissue tolerance. Front Radiat Ther Oncol 23:113, 1989.
17. Hall EJ. Radiobiology for the radiologist. Third Edition. Philadelphia, JB Lippincott, 1988.
18. Rubin P, Casseret GW, Clinical Radiation Pathology. Vol. 1. Philadelphia, WB Saunders, 1968, p. 423.
19. van den Brenk HAS. Radiation effects on the pulmonary system. *In:* Pathology of Irradiation. Berdjis CC (Ed). Baltimore, Williams & Wilkins Co., 1971, p. 569.
20. Phillips TL. Radiation fibrosis. *In:* Pulmonary Diseases and Disorders. Fishman AP (Ed). New York, McGraw-Hill. 2nd Ed. Vol. 1, 1988, p. 773.
21. McDonald S, Rubin P, Maasilta P. Response of normal lung to irradiation. Front Radiat Ther Oncol 23:255, 1989.
22. Travis EL, Terry NHA. Cell depletion and initial and chronic responses in normal tissues. Front Radiat Ther Oncol 23:41, 1989.
23. Penney DP, Rubin P. Specific early fine structural changes in the lung following irradiation. Int J Radiat Oncol Biol Phys 2:1123, 1977.
24. Penney DP, Siemann DW, Rubin P, et al. Morphologic changes reflecting early and late effects of irradiation on the distal lung of mouse. Scanning Electron Micros. 1:413, 1982.
25. Bertalanffy FD, Leblond CP. The continuous renewal of the two types of alveolar cells in the lungs of the rat. Anat Rec 115:515, 1953.
26. Rubin P, Finklestein JN, Siemann DW, et al. Predictive biochemical assays for late radiation effects. Int J Radiat Oncol Biol Phys 12:469, 1986.
27. Hopewell JW, Calvo W, Campling D, et al. Effects of radiation on the microvasculature. Front Radiat Ther Oncol 23:85, 1989.
28. Gross NJ. Pulmonary effects of radiation therapy. Ann Intern Med 86:81, 1977.
29. Jennings FL, Arden A. Development of radiation pneumonitis. Arch Path 74:101, 1962.
30. Hellman S, Kligerman, MM, von Essen CF, Scibetta MP. Sequelae of radical radiother-

apy of carcinoma of the lung. Radiology 82:1055, 1964.
31. Mah K, van Dyk J, Keane T, Poon PY. Acute radiation-induced pulmonary damage: A clinical study on the response to fractionated radiation therapy. Int J Radiat Oncol Biol Phys. 13:179, 1987.
32. Perez CA, Stanley K, Rubin P, et al. A prospective randomized study of various irradiation doses and fractionation schedules in the treatment of inoperable non-oat-cell carcinoma of the lung. Cancer 45:2744, 1980.
33. Cox JD, Azarnia N, Byhardt RW, et al. A randomized phase I/II trial of hyperfractionated radiation therapy with total doses of 6000 cGy to 7920 cGy: Possible survival benefit with ≥ 6960 cGy in favorable patients with Radiation Therapy Oncology Group stage III non-small-cell lung carcinoma: Report of Radiation Therapy Oncology Group 83-11. J Clin Oncol 8:1543, 1990.
34. Mancini A, Corinaldes V, Tison C, et al. Immunological aspects of experimental pulmonary sclerosis due to ionizing radiation. Lancet 1:1397, 1965.
35. Bennett DE, Millon RR, Ackerman LV. Bilateral radiation pneumonitis, a complication of the radiotherapy of bronchogenic carcinoma. Cancer 23:1001, 1969.
36. Gibson PG, Bryant DH, Morgan GW, et al. Radiation-induced lung injury: A hypersensitivity pneumonitis? Ann Intern Med 109:288, 1988.
37. Moss WT, Haddy FJ. The relationship between oxygen tension of inhaled gas and severity of acute radiation pneumonitis. Radiology 75:55, 1960.
38. Wara WM, Phillips TL, Margolis LW, Smith V. Radiation pneumonitis: A new approach to the derivation of time-dose factors. Cancer 32:547, 1973.
39. van Dyk J, Keane TJ, Kan S, et al. Radiation pneumonitis following large single dose irradiation: A re-evaluation based on absolute dose to lung. Int J Radiat Oncol Biol Phys 7:461, 1981.
40. Emirgil C, Heinemann HO. Effects of irradiation of chest on pulmonary function in man. J Appl Physiol 16:331, 1961.
41. Brady LW, German PA, Cander L. The effects of radiation therapy on pulmonary function in carcinoma of the lung. Radiology 85:130, 1965.
42. Teates D, Cooper G. Some consequences of pulmonary irradiation. Am J Roentgenol 96:612, 1966.
43. Cudkowicx L, Cunningham M, Haldane EV. Effects of mediastinal irradiation upon respiratory function following mastectomy for carcinoma of the breast. Thorax 24:359, 1969.
44. Choi NC, Kanarek DJ, Kazemi H. Physiologic changes in pulmonary function after thoracic radiotherapy for patients with lung cancer and role of regional pulmonary function studies in predicting postradiotherapy pulmonary function before radiotherapy. Cancer Treat Symp 2:119, 1985.
45. Curran WJ, Moldofsky PJ, Solin LJ. Analysis of the influence of elective nodal irradiation on postirradiation pulmonary function. Cancer 65:2488, 1990.
46. Ellis F. Dose, time and fractionation: A clinical hypothesis. Clin Radiol 20:1, 1969.
47. Fowler JF. What next in fractionated radiotherapy? Br J Cancer 49(Suppl VI):285, 1984.
48. Sostman HD, Matthay RA, Putman CE. Cytotoxic drug-induced lung disease. Am J Med 62:608, 1977.
49. Demeter SL, Ahmad M, Tomashefski JF. Drug-induced pulmonary disease. Cleveland Clinic Quarterly 46:113, 1979.
50. Muggia FM, Willson JKV, Weiss RB. Respiratory complications during cancer therapy: Diagnosis and management. *In:* Medical Complications in Cancer Patients. Klastersky, Staquet (Eds). New York, Raven Press, 1981, p. 171.
51. Morrison DA, Goldman AL. Radiographic patterns of drug-induced lung disease. Diagnostic Radiology 131:299, 1979.
52. Ginsberg SJ, Comis RL. The pulmonary toxicity of antineoplastic agents. Semin Oncol 9:34, 1982.
53. Schein PS, DeVita VT, Hubbard S, et al. Bleomycin, adriamycin, cyclophosphamide, vincristine and prednisone (BACOP) combination chemotherapy in the treatment of advanced diffuse histiocytic lymphoma. Ann Intern Med 85:417, 1976.
54. Comis RL. Bleomycin pulmonary toxicity. *In:* Bleomycin. Current Status and New Developments. New York, Academic Press, Inc., 1978, p. 179.
55. Sikic BI. Pulmonary toxicity of bleomycin. *In:* Bleomycin Chemotherapy. Sikic BI, Rosencweig M, Carter SK (Eds). Orlando, Academic Press Inc., 1985, p. 247.
56. Cantane R, Schwade JG, Turrisi AT, et al. Pulmonary toxicity after radiation and bleomycin: A review. Int J Radiat Oncol Biol Phys 5:1513, 1979.
57. Dalgleish AG, Woods RL, Levi JA. Bleomycin pulmonary toxicity: Its relationship to renal dysfunction. Med Pediat Oncol 12:313, 1984.
58. Levi JA, Thomson D, Sandeman T, et al. A prospective study of cisplatin-based combi-

nation chemotherapy in advanced germ cell malignancy: Role of maintenance and long-term follow-up. J Clin Oncol 6:1154, 1988.
59. Macdonald JS, Weiss RB, Poster D, Hammershaimb L. Subacute and chronic toxicities associated with nitrosourea therapy. *In:* Nitrosoureas, current status and new developments. Prestayko AW (Ed). New York, Academic Press, Inc., 1981, p. 145.
60. Durant JR, Norgard MJ, Murad TM, et al. Pulmonary toxicity associated with Bischloroethylnitrosourea (BCNU). Ann Intern Med 90:191, 1979.
61. Aronin PA, Mahaley MS, Rudnick SA, et al. Prediction of BCNU pulmonary toxicity in patients with malignant gliomas. N Engl J Med 303:183, 1980.
62. O'Driscoll BR, Hasleton PS, Taylor PM, et al. Active lung fibrosis up to 17 years after chemotherapy with Carmustine (BCNU) in childhood. N Engl J Med 323:378, 1990.
63. Patel AR, Shah PC, Rhee HL, et al. Cyclophosphamide therapy and interstitial pulmonary fibrosis. Cancer 38:1542, 1990.
64. Sostman HD, Matthay RA, Putman CE, Smith GJW. Methotrexate-induced pneumonitis. Medicine 55:371, 1976.
65. Chang AY, Kuebler JP, Pandya KJ, et al. Pulmonary toxicity induced by Mitomycin C is highly responsive to glucocorticoids. Cancer 57:2285, 1986.
66. Weissberg JB, Son YH, Papac RJ et al. Randomized clinical trial of mitomycin C as an adjunct to radiotherapy in head and neck cancer. Int J Radiat Oncol Biol Phys 17:3, 1989.
67. Philip HK, Aisner J, Sutherland JC, Wiernik PH. Possible pulmonary toxicity secondary to vinblastine. Cancer 50:2771, 1982.
68. Phillips TL, Fu KK. Quantification of combined radiation therapy and chemotherapy effects on critical normal tissues. Cancer 37:1186, 1976.
69. Phillips TL. Chemical modifiers of normal-tissue radiation injury. Front Radiat Ther Oncol 23:177, 1989.
70. von der Maase H, Overgaard J, Vaeth M. Effect of cancer chemotherapeutic drugs on radiation-induced lung damage in mice. Radiother Oncol 5:245, 1986.
71. von der Maase H. Experimental drug-radiation interactions in critical normal tissues. *In:* Antitumor Drug-Radiation Interactions. Hill BT, Bellamy AS (Eds). Boca Raton, CRC Press, Inc., 1990, p. 192.
72. Colman M, Zabilansky E, Redpath JL. Modification of the radiation response of mouse lung by Actinomycin D: Dependence on interval between radiation and drug treatments. Int J Radiat Oncol Biol Phys 8:511, 1982.
73. Sherman DM, Carabell SC, Belli JA, Hellman S. The effect of dose rate and adriamycin on the tolerance of thoracic radiation in mice. Int J Radiat Oncol Biol Phys 8:45, 1982.
74. Redpath JL, David RM, Colman M. The effect of adriamycin on radiation damage to mouse lung and skin. Int J Radiat Oncol Biol Phys 4:229, 1978.
75. Overgaard J, Grau C. Interactions between bleomycin and x-irradiation. *In:* Antitumor Drug-Radiation Interactions. Hill BT, Bellamy AS (Eds). Boca Raton, CRC Press, Inc., 1990, p. 54.
76. Tanabe M, Godat D, Kallman RF. Effects of fractionated schedules of irradiation combined with cis-diamminedichloroplatinum II on the SCCVII/ST tumor and normal tissues of the C3H/KM mouse. Int J Radiat Oncol Biol Phys, 13:1523, 1987.
77. Collis CH, Steel GG. Lung damage in mice from cyclophosphamide and thoracic irradiation. The effect of timing. Int J Radiat Oncol Biol Phys 9:685, 1983.
78. Kallman RF, Rapacchietta D, Zaqghloul MS. Schedule-dependent therapeutic gain from the combination of fractionated irradiation plus c-DDP and 5-FU or plus c-DDP and cyclophosphamide in C3H/Km mouse model systems. Int J Radiat Oncol Biol Phys 20:227, 1991.
79. Keane TJ, Van Dyk J, Rider WD. Idiopathic interstitial pneumonia following bone marrow transplantation: The relationship with total body irradiation. Int J Radiat Oncol Biol Phys 7:1365, 1981.
80. Broun ER, Tricot G, Akard L, et al. Treatment of refractory lymphoma with high dose cytarabine, cyclophosphamide and either TBI or VP-16 followed by autologous bone marrow transplantation. Bone Marrow Transplantation 5:341, 1990.
81. Peters LJ, Withers R, Cundiff JH, Dicke KA. Radiobiologic considerations in the use of total-body irradiation for bone marrow transplantation. Radiology 131:243, 1979.
82. O'Donoghue JA, Wheldon TE, Gregor A. The implications of in vitro radiation-survival curves for the optimal scheduling of total body irradiation with bone marrow rescue in the treatment of leukemia. Brit J Radiol 60:279, 1987.
83. Thomas ED. Total body irradiation regimens for marrow grafting. Int J Radiat Oncol Biol Phys 19:1285, 1990.
84. Socie G, Devergie A, Girinsky T, et al. Influence of the fractionation of total body irradiation on complications and relapse rate for

chronic myelogenous leukemia. Int J Radiat Oncol Biol Phys 20:397, 1991.

85. Goodman GE, Crowley J, Livingston RB, et al. Treatment of limited small-cell lung cancer with concurrent etoposide/cisplatin and radiotherapy followed by intensification with high-dose cyclophosphamide: A Southwest Oncology Group Study. J Clin Oncol 9:453, 1991.
86. Mornex F, Trillet V, Chauvin F, et al and the Group Lyonnais d'Oncologie Thoracique. Hyperfractionated radiotherapy alternating with multidrug chemotherapy in the treatment of limited small cell lung cancer (SCLC). Int J Radiat Oncol Biol Phys 19:23, 1990.
87. McCracken D, Janaki LM, Crowley JJ, et al. Concurrent chemotherapy/radiotherapy for limited small-cell lung carcinoma: A Southwest Oncology Group Study. J Clin Oncol 8:892, 1990.
88. Pater J, Coy P, Murray N, et al. Safety of concurrent chemotherapy (CT) and thoracic irradiation (TI) in patients with small cell lung cancer (SCLC): Results of a National Cancer Institute of Canada Clinical Trials Group (NCIC-CTG) study. (Abstract 866). Proc Am Soc Clin Oncol 8:223, 1989.
89. Coy P, Hodson I, Payne DG, et al. The effect of dose of thoracic irradiation on recurrence in patients with limited stage small cell lung cancer. Initial results of a Canadian multicenter randomized trial. Int J Radiat Oncol Biol Phys 14:219, 1988.
90. Perez CA, Einhorn L, Oldham RK, et al. Randomized trial of radiotherapy to the thorax in limited small-cell carcinoma of the lung treated with multiagent chemotherapy and elective brain irradiation: A preliminary report. J Clin Oncol 2:1200, 1984.
91. Shank B, Natale RB, Hilaris BS, Wittes RE. Treatment of small cell carcinoma of lung with combined high dose mediastinal irradiation, whole brain prophylaxis and chemotherapy. Int J Radiat Oncol Biol Phys 7:469, 1981.
92. Maurer LH, Tulloh M, Weiss RB, et al. A randomized combined modality trial in small cell carcinoma of the lung. Cancer 45:30, 1980.
93. Hornback NB, Einhorn L, Shindia H, et al. Oat cell carcinoma of the lung. Cancer 37:2658, 1976.
94. Recine D, Rowland K, Reddy S, et al. Combined modality therapy for locally advanced non-small lung carcinoma. Cancer 66:2270, 1990.
95. Weitberg A, Posner M, Yashar J, et al. Combined modality therapy for stage IIIA non-small cell carcinoma of the lung (NSCCL). (Abstract 872). Proc Am Soc Clin Oncol 9:1990.
96. Mirimanoff RO, Alberto P, Leyvraz S, et al. Alternating accelerated radiotherapy (ART) and chemotherapy (CT) for inoperable, non-metastatic, non-small cell lung carcinoma (NSCLC): A phase II collaborative study. The third international conference on the interaction of radiation therapy and systemic therapy. (Abstract 2-10). March 1990.
97. Pincus M, Reddy S, Lee MS, et al. Preoperative combined modality therapy for stage III M_o non-small cell lung carcinoma. Int J Radiat Oncol Biol Phys 15:189, 1988.
98. Sadeghi A, Payne D, Rubinstein L, Lad T. Lung Cancer Study Group. Combined modality treatment for resected advanced non-small cell lung cancer: Local control and local recurrence. Int J Radiat Oncol Biol Phys 15:89, 1988.
99. Friess GG, Baikadi M, Harvey WH. Simultaneous cisplatin and etoposide with radiation therapy in locoregional non-small cell lung cancer. Final results of a pilot trial. Gralla RJ, Einhorn L (Eds). Small cell lung cancer and non-small cell lung cancer. Royal Society of Medicine Services International Congress and Symposium Series No. 150. Royal Society of Medicine Services Limited, 1989, p. 121.
100. van Harskamp G, Boven E, Vermorken JB, et al. Phase II trial of combined radiotherapy and daily low-dose cisplatin for inoperable, locally advanced non-small cell lung cancer (NSCLC). Int J Radiat Oncol Biol Phys 13:1735, 1987.
101. Crowley T, Jensen B, Phillips T, et al. Radiation Therapy (RT) sandwiched between cycles of combination chemotherapy in inoperable non-small cell carcinoma of the lung (NCOG Pilot Study P-2N-82-2). (Abstract C-711). Proc Am Soc Clin Oncol 4:182, 1985.
102. Madej PJ, Bitran JD, Golomb HM. Combined modality therapy for stage III M_o non-small cell lung cancer. Cancer 54:5, 1984.
103. Chan PYM, Byfield JE, Kagan AR, Aronstam EM. Unresectable squamous cell carcinoma of the lung and its management by combined bleomycin and radiotherapy. Cancer 37:2671, 1976.
104. Santoro A, Viviani AM, Pagnoni R, et al. Long-term therapeutic and toxicologic results of MOPP-RT-MOPP vs ABVD-RT-ABVD in PS IIB-III (A,B) Hodgkin's disease (HD). Proceedings of Am Soc Clin Oncol (Abstract C-777) 4:199, 1985.
105. Cosset JM, Henry-Amar J, Thomas P, et al. Increased pulmonary toxicity in the ABVD arm of the EORTC H6-U trial. Proceedings of

Am Soc Clin Oncol (Abstract 985) 8:253, 1989.

106. Horning SJ, Hoppe RT, Hancock SL, et al. Bleomycin, and methotrexate: An effective adjuvant in favorable Hodgkin's disease. J Clin Oncol 6:1822, 1988.

107. Thompson EI, Stokes JA, Wilimas JA, et al. Serial lung function in pediatric Hodgkin's disease (HD) patients treated with COP-ABVD and mantle irradiation (RT). (Abstract 1121). Proc Am Soc Clin Oncol 7:289, 1988.

108. Fryer CJ, Hutchinson RJ, Krailo M, et al. Efficacy and toxicity of 12 courses of ABVD chemotherapy followed by low-dose regional radiation in advanced Hodgkin's disease in children: A report from the Children's Cancer Study Group. J Clin Oncol, 8:1971, 1990.

Chapter 34

GYNECOLOGIC TOXICITY

ANTHONY H. RUSSELL AND SIDNEY A. SCUDDER

Few areas in oncology offer as rich or diverse opportunities for the intelligent coordination of radiation and chemotherapy as the treatment of patients with gynecologic cancer. Squamous cancers involving the cervix (1,2), vagina (3,4) and vulva (5), whose patterns of failure following conventional therapies commonly include locoregional tumor persistence, offer an attractive arena in which to attempt to emulate the success achieved with chemoradiation in the treatment of squamous cancers of the anal canal (6–8) and esophagus (9).

Careful analysis of patients relapsing after radical hysterectomy for FIGO Stage IB and IIA cancer of the cervix has resulted in the description of adverse histopathologic factors, which identify a subset of patients at comparatively high risk of both locoregional and systemic recurrence (10–12). The patterns of failure in more advanced cervical cancer treated by conventional radiotherapy have remained unchanged since the advent of megavoltage teletherapy. Persistence of pelvic tumor remains a challenge, as does distant dissemination. Appropriately, multimodality strategies are increasingly employed in an effort to address the ineffectiveness of conventional locoregional therapy.

Modern combinations of surgery and radiation in the treatment of patients with endometrial cancers have achieved very high pelvic cancer control rates (13–15). Histologic variants of endometrial cancers, such as papillary serous and clear cell carcinomas, have been identified as being prone to recurrences frequently involving the upper abdominal cavity or remote, extra-abdominal sites (16–21). The addition of chemotherapy to pelvic and extended volume radiation portals requires rigorous, prospective evaluation. Similar considerations apply to the surgical adjuvant therapies employed in the treatment of uterine sarcomas (22–26).

The overall poor prognosis of patients with epithelial ovarian cancer has inevitably led to rational efforts to improve salvage rates by the combination of treatment modalities (surgery followed by chemotherapy and subsequent radiation), each of which possesses only modest efficacy (27–40).

Concern to control an initial life-threatening malignancy must be the major priority in the selection of initial treatment modality and the design of sensible treatment protocols integrating more than one modality of therapy. However, efforts to increase probability of cure in gynecologic cancer by the combined use of radiation and chemotherapy (concurrently or sequentially) must be tempered by the realization that both acute and late toxicities may be augmented with this approach. The therapeutic index will only be increased if the impact of these efforts on cancer control substantially exceeds any enhancement of major acute or chronic iatrogenic complications. Quantification of net benefit requires candid reporting of both acute and late injuries, and therefore necessitates years of meticulous surveillance of patients thought to be cured of their cancer.

Certain complications of radiation therapy such as radiation vaginitis and rectovaginal and vesicovaginal fistulae are rarely seen except in patients treated with intracavitary or interstitial brachytherapy for gynecologic cancer (41–52). Wide-field high dose irradiation, encompassing pelvic and para-aortic nodal volumes (53–67) and/or the entire abdominal cavity (68–75) is frequently employed in gynecologic cancer. Thus toxicity information for normal tissues, such as the liver, is often available (76–79). The toxic effects of radiation and chemotherapy on many of the abdominal viscera are comprehensively described elsewhere in this text, and will not be reiterated here. This chapter focuses on toxicity issues of particular concern in the management of patients with gynecologic cancer. Emphasis is placed on the following.

1. The effects of treatment on endocrine function and reproductive capacity.
2. The impact of cancer treatment on sexual function.
3. The vaginal complications associated with intracavitary and interstitial brachytherapy in the pelvis.
4. The special considerations in the management of the patient with coexistent pelvic malignancy and pregnancy.
5. The potential induction of second neoplasms in patients successfully treated by radiation and chemotherapy.
6. The consequences of treatment of large volumes of normal tissue.
7. The information currently available concerning reported toxicities in gynecologic cancer patients treated with curative intent with radiation and chemotherapy, sequentially or concurrently.
8. The avenues which may be profitably explored to decrease known toxicities of multimodality therapy.

ENDOCRINE AND REPRODUCTIVE INTEGRITY

Ovaries are sensitive to radiation. Historically, ovarian endocrine radio-ablation or radiocastration has been used in the treatment of menorrhagia, endometriosis with pain, and metastatic breast cancer. A fractionated dose of 2000 cGy will virtually assure permanent cessation of menses in premenopausal women (80), a frequent consequence of radical radiation for cancers of the cervix, vagina and uterus. The consequences of endocrine insufficiency (vasomotor instability, accelerated bone demineralization, and potential premature cardiovascular disease) are well known (81–86). Although hormonal replacement can easily be accomplished with oral medication, reproductive capacity can be preserved only with foresight and careful planning.

Gynecologic cancer frequently afflicts premenopausal women at an age when they may not have had children or completed a family of planned size. Technologic advances in reproductive medicine, such as in vitro fertilization and the use of a "surrogate" uterus, offer hope of biologic parenthood to women whose reproductive capacity has been crippled by cancer or its treatment. Although pioneering work in this arena with noncancer patients has raised unprecedented ethical dilemmas and has resulted in celebrated courtroom confrontations, the very existence of such biotechnologic prowess virtually ensures its eventual use for the benefit of women who are reproductively disabled because of prior treatment for cancer.

Effects of Ovarian Irradiation on Progeny

In the not-too-distant past, low-dose radiation to the ovaries and pituitary was employed in the "treatment" of women thought to be infertile. Such "P and O" treatment delivered up to 150 cGy in divided doses to both ovaries and 90 cGy to the pituitary in a bizarre effort to stimulate ovulation, somewhat analogous to kicking the malfunctioning television set to improve a fuzzy picture. Not infrequently, pregnancy followed such treatment (although causality is improbable). Numerous healthy progeny are reported to have been the result (87).

Women irradiated for early-stage Hodgkin's disease have conceived and delivered full-term infants (88). The rate of spontaneous abortion and congenital malformations complicating such pregnancies does not appear to be noticeably different than the background level in the general population. However, the numbers of such women and the numbers of their children available for longitudinal study are small.

Cancer risk among 72,216 children conceived by parents, one or both of whom involuntarily received gonadal radiation exposure at Hiroshima or Nagasaki, is not detectably different from that of children of nonexposed parents (89). However, consequences seen in survivors and their subsequent progeny following a single large radiation exposure to the ovaries must be extrapolated with caution to individuals whose ovaries are exposed to comparable total dose in multiple smaller fractions.

Chemotherapy Effects on Ovarian Function

Administration of cytotoxic chemotherapeutic agents, concurrently or sequentially, is likely to augment adverse effects on ovarian function. Chemotherapy-induced ovarian failure has been reported with a variety of single agents, including busulfan, chlorambucil, vinblastine, and cyclophosphamide (90–99). The use of multiple agents, such as in the MOPP regimen employed for the treatment of Hodgkin's disease, has also been reported to produce ovarian failure as confirmed by decreased estradiol levels and elevations of serum gonadotropins (100–104).

Chemotherapy-associated cessation of menses may be temporary, and menstruation may return several months following cessation of treatment. The effect of chemotherapy is strongly age-dependent, with age over 25 being predictive of a substantially higher risk of chemotherapy-induced amenorrhea, and age over 30 associated with a 12-fold increased risk of menstrual irregularities in women treated for Hodgkin's disease (103,104).

Potentially heritable genetic damage has been studied by Li and colleagues in adult survivors of childhood cancers treated with chemotherapy. Two hundred and eighty-six pregnancies were studied, the aggregate experience of 84 female and 62 male parents. No increase in birth defects was apparent. Karyotyping in 23 of 24 children studied was normal (105). Holmes and Holmes reported on pregnancies in patients treated for Hodgkin's disease with chemotherapy or chemotherapy plus radiation (106). In a small subset (women treated with both radiation and chemotherapy), an increase in congenital anomalies was appreciated. van Thiel and colleagues have pointed out that the recessive nature of most mutations would make chemotherapy induced DNA damage in germ cells difficult to detect, unless inflicted on the X chromosome (sex-linked) (107).

Preservation of ovarian function, both endocrine and potentially reproductive, in women treated for cancer with curative intent requires careful planning prior to initiation of the first therapeutic interventions. The addition of sequential modalities of therapy must be anticipated from the start and the intelligent combination of treatments tailored to specific stages of disease and probable patterns of failure and dissemination. Ovarian function may be preserved in many women successfully treated for gynecologic cancer, but only if the need is anticipated.

SEXUAL DYSFUNCTION

Sexual dysfunction in gynecologic patients may antedate the diagnosis and treatment of cancer. This may be the consequence of symptoms related to the presence of cancer, including malodorous vaginal discharge, vaginal or perineal pruritus, intermenstrual or postcoital bleeding, and dyspareunia (108).

The diagnosis of cancer at any anatomic site may result in profound emotional distress and depression with consequent diminution of libido and sexual interest (109). For the woman afflicted with gynecologic cancer, site-specific symptoms, treatment factors, and physical and psychologic sequelae may add substantially to the burden already imposed by the sense of helplessness and loss of personal esteem frequently experienced by other cancer patients (109–122).

In women with cancer of the genital tract, avoidance of sexual contact may be the consequence of feelings of guilt provoked by the knowledge that some genital tract cancers have been epidemiologically related to coital activity. Information available to patients through the lay press may reinforce the idea that cervical cancer is a "venereal disease." Patients may interpret their development of cervical cancer as retribution for promiscuous sexual behavior or punishment for premarital or extramarital sexual encounters. Lingering, unresolved conflicts precipitated by a prior abortion (often in the distant past) may further compound feelings of guilt. Guilt may also be experienced by women who have ignored signs and symptoms of genital cancer, or who have not sought periodic gynecologic surveillance care, such as cytologic screening (110). A patient's sexual partner may harbor similar feelings of guilt and feel responsible for giving his partner the cancer.

Fears that sexual contact may transmit the cancer from the afflicted female to her partner are not uncommon (114), as well as concerns that the radiation or chemotherapy used in treating the cancer may be "contagious." Such concerns are occasionally encountered by the inquiring physician, but are rarely voluntarily raised by the patient or sexual partner.

Determining a diagnosis may entail multiple sequential pelvic examinations from multiple (frequently male) physicians with the possibility that such examinations constitute a perceived violation of personal privacy and dignity or embarrassment. Examinations, biopsies, and minor diagnostic surgical procedures inflict pain from that quarter of the anatomy which previously may have been (and hopefully will remain) the source of pleasurable physical sensations and a focal point for interpersonal intimacy. The donning of rubber gloves by physicians performing pelvic examinations may unavoidably reinforce the impression that cancer is contagious, or that the genital tract is, in some sense, contaminated and unclean.

Anger provoked by the diagnosis of cancer may be focused on the healthy sexual partner assumed to be the source of the "infection." Fear of again acquiring or transmitting the infection (cancer) following successful treatment can inhibit resumption of sexual activity by both the patient and her sexual partner (109,114).

Radiation therapy is thought by some patients to be palliative treatment. Cancer that cannot be removed surgically may be perceived to be incurable. The consequent depression may be a profound inhibitor of sexual interest. Retention of the organ harboring the primary site (uterus) in patients treated primarily with radiation may prove a source of ongoing anxiety and may impede sexual rehabilitation. Surgical removal of the primary cancer, in contrast, may provide some women with a comforting sensation of distance and separation from the diagnosis (112).

Patients treated in whole or part by radiation may believe that portions of their anatomy become radioactive following treatment. This particular misconception is frequently encountered among patients undergoing intracavitary or interstitial brachytherapy at conventional low dose rates. Such patients are subject to interactions with physicians, nurses, and other hospital workers qualitatively similar to those experienced by patients harboring communicable disease. Hospitalization for diagnostic or therapeutic surgery may be associated with semiprivate accommodation. In contrast, hospitalization for intracavitary or interstitial brachytherapy is invariably accomplished with private accommodation, which achieves isolation for purposes of protection of other patients and hospital staff. The sensation of being in quarantine may persist for some time following removal of radioactive sources and subsequent hospital discharge.

Radiation itself is poorly understood by the average patient. It may be (correctly) thought of as carcinogenic, but the magnitude of this effect may be seriously overestimated. The perception that the genitalia themselves become radioactive following radiation treatment may inhibit subsequent sexual expression. Anxieties on this account may be experienced by sexual partners as well.

Side effects during the course of radiation therapy may profoundly inhibit sexual expression. Cramps, diarrhea, urinary frequency, dysuria, and vaginal pruritus may all be encountered. Depending on the location of the cancer being treated and the placement and design of radiation portals, reaction in the vulva and perineal skin may encompass the full spectrum from little or no reaction to moist desquamation.

The addition of systemic chemotherapy to radiation may enhance many of the psychologic burdens previously described. Some patients misperceive chemotherapy to be a terminal intervention for categorically incurable cancer, thus heightening feelings of anxiety and depression. Administration of chemotherapy, in either the outpatient or inpatient setting, is likely to bring the patient in closer and more frequent contact with other patients receiving chemotherapy who are indeed approaching the terminal phase of incurable illness, further reinforcing these fears. The addition of chemotherapy before or after radiation will lengthen a course of treatment, delaying the time at which a woman may feel recovered from treatment and may put, as far as is possible, the illness behind her. The simultaneous administration of chemotherapy enhances many of the acute side effects of radiation and may add others, contributing to a sense of illness and diminishing both interest in, and capacity for, sexual enjoyment. Synchronous radiation and chemotherapy may result in greater longterm adverse complications in critical normal tissues (vagina, bladder, rectum) unless significantly enhanced probability of cancer control permits reduction in intensity of radiation applied.

Following radiation treatment, each follow-up examination entails disrobing and pelvic examination. Each examination may be the source of both significant anticipatory anxiety, as well as suspense, while the patient is subsequently awaiting the results of surveillance cytologic smears, x-rays, and blood work (116). Each visit may be a reminder of the uncertainty which clouds the future for patients treated for cancer, and the pain and loss of personal dignity associated with treatment.

Loss of procreative capacity may have unpredictable consequences for sexual function. For some women, a sense of personal worth and sexual enjoyment are inextricably linked to reproductive function. Religious convictions and cultural background are of critical importance in this regard. Unfortunately, in some societies, a woman's worth is largely a function of her capacity to bear and raise children. For other women, treatment-induced infertility may be liberating (117). Freedom from the need to observe contraceptive precautions may enhance the spontaneity and enjoyment of sexual encounters. However, loss of ovarian endocrine function by surgical castration or radioablation may be perceived by some patients to accelerate the aging process and decrease their sexual desirability. Loss of sexual self-confidence may be further aggravated by largely cosmetic changes (temporary or permanent) induced by treatment (loss of scalp or pubic hair, permanent skin tattoos defining radiation portals). Endocrine replacement may aid in psychologic rehabilitation as well as in the prevention of osteoporosis, cardiac disease, and atrophic vaginitis (81–86).

For multiple potential reasons, more than one of which may be important for any one patient or couple, sexual dysfunction following radiation therapy for cervical and vaginal cancer is the rule rather than the exception. Many of the same considerations apply to patients treated for other gynecologic cancer, and sexual adjustment problems must be considered and anticipated by physicians if early and successful intervention is to be achieved (122).

VAGINAL SEQUELAE

Gross and microscopic changes of "radiation vaginitis" have been described by Abitol and Davenport (44) and Pitkin and Bradbury (42) based on clinical examination, cytologic smears, and sequential biopsies. Gross abnormalities may vary in severity from a chronically pale and atrophic vaginal mucosa to severe inflammation, tissue necrosis with ulceration (which can progress to fistula formation), and formation of adhesions which (in severe form) may obliterate a portion or all of the vaginal canal. Narrowing and shortening of the vaginal caliber are common, often in conjunction with parametrial or generalized pelvic fibrosis. Microscopically, changes evolve over time. As an immediate response to radiation, there is a loss of most or all of the vaginal epithelium in areas in proximity to brachytherapy sources. This may persist for 3 to 6 months. Subsequent re-epithelialization consists of a thin layer of basal cells with progressive maturation after approximately 2 years. However, in none of the patients studied by Pitkin and Bradbury did a fully developed stratified squamous epithelium regenerate (42).

The use of topical (intravaginal) estrogen following completion of radiotherapy appeared to stimulate epithelial regeneration, both in the immediate post-treatment period and, most significantly, 3 or more months following radiation. "Nearly all estrogen treated subjects exhibited fully developed epithelium . . . A concomitant decrease in inflammatory reaction was also observed" (42). In contrast, low-dose systemic estrogen administration did not appear to stimulate epithelial maturation in patients treated 1 year or longer following irradiation for cervical cancer (44). Systemic (oral) as well as topical hormonal replacement may both be indicated to optimally protect the irradiated vagina, as well as to prevent the systemic consequences of estrogen withdrawal (vasomotor instability, bone demineralization, accelerated atherosclerosis). Patient compliance with oral medication may be a more predictable means of hormone replacement than reliance on potentially erratic systemic absorption of topically administered estrogen from a heavily irradiated vagina.

Microscopic examination of the submucosa and muscular layer of the vagina following radiation reveals hyalinization and collagenization of connective tissue, absence of the small glands important for vaginal lubrication, marked narrowing or obliteration of the luminae of small blood vessels, and hyalinization and replacement of muscle fibers by fibrosis (44). The unirradiated vagina is an elastic, distensible structure (permitting passage of an infant's head). Following high-dose radiation, shortening and narrowing of the vagina are not uncommon, and the vagina may become substantially less elastic and distensible. This may result in inability to engage in vaginal intercourse, and may substantially hamper physicians in their ability to perform pelvic examination for purposes of cancer surveillance.

These complications of radiation therapy are much more effectively prevented than treated. Regular (daily) use of a vaginal dilator, topical estrogen, and periodic examination to ensure compliance are the best mechanisms available to prevent untreatable complications. Premarin vaginal cream in a daily dose of 1 to 2 g intravaginally is an effective and practical regimen for topical estrogen therapy. Following healing, a reduction in dose and frequency of application to a maintenance schedule of approximately 1 g three times weekly is often sufficient to preserve reconstituted vaginal epithelium. In the absence of regular intercourse, daily use of a vaginal dilator is encouraged. For some patients, the use of a dilator carries a stigma of masturbation, and is a source of embarrassment and noncompliance that can be overcome only through sensitive counseling by the physician.

In some patients, severe radiation sequelae in the vagina may progress to fistulization (vesicovaginal, urethrovaginal, ureterovaginal, ileovaginal, or rectovaginal fistulae) (45–52). Some respond to conservative treatment with antibiotics and debulkment of necrotic tissue. Others require diversion of the urinary or fecal stream. In an occasional patient, repair of a fistula may be attempted employing a myocutaneous graft with independent, unirradiated vascular supply, or by excision of necrotic tissue and reestablishment of organ continuity. For example, a high recto-vaginal fistula may occasionally be repaired by low anterior rectal resection and anastomosis of sigmoid to distal rectal stump. Such interventions must be considered high risk and appropriately reserved for carefully selected patients.

In patients with severe, nonhealing radiation vaginitis with ulceration and necrosis, it may be more appropriate to cease efforts intended to help the vagina remain patent, and to allow progressive vaginal agglutination to obliterate the canal. Although it precludes vaginal intercourse and significantly hampers surveillance pelvic examination, this may be a preferable outcome to fistulization.

GENITAL CANCER AND PREGNANCY

Invasive cancers of the cervix (123–137), vulva, vagina (138), endometrium (139), and ovary (140,141) have been described complicating pregnancy. Barber and Brunschwig (133) reviewed a 25-year experience at Memorial James Ewing Hospitals in New York in 1962, noting 47 cases of invasive carcinoma of the cervix and 15 cases of other gynecologic cancers diagnosed during pregnancy or within 1 year of pregnancy. Lutz and colleagues (132), reviewing a 20-year experience at the Medical University of South Carolina, reported 90 genital malignancies associated with pregnancy. Of these patients, 50 had cervical intraepithelial neoplasia (CIS) and 30 had invasive cervical cancer. The rarity of invasive cancers of the endometrium, vulva, vagina, and ovary during pregnancy precludes making any coherent statements concerning management with much foundation. In contrast, pregnancy complicating management of cervical cancer was observed in approximately 1 of 29 patients with cervical cancer at the Medical University of South Carolina, and has been estimated by Waldrop and Palmer to constitute a complicating factor in 1.4% of patients with cervical carcinomas based on a comprehensive literature review in 1963 (130).

Considerable controversy exists concerning the impact of pregnancy on prognosis in cervical cancer, as well as concerning optimal management. Substantially different therapeutic strategies have been employed during the same period, even within the same state. Waldrop and Palmer (130) concluded, "We have tried to review the literature very thoroughly and have found it to be thoroughly confusing and contradictory"—a finding that we would not dispute.

Greer and colleagues have pointed out that both maternal and fetal outcomes should be considered when counselling the pregnant patient with invasive cervical cancer, but noted that "The decision to treat or delay treatment of cervical cancer during pregnancy is not difficult if the pregnancy is unwanted prior to 24 weeks, if the cancer is diagnosed when fetal maturity has been obtained, or if the cancer is far advanced and a delay will not change the maternal prognosis. The difficult decision arises when the pregnancy is wanted and the fetus is not mature." (142).

Results of surgical treatment of FIGO Stages IB and IIA cervical cancer in pregnancy do not differ noticeably from results surgically achieved in nongravid patients. Surgical management, therefore, seems appropriate for these patients (126). During the first two trimesters of pregnancy, invasive cancer of the cervix to be treated primarily with radiation may be managed without significant alteration in treatment strategy, provided that the patient does not wish to carry the pregnancy to term. Treatment is initiated with external beam, and most authors report that spontaneous abortion almost invariably follows 3 to 6 weeks following initiation of treatment (123–128). Only in rare instances has spontaneous abortion failed to follow pelvic radiation, necessitating hysterectomy or curettage for evacuation of nonviable fetal tissue. Radiation-induced abortion in the presence of cervical cancer has not been associated with increased risk of excessive or life-threatening hemorrhage, disseminated intravascular coagulation with hypofibrinogenemia, or infection.

Management of invasive cancer diagnosed during the third trimester of pregnancy can be delayed long enough to ensure fetal maturity with no apparent major decrement in maternal prognosis (142). A delay of 8 to 10 weeks to achieve fetal maturity in a desired pregnancy would appear to substantially outweigh a theoretical decrement in prognosis which cannot reliably be quantitated (142,143).

The mode of delivery in the presence of invasive cervical cancer remains controversial. Several authors have raised concern that vaginal delivery causes tumor dissemination, whereas others have not detected any difference in maternal prognosis in individuals delivered transvaginally as opposed to delivery by hysterectomy. Patient and physician bias, as well as tumor size and location, play important roles in selecting the mode of delivery, thus rendering comparison of outcomes difficult to interpret. The occasional reports of cervical dystocia complicating labor in the setting of cervical cancer argue in favor of delivery by section. The opportunities additionally afforded to assess the status and level of involvement of retroperitoneal lymph nodes, and the potential for lateral ovarian transposition, render this approach significantly more attractive than vaginal delivery.

The historically employed partial treatment by radiation of invasive cervical cancer in the third trimester of pregnancy or earlier is described here only to be condemned. Use of transvaginal cone irradiation or limited intravaginal brachytherapy for purposes of hemostasis unavoidably results in significant in utero fetal exposure. Although this is less likely to result in congenital malformations in patients treated during the third trimester of pregnancy, potential longterm risks of subtle neurologic injury and neoplasia are difficult to justify. Jones and Neill treated 11 pregnant women with cervical cancer with small doses of radium and allowed as many as possible to go to term (134). This treatment produced seven living children, two of whom were microcephalic. Plummer published data on children exposed in utero to radiation from the atom bomb on Hiroshima (144). Fourteen percent of the children had one or more significant congenital anomalies, with the probability of microcephaly or mental retardation closely related to the distance of the mother to the hypocenter. The literature on the deleterious consequences of in utero radiation exposure is voluminous (145–151).

The use of chemotherapy in pregnancy should be avoided if at all possible. It is hard to imagine a situation in which one might need to employ antineoplastic agents for the treatment of gynecologic cancer during pregnancy. There is experience in the use of cytotoxic agents during pregnancy, but the majority of patients are women with leukemias or lymphomas who refuse a therapeutic abortion (152–154). Under these circumstances, the physician cannot delay therapy until fetal maturity without jeopardizing the mother's survival.

During the first trimester of pregnancy, when organogenesis is occurring, all antineoplastic agents should be avoided, as they are all mutagenic, but in particular antimetabolites which carry a high risk of congenital malformations. Antifolates, such as methotrexate and aminopterin, are associated with a high risk of cranial anomalies in the first trimester.

In the second and third trimesters, chemotherapy has been given in life-threatening situations with no obvious increase in the rate of congenital malformations and with morphologically normal children (153,154). However, one cannot be cavalier about this time period because the majority of neurogenesis and brain development is ongoing. The longterm side effects of antineoplastic drugs on brain development and intelligence are unknown and would be difficult to assess quantitatively.

The use of sporadic low-dose chemotherapy to control a neoplasm until fetal maturity should never be done because there are risks to both mother and fetus. Use of suboptimal drug doses in an erratic, unscheduled regimen could lead to drug resistance, making definitive therapy postpartum more difficult. There are no data on concurrent use of chemotherapy and radiation therapy in pregnancy. If a decision has been rendered to delay definitive cancer therapy in the interest of fetal maturity and viability, neither future cancer therapy nor long-term infant health should be compromised by treatment with radiation or chemotherapy.

Invasive cancer complicating the first or second trimester of pregnancy, when pregnancy continuation is desired, represents a more difficult therapeutic decision. Counselling such a patient must take into consideration the patient's and family's moral and religious beliefs and traditions, the patient's parity and prior reproductive history, and the patient's underlying health and prospects for carrying a normal pregnancy to term. Candor requires that the patient be informed that the risk of treatment delay cannot be accurately quantitated. In the event that the patient elects continuation of pregnancy, a decision need not be final. Serial determinations of tumor size by pelvic examination, ultrasound, or MRI may detect rapid tumor progression, suggesting advisability of earlier treatment intervention at the cost of termination of the pregnancy.

SECONDARY NEOPLASMS

Radiation Effects

Radiation exposure of non-neoplastic (but not necessarily normal) tissue carries a risk of induction of neoplasia. Risk of induction of neoplasia is probably a function of absorbed dose, dose rate, multiplicity and frequency of exposures, and quality of radiation. Precise quantitation of risk remains an unresolved area of controversy in environmental health (155).

Development of an otherwise rare second malignancy (often sarcoma) within the tissue volume exposed to radiation for treatment of a histologically distant initial malignancy (frequently of epithelial histology) is the clearest evidence for the carcinogenic potential of radiation applied in the doses and fraction sizes conventionally utilized in the treatment of malignant disease (156–158). A slightly increased risk of development of a common epithelial malignancy (colon, rectal, bladder cancers, etc.) may be subsequently more difficult to detect and quantitate (159). Concerns about the carcinogenic potential of transmitted or scattered radiation incidentally delivered to tissues adjacent to, or remote from, the intended target volume have stimulated international effort to assess the magnitude of risk (160). What has become clear is that therapeutic radiation by fractionated external beam therapy or intracavitary or interstitial brachytherapy techniques, although clearly capable of causing malignancy, is a relatively inefficient inducer of neoplasia (161,162). Estimation of risk therefore, requires studies of large populations over long periods of time. As a practical matter, such work often involves data retrieval from population-based tumor registries with frequently incomplete information concerning details of initial and secondary treatment with radiation and other modalities, as well as imprecise information concerning the nature of second neoplasms which, in some instances, may actually represent recurrence of the original cancer. For example, a follow-up study of women treated for cancer of the cervix based on data in the Ontario Cancer Registry found that an independent physician review of the medical charts of patients with second primary tumors with the same cell type as the cervical cancer resulted in reclassification of 31% of the potential second primary cancers as metastatic from the original cancer of the cervix (163).

Identification of the appropriate control population is essential to precision in risk estimation (159). Multiple cancers in an individual may reflect common risk factors or hazardous lifestyle choices rather than the consequence of radiation or chemotherapy. For example, curative management of cervical cancer has historically depended exclusively on radiation or surgery, alone or in combination. Although radiation has long been known to carry a risk of tumor induction, no such stigma has been plausibly associated with surgery. Longterm survivors of treatment for cervical cancer are at significantly increased risk for the development of lung cancer, based on data from the Danish Cancer Registry (164) and the Ontario Cancer Registry (163). Segregation of patients into two groups—those receiving radiation and those not receiving radiation as part of their initial management—revealed no difference between the groups, both of which reflected increased risk of lung cancer, presumably on the basis of a common risk factor (tobacco consumption) rather than as a consequence of radiation exposure.

In an investigation that studied the largest number of women (182,040) treated for cervical cancer (invasive and in-situ) with long follow-up surveillance (1,278,951 woman-years of observation), Boice and colleagues estimated the risk of second malignancies based on data from 15 population-based registries, with refined analysis based on initial treatment modality and elapsed time since treatment (160). Tissues were divided into those close to the cervix and presumably within the intentionally irradiated volume (urinary bladder, colon and rectum, uterine corpus, ovaries, bone and connective tissue) and receiving doses in the thousands of cGy, tissues an intermediate distance from the target volume (stomach, pancreas, kidney, gallbladder and liver), estimated to receive doses in the hundreds of cGy, and tissues distant from the cervix and presumed to receive doses in the tens of cGy (lung, buccal cavity, breast, brain, thyroid and salivary glands). In this study, 82,616 women with invasive cancer received treatment with radiation and 14,173 did not. Also, 85,251 women with in-situ cancer were treated primarily with surgery, only a few receiving radiation treatment. The magnitude of risk of second cancers and the site distribution of second cancers were comparable between patients treated for in-situ cancer and patients treated for invasive cancer without radiation. In contrast, patients treated with radiation were found to have an overall increased risk of second cancers beginning 10 years following treatment and remaining increased after 30 or more years of surveillance, a trend not paralleled by the experience of unirradiated patients. A 20% increased risk of second cancers in close and intermediate sites was observed, and rose to 40% after 10 years following treatment. In remote tissues, excess risk was observed only for smoking-associated sites, such as the lung. In the entire cohort (irradiated and unirradiated women) elevated risks of second cancers were found for the lung, buccal cavity, urinary bladder, and other genital sites (vulva, vagina, and otherwise not specified). These sites possibly reflect common risk factors (tobacco use) and lifestyle choices (exposure to sexually transmitted disease and potentially oncogenic viruses). Interestingly, a decreased risk of breast cancer was observed, possibly the consequence of surgical or radiotherapeutic ovarian ablation, a finding that has been reported in other studies (163,164).

A study from the Institute of Oncology in Warsaw (157) of 8043 women irradiated for cervical cancer described an excess risk of uterine sarcoma (relative risk 5.38), an observation echoed in a study of uterine malignancies following pelvic irradiation from the Ohio State University Registry (158). Adenocarcinomas of the uterine corpus and uterine sarcomas following therapeutic radiation of cancer of the cervix have been described as presenting with advanced stage at diagnosis and poor prognosis (165,166). This has been attributed to delayed diagnosis due to the comparative infrequency of vaginal bleeding as a presenting symptom, possibly related to stenosis or obliteration of the cervical canal or agglutination of the upper vagina after radiation treatment. Treatment of these radiation-associated malignancies has achieved poor results in comparison to the treatment of patients not previously irradiated.

Boice and associates conducted an international case control study estimating leukemia risk from therapeutic radiation in the setting of cervical cancer (167). Estimates of absorbed dose to active bone marrow were prepared following review of original treatment records. The relative risk of chronic lymphocytic leukemia was not increased, but the estimated relative risk for all other forms of leukemia combined was 2.0. Risk increased with increasing dose to approximately 400 cGy and then decreased, fitting the best in linear exponential function, including a positive linear induction term and a negative exponential term and consistent with a model that postulates leukemic transformation at low dose and killing of potentially transformed cells at higher dose.

Chemotherapy Effects

Chemotherapeutic agents have long been appreciated to carry a risk of secondary malignant neoplasms (SMNs). The first reports surfaced from patients treated with curative therapy for Hodgkin's disease and leukemia, in whom sufficient longterm survivors were available for the development of a SMN. Patients treated successfully for Hodgkin's disease have a risk of developing leukemia, lymphoma, and solid tumors at a higher rate than would be expected (168–173). In the Stanford series, such patients experienced a 17.6% risk of SMN (168). The overall risk of leukemia was 3.3% with a median time to diagnosis of 4.5 years. However, the risk with radiation alone was only 0.6%. When chemotherapy and radiation were both used, the risk rose to 6.1%, which was not significantly different from the rate for chemotherapy alone. Solid tumors were also seen, but the incidence was the same in patients who received radiation alone and radiation plus chemotherapy. The impact of single and combined modality therapies on the induction of SMN in patients treated for Hodgkin's disease is summarized in Table 34–1.

SMNs have been reported in patients treated for multiple myeloma, acute and chronic leukemia, and non-Hodgkin's lymphoma (174). Many of these patients had received both chemotherapy and radiation, but the most common pattern seen was prolonged use of alkylating agents such as melphalan and chlorambucil. Data are now available to suggest that SMNs occur following chemotherapy for ovarian cancer (175–177), in patients receiving adjuvant chemotherapy for breast cancer, gastrointestinal cancer (178), and sporadic cases after lung cancer, bladder cancer, head and neck cancer, melanoma, and others (174).

Clearly, antineoplastic agents are mutagenic, some more so than others. Chemotherapeutic agents most commonly associated with the development of SMNs are listed in Table 34–2. Alkylating agents, procarbazine, and nitrosoureas are the most mutagenic, with abundant animal data supporting their neoplastic potential. It is possible that the combination of chemotherapy and radiation therapy may carry a substantially higher risk of secondary neoplasia. However,

Table 34–1. Effects of Radiotherapy and Chemotherapy on Secondary Neoplasms in Hodgkin's Disease at 15 Years.

	Cumulative Percentage	Peak Incidence
A. *Leukemia*	3–4	3–8 years after treatment
Radiation alone	<1.0	
Combined modality	5–17	
Chemotherapy alone	2–12	
B. *Solid Tumor and Lymphomas*	13–14	13–15 years after treatment
Radiation alone	13–14	
Combined modality	13–14	

Table 34–2. Chemotherapeutic Agents Associated with Secondary Malignant Cancer (SMN)

Alkylating Agents:
Nitrogen mustard
Chlorambucil
Melphalan
Cyclophosphamide
Nitrosoureas:
BCNU
CCNU
Methyl-CCNU
Procarbazine
Etoposide (VP-16)
Chromic phosphate P32

it also appears that the risk changes according to which drugs are used. When patients with Hodgkin's disease receive radiation therapy and drugs that do not include alkylating agents, the risk of leukemia is substantially reduced.

Chemoradiation Effects

Intelligent selection of effective treatment modalities and their successful integration in a manner avoiding prohibitive acute toxicity are the principal goals in the management of an initial life-threatening malignancy. A theoretical worry about late induction of a secondary cancer is generally low in the hierarchy of concerns when one is designing a therapeutic strategy. However, when defining a treatment policy for a group of patients whose overall prognosis is somewhat favorable, some thought must be given to the implications of combining modalities, each of which alone has the capacity to induce neoplasia. For example, women treated for Stage IB or IIA squamous cancer of the cervix by radical hysterectomy and pelvic lymphadenectomy who are found to have metastases to pelvic lymph nodes are generally acknowledged to be at "high risk" of recurrence. Adjuvant pelvic radiation has been historically employed in such patients with no discernible effect on survival (11). However, in retrospective analyses, no discernible effect on survival can be appreciated for two reasons: pelvic radiation in maximally "tolerable" doses is only partially effective in preventing pelvic recurrence (179), and the modest reductions achieved in pelvic recurrence rates have not appeared to affect the rate of distant dissemination (11).

The combination of radiation and synchronous or sequential chemotherapy in gynecologic cancer has been a recent development. The past experience has focused on patients with poor prognosis, most of whom do not survive their initial malignancy. This approach has been employed in individual institutions and is under investigation in the multi-institutional clinical cooperative group setting by the Gynecological Oncology Group (GOG) and the Southwest Oncology Group (SWOG). Although this escalation in treatment intensity seems entirely reasonable, it must be borne in mind that approximately 60% of the patients who will be entered in this Intergroup trial can be expected to survive cancer-free for 5 or more years, even if the adjuvant therapies have no beneficial impact on survival probability.

The experience from the treatment of Hodgkin's disease suggests caution and prudent selection of chemotherapeutic agents when extrapolating combined modality therapy to the adjuvant setting, or to the treatment of patients who enjoy a relatively favorable prognosis when treated with conventional therapies.

LARGE FIELD IRRADIATION

Gynecologic cancers originate in pelvic structures. Largely coincident with the rise of the surgically oriented clinical specialty of gynecologic oncology, understanding of the natural history of pelvic cancers has improved due to more aggressive surgical staging, surgical restaging (second-look laparotomy) and disciplined analysis of patterns of disease relapse and treatment failure (180–193). Understanding the natural history of the disease processes has led to efforts to "get one step ahead" of the disease by elective/adjuvant/prophylactic treatment of tissue volumes at risk of harboring microscopic or occult disease dissemination (57).

The propensity of squamous cancers of the cervix to spread regionally in a somewhat predictable, sequential fashion, to involve pelvic, common iliac, and para-aortic nodes has long been recognized, and has led to benchmark surgical staging studies (194), which in turn have helped create the rationale for the systematic study of extended field radiation for this disease. The curative potential of extended field (pelvic plus para-aortic volume) radiation for patients with histologically verified para-aortic lymph node involvement has been appreciated for some time (60–67). Although substantial salvage has been reported, particularly when lymph node metastases are surgically defined to be microscopic and clinically occult, such salvage has been achieved at the price of substantial radiation bowel morbidity. Refinement in treatment technique appears to substantially reduce radiation-related morbidity and mortality (65). Despite delivery of an aggressive dose, many of these patients develop cancer relapse within the treatment volume, as well as dissemination to remote sites. This has led to attempts to deliver concurrent systemic chemotherapy, both for purposes of radioenhancement and for potential impact on hematogenous cancer spread. Extended field radiation has been delivered with concurrent 5-FU, with 5-FU and cisplatinum, and with 5-FU and mitomycin C (195,196).

At the Radiation Oncology Center in Sacramento, California, pelvic and para-aortic volume have been treated concurrently, using portals that extend from the ischial rami to the top of the 12th thoracic vertebra (196). External radiation dose to the extended volume has ranged from 4500 cGy to 5400 cGy. 5-FU has been administered as a prolonged infusion, generally at 1000 mg/m^2/24 hours for 72 to 96 hours. A second drug, either mitomycin C at 10 mg/m^2 or cisplatinum at 100 mg/m^2 has also been given. Twenty-six patients have been treated for carcinoma of the cervix with radiographically apparent and frequently histologically confirmed metastases to high common iliac or para-aortic nodes. Acute toxicity has been substantial, with several patients requiring hospitalization for dehydration secondary to watery uncontrolled diarrhea, sometimes complicated by nausea and vomiting. Two patients (8%) have died from myelosuppression, one with neutropenia and sepsis, the other with thrombocytopenia and intracerebral hemorrhage. Although several patients are alive and cancer-free for several years following treatment, results are too preliminary to permit comparison of the efficacy of this approach to extended field radiation alone, or to intelligently assess potential increases in late morbidity. It must be emphasized that acute gastrointestinal toxicity has necessitated treatment interruption and prolongation in several patients. However, only one patient treated following radical hysterectomy has required multiple laparotomies for bowel obstruction. Potential concurrent use of bone marrow stimulating factors (G-CSF, GM-CSF, IL-3) may mitigate against the acutely limiting toxicity, which has been myelosuppression (197–199). Use of lower dose per fraction and/or limitation of chemotherapy intensity may be methods of reducing acute toxicity while retaining potential benefits of the synergistic radiation and chemotherapy interaction.

Epithelial cancers of the ovary (182,183) as well as papillary serous and clear cell cancers of the endometrium (16–21) have a propensity to disseminate widely in the abdominal cavity to involve retroperitoneal nodes, as well as peritoneal surfaces (peritoneal seeding). Whole-abdomen radiation has been historically utilized as primary therapy for such tumors (69–75). It has been delivered by the so-called "moving strip" technique (71–74), as well as by open fields. Following the report from Toronto of a randomized trial comparing moving strip with open field radiation in the treatment of ovarian cancer which confirmed comparable efficacy but decreased toxicity employing open fields (200), strip radiation has largely been abandoned and relegated to a historical curiosity. Much of our current knowledge of clinical radiation hepatitis and its dependence on fraction size is derived from patients treated with abdominal radiation for ovarian cancer (76–79).

Schray and co-workers (201,202) have meticulously analyzed the complications of open-field whole-abdomen radiation as sole postoperative treatment for 77 patients with gynecologic cancer, 41 endometrial cancers, 25 ovarian cancers, five nonendometrial uterine cancers, four fallopian tube cancers, and two cervical cancers. A dose of 3000 cGy in 20 fractions was prescribed to the whole abdomen with liver dose limited to 2250 cGy and kidney dose to 1950 cGy. The para-aortic area and medial leaves of the diaphragm were boosted to 4200 cGy and the pelvic volume carried to 5100 cGy with progressively shrinking target volumes. In several patients, small volumes were carried to a cumulative dose of 5600 cGy to 6000 cGy to encompass the vagina or localized areas of suspected residual disease. Fifteen patients judged to be at high risk of bowel injury because of a prior history of bowel disease or obstruction, extensive adhesions, or multiple prior laparotomies, received somewhat reduced doses (2550 cGy to the whole abdomen, 4050 cGy to the medial leaves of the diaphragm, 4950 cGy to the pelvis). Seven patients (9%) required interruption of treatment due to gastrointestinal side effects; of these, three required hospitalization for rehydration. Twenty-one patients (27%) required generally short (2 weeks or less) cumulative treatment interruption due to myelosupression. One patient's treatment was discontinued secondary to thrombocytopenia. Eleven patients developed bowel obstruction, which was clearly related to progressive intra-abdominal cancer in five. Four developed chylous ascites, which resolved in three. Twenty-four (63%) of 38 patients monitored with serial determinations developed elevated hepatic enzymes, 80% of which fell to normal within 2 years. No patient developed a clinical picture of radiation hepatitis.

The use of open-field whole-abdomen irradiation for ovarian cancer has declined with the advent of cisplatinum-based chemotherapy (203,204). In special circumstances such as persistent small-volume disease at second laparotomy, or in an effort to consolidate chemotherapy induced complete remission, whole-abdomen radiation has been used sequentially, generally following 6 or more cycles of cisplatinum-based chemotherapy (27–40). In contrast with the somewhat favorable toxicity experience reported by Schray and colleagues for whole-abdomen radiation alone, whole-abdomen radiation as second-line or consolidative therapy for epithelial ovarian cancers has proven to be both acutely and chronically toxic, with major morbidities equalling or exceeding the salvage rates. Goldhirsch and colleagues (30) reported on 50 patients undergoing salvage or consolidation whole-abdomen radiation (either by strip or by open fields) following chemotherapy-induced complete remission with regimens containing cisplatinum and melphelan. Forty-two percent completed treatment as planned, 11 (22%) could not complete the planned program, and the remainder completed with interruption. Of 24 patients who were treated for consolidation of laparotomy-assessed complete response, 4 could not complete treatment and an additional 8 required treatment interruption. One patient developed chronic malabsorption, and one developed acute myelocytic leukemia.

Hacker and colleagues reported 30 patients who underwent salvage whole-abdomen radiation following second or third look laparotomy documentation of residual disease following extensive prior chemotherapy including intraperitoneal cisplatinum in two patients and intraperitoneal Corynebacterium parvum in three patients (31). The whole abdomen was treated with 120 cGy fractions to 3000 cGy followed by treatment to the pelvic volume to a cumulative dose of 5000 cGy with 180 cGy fractions. Nine patients (30%) could not complete therapy, four due to myelosuppression and five due to disease progression, and seven patients (23%) required treatment interruption ranging from 1 to 4 weeks due to myelosuppression. Eight of 27 patients (30%) surviving 4 or more months from completion of radiation required laparotomy for small bowel obstruction; of these five had no obvious intraperitoneal disease recurrence and three had evidence of residual cancer thought unrelated to the obstruction. At the time of that report, 24 patients had developed recurrence (22 within the abdomen) and 6 patients survived clinically disease-free for 19 to 41 months.

Kuten and colleagues reported on 43 patients undergoing whole-abdomen radiation for minimal residual (less than 2 cm) or microscopic disease following second look laparotomy after 6 to 11 cycles of cisplatinum and Adriamycin (34). Myelosuppression was the major acute toxicity. The initial 26 patients were treated with whole-abdomen open fields for 3000 cGy for 4 weeks. Fifty percent of these patients could not complete the planned course of radiation due to myelosuppression. Seventeen subsequent patients received whole-abdomen radiation via a split field technique, with the lower abdomen receiving 3000 cGy for 3 weeks followed by the same dose delivered to the upper abdomen. Utilizing this approach, 16 of 17 patients (94%) were able to complete the planned course of treatment.

Schray and colleagues reported on 35 patients with advanced epithelial ovarian cancer who underwent 6 to 25 cycles of combination chemotherapy (median 11 cycles), which contained cisplatinum in 30 patients (202). Whole-abdomen radiation was delivered as salvage therapy following second laparotomy in 33 patients. Twenty-four patients had three or more laparotomies. Radiation treatment was intended to deliver 3000 cGy to the whole abdomen at 150 cGy per fraction with sequential boost to the para-aortic nodes and diaphragm to 4200 cGy and the pelvis to 5100 cGy. Nine patients failed to complete the treatment. In 7 patients (20%), this was due to hematologic toxicity. Five patients (14%) developed treatment-related bowel obstruction requiring laparotomy in the absence of disease. Seven additional patients developed bowel obstruction with progressive disease.

Although clearly capable of inducing long-term remission in the occasional patient with documented small volume or microscopic disease detected at second laparotomy, the toxicity of sequential chemotherapy followed by whole-abdomen radiation therapy is substantial. The integration of systemic chemotherapy with wide-field radiation, often in patients who have had prior abdominal surgery, is a risky venture justifiable only in the treatment of patients for whom conventional modalities offer little or no chance for cure. Both patient and treating physician must be prepared for substantial acute toxicity and major late sequelae if treatment affords prolonged survival.

CHEMORADIATION: PRELIMINARY REPORTS OF TOXICITY

Chemotherapy and radiation have been used, both sequentially (adjuvant or neoadjuvant chemotherapy) and synchronously (chemosensitization or chemopotentiation) in the treatment of female pelvic cancers. In general, the acute toxicity of sequential efforts has been characterized by the addition of non-overlapping toxicities of each treatment modality. Sequential treatments are likely to have the most predictable toxicities, except in instances in which chemotherapeutic agents that have organ-specific toxicities (e.g., cyclophosphamide-induced bladder injury) (205) are used for sites which lie within the radiation treatment volume, or when agents are employed that can sensitize normal tissues to radiation effect or reactivate or recall latent radiation injury (Adriamycin, actinomycin D) (206,207).

Many chemoradiation efforts have centered on the treatment of squamous cancers (cervix, vagina, vulva) because of encouraging results with synchronous chemotherapy and radiation in the treatment of squamous cancers of the esophagus and anal canal (6–9). The largest controlled experience employing radiation and concurrent chemotherapy in the treatment of cervical cancer has been with **hydroxyurea** (Hydrea) (208–210). Sinclair established the radiobiologic rationale for this effort by demonstrating, in vitro, that Chinese hamster cells are more radioresistant in G_1 and G_2 phases of the cell cycle than in S-Phase (211). Sinclair demonstrated the hydroxyurea preferentially killed radioresistant S-Phase cells, and arrested cycling cells at the radiosensitive G_1-S interphase (212). Phillips and Tolmach demonstrated in HeLa cells (human cervical cancer cell line) that hydroxyurea inhibits repair of sublethal radiation injury (213).

The Gynecology Oncology Group (GOG) conducted a prospective randomized trial of conventially fractionated external and intracavitary radiation alone versus radiation plus hydroxyurea, which indicated that survival was better in the patients receiving hydroxyurea (208). The large number of ineligible or inevaluable patients reported has rendered interpretation of this trial somewhat controversial. Acute toxicity from hydroxyurea was limited to myelosuppression. Of 47 patients receiving radiation alone, 16 (34%) had Grade I or II myelosuppression as maximum reported toxicity. In contrast, 30 of 57 (53%) of patients receiving hydroxyurea had Grade I or II myelosuppression, 5 had Grade III myelosuppression and 2 had Grade IV (life-threatening) myelosuppression.

Piver and co-workers studied 40 patients with FIGO Stage IIB carcinoma of the cervix following pretreatment laparotomy, which established the absence of overt, extrapelvic nodal metastases (209). Patients were randomized to receive hydroxyurea at 80 mg/kg every third day for 12 weeks during and after conventionally fractionated external and intracavitary radiation, or to receive a placebo.

Survival was statistically improved in the population receiving hydroxyurea. Acute toxicity was primary myelosuppression, with leukopenia (WBC < 2,500/mm^3) observed in 80% of the hydroxyurea group, in contrast to 15% of the placebo group. Severe diarrhea was seen in two patients receiving hydroxyurea, and in none of the placebo group. Seven late complications requiring surgical correction were seen in 25% (5 patients) given hydroxyurea, and 40% (8 patients) given placebo. However, four of five hydroxyurea patients died postoperatively without evidence of cancer following surgical intervention for treatment of late treatment sequelae (1 peritonitis, 1 pelvic abscess, 1 short bowel syndrome, 1 intestinal fistula). Two of eight placebo patients requiring surgical intervention for treatment complications died postoperatively, both of "shock lung."

Piver and colleagues reported on a randomized prospective trial of conventional radiation versus radiation plus hydroxyurea in patients with FIGO Stage III-B carcinoma of the cervix following pretherapy staging para-aortic lymphadenectomy (210). Twenty patients received hydroxyurea administered at 80 mg/kg every third day for 12 weeks, continuing for approximately 4 weeks following completion of radiation, and 25 patients received placebo. Leukopenia (WBC < 2,500,m^3) was seen in 16 patients receiving hydroxyurea (80%), but in none of the placebo group. No significant differences were reported in other acute toxicities or late sequelae.

The Radiation Therapy Oncology Group (RTOG) conducted a Phase III trial of radiotherapy alone or in combination with hypoxic cell sensitizer **misonidazole** (214). One hundred and nineteen patients with FIGO Stages III-B and IV-A cervical cancer were randomized to conventional radiation alone or radiation plus misonidazole at 400 mg/m^2 daily 2 to 4 hours prior to radiation. misonidazole toxicity was limited to severe nausea and vomiting in two patients. Peripheral neuropathy developed in 9 patients. No severe or fatal complications associated with misonidazole were encountered, and no increase in late radiation complications were reported.

Belloni and colleagues reported on a double-blind randomized study of radiation plus placebo versus radiation plus **ICRF-159** in patients with limited cervical cancer (215). Surgery was performed six weeks after 4500 cGy at 150 cGy per fraction. Toxicity attributable to the experimental drug was primarily myelosupression leading to withholding 18 of 170 cycles of ICRF-159 planned 4 leukopenias, 9 thrombocytopenias recorded among 34 patients in the placebo group. Unfortunately, as used in this study, ICRF-159 had no therapeutic benefit.

Cisplatinum (CDDP), used alone or in combination with other drugs, has been the subject of several reports (216–225). Monyak and colleagues reported on 49 patients receiving weekly CDDP initially (4 patients) at 10 mg/m^2 , and subsequently at 20 mg/m^2 concurrently with pelvic radiation in 7 patients, pelvic and low para-aortic node radiation in 14 patients, pelvic and para-aortic node radiation in 21 patients and with whole abdomen radiation in 6 patients (218). Thrombocytopenia was observed in 6 patients with nadir platelet counts of less than 150,000/mm^3, of whom 4 patients had nadir platelet counts less than 100,000/mm^3. One patient experienced a transient, reversible rise in BUN and creatinine. Runowicz and colleagues described myelosuppression as the major acute toxicity in their series of patients receiving CDDP at 20 mg/m^2 for 5 days every 21 days (217). Twenty-one of 43 patients required transfusion of red cells, and two patients required platelet transfusions. Sixty percent of patients experienced nausea and vomiting. One patient suffered renal injury attributable to CDDP. Encouraging preliminary tumor responses were noted.

Wong and colleagues reported on patients with advanced cervical carcinoma randomized to radiation alone (25 patients), radiation plus concurrent weekly CDDP at 25 mg/m^2 (22 patients) or radiation plus concurrent twice-weekly CDDP at 25 mg/m^2/dose (17 patients) (219). Acute side effects attributable to CDDP included nausea, vomiting, and myelosuppression. Diarrhea was noted to be more common in patients receiving CDDP. Seven of 39 patients receiving CDDP required transfusion for hemoglobin < 8g%. Leukopenia necessitating temporary treatment interruption (14 to 18 days) developed in 12 of 39 patients receiving CDDP, and thrombocytopenia, platelets < 100,000/mm^3, was seen in 7 patients receiving the drug. Three patients developed transient mild peripheral neuropathy. All Grade II, III or IV (WHO criteria) acute gastrointestinal or hematologic toxicities were seen in patients receiving CDDP. Unfortunately, no longterm survival advantage was observed in patients receiving CDDP to offset the increased acute toxicity. No significant difference in longterm adverse effects was reported.

Cisplatinum has been given by constant intra-arterial infusion in order to minimize systemic toxicity, maximize tumor exposure to drug, and provide prolonged exposure to drug during multiple fractions of radiation. Rettenmaier and colleagues reported on seven patients with advanced primary or locally recurrent squamous cancer of the cervix treated by constant intra-arterial CDDP infusion via the internal iliac arteries using a totally implantable infusion device infusing at a dose of 50 mg/week in conjunction with conventional external radiation supplemented by interstitial implantation (Syed/Neblett template) (226). No renal or hematologic toxicity was observed. Reversible neurotoxicity was observed in all patients consisting of lower extremity pain.

Methotrexate and **Adriamycin** have also been given as prolonged (8 to 12 days) internal iliac artery infusions during radiation for advanced cervical cancer FIGO Stages III-B and IV (227). Ten mg of either drug was used in 24 hours, sequentially for 5 days, followed by 5 days of the other drug. Infusion was interrupted or discontinued for signs of systemic toxicity. Three patients with prior evidence of liver insufficiency showed worsening of hepatic function and elevation of enzymes and bilirubin. Leukopenia and thrombocytopenia were described as mild and of short duration. No late radiation sequelae were reported, but radiation dose to bladder and rectum was limited to 5000 cGy.

The combination of **cisplatinum** and **5-FU** with concurrent radiation has been the subject of several investigations. Roberts and colleagues reported on 23 patients with advanced squamous cancers of the lower female genital tract (21 cervical, 1 vaginal, 1 vulvar) who received two courses of CDDP and 50 mg/m^2 and 5-FU at 1000 mg/m^2/24 hrs for 96 hours (225). External radiation dose was 4500 cGy in 180 cGy fractions with a planned 14-day rest. Six patients received 3600 cGy to the para-aortic volume in addition to pelvic radiation. All patients subsequently received intracavitary or interstitial brachytherapy. In only one patient was treatment delayed (due to acute enteritis). No significant hematologic, renal, or neurologic toxicity was observed. Three patients had late radiation sequelae. A severe radionecrosis developed in an area of interstitial implantation in a patient with vulvar cancer. Two patients required colostomies, one for rectovaginal fistula and one for severe stenosis of the sigmoid.

Kuske and colleagues reported on 23 patients with advanced gynecologic cancers (15 primary cervical cancers, 4 postsurgical recurrent cervical cancers, 2 endometrial adenocarcinomas, 2 vulvar cancers) treated with conventional radiation in combination with IV bolus cisplatinum at 50 mg/m^2 and 5-FU at 750 mg/m^2/24 hrs for 120 hours (222). Three cycles were planned over 7 to 8 weeks, timed to coincide with both external and intracavitary radiation. Nine patients had radiation treatment interruptions of 1 to 9 weeks because of moist desquamation of the perineum (including 2 patients with vulvar cancers), pulmonary embolus, nausea and vomiting, fistula development, or noncompliance. Eight patients required delays of one week in chemotherapy due entirely or partly to myelosuppression. Severe complications were seen in five patients (one rectosigmoiditis; one vesicovaginal fistula; one bowel obstruction; two pulmonary emboli, of which one was fatal).

It should be noted that pulmonary embolus is a recognized complication of low-dose-rate (conventional) intracavitary and interstitial pelvic brachytherapy attributed to the presence of a foreign object in the pelvis and prolonged enforced bed rest. However, Kuzel and colleagues have reported that 5-FU delivered by continuous infusion (1000 mg/m^2/24 hrs for 4 days) is associated with increased levels of fibrinopeptide A (a peptide cleaved from fibrogen by thrombin) consistent with activation of coagulation (223). Prolonged infusion of 5-FU during intracavitary or interstitial brachytherapy could, in theory, result in an increased risk of thromboembolic complications.

The regimen of 5-FU at 1000 mg/m^2/24 hrs for two cycles of 96 hours each in conjunction with two IV bolus doses of cisplatinum at 100 mg/m^2 has been used in conjunction with adjuvant pelvic radiation (4500 cGy in 25 fractions of 180 cGy) supplemented by intravaginal brachytherapy (2000 cGy mucosal dose) for patients with high risk cervical cancer FIGO Stages I-B and II-A treated by radical hysterectomy and pelvic lymphadenectomy (228). Twenty-three patients have been treated according to a protocol employed at the Radiation Oncology Center in Sacramento principally consisting of patients with one or more nodal metastases. Acute toxicity has consisted of myelosuppression and increased gastrointestinal side effects (cramps, diarrhea), compared to the toxicity in individuals receiving adjuvant pelvic radiation alone. Two patients developed bowel obstruction requiring corrective surgery. Three patients had chronic leg lymphedema. In one, it was mild and in another, asymptomatic. In the third patient, unilateral leg edema was significantly disabling. It is not clear whether these complications represent an increase over what would be expected from adjuvant pelvic radiation alone following radical hysterectomy.

Radiation and concurrent 5-FU, with or without cisplatinum, has been delivered in a planned split-course fashion in Sacramento for locally advanced or recurrent vulvar cancer (229). The 5-FU is administered at 1000 mg/m^2/24 hrs. Cisplatinum, used in a minority of patients, has been given at 100 mg/m^2 IV bolus. To maximize radiation drug synergism, radiation has been delivered twice daily in fractions of 180 cGy (1800 cGy in 5 days). Planned 2-week treatment interruptions have separated each cycle of concurrent radiation and chemotherapy. Radiation dose to areas of potential microscopic involvement has comprised 3600 cGy with two cycles of concurrent chemotherapy. Radiation dose to initial areas of gross involvement (primary and nodal involvement) totalled 5400 cGy with three cycles of concurrent chemotherapy. One of 11 previously untreated patients died during treatment of aspiration pneumonia, her condition possibly aggravated by relative leukopenia. All patients experienced patchy moist desquamation of perineal skin, in several instances progressing to severe confluent moist desquamation. All healed uneventfully. Late sequelae have been limited to skin atrophy and telangiectasis within the high dose radiation volume resulting in dyspareunia in one patient. Late bowel, bladder, or rectal injuries have not been encountered. Among 10 previously untreated patients completing treatment, complete clinical response has been observed in nine, confirmed by repeat biopsy in six. Because of encouraging preliminary results, work continues in this area despite the severity of the acute skin reaction.

Mitomycin C has also been used in conjunction with 5-FU concurrently with radiation in the treatment of both cervical and vulvar cancer. Ludgate and colleagues reported treating 38 patients with locoregionally advanced squamous carcinoma of the cervix with conventionally fractionated radiation and two concurrent 4-day infusions of 5-FU at 1000 mg/m^2/24 hrs for 96 hours each (230). Mitomycin C at 10 mg/m^2 was given on the first day of external beam radiation. External radiation and chemotherapy were delivered following an initial intracavitary insertion. The principal acute toxicity was gastrointestinal, with 17 patients experiencing diarrhea. Thrombocytopenia (platelets less than 80,000/mm^3) occurred in three patients without associated hemorrhage. Six patients developed neutropenia (polymorphonuclear leukocytes $< 2{,}000$/mm^3) complicated by Escherichia coli septicemia in one patient successfully treated with antibiotics. Six patients did not receive the planned second course of 5-FU for various reasons. Late complications consisted of proctitis in 12 patients (32%), and rectovaginal fistulae in 2. Three patients developed vaginal stenosis and dyspareunia as a late manifestation of treatment.

Thomas and colleagues have reported on 200 patients with advanced cervical cancer treated on sequential phase I/II studies employing 5-FU at varying doses, alone or in combination with Mitomycin C at 6 mg/m^2 concurrently with radiation (195). Thirteen patients developed severe but transient oral mucositis with inability to swallow solid food for 1 to 3 days. Seven patients developed acute enteritis requiring either unscheduled interruption of radiation or hospitalization for fluid support. Late complications included radiation cystitis or vesicovaginal fistula in 6 patients, bowel complications unassociated with tumor recurrence in 17 patients (defined as obstruction requiring hospitalization or bowel obstruction, stricture or perforation requiring interventional surgery, or bleeding requiring transfusion or development of fistulae). Death was attributed to treatment complications in three patients. The development of serious late bowel complications correlated with the administration of Mitomycin C, with 17 of 78 patients (21.8%) receiving Mitomycin C developing bowel complications compared to only 8 of 122 (6.6%) receiving 5-FU alone ($p = 0.0046$).

Thomas and co-workers reported on the combination of 5-FU alone or in combination with Mitomycin C with radiation therapy in the treatment of vulvar cancer (231). Thirty-three patients were studied, of whom nine were treated in the adjuvant postsurgical setting, 15 for locoregionally recurrent disease after surgery and 9 as definitive initial treatment. Two late complications were observed, including proctitis requiring colostomy, and avascular hip necrosis.

Bleomycin has been used concurrently with radiation in the treatment of initially inoperable or recurrent vulvar cancer. Iverson reported on 15 patients treated with bleomycin 30 mg three times weekly in conjunction with 300 cGy radiation fractions (1500 cGy and 90 mg bleomycin in 5 days) (232). Two cycles were administered with preoperative intent, but with most patients continuing to a cumulative radiation dose of 3600 to 4000 cGy. Three patients developed signs of pulmonary fibrosis. Only one patient enjoyed prolonged survival following treatment.

As is frequently the case with new or innovative combinations of treatments, initial work with chemoradiation in gynecologic cancer has focused on the treatment of patients for whom conventional strategies yield poor results. Interpretation of toxicity of treatment is compromised by the fact that some patients suffer complications that reflect, in part, the progression of disease that could be expected in the setting of conventional therapies. Patients expiring of local or distant cancer recurrence cannot often be assessed for late morbidity of treatment. Variation in radiation dose, fractionation, and technique, as well as modification or deletion of scheduled chemotherapy, represent efforts to individualize care for patient benefit. Unfortunately, the lack of uniformity of treatment hinders interpretation of toxicity data. Reports to date are valuable primarily in estimating acute toxicities and defining acutely "tolerable" treatment. Meaningful assessment of the full spectrum of acute and late toxicities must await larger numbers of patients, longer follow-up, and comparison with control patients concurrently treated by conventional modalities.

METHODS TO MINIMIZE TOXICITIES

Ovarian Conservation and Reproductive Integrity

The first and most critical step is the recognition by the treating physician that endocrine conservation and potential partial conservation of reproductive capacity are both desirable and potentially achievable goals in selected patients. Lateral transposition of an ovary into the paracolic gutter has been used as a technique for ovarian conservation for patients in whom pelvic radiation is anticipated (233–235). Often the strategy is successful in preserving ovarian endocrine function if the transposed ovary is marked with radio-opaque clips and the radiation portals are designed to exclude the ovary from the direct path of the beam. The presence of metastatic disease in pelvic or extrapelvic lymph nodes, which may require extended volume or lateral portals, may render lateral ovarian transposition ineffective. When pelvic radiation is delivered, the scatter dose delivered to a transposed ovary depends on the distance from the target volume, portal sizes and arrangement, patient size, and beam energy. Belinson and colleagues (234) calculated cumulative scattered dose to transposed ovarian tissue under various clinical conditions, using a 6 MeV linear accelerator to treat a "conventional" pelvic volume to 4500 cGy. In a patient with a 17 cm anteroposterior separation, ovarian dose would be 158 cGy using a 15 cm × 15 cm anteroposterior pelvic fields, 219 cGy using four fields (30 cm lateral separation), and 460 cGy if treating pelvic and para-aortic volumes with anterior and posterior fields. These doses are slightly higher in patients with larger dimensions.

Heterotopic ovarian transplantation prior

to pelvic radiation has been described in a young woman with subdiaphragmatic Hodgkin's disease. Transplantation of an ovary to a subcutaneous site in the inner aspect of the upper arm was described with subsequent observation, by ultrasound, of normal follicular growth and ovulation, and aspiration of a postmature oocyte following ovulation (236). This location for ovarian transplantation has the advantage of being maximally remote from potential radiation fields for gynecologic radiotherapy, as well as being a site easily monitored for ovulation and accessible for potential ovarian harvest for in vitro fertilization. The small risk of simultaneous cancer transplantation in the transplanted ovary—which is usually only detected as a substantial flank tumor recurrence when the ovary is laterally transposed in the abdomen—is also mitigated by the accessibility of this site to noninvasive and inexpensive monitoring.

In this location, the possible adverse impact of systemic chemotherapy on ovarian function might be minimized by the use of a temporary tourniquet around the upper arm to decrease drug delivery to the transplanted ovary when chemotherapeutic agents are used which have a short half-life (rapidly degraded or excreted by liver, kidneys, or peripheral soft tissues). Protection of ovarian function from chemotherapy may also possibly be achieved by temporary suppression of ovarian function by exogenous administration of hormones (237).

Sexual Function

The most important steps in minimizing sexual dysfunction following therapy for gynecologic cancer are the recognition by the physician that sexual dysfunction is the rule rather than the exception, and recognition that early intervention and counseling may be effective in reducing the probability of this outcome. Early, candid conversations with the patient, preferably also including the sexual partner, will allow the patient and partner to understand that anxieties about sexual function are expected and normal and are considered reasonable subject matter for discussion with the treatment team. Gentle exploration of premorbid sexual experience and satisfaction may yield clues as to how to best counsel couples during and after illness and treatment. The treating physicians must inquire about sexual function following therapy because patients may not initiate conversation on this subject. The physician whose surveillance follow-up examination addresses only the presence or absence of cancer will miss opportunities for positive intervention in an area with substantial impact on quality of life and the successfully treated patient's capacity for personal relationships and intimacy.

The importance of the use of vaginal dilators and topical estrogen cannot be overemphasized in preventing permanent symptomatic sequelae of high dose vaginal irradiation. In some patients, these efforts are of little avail, and dyspareunia is the consequence of a shortened or narrow vagina with or without pelvic fibrosis. Under such circumstances, sexual positions other than the so-called "missionary position" may afford couples continued capacity for mutually satisfactory sexual intimacy. The woman superior/astride position may allow the patient more control over the depth of vaginal penetration and pelvic thrusting. Women with shortened vaginal canals may have satisfactory relations with thighs adducted to provide male partners with the sensation of greater vaginal depth. Rear entry, male posterior positioning, may also be a comfortable alternative for both partners when the vaginal depth is shorter than normal. A trial-and-error approach, accompanied by an attitude of patience and realistic expectations, is required. Alternative forms of sexual expression and intimacy may be encouraged in patients unable to have vaginal intercourse, such as digital clitoral stimulation and anoreceptive intercourse. The physician may not be the best qualified individual to assist patients in this regard, but may be the critical individual in recognizing when problems exist and arranging referral to specialists (physician or nonphysician) when appropriate. The attitude of the treating physician in handling the patient's and partner's concerns and questions may be of vital importance in their successful adaptation. A receptive, tactful, and sympathetic manner is generally the most appropriate and effective.

Secondary Neoplasia

In the treatment of Hodgkin's disease, both radiation and chemotherapy have the capacity to induce second cancers (including leukemia). The secondary leukemia experience in advanced Hodgkin's disease suggests that radiation plus limited chemotherapy may carry a risk substantially greater than that of radiation alone. The experience with combined radiation and chemotherapy in gynecologic cancer is too limited for any realistic assessment of possible increases in second neoplasms. Too few patients have been treated, and surveillance follow-up of these patients has been of limited duration. The hazard is theoretical. This hazard of chemoradiation is likely to be kept minimal if the duration and intensity of chemotherapy are kept minimal (see below).

Acute and Chronic Radiation Injury

In the curative management of gynecologic cancer, chemotherapy may be delivered for two reasons: its independent cytotoxic effect and possible impact on the development of distant metastases and its capacity to sensitize cells to radiation and achieve local therapeutic synergism. One must clearly distinguish between these two effects in the design of new therapeutic strategies. If reduction in distant metastases is a goal and systemic chemotherapy appears to have significant activity in the setting of advanced disease, a prolonged course of multiple cycles of multiple agents may be an appropriate strategy. If, conversely, the drugs to be employed do not have significant independent activity against the target cancer, but are being employed as enhancers of radiation response, both acute toxicity and the potential for late sequelae will be minimized if the drugs are given in such a fashion as to maximize the radiation-drug synergism while minimizing systemic drug exposure. Strategies that might be profitably explored include: regional administration of radiosensitizing drugs (intra-arterial or intra-lesional), maximization of radiation-drug interaction by delivery of multiple daily radiation doses during drug delivery (accelerated radiation dose delivery), and the delivery of chemotherapy during intracavitary or interstitial brachytherapy (the ultimate combination of hyperfractionation and accelerated dose delivery). If true synergism is achieved, a reduction in late radiation morbidity may be achieved by a reduction in radiation dose, in a fashion analogous to the manner in which the treatment of anal canal cancer has evolved. Although anal cancers can be readily cured with high-dose radiation alone, equal or better cure rates can be achieved with radiation and very limited, synchronous chemotherapy with lower rates of later morbidity and no obvious induction of secondary neoplasms.

Decreasing acute normal tissue side effects consequent to the effect of unavoidable irradiation of normal tissues may, in theory, be accomplished by the concurrent use of radioprotective agents such as WR-2721, which may selectively protect normal tissues from acute radiation effect (238). Reduction in the dosage of chemotherapeutic drugs used for radioenhancement may have a similar impact. Prospective work needs to be accomplished to define, under clinical circumstances, the minimal dose and optimum schedule of commonly used agents (such as 5-FU) required to obtained genuine supra-additive enhancement with minimum systemic toxicity.

Ultimately, late sequelae of radiation may be minimized if the addition of concurrent chemotherapy selectively affects cells (both cancerous and in normal tissue) that are important for acute radiation response (cycling cell populations) while leaving cells that are important for late radiation injury (which are thought to be infrequently cycling) comparatively unaffected (239). In this regard, use of cycle-specific agents may be the most effective strategy to achieve selective radiosensitization. If a substantially increased tumor cell kill can be achieved acutely, a reduction in total radiation dose may be reflected in substantially lower rates of late radiation injury.

Hematologic Tolerance

Acute hematologic morbidity is the inevitable consequence of combining cytotoxic chemotherapy with radiation fields which unavoidably include a portion of the patient's bone marrow. Neutropenia and thrombocytopenia may be the source of complicating infection or hemorrhage, but may also significantly delay completion of a course of fractionated external radiation. Potential tumor clonogen repopulation during an unplanned treatment interruption necessitated by low blood counts may outweigh the beneficial effect of chemoradiation synergism. In courses of treatment requiring months to complete, red cell transfusion may be required even in the absence of ongoing external blood loss. Concurrent use of hematopoietic growth factors such as granulocyte-colony-stimulating-factor (G-CSF), granulocyte macrophage-colony-stimulating-factor (GM-CSF), interleukin-3 (IL-3), and erythropoietin may be a way to reduce the length of treatment interruptions or avoid them altogether (201–203).

CONCLUSION

Our experience with sequential or concurrent combinations of radiation and chemotherapy is too new to permit assessment of much more than acute toxicities. Hematologic tolerance, acute gastrointestinal side effects, and complications requiring operative intervention are the issues most commonly addressed in the literature published to date. Full assessment of the impact of these combined modalities on normal tissues will require prospective evaluation of large numbers of patients compared to appropriate controls. Candid reporting is essential to a rational evaluation of impact on therapeutic index. Combining modalities without a reduction in the intensity of treatments can only yield additive or supra-additive adverse effects. The excitement of continued investigation in this arena is the potential for increased tumor control with possible equivalent or diminished late effects through the intelligent combination of two therapies, each modulated to account for the actions and toxicities of the other.

REFERENCES

1. Jampolis S, Andras J, Fletcher GH. Analysis of sites and causes of failure of irradiation in invasive squamous cell carcinoma of the intact uterine cervix. Radiology 115:681, 1975.
2. Perez CA, Breaux S, Madoc-Jones H, et al. Radiation therapy alone in the treatment of carcinoma of the uterine cervix: I. Analysis of tumor recurrence. Cancer 51:1393, 1983.
3. Marcus RB, Million RR, Daly JW. Carcinoma of the vagina. Cancer 42:2507, 1978.
4. Perez CA, Camel HM. Long term follow-up in radiation therapy of carcinoma of the vagina. Cancer 49:1308, 1982.
5. Frischbier JH, Thomsen K. Treatment of cancer of the vulva with high energy electrons. Am J Obstet Gynecol 111:431, 1971.
6. Cummings B, Keane T, Thomas G, et al. Results and toxicity of the treatment of anal canal carcinoma by radiation therapy or radiation therapy and chemotherapy. Cancer 54:2062, 1984.
7. Sischy B. The use of radiation therapy combined with chemotherapy in the management of squamous cell carcinoma of the anus and marginally resectable adenocarcinoma of the rectum. Int J Radiat Oncol Biol Phys 11:1587, 1985.
8. Flam MS, John MJ, Mowry PA, et al. Definitive combined modality therapy of carcinoma of the anus. Dis Colon Rectum 30:495, 1987.
9. John MJ, Flam MS, Mowry PA, et al. Radiotherapy alone and chemoradiation for nonmetastatic esophageal carcinoma. A critical review of chemoradiation. Cancer 63:2397, 1989.
10. Boyce J, Fruchter RG, Nicastri AD, et al. Prognostic factors in stage I carcinoma of the cervix. Gynecol Oncol 12:154, 1981.
11. Figge DC, Tamimi HK. Patterns of recurrence of carcinoma following radical hysterectomy. Am J Obstet 140:213, 1981.
12. Fuller AF, Elliot N, Kosloff C, et al. Determinants of increased risk for recurrence in patients undergoing radical hysterectomy for stage IB and IIA carcinoma of the cervix. Gynecol Oncol 33:34, 1989.
13. Salazar OM, Feldstein ML, DePapp EW, et al. Endometrial carcinoma: Analysis of failures with special emphasis on the use of initial preoperative external pelvic radiation. Int J Radiat Oncol Biol Phys 2:1101, 1977.
14. Grigsby PW, Perez CA, Camel HM, et al. Stage III carcinoma of the endometrium: Results of therapy and prognostic factors. Int J Radiat Oncol Biol Phys 11:1915, 1985.
15. Stokes S, Bedwinek J, Kao MS, et al. Treatment of stage I adenocarcinoma of the endometrium by hysterectomy and adjuvant irradiation: A retrospective analysis of 304 patients. Int J Radiat Oncol Biol Phys 12:339, 1986.
16. Silverberg SG, DeGiorg LS. Clear cell carcinoma of the endometrium. Clinical pathologic and ultrastructural findings. Cancer 31:1127, 1973.
17. Hendrickson M, Ross J, Eifel P, et al. Uterine papillary serous carcinoma: A highly malignant form of endometrial adenocarcinoma. Am J Surg Pathol 6:93, 1982.
18. Walker A, Mills S. Serous papillary carcinoma of the endometrium. A clinicopathologic study of 11 cases. Diag Gynecol Obstet 4:261, 1982.

19. Sato Y, Ozaki M, Veda G, et al. A clinicopathologic study of endometrial carcinoma with special reference to new histologic variants. Acta Obstet Gynaec Jpn 37:1015, 1985.
20. Chambers JT, Merino M, Kohorn EI, et al. Uterine papillary serous carcinoma. Obstet Gynecol 69:109, 1987.
21. Kurman RG, Scully RE. Clear cell carcinoma of the endometrium. An analysis of 21 cases. Cancer 37:872, 1976.
22. Belgrad R, Elbadau N, Rubin P. Uterine sarcoma. Radiology 102:159, 1972.
23. Salazar OM, Bonfiglio TA, Pattern SF, et al. Uterine sarcomas. Analysis of failures with special emphasis on the use of adjuvant radiation therapy. Cancer 42:1161, 1978.
24. Vongtama V, Karlen JR, Piver SM, et al. Treatment, results and prognostic factors in stage I and II sarcomas of the corpus uteri. Am J Roentgenol 126:139, 1976.
25. Perez CA, Askin F, Baglan RJ, et al. Effect of irradiation on mixed mullerian tumors of the uterus. Cancer 43:1274, 1979.
26. Echt G, Jepson J, Steel J, et al. Treatment of uterine sarcoma. Cancer 66:35, 1990.
27. Cain JM, Russell AH, Greer BJ, et al. Whole abdominal radiation for minimal residual epithelial ovarian carcinoma after surgical resection and maximal first-line chemotherapy. Gynecol Oncol 29:168, 1988.
28. Coltart RS, Nethersell ABW, Brown CH. A pilot study of high dose abdominopelvic radiotherapy following surgery and chemotherapy for stage III epithelial carcinoma of the ovary. Gynecol Oncol 23:195, 1986.
29. Fuks Z, Rizel S, Biran S. Chemotherapeutic and surgical induction of pathological complete remission and whole abdominal irradiation for consolidation does not enhance the cure of stage III ovarian carcinoma. J Clin Oncol 6:509, 1988.
30. Goldhirsch A, Grenier R, Drether E, et al. Treatment of advanced ovarian cancer with surgery, chemotherapy and consolidation of response by whole abdominal radiotherapy. Cancer 62:40, 1988.
31. Hacker NF, Berek JS, Burnison CM, et al. Whole abdominal radiation as salvage therapy for epithelial ovarian carcinoma. Obstet Gynecol 65:60, 1985.
32. Hainsworth JD, Malcolm A, Johnson DH, et al. Advanced minimal residual ovarian carcinoma. Abdominopelvic irradiation following combination chemotherapy. Obstet Gynecol 61:619, 1983.
33. Hoskins WJ, Lichter AS, Whittington R, et al. Whole abdominal and pelvic irradiation in patients with minimal disease at second-look surgical reassessment for ovarian carcinoma. Gynecol Oncol 20:271, 1985.
34. Kuten A, Stein M, Steiner M, et al. Whole abdominal irradiation following chemotherapy in advanced ovarian carcinoma. Int J Radiat Oncol Biol Phys 14:273, 1988.
35. Linstadt DE, Stern JL, Quivey JM, et al. Salvage whole abdominal irradiation following chemotherapy failure in epithelial ovarian carcinoma. Gynecol Oncol 36:327, 1990.
36. Peters WA, Blasko JC, Bagley CM, et al. Salvage therapy with whole abdominal irradiation in patients with advanced carcinoma of the ovary previously treated by combination chemotherapy. Cancer 58:880, 1986.
37. Rosen EM, Goldberg ID, Rose C, et al. Sequential multi-agent chemotherapy and whole abdominal irradiation for stage III ovarian carcinoma. Radiother Oncol 7:223, 1986.
38. Schray MF, Martinez A, Howes AE, et al. Advanced epithelial ovarian cancer: Salvage whole abdominal irradiation for patients with recurrent or persistent disease after combination chemotherapy. J Clin Oncol 6:1433, 1988.
39. Arian-Schad, Kapp DS, Hackl A, et al. Radiation therapy in stage III ovarian cancer following surgery and chemotherapy: Prognostic factors, patterns of relapse, and toxicity: A preliminary report. Gynecol Oncol 39:47, 1990.
40. Homesley HD, Scarantino CW, Muss HB, et al. Concurrent chemotherapy and single high dose plus whole abdominopelvic radiation for persistent ovarian carcinoma. Gynecol Oncol 34:170, 1989.
41. Perez CA, Breaux S, Madoc-Jones H, et al. Radiation therapy alone in treatment of carcinoma of the uterine cervix: II. Analysis of complications. Cancer 54:235, 1984.
42. Pitkin RM, Bradbury JR. The effect of topical estrogen on irradiated vaginal epithelium. Am J Obstet Gynecol 92:175, 1965.
43. Pitkin RM, van Voorhis LW. Postirradiation vaginitis. An evaluation of prophylaxis with topical estrogen. Radiology 99:417, 1971.
44. Abitol MM, Davenport JH. The irradiated vagina. Obstet Gynecol 44:249, 1974.
45. Boronow RC. Management of radiation-induced vaginal fistulas. Am J Obstet Gynecol 110:1, 1971.
46. Piver MS, Lele S. Enterovaginal and enterocutaneous fistulae in women with gynecologic malignancies. Obstet Gynecol 48:560, 1976.
47. Boronow RC, Rutledge F. Vesicovaginal fistula, radiation, and gynecologic cancer. Am J Obstet Gynecol 111:85, 1971.
48. Bricker EM, Johnston WD. Repair of post irradiation rectovaginal fistula and stricture. Surg Gynecol Obstet 148:499, 1979.

49. Stryker JA, Bartholomew M, Velkley DE, et al. Bladder and rectal complications following radiotherapy for cervix cancer. Gynecol Oncol 29:1, 1988.
50. Villasanta U. Complications of radiotherapy for carcinoma of the uterine cervix. Am J Obstet Gynecol 114:717, 1972.
51. van Nagell JR, Parker JC, Maruyama Y. Bladder and rectal injury following radiation therapy for cervical cancer. Am J Obstet Gynecol 119:727, 1974.
52. Strockbine MF, Hancock JE, Fletcher GH. Complications in 831 patients with squamous cell carcinoma of the intact uterine cervix treated with 3,000 rads or more whole pelvis radiation. Am J Roentgenol 108:293, 1970.
53. Ballon SC, Berman ML, Lagasse LD, et al. Survival after extraperitoneal pelvic and paraaortic lymphadenectomy and radiation therapy in cervical carcinoma. Obstet Gynecol 57:90, 1981.
54. Berman ML, Keys H, Creasman W, et al. Survival and patterns of recurrence in cervical cancer metastatic to periaortic lymph nodes (A Gynecologic Oncology Group Study). Gynecol Oncol 19:8, 1984.
55. Hughes RR, Brewington KC, et al. Extended field irradiation for cervical cancer based on surgical staging. Gynecol Oncol 9:153, 1980.
56. Wharton JJ, Jones HW, Day TG, et al. Preirradiation celiotomy and extended field irradiation for invasive carcinoma of the cervix. Obstet Gynecol 49:333, 1977.
57. Rotman M, Moon S, John M, et al. Extended field para-aortic radiation in cervical carcinoma: The case for prophylactic treatment. Int J Radiat Oncol Biol Phys 4:795, 1978.
58. Fletcher GH, Rutledge FN. Extended field technique in the management of cancer of the uterine cervix. Am J Roentgenol 114:116, 1972.
59. Nelson JH, Boyce J, Malasaet M, et al. Incidence, significance and follow-up of paraaortic lymph node metastases in late invasive carcinoma of the cervix. Am J Obstet Gynecol 128:336, 1977.
60. Brookland RK, Rubin S, Danoff BF. Extended field irradiation in the treatment of patients with cervical carcinoma involving biopsy proven para-aortic nodes. Int J Radiat Oncol Biol Phys 10:1875, 1984.
61. Nori D, Valentine E, Hilaris BS. The role of para-aortic node irradiation in the treatment of cancer of the cervix. Int J Radiat Oncol Biol Phys 11:1469, 1985.
62. Piver MS, Barlow JJ, Krishnamasetty R. Five-year survival (with no evidence of disease) in patients with biopsy confirmed aortic node metastasis from cervical carcinoma. Am J Obstet Gynecol 139:575, 1981.
63. Potish R, et al. The morbidity and utility of periaortic radiotherapy in cervical carcinoma. Gynecol Oncol 15:1, 1983.
64. Silverstein AB, Aron BS, Alexander LL. Paraaortic lymph node irradiation in cervical carcinoma. Radiology 95:181, 1970.
65. Russell AH, Jones DC, Russell KJ, et al. High dose para-aortic lymph node irradiation for gynecologic cancer: Technique, toxicity and results. Int J Radiat Oncol Biol Phys 13:267, 1987.
66. Cheung AY. Extended field irradiation for invasive carcinoma of the cervix. Gynecol Oncol 9:280, 1980.
67. Piver MS, Barlow JJ. High dose irradiation to biopsy confirmed aortic node metastases from carcinoma of the uterine cervix. Cancer 39:1243, 1977.
68. Greer B, Hamberger AD. Treatment of intraperitoneal metastatic adenocarcinoma of the endometrium by the whole abdomen moving strip technique boost irradiation. Gynecol Oncol 16:365, 1983.
69. Dembo AJ. Abdominopelvic radiotherapy in ovarian cancer—a 10 year experience. Cancer 55:2285, 1985.
70. Dembo AJ. Radiotherapeutic management of ovarian cancer. Semin Oncol 111:238, 1984.
71. Dembo AJ, van Dyk J, Japp B, et al. Whole abdominal irradiation by a moving strip technique for patients with ovarian cancer. Int J Radiat Oncol Biol Phys 5:1933, 1979.
72. Perez CA, Korba A, Zivnuska F, et al. ^{60}Co Moving strip technique in management of carcinoma of the ovary: Analysis of tumor control and morbidity. Int J Radiat Oncol Biol Phys 4:379, 1978.
73. Delclos L, Smith JP. Ovarian cancer with special regard to types of radiotherapy. Nat Cancer Inst Monogr 42:129, 1975.
74. Delclos L, Dembo AJ. Ovaries. *In:* Textbook of Radiotherapy. Fletcher GH (Ed). Philadelphia, Lea & Febiger, 1978, p. 834.
75. Townsend R, Glassburn JR, Brady LW, et al. Whole abdominal irradiation for carcinoma of the ovary. Cancer Clin Trials 2:351, 1979.
76. Ingold JA, Reed GB, Kaplan HS, Bagshaw MA. Radiation hepatitis. Am J Roentgenol 93:200, 1965.
77. Wharton JT, Delclos L, Gallagher S, et al. Radiation hepatitis following whole abdominal irradiation. Clin Radiol 27:449, 1976.
78. Schacter L, Crum E, Spitzer T, et al. Fatal radiation hepatitis: A case report and review of the literature. Gyn Oncol 24:373, 1986.
79. Schacter L, Crum E, Spitzer T, et al. Fatal radiation hepatitis: A case report and review of the literature. Gyn Oncol 24:373, 1986.

Endocrine and Reproductive Systems

80. Rubin P, Casarett GW. Clinical radiation pathology. Vol. 2. Toronto, WB Saunders Co, 1968, p. 396.
81. Cann CE, Genant HK, Ettinger, Gordon GS. Spinal mineral loss of postmenopausal estrogen therapy and coronary heart disease. N Engl J Med 313:1044, 1985.
82. Stampfer MJ, Willett WC, Colditz GA, et al. A prospective study of postmenopausal estrogen therapy and coronary heart disease. N Engl J Med 313:1044, 1985.
83. Stampfer MJ, Willett WC, Colditz GA, et al. Postmenopausal estrogen use and heart disease. N Engl J Med 315:135, 1986.
84. Colditz GA, Willett WC, Stampfer MJ, et al. Menopause and the risk of coronary heart disease in women. N Engl J Med 316:1105, 1987.
85. Campbell S, Whitehead M. Estrogen therapy and the menopausal syndrome. Clin Obstet Gynecol 4:31, 1977.
86. Gambrell RD. The menopause: Benefits and risks of estrogen/progestogen replacement therapy. Fertil Steril 37:457, 1982.
87. Kaplan II. Genetic effects in children and grandchildren of women treated for infertility and sterility by roentgen therapy. Report of a study of 33 years. Radiology 72:518, 1959.
88. Horning SJ, Hoppe RT, Kaplan HS. Female reproductive potential after treatment for Hodgkin's disease. N Engl J Med 304:1377, 1981.
89. Yoshimoto Y. Cancer risk among children of atomic bomb survivors. A review of RERF epidemiologic studies. JAMA 264:596, 1990.
90. Shalet SM. Effects of cancer chemotherapy on gonadal function of patients. Cancer Treat Res 7:141, 1980.
91. Shalet SM. Effects of cancer chemotherapy on gonadal function of patients. A review. Clin Endocrinol 18:637, 1983.
92. Chapman RM. Effect of cytotoxic therapy on sexuality and gonadal function. Semin Oncol 9:84, 1982.
93. Belohorsky B, Siracky J, Sandor L, Klauber E. Comments on the development of amenorrhea caused by myleran in cases of chronic myelosis. Neoplasma 7:397, 1960.
94. Fisher B, Sherman B, Rockett H, et al. L-phenylalanine Mustard (L-PAM) in the management of premenopausal patients with primary breast cancer: Lack of association of disease-free survival with depression of ovarian function. National surgical adjuvant project for breast and bowel cancers. Cancer 44:847, 1979.
95. Rose DP, Davis TE. Ovarian function in patients receiving adjuvant chemotherapy for breast cancer. Lancet 1:1174, 1977.
96. Fosdick WM, Parsons JL, Hill DF. Preliminary report: Long-term cyclophosphamide therapy in rheumatoid arthritis. Arthritis Rheum 11:151, 1968.
97. Miller JJ 3d, Williams GF, Leissring JC. Multiple late complications of therapy with cyclophosphamide, including ovarian destruction. Am J Med 50:530, 1971.
98. Warne GL, Fairly KF, Hobbs JB, et al. Cyclophosphamide induced ovarian failure. N Engl J Med 289:1159, 1973.
99. Koyama H, Wada T, Nishizawa Y, et al. Cyclophosphamide induced ovarian failure and its therapeutic significance in patients with breast cancer. Cancer 39:1403, 1977.
100. Sobrinho LG, Levine RA, DeConti RC. Amenorrhea in patients with Hodgkin's disease treated with antineoplastic agents. Am J Obstet Gynecol 109:135, 1971.
101. Morgenfeld MC, Goldberg V, Parisier H, et al. Ovarian lesions due to cytostatic agents during the treatment of Hodgkin's disease. Surg Gynecol Obstet 134:826, 1972.
102. Chapman RM, Sutcliffe SB, Malpas JS. Cytotoxic induced ovarian failure in women with Hodgkin's disease. I. Hormone function. JAMA 242:1877, 1979.
103. Schilsky RL, Sherins RL, Hubbard SM, et al. Long-term follow-up of ovarian function in women treated with MOPP chemotherapy for Hodgkin's disease. Am J Med 71:552, 1981.
104. Andrieu JM, Ochoa-Molina ME. Menstrual cycle, pregnancies and offspring before and after MOPP therapy for Hodgkin's disease. Cancer 52:435, 1983.
105. Li FP, Fine W, Jaffe N, et al. Offspring of patients treated for cancer in childhood. J Natl Cancer Inst 62:1193, 1979.
106. Holmes GE, Holmes FF. Pregnancy outcome of patients treated for Hodgkin's disease. Cancer 52:435, 1983.
107. van Thiel DH, Ross GT, Lipsett MB. Pregnancies after chemotherapy of trophoblastic neoplasms. Science 169:1326, 1970.
108. Anderson BL. Sexual functioning morbidity among cancer survivors: Current status and future research directions. Cancer 55:1835, 1985.
109. Anderson BL, Hacker NF. Treatment for gynecologic cancer: A review of the effects on female sexuality. Health Psych 2:203, 1983.
110. Harris R, Good RS, Pollack L. Sexual behavior of gynecologic cancer patients. Arch Sex Behav 11:503, 1982.
111. Peck A, Boland J. Emotional reactions to radiation treatment. Cancer 40:180, 1977.

112. Cochran SD, Hacker NF, Wellisch DK, Berek JS. Sexual functioning after treatment for endometrial cancer. J Psychosoc Oncol 5:47, 1987.
113. Adelusi B. Coital function after radiation therapy for carcinoma of the cervix uteri. Brit J Obstet Gynaec 87:821, 1980.
114. Decker WH, Schwartzman E. Sexual function following treatment for carcinoma of the cervix. Am J Obstet Gynec 83:401, 1962.
115. Seibel M, Freeman MG, Graves WL. Sexual function after surgical and radiation therapy for cervical carcinoma. South Med J 68:552, 1975.
116. Vincent CE, Vincent B, Griess FC, Linton EB. Some marital-sexual concomitants of carcinoma of the cervix. South Med J 68:552, 1975.
117. Vasicka A, Popovich NR, Brausch CC. Post radiation course of patients with cervical carcinoma: A clinical study of psychic, sexual, and physical well-being of sixteen patients. Obstet Gynecol 11:403, 1958.
118. Abitol MM, Davenport JH. Sexual dysfunction after therapy for cervical carcinoma. Am J Obstet Gynecol 119:181, 1974.
119. Bertelsen K. Sexual dysfunction after treatment of cervical cancer. Danish Med Bull 30(Suppl 2):31, 1983.
120. Hubbard JL, Shingleton HM. Sexual function of patients after cancer of the cervix treatment. Clin Obstet Gynecol 12:247, 1985.
121. Capone MA, Westie KS, Good RS. Sexual rehabilitation of the gynecologic cancer patient: An effective counseling model. Front Radiat Ther Oncol 14:123, 1980.
122. Donahue VC, Knapp RC. Sexual rehabilitation of gynecologic cancer patients. Obstet Gynecol 49:118, 1977.
123. Bosch A, Marcial VA. Carcinoma of the uterine cervix associated with pregnancy. Am J Roentgenol 96:92, 1966.
124. Hacker NF, Berek JS, Lagasse LD, et al. Carcinoma of the cervix associated with pregnancy. Obstet Gynecol 59:735, 1982.
125. Thompson JD, Caputo TA, Franklin EW, Dale E. The surgical management of invasive cancer of the cervix in pregnancy. Am J Obstet Gynecol 121:853, 1975.
126. Creasman WT, Rutledge F, Smith JP. Carcinoma of the ovary associated with pregnancy. Obstet Gynecol 38:111, 1971.
127. Dudan RC, Yon JL, Ford JH, Averette HE. Carcinoma of the cervix and pregnancy. Gynecol Oncol 1:283, 1973.
128. Creasman WT, Rutledge FN, Fletcher GH. Carcinoma of the cervix associated with pregnancy. Obstet Gynecol 36:495, 1970.
129. Nikser J, Shubat N. Stage IB cervical carcinoma and pregnancy: Report of 49 cases. Am J Obstet Gynecol 145:203, 1983.
130. Waldrop GM, Palmer JP. Carcinoma of the cervix associated with pregnancy. Am J Obstet Gynecol 86:202, 1963.
131. Prem KA, Makowski EL, McKelvey JL. Carcinoma of the cervix associated with pregnancy. Am J Obstet Gynecol 95:99, 1966.
132. Lutz MH, Underwood PB, Rozier JC, Putney FW. Genital malignancy in pregnancy. Am J Obstet Gynecol 129:536, 1977.
133. Barber HR, Brunschwig A. Gynecologic cancer complicating pregnancy. Am J Obstet Gynecol 85:156, 1963.
134. Jones HW, Neill W. The treatment of carcinoma of the cervix during pregnancy. Am J Obstet Gynecol 48:477, 1944.
135. Kinch RAH. Factors affecting the prognosis of cancer of the cervix in pregnancy. Am J Obstet Gynecol 82:45, 1961.
136. Kistner RW, Gorbich AC, Smith GV. Cervical cancer in pregnancy: Review of the literature with presentation of thirty additional cases. Obstet Gynecol 9:554, 1957.
137. McDugg HC, Carney WI, Waterman GW. Cancer of the cervix and pregnancy. Obstet Gynecol 8:196, 1956.
138. Collins CG, Barclay DL. Cancer of the vulva and cancer of the vagina in pregnancy. Clin Obstet Gynecol 6:927, 1973.
139. Karlen JR, Sternberg LB, Abbott JN. Carcinoma of the endometrium co-existing with pregnancy. Obstet Gynecol 40:334, 1972.
140. Novak ER, Lambrou CD, Woodrugg JD. Ovarian tumors in pregnancy. An ovarian tumor registry review. Obstet Gynecol 46:401, 1975.
141. Jubb ED. Primary ovarian carcinoma in pregnancy. Am J Obstet Gynecol 85:345, 1963.
142. Greer BE, Easterine TR, McLennan DA, et al. Fetal and maternal considerations in the management of Stage IB cervical cancer during pregnancy. Gynecol Oncol 34:61, 1989.
143. Vohr BR, Garcia-Coll CT. Neurodevelopmental and school performance of very low birth weight infants: A seven year longitudinal study. Pediatrics 76:345, 1985.
144. Plummer G. Anomalies occurring in children exposed in utero to the atom bomb in Hiroshima. Pediatrics 10:687, 1952.
145. Hammer-Jacobsen E. Congenital malformations induced by radiation. Strahlentherapie 116:152, 1961.
146. Murphy DP. The outcome of 625 pregnancies in women subjected to pelvic radium or roentgen irradiation. Am J Obstet Gynecol. 18:179, 1929.

147. Dekaban AS. Abnormalities in children exposed to x-irradiation during various stages of gestation: Tentative timetable of radiation injury to the human fetus, Part I. J Nucl Med 9:471, 1968.
148. MacMahon B. Prenatal x-ray exposure and childhood cancer. J Natl Cancer Inst 28:1173, 1962.
149. Stewart A, Kneak GW. Radiation dose effects in relation to obstetric x-rays and childhood cancers. Lancet 1:1185, 1970.
150. Sweet DL, Kinzie J. Consequences of radiotherapy and anti-neoplastic therapy for the fetus. J Reprod Med 17:241, 1976.
151. Boice JD. Fetal risk from radiotherapy and chemotherapy exposure in utero. Cancer Bull 38:293, 1986.
152. Nicholson HO. Cytotoxic drugs in pregnancy. Review of reported cases. J Obstet Gynaec Brit Cwlth 75:307, 1968.
153. Gilland J, Weinstein L. The effects of cancer chemotherapeutic agents on the developing fetus. Obstet Gynecol Surv 38:6, 1983.
154. Reynoso EE, Shepherd FA, Messner HA, et al. Acute leukemia during pregnancy: The Toronto leukemia study group experience with long term follow-up of children exposed in utero to chemotherapeutic agents. J Clin Oncol 5:1098, 1987.

Secondary Neoplasms

155. Beebe GW. Developments in assessing carcinogenic risks from radiation. *In:* Radiation Carcinogenesis. Epidemiology and Biological Significance. Boice JD, Fraumeni JF (Eds). New York, Raven Press, 1984, p. 457.
156. Fehr P, Prem KA. Postirradiation sarcoma of the pelvic girdle following therapy for squamous cell carcinoma of the cervix. Am J Obstet Gynecol 6:309, 1978.
157. Czesnin K, Wronkowski Z. Second malignancies of the irradiated area in patients treated for uterine cervix cancer. Gynecol Oncol 6:309, 1978.
158. Meredith RF, Eisert AR, Kaka Z, et al. An excess of uterine sarcomas after pelvic irradiation. Cancer 58:2003, 1986.
159. Messerschmidt GL, Hoover R, Young RC. Gynecologic cancer treatment: Risk factors for therapeutically induced neoplasia. Cancer 48:442, 1981.
160. Boice JD, Day NE, Anderson A, et al. Second cancers following radiation treatment for cervical cancer: An international collaboration among cancer registries. J Natl Cancer Inst 74:955, 1985.
161. Pizzarello DJ, Roses DF, Newall J, Barish RJ. The carcinogenicity of radiation therapy. Surg Gyn Obstet 159:189, 1984.
162. Tucker MA, Fraumeni JF. Treatment-related cancers after gynecologic malignancy. Cancer 60:2177, 1987.
163. Clarke EA, Kreiger N, Spengler RF. Second primary cancer following treatment for cervical cancer. Can Med Assoc J 131:553, 1984.
164. Storm HH. Second primary cancer after treatment for cervical cancer. Late effects after radiotherapy. Cancer 61:679, 1988.
165. Fehr PE, Prem KA. Malignancy of the uterine corpus following irradiation therapy for squamous cell carcinoma of the cervix. Am J Obstet Gynecol 119:685, 1974.
166. Kwon TH, Prempree T, Tang CK, et al. Adenocarcinoma of the uterine corpus following irradiation for cervical cancer. Gynecol Oncol 11:102, 1981.
167. Boice JD, Blettner M, Kleinerman RA, et al. Radiation dose and leukemia risk in patients treated for cancer of the cervix. J Natl Cancer Inst 79:1295, 1987.
168. Tucker MA, Coleman CN, Cox RS, et al. Risk of second malignancies following Hodgkin's disease after 15 years. N Engl J Med 318:76, 1988.
169. Arseneau JC, Sponzo RW, Leven DL, et al. Nonlymphomatous malignant tumors complicating Hodgkin's disease. Possible association with intensive therapy. N Engl J Med 287:1119, 1972.
170. Henry-Amar M. Second cancers after radiotherapy and chemotherapy for early stages of Hodgkin's disease. J Natl Cancer Inst 71:911, 1983.
171. Kaldo JM, Day NE, Clarke EA, et al. Leukemia following Hodgkin's disease. N Engl J Med 322:7, 1990.
172. Valagussa P, Santoro A, Fossati-Bellani F, et al. Second acute leukemia and other malignancies following treatment for Hodgkin's disease. J Clin Oncol 4:830, 1986.
173. Blayney DW, Longo DL, Young RC, et al. Decreasing risk of leukemia with prolonged follow-up after chemotherapy and radiotherapy for Hodgkin's disease. N Engl J Med 316:710, 1987.
174. Kyle RA. Second malignancies associated with chemotherapeutic agents. Semin Oncol 9:131, 1982.
175. Reimer RR, Hoover R, Fraumeni JF, Young RC. Acute leukemia after alkylating agent therapy in ovarian cancer. N Engl J Med 297:177, 1977.
176. Greene MH, Boice JD, Greer BE, et al. Acute nonlymphocytic leukemia after therapy with alkylating agents for ovarian cancer: A

study of five randomized clinical trials. N Engl J Med 307:1416, 1982.
177. Kaldo JM, Day NE, Pettersson F, et al. Leukemia following chemotherapy for ovarian cancer. N Engl J Med 322:1, 1990.
178. Boice JD, Greene MH, Killen JY, et al. Leukemia and preleukemia after adjuvant treatment of gastrointestinal cancer with semustine (Methyl-CCNU). N Engl J Med 309:1079, 1983.
179. Russell AH, Tong D, Figge DC. Adjuvant postoperative pelvic radiation for carcinoma of the uterine cervix: Pattern of cancer recurrence in patients undergoing elective radiation following radical hysterectomy and pelvic lymphadenectomy. Int J Radiat Oncol Biol Phys 10:211, 1984.

Large Field Irradiation

180. Boronow RC, Morrow CP, Creasman WT, et al. Surgical staging in endometrial cancer: Clinical-pathological findings of a prospective study. Obstet Gynecol 63:825, 1984.
181. Creasman WT, Morrow CP, Bundy BN, et al. Surgical pathological spread patterns of endometrial cancer. Cancer 60:2035, 1987.
182. Bagley CM, Young RC, Schein PS, et al. Ovarian cancer metastatic to the diaphragm frequently undiagnosed at laparotomy. A preliminary report. Am J Obstet Gynecol 116:397, 1973.
183. Knapp RC, Fricaman EA. Aortic lymph node metastases in early ovarian cancer. Am J Obstet Gynecol 119:1013, 1974.
184. Buchsbaum HJ, Lifshitz S. Staging and surgical evaluation of ovarian carcinoma. Semin Oncol 11:227, 1984.
185. Ballon SC, Pornuff JC, Sikic BI, et al. Second look laparotomy in epithelial ovarian carcinoma. Precise definition, sensitivity, and specificity of the operative procedure. Gynecol Oncol 17:154, 1985.
186. Barnhill DR, Hoskins JW, Heller PB, Park RC. The second look surgical reassessment for epithelial ovarian carcinoma. Gynecol Oncol 19:148, 1984.
187. Roberts WS, Hodel K, Rich WM. Second look laparotomy in the management of gynecologic malignancy. Gynecol Oncol 13:345, 1982.
188. Smirz LR, Stehman FB, Ulbright TM, et al. Second look laparotomy after chemotherapy in the management of ovarian malignancy. Am J Obstet Gynecol 152:661, 1985.
189. Smith JP, Delgado G, Rutledge F. Second look operation in ovarian cancer. Cancer 38:1438, 1976.
190. Webb JG, Snyder JA, William RJ, Decker DG. Second look laparotomy in ovarian cancer. Cancer 38:1438, 1976.
191. Lagasse LD, Creasman WT, Shingleton HM, et al. Results and complications of operative staging in cervical cancer. Experience of the Gynecologic Oncology Group. Gynecol Oncol 9:90, 1980.
192. Sundersanam A, Charyulu K, Belinson J, et al. Influence of exploratory celiotomy on the management of carcinoma of the cervix. Cancer 41:1049, 1978.
193. Welander CE, Pierce VK, Nori D, et al. Pretreatment laparotomy in carcinoma of the cervix. Gynecol Oncol 12:336, 1987.
194. Buchsbaum HJ. Extrapelvic lymph node metastases in cervical carcinoma. Am J Obstet Gynecol 133:814, 1979.
195. Thomas G, Dembo A, Fyles A, et al. Concurrent chemoradiation in advanced cervical cancer. Gynecol Oncol 38:446, 1990.
196. Russell AH, Mesic JB, Scudder SA, et al. Extended volume irradiation and synchronous cytotoxic chemotherapy for treatment of cervical cancer with metastases to retroperitoneal lymph nodes (in preparation).
197. Gabrilove JL. Introduction and overview of hematopoietic growth factors. Semin Hematol 26(Suppl 2):1, 1989.
198. Garnick MB, O'Reilly RJ. M-CSF, IL-3, IL-4, IL-6: Clinical promise. Hematol Oncol Clin N Am 3:495, 1989.
199. Golde DW, Glasply JA. The colony-stimulating factors: Biology and clinical use. Oncology 4:25, 1990.
200. Dembo AJ, Bush RS, Beale HA, et al. A randomized clinical trial of moving strip versus open field whole abdominal irradiation in patients with invasive epithelial cancer of ovary (Abstr). Int J Radiat Oncol Biol Phys 9(Suppl):97, 1983.
201. Schray MF, Martinez AS, Howes AE. Toxicity of open-field whole abdominal irradiation as primary postoperative treatment in gynecologic malignancy. Int J Radiat Oncol Biol Phys 16:397, 1989.
202. Schray MF, Martinez A, Howes AE, et al. Advanced epithelial ovarian cancer: Toxicity of whole abdominal irradiation after operations, combination chemotherapy, and reoperation. Gynecol Oncol 24:68, 1986.
203. Wiltshaw E, Kroner T. Phase II study of Cis-Dichlorodiamine Platinum (NSC-119875) in advanced adenocarcinoma of the ovary. Cancer Treat Rep 60:55, 1976.
204. Ehrlich CE, Einhorn L, Williams SD, et al. Chemotherapy for stage III-IV epithelial ovarian cancer with Cis-Dichlorodiammine Platinum (II), Adriamycin and Cyclophos-

phamide: A preliminary report. Cancer Treat Rep 63:281, 1979.

Chemoradiation Toxicity

205. Sell A, Bertelson K, Andersen JE, et al. Randomized study of whole abdomen irradiation versus pelvic irradiation plus cyclophosphamide in treatment of early ovarian cancer. Gynecol Oncol 37:367, 1990.
206. Donaldon SS, Glick JM, Wilbur JR. Adriamycin activating a recall phenomenon after radiation therapy. Ann Intern Med 81:407, 1974.
207. Stein RS. Radiation recall enteritis after Actinomycin-D and Adriamycin therapy. South Med J 71:960, 1978.
208. Hreshchyshyn JM, Aron BS, Boronow RC, et al. Hydroxyurea or placebo combined with radiation to treat stages III-B and IV cervical cancer confined to the pelvis. Int J Radiat Oncol Biol Phys 5:317, 1979.
209. Piver MS, Barlow JJ, Vongtama V, Blumenson L. Hydroxyurea: A radiation potentiator in carcinoma of the uterine cervix. Am J Obstet Gynecol 147:803, 1983.
210. Piver MS, Vongtama V, Emrich LJ. Hydroxyurea plus pelvic radiation versus placebo plus pelvic radiation in surgically staged Stage III-B cervical cancer. J Surg Oncol 35:129, 1987.
211. Sinclair WK. Hydroxyurea: Effect on chinese hamster cells grown in culture (part I). Cancer Res 27:297, 1967.
212. Sinclair WK. The combined effect of hydroxyurea and x-rays in Chinese hamster cells in vitro. Cancer Res 28:198, 1968.
213. Phillips RA, Tolmach LJ. Repair of potentially lethal damage in x-irradiated HeLa cells. Radiat Res 29:413, 1966.
214. Leibel S, Bauer M, Wasserman T, et al. Radiotherapy with or without misonidazole for patients with stage IIIB or stage IVA squamous cell carcinoma of the uterine cervix: Preliminary report of a Radiation Therapy Oncology Group randomized trial. Int J Radiat Oncol Biol Phys 13:541, 1987.
215. Belloni C, Mangioni L, Bortolozzi G, et al. ICRF 159 plus radiation versus radiation therapy alone in cervical carcinoma: A double blind study. Oncology 40:181, 1983.
216. Haie C, George M, Pejovic MH, et al. Feasibility study of an alternating schedule of radiotherapy and chemotherapy in advanced uterine cervical carcinoma. Radiother Oncol 12:121, 1988.
217. Runowicz CD, Wadler S, Rodriguez-Rodriquez L, et al. Concomitant cisplatin and radiotherapy in locally advanced cervical carcinoma. Gynecol Oncol 34:395, 1989.
218. Monyak DJ, Twigg LB, Potish RA, et al. Tolerance and preliminary results of simultaneous therapy with radiation and cisplatin for advanced cervical cancer. NCI Monogr 6:369, 1988.
219. Wong LC, Choo YC, Choy D, et al. Long term follow-up of potentiation of radiotherapy by cisplatinum in advanced cervical cancer. Gynecol Oncol 35:159, 1989.
220. Goldhirsch A, Greiner R, Bleher A, et al. Combination of chemotherapy with methotrexate, bleomycin and cis-platinum, and radiation therapy for locally advanced carcinoma of the cervix. Am J Clin Oncol 9:12, 1986.
221. John M, Flam M, Sikic B, et al. Preliminary results of concurrent radiotherapy and chemotherapy in advanced cervical carcinoma: A Phase I-II prospective intergroup NCOG-RTOG study. Gynecol Oncol 37:1, 1990.
222. Kuske RR, Perez CA, Grigsby PW, et al. Phase I/II Study of definitive radiotherapy and chemotherapy (cisplatin and 5-fluorouracil) for advanced or recurrent gynecologic malignancies: Preliminary report. Am J Clin Oncol 12:467, 1989.
223. Kuzel T, Esparaz B, Green D, Kies M. Thrombogenicity of intravenous 5-Fluorouracil alone or in combination with cisplatin. Cancer 65:885, 1990.
224. Friedlander ML, Atkinson K, Coppleson JVM, et al. The integration of chemotherapy into the management of locally advanced cervical cancer: A pilot study. Gynecol Oncol 19:1, 1984.
225. Roberts WS, Kavanagh JJ, Greenberg H, et al. Concomitant radiation therapy and chemotherapy in the treatment of advanced squamous carcinoma of the lower female genital tract. Gynecol Oncol 34:183, 1989.
226. Rettenmaier MA, Moran MF, Ramsinghani NF, et al. Treatment of advanced and recurrent squamous carcinoma of the uterine cervix with constant intra-arterial infusion of cisplatin. Cancer 61:1301, 1988.
227. Falappa P, Trodella L, Cotronco AR, Turriziani A. Advanced carcinoma of the cervix treated by continuous pelvic arterial infusion with cytostatics and radiation therapy. Eur J Radiol 2:307, 1982.
228. Russell AH, Mesic JB, Scudder SA, et al. Pelvic radiation with synchronous cytotoxic chemotherapy as adjuvant treatment for high risk cervical cancer following radical hysterectomy and pelvic lymphadenectomy (in preparation).
229. Russell AH, Mesic JB, Scudder S, et al. Synchronous radiation and cytotoxic chemotherapy for locally advanced or recurrent

squamous cancer of the vulva. Gynecol Oncol 47:14, 1992.

230. Ludgate SM, Crandon AJ, Hudson CN, et al. Synchronous 5-Fluorouracil, Mitomycin C and radiation therapy in the treatment of locally advanced carcinoma of the cervix. Int J Radiat Oncol Biol Phys 15:389, 1988.
231. Thomas G, Dembo A, DePetrillo A, et al. Concurrent radiation and chemotherapy in vulvar carcinoma. Gynecol Oncol 34:263, 1989.
232. Inverson T. Irradiation and bleomycin in the treatment of inoperable vulvar carcinoma. Acta Obstet Gynecol Scand 61:195, 1982.

Minimizing Toxicities—Methodology

233. Hoden K, Rich WM, Austin P, DiSaia PJ. The role of ovarian transposition in conservation of ovarian function in radical hysterectomy followed by pelvic radiation. Gynecol Oncol 13:195, 1981.
234. Belinson JL, Doherty M, McDay JB. A new technique for ovarian transposition. Surg Gynecol Obstet 159:157, 1984.
235. Husseinzadeh N, Nahhas SW, Velkley DE, et al. The preservation of ovarian function in young women undergoing pelvic radiation therapy. Gynecol Oncol 18:373, 1984.
236. Leporrier M, von Theobald P, Roffe JL, Muller G. A new technique to protect ovarian function before pelvic irradiation. Heterotopic ovarian autotransplantation. Cancer 60:2201, 1987.
237. Chapman RM, Sutcliffe SB. Protection of ovarian function by oral contraceptives in women receiving chemotherapy for Hodgkin's disease. Blood 58:849, 1981.
238. Yuhas JM, Storer JB. Differential chemoprotection of normal and malignant tissues. J Natl Cancer Inst 42:331, 1969.
239. Rubin P. The Franz Buschke lecture: Late effects of chemotherapy and radiation therapy: A new hypothesis. Int J Radiat Oncol Biol Phys 10:5, 1984.

Chapter 35

CARDIAC TOXICITY

MOHAMED K. ALI AND SEWA S. LEGHA

The ultimate goal of the treatment of cancer is an uncomplicated cure rather than a simple increase in survival. It is therefore imperative to avoid treatments associated with severe irreversible damage, particularly to vital organs. Consequently, the concept of relapse-free survival should be expanded to include complication-free survival rates in determining the true therapeutic efficacy of cancer therapy. Such a therapeutic goal is therefore highly desirable because it represents both quantitative and qualitative outcome of any oncologic treatment program.

In the past, single-modality treatments such as surgery, radiation therapy, or chemotherapy were heavily emphasized. With the more frequent use in recent years of combined modality approaches, increasingly more patients have been cured of their cancer in terms of control of local, regional and disseminated disease. When chemotherapeutic agents are added to radiotherapy, they can increase or decrease the therapeutic ratio depending on the balance between the antitumor action and the acute as well as chronic toxicity of the combination utilized. Although much information is available as to the therapeutic effects and undesirable consequences of single agents, data on complications of combined modality programs are scanty and fragmented. In addition, the testing of chemotherapeutic agents for their potential enhancement of radiation injury to normal tissues is usually not part of their pretherapeutic evaluation. Planning for safe and effective use of this combination concomitantly or sequentially in various oncologic scenarios still remains a challenging task.

In this chapter, data concerning the cardiac complications of radiation and chemotherapy, separately and in combination will be presented.

PATHOGENESIS OF RADIOTHERAPY- AND CHEMOTHERAPY-INDUCED INJURY TO CARDIAC TISSUES

The acute clinical effects of radiotherapy and chemotherapy have been well delineated. As the combination of these two modalities becomes more successful, late effects dominate the therapeutic equation. These late toxicities were initially believed to be exclusively due to radiotherapy because the main concern for tolerance of most chemotherapeutic agents has been their acute toxicity, which usually affects the rapidly proliferating cells (1). In contrast, mature postmitotic cells have been thought to be insensitive to drugs and therefore immune to acute and late effects of chemotherapy. Although this selective effect of drugs can explain their therapeutic activity, the clinical evidence no longer supports this view as it applies to normal tissues (2). The cardiotoxic effect of Adriamycin (doxorubicin; ADR) is a notable example of the effect of a chemotherapeutic agent on the mature nonproliferating myocytes (3).

In general, tissue vulnerability to the effects of drugs depends on the capacity of the tissues to absorb, concentrate or metabolize these agents or their derivatives and may be dependent on cell mitotic behavior and maturation (4). Similarly, parenchymal tissues that normally undergo frequent renewal by mitotic division are at higher risk for direct radiation injury than those that normally renew very slowly or not at all (5). Patients in the pediatric age, whose normal tissues are still proliferating, are therefore more vulnerable to the injurious effects of both chemotherapy and radiotherapy than adults whose organs are, to a large extent, in a mature state. These early primary parenchymal injuries can prevent effective cell renewal and/or growth and may manifest as late functional and structural abnormalities in the affected organ systems. This might explain the findings in recent reports of a high incidence of late myocardial dysfunction among patients who were treated with ADR during their early years and the paucity of such changes among those who received this drug during adult years (6,7).

It also has to be recognized that both the acute and late effects of radiotherapy and chemotherapy have different cellular targets within various organs as well as different time courses of pathological and clinical expression. These differences can be largely explained by variations in cell kinetics, radiosensitivity, and pharmacosensitivity between the parenchymal component and vasculoconnective tissue components of different organs. One of the unique features of radiation injury to normal tissues is an intermediate sensitivity of the small blood vessels and intraparenchymal connective tissue. These structures are not as sensitive as the renewing parenchymal tissues but are more sensitive than slowly renewable or nonrenewable tissues (8). The vasculoconnective tissue changes start with injury to the capillary endothelial cells, resulting in increased permeability which occurs soon after irradiation and results in plasma transudation into the vessel wall and parenchymal interstices. This initiates a sequence of events in such tissues which lead to increased fibroblastic activity and increase in the collagenous content and density of the vascular, perivascular and interstitial connective tissues. These fibrotic changes progress with time, leading to a decrease in the effective microcirculation. The resultant ischemia eventually leads to secondary deterioration in the functional capacity and cellular content of parenchymal tissues. Such progression varies in rate and severity in various parts of the irradiated organ and this may explain the significant variation in the latent period and in the onset of various clinical manifestations of these fibrotic changes. The very late onset of heart block (5 to 23 years) and the earlier onset of pericardial and myocardial abnormalities exemplifies the significant variation in the progression of the fibrotic changes within the human heart following its exposure to ionizing irradiation (9). These postirradiation cardiac abnormalities also confirm the experimental data indicating that vasculoconnective tissue fibrosis is qualitatively common to virtually all organs and is relatively independent of the radiosensitivity of the associated parenchymal tissue because the myocyte itself is known to be radioresistant.

It is therefore clear that radiation injury to various organs includes a permanent and progressive component similar and additive to the basic aging process (8). These premature aging changes tend to reduce the tolerance of tissues to various physical, functional, and chemical stresses and injuries.

Chemotherapeutic agents can cause tissue injury directly or enhance the injury caused by radiotherapy. The antibiotic class of chemotherapeutic agents tops the list of drugs that can enhance radiation injury with increased toxicity reported in all tissues except the central nervous system (10–13). The second most common type of injury with the combination of radiotherapy and chemotherapy appears to occur with drugs causing injury to normal tissues on their own such as ADR to the heart and methotrexate (MTX) to the central nervous system (14). Because this chapter deals with the cardiac toxicity of the combined modality, the following discussion will be, to a large extent, devoted to the clinical manifestations of cardiac injury resulting from ADR and ionizing irradiation.

CARDIAC COMPLICATIONS OF CHEMOTHERAPY

Mechanisms of Injury

The myocardial cell, which lacks the property of rapid mitosis, was once considered not to be at risk for injury due to chemotherapy. Unfortunately, this notion is untrue, and the number of chemotherapeutic agents associated with cardiac toxicity is gradually increasing. The mechanisms of injury from these agents include hypersensitivity, ischemic effects, and direct toxic damage. Cyclophosphamide in large doses (5 g/m^2) can cause acute hemorrhagic myocardial necrosis and recent evidence suggests that other agents such as 5-fluorouracil might also cause or modify latent cardiomyopathy by adding an ischemic insult (15–18).

Of the chemotherapeutic agents known to cause cardiomyopathy, by far the most important and best studied are the anthracycline antibiotics, daunomycin and ADR. These drugs cause a dose-related, transient inhibition of DNA-dependent RNA synthesis at the nuclear and mitochondrial level which affects functional and structural proteins (19). The cardiac expression of this action is a direct damage to the myocytes, which is characterized by loss of contractile elements in the form of myofibril degeneration and/or sacrotubular vacuolization (20). Severe changes result in cell necrosis with both mitochondrial and nuclear degeneration resulting in diffuse patches of replacement fibrosis.

Quantitative Evaluation of Adriamycin Cardiac Toxicity

A system of grading the severity of histopathologic and ultrastructural changes has been derived from extensive experience with human endomyocardial biopsies (21–24). The original grading method developed by Billingham used a four-point (0–3) scale and showed a good correlation between a high grade (2–3) injury and the risk of developing congestive heart failure (23). These findings led to the recommendation that ADR be discontinued in patients who developed grade 2 changes in the cardiac biopsy. The Billingham classification was further refined by Benjamin et al, who devised a five-point scale with intermediate grades (0.5 and 1.5) of toxicity. (22) The clinical experience using this scale demonstrated a good correlation between the biopsy grade and risk of heart failure; a 20% risk in association with a biopsy score of 1.5 indicated that this toxicity grade should be considered the upper limit of tolerance for ADR administration (20,24). A good correlation of the grade of cardiac toxicity with both total dose administered and clinical features of ADR-induced cardiomyopathy has been shown in several studies (3,22–25). Cardiac biopsy has also proven to be a valuable tool for investigating the cardiac effects of new anthracycline analogues (3,22–25).

Although cardiac biopsy has been universally accepted as the standard method of classifying structural damage, many invasive and noninvasive techniques for monitoring the myocardial function of patients receiving ADR have been utilized. The most widely used functional parameter, so far, has been the ejection fraction (EF) determined by either echocardiography or nuclear scanning techniques. One limitation of using serial ejection fractions is the lack of standardization and the variability of techniques and normal values from one institution to another. Despite these limitations, ejection fractions can help separate patients considered for ADR therapy into very low risk (EF $\geq$ 65%), high risk (EF 50%), and intermediate risk (EF 50% to 64%) for developing congestive failure (24). Other investigators believe that the change in ejection fraction with a drop of 10 to 15 points from the baseline is of greater prognostic significance than the absolute value (25). Cardiac monitoring by means of electrocardiogram (EKG), although commonly used, fails to provide any useful guidelines and has not proven to be sensitive or specific for the cardiac toxicity of ADR (26).

Risk Factors for Adriamycin Cardiac Toxicity

The clinical manifestations of ADR cardiomyopathy represent the consequences of diffuse myocardial dysfunction that culminates in right and left ventricular decompensation (27). The development of congestive heart failure may be rapid and difficult to predict by most of the commonly used methods of cardiac monitoring, including ejection fractions. Fortunately, intensive ongoing clinical research has led to the identification of specific risk factors for increased cardiac toxicity. Among the most significant risk factors are the cumulative dose of the drug, the rate of its infusion, prior significant cardiac disease, extremes of age, and prior or concomitant irradiation of major portions of the heart (28–33).

Cumulative Dose

The most important contribution to minimizing the risk of ADR-induced congestive heart failure was the discovery of its cumulative dose relationship. In an analysis of risk factors for developing cardiac toxicity, von Hoff et al found that the incidence of this complication was clearly related to the cumulative dose of ADR received (33). Their report indicated that the incidence of congestive heart failure for a total dose below 550 mg/m^2 was low (1 to 5%) with a steep increase (25 to 30%) with dose levels exceeding 550 mg/m^2. Although the analysis indicated that cardiac toxicity at a total dose traditionally considered safe occasionally occurred, the data provided reasonable rationale for limiting the cumulative dose of ADR given by the bolus method to 550 mg/m^2.

Schedule of Adriamycin Administration

Other risk factors identified by von Hoff et al were related to the schedule of ADR administration. The data indicated that weekly ADR administration was less cardiotoxic than the standard 3 weekly administration; the overall incidence of congestive heart failure being 0.8 and 2.9% for the two methods, respectively (33). A more important development in the efforts to reduce ADR cardiac toxicity, however, has been the salutary effect of prolonged continuous infusion delivery over 24 to 96 hours instead of its administration as an intravenous bolus (28). Because a reasonable explanation for the lower cardiac toxicity of weekly schedule of ADR is lower peak plasma levels, minimizing such peaks by continuous infusion appeared to be a logical approach to further reduction of cardiac toxicity. That lowering the peak plasma level can reduce the amount of ADR entering the myocytes has been experimentally shown in mice given small frequent doses of the drug which resulted in a significantly lower concentration compared to that observed when the same total dose was injected as a single bolus (34). A direct relationship has also been demonstrated between the relative amounts of ADR metabolites accumulating in the myocardium and the degree of cardiac toxicity (35).

Preexisting Heart Disease

The importance of pre-existing heart disease as a risk factor for ADR cardiac toxicity has been cited in several reports (33). Conditions often associated with increase in left ventricular and end-diastolic pressure, such as hypertension, aortic stenosis, and cardiomyopathies of all types, can cause heart failure at a lower-than-usual cumulative dose of ADR.

Patient's Age

Patients at extremes of age are also considered at higher risk for cardiac dysfunction following standard doses of ADR (31–33). Although the increase in left ventricular end-diastolic pressure often found in the elderly patients can account for increased ADR cardiac toxicity, the inhibition of the growth of cardiac myocytes has been blamed for the increased risk in the pediatric age group.

Mediastinal Irradiation

Irradiation of major portions of the heart, which often occurs in the course of treating patients who have breast cancer, lung cancer, or lymphomas, also potentiates the development of ADR-induced cardiomyopathy, which is detailed in the following section. The recognition of all the aforementioned risk factors may improve the chances for early detection of cardiac decompensation in its incipient and potentially reversible stage. In addition, several studies have shown that a gradual recovery of myocardial function usually occurs after discontinuation of ADR and that many patients who develop frank congestive heart failure have a good chance of recovery with the use of conventional medical therapy (28,36,37). These optimistic reports add further encouragement to the ongoing efforts devoted to further elucidation and better quantitation of the cardiac toxicity in cancer patients treated with the combination of radiotherapy and ADR.

CARDIAC COMPLICATIONS OF RADIOTHERAPY

During the orthovoltage era of radiation therapy, with equipment delivering voltages between 140 and 400 kilovolts, the maximal dose that was delivered was largely absorbed at the skin surface. The absence of cardiac complications related to mediastinal irradiation using these old techniques was misinterpreted as radioresistance of all cardiac structures. With the introduction of megavoltage techniques, which are more skin-sparing, higher radiation doses could be delivered to deeper structures. Reports of cardiac damage soon followed the widespread clinical use of these updated techniques (38).

High doses of mediastinal irradiation are frequently given to patients with carcinomas of the lung and esophagus, as well as other mediastinal tumors. However, cardiac damage is most commonly seen in patients irradiated for Hodgkin's disease, as mantle irradiation often involves a much greater cardiac volume (39,40). The longer survival of these patients also provides more time for the results of the tissue injury to become clinically apparent. Although individual susceptibility may play some role, both postirradiation cardiac injury and rates of cure of Hodgkin's disease are dose- and schedule-related. The composite data from world literature indicate that the local recurrence rate decreases from 60 to 80% when a single tumor dose of 1000 cGy was used, to 1.3% for tumor doses of approximately 4400 cGy delivered over a 4½-week period. Doses of this magnitude, when delivered to the entire mediastinum, resulted in a 6.7% incidence of cardiac disease (39).

Acute Manifestations

Experimental animal data and clinical reports indicate that radiation-induced cardiac injury can be classified into an acute inflammatory and a chronic fibrotic phase, with a latent stage in between (41). The initial phase represents an acute, self-limited, generally reversible pancarditis that occurs within days or weeks after irradiation. The clinical manifestations of this phase are usually those of acute pericarditis such as chest pain, friction rub, fever, electrocardiographic S-T segment elevation, and sometimes pericardial effusion (Fig. 35–1) (42). These patients almost always respond to conservative management such as a brief hiatus in the course of radiotherapy and/or short courses of ibuprofen, indomethacin, or corticosteroids, without any lasting cardiac sequelae.

Late Manifestations

After a latent period that varies from months to years following treatment, radiation-related chronic cardiac injury may appear (Fig. 35–2). The clinical syndromes most noticeable during this phase include pericardial effusion and tamponade, constrictive pericarditis, myocardial fibrosis, coronary artery disease, chronic valvulitis, and abnormalities of cardiac conduction (43).

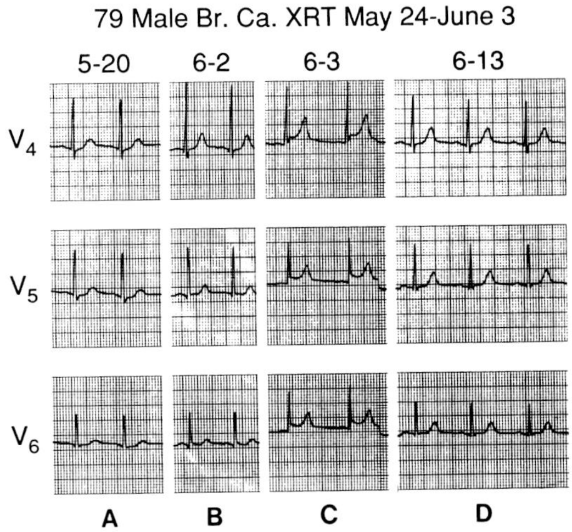

Fig. 35–1. Electrocardiographic manifestations of radiation-induced acute pericarditis. A: Preradiation; B: onset of chest pain following 7 days of mediastinal irradiation; C: significant S–T segment elevation 24 hours following onset of chest pain; D: normalization of S–T segment following 10 days of indomethacin therapy.

Postirradiation Chronic Pericarditis

In contrast to the infrequently described acute pericarditis, chronic effusive or constrictive pericarditis is the most commonly reported cardiac complication following mediastinal irradiation (44, 45). Although small to moderate-sized effusions are occasionally encountered within a few days or weeks of completing mediastinal irradiation, the majority of postirradiation pericardial effusions occur months or years later. If they are symptomatic, medical therapy with nonsteroidal anti-inflammatory agents or steroids and close follow-up are appropriate. Large effusions can cause cardiac tamponade and require emergency pericardiocentesis. The definitive treatment of persistent or recurrent pericardial effusion as well as effusive-constrictive pericarditis requires extensive parietal pericardiectomy. Although limited pericardial window has been used as the initial therapy, it often results in later development of constrictive pericarditis (46,47).

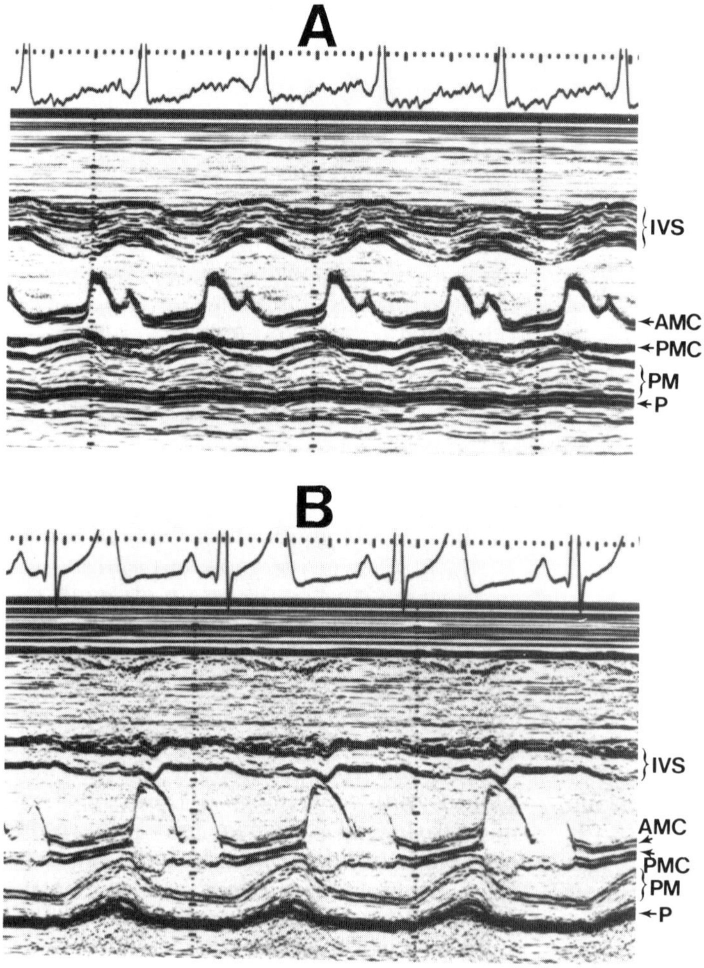

Fig. 35–2. A. Chronic postirradiation pancarditis. M-Mode echocardiogram of a 38-year-old woman who received mediastinal and left hilar irradiation at ages 17 and 21 years, respectively, for Hodgkin's disease. Notice thickening and fibrosis of the interventricular septum (IVS), posterior myocardium (M), anterior and posterior mitral cusps (AMC and PMC), as well as the pericardium (P), which is also immobile, a finding highly suggestive of constrictive pericarditis. B. M-Mode echocardiogram of a healthy adult at the same level as that of Figure 2A showing normal structures for comparison.

The hemodynamic changes and clinical manifestations of constrictive pericarditis can be easily confused with those of cardiac tamponade or restrictive cardiomyopathy, and surgical exploration may occasionally be necessary to differentiate between these entities (48,49). In symptomatic patients, pericardial stripping with removal of both layers of the adherent pericardium is required. This is a more difficult and risky procedure than parietal pericardiectomy, but the availability of cardiopulmonary bypass techniques has significantly enhanced the success and safety of the procedure.

Postirradiation Cardiomyopathy

Both human and animal studies have shown that the myocardium is the most frequent site of postirradiation cardiac injury. The pathologic changes include hyaline degeneration secondary to interstitial fibrosis, which has been recognized as the most characteristic feature (50–53). Although frank congestive heart failure is rare, recent studies utilizing echocardiography and nuclear cardiac scanning techniques have revealed a high incidence of late subclinical cardiac dysfunction among patients previously treated with mantle irradiation (54,55). All published reports, however, are retrospective, and wider application of such noninvasive techniques in prospective protocols is desirable to further elucidate the true incidence and clinical significance of this complication.

Postirradiation Coronary Artery Disease

Several investigators have reported patients who developed evidence of coronary artery disease following mediastinal irradiation which varied in severity from stable angina pectoris to myocardial infarction and, on rare occasions, sudden cardiac death (56–62). The increasing frequency of these reports may be largely due to the availability of better diagnostic facilities including exercise electrocardiography, nuclear techniques, and coronary angiography. Several reports of successful treatment of such patients with either bypass grafting or balloon angioplasty have been published (63,64).

Postirradiation Abnormalities of Impulse Conduction

Several electrocardiographic changes have been described during and after mediastinal irradiation. These include abnormalities of the P wave and P-R interval and a variety of intraventricular conduction abnormalities. These electrocardiographic changes were once thought to be incidental with no obvious clinical significance. A few pathologic reports, however, have described extensive fibrotic replacement of the specialized conduction structures within the heart (9,65). Electrophysiologic studies on the bundle of His have demonstrated proximal failure of impulse transmission at the level of the atrioventricular node as well as at distal infranodal sites in some patients. In addition, several reports of complete heart block occurring as a late sequel of radiation therapy have been published. The latent period between radiation and heart block ranged from 5 to 23 years and the treatment of many of these patients by inserting a permanent cardiac pacemaker was successful (9, 61, 66). This potential for successful management should encourage the close monitoring of patients who have received mediastinal irradiation. An electrocardiogram should be obtained at the time of each follow-up visit, and detailed electrocardiographic studies should be undertaken if signs or symptoms indicate the possibility of progressive conduction abnormalities.

COMBINED CARDIOTOXICITY OF ADRIAMYCIN AND RADIATION THERAPY

Several clinical reports have described enhancement of acute toxicity and a recall phenomenon when the combination of ADR and ionizing radiation is used concomitantly or sequentially. These reactions have been reported in different organs and tissues, but mainly involve the skin, esophagus, lung, oral mucosa, and heart (13, 67, 68). Although the usual outcome of the majority of these acute reactions is complete healing, the potential for severe long-term complications exists. The combined effects of radiation and ADR on the heart result in injury to different target cells by each mode of therapy, namely, the damaging effect of radiation on the microvasculature, and that of ADR on the myocytes. In addition, synergy of the cardiotoxic effects of combined heart irradiation and ADR has been demonstrated histologically by both light and electron microscopy in New Zealand white rabbits as well as in human cardiac biopsies (69,70). Fajardo et al have documented qualitative and quantitative differences between the cardiac damage in rabbits receiving low doses of either ADR or radiation alone and that in those receiving the combination (71). The lesions produced by the combination were more severe than those produced individually by each agent. Because the combined effect was greater in magnitude than the algebraic sum of the individual effects, they concluded that the combined effect is not merely additive but probably synergistic. These workers also demonstrated a potentiation of ADR-associated functional abnormalities in the irradiated rabbits as assessed by the incidence of pleural effusions and ascites. The results of other animal studies, however, indicated a weaker interaction between the two modalities and that additive toxicity, without evidence of potentiation, occurred (72).

Published clinical reports provide more convincing evidence for the potentiation of ADR cardiac toxicity by prior cardiac irradiation (3,31,70,73–75). Billingham et al examined the cardiac biopsies of patients who received total ADR doses of 90 to 445 mg/m^2 and prior mediastinal irradiation (70). The radiation dose varied from 4600 to 5700 cGy and the therapy was completed 6 to 14 years prior to ADR administration. The severity of pathologic changes was compared with that of dose-matched control patients who had not received mediastinal irradiation. The investigators found that the grades of histopathologic changes were significantly higher for the group irradiated (mean 2.0 ± 0.98) compared to the score in those not irradiated (1.8 ± 0.23) ($p < 0.01$). They concluded that ADR cardiac toxicity was potentiated by previous mediastinal irradiation. This effect was also demonstrated functionally by an increase in the incidence of heart failure in previously irradiated patients. Furthermore, the finding of lower pathologic grades among patients who had subcarinal blocks compared to those without cardiac protection suggests a possible relation between the dose of cardiac irradiation and the degree of potentiation of ADR-induced cardiac damage. The majority of published reports so far indicate that such potentiation is relatively independent of the length of time between cardiac irradiation and ADR chemotherapy. The time interval between the two modalities was, in some instances, so long that the unexpected cardiac decompensation was erroneously attributed solely to the late effects of ADR (76,77).

In addition to the wide variation in time interval separation, the dose fractionation and treatment portals for radiotherapy are so variable in the reported studies that quantitative evaluation of the contribution of each modality to the development of cardiomyopathy has been difficult. Eltringham et al (72) used experimental animals given different dose schedules of ADR and explored its interaction with radiotherapy to calculate equivalent cardiotoxic units. On the basis of doses and intervals used in these experiments and his own experience, Rubin found 25 cGy to be equivalent to 1 mg/m^2 of adriamycin and the threshold of 450 to 500 mg/m^2 of the latter to be parallel to a 4500 to 5000 cGy dose of radiation therapy (78). Although the pathologic lesions produced by ADR were different from those produced by radiation, they were considered pathophysiologically additive.

CHEMORADIATION CARDIOTOXICITY—GUIDELINES FOR ITS REDUCTION

In an effort to make available experimental and clinical data useful in planning safer combination schedules, Phillips and Fu proposed the calculation of the dose effect factor (DEF) (79). The authors compiled published clinical and experimental data on the relative augmentation of injury to various normal tissues that occurs when radiotherapy and chemotherapy were combined. Although clinical and/or experimental DEF values were established for skin and mucous membranes, esophagus, lung, and the gastrointestinal tract, no numerical values for cardiac injury are currently available.

Based on clinical observations, Mayer et al proposed that the dose of radiotherapy be reduced by 1000 cGy if used simultaneously or shortly after ADR (67). Likewise, it is prudent to decrease the dose of ADR by 25 to 50% for each course given during or immediately following radiotherapy. To devise clinical guidelines for adjusting cumulative dose to avoid cardiac toxicity, we have reviewed the published clinical literature on cardiac toxicity following ADR in patients who had previously received radiotherapy to the mediastinum or to the left anterior chest wall (Table 35–1) (3,29,31,32,67,73,74,77, 80–83). Taking into consideration the equation suggested by Rubin of 1 mg/m^2 of ADR being equivalent to 25 cGy as well as the data shown in Table 35–1 we propose that patients with incidental cardiac irradiation should have a reduction in their cumulative ADR dose by 150 to 200 mg/m^2 to minimize the risk of heart failure (67,73–83). This translates into a cumulative ADR dose limit of 400 to 450 mg/m^2 for such patients for the same risk of cardiac toxicity expected from a cumulative dose of 550 to 600 mg/m^2 for a person with an unirradiated heart.

In addition to limiting the cumulative dose, attempts to decrease the cardiac toxicity of chemoradiation has included continuous infusion ADR therapy, the use of cardioprotective agents, the development of less toxic anthracycline analogues, and modification of radiotherapeutic techniques.

Continuous Infusion Adriamycin Therapy

Legha et al compared the functional and cardiac biopsy findings in 21 patients who received ADR over 48 or 96 hours to those of 30 control patients treated by standard bolus intravenous injection (28). Both groups were studied prospectively and were well matched by known risk factors for developing ADR cardiomyopathy. The median cumulative dose for those receiving continuous infusion was 600 mg/m^2 compared with 465 mg/m^2 in the control group. Despite a lower cumulative dose, 14 of the 30 patients in the control group showed severe

Table 35–1. Summary Reports Indicating Additive or Synergistic Cardiotoxicity of Adriamycin (ADR) and Incidental Cardiac Irradiation (RT)

Source (Ref)	Features of Patients Who Developed Heart Failure	Implications
Gilladoga et al (31)	50 children treated with ADR >500 mg/m^2 heart failure in 4/8 (50%) with RT versus 4/42 (10%) without RT (p = 0.02)	Recommended: limit cumulative ADR to 500 mg/m^2 if RT to heart; 600 mg/m^2 if no RT
Pratt et al (32)	Literature review: median ADR dose causing heart failure in 13 children who had RT, 470 mg/m^2 (range 350–720 mg/m^2) versus 550 mg/m^2 (range 360–1695) in 10 without RT	Limit cumulative ADR dose to 450 mg/m^2 if patient had RT to heart
Minow et al (75)	Four patients with prior RT developed heart failure after an ADR dose of 450–550 mg/m^2	Limit dose to 450 mg/m^2 with RT versus 55 mg/m^2 in orders
Kinsella et al (74)	80 patients treated with ADR, dose range, 100–540 mg/m^2 (median, 400 mg/m^2), 3 developed heart failure at 420, 465 and 490 mg/m^2	Recommend ADR dose limit of 400 mg/m^2 in cases of prior RT
Bristow et al (3)	3 patients, ADR dose, 330, 395, 445 mg/m^2	—
Cortes et al (29)	2 patients, ADR dose of 450 and 500 mg/m^2	—
Merrill et al (73)	2 patients, ADR dose, 400 and 470 mg/m^2	—
Rosen et al (81,82)	2 patients, ADR dose, 600 mg/m^2 and 720 mg/m^2	—
Mayer et al (67)	1 patient, ADR dose, 525 mg/m^2	—
Gerber et al (80)	1 patient, ADR dose, 350 mg/m^2	—
Friedman et al (83)	1 patient, ADR dose, 400 mg/m^2	—
Gottlieb et al (76)	1 patient, ADR dose, 580 mg/m^2	—
Freter et al (77)	1 patient, ADR dose, 450 mg/m^2	—
Overall Results	Median dose of ADR causing heart failure: 470 mg/m^2 (range, 330–720 mg/m^2)	Conclusion: Limit cumulative ADR dose to 400 mg/m^2 in patients with incidental RT to heart

cardiac damage in the form of grade 2 or 3 changes in their cardiac biopsies, which precluded further ADR therapy, in comparison with 2 of 21 patients from the continuous infusion group. Even though 24-hour infusion caused less cardiac damage compared to the bolus administration, the study clearly demonstrated that the best protection occurred with 48- and 96-hour infusions. Most importantly, the prospective follow-up of both patient groups convincingly indicated that the antitumor activity of ADR was not compromised by its delivery as a continuous infusion. The data of this study were validated by others, and it is now believed that one can deliver twice as much ADR by 96-hour infusion with lesser cardiac toxicity than that encountered following standard delivery by the bolus method. Specifically, a cumulative dose of 600 mg/m^2 by 48-hour infusion and 800 mg/m^2 by 96-hour infusion can be given to patients who have no cardiac risk factors, with less risk of cardiac toxicity than with 450 mg/m^2 of ADR given by the bolus schedule (24).

Cardioprotective Agents

Among promising cardioprotective agents is ICRF-187, which was found effective in a chronic beagle-dog study (84). More recently, a clinical trial in patients receiving ADR has confirmed the cardioprotective effect of ICRF-187 (85). Further clinical trials should provide better definition of the extent and duration of the cardiac protection provided by this agent.

Anthracycline Analogues

A large number of anthracycline analogues have been developed and have been claimed to be less cardiotoxic than ADR. So far, only one has had sufficient clinical evaluation in this regard, namely, **epirubicin.** A statistically significant decrease in the incidence of both congestive heart failure and impairment of ejection fraction for epirubicin compared to ADR, even after correction for decreased potency have been reported (86). The magnitude of the protection, however, is small and appears equal to that observed with weekly or 24-hour infusion schedules of adriamycin. Epirubicin infusion over 48 hours has also been credited for substantial decrease in cardiac toxicity (87). A more recently reported cardiac biopsy study of patients who received epirubicin has indicated that the histopathologic and ultrastructural changes were similar to those caused by other anthracyclines (88). A strong correlation was demonstrated between the total dose of epirubicin and the quantitative pathologic changes using Billingham's scale. The investigators identified the total epirubicin dosage of 300 mg/m^2 as the starting point beyond which there were detectable histopathologic changes similar to those observed after a cumulative ADR dose of 200 mg/m^2.

Mitoxantrone is an anthraquinone lacking the aminosugar group of the anthracycline antibiotics. The morphologic changes noted in the myocardial cells of mitoxantrone-treated patients, however, are qualitatively similar to those noted with ADR therapy and indicate the DNA-reactive nature of both drugs (89). The studies reported so far indicate that the cardiac toxicity of mitoxantrone at lower cumulative doses ($<$ 100 mg/m^2) is mild and hemodynamically insignificant, and may not be of any clinical relevance. Patients who have been treated previously with ADR are at higher risk for the development of congestive heart failure with mitoxantrone therapy, particularly if other cardiac risk factors are present. Such patients, as well as those receiving higher cumulative doses of mitoxantrone ($>$ 100 mg/m^2), should be closely monitored by serial cardiac ejection fractions and, if indicated, by endomyocardial biopsy. The risk of cardiac toxicity due to mitoxantrone exceeds 10% beyond a cumulative dose of 160 mg/m^2, which is the current upper limit of recommended dose.

Modification of Radiotherapeutic Techniques

Prior to effective chemotherapy, Hodgkin's disease of the mediastinum was treated with radiotherapy only. To avoid late cardiac and pulmonary complications in treating patients with large mediastinal masses, the lateral borders of the fields were reduced, along with shrinkage of the tumor mass at weekly to biweekly intervals. Currently, such patients are initially treated with chemotherapy in an effort to reduce the tumor masses prior to the initiation of radiotherapy. Further reduction of tumor size during subsequent radiotherapy is usually slow and therefore does not require progressive reduction of the irradiation field. The use of electron beams for treating chest wall tumors has also proven to be more cardioprotective than other methods of irradiation.

SUMMARY

It is therefore self-evident that, although the cardiac injury produced by ADR and radiotherapy affect different tissues within the heart, the net result, even without potentiation or augmentation, represents the sum of the pathophysiologic effects of direct myocyte damage and injury to the vasculoconnective tissue. These cardiac effects appear to be dependent on the dose of each modality but relatively independent of their chronologic usage. Patients receiving the combination therapy are clearly at an increased risk for severe cardiac toxicity. Challenging research questions concerning the safe use of the combination are still unanswered, and well controlled prospective clinical and experimental studies designed to provide more accurate quantitation of the interaction between the two treatment modalities are needed. Until such data become available, dose limitation, close monitoring of cardiac function by noninvasive methods, and if necessary, endomyocardial biopsy are warranted for patients receiving a combination of ADR and radiation therapy.

REFERENCES

1. Holland JF, Frei E. Cancer Medicine. Philadelphia, Lea & Febiger, 2nd Ed., 1982, p. 685.
2. Brady LW. Long term normal tissue effects of cancer treatment. Can Clin Trials 4(Suppl) 7:9, 1981.
3. Bristow MR, Mason JW, Billingham ME, Daniels JR. Doxorubicin cardiomyopathy: Evaluations by phonocardiography, endomyocardial biopsy, and cardiac catheterization. Ann Intern Med 88:168, 1978.

4. Chabner BA, Myers CE, Oliverio VT. Clinical pharmacology of anticancer drugs. Semin Oncol 4:217, 1977.
5. Hall EJ. Radiobiology for the Radiologist. New York, Harper and Row, 1978, p. 195.
6. Lipshultz SE, Colan SD, Gelber RD, et al. Late cardiac effects of doxorubicin therapy for acute lymphoblastic leukemia in childhood leukemia. J Am Coll Cardiol 11:135A, 1988.
7. Ali MK, Ewer MS, Balakrishnan PV, et al. Late effect of adriamycin chemotherapy on myocardial function. Chest 94:16S, 1988.
8. Casarett GW. Similarities and contrasts between radiation and time pathology. *In:* Advances in Gerontological Research. Strehler B (Ed). New York, Academic Press, 1964, p. 109.
9. Cohen SI, Bharati S, Glass J, Lev M. Radiotherapy as a cause of complete atrioventricular block in Hodgkin's disease. Arch Intern Med 141:676, 1981.
10. D'Angio GJ, Farber S, Maddock CL. Potentiation of x-ray effects by actinomycin D. Radiology 73:175, 1959.
11. D'Angio GJ. Clinical and biologic studies of actinomycin D and roentgen irradiation. Am J Roentgenol 87:106, 1962.
12. Liebner EJ. Actinomycin D and radiation therapy. Am J Roentgenol 87:94, 1962.
13. Donaldson SS, Glick JM, Wilbur JR. Adriamycin activating a recall phenomenon after radiation therapy. Ann Intern Med 81:407, 1974.
14. Jaffe N, Farber S, Traggis D, Geiser C, et al. Favorable response of metastatic osteogenic sarcoma to pulse high-dose methotrexate with citrovorum rescue and radiation therapy. Cancer 31:1367, 1973.
15. Buckner CK, Rodolph RH, Fefer A. High-dose cyclophosphamide therapy for malignant disease. Toxicity, tumor response, and the effects of stored autologous marrow. Cancer 29:357, 1972.
16. O'Connell TX, Berenbaum NC. Cardiac and pulmonary effects of high-dose cyclophosphamide and isophosphamide. Cancer Res 34:1586, 1974.
17. Mancuso L, Bondi F, Marchi S, et al. Cardiac toxicity of 5-fluorouracil. Report of a case of spontaneous angina. Tumori 72:121, 1986.
18. Kleiman NS, Lehan DE, Geyer CE, et al. Prinzmetal's angina during 5-fluorouracil chemotherapy. Am J Med 82:566, 1987.
19. Arena E, Biondo F, D'Alessandro N, et al. DNA, RNA and protein synthesis in heart, liver and brain of mice treated with daunomycin or adriamycin. IRCS Medical Science Cancer 2:1053, 1974.
20. Billingham ME, Mason JW, Bristow MR, Daniels JR. Anthracycline cardiomyopathy monitored by morphologic changes. Cancer Treat Rep 62:865, 1978.
21. Bristow MR, Thompson PD, Martin RP, et al. Early anthracycline cardiotoxicity. Am J Med 65:823, 1978.
22. Benjamin RS, Ewer MS, MacKay B, et al. An endomyocardial biopsy study of anthracycline-induced cardiomyopathy—detection, reversibility and potential amelioration. Proc Am Assoc Cancer Res/Am Soc Clin Oncol 20:372, 1979.
23. Bristow MR, Mason JW, Billingham ME, Daniels JR. Dose-effect and structure-function relationships in doxorubicin cardiomyopathy. Am Heart J 102:709, 1981.
24. Benjamin RS, Chawla SP, Ewer MS, et al. Organ directed toxicities of anticancer drugs. *In:* Assessment of Approaches to Cardiac Monitoring and Cardio Protection. Hacker MP, Lazo JS (Eds). Boston, Martinus Nijhoff Publishers, 1988, p. 41.
25. Alexander J, Dainiak N, Berger HJ, et al. Serial assessment of doxorubicin cardiotoxicity with quantitative radionuclide angiocardiography. N Engl J Med 300:278, 1978.
26. Ali MK, Soto AP, Maroongroge D, et al. Electrocardiographic changes after adriamycin chemotherapy. Cancer 43:465, 1979.
27. Haq MM, Legha SS, Choksi J, et al. Doxorubicin-induced congestive heart failure in adults. Cancer 56:1361, 1985.
28. Legha SS, Benjamin RS, Mackay B, et al. Reduction of doxorubicin cardiotoxicity by prolonged continuous intravenous infusion. Ann Intern Med 96:133, 1982.
29. Cortes EP, Gupta M, Chou C, et al. Adriamycin cardiotoxicity: Early detection by systolic time interval and possible prevention by coenzyme Q_{10}. Cancer Treat Rep 62:887, 1978.
30. Cortes EP, Lutman G, Wanka J, et al. Adriamycin (NSC-123127) cardiotoxicity: A clinicopathologic correlation. Cancer Chemother Rep 2:215, 1975.
31. Gilladoga AC, Manuel C, Tan C. Cardiotoxicity of adriamycin (NSC 123127) in children. Cancer Chemother Rep 6:209, 1975.
32. Pratt CB, Ranson JL, Evans WE. Age related adriamycin cardiotoxicity in children. Cancer Treat Rep 62:1381, 1978.
33. von Hoff DD, Layard MW, Basa P, et al. Risk factors for doxorubicin-induced congestive heart failure. Ann Intern Med 91:710, 1979.
34. Pacciarini MA, Barbieri B, Colombo T, et al. Distribution and antitumor activity of adriamycin given in a high-dose and a repeated low-dose schedule in mice. Cancer Treat Rep 62:791, 1978.
35. Jaenke RS, Deprex-Deampeneeve D, Trouet A. Cardiotoxicity and comparative pharma-

cokinetics of six anthracyclines in the rabbit. Cancer Res 40:3530, 1980.
36. Goorin AM, Borow KM, Goldman A, et al. Congestive heart failure due to adriamycin cardiotoxicity: Its natural history in children. Cancer 47:2810, 1981.
37. Saini J, Rich MW, Lyss AP. Reversibility of severe left ventricular dysfunction due to doxorubicin cardiotoxicity. Ann Intern Med 106:814, 1987.
38. Stewart JR and Fajardo LF. Radiation-induced heart disease: Clinical and experimental aspects. Radiol Clin North Am 9:511, 1971.
39. Kaplan HS. Radiotherapy. *In:* Hodgkin's Disease. Kaplan HS (Ed). Cambridge, Harvard University Press, 1972, p. 279.
40. Kaplan HS, Stewart JR. Complications of intensive megavoltage radiotherapy for Hodgkin's disease. NCI Monogr 36:439, 1973.
41. Fajardo LF, Stewart JR. Experimental radiation induced heart disease. I. Light microscopic studies. Am J Pathol 59:299, 1970.
42. Glicksman AS, Nickson JJ. Acute and late reactions to irradiation in the treatment of Hodgkin's disease. Arch Intern Med 131:369, 1973.
43. Ali MK, Ewer MS. Cancer and the cardiopulmonary system. New York, Raven Press, 1984, p. 101.
44. Blumenfeld H, Thomas SF. Chronic massive pericardial effusion following roentgen therapy for carcinoma of the breast with a case report. Radiology 44:335, 1945.
45. Martin RG, Ruckdeschel JC, Chang P, et al. Radiation-related pericarditis. Am J Cardiol 35:216, 1975.
46. Morton DL, Glancy DL, Joseph WL, Adkins PC. Management of patients with radiation-induced pericarditis with effusion: A note on the development of aortic regurgitation in two of them. Chest 64:291, 1973.
47. Morton DL, Kagan AR, Roberts WC, et al. Pericardiectomy for radiation-induced pericarditis with effusion. Ann Thorac Surg 8:195, 1969.
48. Muggia FM, Cassileth PA. Constrictive pericarditis following radiation therapy. Am J Med 44:116, 1968.
49. Steinberg I. Effusive-constrictive radiation pericarditis. Two cases illustrating value of angiocardiography in diagnosis. Am J Cardiol 19:434, 1967.
50. Rubin E, Camara J, Grayzel DM, Zak FG. Radiation-induced cardiac fibrosis. Am J Med 34:71, 1963.
51. Botti RE, Driscol TE, Pearson OH, Smith JC. Radiation myocardial fibrosis simulating constrictive pericarditis. A review of the literature and a case report. Cancer 22:1254, 1968.
52. Brosius FC, Waller BF, Roberts WC. Radiation heart disease. Analysis of 16 young (aged 15 to 33 years) necropsy patients who received over 3,500 rads to the heart. Am J Med 70:519, 1981.
53. Applefeld MM, Slawson RG, Spicer KM, et al. Long-term cardiovascular evaluation of patients with Hodgkin's disease treated by thoracic mantle radiation therapy. Cancer Treat Rep 66:1003, 1982.
54. Gomez GA, Park JJ, Panahon AM, et al. Heart size and function after radiation therapy to the mediastinum in patients with Hodgkin's disease. Cancer Treat Rep 67:1099, 1983.
55. Perrault DA, Levy M, Herman JD, et al. Echocardiographic abnormalities following cardiac radiation. J Clin Oncol 3:546, 1985.
56. Cohn KE, Stewart JR, Farjardo LF, Hancock EW. Heart disease following radiation. Medicine (Baltimore) 46:281, 1967.
57. Dollinger MR, Lavine DM, Faye LV Jr. Myocardial infarction due to postirradiation fibrosis of the coronary arteries. JAMA 195:316, 1966.
58. Hamilton DV, Reed PI. Myocardial infarction following radiotherapy for Hodgkin's disease. Br J Clin Pract 32:181, 1978.
59. Huff H, Sanders EM. Coronary-artery occlusion after radiation. N Engl J Med 286:780, 1974.
60. Prentice RTW. Myocardial infarction following radiation. Lancet 2:388, 1965.
61. Rasmussen S, Dossing M, Walbom-Jorgesen S. Coronary heart disease—a possible risk in megavoltage therapy? Acta Med Scand 203:237, 1978.
62. Rodgers DL. Precocious myocardial infarction after radiation treatment for Hodgkin's disease. Chest 70:675, 1976.
63. Ali MK, Fuller KG, Leachman RD, et al. Radiation-related myocardial injury. Management of two cases. Cancer 38:1941, 1976.
64. Iqbal SM, Hanson EL, Goffredo GG. Bypass graft for coronary arterial stenosis following radiation therapy. Chest 71:664, 1977.
65. Phillips SJ, Macken DL, Rugh R. Pathological sequelae of acute cardiac irradiation in monkeys. Am Heart J 81:528, 1971.
66. Tzivoni D, Ratzkowski E, Biran S, et al. Complete heart block following therapeutic irradiation of the left side of the chest. Chest 71:231, 1977.
67. Mayer EG, Poulter CA, Aristizabal SA. Complications of irradiation related to apparent drug potentiation by adriamycin. Int J Radiat Oncol Biol Phys 1:1179, 1976.
68. Cassady JR, Richter MP, Piro AJ, Jaffe N. Radiation-adriamycin interactions: Preliminary clinical observations. Cancer 36:946, 1975.

69. Eltringham JR, Fajardo LF, Stewart JR. Adriamycin cardiomyopathy-enhanced cardiac damage in rabbits with combined drug and cardiac irradiation. Radiology 115:471, 1975.
70. Billingham ME, Bristow MR, Glatstein E, et al. Adriamycin cardiotoxicity: Endomyocardial biopsy evidence of enhancement by irradiation. Am J Surg Pathol 1:17, 1977.
71. Fajardo LF, Eltringham JR, Stewart JR. Combined cardiotoxicity of adriamycin and x-radiation. Lab Invest 34:89, 1976.
72. Eltringham JR, Fajardo LF, Stewart JR, Klauber MR. Investigation of cardiotoxicity in rabbits from adriamycin and fractionated cardiac irradiation: Preliminary results. Front Radiat Ther Oncol 13:21, 1979.
73. Merrill J, Greco FA, Zimber H, et al. Adriamycin and radiation: Synergistic cardiotoxicity. Ann Intern Med 82:122, 1975.
74. Kinsella TJ, Ahmann DL, Giuliani ER, Lie JT. Adriamycin cardiotoxicity in stage IV breast cancer: Possible enhancement with prior left chest radiation therapy. Int J Radiat Oncol Biol Phys 5:1997, 1979.
75. Minow RA, Benjamin RS, Gottlieb JA. Adriamycin (NSC-123127) cardiomyopathy—An overview with determination of risk factors. Cancer Chemother Rep 2:195, 1975.
76. Gottlieb SL, Edmiston WA, Haywood LJ. Late, late doxorubicin cardiotoxicity. Chest 78:880, 1980.
77. Freter CE, Lee TC, Billingham ME, et al. Doxorubicin cardiac toxicity manifesting seven years after treatment. Am J Med 80:483, 1986.
78. Rubin P. The Franz Buschke lecture: Late effects of chemotherapy and radiation therapy: A new hypothesis. Int J Radiat Oncol Biol Phys 10:5, 1984.
79. Phillips TL, Fu KK. Quantification of combined radiation therapy and chemotherapy effects on critical normal tissues. Cancer 37:1186, 1976.
80. Gerber MA, Gilbert EM, Chung KJ. Adriamycin cardiotoxicity in a child with Wilms' tumor. J Pediat (87)4:629, 1975.
81. Rosen G, Wollner N, Tan C, et al. Disease-free survival in children with Ewing's sarcoma treated with radiation therapy and adjuvant four-drug sequential chemotherapy. Cancer 33:384, 1974.
82. Rosen G, Tefft M, Martinez A, et al. Combination chemotherapy and radiation therapy in the treatment of metastatic osteogenic sarcoma. Cancer 35:622, 1975.
83. Friedman MJ, Ewy GA, Jones SE, et al. 1-year follow-up of cardiac status after adriamycin therapy. Cancer Treat Rep 63:1809, 1979.
84. Hermann EH, Ferrans VJ, Meyers CE, van Vleet JF. Comparison of the effectiveness of (±)1-1, 2-bis (3,5-dioxopiperazinyl-l-yl) propane (ICRF-187) and N-acetylcysteine in preventing chronic doxorubicin cardiotoxicity in beagles. Cancer Res 45:276, 1985.
85. Speyer JL, Green MD, Kramer E, et al. Protective effect of the bispiperazinedione (ICRF-187) against doxorubicin-induced cardiac toxicity in women with advanced breast cancer. N Engl J Med 319:745, 1988.
86. Jain KK, Casper ES, Geller NL, et al. A prospective randomized comparison of epirubicin and doxorubicin in patients with advanced breast cancer. J Clin Oncol 3:818, 1985.
87. Hortobagyi GN, Yap HY, Kau SW, et al. A comparative study of doxorubicin in patients with metastatic breast cancer. Am J Clin Oncol (CCT) 12:57, 1989.
88. Dardir MD, Ferrans VJ, Mikhael YS, et al. Cardiac morphologic and functional changes induced by epirubicin chemotherapy. J Clin Oncol 7:947, 1989.
89. Benjamin RS, Chawla SP, Ewer MS, et al. Mitoxantrone cardiotoxicity: Evaluation by nuclear angiography and endomyocardial biopsy. *In:* Pharmanual. Smyth JF (Ed). New Jersey, Sieber, McIntyre, 1984, p. 49.

Chapter 36

SKIN AND SOFT TISSUE TOXICITY

MADHU J. JOHN AND REGINA ROCHFORD

Acute skin reactions were the single most frequent factor that inhibited adequate tumor delivery dose in the orthovoltage era of radiotherapy. With current availability of megavoltage radiotherapy machines and judicious application of treatment techniques, such reactions are comparatively infrequent. In fact, when clinical situations require that a high dose be delivered to the skin, as in carcinomas of the skin or postmastectomy chest wall recurrences, special techniques such as tissue-compensator/bolus applications and/or electron beam therapy are required. Nevertheless, the legacy of "radiation burns" from the orthovoltage era is a major residual deterrent to the use of radiotherapy in the minds of surgical and medical oncologists and patients with cancer.

Just as with radiotherapy, chemotherapeutic agents are particularly active against rapidly dividing normal tissues such as the skin. Thus, cutaneous complications of chemotherapy can be provoked by a wide range of drugs and can vary from transient alopecia to widespread exfoliative dermatitis (1).

Cutaneous complications of megavoltage radiotherapy alone or chemotherapy alone are generally not life-threatening or dose-limiting. When the two modalities are combined, sequentially or concurrently, the potential for increased cutaneous reactions is greater. In fact, there are clinical examples of dose limitations being imposed on head and neck and anal canal cancers treated with chemoradiation (2,3). Other problems of chemoradiation-induced cutaneous reactions include the possibility of misdiagnosis of acute-graft-versus-host disease after bone marrow transplantation (4). A differential diagnosis of recurrent cancer may mistakenly be entertained in certain patients. These are patients who have previously received radiotherapy and, when certain cytotoxic agents are administered to them, develop an acute cutaneous flare-up called the "recall phenomenon" at the site of previous radiotherapy (5,6).

CLINICOPATHOLOGIC CLASSIFICATION OF CHEMORADIATION-INDUCED SKIN REACTIONS

The mucocutaneous reactions to cancer chemotherapy alone can vary considerably in clinical manifestation. They may be locoregional, such as alopecia, stomatitis, local cellulitis and/or phlebitis, erythema, nail changes, and radiation recall. Systemic manifestations include hypersensitivity reactions such as urticaria, angioedema, diffuse hyperpigmentation of the skin, and photosensitivity.

Possible acute cutaneous reactions to megavoltage radiotherapy alone consists of two phases of erythema (initial and "proper"), dry and moist desquamation, hyperpigmentation, and finally necrosis (7). With currently employed doses of radiotherapy, skin reactions rarely exceed those of dry desquamation and hyperpigmentation. Cutaneous reactions to chemoradiation may be classified into three categories based on mechanisms of pathogenesis and clinical presentation (Table 36–1).

Class I: Local Cytotoxic Effects

When the two modalities are combined, the local cutaneous effects usually attributable to radiotherapy alone become manifest at lower doses. The side effect of moist

Table 36–1. Clinicopathologic Classification of Cutaneous Reactions to Chemoradiation

Category	Clinical Presentation	Differential Diagnosis	Drugs	Mechanism of Cutaneous Toxicity
I. Local cytotoxic effects	Alopecia Stomatitis Local necrosis Radiation recall Moist desquamation	Local tumor recurrence	MTX, AMD 5-FU, ADR BLM Vinblastine Mitomycin-C Nitrosoureas	Direct cytotoxic effect Interference in nucleic acid and protein synthesis and ribosomal function, suppression of local mononuclear responses of inflammation
II. Pigmentary changes	Localized or linear hyperpigmentation or hypopigmentation, e.g., face, hands, nails, axilla, nipple, areola, general hyperpigmentation Photosensitivity	Graft-versus-host disease Inflammatory breast Ca Addison's disease	Nitrosoureas 5-FU MTX Vinblastine BLM Hormones Hydroxyurea CP, ADR	Direct action on melanocytes resulting in stimulation or reduction of enzymatic activity related to melanin production
III. Hypersensitivity reaction	Local/diffuse rashes or eruptions Urticaria, angioedema Skin or nail atrophy Acral sclerosis/erythema	Subcutaneous/cutaneous Metastatic cancer Graft-versus-host disease	Melphalan Procarbazine MTX AMD, BLM Mithramycin CP, ADR, L-asparaginase DTIC Azathioprine Chlorambucil	Hypersensitivity response

MTX = methotrexate, 5-FU = 5-fluorouracil, ADR = adriamycin/doxorubicin, BLM = bleomycin, CP = cyclophosphamide/cytoxan, AMD = actinomycin-D/dactinomycin

desquamation, for example, which is rarely seen in the megavoltage era below tumoricidal doses between 6000 and 7000 cGy (in 6 to 7 weeks), is often seen with 3600 to 4500 cGy (in 4 to 5 weeks) of pelvic radiotherapy combined with concurrent chemotherapy including 5-fluorouracil (5-FU) and mitomycin C for anal canal carcinoma (8).

Aside from premature moist desquamation, the other cutaneous side effect distinctly associated with radiotherapy-chemotherapy interaction is the phenomenon of "radiation recall." D'Angio initially brought this phenomenon to our attention in 1959 when he noted that the administration of actinomycin D to children who had previously received radiotherapy, provoked a erythematous cutaneous flare confined to the specific irradiated area (Fig. 36–1 A and B) (6). Subsequently, this phenomenon was reported with other chemotherapeutic agents such as Adriamycin (ADR), methotrexate (MTX), hydroxyurea, 5-FU, and bleomycin (9). Patients would have received radiotherapy a few days to several years prior to receiving any of these drugs. The reverse phenomenon, which may be termed a "reverse recall," has been noted only with busulphan. Cutaneous reactions of increased intensity lasting for prolonged periods of time has been noted in patients receiving radiotherapy 30 days or more after busulphan therapy. Vassal et al noted prolonged alopecia and severe erythema and reaction within radiation portals at 1500 cGy in patients previously treated with high-dose busulphan (10).

Both premature moist desquamation and the radiation recall phenomenon are manifestations of direct cytotoxic effects of drugs and radiotherapy. In extreme cases, both reactions may proceed to skin necrosis unless modifications are made in either radiotherapy and/or chemotherapy delivery. With moist desquamation, this may entail a temporary cessation of both drugs and radiotherapy. In the case of radiation recall, the drug provoking the local reaction may have to have another substituted for it. In both cases, these extremes of skin reaction might

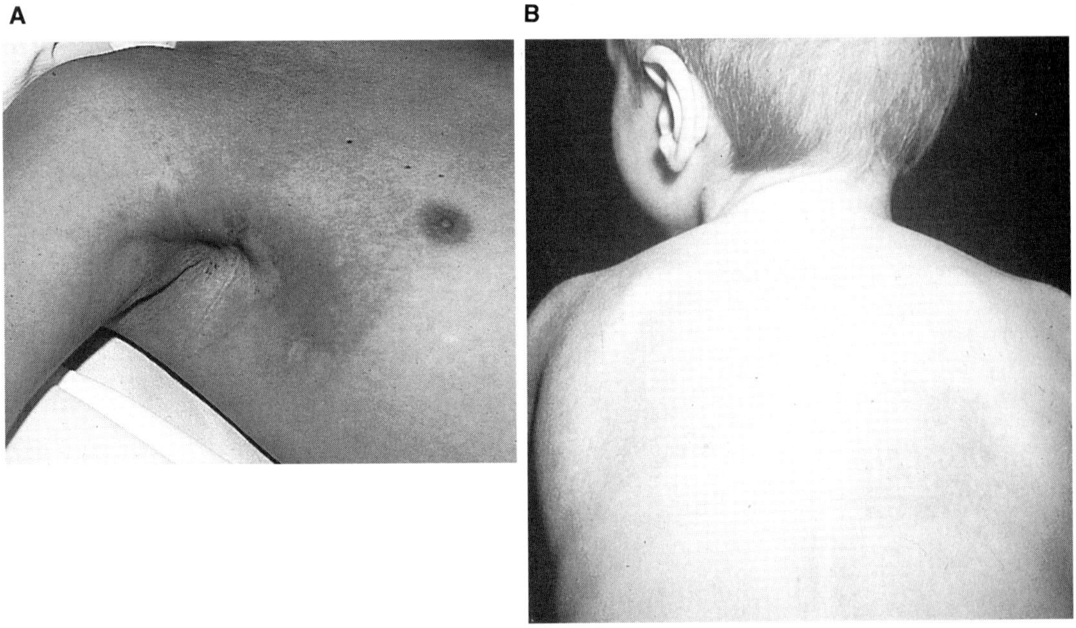

Fig. 36–1. A. This 7-year-old boy with metastatic rhabdomyosarcoma developed discrete erythema in the area of radiotherapy given several weeks prior to a dose of Actinomycin D. B. This 4-year-old boy received RT and Actinomycin D for left midlung and right pericardiac metastases from Wilms' tumor. (From D'Angio GJ. Am J Roentgen Rad Ther Nuc Med 87:106, 1962.) (Figure 36–1 also appears in color in the color section.)

occasionally be mistaken for local tumor recurrence.

Histopathologic changes seen in cutaneous chemoradiation reactions resemble those provoked by radiotherapy alone. Epidermal sloughing, atrophy of epidermal papillae, bullae formation under the epidermis, dermal hyperemia, inflammatory cell infiltration (either lymphocytes or eosinophils) and vascular and connective tissue damage are the features that characterize extreme cutaneous reaction to radiotherapy as well as chemoradiation (7).

Class II: Pigmentary Changes

Local hyperpigmentation or hypopigmentation can be reactions to either radiotherapy alone or to certain drugs such as the nitrosoureas, 5-FU, and some hormones. This is thought to be due to, respectively, either a stimulation or an obliteration of melanin-producing melanocytes situated at the junction of the epidermis and dermis.

Prolonged administration of DES has resulted in hyperpigmentation and erythema around the areola and nipple which could be mistaken for changes related to inflammatory breast cancer (11). When generalized hyperpigmentation occurs secondary to a drug, the pigmentary changes within a concurrent radiation field are not particularly worse than outside the field. This can be explained once again on the basis of melanocyte depletion or stimulation within the skin area in question. In this connection, it may be noted that occasionally widespread hyperpigmentation, particularly of the neck, face, and hands, with symptoms of fatigue, weight loss, and diarrhea, have been noted in patients receiving busulphan and whole body irradiation for chronic myelogenous leukemia (12,13). A differential diagnosis of Addison's disease may be ruled out by documenting normal endocrine chemistries.

Photosensitivity or an accelerated reaction to ultraviolet sunlight is a phenomenon seen with irradiated skin. Generalized photosensitivity is also frequently seen in patients who have received DTIC, 5-fluorouracil, methotrexate, and vinblastine as systemic treatment (1,11).

Kidney transplant recipients receiving azathioprine and prednisone for immunosuppression have been noted to have high incidences of cutaneous infections such as with herpes virus and malignancies such as squamous cell carcinoma of the skin. In vivo studies have suggested that local immune functions on skin are markedly depressed (more than systemic immunosuppression) by interaction between ultraviolet irradiation and azathiprone and prednisone (14).

Class III: Hypersensitivity Reactions

Almost every chemotherapeutic drug currently in use has been reported to have provoked hypersensitivity reactions of one degree or another (1). The usual symptoms and signs of such allergic reactions vary and may include pruritis, urticaria, angioedema, flushing diaphoresis, chest pain, nausea, and vomiting. Extreme reactions simulating the Steven-Johnson syndrome are rarely reported (15). The drugs particularly associated with such anaphylaxis are 5-FU, MTX, bleomycin, actinomycin D, and ADR. Figure 36–2 shows a generalized hypersensitivity reaction to MTX developing 3 days after its administration.

The distinctive syndrome of intense macular acral erythema in patients treated with cyclophosphamide (CP) and whole-body irradiation has been reported in up to 35% of patients receiving bone marrow transplantation (16). It is characterized by the development of nonintense macular well-defined erythema over the palms and sometimes the dorsal surfaces of fingers about 10 days after bone marrow transplantation. Some patients go on to have painful bullae formation in the same areas. Similar reactions in feet have been noted to be less severe. High-dose methotrexate, prolonged infusions of 5-FU, and ADR have been known to produce variations of the syndrome that may be mistaken for acute graft-versus-host disease (1,11).

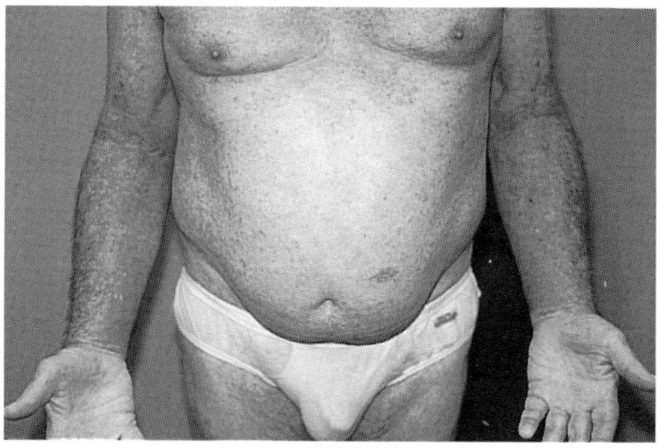

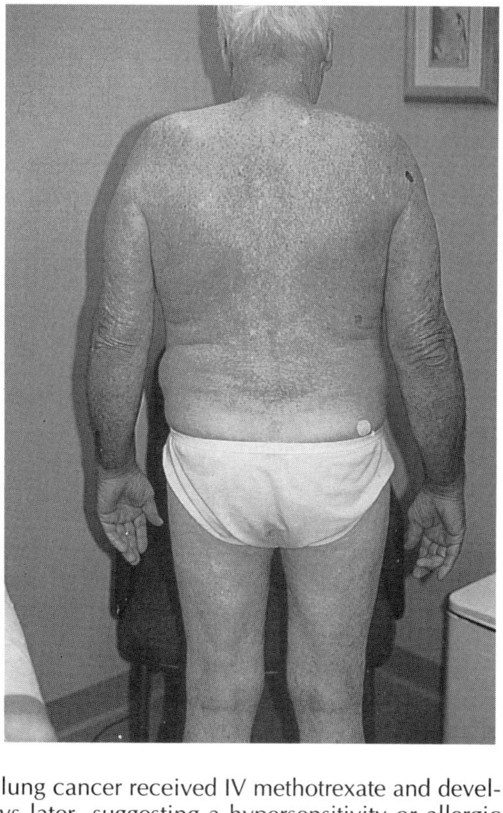

Fig. 36–2. This 69-year-old male with nonsmall-cell lung cancer received IV methotrexate and developed a generalized erythematous, papillary rash 2 days later, suggesting a hypersensitivity or allergic reaction. (Figure 36–2 also appears in color in the color section.)

Also, patients receiving whole-body electron beam irradiation and some drugs have been known to develop a generalized toxic endodermal necrolysis that sometimes ends fatally. Mithramycin and ADR are two drugs that have been thus implicated in combination with radiation (15,17).

CUTANEOUS REACTIONS TO CHEMORADIATION BY DRUG CLASSIFICATION

Antimetabolites and antibiotics are two classes of drugs are particularly associated with cutaneous reactions that may be enhanced by radiotherapy. On account of the wide anti-neoplastic spectrum of these and other classes of drugs as well as radiotherapy in general, it may be worthwhile to note these general and specific interactions manifested by the skin.

Alkylating Agents

This group of drugs includes CP, melphalan, busulphan, thiotepa, and the nitrosoureas (BCNU, CCNU, methyl-CCNU). As a group, these drugs are non-cell-cycle phase-specific and may be considered radiomimetic. CP and irradiation are frequently employed in bone marrow and kidney transplantation to prevent transplant rejection, in several solid tumors, and as lymphomas and leukemias. The nitrosoureas are frequently combined with irradiation of brain tumors. Melphalan is frequently used in breast and ovarian cancer and in multiple myeloma, in which, once again, radiotherapy is frequently used as well. Thiotepa and nitrogen mustard have been used extensively in Hodgkin's disease and mycosis fungoides, both diseases generally treated with radiotherapy as well. Chapter 8 describes alkylating agents in greater detail.

Generally, alkylating agents by themselves are known to have all three types of cutaneous reactions namely, cytotoxic, pigmentary and allergic/hypersensitivity reactions. In combination with radiotherapy, only CP has been implicated in producing a distinct cutaneous phenomenon of acral erythema as described above (4). Nevertheless, with the increasing combined use of these drugs with radiotherapy, the possibility of additive cutaneous reactions exists and should be kept in mind in clinical applications.

Antimetabolites

5-FU and MTX are two drugs in this category that are extensively used in combination with radiotherapy in a wide variety of neoplastic diseases. MTX, for example, has been used in conjunction with radiotherapy, whether sequentially or concurrently, in acute leukemias and head and neck cancers. 5-FU is used extensively in breast and gastrointestinal tumors and has emerged as the single most often used drug combined concurrently with radiotherapy for purposes of radioenhancement.

Both these drugs have been clinically implicated in the radiation recall phenomenon. High-dose MTX given within 3 weeks following radiotherapy was reported to evoke a severe erythema occasionally proceeding to necrosis in irradiated skin (18). Much earlier, in 1962, 5-FU had been known to cause similar cutaneous damage when combined with radiotherapy (19). Both drugs are also known to interact with ultraviolet radiation and sunlight with various different cutaneous reactions such as erythema and hyperpigmentation. Moist desquamation of irradiated skin has been noted to develop with much lower doses of radiotherapy than usual when 5-FU is given concurrently in anal canal cancers and brain tumors.

Antibiotics

This group of drugs also has a wide spectrum of antineoplastic activity and has been used in conjunction with radiotherapy in several solid tumors. The drugs include bleomycin, ADR, actinomycin-D, and mitomycin-C. Actinomycin-D is used extensively in conjunction with radiotherapy in several pediatric neoplasms such as Wilms' tumor, Ewing's sarcoma, and rhabdomyosarcoma. ADR with a broad antineoplastic spectrum by itself, is used with radiotherapy on the treatment of breast and bladder carcinomas, soft tissue sarcomas, and lymphomas. After 5-FU, bleomycin is the most commonly tested drug in advanced head and neck cancer, either preceding or concurrently with radiotherapy. Mitomycin C has been used broadly (and empirically) in recent years in advanced cancers of the esophagus, anal canal, and uterine cervix.

Actinomycin D was the first drug ever to be implicated in the causation of radiation recall by D'Angio et al in 1959 (6). Subsequently, both bleomycin and ADR have been known to cause this fairly unique phenomenon (20,21). These three drugs, as well as Mitomycin C, have been shown to have additive or synergistic activity with radiotherapy in experimental systems.

Severe alopecia almost always occurs in patients receiving ADR and stomatitis is usually the dose-limiting side effect of both bleomycin and actinomycin D. Antineoplastic antibiotics in general, and bleomycin in particular, tend to concentrate in the skin. Consequently, their use with radiotherapy is often tempered by cutaneous toxicity.

Microtubule Function Inhibitors

The drugs in this group, including vinblastine, vincristine, and VP-16, are primarily employed in malignant lymphomas, both Hodgkin's and non-Hodgkin's disease, leukemias, and lung cancers (1). Reversible alopecia and stomatitis are frequent complications of their therapy. Only vinblastine therapy in the group is associated frequently with photosensitivity. As a group, these drugs are unlikely to be restricted or modified in their use in combination with radiotherapy by cutaneous toxicity.

Miscellaneous

Hydroxyurea, an S-phase antineoplastic, is used frequently in chronic myelogenous leukemia and concurrently with radiotherapy in cervical and brain tumors. Cutaneous side effects such as alopecia and hyperpigmentation are usually seen only with longterm maintenance therapy with this drug (22).

L-asparaginase, a drug frequently used in acute lymphocyte leukemia, has notably the highest incidence of hypersensitivity reactions such as urticaria and generalized erythema among all antineoplastic drugs (1). Even so, chemoradiation with this drug is unlikely to result in cutaneous complications.

PRACTICAL CONSIDERATIONS

As stated previously, even though cutaneous complications are rarely dose-limiting in the megavoltage era of radiotherapy, the fairly common manifestation of mucocutaneous toxicity of anti-neoplastic drugs and the expanded employment of chemoradiation (23) obligates an increasing awareness of the effects of interaction of the two modalities on the skin. This perception can aid the oncologist designing treatment regimens employing chemoradiation, particularly in terms of dose modification and timing of administration of either modality. It can also decrease the possibilities of obfuscation of the diagnoses of recurrent cancer or acute graft-versus-host reaction with severe skin reactions by the clinician.

Dose and Timing Modifications

The classic example of the impact of mucocutaneous reactions in the timing or sequencing of modalities is with head and neck cancer studies. Several regimens using chemoradiation simultaneously in this specific site led to reports of prohibitive mucocutaneous toxicity, leading investigators to suggest that sequential use of radiotherapy and chemotherapy should be the preferred method of investigation in the future (24,25). This conclusion may perhaps have been altered with the knowledge that bleomycin (which was frequently used in these combination protocols) had this propensity for accumulation in the skin and not infrequently associated with the "radiation recall" phenomenon (21).

The matter of dose modification due to cutaneous toxicity of chemoradiation is best illustrated by various experiences in anal canal carcinoma. The standard radiotherapy dose for this disease is considered to be 6000 cGy in 6 weeks (26). Multiple investigators, including research groups such as the RTOG, have determined that 4000 cGy to 4500 cGy to the pelvis combined with 5-FU and mitomycin C chemotherapy almost universally result in transient moist desquamation of the perineal skin (3,8,27). The Princess Margaret experience has suggested that 6000 cGy, in combination with the same drugs, can be administered only in split-course fashion, i.e., with a planned rest of 2 or more weeks about halfway through the treatment regimen (3).

Thus, if cutaneous complications are the dose-limiting factor in chemoradiation investigations, it may be particularly advantageous to avoid or minimize the use of drugs that have a proclivity for enhancement or recall of radiation reaction on the skin. For example, the use of bleomycin could be minimized or replaced by cisplatinum in a chemoradiation protocol without compromising adequate radiation delivery. By the same token, if the severe but transient perineal dermatitis is deemed unacceptable by the oncologist, it would follow that 5-FU (which appears to be primarily responsible for radioenhancement of skin reactions) would have to be administered in altered form (low-dose cutaneous infusion), less frequently (once instead of twice) or replaced by another drug. Fortunately, the severe dermatitis in this case is not life-threatening and is consistently transient. Moreover, the dose modification of radiotherapy in this case does not appear to compromise the long-term results.

Differential Diagnosis

With the establishment of bone marrow transplantation for several leukemias and intransigent lymphomas, and its potential use in several solid tumors, the need for differentiating acral erythema associated with immunosuppressive drugs and whole-body irradiation and acute graft-versus-host reactions will take on increasing importance (1,11). Dermal reaction by "recall" can be severe enough to be misdiagnosed as recurrent cancer, with grave repercussions on subsequent treatment.

Cutaneous eruptions, particularly secondary to drugs, may occasionally be confused with subcutaneous metastatic cancers. Finally, pigmentary skin changes on the breast secondary to hormonal therapy may sometimes be misinterpreted as being characteristic of inflammatory breast cancer (11).

Management of Skin Reactions

Because moist desquamation is the only dose-modifying or dose-restricting cutane-

Table 36–2. Management of Various Levels of Cutaneous Reactions to Chemoradiation

Level and Description	Management*
I. *Potential:* for disproproportionate and early reaction	1. *Assessment* of (a) nutritional status, (b) skin: general and local. 2. *Avoidance of irritants:* (a) mechanical: constricting clothes, synthetic fabrics, trauma, massage, shaving. (Use loose cotton clothing, electric shavers). (b) Chemical: soaps, perfumes, deodorants, talcum, rubbing alcohol, creams, ointments (keep local skin clear and dry, gentle soaps up to 2 times/week only). (c) Temperature: extremes of cold or heat, heating pads, ice caps, (skin may be washed with lukewarm water in shower, sitz baths). (d) Ultraviolet radiation: sun exposure.
II. *Erythema/dry desquamation:* Scaling, itching	Hydrocortisone skin ointment (not cream) 1% for erythema; corn starch dusting over itching areas. Hydrophilic topical ointments (Aquaphor, Eucerin, Lubriderm). None of these substances should be left over skin at time of radiotherapy.
III. *Moist desquamation:*	1. Skin care for dry desquamation discontinued, avoid hydrocortisone specifically. 2. Step up efforts to keep skin clean and dry. 3. Irrigate with normal saline, lukewarm water, or weak (1%) hydrogen peroxide solution hydrotherapy for some areas, such as perineum. Dab dry with cotton swabs; use blow dryer for generally inaccessible areas. Open, semi-open or occlusive dressings, depending on site of desquamation, extent of necrotic debris and presence of infection (non-adherent hydrophilic dressing).
IV. *Necrosis:* Ulcerating areas, presence of infection	1. Step up frequency of care as for Level III. 2. Antibiotics of topical/systemic or both (sulphadiazine)
V. *Chronic effects:* Atrophy, fibrosis, telangiectasia, hyperpigmentation (permanent)	1. *Prevention:* Use of multiple radiotherapy fields, avoidance of hypofractionation, increased use of hyperfractionation avoidance or sparing use of drugs with particular tendency for accumulative effects on skin or hyperpigmentation (see Table 36–1). 2. *Precautionary skin care* as in Level I during *and after* chemoradiation. 3. *Local skin emollients* and mild massage (to decrease subcutaneous fibrosis) in post-treatment period particularly in head and neck areas.

*Suggestions with regards to skin care relate generally to area of radiotherapy treatment only unless otherwise specified

ous phenomenon specific to chemoradiation, a few words on its management are appropriate. The principles of managing these extremely uncomfortable complications are the continued precautions against mechanical and chemical irritation to the damaged skin, prevention of infection, and the modification of local conditions that are conducive to rapid healing.

Managing the various degrees of skin reactions to combinations of chemotherapy and radiotherapy is similar to managing reactions related to radiotherapy alone. McNally described three levels of altered skin integrity secondary to radiation therapy and their management (28). Based on this, and some descriptions of combined modality effects, we have classified acute and chronic skin reactions secondary to chemoradiation into five levels with suggested interventions in each (Table 36–2) (29–31). Level I deals with the potential for increased skin reactions when both modalities are combined. Management of these is primarily in terms of making the patient aware of the possibilities of skin reactions to the planned combination treatment, and the means of avoiding or minimizing such reactions.

We believe that local intervention for dry and moist desquamation of the skin is inherently different and have described these interventions in two different levels (II and III). Level IV skin reactions, which are similar to the Grade IV skin reactions described in the Common Toxicity criteria in Chapter 42, require more drastic intervention. Level III and IV types of reactions may result in the modification or even cessation of ongoing radiation and/or chemotherapy. The principles of managing these extremely uncomfortable complications are the prevention of mechanical and chemical irritation of the damaged areas, the treatment or prevention of infection, and the modification of local conditions that are conducive to rapid healing. Level V relates to long-term cutaneous effects of chemoradiation. These are generally untreatable, but may be preventable by modifications of radiotherapy delivery and technique.

REFERENCES

1. Hood FA, Haynes HA. Mucocutaneous complications of cancer chemotherapy. *In:* Dermatology in general medicine. Fitzpatrick TB, Eisen AZ, Wolff K, Freedburg IM, Austin KF (Eds). New York, McGraw-Hill, 1986, p. 80.
2. Fu KK. Normal tissue effects of combined radiotherapy for head and neck cancer. *In:* Frontiers in Radiation Therapy Oncology. Vol. 13. New York, Karger, Basel, 1979, p. 113.
3. Cummings BJ, Keane TJ, Thomas GM, et al. Results and toxicity in the treatment of anal canal carcinoma by radiation therapy or radiation therapy and chemotherapy. Cancer 54:2062, 1984.
4. Crider MK, Jansen J, Norins AL, McHale MS. Chemotherapy-induced acral erythema in patients receiving bone marrow transplantation. Arch Dermatol 122:1023, 1986.
5. Jaffe N, Farber S, Traggis D, et al. Favorable response of metastatic osteogenic sarcoma to pulse high-dose methotrexate with citrovorum rescue and radiation therapy. Cancer 31:1367, 1973.
6. D'Angio GJ, Farber S, Maddock C. Potentiation of x-ray effects by actinomycin-D. Radiology 73:175, 1959.
7. Rubin P, Casarett GW (Eds). Clinical Radiation Pathology. Philadelphia, W.B. Saunders, 1968, p. 62.
8. John M, Flam M, Lovalvo L, Mowry PA. Feasibility of non-surgical definitive management of anal canal carcinoma. Int J Radiat Oncol Biol Phys 13:299, 1987.
9. Phillips TL. Tissue toxicity of radiation-drug interactions. *In:* Radiation-drug Interactions in the Treatment of Cancer. Sokol GH, Maickel RP (Eds). New York, Wiley and Son, 1980, p. 175.
10. Vassal G, Hartmann O, Habraud JL, et al. Radiosensitization after busulphan. Lancet 1:571, 1987.
11. Nixon DW, Prozzi D, York RM, et al. Dermatologic changes after systemic cancer therapy. Cutis 27:181, 1981.
12. Feingold ML, Koss LG. Effects of long-term administration of busulfan. Arch Intern Med 124:66, 1969.
13. Korando FC, Dehmel EM, Kahn G, Penn I. Cutaneous complications in immunosuppressed renal homograft recipients. J Invest Dermatol 229:419, 1974.
14. Kelly GE, Meikle W, Sheil AGR. Scheduled and unscheduled DNA synthesis in epidermal cells of hairless mice treated with immunosuppressive drugs and UVB-UVA irradiation. Brit J Dermatol 117:429, 1987.
15. Purpora D, Ahern MJ, Silverman N. Toxic epidermal necrolysis after mithramycin. N Engl J Med 299:1412, 1978.
16. Lokich JJ, Moore C. Chemotherapy associated palmar-plantar erythrodysethesia syndrome. Ann Intern Med 98:611, 1984.
17. Solberg LA. Doxorubicin-enhanced skin reaction after whole body electron-beam irradia-

tion for leukemia. Cutis Mayo Clin Proc 55:711, 1980.

18. Rosen G, Tefft M, Martinez A, et al. Combination chemotherapy and radiation therapy in the treatment of metastatic osteogenic sarcoma. Cancer 35:622, 1975.
19. Falkson G, Schulz EJ. Skin changes in patients treated with 5-fluorouracil. Br J Dermatol 74:229, 1962.
20. Greco FA, Brereton HD, Kent H, et al. Adriamycin and enhanced radiation reaction in normal esophagus and skin. Ann Intern Med 85:294, 1976.
21. Yagoda A, Mukherji B, Young C, et al. Bleomycin, an antitumor antibiotic. Ann Intern Med 77:861, 1972.
22. Kennedy BJ, Smith LR, Goltz RW. Skin changes secondary to hydroxyurea therapy. Arch Dermatol 111:183, 1975.
23. John MJ, Flam MS, Mowry PA. Clinical potential for synchronous radiotherapy and chemotherapy for advanced squamous cell carcinoma. NCI Monogr 6:375, 1989.
24. Fu KK. Biologic basis for the interaction of chemotherapeutic agents and radiotherapy. Cancer 55:2123, 1985.
25. Vermund H, Kaalhus O, Winther F, et al. Bleomycin and radiation therapy in squamous cell carcinoma of the upper aero-digestive tract. A phase III clinical trial. Int J Radiat Oncol Biol Phys 11:1877, 1985.
26. Cantril ST, Green JP, Schall GL, Schaupp WC. Primary radiotherapy in the treatment of anal carcinoma. Int J Radiat Oncol Biol Phys 9:1271, 1983.
27. Sischy B, Doggett RLS, Krall JM. Definitive irradiation and chemotherapy for radiosensitization in management of anal carcinoma: Interim report RTOG #83-14. J Natl Cancer Inst 81:850, 1989.
28. McNally JC. Skin integrity, impairment of: related to radiation therapy. *In:* Guidelines for Cancer Nursing Practice. McNally JC, Stair JC, Somerville ET (Eds). Orlando, Grune and Stratton, 1985, p. 174.
29. Smith DS, Chamorro TP. Nursing care of patients undergoing combination chemotherapy and radiotherapy. Cancer Nurs 1:129, 1978.
30. Miaskowski C. Potential and actual impairments in skin integrity related to cancer and cancer treatment. Top Clin Nurs 5:64, 1983.
31. O'Rourke ME. Enhanced cutaneous effects in combined modality therapy. Oncol Nurs Forum 14:31, 1987.

Chapter 37

ORAL CAVITY TOXICITY

SOL SILVERMAN JR.

Ionizing radiation delivered for head and neck malignancies and chemotherapy given in doses that kill cancer cells induce unavoidable changes in oral tissues, causing compromises in oral function and host defenses, and potentially severe complications. When radiation and chemotherapy are used in combination, adverse toxic side effects are usually accentuated.

RADIATION THERAPY

Radiation changes associated with treatment of the oral cavity can cause the following: localized skin reactions, intraoral changes including acute mucositis (erythema, pseudomembrane-covered ulcerations, and hyperkeratosis); delayed soft tissue necrosis; damage to the bone that can result in osteonecrosis and sequestration or progressive osteonecrosis; destruction of salivary glands resulting in abnormal saliva, increased caries activity, infections, and other dental defects; and damage to taste buds leading to transient, or sometimes permanent, loss or alteration of taste.

Mucocutaneous Changes

Unless intraoral or interstitial treatment is used, most patients develop some erythema and moderate tanning of the skin in the treatment portal. Rarely, melanocytes are destroyed and vitiligo spots may appear. Hair follicles are radiosensitive; therefore, if hair is in the treatment beam, it will cease to grow and will fall out. This is often transient. Subcutaneous damage can disrupt appearance and function by telangiectasia, fibrosis, and edema.

The acute oral mucosal reaction (mucositis) is secondary to radiation-induced mitotic death of the basal cells in the oral stratified squamous epithelium and inflammation. Because these epithelial cells require about 2 weeks to mature, there is a delay of about this time between the onset of radiation therapy and the appearance of mucositis. If the radiation is delivered at a rate equivalent to the ability of the oral mucosa to regenerate, then only mild mucositis will be seen. When the weekly or daily dose is increased just slightly over conventional dose, destruction will outpace proliferation and a rather marked mucositis will develop (Fig. 37–1). This occurs at doses between 180 and 220 cGy per day, 5 days per week. Thus, patients receiving 170 cGy per day rarely develop mucositis, and those receiving 220 cGy per day almost always develop a marked confluent mucositis. Acute mucositis is not related to late radiation-induced atrophy and telangiectasis of the mucosa (Fig. 37–2). However, this late change often increases the risk of pain and/or necrosis.

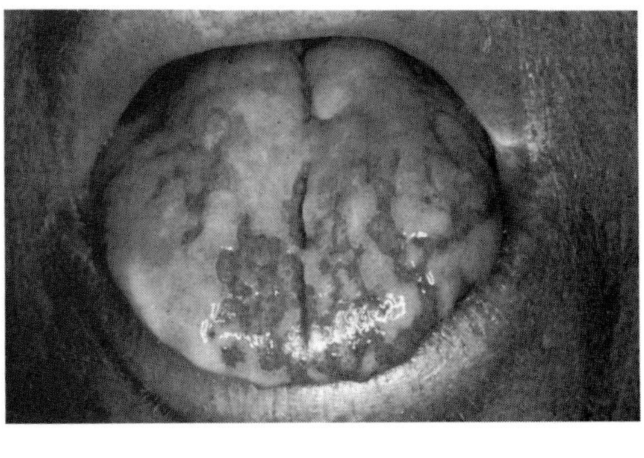

Fig. 37–1. Moderately severe mucositis 3 weeks after irradiation began. Yellow-white pseudomembranes are covering areas of ulcerated mucosa.

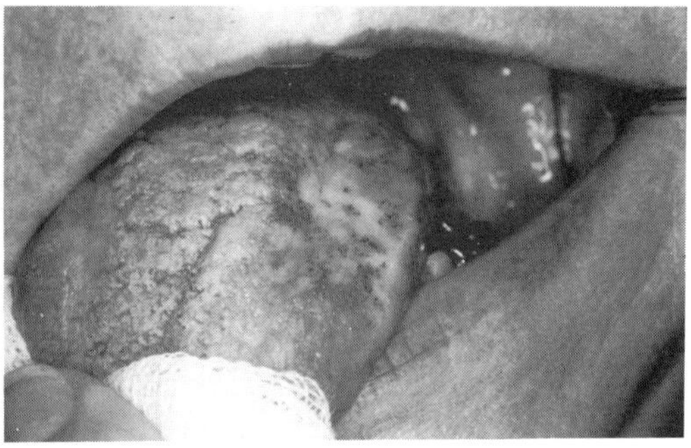

Fig. 37–2. Long-lasting radiation-induced changes in the tongue, including telangiectasia, fibrosis, and atrophy.

Management may sometimes require a 1-week interruption of therapy. Topical anesthetics (viscous xylocaine) may be of some value, but the pain usually requires systemic analgesic drugs. Because infections may be associated, appropriate diagnoses and antimicrobial agents must be considered.

Loss of Taste

Because of the irradiation of the taste buds, patients develop a partial (hypogeusia) or complete (ageusia) loss of taste during treatment (1). The alterations in taste for sweet, sour, bitter, and salt are variable and are caused by damage to the cells in the taste buds and/or their innervating nerve fibers (2). These cells will regenerate within 4 months after treatment in most cases, although permanent impairment may result.

Dietary consultations regarding recipes with pleasing texture and taste are essential to improve intake of food. Failure to eat is often associated with the loss of pleasure in eating and lack of imagination in food preparation. This is further complicated when surgery has also been required as a part of treatment and causes difficulties with mastication and swallowing. Recent trials with zinc supplements far exceeding recommended daily doses appear to be of some help (zinc sulfate capsules, 220 mg twice daily with meals; approximately 100 mg of elemental zinc) (3,4). In addition to improving taste perception in some patients, zinc has occasionally improved saliva production.

Impairment of Salivary Function

Exposure of the salivary glands to the field of ionizing radiation induces fibrosis, fatty degeneration, acinar atrophy, and cellular necrosis within glands. A critical dose level has not been identified (5,6). The serous acini appear to be more sensitive than the mucinous. During irradiation, the glandular secretions are usually diminished, thick, sticky, and very bothersome to the patient. Some patients are unable to produce more than 1 ml of pooled saliva in 10 minutes. The duration of this depressed salivary function varies from one patient to another. In most patients, there is usually regeneration several months after treatment, and the undesirable signs and symptoms of xerostomia (discomfort, difficulty in speech and swallowing) are at least partly reversed. In some patients, recovery of adequate saliva for oral comfort and function may take from 6 to 12 months; in others, the saliva remains inadequate indefinitely and is the source of major posttreatment complaints. When both of the parotid glands are exposed to the treatment beam, saliva diminution is most marked, and the prognosis for recovery is poor.

Frequent sips of water and water rinses are essential for partial control of radiation-induced xerostomia. Sugarless chewing gum and tart candy may be helpful. In some patients, pilocarpine hydrochloride (solution or tablets) has been effective in stimulating saliva production (7). Approximately 5 mg four times daily has been an optimal dosage for most patients. Side effects can include sweating and stomach discomfort, but this usually occurs only at higher dosages.

In a double-blind controlled study of 12 patients irradiated for head and neck cancer at the Oral Medicine Clinic, University of California, San Francisco, pilocarpine administration (15 to 30 mg daily) appeared to be beneficial (8). All 12 patients had marked xerostomia which had failed to improve even though 6 months had elapsed since radiation treatment. After receiving pilocarpine, 9 of 12 improved subjectively, 9 of 12 had increased stimulated parotid flow rates, and 6 of 12 demonstrated improvement in whole saliva volume. While on placebo medication for 3 months, none of the 12 showed objective or subjective benefit. Another salivary gland stimulant, bethanechol (Urecholine, administered as tablets in divided doses varying from 25 to 200 mg daily) has been helpful in many xerostomic patients. Synthetic saliva solutions and saliva substitute lubricants have been of limited help in most patients with dry mouth, although some favorable reports have been published (9,10).

Nutritional Problems

Because of the painful mucositis, loss of taste, and partial xerostomia, the lack of desire (or frank inability) to eat is a common and almost universal complaint in patients receiving external irradiation to the oral cavity. This is particularly the case when the treatment field includes the oropharynx. These changes, in combination with difficulty in mastication and swallowing caused by the tumor and the treatment, result in weight loss. Marked weight loss leads to weakness, inactivity, discouragement, further anorexia, and susceptibility to infection. Therefore, close attention is given to food intake and weight maintenance during treatment and follow-up. Dietary supplements, menu preparation, and encouragement to eat become important factors. Diet may vary depending upon patient attitude, effort, previous surgical intervention, saliva and taste status, food texture, and pain.

A B C

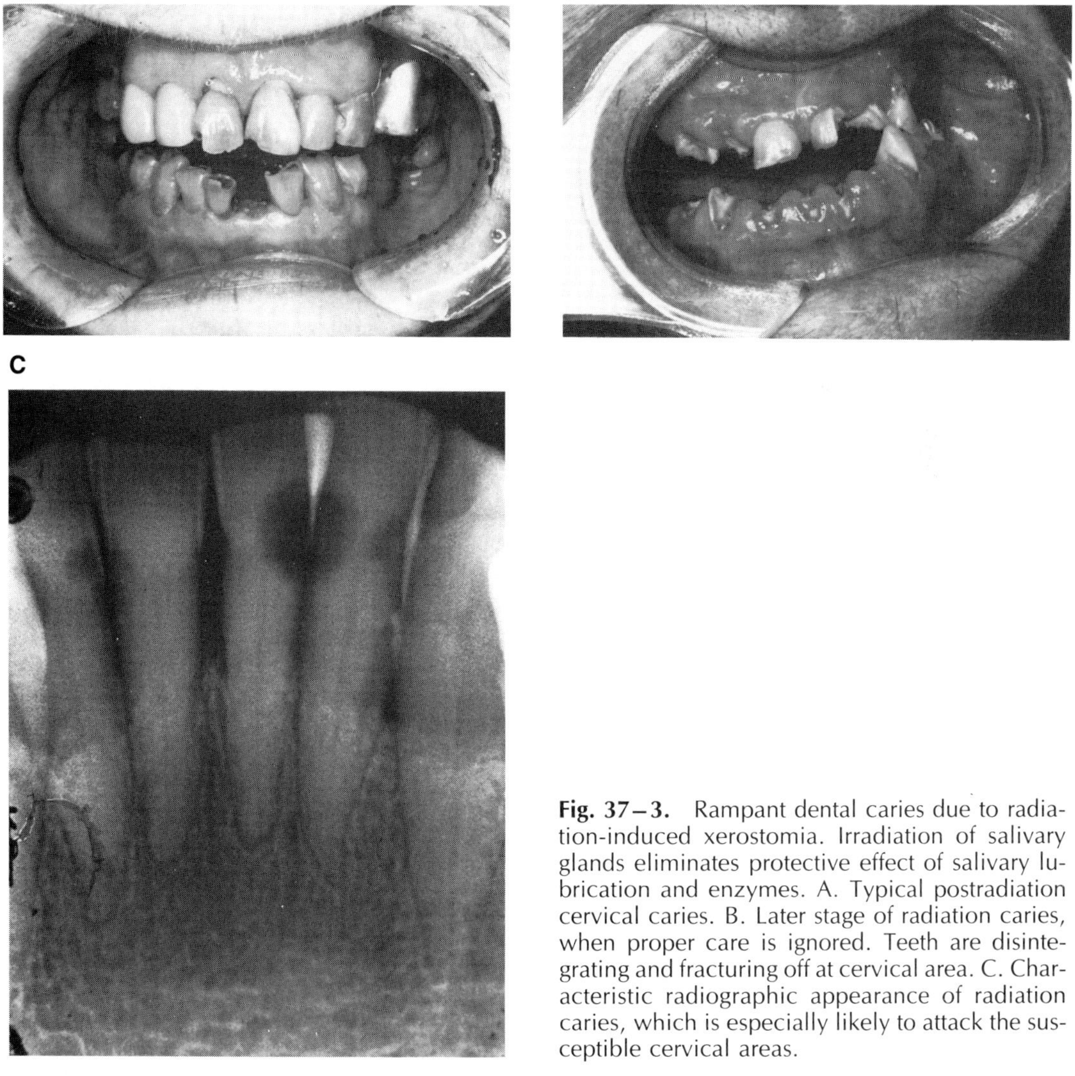

Fig. 37–3. Rampant dental caries due to radiation-induced xerostomia. Irradiation of salivary glands eliminates protective effect of salivary lubrication and enzymes. A. Typical postradiation cervical caries. B. Later stage of radiation caries, when proper care is ignored. Teeth are disintegrating and fracturing off at cervical area. C. Characteristic radiographic appearance of radiation caries, which is especially likely to attack the susceptible cervical areas.

Dental Caries

Patients who have not shown any degree of caries for years may develop dental decay and varying degrees of tooth disintegration after irradiation (Fig. 37–3). The cervical areas are most typically affected. This condition appears to be due to the lack of saliva as well as to changes in its chemical composition (11–14). One result of radiation xerostomia is a pronounced shift toward a highly acidogenic, highly carcinogenic oral microflora (15–17). The protective influence of saliva has been demonstrated by extensive dental destruction found in animals subjected to salivary gland ligation or removal and in patients with xerostomia caused by drugs (e.g., diuretics, antidepressants) or disease (e.g., Sjögren's syndrome) (18).

Radiation-induced dental effects depend on salivary changes and occur when the glands are included in the field of treatment, not upon direct irradiation of the teeth themselves (19). Whether direct irradiation of teeth alters the organic or inorganic components in some manner, making them more susceptible to decalcification, has not been shown clearly (20,21). Remineralization of enamel by a salivary substitute has been reported (22). No clinical or histologic pulpal differences appear to occur in noncarious human adult teeth, whether they have been in or out of the primary field of radiation. Studies in monkeys have also found no dental pulp damage (23,24).

To prevent or at least minimize radiation caries, oral hygiene must be maximal, and include intensive home care and frequent office visits for examination and prophylaxis (25). Mouth rinsing is essential; hydrogen peroxide rinses (3% H_2O_2 and equal parts water) and/or antiseptic mouth rinses, if tolerated, are helpful in eliminating debris and controlling microbial flora. Daily topical fluoride application either as a solution for mouth rinsing or a gel delivered by means of brushing or a tray, is extremely effective (26,27). Attempts should be made to increase salivary flow by either local or systemic means. Foods and beverages containing sucrose should be avoided as much as possible. If carious lesions develop, removal and restoration should take place immediately. Appropriate use of dental x-ray imaging is in order when indicated to monitor caries activity (28).

Candidiasis

Infections of the mouth by Candida albicans are commonly seen in irradiated patients (Fig. 37–4, Table 37–1), and are related to the alterations in saliva (29,30). Clinically, the signs may be confused with radiation mucositis or other sources of infection. Candidiasis is usually painful. Management is primarily with the use of antifungal drugs. Systemic administration (200 mg ketoconazole daily with food) is usually more effective for both response and compliance. Topical administration entails the use of nystatin or clotrimazole tablets dissolved orally. Because of pain from mucositis and dryness, patients may experience difficulty in dissolving tablets topically. Suspensions are another alternative form of treatment, but often this treatment is not as effective as the tablets (possibly because of limited contact time between drug and fungus). These fungal-control approaches are often used in combination. Antiseptic mouth rinses similar to those used for caries control may be helpful if tolerated. In addition, topical (viscous xylocaine) or systemic analgesics may be required.

Osteoradionecrosis

Osteonecrosis is one of the more serious complications of head and neck irradiation for cancer (Fig. 37–5). Bone cells and vascularity may be irreversibly injured (Fig. 37–6) (31,32). Fortunately, in many cases devitalized bone fragments sequestrate and lesions spontaneously heal. However, when radiation osteonecrosis is progressive, it can lead to intolerable pain or fracture and may necessitate jaw resection. The preventive and therapeutic use of antibiotics and hyperbaric oxygen can be effective, but reproducible beneficial results remain uncertain (32–35).

The incidence of osteoradionecrosis varies according to the reporting institution, aggressiveness of radiotherapy, and follow-up time (Tables 37–2 through 37–4) (36–40). The risk for developing a spontaneous osteoradionecrosis is somewhat unpredict-

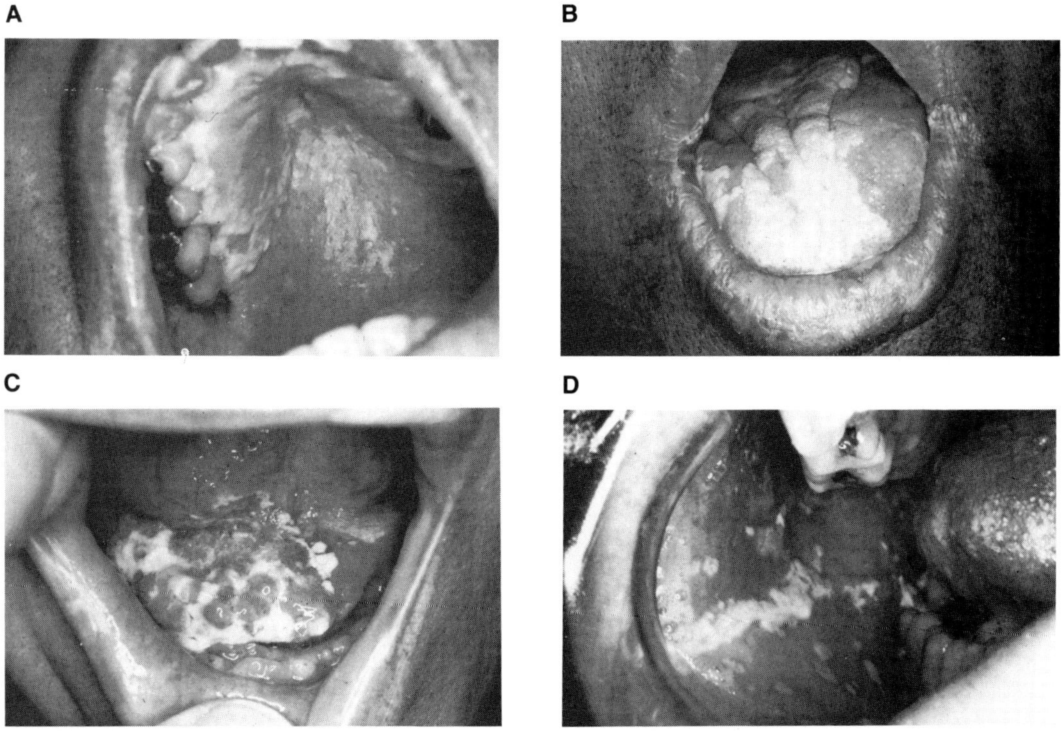

Fig. 37–4. Candidiasis following radiation-induced xerostomia. This infection can take many forms and is often confused with mucositis. A. Candidiasis of the palate after 5 weeks of irradiation. B. Lingual candidiasis at the end of radiation. Note angular cheilitis. C. Acutely painful candidiasis after 3 weeks of irradiation. D. Mucositis complicated by candidiasis at the end of the 4 weeks of radiation (approximately 3000 cGy). The patient also complained of dryness.

able, but is related to the dose of radiation delivered and the bone volume. The risk is increased in dentulous patients, even more if teeth within the treatment field are removed after therapy. When spontaneous bone exposure occurs, it usually takes place more than 1 year after radiation is completed.

Table 37–1. Occurrence of Oral Candida in 109 Irradiated Oral Cancer Patients*

	Candida Culture		
Percent of Patients	Before Therapy	End of Therapy	After Therapy†
41	Negative	Negative	Negative
10	Negative	Negative	Positive
27	Negative	Positive	Positive
22	Positive	Positive	Positive

*Data with permission from Silverman S Jr, et al. J Oral Med 39:194, 1984.
†Mean time, 14 months.

Animal models to study the effects of ionizing radiation on jaw bones have demonstrated changes similar to those observed in human specimens: marrow vascularity and fatty degeneration; reduction of osteocytes, osteoblasts and osteoclasts; enlarged lacunae; and microfractures.

Based on a detailed study (36) of 100 head and neck patients who underwent radiation therapy for cancers at the University of California, San Francisco, regarding the effects of radiation on the jaw bones, certain facts emerge.

1. Patients who were edentulous at the time of diagnosis of cancer had a relatively low risk of osteonecrosis.
2. Patients who were dentulous had a greater risk.
3. The increased risk in dentulous patients appeared to be associated with

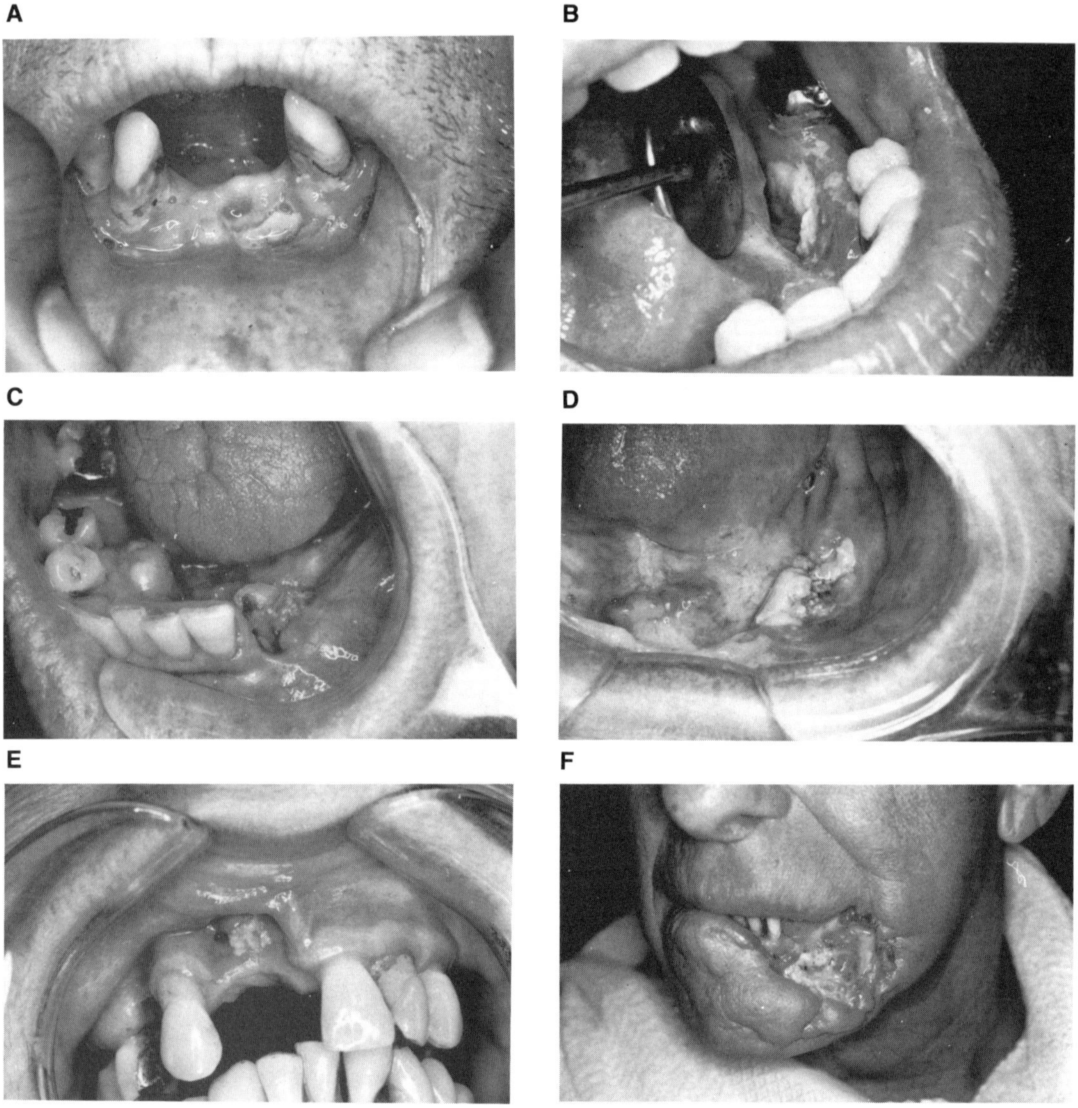

Fig. 37–5. Osteoradionecrosis following irradiation for head and neck cancer. This condition can occur spontaneously or after trauma. A. Spontaneous osteoradionecrosis of the mandible, which developed 3 years after treatment and responded to antibiotics. B. Osteoradionecrosis of the mandible appearing 6 months after treatment and developing after trauma. This did not respond to antibiotics and required mandibular resection. C. Osteoradionecrosis of the mandible developing 1 year after treatment, following extraction of the lower left cuspid. D. Osteoradionecrosis of the left mandible developing 1-½ years after treatment, even though lower denture was not worn. E. Osteoradionecrosis of the maxilla (an infrequent occurrence) developing 2 years after treatment. There had been no known trauma. F. Osteoradionecrosis of the mandible, which was not controlled by antibiotics. Patient refused resection.

tooth extractions after radiation therapy.

4. Dentulous patients with pretreatment extractions or no extractions appeared to have risks similar to those of the edentulous patients.
5. Spontaneous osteoradionecrosis can occur.
6. The most important risk factor for the development of osteonecrosis appeared to be the radiation dose to the bone, particularly in the mandible.

A

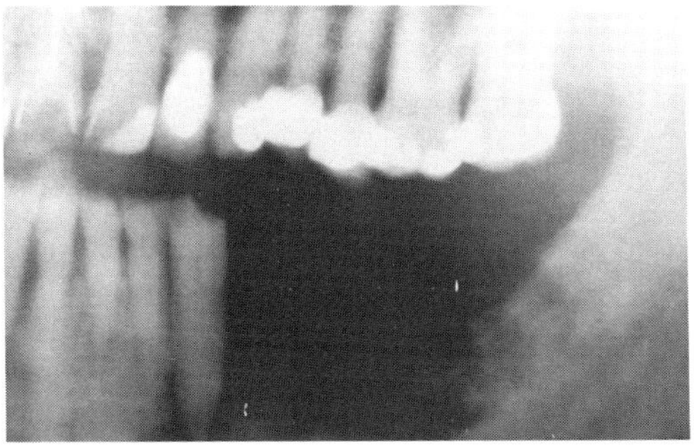

B

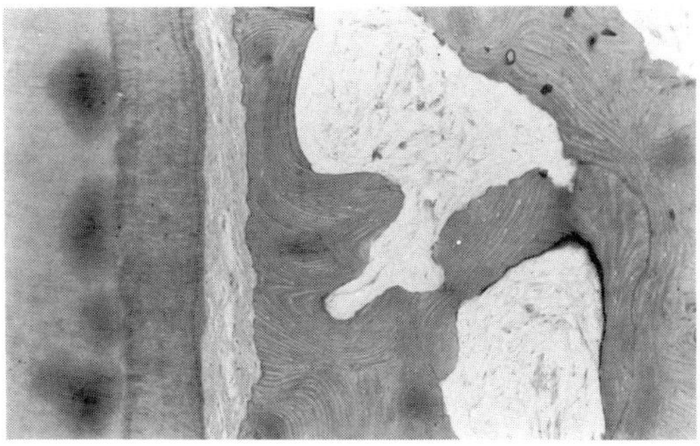

C

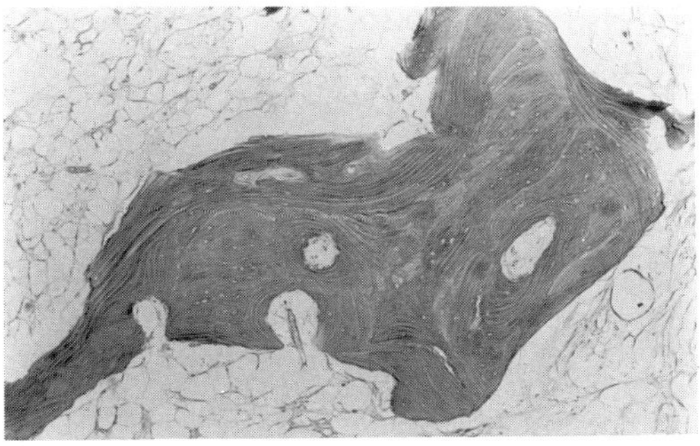

Fig. 37–6. Osteoradionecrosis. Histologic specimens showing devitalization of jawbone by radiation. A. Radiograph of advanced osteonecrosis that progressed to this stage 4 years after radiation (6800 cGy) for a squamous carcinoma of the mouth floor. There was exposed bone and severe pain. B. Dental socket area (left to right): dentin, cementum, periodontal ligament, bone marrow (alveolar bone). C. Higher-power view of an alveolar bone trabecula, showing bone and marrow. Marrow is acellular and shows marked avascularity, lack of fibrous connective tissue, and some fatty degeneration. Note lack of osteocytes, osteoblasts, and osteoclasts.

7. Clinical changes in skin and/or mucosa indicating radiation damage was a risk indicator for osteonecrosis.
8. The risk for osteonecrosis continues indefinitely following radiation therapy.

In our experience, the risk of osteonecrosis is negligible when the bone irradiation dose is less than 6500 cGy, but great when the dose exceeds 7500 cGy. Fortunately for patients' function and appearance, the risk of osteonecrosis related to denture-wearing is small (38). Other investigators have found similar risk factors related to osteonecrosis (32,39,40). Trismus is a rare occurrence and can result from pain, infection, tumor, or connective tissue scar.

Soft-Tissue Necrosis

Soft tissue necrosis may be defined as the occurrence of a mucosal ulcer in irradiated tissue that has no residual cancer (Fig. 37–7). The incidence of soft tissue necrosis is related to dose, time, and volume irradiated. The risk is far greater with interstitial implantation and intraoral techniques because of the higher irradiation doses used.

Soft-tissue necrosis is usually painful. Optimal hygiene is required and analgesics are

Table 37–2. Reported Incidence of Osteonecrosis in Patients Irradiated for Head and Neck Cancers

Source, Year	Hospital	No. of Patients	Years	Dosage (cGy)	Cases of Osteonecrosis
Beumer, 1972	UCSF	278	1961–69	5000–7000	10 (4%)
Bedwinek, 1976	MDAH	381	1966–71	6000–7500	54 (14%)
Murray, 1980	MDAH	397	1971–75	4000–>8000	77 (19%)
Morrish, 1981	UCSF	100	1971–77	5000–7500	22 (22%)

UCSF = University of California, San Francisco
MDAH = M.D. Anderson Hospital (Texas)

Table 37–3. Incidence of Osteonecrosis According to Radiation Dose to Bone*

Dose to Bone (cGy)	Incidence of Osteonecrosis	
	Dentulous Patients	Edentulous Patients
< 6500	0/36 (0%)	0/3 (0%)
6500–7500	8/29 (28%)	1/15 (7%)
> 7500	11/13 (85%)	2/4 (50%)
Total	19/78 (24%)	3/22 (14%)

*Data with permission from Morrish RB, et al. Cancer 47:1980, 1981.

usually helpful, but antibiotics are generally of little help in relieving pain and promoting healing. Because these ulcerations are often at the site of primary tumor, periodic assessment for recurrence is essential until the necrosis heals.

CHEMOTHERAPY

When using cytotoxic chemotherapeutic drugs, it is extremely important to keep patients free from oral foci of infection and pain to minimize local infections and bacteremia, and to enable patients to follow a nutritious diet. The chemotherapeutic agents used to eradicate tumor production also adversely affect normal cells, particularly those that have relatively high turnover rates, such as oral epithelial tissues. The depressant effect of therapy on oral epithelial mitosis can result in thinning and ulceration of those tissues (Fig. 37–8) as well as the salivary gland and cause taste dysfunction (41,42). The oral ulcerations may be due to direct cellular cytotoxicity from the chemotherapeutic agents, to increased susceptibility to microorganisms owing to neutropenia, to trauma, or to a combination of these factors. Commonly used antineoplastic drugs that are specifically toxic to oral mucosa (opposed to those that cause mucositis indirectly by their bone marrow effect) are listed in Table 37–5.

It is important to realize that the ability of oral tissues to resist trauma and to repair themselves is significantly compromised, and even irritation from eating and talking can lead to mucosal breakdown. Because continued therapy further induces myelosuppression, leukopenia, and thrombocytopenia, patients will become even more susceptible to infection and bleeding (42–48).

The increased risk of infection is particularly important. Not only can periodontal and dental infections have serious consequences, but the oral cavity can be the site of infections caused by viruses, fungi, and acquired bacterial pathogens (Fig. 37–9). The reactivation of herpes-family viruses (49,50) such as herpes simplex I and Varicella zoster, can cause significant mucosal breakdown, pain, and hemorrhage, and increase the risk of secondary infection. Fungal infection, caused by Candida and Aspergillus species, in addition to producing local disease, can spread systemically and cause serious infec-

Table 37–4. Association of Dental Extractions and Osteonecrosis in 78 Irradiated Dentulous Patients*

Time of Extraction	Radiation Dose (cGy)		Osteonecrosis	
	Range	Mean	Incidence	Mean Time of Onset After Treatment (mos)
No extractions	6940–9280	(7871)	5/41 (12%)	29
Before radiotherapy	7580–9610	(8500)	3/19 (16%)	41
After radiotherapy	6700–8100	(7346)	11/18 (61%)	20
Total	6700–9610	(7666)†	19/78 (24%)	22

*Data with permission from Morrish RB, et al. Cancer 47:1980, 1981.
†Radiation for dentulous patients without osteonecrosis ranged between 4950 and 9700 cGy (avg. 6450 cGy).

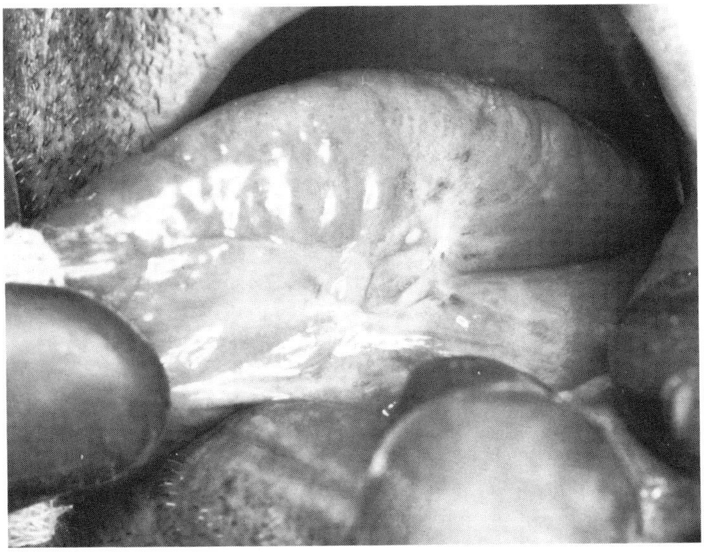

Fig. 37–7. Soft-tissue necrosis. This painful ulcer appeared 6 months after radium needles were implanted for tongue carcinoma (calculated dose, 6800 cGy). Lesion healed in 4 months.

tions (51–54). Bacterial infections can be caused by organisms normally found in the oral cavity, as well as by a number of opportunistic pathogens such as Pseudomonas, Klebsiella, Serratia, Escherichia, and other gram-negative bacteria (55–57). Identification of the source of infection and appropriate selection of antimicrobial agents are critical to effective management.

Marrow transplantation is associated with frequent and significant oral and head and neck complications (58). High doses of chemotherapeutic agents, with or without total body irradiation, can result in severe oral and pharyngeal mucositis, pain, infections, and hemorrhage. An additional complication of marrow transplantation is graft-versus-host disease (GVHD), which results from the reaction of donor T-lymphocytes against host antigens (59,60). The oral cavity can be the site of both acute and chronic GVHD.

Children who receive chemotherapy and/or radiation therapy to the jaws when permanent teeth are developing may suffer a number of abnormalities involving teeth and jaws: complete or partial dental agenesis, root malformation, and maldevelopment of jaws (61).

ORODENTAL PROPHYLAXIS AND MANAGEMENT—SUMMARY

In view of the risk that accompanies high-dose irradiation and/or chemotherapy, spe-

A **B**

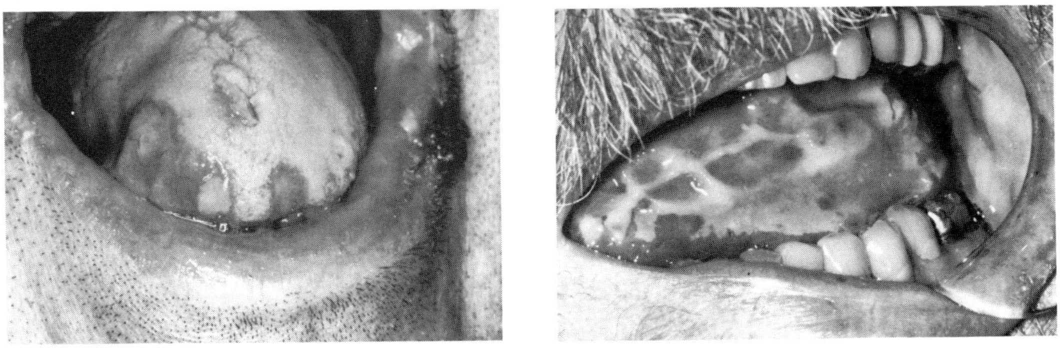

Fig. 37–8. A. Oral ulcerations in a patient with chemotherapy-induced leukopenia (WBC 1000). Ulcers healed as white count rose to about 3000. B. More extensive oral mucositis in a patient who received a combination of chemotherapy and total body radiation for a marrow transplant.

Table 37–5. Commonly Used Antineoplastic Drugs (by Category) that Are Specifically Toxic to Oral Mucosa

Antimetabolites
5-Fluorouracil (5-FU)
Methotrexate (MTX)
Hydroxyurea
Antibiotics
Bleomycin (BLM)
Adriamycin (doxorubicin, ADR), prolonged infusions
Mitomycin C (MMC)
Actinomycin D (dactinomycin)
Plant Alkaloids
Vincristine (VCR)
Vinblastine (VBL)

cial attention to preradiation dental planning appears critical. Factors important to the dental management of these patients include the following.

(1) Anticipated bone dose.
(2) Pretreatment dental status, dental hygiene, and retention of teeth that will be exposed to high-dose irradiation.
(3) Extraction techniques.
(4) Allowance of adequate healing time for teeth extracted before radiotherapy.
(5) Patient motivation and capability of compliance to preventive measures.

Because many infections occur months or years after treatment, it is evident that the tissue changes induced by chemoradiation persist for long periods and may be irreversible. Therefore, extreme care must be taken in evaluating the status of the teeth and periodontium before, during and after treatment, and optimal oral and periodontal hygiene must be maintained because of the lowered biologic potential for healing in response to physical irritation, chemical agents, and microbial organisms (62). Such attention is critical because of the potentially progressive nature of radiation osteonecrosis, which may involve large segments of bone and present a major therapeutic problem, possibly requiring extensive resection.

It is impossible to establish precise formulas for managing prechemoradiation and postchemoradiation dental problems. Extractions are considered primarily for teeth with a poor prognosis due to such conditions as advanced periodontal disease, extensive caries activity, and periapical lesions. Other considerations are sources of chronic soft-tissue irritation (trauma), and the degree of patient cooperation in preventive home care and dental office programs. The decision is modified further for each patient on the basis of the individual's prognosis, age, desires, economic aspects, and chemoradiation delivery. Reported studies and personal experience do not substantiate the advisability of extracting all teeth before treatment as a good preventive measure. For extractions, a minimum of 1 week to 10 days is arbitrarily allowed for initial healing before treatment is instituted. However, if the situation permits, more time is preferable, up to 14 or even 21 days (32,63).

There is no evidence as to how many teeth should be extracted at one time. Therefore, whether before or after irradiation, all of the

A B

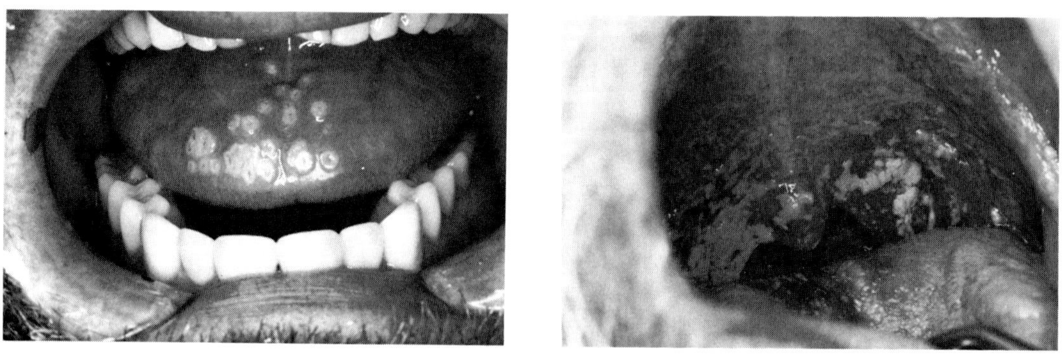

Fig. 37–9. A. Herpes simplex infection of the tongue in an immunosuppressed patient being treated by chemotherapy for lymphoma. B. Florid oral candidiasis in a leukemia patient receiving monthly pulse chemotherapy. Cyclic manifestations were associated with leukopenia.

teeth indicated for removal are extracted as suits the needs of the surgeon and the patient. The use of antibiotics during the healing period is important to minimize infection.

Whenever possible, an attempt is made to retain teeth to support tooth-borne appliances for the tentatively planned rehabilitation of these patients. It must be recalled that many teeth, either primarily or secondarily exposed to radiation, remain relatively free of disease and functional for long periods of time. This significantly facilitates rehabilitation. However, tissue-borne prostheses are not contraindicated (39,64). In general, mucosa that appears fibrosed, telangiectatic, and atrophic is at greater risk.

The periodontium is maintained in optimal condition by periodic routine periodontal procedures. When areas exposed to radiation are treated, extreme care is exercised and antibiotics may be selectively administered. Fluoride applications (daily, in the form of mouth rinses or gels) appear to aid in minimizing tooth decalcification and caries in these patients. There are no unusual contraindications for endodontic procedures (65).

In conclusion, review of the literature and our own experience indicate that carefully controlled studies are necessary before definitive guidelines can be formulated for managing orodental structures that have been or are to be radiated and subjected to chemotherapy (66,67). Until such information is available, each case must be managed individually, based on the patient's needs, the status of the tumor, and the risks known to exist for dental health. An overall "one-type" empirical approach for all patients is contraindicated.

REFERENCES

1. Silverman JE, Weber CW, Silverman S Jr, et al. Zinc supplementation and taste in head and neck cancer patients undergoing radiation therapy. J Oral Med 38:14, 1983.
2. Conger AD, Wells MA. Radiation and aging effects on taste structure and function. Radiation Res 37:31, 1969.
3. Mossman KL, Henkin RI. Radiation-induced changes in taste acuity in cancer patients. Int J Radiat Oncol Biol Phys 4:663, 1978.
4. Silverman S Jr, Thompson JS. Serum zinc and copper in oral/oropharyngeal carcinoma. Oral Surg 57:34, 1984.
5. Eneroth C, Henrickson CO, Jakobsson PA. Effect of fractionated radiotherapy on salivary gland function. Cancer 30:1147, 1972.
6. Buchner JA, Fleming TJ, Fuller LM, et al. Preliminary observations on the effect of mantle field radiotherapy on salivary flow rates in patients with Hodgkin's disease. J Dent Res 67:518, 1988.
7. Fox PC. Systemic therapy of salivary gland hypofunction. J Dent Res 66:689, 1987.
8. Greenspan D, Daniels TE. Effectiveness of pilocarpine in postradiation xerostomia. Cancer 59:1123, 1987.
9. Nakamoto RY. Use of saliva substitute in postradiation xerostomia. J Prosthet Dent 42:539, 1979.
10. Levine MJ, Aguirre A, Hatton MN, et al. Artificial salivas: Present and future. J Dent Res 66:693, 1987.
11. Shannon IL, Starcke EN, Wescott WB. Effect of radiotherapy on whole saliva flow. J Dent Res 56:693, 1977.
12. Dreizan S, Brown LR, Handler SH, et al. Radiation-induced xerostomia in cancer patients. Cancer 38:273, 1976.
13. Makkonen TA, Tenovuo J, Vilja P, et al. Changes in the protein composition of whole saliva during radiotherapy in patients with oral/oropharyngeal cancer. Oral Surg Oral Med Oral Pathol 62:270, 1986.
14. Council on Dental Therapeutics. Consensus: Oral health effects of products that increase salivary flow rate. J Am Dent Assoc 116:757, 1988.
15. Brown LR, Dreizen S, Handler SH, et al. Effect of radiation-induced xerostomia on human oral microflora. J Dent Res 54:740, 1975.
16. Cowman RA, Baron SS, Glassman AH, et al. Changes in protein composition of saliva from radiation-induced xerostomia patients and its effect on growth by oral streptococci. J Dent Res 61:336, 1983.
17. Keene HJ, Fleming TJ. Prevalence of caries-associated microflora after radiotherapy in patients with cancer of the head and neck. Oral Surg Oral Med Oral Pathol 64:421, 1987.
18. Schubert MM, Izutsu KT. Iatrogenic causes of salivary gland dysfunction. J Dent Res 66:680, 1987.
19. Frank RM, Herdly J, Phillippe E. Acquired dental defects and salivary gland lesions after irradiation for carcinoma. J Am Dent Assoc 70:868, 1965.
20. Walker R. Direct effect of radiation on the solubility of human teeth in vitro. J Dent Res 54:901, 1975.
21. Shannon IL, Wescott WB, Starcke EN, et al. Laboratory study of cobalt-60-irradiated human dental enamel. J Oral Med 33:23, 1978.

22. Shannon IL, Trodahl JN, Starcke EN. Remineralization of enamel by a saliva substitute designed for use by irradiated patients. Cancer 41:1746, 1978.
23. Hutton MF, Patterson SS, Mitchell DF, et al. Laboratory study of cobalt-60 radiation on the dental pulps of monkeys. Oral Surg 38:279, 1974.
24. Nickens GE, Patterson SS, El-Kafrawy AH, et al. Effect of cobalt-60 radiation on the pulp of restored teeth. J Am Dent Assoc 94:701, 1977.
25. Carl W, Schaaf NG, Chen TY. Oral care of patients irradiated for cancer of the head and neck. Cancer 30:448, 1972.
26. Dreizen S, Brown LR, Daily TE, et al. Prevention of xerostomia-related dental caries in irradiated cancer patients. J Dent Res 56:99, 1977.
27. Wei SHY. Clinical use of fluorides: A state-of-the-art conference on the uses of fluorides in clinical dentistry (Conference summary). J Am Dent Assn 109:472, 1984.
28. Jones GA, Purdy RB, Stoker HW, et al. Use of dental x-rays on postirradiated patients with head and neck cancer. J Am Dent Assoc 117:599, 1988.
29. Silverman S Jr, Luangjarmekorn L, Greenspan D. Occurrence of oral candida in irradiated head and neck cancer patients. J Oral Med 39:194, 1984.
30. Rossie KM, Taylor J, Beck FM, et al. Influence of radiation therapy on oral *Candida albicans* colonization: A quantitative assessment. Oral Surg Oral Med Oral Pathol 64:698, 1987.
31. Rohrer MD, Kim Y, Fayos JV. The effect of cobalt-60 irradiation on monkey mandibles. Oral Surg 48:424, 1979.
32. Marx RE, Johnson RP. Studies in the radiobiology of osteoradionecrosis and their clinical significance. Oral Surg Oral Med Oral Pathol 64:379, 1987.
33. Hart GB, Mainous EG. The treatment of radiation necrosis with hyperbaric oxygen (OHP). Cancer 37:2580, 1976.
34. Marx RE, Johnson RP, Kline SN. Prevention of osteoradionecrosis: A randomized prospective clinical trial of hyperbaric oxygen versus penicillin. J Am Dent Assoc 111:49, 1985.
35. Fattore LaD, Strauss RA. Hyperbaric oxygen in the treatment of osteoradionecrosis: A review of its use and efficacy. Oral Surg Oral Med Oral Pathol 63:280, 1987.
36. Morrish RB, Chan E, Silverman S Jr, et al. Osteonecrosis in patients irradiated for head and neck carcinoma. Cancer 47:1980, 1981.
37. Beumer J III, Silverman S Jr, Benak SB. Hard and soft tissue necrosis following radiation therapy for oral cancer. J Prosthet Dent 27:640, 1972.
38. Bedwinek JM, Shukovsky LJ, Fletcher GH, et al. Osteonecrosis in patients treated with definitive radiotherapy for squamous cell carcinoma of the oral cavity and naso- and oropharynx. Radiology 119:665, 1976.
39. Murray CG, Herson J, Daly TE, et al. Radiation necrosis of the mandible: A 10-year study. Part I. Factors influencing the onset of necrosis. Int J Radiat Oncol Biol Phys 6:543, 1980.
40. Murray CG, Herson J, Daly TE, et al. Radiation necrosis of the mandible: A 10-year study. Part II. Dental factors; onset, duration and management of necrosis. Int J Radiat Oncol Biol Phys 6:549, 1980.
41. Schum CA, Izutsu KT, Molbo DM, et al. Changes in salivary buffer capacity in patients undergoing cancer chemotherapy. J Oral Med 34:76, 1979.
42. Schubert MM, Izutsu KT. Iatrogenic causes of salivary gland dysfunction. J Dent Res 66:680, 1987.
43. Bodey GP, Rodriguez V, Chang HY, et al. Fever and infection in leukemic patients. Cancer 41:1610, 1978.
44. Greenberg MS, Cohen SG, McKitrick JC et al. The oral flora as a source of septicemia in patients with acute leukemia. Oral Surg Oral Med Oral Pathol 52:32, 1982.
45. Dreizan S, Bodey GP, Valdivieso M. Chemotherapy-associated oral infections in adults with solid tumors. Oral Surg Oral Med Oral Pathol 55:113, 1983.
46. DePaola LG, Peterson DE, Overholser CD, et al. Dental care for patients receiving chemotherapy. JADA 112:198, 1986.
47. Dreizen S, McCredie KB, Bodie GP, Keating MJ. Quantitative analysis of the oral complications of antileukemia chemotherapy. Oral Surg Oral Med Oral Pathol 62:650, 1986.
48. Barrett AP. Clinical characteristics and mechanisms involved in chemotherapy-induced oral ulceration. Oral Surg Oral Med Oral Pathol 63:424, 1987.
49. Rand KH, Kramer B, Johnson AC. Cancer chemotherapy-associated symptomatic stomatitis. Role of herpes simplex virus (HSV). Cancer 50:1262, 1982.
50. Lam MT, Pazin GJ, Armstrong JA, et al. Herpes simplex infection in acute myelogenous leukemia and other hematologic malignancies. Cancer 48:2168, 1981.
51. Rodu B, Carpenter JT, Jones MR. The pathogenesis and clinical significance of cytologically detectable oral candida in acute leukemia. Cancer 62:2042, 1988.
52. Barrett AP. Recognition and management of invasive pharyngeal candidasis in acute leu-

kemia. Oral Surg Oral Med Oral Pathol 67:275, 1989.
53. Dreizen S, Bodey GP, McCredie KB, Keating MJ. Orofacial aspergillosis in acute leukemia. Oral Surg Oral Med Oral Path 59:499, 1985.
54. Schubert MM, Peterson DE, Meyers J, Truelove EL. Head and neck aspergillosis following bone marrow transplantation. Cancer 57:1092, 1986.
55. Dreizen S, Brown LR. Oral microbial changes and infections during cancer chemotherapy. *In:* Oral Complications of Cancer Chemotherapy. Peterson DE, Sonis ST (Eds). Boston, Martinus Nijhoff, 1983, p. 41.
56. Minaw GE, Rednor JL, Peterson DE, et al. Oral succession of gram-negative bacilli in myelosuppressed cancer patients. J Clin Microbiol 26:2105, 1988.
57. Bergmann OJ. Oral infections and septicemia in immunocompromised patients with hematologic malignancies. J Clin Microbiol 26:2105, 1988.
58. Kolbison DA, Schubert MM, Flournoy N, Truelove EL. Early oral changes following bone marrow transplantation. Oral Surg Med Oral Pathol 66:130, 1988.
59. Sale GE, Shulman HM, Schubert MM, et al. Oral and opthalmic pathology of graft-versus-host disease in man: Predictive value of the lip biopsy. Hum Pathol 12:1022, 1981.
60. Rosenberg S, Kolodney H, Wong GY, Murphy ML. Altered dental root development in long-term survivors of pediatric acute lymphoblastic leukemia. Cancer 59:1640, 1987.
61. Rosenberg S, Kolodney H, Wong GY, Murphy ML. Altered dental root development in long-term survivors of pediatric acute lymphoblastic leukemia. Cancer 59:1640, 1987.
62. Beumer J III, Curtis TA, Morrish RB Jr. Radiation complications in edentulous patients. J Prosthet Dent 36:193, 1976.
63. Regezi JA, Courtney RM, Kerr DA. Dental management of patients irradiated for oral cancer. Cancer 38:994, 1976.
64. Starcke EN, Shannon IL. How critical is the interval between extractions and irradiation in patients with head and neck malignancy? Oral Surg 43:333, 1977.
65. Seto BG, Beumer J III, Kagaqwa T, et al. Analysis of endodontic therapy in patients irradiated for head and neck cancer. Oral Surg Oral Med Oral Pathol 60:540, 1985.
66. National Cancer Institute. Oral complications of cancer therapies. Diagnosis, prevention, and treatment. NCI Monogr 9:1990.
67. Jansma J, Vissink A, Spijkervet FK, et al: Protocol for the prevention and treatment of oral sequelae resulting from head and neck radiation therapy. Cancer 70:2171, 1992.

Chapter 38

PEDIATRIC TOXICITY

GIULIO J. D'ANGIO AND NANCY J. BUNIN

The problems associated with organ-specific chemoradiation toxicity are compounded in children. This is because interference with normal growth and development of the individual organ, tissue, or part are added to the potential damage to the functioning and stromal cells (1,2). There is also the related issue of oncogenesis, particularly cogent in children (3). Their expected longevity after cure of the initial cancer far exceeds the latent periods usually entailed for the appearance of second tumors (3). A third and very relevant consideration is the fact that combined modality therapy is common in pediatric oncology. Phillips and Fu, among others, conducted detailed murine laboratory studies of the effects of radiation plus various chemotherapeutic agents on selected vital organs (4). They documented the radiation-enhancing effects of such combinations, and these have been presented elsewhere in this volume. Here, the emphasis will be placed on clinical data derived from pediatric experience.

Certain drugs used frequently in children with cancer, notably actinomycin D (dactinomycin, AMD) and doxorubicin (Adriamycin, ADR), augment radiation responses (5,6). They can also reactivate latent radiation reactions in tissues irradiated weeks before.

These heightened responses are reflected in any tissue or structure in the body. Mucosal reactions are more severe after combined chemoradiation therapy, and reactivation can be a major problem in the upper respiratory tract, the lungs, and the gastrointestinal tract (7,8). Usually, these combined effects occur when the two modalities are used together, or when the chemotherapy follows radiation therapy. Priming of tissues by prior administration is usually not the problem, although it has been reported by Cassady in the case of the esophagus, which apparently can be sensitized by prior chemotherapy (9). The reactivation of latent radiation damage becomes less likely as the time interval from the completion of radiation therapy becomes longer. Severe flare-ups are seldom encountered 3 or more months after the completion of radiation therapy.

It is apparent that every and any structure in the body must be considered vulnerable to the effects of chemoradiation (4). It is of interest that these combined effects can be seen in tissues that are responsive to either of the agents when used alone, and in other structures that are responsive to only one of the two in commonly employed doses. An example of the first of these possibilities is the skin. The original reports of combined chemoradiation effects recorded cutaneous reactions in children given kilovoltage radiation together with AMD (5). AMD by itself can produce tanning of the skin, especially in intertriginous regions, or cause a generalized rash. The agent can therefore be considered dermatopathic in its own right, and skin erythema after kilovoltage radiation is a common experience. Unlike skin changes, pneumonopathy is not a consequence of AMD, although it can follow radiation. The combination of the two can lead to more severe changes (7). Conversely, ADR is a known cardiotoxin, producing changes in the myocardium, whereas radiation therapy usually does not. Myocardial damage is more severe in both animal experiments and human experience when ADR and cardiac radiation therapy are used together (10,11). Still another possibility is demonstrated by the cognitive dysfunctions encountered in children after systemic methotrexate administration and cranial irradiation (12). Both of the modalities are mildly toxic in commonly used doses; their combination produces more impressive damage.

These and other chemoradiation interactions will now be considered in greater detail.

GROWTH AND DEVELOPMENT EFFECTS

Impairments can be secondary to both direct and indirect effects.

Direct

Bones and Soft Tissues

It has been known ever since the classic experiment in chicks reported by Perthes that local radiation can stunt growth (13). These effects are expressed in both the irradiated bone and the associated soft tissues. The severity of the growth anomalies is directly proportional to the dose delivered, and inversely to the age of the child at the time of irradiation (2,14,15). The effects are further modulated by whether ortho- or megavoltage irradiation is used, by time-dose-fraction considerations, and vary according to the part irradiated (16). Studies of tibial growth in young rats have shown, for example, that twice the nominal single dose in the range of 500 to 1500 cGy must be given by fractionated irradiation to produce the same bone-shortening (17). Addition of one or more of such anticancer agents as AMD and ADR can markedly increase radiation-associated injury. Bone and soft-tissue necrosis so severe as to require amputation have been reported under these circumstances, the dose of radiation in itself being insufficient to cause that degree of damage (18). It is therefore probable, but not documented, that combined chemoradiation increases any growth disturbance caused by radiation therapy alone. Several recent reports of longterm orthopedic sequelae in irradiated Wilms' tumor patients do not introduce the chemotherapy variable in the analysis. Because AMD has been used in such patients for 20 or more years, numbers of survivors should now be available for comparison with older cohorts treated before the advent of AMD. It should be noted, however, that Silber et al., in describing a method by which growth impairment can be predicted, state that ". . . addition of a variable to consider radiopotentiating chemotherapy would not add greatly to the explanation of potential height loss." (2).

Tissues and structures other than the axial and appendicular skeleton can be affected. Vessels irradiated in early life can fail to develop at the same pace as nonirradiated segments (15). The result is a narrowed sleeve. It is important to keep in mind that these local effects can have systemic consequences. Coarctation of the aorta at the level of the renal artery, reported after radiation given to children following nephrectomy for Wilms' tumor, can lead to hypertension and its consequent problems. Again, combined chemoradiation can be expected to produce more injury than either modality alone.

Face

Disturbance in normal facial bone growth is among the most disabling of the deformities that can result from local radiation (19,20). Gross facial disfigurement is especially disabling psychologically, particularly in teenagers (Fig. 38–1). Development of the tooth bud can be severely impaired by radiotherapy and chemotherapy, if not completely aborted by local radiation therapy of the jaws (19–21). The resultant imperfect dentition requires skillful continuing dental care as malformed or incompletely erupted teeth make their appearance. Surveillance by a plastic surgeon and an orthodontist should be enlisted early.

Breast

Breast development in girls can be suppressed by radiation therapy. Beyond the psychologic disturbances occasioned by underdevelopment of one or both breasts is the potential for oncogenesis in surviving girls (see below).

Parenchymal Organs

Another associated problem is the aborting of parenchymal organs stimulated to hypertrophy or regenerate. Tefft et al reported that radiation therapy given immediately after partial hepatectomy suppresses the hepatocellular response so that liver regeneration is incomplete (22). As the child grows older,

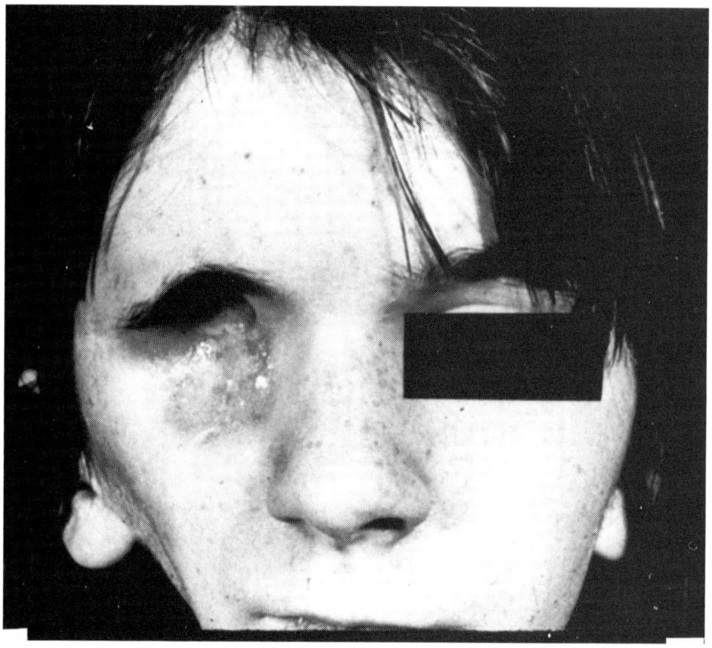

Fig. 38–1. Appearance 5 years after exenteration of the right orbit. Dactinomycin and postoperative radiation therapy (5000 cGy) was given to the tumor bed and to involved upper cervical lymph nodes. Underdevelopment of the right side of the face and mandible is obvious. There were severe problems in dentition as well.

the liver fails to enlarge concurrently, interfering with normal growth and development. This can lead eventually to liver failure if the suppressive effects have been sufficiently pronounced.

Similarly, compensatory hypertrophy of the remaining kidney after unilateral nephrectomy can be inhibited by irradiation and chemotherapy. Sagerman et al long ago reported underdeveloped kidneys after abdominal radiation given to children, and Donaldson and colleagues demonstrated an inhibition of compensatory renal enlargement when the remaining kidney was irradiated in unilaterally nephrectomized weanling mice (23,24). Moskowitz et al studied how various anticancer drugs affected compensatory kidney growth (25). They found that AMD, vincristine (VCR), and ADR in the doses they used (minimal lethal doses) inhibited compensatory kidney enlargement in the same murine system. Resnick and coworkers had shown a similar result after mithramycin (26). Moskowitz and colleagues attributed the renal effect to a delay in the mitotic response that is normally initiated promptly after nephrectomy. These laboratory results do not seem to translate into clinical problems, however. Several studies of Wilms' tumor survivors treated with AMD + other drugs + radiation therapy have been reported at intervals over more than two decades. They fail to demonstrate interference with renal compensatory enlargement, or indicate major problems with renal failure (23,27,28). The most recent of these are from the National Wilms' Tumor Study. In one, hypertension was more prevalent in survivors; but in another, no suggestive signs or symptoms were reported in questionnaires designed to detect major late effects (27,28).

Indirect

Glands that are responsible for the hormonal regulation of growth and development can also be adversely affected by treatment (1). The pituitary, thyroid, and gonads are all vulnerable. Suppression of growth hormone from direct irradiation of the pituitary can occur after relatively high doses delivered to the region (29). However, growth hormone deficiency can be detected in surviving irradiated leukemic patients given relatively low doses (e.g., 2400 cGy) when combined with methotrexate, especially when the drug is given systemically (30). Radiation by itself given in higher doses (e.g. 3000 cGy) to children with medulloblastoma has produced similar effects (31). It remains to be seen whether new combined chemoradiation regimens for medulloblastoma will augment these already manifest effects.

Irradiation of the neck, as for Hodgkin's disease, can lead to hypothyroidism, but this is not known to be more pronounced in children receiving both chemotherapy and radiation therapy (29). Growth stunting is avoided by administering exogenous hormone. Hypogonadism delays growth and development and affects distribution of body tissues at any age. These issues are considered at length below.

GONADAL EFFECTS

Advances in the treatment of pediatric solid tumors and leukemia have greatly increased the potential for long-term survival and cure for many diseases (1). However, this improvement in survival has directed more attention to the long-term effects of radiation and chemotherapy on gonadal function and reproduction. An increasing amount of information is available on hormonal and reproductive function in survivors of pediatric malignancies, and these issues are under active investigation. These issues were considered in considerable depth at a recent conference (32). In the cancers that have met with the greatest treatment success, such as Wilms' tumor, Hodgkin's disease, and acute lymphoblastic leukemia, more opportunity is afforded to study the longterm effects of chemotherapy and radiotherapy. Therapy has become more aggressive in the recent years, and there is greater potential for the cure of other childhood cancers as well. Because different drugs and drug combinations are used, other as yet unknown longterm side effects on gonadal function may become manifest. Prolonged follow-up studies of all survivors is mandatory (32).

Males

Depletion of the germinal epithelium lining the seminiferous tubules is the primary lesion caused by chemotherapy and radiotherapy. The interstitial Leydig cells remain normal, but there is complete aplasia of germinal cells (33–38). Clinically, this is characterized by a decrease in testicular volume, oligospermia or azoospermia, and infertility. In boys, however, permanent Leydig cell damage may result, with arrested pubertal development requiring testosterone supplementation (39,40). Chemical markers of gonadal dysfunction include elevated follicle stimulating hormone (FSH) and luteinizing hormone (LH), and decreased serum testosterone. However, a more sensitive chemical test in boys may be the response of FSH and LH to luteinizing hormone releasing hormone (39). Impairment of testosterone response to human chorionic gonadotrophin (HCG) may also help define Leydig cell dysfunction in boys (39).

Direct information on radiation effects on human fertility is available from reports of the longterm damage caused by therapeutic exposure and deliberate experimental exposures to acute radiation. These experimental studies involved single-exposure delivery to the testes of normal men (33,41). In general, the duration and severity of damage to spermatogenesis depend on radiation dosage. Briefly, spermatogonia are the most sensitive cell type, followed by spermatocytes, which are damaged at doses of 200 to 300 cGy. Spermatocytes are damaged at doses of 400 to 600 cGy; the resultant spermatozoa were significantly decreased, indicating that covert damage had occurred. Testicular depletion occurs in 46 days, with an additional 21 days for the sperm count to drop to azoospermia at all dose levels greater than 78 cGy. At higher doses (400 to 600 cGy), the sperm concentration decreases prior to 46 days because of damage to spermatids (41).

Recovery of testicular function may occur in a dose-dependent manner. There is a time lag between initiation of testicular recovery and an increase in the sperm count. The beginning of recovery is evident from the increase in germ cell numbers, which precedes the show of sperm or increase in sperm numbers. The length of complete recovery varies with the amount of radiation received. It is 9 to 18 months following < 100 cGy, 30 months following 200 to 300 cGy, and > 5 years following 400 to 600 cGy (41).

There is evidence to suggest that fractionated doses may be more harmful to the adult testis than acute doses (42–44). Marked temporary reduction in sperm count may be induced by fractionated doses as low as 35 cGy. Fractionation may prolong the recovery time. In addition, the length of the sterile period varies with total exposure, size and sequence of fractions, and the time intervals between fractions. In a recent study of male reproductive function in longterm survivors, interpatient variability was noted from the effects of radiation therapy and chemotherapy. Recovery of testicular function was not observed after 30 months when the testes received more than 50 cGy (38). In general, however, sterile patients had received large scatter doses of radiation; boys receiving > 250 cGy, albeit in fractions, developed azoospermia (38).

Much of the information regarding the direct effects of fractionated radiation therapy on fertility and hormonal function in boys comes from studies of survivors of testicular relapse in acute lymphoblastic leukemia. Whereas endocrine disturbances appear to be relatively uncommon in patients given uncomplicated therapy for ALL, (45) this is not the case for the approximately 6% of boys who develop a testicular relapse. In general, therapy for gonadal recurrence includes systemic reinduction chemotherapy and 2400 cGy to both testes, with significant testicular dysfunction ensuing (39,40,46). In a study by Leiper et al, testicular irradiation given before puberty was found to cause permanent Leydig cell damage (39). Fifty-four percent of boys showed evidence of complete pubertal delay or arrested development in Tanner stage II, with absence of the pubertal growth spurt and delayed bone age. Basal gonadotrophins were high in all the boys studied, even in those with normal growth velocities and pubertal stages. Of interest is that boys showing normal adolescent development received testicular radiation at a mean age of 9.8 years compared with a mean of 7.9 years in those progressing no further than Tanner stage II. This suggests that there may be a greater risk of permanent Leydig cell failure if radiation is given earlier in childhood. Brauner et al found that impaired testosterone secretion commonly results from testicular irradiation (46). There were, however, some patients capable of maintaining compensated Leydig-cell activity, with only high plasma concentrations of luteinizing hormone. A diminished testicular volume, indicating tubular atrophy, was found in all pubertal patients, including three who had not received drugs implicated in gonadal damage.

It is evident from these studies that, in boys, the Leydig cell sustains significant and, in some instances, permanent damage after fractionated testicular radiotherapy. However, the severity appears to be variable and may be related to the time elapsed since irradiation. Prepubertal testicular irradiation may damage the Leydig cells, although it may not become evident until the patient is postpubertal. This was confirmed by Shalet et al (47); men who during childhood had received scattered irradiation to the testes (between 270 and 980 cGy) were studied. They had small testes, were oligo- or azoospermic, and had high FSH levels. A similar group of males, who were still prepubertal at the time of the investigation, were also studied. These boys had normal FSH levels, implying that irradiation-induced damage to the germinal epithelium may not become apparent until after puberty. The Leydig cells appeared to be relatively resistant, as evidenced by normal testosterone levels in all but one patient. Another small study investigating 7 boys with testicular relapse found delayed sexual maturation in addition to elevated FSH concentrations and low testosterone levels in three of four boys with bilateral involvement (45). This raises the possibility that the Leydig cell dysfunction may be due to replacement of the testicular interstitium by leukemic cells, but additional study regarding the relative contributions of radiotherapy and chemotherapy is needed.

The effects of treatment on fertility has been studied extensively in male survivors of childhood Hodgkin's disease. Besides radiation, drugs implicated in the causation of sterility, such as alkylating agents, have been generally used in children with advanced Hodgkin's disease. It is therefore difficult to separate the effects of these two modalities. The evaluation of pediatric survivors is additionally complex because of the diversity of therapeutic regimens used. In men, "inverted Y" irradiation therapy to para-aortic and iliac nodes has been reported to produce 70 to 100% azoospermia despite testicular shielding. The dosage to the testes is closely related to their position relative to the inferior border of the field. The scatter dose to the testes that may result from subdiaphragmatic irradiation without testicular shielding may range from 18 to 36 cGy, or up to 1% of the total dose to a para-aortic field. From a pelvic field, the scatter dose may range up to 10% of the total, or 360 cGy (48). In a study by Speiser reviewing total nodal irradiation with estimated scatter of 140 to 300 cGy, all men had azoospermia at 2 to 40 months of follow-up (44). It is questionable whether this is adequate time for recovery, as shown in other studies. Pedrick and Hoppe reviewed 18 men who had pelvic radiotherapy for Hodgkin's disease (43). Even with meticulous testicular shielding, which reduces scatter, the patients received 28 to 135 cGy to the testes. Sixty-six percent had normal sperm counts when studied more than 18 months later, and 88% were fertile after 12 months. Finally, Kinsella determined that low doses of 10 to 70 cGy of scattered radiotherapy caused transient injury, as demonstrated by elevations of FSH and oligospermia (48). There was no discernible effect on Leydig cell function in this dose range. Also, FSH levels remained in the normal range for doses less than 200 cGy. What is unclear, however, is whether the prepubertal testis may be more sensitive to these lower doses than the adult testis.

The effects of radiation may be difficult to separate from those of chemotherapy. However, in one such study by Byrne et al, the effects of these different components on fertility were analyzed in longterm (at least 5 years) survivors of pediatric and adolescent cancer (49). Hodgkin's disease was the most common entity in their study. Fertility was assessed by pregnancy status and impregnation frequency. Subdiaphragmatic radiotherapy depressed fertility by approximately 25% in both sexes, probably attributable to scatter. Alkylating agents were even more detrimental in men, whether or not the drugs were combined with radiotherapy. The implications of this study should influence the development of new therapies because most of these children are cured of the disease.

However, the effects of chemotherapy may vary according to when drugs are given relative to puberty, and when the effects are evaluated relative to puberty. Alkylating agents are used to treat a wide variety of pediatric neoplasms. This drug class includes cyclophosphamide, busulfan, and melphalan; the most common testicular dysfunction affects late spermatogonia and spermatocytes. Combination chemotherapy has made it difficult to evaluate the role of individual agents with precision. There is, however, much information available regarding the gonadal effects of cyclophosphamide alone. This is derived from studies of boys treated with this agent for the nephrotic syndrome, and has revealed dysfunction independent of timing of administration in relation to puberty (49–52). This contrasts with earlier reports that suggested a difference in testicular sensitivity dependent upon age. Byrne et al noted spermatogenic dysfunction in 6 of 15 boys given the drug before or during puberty, when all boys were evaluated following complete pubertal development (49). Toxicity was probably dose-related, but all boys treated after puberty demonstrated gonadal dysfunction. Penso et al noted oligo- or azoospermia in 5 of 7 young males treated with cyclophosphamide, examined at least 12 months following discontinuation of the drugs (50). The patients had received between 18 and 39 g of cyclophosphamide, and absence of spermatogenesis was confirmed by testicular biopsy. Pennisi et al found normal FSH, LH, and testosterone levels in 16 boys treated prior to puberty, but testicular biopsies were abnormal in 4 of 5 boys (52). Evidence for a dose-response relationship between fertility and alkylating agents in prepubertal boys is apparent from other studies of nephrotic boys. Etteldorf et al evaluated eight males aged 7.5 to 13 years (53). All had been off therapy for at least 6.5 years. Those who had received under 10.5 g of cyclophosphamide had normal sperm counts, testicular histology, and serum gonadotropins. However, boys given more than 11 g were azoospermic, with testicular biopsies demonstrating germinal aplasia. This evidence suggests that the prepubertal testis may be more tolerant to moderate doses of alkylating agents than the pubertal testis, but that large doses have significant effects on both hormonal function and fertility.

The recovery of spermatogenesis is unpredictable, and it is unclear whether the degree of damage is related to the duration of therapy. Buchanan et al studied 26 adult male patients who developed azoospermia within 6 months of starting cyclophosphamide therapy for the nephrotic syndrome (54). In 12, spermatogenesis returned within 15 to 49 months after stopping the drug. In this study, the return of spermatogenesis was not significantly related to the duration of therapy, total dose, or length of follow-up after stopping treatment. However, the amount of drug given was not specified in their report.

Additional confirmation that the prepubertal state may not protect fertility in males following alkylating agent therapy comes from a study by Aubier et al (55). They evaluated 30 males who had received combination chemotherapy for solid tumors. All patients who were prepubertal or intrapubertal at the time of therapy achieved normal puberty. Prepubertal status did not, however, protect 12 of 19 boys treated with alkylating agents, all of whom became sterile. A dose relationship for these drugs was confirmed; all boys who received > 9 g/m^2 of cyclophosphamide became sterile. Jaffe et al also noted sterility with large doses of single alkylators or reduced doses when combined with other agents in boys treated both prior to and during puberty (56). However, the response of individual patients varied. Some of the controversy regarding the importance of timing of the alkylating agents relative to puberty can be attributed to the reliance on hormonal tests to define the extent of damage. It is clear from the results of Shalet et al, as well as those of Pennisi and Aubier mentioned above, that current hormonal tests of testicular function may not detect moderately severe damage to the tubular system in prepubertal boys when unassociated with Leydig cell impairment (52,55,57). Although an increase in basal follicle-stimulating hormone levels may give a good indication of testicular damage, normal levels do not rule out the possibility of azoospermia. It is therefore apparent that future studies must take this into consideration, and sperm evaluation or testicular biopsy as well as hormone levels may be necessary for adequate follow-up studies.

Treatment with combination chemotherapy may produce more long-lasting azoospermia or gonadal function than treatment with single agents. Evidence for this stems from studies of patients treated with combination chemotherapy for Hodgkin's disease. MOPP therapy, consisting of mechlorethamine, vincristine, procarbazine, and prednisone, is one of the most commonly used regimens. Both mechlorethamine (nitrogen mustard) an alkylator, and procarbazine have been implicated in causing germinal aplasia of the seminiferous tubules. Procarbazine has demonstrated toxicity to the germinal epithelium of adult male monkeys (58,59). The hormonal and fertility effects of therapy for Hodgkin's disease have been studied extensively in adult patients, and more information is currently becoming available regarding the pediatric age group. Sherins et al assessed 19 boys with Hodgkin's disease who had received MOPP therapy. Nine of the 13 pubertal boys developed gynecomastia and germinal aplasia, with an increase in gonadotropins and decreased serum testosterone, whereas six prepubertal boys did not (60). This is evidence that the Leydig cells of adolescent testes can be injured by MOPP therapy, but it remains unclear whether prepubescent boys are spared. Additional follow-up is necessary to determine whether testicular injury will become manifest at a later age. A contradictory result was obtained by Whitehead and colleagues, who evaluated 12 males given MOPP during childhood (61). Nine had small testes, but gynecomastia was found in only one. All six patients studied 2.4 to 8 years after discontinuation of therapy were azoospermic. Most late pubertal patients in this study had increased FSH, reflecting germinal epithelium damage. The Leydig cells were more resistant to cytotoxic induced damage, and normal pubertal development ensued. In general, it was apparent that prepubertal boys did sustain testicular damage from MOPP therapy. In the study by Aubier et al, only those boys who received < 3 courses of MOPP retained fertility when examined 2 to 16 years after completion of therapy (55). This includes 5 who were prepubertal at the time of therapy.

Vincristine, methotrexate, and mercaptopurine are among the drugs most commonly used in antileukemic chemotherapy. According to Blatt et al, they do not appear to damage testicular development, at least as estimated by testicular volume, serum gonadotropin and testosterone levels, and semen analysis (45). A different result is recorded by Shalet et al, who evaluated testicular function after ALL chemotherapy using testicular biopsies and measurements of LHRH and HCG stimulation tests. Most boys showed a normal Leydig cell response to HCG stimulation, but it was predicted that many boys would be oligospermic or azoospermic at the end of puberty (47). Lendon et al reported the testicular histology of 44 boys treated with combination chemotherapy for ALL, most of whom had received therapy when prepubertal (62). The mean tubular fertility index (TFI) (percentage of seminiferous tubules containing identifiable spermatogonia) was 50% less than that in age-matched controls. Previous therapy with cyclophosphamide or cytarabine (> 1 g/m^2) appeared to depress the TFI, but it appeared to improve after completion of chemotherapy. This is an unusual report in that cytarabine has not previously been associated with depression of male gonadal function. Finally, in adult males with acute or chronic leukemias, the amount of testicular damage was dependent upon the length of therapy rather than the specific regimen used (36). Only Sertoli cells remained in patients treated for more than three months. However, the longterm effects of therapy and return of fertility were not evaluated in this study. Fertility does not appear to be affected in boys who receive antileukemic therapy without an alkylator, and there have been reports of successful paternity following such therapy for ALL (63).

The effects on male gonadal function of other classes of chemotherapeutic agents have been less well studied; it is difficult because of the combination therapy employed for most neoplastic diseases. Doxorubicin has been shown to affect the primitive spermatogonia of mouse testes (64), but it appears that the drug is less toxic to the human testis (65); and dactinomycin, vinblastine, and vincristine do not appear to be testicular toxins in boys (55). There is currently no information regarding gonadal damage following some of the newer agents, such as cisplatin, carboplatinum, and ifosfamide. Ifosfamide is an alkylator, however, so that effects similar to those described for cyclophosphamide can be expected.

In summary, earlier studies have suggested that the prepubertal testis may be less sensitive to the effects of chemotherapy and radiation therapy, but more recent data have failed to verify this. The germinal epithelium appears to be more vulnerable to the effects of therapy, and azoospermia may be irreversible. The Leydig cells are less susceptible to cytotoxic therapy, but the effects may vary depending on when the therapy was given relative to puberty, and the notion that the prepubertal testis is more resistant again remains unproven. It is difficult to come to any specific conclusions regarding the impact of combined radiation and chemotherapy on the juvenile testis, given these conflicting and inconclusive data, and the sensitivity of the germinal epithelium to both radiation and the alkylating agents. Ablation of both hormonal and spermatogenic functions is most likely to occur, however, after the converging damage produced by alkylators and radiation.

Females

The normal development of the ovary during childhood is characterized by follicle growth and atresia, but comparatively little information is available regarding the effects of chemotherapy and radiotherapy on ovarian development and function. Reasons for this include the inaccessibility of the ovary to biopsy, and dependence on menstrual and fertility history for evaluation. The radiation sensitivity of the human ovary has not been well defined. Although it has been thought to be relatively radioresistant (66), there is substantial evidence that this may not be the case. In fact, radiation therapy may play a more profound role in the disturbance of fertility and gonadotrophin levels than chemotherapy in girls undergoing treatment.

In a study by Himelstein-Braw et al (67), the ovaries of 12 girls with abdominal tumors were studied and compared to control samples. Although normal ovaries were found in girls who had received only a short course of chemotherapy, all patients who had received radiation therapy alone or in combination with drugs had severely damaged ovaries, with inhibition of follicle growth. Stillman et al. investigated ovarian failure among 182 longterm survivors of childhood cancer (68). Overall, ovarian failure was found in 12%, all of whom had received whole abdominal radiation with a calculated mean ovarian tissue dose (OTD) of 3200 cGy (range, 1200 to 5000) with one ovary included in the port. The incidence was much higher (68%) in girls who had both ovaries within abdominal radiotherapy fields, and it was 14% in five of 35 patients whose ovaries were at the edge of the treatment field. These five patients had a mean OTD of 290 cGy. None of 122 patients with one or both ovaries outside of the treatment field developed ovarian failure. The location of the ovaries relative to radiation treatment fields was the only risk factor for subsequent ovarian dysfunction, even accounting for the chemotherapeutic agents administered and cumulative doses. The importance of location of radiation therapy in treatment of girls with ALL was also shown by Hamre et al (69). The incidence of ovarian failure was 93% for girls who received craniospinal radiation plus 1200 cGy to the abdomen for ALL, as compared to 49% for those treated with craniospinal radiation alone, and 9% for those treated only with cranial radiation. Shalet et al reviewed the effects of abdominal radiation in 18 girls evaluated between 1 and 26 years after irradiation (70). The serum gonadotropins and estrogen levels were consistent with ovarian failure in each patient, but there was a disproportionate elevation in serum follicle stimulating hormone (FSH) compared to LH in 16 patients.

Girls who are to receive subdiaphragmatic radiotherapy for Hodgkin's disease often undergo oophoropexy at the time of staging laparotomy. This entails relocating the ovaries in the midline, and a 10-cm-thick lead block is used to shield the ovaries during irradiation. With this technique, up to two thirds of women may retain ovarian function (71,72). The minimum radiation dose to the ovaries is 350 to 400 cGy over 29 to 46 days due primarily to scattered radiation.

There has been relatively little research on the effects of cytotoxic drugs on gonadal function in the prepubertal and pubertal female. The effects of akylating agents are the best understood. There appears to be no delay in menarche or interruption of menses in girls treated with the single agent cyclophosphamide (CPM) (49,73,74), although low cumulative doses were used in some of these studies. Evaluation of women who had received CPM during childhood for renal disease found no evidence of menstrual dysfunction, and pregnancies have been documented. However, Miller et al report ovarian destruction in a girl treated for a prolonged period (29 months) with CPM for arthritis (75). It is possible that the timing of drug administration relative to puberty may be important; ovarian failure following CPM administration in women has been documented (76,77).

The acute effects of antileukemic therapy on the ovaries has been recently reported by Himelstein-Braw et al, who studied the gonads of 31 patients at autopsy (78). Follicle development was inhibited in almost all; and in those in whom follicle development had occurred, the number and size of follicles was reduced. The ovaries of girls treated for less than 1 week were normal, whereas all those treated for more than 2 months showed inhibition of follicle growth. This suggests that the treatment, and not the disease, inhibited follicle development. The impaired follicular maturation in these patients may prove reversible; but if a serious depletion of primordial follicles occurred following exposure to cytotoxic drugs, then long-term sequelae on fertility could well ensue. Siris et al examined the effects of childhood leukemia and chemotherapy in 35 girls and women (79). Most patients had received combinations of steroids, vincristine, methotrexate, and 6-mercaptopurine, but a minority had received cyclophosphamide in addition, or busulfan. Pubertal progression and reproductive function were normal in 80% of these patients when studied at a median time of 49 months from discontinuation of therapy. The findings in seven patients were abnormal, with four exhibiting hypothalamic-pituitary dysfunction and three with evidence of primary ovarian dysfunction. Normal pubertal development correlated best with pubertal status at onset of leukemia; abnormalities appeared in 6 of 18 with diagnosis of leukemia during puberty or after menarche compared to only 1 of 17 patients diagnosed prior to puberty (47). The majority of patients treated with cyclophosphamide had normal pubertal development, but demonstrated abnormal progressions. However, these two patients did not show primary ovarian dysfunction, a condition generally observed in women receiving the alkylator. Shalet et al found biochemical evidence of ovarian failure in 2 of 7 prepubertal girls who had received combination chemotherapy for ALL (80). These girls had all received cyclophosphamide. Data are insufficient to relate cytotoxic-induced ovarian damage to the total drug dosage and duration of therapy. However, there is pathologic evidence that gonadal damage does occur in girls.

Hodgkin's disease per se does not impair ovarian function, but many studies document impairment of gonadal function in women receiving chemotherapy for the condition. Commonly used agents, including mechlorethamine (mustard) and procarbazine, may have deleterious effects on the ovary (81). The incidence of amenorrhea in women receiving these agents for Hodgkin's disease is reported between 15% and 62% (82,83). The ovarian failure is age-related, with many women < 30 years old retaining or regaining full function (81,84). There have been reports of oral contraceptives having a protective effect against chemotherapy-induced ovarian damage, but this has not been confirmed in more recent studies (84). Radiotherapy also has an influence on gonadal function in girls and young women treated for Hodgkin's disease. Infertility in those treated with combined modality therapy appears to be directly related to the gonadal dose and the age at treatment (82). Many young women retained or recovered reproductive capacity despite temporary amenorrhea and premature menopausal symptoms, but no woman with permanent amenorrhea or menopausal symptoms became pregnant. In general, the effects of Hodgkin's disease therapy on fertility appear to be less profound than in males. Alkylating agents alone produce no demonstrable effects, and combined chemoradiation does not alter fertility when compared to radiotherapy alone, unlike what is observed in males (49). Again, although shielding was used in these girls, the scatter dose was sufficient to have a detectable effect on fertility.

Pregnancy

The longterm effects of radiation and chemotherapy on the outcome of pregnancy have also been studied in the female survivors of cancer who were treated when adults. These analyses are limited by the survival rates of patients with a particular diagnosis. Most reports, therefore, involve small numbers of patients, nor is there much relevant information regarding survivors of childhood cancer. Again, the two malignant neoplasms with the most data and follow-up are Hodgkin's disease and Wilms' tumor. Pregnancy following therapy for Hodgkin's disease has been well documented (71,85,86). Oophoropexy has helped preserve ovarian function in patients receiving subdiaphragmatic radiation (71,72,87). In general, studies of pregnancies following therapy for Hodgkin's disease demonstrate no differences in spontaneous abortions or abnormal offspring when compared with control groups (88). Horning et al described 20 women who became pregnant following total nodal irradiation and/or chemotherapy (82). No birth defects or fetal wastage was seen in the 24 conceptions. Another retrospective study was done of patients under 20 years old at the time of diagnosis in whom the spontaneous abortion rate was 2.9% (less than that reported in the general population) (89). However, the frequency of stillbirth was 14.2% among women treated only with radiation therapy and 9.9% among those treated with combined modality therapy; both incidences are higher than the incidence reported in the general population (1.9%). None of the three women who experienced a stillbirth received abdominal radiation, and only one was treated with combined modality therapy. The significance of this study is unknown and awaits further confirmation. The incidence of congenital anomalies was reported as 9%, similar to that encountered in the general population. The anomalies included lacrimal duct blockage, hydrocele, and ventricular septal defect.

There have been reports of successful normal pregnancies following therapy for leukemia (90), and the effect of leukemia and its treatment on fetuses exposed in utero has been recorded (91). When leukemia was diagnosed in the first or second trimester, there was a high incidence of abortion and premature delivery. Four of the babies of six patients who were on maintenance chemotherapy for leukemia at the time of pregnancy were born prematurely, and three at term; all seven were of low birth weight. There was one instance of congenital abnormalities present in the offspring of a mother who had received daily cyclophosphamide and intermittent steroids. However, there were no other documented cases, even in those babies exposed to cytotoxic agents during the first trimester. In addition, there were no congenital anomalies detected in the fetuses examined following spontaneous or induced abortion or stillbirth.

Female survivors of Wilms' tumor have been the subject of recent investigation. Li et al reported the outcome of pregnancy in 99 patients cured of Wilms' tumor (92). An adverse outcome occurred in 30% of the 114 pregnancies in women who had received abdominal radiation. There were 17 perinatal deaths, five of them in premature infants. Another 17 infants had low birth weights. An adverse outcome was found in only 3% of 77 pregnancies among nonirradiated women and wives of male patients. It was therefore significant that radiation, not chemotherapy, emerged as the predominant feature in determining outcome of pregnancy. It is, however, especially noteworthy that no increase in congenital anomalies was noted in either group. It was speculated that radiation may induce somatic damage in abdominal pelvic structures, but little is known about possible radiation-induced uterine damage. We theorize that uterine fibrosis and abnormal uterine musculature and blood supply could result and thus play a role. Byrne et al retrospectively reviewed 47 female Wilms' tumor survivors and their sibling controls (93). They found a fourfold excess risk for any adverse live birth outcome, including birth defects when compared to their siblings. In this study, 27 survivors received surgery and radiation and 16 received combined modality therapy. More female survivors had a low-birthweight infant or premature infant than controls. No difference was detected in this study as to outcome and whether the female survivors received radiotherapy alone or combined with chemotherapy.

The teratogenicity or mutagenicity of chemotherapy is difficult to demonstrate. Few patients have children during or following chemotherapy, and many who conceive have elective abortions. There is nothing to suggest that chemotherapy administered to a woman before conception or after the first trimester has an effect on outcome (94). Radiation can cause both dominant and recessive mutations. A dominant mutation is likely to result in an abortion, whereas a recessive mutation may not be detected in the first generation (95). Currently, no data support adverse genetic effects after high-dose therapeutic radiation. Unique relevant experience was reported by Kaplan, who irradiated women for menstrual dysfunction and sterility (96). This was done prior to 1960, and total doses of 65 cGy were given to the ovaries. No radiation-induced genetic damage was detected in the first or second generation offspring, albeit the numbers are small. Also, no significant increase in malformations or leukemia has been documented in the larger numbers of children born to mothers exposed to radiation from the nuclear explosions in Hiroshima and Nagasaki (35,97).

Special Considerations

Cranial radiation is used in pediatric oncology to treat primary brain tumors and acute lymphoblastic leukemia, either prophylactically or for meningeal disease. Although 3500 cGy has been shown to produce gonadotropin deficiency at the time of puberty, children who have undergone cranial irradiation with doses in the range of 2400 cGy appear to undergo normal pubertal development and to have normal gonadotropin levels (69). It has nonetheless been suggested by Shalet et al that cranial radiation may have been a contributing factor in the development of ovarian failure in three prepubertal girls (80).

Research into the gonadal effects of therapy for children with brain tumors has just begun. Cranial or craniospinal radiation may play a role in producing these effects. Rappaport et al studied 45 children of pubertal age who had received cranial radiation for medulloblastoma (98). These children had received between 2500 and 5000 cGy to the pituitary gland and hypothalamus, and puberty progressed normally in 31 of the 45. Severe gonadotropin deficiency was seen in five patients, and secondary amenorrhea in five girls. These patients usually had associated growth hormone deficiency as well. Results in children treated with craniospinal radiation for medulloblastoma were analyzed by Brown et al (99). Doses to the pituitary-hypothalamic axis were estimated to be between 4170 and 5000 cGy. Despite gonadal damage, evidenced by abnormal FSH response to gonadotropin releasing hormone, all but one child had normal pubertal progression. Adjuvant chemotherapy has been more widely used during the past 10 years for the therapy of brain tumors, and may play a larger role in gonadal dysfunction than cranial or craniospinal radiotherapy. The agents most commonly used are procarbazine and the nitrosoureas BCNU or CCNU; they are known to cause gonadal damage (100–102). It can be predicted that all boys under 16 years of age who receive one of the nitrosoureas will develop permanent testicular dysfunction, as evidenced by abnormal gonadotropin levels, but pubertal progression will proceed normally (101). Similar effects can be anticipated in girls treated with craniospinal radiation and chemotherapy containing nitrosoureas with or without procarbazine. Evaluation of girls is complicated by the fact that their ovaries may receive a scatter dose of 90 to 1000 cGy from spinal fields.

Bone marrow transplantation (BMT) methods have been adapted for leukemia and solid tumors, and their use has increased greatly over the past 10 years. The extremely intensive therapies given prior to transplant, including high dose chemotherapy and radiation therapy, have significant effects on gonadal function in children. Alkylating agents, particularly cyclophosphamide, are commonly used in many preoperative regimens, and are known causes of gonadal dysfunction. Gonadal function following high-dose cyclophosphamide was studied in 94 patients with transplants for aplastic anemia (103). Prepubertal girls had normal gonadotrophin levels and normal menarcheal development, and women under 26 years of age usually had return of menses following transplantation. Similarly, of 19 boys who were prepubertal at the time of transplant, all developed normally at puberty and had normal gonadotropin levels. Normal outcomes to pregnancy have been reported in these patients.

Patients receiving transplants for leukemia are generally prepared with total body irradiation (TBI) in addition to chemotherapy. TBI has been shown to produce gonadal failure in nearly all postpubertal patients at the time of BMT. There may be a slightly better outlook for pediatric patients. Among 142 children receiving transplants in Seattle, 68% of prepubertal patients had delayed development of secondary sexual characteristics, and gonadal failure occurred in nearly all who were postpubertal at the time of BMT (104). Four of 14 girls transplanted before puberty had recovery of ovarian function, but in general, gonadal recovery occurs in only a minority of young females after cyclophosphamide and TBI (103,104).

The improvement in survival for many children with cancer has led to a focus on longterm effects, including gonadal function. It is apparent that detailed, longitudinal studies of many patients are still necessary before the gonadal effects of aggressive chemotherapy and radiation in children are completely understood.

PULMONARY EFFECTS

Longterm effects on pulmonary function from chemotherapy and radiation, alone and in combination, are becoming evident as both the intensity of therapy and the number of survivors increase.* Technical improvements in the administration of radiation therapy, such as shielding and the use of shrinking field techniques, have avoided some of the complications (105). Subtle late effects nonetheless become evident in some children who are serially and thoroughly evaluated.

Radiation Effects

The damage produced by lung radiation may differentially affect the major cell populations in the lung (106). Type I pneumocytes, which form the major portion of the alveolar epithelium, are postmitotic cells and do not enter mitosis or regenerate. Type II pneumocytes, which are the principal source of pulmonary surfactant, are capable of rapid division and may differentiate into type I cells in response to injury. Capillary endothelial cells are also capable of division. It is therefore likely that radiation damage is most marked in the bronchial epithelial cells, capillary endothelial cells and type II pneumocytes, because these cell types have the highest mitotic rates. The severity of radiation damage depends on several factors, including the volume of lung irradiated, the dose rate, and possibly the age of the child. Growth and development of the lung in infancy and childhood is characterized by proliferation of alveoli with an increase in the

*Pulmonary toxicity of chemoradiation is discussed further in Chapter 33.

numbers of respiratory bronchioles and alveolar ducts. Adult values are reached by approximately 8 years of age. The existing alveoli continue to increase in size until the growth of the chest wall is completed in puberty. The increase in lung vasculature parallels alveolar development. It is therefore possible that irradiation of the lungs of young children interferes with pulmonary vasculature growth, and this factor accounts for the deleterious effects on lung function seen in young children so treated.

Overt manifestations of radiation damage include the development of pneumonopathy. Symptoms usually become apparent 2 to 3 months after completion of radiation therapy, and may include dry cough, fever, dyspnea, chest pain, and rarely, hemoptysis (107). Such patients almost all eventually develop radiologic and laboratory evidence of pulmonary fibrosis, even though the signs and symptoms may subside over weeks or months. The adult respiratory distress syndrome (ARDS) can develop in patients given lung radiation, even without added drugs, and appear 2 to 10 weeks after completion of whole thoracic radiation (108). Moderately high doses of radiotherapy alone, e.g., 4000 cGy, are required, but lower doses, such as 1200 cGy, suffice when combined with chemotherapy (see below).

Chest radiographs may demonstrate progressive interstitial changes. Recently, computerized axial tomography (CT) has been found to be a sensitive measure of these effects. Patchy consolidation on CT correlates with radiation pneumonopathy, solid consolidation suggests radiation fibrosis (109,110), and blood vessel shrinkage and pleural thickening are well delineated (111). Defects in perfusion are sensitively detected with SPECT, and pulmonary function tests reveal decreases in lung volume and impairments of gas exchange.

Lung damage following irradiation is compounded in children by the underdevelopment of the irradiated thorax, which in turn further restricts pulmonary function. Hence, the higher the dose, the younger the age, the more pronounced the resultant pulmonary deficit (Fig. 38–2).

Most of the data regarding the long-term effects of pulmonary irradiation in children come from Hodgkin's disease and Wilms' tumor patients. In general, the incidence of pulmonary damage from mantle-field irradiation for Hodgkin's disease is no greater in children than in adults (112,113). Kadota et al studied 12 patients years after mantle radiation (median 3500 cGy; range 1950 to 5500) given during childhood (114). Freedom from symptoms did not ensure normalcy on testing. One of the 12 was symptomatic but had pericarditis, and three had mild pulmonary fibrosis seen on chest radiographs. Pulmonary function tests were normal in six patients, but five had evidence of restrictive lung disease, with normal carbon monoxide diffusing capacity (DLCO), and one developed obstructive lung disease. Six of 12 patients had normal exercise tolerance on testing, but six had reduced capacity. Patients who had received more than 4900 cGy or who had large mediastinal masses resulting in larger radiation fields, appeared to be at greater risk for long-term effects, but less intensive therapy did not guarantee freedom from abnormalities. This experience apparently differs from that in adults (115,116), in whom minimal or no significant pulmonary late effects have been observed, but comprehensive follow-up studies of these patients are lacking.

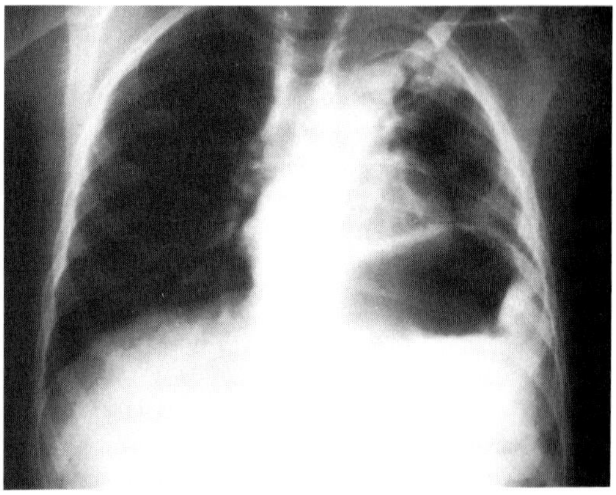

Fig. 38–2. Chest x-ray film. The patient was treated for non-Hodgkin's lymphoma 9 years before. 1200 cGy was delivered to the left hemithorax and an additional 2600 cGy was delivered to the mediastinum. The left lung is nonfunctional secondary to pulmonary fibrosis, carnification superiorly, and failure of the left upper trunk to develop. A shift of the mediastinum to the left and a high left hemidiaphragm reflect the poor air exchange. Bronchiectasis is a frequent complication in settings such as this.

Adverse effects of pulmonary irradiation in children with Wilms' tumor (WT) metastatic to the lung have been reported over the years. Age may play a role in the late effects seen because the median age of treated children was 3.5 years (117–119). Wohl et al described 12 children with WT followed 7 to 17 years after irradiation for pulmonary metastases (117). They were, on the average, 43 months old at the time of radiation, and had received between 850 and 1240 cGy at the midplane of the chest. A decrease in total lung capacity and diffusing capacity was documented; abnormalities were not found after Actinomycin-D therapy alone. In another study, children who had received orthovoltage lung irradiation for metastatic disease (10 patients) or prophylaxis (5 patients) were compared with 18 who had not (120). The dosage ranged from 1160 to 1370 cGy. Patients treated for metastatic disease had a moderate decrease in lung volume, with possible obstruction of large airways, whereas those given prophylactic radiation had normal lung volumes. The latter group also demonstrated obstruction of large airways. Only two patients were symptomatic; both had received radiation for metastatic disease. In a larger study by Benoist et al, 48 children given 2000 cGy and actinomycin D for pulmonary metastases were evaluated with pulmonary function tests prior to therapy and yearly thereafter from ages 2 to 17 years (121). A decrease in lung volume and dynamic compliance was detected. This generally progressed in severity over a longer period of time than the first few post-therapy months. Pressure volume curves, blood gases, and carbon monoxide transfer were normal. Two of the patients had acute pneumonitis. A decrease in sagittal and frontal thoracic diameters was another of the late effects. A possible explanation for the decreased volume is injury to developing alveoli and peripheral airways rather than pulmonary fibrosis. Thoracic hypoplasia may also account for the abnormal pulmonary tests (121,122).

Review of the second National Wilms' Tumor Study (NWTS) revealed 23 patients with iatrogenic toxic events (123). Four who had 1400 cGy whole-lung irradiation developed pulmonary complications. Mortality was significant, with three deaths, including one with combined hepatic and pulmonary toxicity. NWTS-3 patients with metastatic Wilms' tumor were given 1200 cGy pulmonary radiation, and diffuse interstitial pneumonitis was reported in 19 of 153 patients (12%), of unknown etiology in 15 (124). Pneumonitis occurred a median of 67 days after the completion of radiation. Three patients with Pneumocystis carinii were treated successfully and survived, but outcome was poor in those with pneumonopathy of unknown etiology (27%).

The pulmonary effects of radiation are also evident after total body irradiation (TBI). It has been given in various doses and schedules, and combined with high dose chemotherapy in preparatory regimens for bone marrow transplantation. Diffuse interstitial pneumonitis (DIP) occurring after transplant was a frequent fatal complication when TBI was given in single doses of 1000 cGy or more. Correct determination of contributing factors was complicated by different radiation dosimetry standards, dose rate considerations, and the status of the lungs before the high doses of chemotherapy and TBI given at the time of the transplant. Serota et al found in a prospective study that the pulmonary function status of ALL patients before transplant varied considerably (125). About half of the children had subnormal levels before the conditioning treatments for BMT, presumably due to prior chemotherapy, infections or both. It is therefore clear that the lungs of BMT patients can be damaged by combined therapy given at the time of the transplant itself, but the extent can be aggravated because it is superimposed on injury residual from antecedent therapies. Radiation as currently given may still contribute to the development of DIP, but other factors, such as concomitant very-high-dose chemotherapy, infection, and graft-versus-host disease also play a role in its etiology (126,127). In any case, radiation pneumonopathy lessened as lower single doses were used, or doses of 1000 cGy or even more were given in fractionated and hyperfractionated schedules. Thomas has recently reviewed these issues (128).

Chemotherapy Effects

Various cytotoxic drugs are well known to cause pulmonary damage. Bleomycin, the most commonly implicated agent, is used in pediatrics primarily for Hodgkin's disease, germ cell tumors, and less commonly, non-Hodgkin's lymphoma. In animal models, bleomycin causes endothelial blebs in the alveolar capillary endothelium followed by interstitial fibrinous edema and hyaline membrane formation (129). There is a decrease in Type I pneumocytes and a change in Type II pneumocytes, with proliferation and migration into alveolar sacs. The alveolar septae become thickened, with an overall decrease in their number (129,130). In humans, the overall effect is one of pulmonary fibrosis, with a decrease in carbon monoxide diffusing capacity (131). Clinically, cough, dyspnea, and low-grade fever may develop 1 to 3 months after the drug is discontinued, and herald bleomycin toxicity. Serial breath DLCO seemed to be the most sensitive indicators of subclinical pulmonary toxicity (132).

Bleomycin toxicity risk factors include high dose, age, prior pulmonary disease, and radiotherapy. The elderly are very prone, but there have been a few reports of bleomycin toxicity in very young children as well. Patients under age 3 at the time of diagnosis were reported to be more likely to have abnormalities on pulmonary function testing. Forced vital and total lung capacities were limited in a study by Miller et al (133). The method of administration may also affect the development of pulmonary toxicity; continuous infusion is said to reduce complications (134). In adults given < 500 units of bleomycin, the incidence of clinically detectable pulmonary injury is 5 to 10%, with a mortality of 1 to 2% (135). However, toxicity and even death have been reported with dosages as low as 30 units when the drug was given prior to or concomitantly with radiation therapy (136). The true extent of bleomycin-related lung damage in children is unknown because studies are few and results inconsistent. One review of children given combined modality therapy for Hodgkin's disease found that prior radiation did not predict abnormalities in post-therapy DLCO. All children had received prior mantle radiation, and 80% of patients with normal post-therapy DLCO had received mantle radiation with doses of 1500 to 2900 cGy. The maximum dose of bleomycin given in this study was 93 units (137).

Both dactinomycin (AMD) and doxorubicin (ADR) modify radiation responses, and studies in mice demonstrate increased cytotoxicity when AMD is combined with radiation therapy (138). It is possible that the AMD induces partial synchrony of dividing cells, resulting in a larger fraction being in the sensitive phase of the cycles at the time of radiation exposure (139). In any event, AMD has been found to sensitize the lung and lower the threshold for the development of radiation pneumonitis (140). Both AMD and ADR may cause radiation "recall" or reactivation of radiation damage (124,141,142). This has important implications for treatment plans, and these drugs should be administered cautiously following pulmonary radiation.

Other pulmonary toxic agents include the nitrosoureas and alkylating agents. Pulmonary fibrosis has been reported, sometimes after long delays, in patients receiving carmustine and busulfan with histologic changes similar to those reported for bleomycin (143,144). O'Driscoll et al have reported BCNU-related pulmonary fibrosis becoming manifest more than 15 years after discontinuing the drug (145). Signs of cyclophosphamide (CP) toxicity include dyspnea, fever, cough, and interstitial infiltrates, and do not appear to be schedule- or dose dependent (146). Similar events have been reported by Baker et al following ifosfamide therapy, with fatal outcome in these patients (147). Methotrexate (MTX) may also produce pulmonary symptoms with hypoxemia and development of interstitial infiltrates. Unlike that of CP, MTX toxicity may be schedule-dependent because daily or weekly administration seems to result in more toxicity than administration every 2 to 4 weeks (146). However, recovery from toxicity does occur following withdrawal of MTX, unlike the other agents discussed.

In summary, early and late pulmonary effects from radiation and chemotherapy have been documented in children, but the results do not demonstrate clear-cut dose responses except in broad terms. Combined effects with specific chemoradiation combinations are not universal and are unpredictable from one child to the next. More studies of specific chemoradiation combinations, serial testing, and longer follow-up are indicated to define potential toxicity in the pediatric age group more accurately and completely.

CARDIAC EFFECTS

The effects of thoracic radiation therapy (RT) and certain chemotherapeutic agents on the heart in survivors of childhood cancer are still largely unknown. Extensive serial evaluation of these young patients is necessary, much of what is currently known is based on studies of adults.

The effects of RT on cardiac function have been documented most extensively in patients undergoing mediastinal irradiation for Hodgkin's disease. As more sophisticated methods have become available for the evaluation of the heart and its coverings, more RT sequelae have become evident.

Cardiac effects of thoracic RT include both acute and delayed pericarditis (148,149). Acute pericarditis is an infrequent occurrence, with symptoms of chest pain, fever, and occasionally, changes on the EKG. Delayed pericarditis occurs more frequently with an onset several months to years following irradiation. This may present as an acute process, or as a chronic pericardial effusion, often in an asymptomatic patient. Some degree of tamponade occurs in up to 50% of patients, and echocardiographic changes are common. Pancarditis, which may be more common in those who have received > 6000 cGy, is the most severe form of radiation-related cardiac disease. Fibrosis can develop in both the myocardium and pericardium, leading to congestive heart failure. Other RT-related sequelae include functional valvular and conduction defects. Recent reports have documented a high incidence of post-RT endocardial changes resembling fibroelastosis with focal valvular thickening (150). Mitral insufficiency has been the most commonly seen valvular lesion. Conduction defects, such as right bundle branch block or even complete heart block, have been reported in patients who receive mantle radiation for Hodgkin's disease (151). The right bundle lies close to the endocardium, on the right side of the septum, so it may be at greater risk of radiation exposure (152). The time to development of heart block has ranged from 5 to 23 years (153). Whether radiation causes coronary artery disease is controversial. Corn et al have recently reviewed the evidence (154). They conclude that, whatever may have been true in past years, modern radiation methods seem to have been successful in avoiding this complication. It is known that radiation causes endothelial damage and thus may accelerate the development of atherosclerosis (155,156). McEniery et al described radiation-associated pathology as characterized by stenosis of the ostia of the left and right coronary vessels (157). Necropsy studies of young patients who had received over 3500 cGy to the heart, showed significant narrowing of pericardial coronary arteries by fibrous tissue (150). Longterm studies are necessary in children who have received mediastinal radiation in order to evaluate the frequency and severity of this potential complication from RT alone. Those analyses will be made difficult because almost all children receive combined chemoradiation.

Pathologic studies of irradiated hearts demonstrate a transient exudate of granulocytes, pericardial thickening, and pericardial exudate. The myocardium may show diffuse interstitial fibrosis, and intramural arteries may demonstrate endothelial proliferation with thickening of the media and adventitia (150,152).

The incidence of a symptomatic cardiac injury has been reported to be as high as 50% in adults who received < 4000 cGy of mediastinal radiation for Hodgkin's disease (158), and up to 68% of patients, most of whom received > 4000 cGy, showing cardiac abnormalities (159). However, it is apparent that many asymptomatic patients will have abnormal findings on detailed cardiac evaluation. This includes a decrease in left ventricular ejection fraction (151,159,160), increase in right ventricular wall thickness (151), thickening of aortic and mitral valves (161) and a constrictive or occult pericarditis or abnormal hemodynamic response to a fluid challenge (152). Coronary artery disease was found in 15 adults at a mean of 16 years after chest radiation (157). They had received a mean dose of 4200 cGy, and were treated at a median age of 40 years. Narrowing of the left main coronary artery was noted in 50%, with complete heart block in

25%. In general, there was a high incidence of left main and right ostial coronary disease, noted in 3 patients. One of the 3 was a 12-year-old boy who underwent mantle radiation for Hodgkin's disease 7 years earlier (152). The boy developed angina pectoris, and suffered an acute infarction with sudden death.

The incidence of symptomatic cardiac injury in children has been reported to be as high as 13% following mediastinal radiation for Hodgkin's disease (162). This has led to refinements in technique, including opposed-field methods rather than a single anterior field (163), cardiac and subcarinal blocks (161), and dose modifications. Symptomatic cardiac dysfunction is an infrequent sequela after mediastinal irradiation using equally weighted anterior-posterior fields (both treated daily) and megavoltage apparatus (154). In a more recent study by Green et al, 28 patients who had received mediastinal radiation during childhood or adolescence for Hodgkin's disease were evaluated for a median of 90 months (19 to 182) following therapy (164). The median midplane dose was 3065 cGy. All patients were asymptomatic, and all had normal cardiothoracic ratios on x-ray films. Neither the voltage nor the rhythm was abnormal on EKG, and there was no impairment of left ventricular function. Left ventricular end diastolic (LVED) volume was increased in 19% however, and left ventricular ejection fraction (LVEF) in 15%. Pericardial thickening on echocardiography was noted in 12 (43%). This finding was more frequent in patients observed > 72 months following therapy. This illustrates the importance of serial evaluation in children who have received radiation to the chest.

The anthracyclines are the most common chemotherapeutic agents implicated in the development of cardiotoxicity. Acute effects of administration includes ST-segment elevation, and atrial dysrhythmias (165). Subacute effects include the pericarditis-myocarditis syndrome caused by a large intravenous drug bolus. Chronic effects include right or left ventricular dysfunction, with cardiomyopathy. Histologic changes have been well documented. Initially, there is accumulation of contraction bands and granulation of the cytoplasm (166). Dramatic changes are also seen in nuclear and nucleolar morphology that return to normal within 24 hours after therapy (167). Focal cellular changes throughout the thickness of the left ventricular wall and intraventricular septum are chronic changes. There is vacuolar degeneration within the cytoplasm and myofibrillar loss within the myocyte (166). The exact cause of the anthracycline damage is unclear, but one theory is that free radical formation and the release of cardio/vasoactive substances mediate the damage.

The incidence of congestive heart failure and concomitant histologic damage rises with the cumulative dose of an anthracycline, but there is a great degree of variability among patients. In adults, the incidence of ADR cardiotoxicity has been reported to be 0.27% after total doses of < 550 mg/m^2 (167). The incidence of congestive heart failure (CHF), by contrast, has been reported as high as 55% in unirradiated adults receiving more than 600 mg/m^2 (158). Comprehensive long-term studies in children are lacking, but available data suggest that children, particularly those under 1 year of age (168), may be more sensitive to the effects of anthracyclines when doses exceed 300 mg/m^2 (168–171). Lower doses appear to be well tolerated in children followed for 5 or more years (28). There is a recent review of the effects of anthracyclines on children with acute lymphoblastic leukemia who had received doses of from 225 to 470 mg/m^2 (172). The most important factors contributing to the development of CHF included age and dose rate. All 12 children who developed CHF were < 7 years of age at diagnosis, and 50% were between 1 and 3. The cardiomyopathy associated with anthracycline toxicity in children is frequently fatal, but up to 80% of children can survive an acute episode of congestive failure (173). It is impossible to predict from echocardiographic evidence alone which children will recover. Biancaniello et al found that cardiac dysfunction, if it occurred, generally developed within 5 months following cessation of the anthracycline (174). Discontinuing anthracycline therapy in patients with a left ventricular shortening fraction < 20% without signs of failure resulted in an improvement in the shortening fraction.

It is well known that mediastinal RT potentiates the effects of the anthracyclines. Most of the children reported by Pratt et al who developed cardiomyopathy had also received chest irradiation (170). The newer regimens that utilize low-dose mediastinal radiation for Hodgkin's disease in conjunction with anthracyclines probably reduce the risk for cardiac complications (159), but longterm studies in children are lacking.

Additional evidence is being gathered by the Late Follow-Up Study of the National Wilms' Tumor Study (28). Questionnaire data are obtained from children surviving 5 or more years. Evans et al reported the frequency of cardiovascular abnormalities to be 2.4 for 100 person-years at risk for children who received ADR; it was 1.1 for matched counterparts who did not. Reanalysis showed that the reported cardiovascular problems, when real, often antedated ADR therapy, eliminating the apparent increase in frequency.

CP has also been implicated in cardiotoxicity after very high doses such as those used in bone marrow transplantation regimens. The cardiac histopathology is similar to that caused by the anthracyclines. The true incidence of this effect is unknown because many BMT regimens are currently in use, employing different doses of the drug with or without irradiation. Little short-term toxicity was encountered by Mason et al (175) in 28 patients given 90 mg/kg of cyclophosphamide; whereas Cazin et al reported 6 fatal cases of cardiomyopathy and/or pericarditis among 63 transplant patients who had received cyclophosphamide in addition to total-body irradiation (176). Other complications included pericarditis and arrhythmias. The potentiating effect of the total body irradiation needs to be taken into account when evaluating the effect of high-dose cyclophosphamide in transplant preoperative regimens.

Effective methods for following patients receiving anthracyclines and/or mediastinal radiation are the subject of much research. Changes on EKG have been described, and include decrease in QRS voltage, or QT interval prolongation. In one study of children, a prolongation of the QT interval preceded the decline in shortening fraction by as much as four months (177); but EKG changes in themselves are not reliable predictors of subsequent cardiomyopathy (20). Echocardiography may demonstrate decrease in left ventricular ejection fraction or end diastolic volume; and a change in the shortening fraction is often used as a signal to discontinue anthracycline therapy (178). In general, a shortening fraction less than 28% is considered abnormal. M-mode scans of contraction and thickening and thinning curves of the left posterior ventricular wall may be more sensitive indicators than shortening fraction estimation (178). Nuclear gated heart scans seem to be more reliable than echocardiography, particularly when exercise testing is introduced (179). The most sensitive means of assessing cardiac damage, however, is endomyocardial biopsy (180,181), but this has the obvious disadvantage of being an invasive procedure. It may be particularly useful in patients who have reached the tolerable limits of total cumulative dosage, but who require still more anthracyclines for optimal therapy.

Recent interest has focused on prevention of cardiotoxicity from anthracyclines. N-acetylcysteine has been proposed as a protective agent to prevent damage through quenching of doxorubicin-generated free radical formation, but it does not alter acute nuclear effects (167) or cardiomyopathy (182). Studies in both animals and humans suggest that the bispiperzinedione ICRF-187 can prevent the development of dose-related cardiac toxicity in many patients without interfering with antitumor effects (183). The mechanism is not completely understood.

Other methods to prevent cardiotoxicity include alterations of the dosing schedule or route of administration of anthracycline. Weekly regimens have been reported to have decreased toxicity (184), as have infusions over 48 to 96 hours (185). There have been no pediatric studies to document this, nor of the effects of these changes in drug delivery on the chemotherapy-radiotherapy interaction.

Considerable hope has also been attached to the use of the doxorubicin congener epirubicin. Experience in women with breast cancer is sobering (186). Total cumulative doses under 500 mg/m^2 were well tolerated, but cardiotoxicity became more frequent when doses exceeded that value. Eleven of 20 patients given more than 1000 mg/m^2 showed evidence of heart damage; seven of the 11 developed congestive heart failure, and four of the seven died. The authors did not find measurements of the left ventricular ejection fraction to be a reliable predictor of severe difficulty.

GASTROINTESTINAL TRACT AND LIVER

Pronounced mucositis is a common effect after high-dose RT of mucosal surfaces, such as the oral cavity, esophagus, and intestine. Children rarely receive doses high enough to produce these direct effects. Some chemotherapeutic agents also cause severe mucositis if given in sufficiently high doses. The combination of the two can produce extremely severe reactions, especially when AMD or ADR is added to RT. Incapacitating mucositis of the upper respiratory pathways and upper esophagus was almost universal when the combination chemotherapy of a recent IRS protocol that included ADR was used with local RT. Inability to swallow, drooling, and refusal to eat persisted for many months, even after apparent healing of the mucosa. As in other areas of the body, the most pronounced toxicity results when the drugs and RT are given at the same time, or when chemotherapy administered after completion of the RT course reactivates the latent radiation damage. The drugs usually do not "prime" the body part to increase subsequent RT toxicity. Cassady et al have reported an exception, however, in the case of the esophagus (187). Children receiving ADR prior to radiation developed severe esophagitis after RT doses that are usually well tolerated. The same may hold elsewhere in the intestine. In either event, pronounced acute enteritis, sometimes with perforation, can result. The longterm effect is a pipe-stem segment or segments of gut that had been included in the RT field. Resultant loss of function, intestinal obstruction, and impaired nutrition necessitate bowel resections and other surgical maneuvers to get around the problem area.

Several of the chemotherapeutic agents used in pediatric oncology are hepatotoxins (188). The clinical experience accumulated with such hepatotoxins as methotrexate has enabled chemotherapists to devise drug regimens that rarely produce profound or lasting liver damage. Some agents are metabolized in the liver and recirculated via reabsorption of the bile. The antitumor antibiotics and vincristine are prime examples. AMD by itself can produce a hepatotoxic picture similar to veno-occlusive disease, and vincristine has been reported to do the same (189,190). Recent experience in the NWTS appears to substantiate that children assigned to receive only postoperative AMD and vincristine develop chemical and clinical signs of hepatopathy (191–193). These toxic effects seem to have increased in recent years; the matter is discussed in greater detail elsewhere (193). Radiation therapy is a known hepatotoxin, too. Usually, doses to the whole organ in excess of 3000 cGy are needed to cause hepatic dysfunction (194). A combination of chemotherapy and RT augments the effects of either. One of the major and early signs is a selective thrombocytopenia in association with swelling of the organ, and a decrease in hepatic cell function as demonstrated by radionuclear imaging studies of function (195). These changes can be misinterpreted as evidence of metastatic disease, and the supervising physician should be aware of these physical and laboratory findings as a help in distinguishing between the two. Usually, the liver returns to normal, and the lethality rate is low; but occasionally, hepatic cirrhosis supervenes, with the secondary consequences associated with that condition (196). Splenorenal shunts have been needed in occasional patients to mitigate the risks associated with esophageal varices. The regenerating liver after partial nephrectomy is vulnerable to chemoradiation therapy effects; these have been discussed above.

URINARY TRACT*

Compensatory hypertrophy of the kidney can be adversely affected by chemotherapy and irradiation. This has been discussed under Growth and Development. The kidneys and bladder are sensitive to radiation and to different chemotherapeutic changes.

Kidneys

Radiation nephropathy is a well recognized complication of kidney irradiation, and can be expected with greater frequency when doses of 2000 cGy in 200 cGy daily

*Refer to Chapter 39 for further details of urinary tract toxicity.

fractions are exceeded (197). Until recently, most of the chemotherapeutic agents in the doses ordinarily used in pediatric oncology have not been associated with renal toxicity. Kidney damage can occur, however, when standard drugs are given in high doses. Potentially nephrotoxic drugs that fit this category include methotrexate (MTX) in gram amounts, even with citrovorum "rescue," and the nitrosoureas; e.g., BCNU or methyl CCNU in doses exceeding 1.5 g/m^2, according to Schacht et al (198,199). Cisplatinum (CDDP) and ifosfamide (IFM) are relatively recent additions to the oncologic armamentarium, and both are renal toxins (200–203). CDDP affects the glomerular unit, and IFM, the tubular component of the kidney. Cumulative doses of CDDP in excess of 1 g/m^2 can produce severe and persistent renal damage. The same is true of IFM when a total dose in the range of 100 to 120 g/m^2 is exceeded, although renal damage has been reported after lower doses. Jaffe et al have recorded impaired MTX excretion in children with osteosarcoma given high-dose MTX along with CDDP as the amounts of the latter drug accumulated (204).

CDDP and IFM given together have predictably dire results (202). It would be anticipated that superimposed RT would precipitate further difficulties. Stewart et al reported increased damage to the mouse kidney from CDDP plus radiation, but there are no substantial clinical data except for those reported in bone marrow transplantation patients (205). They, of course, receive high doses of all agents (see below). By contrast, the radiation-enhancing and reactivating agents AMD and ADR have not been associated with prohibitive renal toxicity when given in association with 1500 cGy (150 cGy/d) to the kidney. This has been established through the follow-up of NWTS-treated children, in which these chemoradiation combinations have been used over many years (28). Caution is nonetheless the key word. It is not known what would happen if higher doses of the agents mentioned were to be employed in any combination. Some hints can be derived from experience in survivors of bone marrow transplantation (BMT). Tarbell et al reported their experience with 29 such children who underwent high dose chemotherapy plus TBI for ALL or neuroblastoma (NBL) prior to BMT (206). Eleven of the 29 surviving 3 months or longer developed renal dysfunction 3 to 7 months after BMT. TBI doses ranged from 850 cGy × 1 (one pt) to 1200 to 1400 cGy in b.i.d. fractions of 175 to 216 cGy each at rates of 5 cGy/min for the one given 850 cGy and 10 cGy/min for the others. The multiple drug regimens used for ALL included tenoposide plus cytarabine plus CP; and the four drugs tenoposide, CDDP, melphalan and CP for the NBL patients, all of whom had received prior CDDP. Tarbell et al point out that the circumstances were exceptional, but the renal findings were nonetheless very similar to those associated with the acute phase of radiation nephropathy. Here, the changes were secondary to combined therapy damage in all probability (206).

Bladder

Radiation cystitis is a well-known complication after 5000 or more cGy given to the bladder, but such doses are seldom used in pediatric oncology (207). Cyclophosphamide and ifosfamide, even when covered by the uroprotector mercaptoethane sulponate (MESNA), can also result in a severely damaged bladder. Small capacity, urgency, tenesmus, and hematuria can be so pronounced from these causes as to require cystectomy for relief (208). It is disappointing that MESNA is not totally effective in preventing this devastating complication. Lower doses of RT given before or during therapy with these cytotoxic drugs often lead to bladder damage. Brugières et al described their experience in patients undergoing BMT following high-dose CP (209). Previous irradiation of the bladder was one of the predisposing factors among 19 children who had varying degrees of difficulty. Data from the Intergroup Rhabdomyosarcoma Study are similar, though cyclophosphamide preceded radiation in that study.

The proportion of children suffering disabling cystitis is nonetheless small. Few require cystectomy for intractable cystitis. Most are managed by conservative measures such as intravesical instillation of phenol, which can cause its own secondary effects, e.g., hydronephrosis because of ureteral strictures from reflux (208).

BONE MARROW TRANSPLANTATION EFFECTS

The epitome of combined chemoradiation toxicity is encountered in the regimens used to "condition" patients for bone marrow transplantation. The objective of these treatments given to children with malignant conditions is not only to suppress the immunologic response to allogeneic marrow but also to achieve total kill of the malignant cells. Therefore, both drugs and total body irradiation are often given in supralethal doses, with the infused autologous or donor bone marrow expected to "rescue" the patient, who would otherwise die of the treatments given. Beside the bone marrow, the gastrointestinal tract and the lungs are the most vulnerable tissues, but no organ or structure is spared.

Doses of more than 1000 cGy given in various fractionation schemes are well tolerated; for example, a 20% higher dose can be given in 6 individual fractions administered twice a day (nominal 200 cGy b.i.d. × 6) (210). Pulmonotoxic drugs like CP are also used in conditioning regimens, as are drugs that are radiation enhancers but are not commonly considered direct pulmonary toxins; e.g., ADR. The combination of total body irradiation and chemotherapeutic agents, even though within tolerance limits for the lung, can produce pronounced changes in other tissues and structures. An invariable result is mucositis of varying intensity affecting the mouth, throat, and gastrointestinal tract. These changes can be so pronounced as to be incapacitating when children surviving the procedure and the underlying disease become anorectic for long periods for reasons that are not entirely clear (210). The initial discomfort associated with swallowing seems to be the initiating factor. Exsanguinating bloody diarrheas require massive replacement of blood and blood components. Sometimes even this is inadequate, and death results.

Severe changes in the skin, liver, kidneys, brain, and bladder are common. An extraordinary fact is the almost total reconstitution of the affected organ systems after such massive, encompassing damage. Obviously, the choice of drugs and dose levels is critically important in achieving this happy result. Even then, growth and development are severely curtailed, and most of the surviving children fail to develop to their full height and weight potential, apparently because of hormonal dysfunctions (211–213). Sanders et al studied longterm survivors of BMT. Thyroid, pituitary and gonadal endocrinopathies were found in patients treated with high-dose cyclophosphamide (HD/CP) and TBI, but not after HD/CP alone (211). Hormonal replacement from exogenous sources alleviates some of these problems (214). Growth hormone has become available, and its efficacy in restoring normal patterns is being tested in various transplant centers.

Death can occur from compromise of any individual organ, usually the lung, but also from two or more organs failing together. The margin of safety for pulmonary toxicity after single-dose irradiation has been reported by van Dyk et al (215). They found that lung doses of 500 cGy, corrected for air transmission, resulted in 3% of pneumonopathy. An increase in dose to 1000 cGy raised the pneumonopathy rate to 80%. Those who survive display dysfunction ranging from disabling dyspnea to changes appreciable only on laboratory tests (216).

Nervous System

Cancer treatment can disrupt the central nervous system (CNS) in any of many ways (217,218). Both the brain and the spinal cord are vulnerable to the direct effects of irradiation, and some of the chemotherapeutic agents used in pediatric oncology are neurotoxins. Combinations of the two in some cases augment predictable effects; in others, unanticipated events result. The diagnosis of cancer itself can lead to psychologic upset, and to the Damocles syndrome in the longterm survivor (219). This discussion will not encompass these admittedly important aspects of cancer, but will concentrate on the more direct effects of chemoradiation on the brain and spinal cord.

First, a brief overview is needed of the effects of RT and of the various chemotherapeutic agents used in pediatrics.

There is abundant literature covering the complications caused by RT itself; these have been known for many years (220). Spinal cord effects range from transient myelopathy (Lhermitte's syndrome) to transverse myelitis (221,222). In the brain, the spectrum ranges from temporary somnolence after whole-brain RT to frank necrosis (218,220). Brain necrosis after radiation is well documented and is dose-dependent. Although there can be direct neuronal damage, it is the glial apparatus and other supporting structures that are more vulnerable. Fraction size appears to be one of the major modulating factors; less damage is produced by smaller individual cGy fractions than the same total dose attained by larger fractions. Tolerance levels for critical CNS structures in adults have been published (220,222) and their applicability to children has been assumed. Even these levels have been called into question recently insofar as the cervical cord is concerned (224,225). Also, limits are being explored in clinical trials of adults and children using b.i.d. fractionation schemes, starting with the pioneering work of the San Francisco group in brain stem tumors (226). These are based on the differential sensitivities of neural and supporting tissues, as expressed in the "neuroret" concept by Sheline (220). Doses of 100 cGy b.i.d. to totals of 6600 to 7800 cGy have not caused brain stem necrosis in the small number of patients tested. The same investigators have used this approach in children, as have others (227,228).

The list of chemotherapeutic agents responsible for similar problems grows longer. Often, the CNS adversities come as a surprise once the drugs are employed clinically and experience with humans grows. An example is the report by Kay et al in 1972 of leukoencephalopathy associated with intrathecal MTX (229). Usually reversible signs of encephalopathy, e.g., confusion, were reported by Oettgen et al after L-asparaginase was given to children (230). They can occasionally be more severe and more protracted, but are not clearly dose-related.

Interactions among some drugs coming into increased use are now also being reported. Pratt et al found that the neurotoxicity of IFM was enhanced when it followed CDDP therapy (231). These kinds of interplays make it difficult to define the role of RT when it is added to the multidrug chemotherapy regimens being explored in the treatment of brain tumor patients and other children given cranial irradiation. The analyses are further confounded when chemoradiation sequencing factors are considered. Kretschmar et al found that CDDP toxicity was not increased if the drug was given before RT, Walker and colleagues have reported enhancement of this complication when RT was given simultaneously with or before CDDP (232,234).

Of the various drugs used commonly in pediatric oncology, methotrexate (MTX) has been the one most often implicated in iatrogenic leukoencephalopathy. The anatomic bases for brain and spinal cord changes were definitively described by Price and his coworkers (234,235). Many of the reports deal with children with leukemia and are therefore clouded because of possible complicating leukemic involvement of the meninges. Some patients also had cranial RT in varying doses. Nonetheless, it is clear from patients with other malignant diseases that MTX, especially when given in high doses systemically, can lead to objective signs of leukoencephalopathy. These have been demonstrated by Fusner et al for patients with rhabdomyosarcoma (236), and by Lien et al for osteogenic sarcoma (237). Associated MTX changes range widely. Least ominous are the subtle decreases in white matter and scattered calcifications, sometimes long delayed, visible on imaging studies without clinical signs or symptoms (238). Some patients, however, develop life-threatening alterations in consciousness and focal neurologic deficits (239). These have been reversible in most cases, but not all, as was noted by Kay et al in their original report (229). Many of their affected patients received intrathecal (IT) as well as systemically administered drugs, emphasizing the importance of the IT route in producing CNS problems. The neurotoxic effects of MTX can be augmented when it is used in conjunction with radiation. The more usual pattern is a mixture of leukoencephalopathy with focal areas of necrosis. The combined effect is more marked when the two are given together, or when methotrexate follows irradiation. Cytarabine mimics many of the effects produced by MTX when given in high doses intravenously, or when administered intrathecally (240).

Agents other than MTX and cytarabine introduced into the ventricular or subarachnoid pathways can produce profound changes. Vincristine so given is lethal. There has been a report of a girl inadvertently given

ADR intrathecally (241). In 12 hours she developed nonspecific signs that progressed to major neurotoxicity including coma in 2 weeks. Fortunately these changes proved reversible.

Diffuse encephalopathy has also been reported after systemic treatments with many drugs including the nitrosoureas, CP, and recently after interleukin-2 was given to an adult (218,242). Dose-dependent neurotoxicity manifested as seizures follows busulfan in children (243).

Focal rather than diffuse neurologic and encephalopathic changes can be associated with intravenous CDDP therapy. Blindness has been reported, and deafness is common (218,244). Also well documented are peripheral manifestations including paresthesias and autonomic neuropathies resembling those associated with vincristine (218).

Cranial and spinal cord irradiation in high doses can cause brain and cord necrosis (220,222). Such high doses ($>$ 6000 cGy to the brain and $>$ 4500 cGy to the cord in daily fractions of $>$ 180 cGy) are seldom delivered to children. Lower doses can, however, augment some of the chemotherapy-associated neurologic deficits described. CDDP-related deafness is made more profound when RT includes the ear, and MTX leukoencephalopathy is worse, especially when RT is given after rather than before the MTX (234,245).

Transverse myelitis is a well-recognized sequel of radiation. An extensive review by Goldwein suggests that age, fraction size, length of cord irradiated, and total dose delivered are all relevant (223). A dose of 4500 cGy given in 150 cGy daily fractions to a few segments of the cord of an older individual is considered to be within tolerance limits. The same dose given in 250 cGy fractions to 5 or more segments of the cord of a young patient might eventually lead to transverse myelitis.

Transverse myelopathy was reported some years ago by Littman et al in two of four children (one with ependymoblastoma and three with medulloblastomas) given systemic dactinomycin in addition to standard doses of craniospinal radiation (3700 to 4000 cGy to the axis and 4500 to 5600 cGy to the posterior fossa) (246). No similar reports have followed, but a puzzling and reminiscent problem has been reported by Raney et al (247). Patients who entered in the Intergroup Rhabdomyosarcoma Study at high risk for intracranial extension received cranial $\pm$ spinal RT of 3000 cGy and intrathecal (IT) medications as well as systemic chemotherapy. Ascending myelopathy was encountered in 5 of 149 children so treated. The IT drugs were cytarabine, MTX, and hydrocortisone. The drugs given systemically were vincristine, AMD, ADR, CP $\pm$ etoposide $\pm$ CDDP. The neurologic signs did not coincide entirely with the RT fields used. Raney et al state that no additional cases have been encountered because the number of courses of IT drugs was kept to not more than 4, although the same medications were used (247). It is difficult to sort out what was responsible for the myelopathies, but the chemotherapy appears to have had played a major role because the RT doses are below tolerance levels. Transverse myelitis has been reported for both MTX and cytarabine given intrathecally without RT (240,248). The fact that Raney et al have seen no additional cases since the number of IT courses was decreased points in the same direction (247). It is still entirely possible that the three therapies interacted to produce the problem, and that the drugs used systemically were additional contributors.

Cognitive and neuro-psychologic dysfunction are among the most troublesome of the complications encountered. Radiation alone can be responsible, apparently even after very low doses. The experience reported by Ron et al is indicative (249). Israeli children who had been given scalp RT for tinea capitis were tested when they became young adults, and were found to function less well than controls. The estimated doses to the cerebral cortex were in the 100 to 200 cGy range. Many subsequent studies implicate RT alone for varying decrees of neuropsychologic difficulties demonstrated in brain tumor survivors. Neuropsychologic testing has revealed a fairly consistent pattern, more marked in children under age 6 when irradiated. Decreases in IQ, short-term memory loss, and disturbances in visual-motor integration are often seen (250–257). Other deficits can also become apparent in the children who survive doses in the 3000 to 4000 cGy range given to the whole brain. A similar dysfunctional pattern has been reported in leukemic children given lesser doses (1800 to 2400 cGy) together with systemic MTX. Such analyses are always confounded by the direct and secondary disturbances caused by the brain tumors themselves (e.g., hydrocephalus) and by surgery. Hirsch et al attempted to correct for these factors by comparing two sets of survivors of posterior fossa tumors (250). One set, those with cerebellar astrocytomas, were nonirradiated. They fared well compared with a cohort of children with medulloblastoma who had received 3500 cGy to the whole brain and spinal cord and 5000 cGy to the posterior fossa.

Children in the medulloblastoma group had varying degrees of difficulty, including IQs below 70 in about a third, and emotional and behavioral problems as well as neurologic dysfunctions. These included speech, writing, and reading disorders, and spatial disorientations. Experience with these same patients was updated by the same investigators, and the results were far from encouraging (251). The neuropsychologic problems became more severe with time. None of those surviving 10 years were normally employed, for instance, and 85% had IQs less than 80. The depth of dysfunction was inversely correlated with age at the time of treatment, especially for those under 6. Lannering et al have reported generally confirmatory data, as have others, including the age factor (252,253). Packer et al record discouraging preliminary studies of three children who were under three years of age when treated and therefore given 2400 cGy rather than 3600 cGy. Their cognitive deficits were not mitigated by the lower dose (253). It should be noted that survivors of brain tumors in general, regardless of treatment, are dysfunctional compared with sibling controls, as is made clear in the balanced report by Mostow et al (217).

Most of these confounding factors are absent in children with acute lymphocytic leukemia (ALL) given "prophylactic" cranial RT. They are usually free of neurologic problems even though subtle leukemic CNS lesions cannot be excluded from consideration. More important in evaluating the long-term effects of cranial RT given these children are the systemic and intrathecal drugs used before, during, and after RT. They are probably cofactors. At least two of the agents commonly employed—MTX and cytarabine—have their own direct effects on the brain and spinal cord (see above). Consequently, most of the voluminous literature on this topic must be considered reports of combined chemoradiation. An article by Bleyer et al points up the increase in neuropsychologic disturbances observed when both IT/MTX and 2400 cGy cranial RT are used as opposed to cranial RT alone, although both groups were affected (254). Ochs et al compared neuropsychologic function in two groups, one randomized to receive 1800 cGy cranial RT, and the other only high-dose systemic MTX for CNS "prophylaxis" (255). The deficits were comparable in the two groups. These two papers serve to emphasize the complex interplays of drugs and RT in the genesis of similar functional disorders. The reference lists of those articles should be consulted for additional reading on the topic. Of the many worthy reports, perhaps that of Meadows et al deserves special attention (256). It has particular value because it was a prospective study of 31 children with acute lymphocytic leukemia given 2400 cGy cranial RT and only 6 doses of intrathecal methotrexate. It has additional interest because the same group of investigators studied and defined the specific learning problems in affected children, and suggested remedial teaching methods (257). Meadows and her colleagues found functional deficits that could not be defined by IQ tests, as well as documenting drops in overall IQ scores (256,257). These changes required 3 or more years to become manifest, and were again age-related, being most marked in children under 6 years of age when irradiated. An earlier group of six ALL patients treated similarly at the same institution, who did not receive cranial RT, did not develop similar difficulties, nor did six Wilms' tumor patients. Of interest was the observation that the most pronounced drops in IQ (20 or more points) occurred in children with initial scores in the 110 to 130 range.

Peripheral Nerves

These are resistant to radiation therapy. Peripheral neuropathy is an accepted, reversible complication of vincristine chemotherapy. Tingling in the extremities has also been reported after CDDP therapy, and similar sensory changes are occasionally seen with other chemotherapeutic agents, especially those that are lipid-soluble. To date, no major enhancement of peripheral nerve damage has been recorded when any of these drugs are used in combination with radiation therapy in children. Direct radiation effects on relatively sensitive regions such as the brachial plexus are seldom encountered in children. This is probably because doses given to adults who eventually develop brachial plexopathy are seldom delivered to the supraclavicular regions of children, i.e., in the 6000-cGy range.

Cranial nerve dysfunctions can occur; notably, optic nerve damage has been reported in patients given 5000 to 6000 cGy of radiation to the region of the optic chiasm. The other cranial nerves seldom demonstrate damage even after relatively high doses. However, when CDDP, an ototoxic drug, is used with irradiation of the base of the skull, deafness is an almost invariable result after usually tolerable radiation doses in the 3000-cGy range (218).

Peckham et al found that, rather than global difficulties, each affected child developed a particular problem, and the level of dysfunction varied (257). Performance could be improved by tutoring and parental support.

In summary, both radiation therapy and certain anticancer drugs can produce anatomic and functional adversities. Interactions between drugs can magnify their individual effects, or produce new syndromes. Combined chemoradiation regimens can do the same, especially in the realm of neuropsychologic and cognitive difficulties.

ONCOGENESIS

Both benign and malignant neoplasms are associated with the treatments given to children with cancer.

Benign Neoplasms

These can take many forms, but the majority are of cartilaginous origin. Exostoses (osteochondromas) (Fig. 38– 3) are the most common benign lesion following irradiation. They accounted for 19 of the 47 benign conditions (40%) encountered by Evans et al. in their report of the Late Follow-up Study component of the NWTS (28). All but two were in irradiated fields. Other benign lesions reported by Evans et al include 12 nevi,

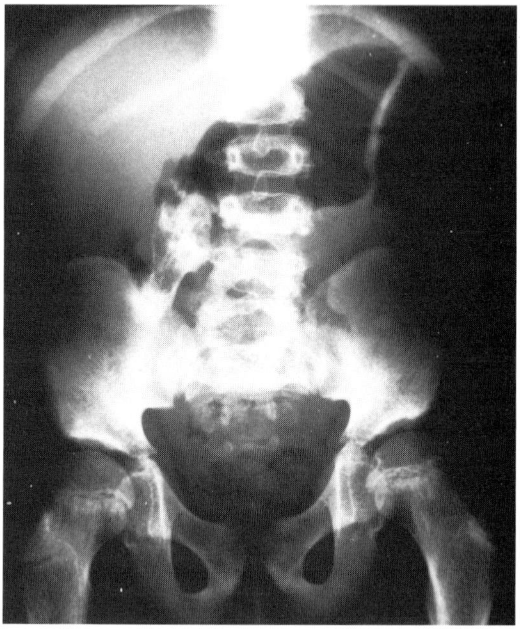

Fig. 38–3. X-ray film: lumbar spine and pelvis. There is a large exostosis (osteochondroma) arising from the region of the right sacroiliac joint. This bony outgrowth interfered with lateral bending; it was amputated at the base, which solved the problem.

seven lipomas and other soft tissue lesions, two breast nodules, two thyroid adenomas, and five assorted others. Ten of the 28 (36%) were not in the RT portals, including one of the two thyroid nodules. The cause-and-effect relationships are therefore more tenuous than is the case for exostoses. Evans and colleagues found no influence of the chemotherapies used in the NWTS, viz., dactinomycin, vincristine, and doxorubicin.

Simple surgical excision suffices for the control of most of these lesions. When an osteochondroma interferes with function because of impingement on adjacent structures at a joint, amputation at the base is indicated. Malignant degeneration in these lesions is very rare, if it ever occurs.

Histologically benign tumors in the brain and its coverings, as well as in the parotid and thyroid glands, have been reported after low-dose RT. One such report is by Modan et al, who followed children given scalp RT for tinea capitis (258). An excess number of meningiomas and tumors of the brain and the parotid and the thyroid glands were found in the treated patients compared with their siblings and case controls. The estimated doses ranged from 6.5 cGy to the thyroid to 140 cGy to the surface of the brain. This experience has updated by Ron et al insofar as tumors of the nervous system are concerned, and both benign and malignant lesions continue to be identified (259).

Except for that of Evans et al, there is no systematic study of treatment-associated benign tumors where the possible influence of anticancer chemotherapy can be assessed; none was apparent in their report as noted above (28).

Malignant Neoplasms

There have been numerous reports of second malignant neoplasms (SMNs) developing in long-term survivors of childhood cancer (260–263). RT has been implicated in many cases (260–264). The RT-associated SMNs include examples of virtually every species of cancer, ranging from brain tumors through leukemia and sarcomas to epithelial growths (260).

Members of the Late Effects Study Group (LESG) and their collaborators, and others before them, have issued several reports of the second malignant neoplasms (SMNs) encountered in long-term survivors of childhood cancer. The study by Miké et al was based on 15,000 children with cancer (260).

A sevenfold increase in the risk of developing an SMN in the first 5 years after treatment was found (when the general pediatric population cancer incidence rates were used for comparison). The risk rose to 10 for 5- to 15-year survivors. The investigators ascribe the initial sevenfold risk to the increased susceptibility to malignant disease of cancer patients, especially those with predisposing conditions such as the hereditary forms of retinoblastoma and Wilms' tumor, and to the phacomatosis (260,264). Miké et al suggest that the rise to the tenfold level might be caused by the therapy given. In fact, almost three out of four of the SMNs developed in irradiated tissues. Sarcomas of the supporting structures, i.e., bone and soft tissues, were the most frequent SMNs encountered (N = 39), even though retinoblastoma (RBL) survivors were excluded from the study, and the association between bone sarcomas and familial RBL is well known. Cancers of the thyroid were also frequent (N = 17), reflecting the sensitivity of this gland to RT oncogenesis; leukemias followed (N = 13). Miké and colleagues could not address the RT-chemotherapy interaction issue, but an earlier LESG report based on some of the same study population had done so. There it was found that dactinomycin (AMD)—an oncogen in animal systems—appeared to decrease the risk of RT-associated SMNs by a factor of 7 (265). Subsequent reports from the LESG and others have failed to substantiate the "protective" effect of AMD. It is nonetheless intriguing to note the decreased frequency of acute nonlymphoblastic leukemia in ABVD*-treated adults with Hodgkin's disease, whether irradiated or not (266). The ABVD drug combination contains doxorubicin, which shares some of the same RT interactions as AMD, as pointed out earlier.

A few other reports suggest either a protective or enhancing relationship between RT and the drugs commonly used in pediatric oncology. Strong et al. found that intensive chemotherapy appeared to augment the cumulative risk of osteosarcoma developing in the irradiated bones of Ewing's tumor survivors (267). It was estimated to be 25% over 20 years for patients treated primarily with RT, and 70% over 10 years for those given combined therapy. Moreover, the SMN appeared after a shorter latent period. The alkylating agent CP and the mitotic inhibitor vincristine were the two drugs implicated by them. Alkylating agents as well as RT were documented by the LESG to increase the risk of SMNs in bone in a dose-response relationship (267). Irradiated children had a 1.7-fold increase in risk, rising to 40-fold for those receiving more than 6000 cGy. The relative risk ascribed to alkylating agents was 4.7; it increased with cumulative drug dose. No other anticancer drugs used shared in osteooncogenesis, nor was there any apparent interaction between RT and alkylators.

Newton et al of the LESG have reviewed these issues (269). Their report confirms the relevance of RT in the genesis of bone sarcomas as SMN, but not the independent role

*A = Adriamycin, B = bleomycin, V = vincristine, D = dacarbazine.

of alkylators. They found that anthracyclines, and perhaps alkylating drugs, too, shortened the latent period to the appearance of the SMN. Although they could not demonstrate any enhancing RT oncogenic effect, they postulate that ". . . agents that shorten the interval to SMN must play a role in the carcinogenic process, whether it be as initiators, promoters, or cocarcinogens." Such a role for the anthracycline doxorubicin is given some support by the observations made by Tucker et al in a study of SMNs, where the drug appeared to be an independent, albeit not strong, leukemogen (270).

In summary, no compelling data indicate that any chemotherapeutic agent or combination of agents either augments or protects against the undisputed carcinogenic effects of irradiation. The possible exception is the special case of Hodgkin's disease (HD). Many reports describe secondary acute nonlymphoblastic leukemia (ANLL) and "solid" cancers of various histologies. It is well to keep these separate.

It should be recalled that, for some years, ANLL in HD patients was considered to be caused by RT, which was the only treatment available in that era (270). RT has been exonerated in more recent reviews (266,271). Cimono et al for example, record their experience with different chemoradiation regimens (266). They find, as did Valagussa et al. before them, that the agents in MOPP, namely, mechlorethamine, Oncovin, procarbazine, and prednisone, appear to be the offenders (273). Because ANLL is found rarely in HD patients before or concomitant with the diagnosis of HD, and because ANLL was recognized before the advent of chemotherapy, it seems indisputable that the two diseases are intrinsically associated. By this construct, some treatments can be said to suppress the appearance of the leukemia more effectively than others. The notion that any therapy *causes* ANLL must be accepted with caution. Tucker et al found no difference in the risk of leukemia in adults given multidrug regimens with and without RT, for example (274).

Solid tumors are a separate matter. The LESG reports that the risk of bone tumors in children surviving HD is higher than that of leukemia and that skin and thyroid cancers are also frequent, thus following the general tendencies in all long-term survivors of childhood cancer (275).

Before concluding this section, a word must be said about the second cancers appearing in immunocompromised children, such as those who survive bone marrow transplantation. Lymphomas predominate in patients who are immunodeficient for whatever reason, so that chemoradiation plays an indirect although initiating role under such circumstances (276).

REFERENCES

1. Waterhouse DO, Meadows AT. Late effects of childhood cancer therapy. *In:* Complications of Cancer Management. Plowman PN, McElwain T, Meadows A (Eds). Oxford, Butterworth, 1991, p. 95.
2. Silber JH, Littman PS, Meadows AT. Stature loss following skeletal irradiation for childhood. J Clin Oncol 8:304, 1990.
3. Meadows AT, Krejmas NL, Belasco JB. The medical cost of cure. Sequelae in survivors of childhood cancer. *In:* Status of the Curability of Childhood Cancer. van Eys J, Sullivan MP (Eds). New York, Raven Press, 1980, p. 263.
4. Phillips TL, Fu KK. Quantification of combined radiation therapy and chemotherapy effects on critical normal tissues. Cancer 37:1186, 1976.
5. D'Angio GJ, Farber S, Maddock CL. Potentiation of x-ray effects by actinomycin-D. Radiology 73:175, 1959.
6. Donaldson SS, Glick J, Wilbur J. Adriamycin activating a recall phenomenon after radiation therapy (Letter). Ann Intern Med 81:407, 1974.
7. Green DM, Finklestein JZ, Tefft ME, Norkool P. Diffuse interstitial pneumonitis after pulmonary irradiation for metastatic Wilms' tumor. Cancer 63:450, 1989.
8. McInerney DP, Bullimore J. Reactivation of radiation pneumonitis. Br J Radiol 73:175, 1977.
9. Cassady JR, Richter MP, Prio AJ, Jaffe N. Adriamycin interactions. Preliminary clinical observations. Cancer 36:946, 1975.
10. Stewart JR, Fajardo LF, Cohn KE, et al. Experimental radiation-induced heart disease in rabbits. Radiology 91:814, 1968.
11. Makinen K, Makipernaa A, Rautonen J, et al. Long-term cardiac sequelae after treatment of malignant tumors with radiotherapy or cytostatics in childhood. Cancer 65:1913, 1990.
12. Meadows AT, Gordon J, Massari DJ, et al. Declines in IQ scores and cognitive dysfunc-

tion in children with acute lymphocytic leukaemia treated with cranial irradiation. Lancet ii:1015, 1981.
13. Perthes G. Ueber den einfluss der roentgenstrahlen auf epithelial gewebe insbensondere auf das carcinom. Archiv Fuer Klinische Chirurgie 71:955, 1903.
14. Neuhauser EBD, Wittenborg MH, Berman CZ, Cohen J. Irradiation effects of roentgen therapy on the growing spine. Radiology 59:637, 1952.
15. Littman PS, D'Angio GJ. Growth considerations in the radiation therapy of children with cancer. Ann Rev Med 30:405, 1979.
16. Rate WR, Butler MS, Robertson WW Jr, D'Angio GJ. Late orthopedic effects in children with Wilms' tumor treated with abdominal irradiation. Med Pediatr Oncol 19:265, 1991.
17. Hahn EW, Feingold S, D'Angio GJ. A study of the equivalent single irradiation dose for growing bone in rats. (Abstract). Proc Am Assoc Cancer Res 14:95, 1973.
18. Tefft M, Lattin PB, Jereb B, et al. Acute and late effects on normal tissue following combined chemo-radiotherapy for childhood rhabdomyosarcoma and Ewing's sarcoma. Cancer 137:1201, 1976.
19. Jaffe N, Toth BB, Hoar RE, et al. Dental and maxillofacial abnormalities in long-term survivors of childhood cancer. Effects of treatment with chemotherapy and radiation to the head and neck. Pediatrics 73:816, 1984.
20. Fromm M, Littman P, Raney RB, et al. Late effects after treatment of twenty children with soft tissue sarcomas of the head and neck. Cancer 57:2070, 1986.
21. Maguire A, Craft AW, Evans RGB, et al. The long-term effects of treatment on the dental condition of children surviving malignant disease. Cancer 60:2570, 1987.
22. Tefft M, Mitus A, Das L, et al. Irradiation of the liver in children. Review of experience in the acute and chronic phases, and in the intact normal and partially resected. Am J Roentgenol 108:365, 1970.
23. Sagerman RH, Berdon WE, Baker D. Renal atrophy without hypertension following abdominal irradiation in infants and children. Ann Radiol 12:278, 1969.
24. Donaldson SS, Moskowitz PS, Canty EL, Efron B. Radiation-induced inhibition of compensatory renal growth in the weanling mouse kidney. Radiology 128:491, 1978.
25. Moskowitz PS, Donaldson SS. Chemotherapy-induced inhibition of compensatory renal growth in the immature mouse. Am J Roentgenol 134:491, 1980.
26. Resnick MI, Albert DJ, Persky L. Inhibition of compensatory renal hypertrophy with Mithromycin. J Urol 108:194, 1972.
27. Finklestein JZ, Norkool P, Green DM, et al. Diastolic hypertension in Wilms' tumor survivors. A late effect of treatment? A report from the National Wilms' Tumor Study Group. Am J Clin Oncol (In Press).
28. Evans AE, Norkool P, Evans I, et al. Late effects of treatment for Wilms' tumor. A report from the National Wilms' Tumor Study Group. Cancer 67:331, 1991.
29. Fuks Z, Glatstein E, Marsha GW, et al. Long-term effects of external radiation on the pituitary and thyroid glands. Cancer 37:1152, 1976.
30. Costin G. Effects of low-dose cranial radiation on growth hormone secretory dynamics and hypothalamic-pituitary function. Am J Dis Child 142:847, 1988.
31. Packer RJ, Meadows AT, Rorke LB, et al. Long-term sequelae of cancer treatment on the central nervous system in childhood. Med Pediatr Oncol 15:241, 1987.
32. Green DM, D'Angio GJ. Late Effects of Treatment for Childhood Cancer. New York, Wiley-Liss, 1992.
33. Ash P. The influence of radiation on fertility in man. Br J Radiol 53:535, 1983.
34. Chapman RM. Effect of cytotoxic therapy on sexuality and gonadal function. Semin Oncol 9:84, 1982.
35. Joblon S. The late effects of acute external exposure to ionizing radiation in man. Radiat Res 59:146, 1974.
36. Maguire LC, Dick FR, Sherman BM. The effects of antileukemic therapy on gonadal histology in adult males. Cancer 48:1967, 1981.
37. Shalet SM. Effects of cancer chemotherapy on gonadal function of patients. Cancer Treat Rev 7:141, 1980.
38. Shapiro E, Kinsella TJ, Makuch RW, et al. Effects of fractionated irradiation on endocrine aspects of testicular function. J Clin Oncol 3:1232, 1985.
39. Leiper AD, Grant DB, Chessells JM. The effect of testicular irradiation on Leydig cell function in prepubertal boys with acute lymphoblastic leukaemia. Arch Dis Child 58:906, 1983.
40. Blatt J, Sherins RJ, Niebrugge D, et al. Leydig cell function in boys following treatment for testicular relapse of acute lymphoblastic leukemia. J Clin Oncol 3:1227, 1985.
41. Rowley MJ, Leach DR, Warner GA, Heller CG. Effect of graded doses of ionizing radiation on the human testis. Rad Res 59:665, 1974.
42. Lushbaugh CC, Casarett GW. The effects of gonadal irradiation in clinical radiation therapy: A review. Cancer 37:1111, 1976.

43. Pedrick TJ, Hoppe RT. Recovery of spermatogenesis following pelvic irradiation for Hodgkin's disease. Int J Radiat Oncol Biol Phys 12:117, 1986.
44. Speiser B, Rubin P, Casarett G. Aspermia following lower truncal irradiation in Hodgkin's disease. Cancer 32:692, 1973.
45. Blatt J, Poplack DG, Sherins RJ. Testicular function in boys after chemotherapy for acute lymphoblastic leukemia. N Engl J Med 304:1121, 1981.
46. Brauner R, Czernichow P, Cramer P, et al. Leydig-cell function in children after direct testicular irradiation for acute lymphoblastic leukemia. N Engl J Med 309:25, 1983.
47. Shalet SM, Beardwell CG, Jacobs NS. Testicular function following irradiation of the human prepubertal testis. Clin Endocrinol 9:483, 1978.
48. Kinsella TJ, Trirette G, Rowland J, et al. Long-term follow-up of testicular function following radiation therapy for early-stage Hodgkin's disease. J Clin Oncol 7:718, 1989.
49. Byrne J, Mulvihill JJ, Myers MH, et al. Effects of treatment on fertility in long-term survivors of childhood or adolescent cancer. N Engl J Med 317:1315, 1987.
50. Penso J, Lippe B, Ehrlich R, et al. Testicular function in prepubertal and pubertal male patients treated with cyclophosphamide for nephrotic syndrome. J Pediatr 84:831, 1974.
51. Rapola J, Kodkimies O, Huttunen NP, et al. Cyclophosphamide and the pubertal testis. Lancet i:88, 1973.
52. Pennisi AJ, Crushkin CM, Lieberman E. Gonadal function in children with nephrosis treated with cyclophosphamide. Am J Dis Child 129:315, 1975.
53. Etteldorf JN, West CD, Pitcock JA, et al. Gonadal function, testicular meiosis following cyclophosphamide therapy in patients with nephrotic syndrome. J Pediatr 88:206, 1976.
54. Buchanan JD, Fairley KF, Barrie JU. Return of spermatogenesis after stopping cyclophosphamide therapy. Lancet i:156, 1975.
55. Aubier F, Flamant F, Brauner R, et al. Male gonadal function after chemotherapy for solid tumors in childhood. J Clin Oncol 7:304, 1989.
56. Jaffee N, Sullivan MP, Ried H, et al. Male reproductive function in long-term survivors of childhood cancer. Med Ped Oncol 16:241, 1988.
57. Shalet SM, Hann IM, Lendon M, et al. Testicular function after combination chemotherapy in childhood for acute lymphoblastic leukaemia. Arch Dis Child 56:275, 1981.
58. Sieber SM, Adamson RH. Toxicity of antineoplastic agents in man: Chromosomal aberrations, antifertility effects, cogenital malformations and carcinogenic potential. Adv Cancer Res 22:57, 1975.
59. Sieber SM, Correa P, Dalgard W, et al. Carcinogenic and other adverse effects of procarbazine in nonhuman primates. Cancer Res 38:2125, 1978.
60. Sherins RJ, Olweny CLM, Ziegler JL. Gynecomastia and gonadal dysfunction in adolescent boys treated with combination chemotherapy for Hodgkin's disease. N Engl J Med 299:12, 1978.
61. Whitehead E, Shalet SM, Morris Jones PH, et al. Gonadal function after combination chemotherapy for Hodgkin's disease in childhood. Arch Dis Child 47:287, 1982.
62. Lendon M, Hamm IM, Palmer MK, et al. Testicular histology after combination chemotherapy in childhood acute lymphoblastic leukaemia. Lancet ii:439, 1978.
63. Lilleyman JS. Male fertility after successful chemotherapy for lymphoblastic leukaemia. Lancet ii:1125, 1979.
64. Lu CC, Meistrich ML. Cytotoxic effects of chemotherapeutic drugs on mouse testis cells. Cancer Res 39:3575, 1979.
65. deCunha MF, Meistrich ML, Reid HL, et al. Effect of chemotherapy on human sperm production. Proc Am Assoc Cancer Res 20:100, 1979.
66. Baker TG. Radiosensitivity of mammalian oocytes with particular reference to the human female. Am J Obstet Gynceol 110:746, 1971.
67. Himelstein-Braw R, Peters H, Faber M. Influence of irradiation and chemotherapy on the ovaries of children with abdominal tumours. Br J Cancer 36:269, 1977.
68. Stillman RJ, Schinfeld JS, Schiff I, et al. Ovarian failure in long-term survivors of childhood malignancy. Am J Obstet Gynecol 139:62, 1981.
69. Hamre MR, Robison LL, Nesbit ME, et al. Effects of radiation on ovarian function in long-term survivors of childhood acute lymphoblastic leukemia: A report from the CCSG. J Clin Oncol 5:1759, 1987.
70. Shalet SM, Beardwell CG, Jones PH, et al. Ovarian failure following abdominal irradiation in childhood. Br J Cancer 33:655, 1976.
71. LeFloch O, Donaldson SS, Kaplan HS. Pregnancy following oophoropexy and total nodal irradiation in women with Hodgkin's disease. Cancer 38:2263, 1976.
72. Baker JW, Morgan RL, Peckham MJ, et al. Preservation of ovarian function in patients requiring radiotherapy for para-aortic and pelvic Hodgkin's disease. Lancet 1:1307, 1972.
73. Chiu J, Drummon KN. Long-term follow-up of cyclophosphamide therapy in frequent re-

lapsing minimal lesion nephrotic syndrome. J Pediatr 84:825, 1974.
74. DeGrott GW, Faiman C, Winter JSD. Cyclophosphamide and the prepubertal gonad: A negative report. J Pediatr 84:123, 1977.
75. Miller JJ, Williams GF, Leissring JC. Multiple late complications of therapy with cyclophosphamide, including ovarian destruction. Am J Med 50:530, 1971.
76. Warne GL, Fairley KF, Hobbs JB, et al. Cyclophosphamide induced ovarian failure. N Engl J Med 289:1159, 1973.
77. Kumar R, Biggart JD, McEvoy, et al. Cyclophosphamide and reproductive function. Lancet ii:1212, 1972.
78. Himelstein-Braw R, Peters H, Faber M. Morphological study of the ovaries of leukaemic children. Br J Cancer 38:82, 1978.
79. Siris ES, Leventhal BG, Vailukaitis JL. Effects of childhood leukemia and chemotherapy on puberty and reproductive function in girls. N Engl J Med 294:1143, 1976.
80. Shalet SM, Beardwell CG, Twomey JA, et al. Endocrine function following the treatment of acute leukemia in childhood. J Pediatr 90:920, 1977.
81. Chapman RM, Sutcliff SB, Malpas JS. Cytotoxic-induced ovarian failure in women with Hodgkin's disease. I. Hormone function. JAMA 242:1877, 1979.
82. Horning SJ, Hoppe RT, Kaplan HS, et al. Female reproductive potential after treatment for Hodgkin's disease. N Engl J Med 304:1377, 1981.
83. Schilsky RL, Sherins RJ, Hubbard SM, et al. Long term follow-up of ovarian function in women treated with MOPP chemotherapy for Hodgkin's disease. Am J Med 71:552, 1981.
84. Whitehead E, Shalet SM, Blackledge G, et al. The effect of combination chemotherapy on ovarian function in women treated for Hodgkin's disease. Cancer 52:988, 1983.
85. Johnson SA, Goldman JM, Hawkins DF. Pregnancy after chemotherapy for Hodgkin's disease. Lancet ii:93, 1979.
86. Holmes GE, Holmes FF. Pregnancy outcome of patients treated for Hodgkin's disease. Cancer 41:1317, 1978.
87. Thomas PR, Winstanley D, Peckham MJ. Reproductive and endocrine function in patients with Hodgkin's disease: effects of oophoropexy and irradiation. Br J Cancer 33:226, 1976.
88. Andrieu JM, Ochoa-Molina ME. Menstrual cycle, pregnancies and offspring before and after MOPP therapy for Hodgkin's disease. Cancer 52:435, 1983.
89. Green DM, Hall B. Pregnancy outcome following treatment during childhood or adolescence for Hodgkin's disease. Ped Hematol Oncol 5:269, 1988.
90. Estiu M. Successful pregnancy in leukaemia. Lancet i:433, 1977.
91. Reynoso EE, Shepard FA, Messner HA, et al. Acute leukemia during pregnancy: The Toronto Leukemia Study Group experience with long-term follow-up of children exposed in utero to chemotherapeutic agents. J Clin Oncol 5:1098, 1987.
92. Li FP, Gimbrere K, Gelber RD, et al. Outcome of pregnancy in survivors of Wilms' tumor. JAMA 257:216, 1987.
93. Byrne J, Mulvilhill JJ, Connelly RR, et al. Reproductive problems and birth defects in survivors of Wilms' tumor and their relatives. Med Ped Oncol 16:233, 1988.
94. Blatt J. Mulvihill JJ, Ziegler JL, et al. Pregnancy outcome following cancer chemotherapy. Am J Med 69:828, 1980.
95. Lewis EB. Possible genetic consequences of irradiation of tumors in childhood. Radiology 114:147, 1975.
96. Kaplan H. Genetic effects in children and grandchildren, or women treated for infertility and sterility by roentgen therapy. Report of a study of thirty-three years. Radiology 72:518, 1959.
97. Hoshino T, Lato H, Finch SC, et al. Leukemia in offspring of atomic bomb survivors. Blood 30:719, 1967.
98. Rappaport R, Brauner R, Czernichow P, et al. Effect of hypothalamic and pituitary irradiation on pubertal development in children with cranial tumors. J Clin Endocrinol Metab 54:1164, 1982.
99. Brown IH, Lee TJ, Eden OB, et al. Growth and endocrine function after treatment for medulloblastoma. Arch Dis Child 58:722, 1983.
100. Ahmed SR, Shalet SM, Campbell RA, et al. Primary gonadal damage following treatment of brain tumors. J Pediatr 103:562, 1983.
101. Clayton PE, Shalet SM, Price DA, et al. Testicular damage after chemotherapy for childhood brain tumors. J Pediatr 112:922, 1988.
102. Clayton PE, Shalet SM, Price DA, et al. Ovarian function following chemotherapy for childhood brain tumors. Med Pediatr Oncol 17:92, 1989.
103. Sanders JE, Buckner CD, Amos D, et al. Ovarian function following marrow transplantation for aplastic anemia or leukemia. J Clin Oncol 6:813, 1988.
104. Sanders JE, Pritchard S, Mahoney P, et al. Growth and development following marrow transplantation for leukemia. Blood 88:1129, 1986.

105. Hoppe RT. The management of Stage II Hodgkin's disease with a large mediastinal mass. A prospective program emphasizing irradiation. Int J Radiat Oncol Biol Phys 11:349, 1985.
106. Gross NJ. Pulmonary effects of radiation therapy. Ann Intern Med 86:81, 1977.
107. Isaacs RD, Wattie WJ, Wells AU, et al. Massive haemoptysis as a later consequence of pulmonary irradiation. Thorax 42:77, 1987.
108. Fulkerson WJ, McLendon RE, Prosnitz LR. Adult respiratory distress syndrome after limited thoracic radiotherapy. Cancer 57:1941, 1986.
109. Libshitz HI, Shuman LS. Radiation-induced pulmonary change: CT findings. J Comp Assoc Tomogr 8:15, 1984.
110. Mah K, Poon PY, van Dyk J, et al. Assessment of acute radiation-induced pulmonary changes using computed tomography. J Comp Assoc Tomogr 10:736, 1986.
111. McGivern ND, Bullimore J, Hill J, Davies ER, Goddard P. Diagnostic imaging of post-irradiation changes in the chest. Clin Radiol 39:109, 1988.
112. Donaldson SS, Kaplan HS. Complications of treatment of Hodgkin's disease in children. Cancer Treat Rep 66:977, 1982.
113. Kinsella TJ, Fraaxx BA, Glatstein E. Late effects of radiation therapy in the treatment of Hodgkin's disease. Cancer Treat Rep 66:991, 1982.
114. Kadota RP, Burgert EO, Driscoll DJ, Gilchrist GS. Cardiopulmonary function in long-term survivors of childhood Hodgkin's lymphoma: A pilot study. Mayo Clin Proc 63:362, 1988.
115. Smith LM, Mendenhall NP, Cicale MN, et al. Results of a prospective study evaluating the effects of mantle irradiation on pulmonary function. Int J Radiat Oncol Biol Phys 16:79, 1989.
116. Morgan GW, Freeman AP, McLean RG, et al. Late cardiac, thyroid and pulmonary sequelae of mantle radiotherapy for Hodgkin's disease. Int J Radiat Oncol Biol Phys 11:1925, 1985.
117. Wohl MEB, Griscom NT, Traggis DG, Jaffe N. Effects of therapeutic irradiation delivered in early childhood upon subsequent lung function. Pediatrics 55:507, 1975.
118. Miller RW, Fusner JE, Fink RJ, et al. Pulmonary function abnormalities in long-term survivors of childhood cancer. Med Pediatr Oncol 14:202, 1986.
119. Makipernaa A, Heino M, Laitnen LA, Siimes MA. Lung function following treatment of malignant tumors with surgery, radiotherapy, or cyclophosphamide in childhood. Cancer 63:625, 1989.
120. Littman P, Meadows AT, Polgar G, et al. Pulmonary function in survivors of Wilms' tumor. Cancer 37:2773, 1976.
121. Benoist MR, Lemerle J, Jean R, et al. Effects of pulmonary function of whole lung irradiation for Wilms' tumor in children. Thorax 37:175, 1982.
122. Kinsella JP, Brasch RC, Ablin AA. Unilateral hypoplasia of the hemithorax causing "pseudoscoliosis" after lung irradiation in a child with Wilms' tumor. Pediatr Radiol 15:340, 1985.
123. Thomas PRM, Tefft M, D'Angio GJ, Norkool P. Acute toxicities associated with radiation in the second National Wilms' Tumor Study. J Clin Oncol 6:1694, 1988.
124. Green DA, Finklestein JZ, Tefft ME, Norkool P. Diffuse interstitial pneumonitis after pulmonary irradiation for metastatic Wilms' tumor. Cancer 63:450, 1989.
125. Serota FT, August CS, Koch PA et al. Pulmonary function in patients undergoing bone marrow transplantation. Med Pediatr Oncol 12:137, 1984.
126. Cardozo BL, Zoetelieff H, van Bekkum DW, et al. Lung damage following bone marrow transplantation: The contribution of irradiation. Int J Radiat Oncol Biol Phys 11:907, 1985.
127. Sutedja YG, Apperley JF, Hughes JMB, et al. Pulmonary function after bone marrow transplantation for chronic myeloid leukaemia. Thorax 42:163, 1988.
128. Thomas ED. Total body irradiation for marrow grafting. Int J Radiat Oncol Biol Phys 19:1285, 1990.
129. Ginsburg SJ, Comis RL. The pulmonary toxicity of antineoplastic agents. Semin Oncol 9:34, 1982.
130. Adamson IYR, Bowden DH. The pathogenesis of bleomycin-induced pulmonary fibrosis in mice. Am J Pathol 77:185, 1974.
131. Pascual RS, Mosher MB, Sikand RS, et al. Effects of bleomycin on pulmonary function in man. Am Rev Resp Dis 108:211, 1973.
132. Comis RL. Bleomycin pulmonary toxicity. *In:* Bleomycin Current Status and New Developments. Carter SK, Crooke ST (Eds). New York, Academic Press, 1978, p. 279.
133. Miller R, Fusner J, Fink R, et al. Pulmonary function abnormalities in long-term survivors of childhood cancer. Med Pediatr Oncol 14:202, 1986.
134. Sikic BI, Collins JM, Mimnaugh EG, Gram TE. Improved therapeutic index of bleomycin when administered by continuous infusion in mice. Cancer Treat Rep 62:2011, 1978.

135. Bauer KA, Skarin AT, Balikian JP, et al. Pulmonary complications associated with combination chemotherapy programs containing bleomycin. Am J Med 74:557, 1983.
136. Samuels ML, Johnson DE, Holoye PY, Lanzotti VJ. Large-dose bleomycin therapy and pulmonary toxicity. JAMA 235:1117, 1976.
137. Mefferd JM, Donalson SS, Link MP. Pediatric Hodgkin's disease: Pulmonary, cardiac, and thyroid function following combined modality therapy. Int J Radiat Oncol Biol Phys 16:679, 1989.
138. Phillips TL, Wharam MD, Margolis LW. Modification of radiation injury to normal tissues by chemotherapeutic agents. Cancer 35:1678, 1975.
139. Concannon JP, Dalbow MH, Hagemann RF, et al. Radiation and actinomycin D mortality studies in C57BL/6 mice. II. Combined treatment and gastrointestinal lethality. Cancer 32:5533, 1973.
140. Wara WM, Phillips TL, Margolis LW, Smith V. Radiation pneumonitis: A new approach to the derivation of time-dose factors. Cancer 32:547, 1973.
141. McIvery DP, Bullimore J. Reactivation of radiation pneumonitis by adriamycin. Br J Radiol 50:224, 1977.
142. Cohen IJ, Loven D, Schoenfeld T, et al. Dactinomycin potentiation of radiation pneumonitis: A forgotten interaction. Pediatr Hematol Oncol 8:187, 1991.
143. Weinstein AS, Diener-West M, Nelson DF, Pakuris E. Pulmonary toxicity of carmustine in patients treated for malignant glioma. Cancer Treat Rep 70:943, 1986.
144. Littler WA, Ogilvie C. Lung function in patients receiving busulphan. Br Med J 4:530, 1970.
145. O'Driscoll RN, Haselton PS, Taylor PM, et al. Active lung fibrosis up to 17 years after chemotherapy with carmustine (BCNU) in childhood. N Engl J Med 323:378, 1990.
146. Ginsberg SJ, Comis RL. The pulmonary toxicity of antineoplastic agents. Semin Oncol 9:34, 1982.
147. Baker WJ, Fistel SJ, Jones RV, Weiss RB. Interstitial pneumonitis associated with ifosfamide Therapy. Cancer 65:2217, 1990.
148. Steward JR, Fajardo LF. Radiation-induced heart disease: An update. Prog Cardiovasc Dis 27:173, 1984.
149. Applefeld MM, Wiernik PH. Cardiac disease after radiation therapy for Hodgkin's disease: Analysis of 48 patients. Am J Cardiol 51:1679, 1983.
150. Brosins FC III, Waller BF, Roberts WC. Radiation heart disease: Analysis of 16 young (aged 15 to 33) necropsy patients who received over 3,500 cGy to the heart. Am J Med 70:519, 1981.
151. Gomez SA, Park JJ, Panahon AM, et al. Heart size and function after radiation therapy to the mediastinum in patients with Hodgkin's disease. Cancer Treat Rep 67:1099, 1983.
152. Totterman KJ, Pesonen E, Siltanen P. Radiation-related chronic heart disease. Chest 83:875, 1983.
153. Cohen SI, Bharati S, Glass J, Lev M. Radiotherapy as a cause of complete atrioventricular block in Hodgkin's disease. Arch Intern Med 141:676, 1981.
154. Corn BW, Trock BJ, Goodman RL. Irradiation-related ischemic heart disease. J Clin Oncol 8:741, 1990.
155. Mittal B, Deutsch M, Thompson M, Lee Dameshek H. Radiation-induced accelerated coronary arteriosclerosis. Am J Med 81:183, 1986.
156. Radwaner BA, Geringer R, Goldmann AM, et al. Left main coronary artery stenosis following mediastinal irradiation. Am J Med 82:1017, 1987.
157. McEniery PT, Dorosti K, Schiavone WA, et al. Clinical and angiographic features of coronary artery disease after chest irradiation. Am J Cardiol 60:1020, 1987.
158. Gottdiener JS, Katin MJ, Borer JS, et al. Late cardiac effects of therapeutic mediastinal irradiation. N Engl J Med 308:569, 1987.
159. Pohjola-Sintonen S, Totterman K, Salmo M, Siltanen P. Late cardiac effects of mediastinal radiotherapy in patients with Hodgkin's disease. Cancer 60:31, 1987.
160. LaMonte CS, Yeh SDJ, Straus DJ. Long-term follow-up of cardiac function in patients with Hodgkin's disease treated with mediastinal irradiation and combination chemotherapy including doxorubicin. Cancer Treat Rep 70:439, 1986.
161. Perrault DJ, Levy M, Herman JD, et al. Echocardiographic abnormalities following cardiac radiation. J Clin Oncol 3:546, 1985.
162. Carmel RJ, Kaplan HS. Mantle irradiation in Hodgkin's disease. An analysis of technique, tumor eradication, and complications. Cancer 37:2813, 1976.
163. Coltart RS, Roberts JT, Thom CH, Petch MC. Severe constrictive pericarditis after single 16MeV anterior mantle irradiation for Hodgkin's disease. Lancet 1:488, 1985.
164. Green DM, Gingell RL, Pearce J, et al. The effect of mediastinal irradiation on cardiac function of patients treated during childhood and adolescence for Hodgkin's disease. J Clin Oncol 5:239, 1987.
165. Minow RA, Benjamin RS, Gottlieb JA. Adriamycin (NSC-123127) cardiomyopathy. An

overview with determination of risk factors. Cancer Chemother Rep 6:195, 1975.
166. Kantrowitz NE, Bristow MR. Cardiotoxicity of antitumor agents. Prog Cardiovasc Dis 27:195, 1984.
167. Unverferth JB, Magorien RD, Balcerzak SP, et al. Early changes in human myocardial nuclei after doxorubicin. Cancer 52:215, 1983.
168. Mosijczuk AD, Ruymann FB, Mease AD, Bernier RD. Anthracycline cardiomyopathy in children. A report of two cases. Cancer 44:1582, 1979.
169. von Hoff DD, Rozencweig M, Layard M, et al. Daunomycin-induced cardiotoxicity in children and adults. Am J Med 62:200, 1977.
170. Pratt CB, Ransom JL, Evans WE. Age-related adriamycin cardiotoxicity in children. Cancer Treat Rep 62:1381, 1978.
171. Smith PH, Ekert H, Waters KD, et al. Letter: High incidence of cardiomyopathy in children treated with adriamycin and DTIC in combination chemotherapy. Cancer Treat Rep 61:1736, 1977.
172. Sallan SE, Clavell LA. Cardiac effects of anthracyclines used in the treatment of childhood acute lymphoblastic leukemia: A 10-year experience. Semin Oncol 11:19, 1984.
173. Goorin AM, Borow CM, Goldman A, et al. Congestive heart failure due to adriamycin cardiotoxicity: Its natural history in children. Cancer 47:2810, 1981.
174. Biancaniello T, Meyer RA, Wong KY, et al. Doxorubicin cardiotoxicity in children. J Pediatr 97:45, 1980.
175. Mason JW, Bristow MR, Billingham ME, Daniels JR. Invasive and noninvasive methods of assessing adriamycin cardiotoxic effects in man: Superiority of histopathologic assessment using endomyocardial biopsy. Cancer Treat Rep 62:857, 1978.
176. Cazin B, Gorin NC, Laporte JP, et al. Cardiac complications after bone marrow transplantation. Cancer 57:2061, 1986.
177. Bender KS, Shematex JP, Leventhal BG, Kan JS. QT interval prolongation associated with anthracycline cardiotoxicity. J Pediatr 105:442, 1984.
178. Goldberg SJ, Hutter JJ, Feldman L, Goldberg SM. Two sensitive echocardiographic techniques for detecting doxorubicin toxicity. Med Pediatr Oncol 11:172, 1983.
179. Ritchie JL, Singer JW, Thaming D, et al. Anthracycline cardiotoxicity: Clinical and pathologic outcomes assessed by radionuclide ejection fraction. Cancer 46:1109, 1980.
180. Pegelow CH, Popper RW, deWit SA, et al. Endomyocardial biopsy to monitor anthracyline therapy in children. J Clin Oncol 2:443, 1984.
181. Billingham ME, Mason JW, Bristow MR, Daniels JR. Anthracycline cardiomyopathy monitored by morphologic changes. Cancer Treat Rep 62:865, 1978.
182. Doroshaw JH, Locker GY, Ifrim I, Myers CE. Prevention of doxorubicin cardiac toxicity in the mouse by N-acetylcysteine. J Clin Invest 68:1053, 1981.
183. Speyer JL, Green MD, Kramer E, Rey M, et al. Protective effect of the bispiperazinedione ICRF-187 against doxorubicin-induced cardiac toxicity in women with advanced breast cancer. N Engl J Med 319:745, 1988.
184. Weiss AJ, Metter GE, Fletcher WS, et al. Studies on adriamycin using a weekly regimen demonstrating its clinical effectiveness and lack of cardiac toxicity. Cancer Treat Rep 60:813, 1976.
185. Legha SS, Benjamin RS, Mackay B, et al. Reduction of doxorubicin cardiotoxicity by prolonged continuous intravenous infusion. Ann Intern Med 96:133, 1982.
186. Jain KK, Casper ES, Geller NL, et al. A prospective randomized comparison of epirubicin and doxorubicin in patients with advanced breast cancer. J Clin Oncol 3:818, 1985.
187. Cassady JR, Richter MP, Piro AJ, Jaffe N. Radiation–adriamycin interactions: Preliminary clinical observations. Cancer 36:946, 1975.
188. Zimmerman HJ. Hepatotoxic effects of oncotherapeutic agents. *In:* Popper H, Schaffner F (Eds). Progress in liver diseases, Philadelphia, Grune & Stratton, 1986, p. 621.
189. Oberlin O, Tournade MF, Daltroff G, et al. Hepatic toxicity compatible with veno-occlusive disease (VOD) after actinomycin D in non-irradiated Wilms' tumor. (Abstract). Med Pediatr Oncol 17:317, 1989.
190. Bhannon RA, Miller DG, Diamond HD. Vincristine in treatment of lymphomas and leukemias. Cancer Res 23:613, 1963.
191. Green DM, Finklestein JZ, Norkool P, et al. Severe hepatic toxicity after treatment with single-dose dactinomycin and vincristine. Cancer 62:270, 1988.
192. D'Angio GJ. Hepatotoxicity and actinomycin D. Lancet i:1290, 1990 (letter).
193. Green DM, Norkool P, Breslow NE, et al. Severe hepatic toxicity after treatment with vincristine and dactinomycin using single-dose or divided dose schedules. A report from the National Wilms' tumor study. J Clin Oncol 8:1525, 1990.
194. Ingold JA, Reed GB, Kaplan HS, Bagshaw MA. Radiation hepatitis. Am J Roentgenol 93:200, 1965.
195. Tefft M, Traggis D, Filler RM. Liver irradiation in children. Acute changes with tran-

sient leukopenia and thrombocytopenia. Am J Roentgenol 106:750, 1969.
196. Reed GB Jr, Cox AJ Jr. Human liver after radiation injury: form of veno-occlusive disease. Am J Pathol 48:597, 1966.
197. Rubin P. Law and order of radiation sensitivity. Absolute versus relative. tolerance of normal tissues. Front Radiat Ther Oncol 23:7, 1989.
198. Abelson HT, Fosburg MT, Beardsley GP, et al. Methotrexate-induced renal impairment. Clinical studies and rescue from systemic toxicity with high-dose leucovorin and thymidine. J Clin Oncol 1:208, 1983.
199. Schacht RG, Feiner HD, Gallo GR, et al. Nephrotoxicity of nitrosoureas. Cancer 48:1328, 1981.
200. Vogelzang NJ. Nephrotoxicity from chemotherapy. Prevention and management. Oncology 5:97, 1991.
201. Dentino M, Luft FC, Moo NY, et al. Long term effect of cisdiamminedichloride platinum (CDDP) on renal function and structure in man. Cancer 41:1274, 1978.
202. Goren MP, Wright RK, Pratt CB, et al. Potentiation of ifosfamide neurotoxicity. Hematotoxicity and tubular nephrotoxicity by prior cis-diamminedichloroplatinum (II) therapy. Cancer Res 47:1457, 1987.
203. Groth S, Neilsen H, Sorensen JB, et al. Acute and long-term nephrotoxicity of cis-platinum in man. Cancer Chemother Pharmacol 17:191, 1986.
204. Jaffe N, Keifer R, Robertson R, et al. Renal toxicity with cumulative doses of cis-diammine-dichloroplatinum-II in pediatric patients with osteosarcoma. Cancer 59:1577, 1987.
205. Stewart FA, Bartelink H, van der Voet GB, de Wolff FA. Renal damage in mice after sequential cisplatin and irradiation. The influence of prior irradiation on platinum elimination. Radiother Oncol 21:277, 1991.
206. Tarbell NJ, Guinan EC, Chin KL, et al. Renal insufficiency after total body irradiation for pediatric bone marrow transplantation. Radiother Oncol 1 (Suppl):139, 1990.
207. Cox R. II. Treatment by 2 MeV x rays. A contribution to the symposium on "Treatment of Carcinoma of the Bladder" at the British Institute of Radiology. January 14, 1960.
208. Ross AJ III, O'Neill JA. Surgical emergencies. *In:* Practical Pediatric Oncology. D'Angio GJ, Sinniah D, Meadows AT, et al (Eds). London, Edward Arnold, 1992, p. 64.
209. Brugières L, Hartmann O, Travagli JP, et al. Hemorrhagic cystitis following high dose chemotherapy and bone marrow transplantation in children with malignancies. Incidence, clinical course, and outcome. J Clin Oncol 7:194, 1989.
210. Kamani NR, August CS. Management of problems of bone marrow transplantation. *In:* Practical Pediatric Oncology. D'Angio GJ, Sinniah D, Meadows AT, et al (Eds). London, Edward Arnold, 1992, p. 114.
211. Sanders JE. Late effects in children receiving total body irradiation for bone marrow transplantation. Radiother Oncol 1(Suppl):82, 1990.
212. Sanders JE, Buckner CD, Leonard JM, et al. Late effects on gonadal function of cyclophosphamide, total-body irradiation, and marrow transplantation. Transplantation 36:252, 1983.
213. Leiper AD, Stanhope R, Lau T, et al. The effect of total body irradiation and bone marrow transplantation during childhood and adolescence on growth and endocrine function. Br J Haematol 67:419, 1987.
214. Carter MC, Thompson EI, Simone JV. The survivors of childhood solid tumors. Pediatr Clin North Am 38:505, 1991.
215. van Dyk J, Keane TJ, Kan S, et al. Radiation pneumonitis following large single dose irradiation. A re-evaluation based on absolute dose to lung. Int J Radiat Oncol Biol Phys 7:461, 1981.
216. Serota FT, August CS, Koch PA, et al. Pulmonary function in patients undergoing bone marrow transplantation. Med Pediatr Oncol 12:137, 1984.
217. Mostow EN, Byrne J, Connelly RR, Mulvihill JJ. Quality of life in long-term survivors of CNS tumors of childhood and adolescence. J Clin Oncol 9:592, 1991.
218. Packer RJ, Meadows AT, Rorke LB, et al. Long-term sequelae of cancer treatment on the central nervous system in childhood. Med Pediatr Oncol 15:241, 1987.
219. Koocher GP, O'Malley JE. The Damocles Syndrome: Psychosocial consequences of surviving childhood cancer. New York, McGraw-Hill, 1981.
220. Sheline GE. Irradiation injury of the human brain: A review of clinical experience. *In:* Radiation Damage to the Nervous System. Gilbert MA, Kagan AR (Eds)., New York, Raven Press, 1980, p. 39.
221. Jones A. Transient radiation myelopathy (with reference to Lhermitte's sign of electrical paresthesia). Br J Radiol 37:727, 1964.
222. Abbatucci JS. Radiation myelopathy of the cervical spinal cord: Time, dose and volume factors. Int J Radiat Oncol Biol Phys 4:239, 1978.
223. Goldwein JW. Radiation myelopathy: A review. Med Pediatr Oncol 15:89, 1987.

224. Marcus RB Jr., Million RR. The incidence of myelitis after irradiation of the cervical spinal cord. Int J Radiat Oncol Biol Phys 19:3, 1990.
225. Schultheiss TE. Spinal cord radiation "tolerance": Doctrine vs. data. Editorial. Int J Radiat Oncol Biol Phys 19:219, 1990.
226. Linstadt DE, Edwards SB, Prados M, et al. Hyperfractionated irradiation for adults with brainstem gliomas. Int J Radiat Oncol Biol Phys 20:757, 1991.
227. Wara WM, Edwards MSB, Levin VA, et al. A new treatment regimen for brainstem glioma: A pilot study of the Brain Tumor Research Center and Childrens Cancer Study Group (Abstract). Int J Radiat Oncol Biol Phys 12(S1):143, 1985.
228. Packer RJ, Littman PA, Sposto RM, et al. Results of a pilot study of hyperfractionated radiation therapy for children with brain stem gliomas. Int J Radiat Oncol Biol Phys 13:1647, 1987.
229. Kay HEM, Knapton PJ, O'Sullivan JP, et al. Encephalopathy in acute leukaemia associated with methotrexate therapy. Arch Dis Child 47:344, 1972.
230. Oettgen HF, Stephenson PA, Schwartz, MK, et al. Toxicity of E. coli L-asparaginase in man. Cancer 25:253, 1970.
231. Pratt CB, Marshall PG, Meyer WH, et al. Ifosfamide neurotoxicity is related to previous cisplatin treatment for pediatric solid tumors. J Clin Oncol 8:1399, 1990.
232. Kretschmar CS, Warren MP, Lavally BL, et al. Ototoxicity of preradiation cisplatin for children with central nervous system tumors. J Clin Oncol 8:1191, 1990.
233. Walker DA, Pillow J, Waters KD, Keir E. Enhanced cis-platinum ototoxicity in children with brain tumors who have received simultaneous or prior cranial irradiation. Med Pediatr Oncol, 17:48, 1989.
234. Price RA, Jamieson PA. The central nervous system in childhood leukemia II. Subacute leukoencephalopathy. Cancer 35:306, 1978.
235. Price RA, Birdwell DA. The central nervous system in childhood leukemia. III. Mineralizing microangiopathy and dystrophic calcification. Cancer 42:717, 1978.
236. Fusner JE, Poplack DG, Pizzo PA, Di Chiro G. Leukoencephalopathy following chemotherapy for rhabdomyosarcoma: Reversibility of cerebral changes demonstrated by computed tomography. J Pediatr 91:77, 1977.
237. Lien HH, Blomlie V, Saeter G, et al. Osteogenic Sarcoma: MR signal abnormalities of the brain in asymptomatic patients treated with high-dose methotrexate. Radiology 179:547, 1991.
238. Riccardi R, Brouwers P, Di Chiro, G, Poplack DG. Abnormal computed tomography brain scans in children with acute lymphoblastic leukemia: Serial long-term follow-up. J Clin Oncol 3:12, 1985.
239. Packer RJ, Grossman RI, Belasco JB. High dose systemic methotrexate-associated acute neurologic dysfunction. Med Pediatr Oncol 11:159, 1983.
240. Baker WJ, Royer GL Jr, Weiss RB. Cytarabine and neurologic toxicity. J Clin Oncol 9:679, 1991.
241. Arico M, Nespoli L, Porta F, et al. Severe acute encephalopathy following inadvertent intrathecal doxorubicin administration. Med Pediatr Oncol 18:261, 1990.
242. Vecht CJ, Keohane C, Menon RS, et al. Acute fatal leukoencephalopathy after interleukin-2 therapy (Letter to Editor). N Engl J Med 321:1146, 1990.
243. Vassal G, Deroussent A, Hartmann O, et al. Dose-dependent neurotoxicity of high-dose busulfan in children: A clinical and pharmacological study. Cancer Res 50:6203, 1990.
244. Ruiz L, Gilden J, Jaffe N, et al. Auditory function in pediatric osteosarcoma patients treated with multiple doses of cis-diamminedichloroplatinum (II). Cancer Res 49:742, 1990.
245. Granowetter I, Rosenstock JG, Packer RJ. Enhanced cisplatinum neurotoxicity in pediatric patients with brain tumors. J Neuro Oncol 1:293, 1983.
246. Littman P, Rosenstock JG, Bailey C. Radiation myelitis following craniospinal irradiation with concurrent actinomycin-D therapy. Med Pediatr Oncol 5:145, 1978.
247. Raney RB, Tefft, Heyn R, et al. Ascending myelitis after intensive chemotherapy and radiation therapy in children with cranial parameningeal sarcoma. Cancer 69:1498, 1992.
248. Thompson SW, Saiki J, Kornfeld M. Paraplegia following intrathecal antileukemic therapy. Proc Am Acad Neurol 21:454, 1971.
249. Ron E, Modan B, Flor S, et al. Mental function following scalp irradiation. Am J Epidemiol 116:149, 1982.
250. Hirsch JF, Reinier D, Czernichow P, et al. Medulloblastoma in childhood. Survival and functional results. Acta Neurochir 48:1, 1979.
251. Hoppe-Hirsch E, Reinier D, Lellouch-Tubiana A, et al. Medulloblastoma in childhood: Progressive intellectual deterioration. Child Nerv Syst 6:60, 1990.
252. Lannering B, Ildiko M, Lundberg A, Olsson E. Long-term sequelae after pediatric brain tumors: Their effect on disability and quality of life. Med Pediatr Oncol 18:304, 1990.

253. Packer RJ, Sutton LN, Atkins TE, et al. A prospective study of cognitive function in children receiving whole-brain radiotherapy and chemotherapy: 2-year results. J Neurosurg 70:707, 1989.
254. Bleyer WA, Fallavollita J, Robison L, et al. Influence of age, sex and concurrent intrathecal methotrexate therapy on intellectual function after cranial irradiation during childhood: A Report from the Children's Cancer Study Group. Pediatr Hematol Oncol 7:329, 1990.
255. Ochs J, Mulhern R, Fairclough D, et al. Comparison of neuropsychologic functioning and clinical indicators of neurotoxicity in long-term survivors of childhood leukemia given cranial radiation or parenteral methotrexate: A prospective study. J Clin Oncol 9:145, 1991.
256. Meadows AT, Gordon J, Massari DJ, et al. Declines in IQ scores and cognitive dysfunctions in children with acute lymphocytic leukaemia treated with cranial irradiation. Lancet ii:1015, 1981.
257. Peckham VC, Meadows AT, Bartel N, Marrero O. Educational late effects in long-term survivors of childhood acute lymphocytic leukemia. Pediatrics 81:127, 1988.
258. Modan B, Baidatz D, Mart H, et al. Radiation-induced head and neck tumours. Lancet i:277, 1974.
259. Ron E, Modan B, Boice JD, et al. Tumors of the brain and nervous system after radiotherapy in childhood. N Engl J Med 319:1033, 1988.
260. Miké V, Meadows AT, D'Angio GJ. Incidence of second malignant neoplasms in children. Results of an international study. Lancet ii:1325, 1982.
261. Tucker MA, Meadows AT, Boice JD, et al. Cancer risk following treatment of childhood cancer. *In:* Radiation Carcinogenesis: Epidemiology and Biological Significance. Boice JD, Fraumeni JF (Eds). New York, Raven Press, 1984, p. 211.
262. Hawkins MM, Draper GJ, Kingston JL. Incidence of second primary tumours among childhood cancer survivors. Br J Cancer 56:339, 1987.
263. Kingston JE, Hawkins MM, Draper GJ, et al. Patterns of multiple primary tumours in patients treated for cancer during childhood. Br J Cancer 56:331, 1987.
264. Draper GJ, Sanders BM, and Kingston JE. Second primary neoplasms in patients with retinoblastoma. Br J Cancer 53:661, 1986.
265. D'Angio GJ, Meadows A, Miké V, et al. Decreased risk of radiation associated second malignant neoplasms in actinomycin-D treated patients. Cancer 37(Suppl):1177, 1976.
266. Cimino G, Papa G, Tura S, et al. Second primary cancer following Hodgkin's disease. Updated results of an Italian multicentric study. J Clin Oncol 9:432, 1991.
267. Strong LC, Herson J, Osborne BM, Sutow WW. Risk of radiation-related subsequent malignant tumors in survivors of Ewing's sarcoma. J Natl Cancer Inst 62:1401, 1979.
268. Tucker MA, D'Angio GJ, Boice JD Jr, et al. Bone sarcomas linked to radiotherapy and chemotherapy in children. N Engl J Med 317:588, 1987.
269. Newton WA, Meadows AT, Shimada H, et al. Bone sarcomas as second malignant neoplasms following childhood cancer. Cancer 67:193, 1991.
270. Tucker MA, Meadows AT, Boice JD Jr, et al. Leukemia after therapy with alkylating agents for childhood cancer. J Natl Cancer Inst 78:459, 1987.
271. Rosner F. Acute leukemia as a delayed consequence of cancer chemotherapy. Cancer 37:1033, 1976.
272. Kaldor JM, Day NE, Clarke EA, et al. Leukemia following Hodgkin's disease. N Engl J Med 322:7, 1990.
273. Valagussa P, Santoro A, Kenda R, et al. Second malignancies in Hodgkin's disease. A complication of certain forms of treatment. Br Med J 280:216, 1980.
274. Tucker MA, Coleman CN, Cox RS, et al. Risk of second malignancies after treatment for Hodgkin's disease. N Engl J Med 317:76, 1988.
275. Meadows AT, Obringer AC, Marrero O, et al. Second malignant neoplasms following childhood Hodgkin's disease. Treatment and splenectomy as risk factors. Med Pediatr Oncol 17:477, 1989.
276. Penn I. Cancers complicating organ transplantation. N Engl J Med 1323:767, 1990.

Chapter 39

GENITOURINARY TOXICITY*

KEVIN P. BARTON AND RICHARD L. SCHILSKY

RENAL TOXICITY

Renal dysfunction is a frequent complication of cancer and its therapy. Abnormalities of renal function may result from tumor infiltration of the renal parenchyma (1), ureteral or urethral obstruction, tumor lysis syndrome (2) accompanied by hyperuricemia and extreme hyperphosphatemia (3), or, rarely, xanthine nephropathy (4) following allopurinol therapy. Many tumor-associated nephropathies result from the toxic effects of paraproteins (5), immune-complexes, lysozymuria (6), and hypercalcemia. The renal function of cancer patients is often further compromised by hypotension, sepsis, intravascular volume depletion, or the use of other nephrotoxic drugs such as the aminoglycosides, amphotericin B, or cyclosporin A.

This section will review the renal toxicity of chemotherapy, radiotherapy, and combined chemoradiation.

Chemotherapy-Induced Nephritis

Cisplatinum

Cisplatinum (cis-diammine dichloroplatinum II) is an inorganic platinum coordination complex that is effective in treatment of many human tumors. Its renal toxicity was quickly recognized in preclinical and early clinical studies (7,8). Cisplatinum is excreted primarily via the kidney. In animals, it undergoes an initial distribution phase with a half-life of less than 1 hour followed by a slower elimination phase with a half-life of one to several days (9). Approximately 50% of a dose is excreted within 4 hours and 76% within 48 hours. Cisplatinum is highly bound to serum proteins.

The precise mechanism of cisplatinum's renal toxicity remains unclear. Although changes in both the proximal and distal tubules have been observed in animals, the major finding in humans following treatment with cisplatinum is necrosis of the distal tubules and collecting ducts (10,11). Despite our incomplete understanding of the mechanism of cisplatinum's renal toxicity, many methods have been developed to minimize toxicity.

CLINICAL MANIFESTATIONS

Renal toxicity, manifested as an elevated serum BUN and creatinine, is common at some point during the course of therapy in most patients receiving cisplatinum. Toxicity appears to be related to both cumulative dose and dose intensity. Rossof and colleagues reported a serum BUN greater than 25 mg/dL in 6 of 25 patients who received 50 mg/m^2 , and in all who received 200 mg/m^2 (12). Serum BUN and creatinine are less sensitive indicators of cisplatinum renal toxicity than the 24-hour urine creatinine clearance. Dentino and colleagues reported a mean fall in creatinine clearance from 112 to 62 mL/minute accompanied by only modest elevations in BUN and creatinine (10). Several investigators have examined excretion of uri-

*Editor's note: The authors have described toxicity to the kidney, urinary bladder, and gonads separately. Description of each site is further elaborated to cover the unique toxicities related to chemotherapy, radiotherapy, and chemoradiation. Some chemotherapy-related toxicities described here may be discussed in some detail in Part II of this book, particularly in Chapters 8 and 9. Chapter 34 on gynecologic toxicity may provide additional insights into ovarian toxicity.

nary enzymes as an indicator of cisplatinum renal toxicity (13–15). Excretion of N-acetyl-β-D-glucosaminidase, alanine aminopeptidase, leucine aminopeptidase, β-glucuronidase, and β_2-microglobulin may be increased in the days following cisplatinum treatment. The increased excretion of these enzymes may correlate with cisplatinum-induced renal tubular dysfunction, but has not been correlated with changes in creatinine clearance.

Cisplatinum frequently produces hypomagnesemia (16), which is sometimes associated with hypocalcemia, and hypokalemia. Hypomagnesemia occurred in 26 of 30 patients (87%) who received cisplatinum along with vinblastine and bleomycin for germ cell tumors, and has been reported to persist for months to years following completion of therapy (17,18).

MANAGEMENT

Hydration with intravenous saline and mannitol to achieve a brisk diuresis following administration of cisplatinum has resulted in decreased toxicity in both animals and man (19–22). The drug should be prepared and administered in hypertonic or normal saline. Renal toxicity is increased in animals treated with cisplatinum that is prepared and administered in distilled water (9,23). Ozols and colleagues demonstrated safe administration of high dose cisplatinum with hypertonic saline (24), although protection of the kidneys may have been the result of the brisk saline diuresis employed rather than the use of hypertonic solutions. The use of hydration, mannitol, and hypertonic saline are believed to decrease nephrotoxicity by decreasing the time of exposure of the renal tubules and collecting ducts to free platinum and by maintaining a high chloride environment in the renal tubules to prevent activation of the drug.

Several investigators have examined the use of furosemide to decrease cisplatinum renal toxicity, and conflicting results have been obtained (25–27). Ostrow and colleagues demonstrated no difference in renal toxicity between patients receiving saline and mannitol and those receiving saline and furosemide (28). Indeed, some studies in animals suggest that furosemide may increase the nephrotoxicity of cisplatinum.

Sodium thiosulfate given intravenously was effective in protecting against renal toxicity in a group of patients with ovarian carcinoma treated with intraperitoneal cisplatinum at doses up to 270 mg/m^2 (29). The concept of "systemic protection" with thiosulfate in the setting of intraperitoneal chemotherapy is appealing. Many other agents including diethyl dithiocarbamate (30), an experimental radioprotective agent, WR-2721 [S-2-(3-amino propylamino) ethylphosphorothioic acid] (31), probenecid (32), and verapamil (33) have been proposed as agents for preventing cisplatinum associated nephrotoxicity. Further studies will be necessary to determine if the clinical use of these agents can improve the therapeutic index of cisplatinum.

Carboplatin

Carboplatin (CBDCA, NSC 241240, diamminecyclobutane dicarboxylatoplatinum, or JM 8) is a second-generation platinum analog. Phase I studies have revealed myelosuppression, particularly thrombocytopenia, as the dose-limiting toxicity (34–36). No significant changes in renal function were seen at the highest tolerated doses. Histopathologic changes are not seen in the kidneys of rats given the LD_{10} dose of carboplatin (37). The role of carboplatin in clinical oncology is presently being defined by ongoing clinical trials. However, it is the preferred agent for patients with underlying renal dysfunction, although dose modification may be required to prevent severe thrombocytopenia in the setting of decreased creatinine clearance.

Methotrexate

Methotrexate (MTX) is an antimetabolite that exerts its cytotoxic effects through inhibition of dihydrofolate reductase. MTX is excreted via renal elimination with over 90% of a standard intravenous dose appearing unchanged in the urine (38). Renal toxicity occurs primarily in patients receiving high-dose MTX (50 to 250 mg/kg IV over 6 hours). Pitman and colleagues reported a rise in serum creatinine by 50% over baseline in 60% of patients within 24 hours after high-dose MTX (39).

During high-dose MTX therapy, there is extensive metabolism of MTX to 7-hydroxymethotrexate (7-OH MTX) (40,41). 7-OH MTX may account for as much as 33% of the MTX appearing in the urine 24 to 48 hours after high-dose therapy. Both MTX and 7-OH MTX are poorly soluble in acidic aqueous solutions, with 7-OH MTX being 3- to 5-fold less soluble than MTX. The renal toxicity of high-dose MTX appears to be mediated primarily by precipitation of MTX and 7-OH MTX in the renal tubules and collecting ducts during production of acid urine (42).

Pathologic changes seen in MTX renal toxicity include necrosis of the proximal renal tubules (43).

MANAGEMENT

The renal toxicity of MTX can be minimized by brisk diuresis and urinary alkalinization during drug administration (44). Renal failure or renal insufficiency secondary to MTX is generally transient, with recovery after 2 to 3 weeks. During the recovery period, MTX elimination may be significantly impaired and plasma levels must be monitored closely. Leucovorin must be administered until plasma MTX levels are below 5×10^{-8} M to protect against severe bone marrow and mucosal toxicity.

Cyclophosphamide and Ifosfamide

Cyclophosphamide and ifosfamide are alkylating agents of the oxazaphosphorine group. These compounds undergo hepatic activation to 4-hydroxyoxazophosphorines, followed by conversion to phosphoramide mustard and acrolein. These alkylating metabolites are renally excreted and are felt to produce both the renal toxicity and urotoxic effects of these drugs (45). The urotoxicity of these agents, hemorrhagic cystitis, will be discussed later in this chapter.

The primary nephrotoxic effect of cyclophosphamide is inappropriate water retention (46–48). This syndrome occurs shortly after cyclophosphamide administration and generally resolves within 24 hours. It is presumed to be mediated by a direct toxic effect of the alkylating metabolites of cyclophosphamide on the distal renal tubules and collecting ducts. Antidiuretic hormone (ADH) may play a role in this syndrome, but its significance is incompletely understood. Furosemide may prevent this toxicity (49).

Ifosfamide occasionally causes severe renal toxicity (50–52). Cohen and colleagues reported elevations of serum BUN to 30 mg/dL in 2 of 14 patients who received doses of 5000 to 7000 mg/m^2 (52). Adult Fanconi's syndrome with progressive renal failure has been described in a patient who received 8 courses of ifosfamide infusions of 8 g/m^2 (53). The nephrotoxicity of ifosfamide appears to be mediated primarily via its 4-hydroxy metabolite, acrolein, and other metabolites (44).

MANAGEMENT

Methods to minimize the nephrotoxicity and urotoxicity of ifosfamide include hydration, urinary acidification, and the use of sulfhydryl compounds such as MESNA and N-acetyl cysteine (45). Sodium-2-mercaptoethane-sulforate (MESNA) is able to completely abrogate the glomerular and tubular necrosis seen in mice given an LD_{10} dose of ifosfamide (50,54). However, its protective effect in humans is largely limited to bladder protection, with no protection against renal toxicity of ifosfamide.

Nitrosoureas

The nitrosoureas, 1,3 bis (2 chloroethyl)-1-nitrosourea (BCNU), 1-(2-chloroethyl)-3-cyclohexyl-1-nitrosourea (CCNU), and 1-(2-chloroethyl)-3-(4-methyl cyclohexyl)-1-nitrosourea (methyl CCNU), are highly lipid-soluble compounds that have alkylating activity.

Preclinical studies demonstrated azotemia in three of four animals given CCNU at a dose of 240 mg/m^2. This azotemia developed more than 3 weeks following therapy and examination of the kidneys revealed interstitial fibrosis (55).

In man, renal toxicity has been a late, insidious event. It occurs primarily in patients who receive multiple courses of therapy with total doses of BCNU or methyl CCNU in excess of 1500 mg/m^2 (56). Schacht and colleagues noted the absence of signs of renal toxicity by urinalysis, or serum chemistries during therapy (56). Harmon and colleagues have reported a decrease in renal size during therapy with methyl CCNU in children (57). Renal tissue is often histologically normal in patients who die from progressive cancer shortly after receiving one or two courses of nitrosourea therapy. Renal tissue from patients with established renal toxicity demonstrates tubular atrophy, interstitial fibrosis with infiltration by chronic inflammatory cells, and glomerular sclerosis (56). Progressive renal dysfunction may develop despite discontinuation of nitrosoureas in patients with early renal dysfunction. The risk of late progressive toxicity must be considered in any decision to give a large cumulative dose of a nitrosourea.

Streptozotocin is a glycosylated nitrosourea that produces nephrotoxicity as its dose-limiting toxicity. Broder and Carter reported evidence of renal toxicity in 65% of patients with 11% having fatal renal toxicity (58). Unlike the other nitrosoureas, streptozotocin frequently produces transient reversible proteinuria as an early manifestation of renal toxicity. Other reported effects of streptozotocin include Fanconi's syndrome, proximal renal tubular acidosis, and hypokalemia (51,59). Renal tissue in patients with streptozotocin toxicity generally shows a diffuse tubulointerstitial nephritis and tubular atrophy (60). Although toxicity may occur at lower doses, severe nephrotoxicity is unusual at doses less than 1.5 g/m^2/week. Discontinuation of streptozotocin upon recognition of proteinuria or a decreasing creatinine clearance may allow recovery of normal renal function.

Mitomycin C

Mitomycin C is an antitumor antibiotic that has been implicated as the cause of an unusual syndrome of renal failure and microangiopathic hemolytic anemia (MAHA) (61–63). This syndrome appears to occur in a dose-dependent manner (61). Valavaara and Nordman reported renal toxicity in 1 of 63 patients (1.6%) who received less than 50 mg/m^2 mitomycin C, 4 of 37 (10.8%) who received 50 to 69 mg/m^2 and 5 of 18 (27.8%) who received more than 70 mg/m^2 (61). Clinically, there is an abrupt onset of azotemia, proteinuria, microscopic hematuria, and hypertension along with the microangiopathic anemia and thrombocytopenia. Pathologic changes in the kidney include fibrin thrombi in the glomeruli, glomerular sclerosis, renal cortical necrosis, and tubulointerstitial atrophy (63–65). This syndrome may be the result of renal endothelial cell injury by the drug (66). Treatment of the nephrotoxicity of mitomycin C has generally been disappointing. Steroids, heparin, and platelet inhibitors have been used without success (64). The value of plasma exchange is controversial.

Mithramycin

Mithramycin is an antitumor antibiotic that inhibits DNA-directed RNA synthesis. Azotemia occurred in 22 of 54 (40%) patients given 25 to 50 μg/kg/day for 5 consecutive days (67). Pathologic changes in the kidney include necrosis of the proximal and distal renal tubules. The mechanism of mithramycin renal toxicity is unclear. However, the drug is now used primarily for treatment of hypercalcemia, and the doses employed are unlikely to cause significant nephrotoxicity.

Interferons

The interferons are naturally occurring glycoproteins that mediate a wide range of biologic responses, including antiviral, antiproliferative, and cytotoxic effects. The interferons undergo glomerular filtration followed by reabsorption and catabolism in the renal tubules (68). The renal toxicity of α interferon consists primarily of proteinuria (69), enzymuria (70), and occasional reports of interstitial nephritis and nephrotic syndrome (71,72).

Averbuch and colleagues reported a patient with mycosis fungoides who developed nephrotic range proteinuria (28 g) during treatment with leukocyte A interferon (100 million units IM three times per week). Renal biopsy revealed normal glomeruli but extensive interstitial infiltrate composed predominantly of lymphocytes, eosinophils, and plasma cells. Tubular dilatation and focal degeneration and necrosis of proximal tubular cells were also observed (71). Kramer and colleagues reported that 8 of 8 renal transplant patients who received recombinant DNA leukocyte A interferon as prophylactic antiviral therapy developed steroid-resistant acute rejection episodes (73). The mechanism of interferon renal toxicity remains unclear.

Interleukin-2

Interleukin-2 (IL-2, T-cell growth factor) is a glycoprotein that is produced by activated T-cells, and mediates immunoregulatory phenomena. Some degree of acute renal dysfunction was observed in over 90% of patients receiving high doses of IL-2 or IL-2/LAK (lymphokine-activated killer cells) (74). Infusions of IL-2 or IL-2/LAK were associated with hypotension, fluid retention, azotemia, oliguria, and low fractional sodium excretion. Renal function returned to baseline within 7 days in 62% of patients, within 14 days in 84%, and within 30 days in 95%.

Christiansen and colleagues reported a patient with recurrent elevation of serum creatinine during IL-2 therapy (75). The following alterations in renal function were observed following IL-2 therapy: decreased creatinine clearance, decreased prostaglandin E_2 excretion, and increased renin and aldosterone. Nonsteroidal anti-inflammatory drugs may exacerbate renal toxicity by further decreasing prostaglandin synthesis. Pretreatment elevation of the serum creatinine or previous nephrectomy have been associated with prolonged time to recovery of renal function (74).

Other Drugs

Many other chemotherapeutic agents may occasionally produce renal toxicity. Vincristine has been associated with the syndrome of inappropriate secretion of ADH (76,77). Severe renal toxicity has been observed following treatment with 2′deoxycoformycin (78), particularly in patients with pretreatment renal impairment. Renal tubular dysfunction has been reported in many patients receiving 5-azacytidine (79).

Radiation Nephritis

Renal toxicity following radiation was described in 1904 by Baermann and Linser (80) and later by Domagk (81). Radiation nephritis, however, remained a poorly described entity until the reports of Luxton and colleagues in the early 1950s (82,83). Luxton reported 27 patients with renal toxicity following abdominal irradiation (2230 to 3250 cGy) for testicular tumors (82). These 27 patients represented approximately 20% (27 of 137) of all patients with testicular tumors who were treated at the Christie Hospital and Holt Radium Institute from 1947 to 1950. Although Luxton divided these patients into acute radiation nephritis (13 cases), chronic radiation nephritis (eight cases), benign hypertension (four cases), and late malignant hypertension (two cases), it is likely that all these syndromes represent different clinical manifestations of radiation nephritis.

The most consistent early effect of radiation on renal function in man is a decrease in renal plasma flow (84). Renal plasma flow decreases progressively during radiotherapy after the first 400 cGy. No consistent changes are seen in blood pressure or other commonly used clinical or laboratory measures of renal function in most patients during radiation therapy. Following radiation therapy, there is a latent period of several months before renal damage is manifest. When radiation is confined to only one kidney or a portion of one kidney, the amount of late renal damage as assessed by decreased creatinine clearance appears to correspond to the percentage of the kidney irradiated (85). Willett and colleagues noted a decreased creatinine clearance in a group of 86 patients who had received radiation to greater than 50% of one kidney at doses of at least 2600 cGy and survived for one year or more. Only one patient developed a clinically significant sequela: malignant hypertension (85). When both kidneys are irradiated, Luxton and colleagues noted postradiation renal damage in one fifth of patients treated with abdominal radiation for testicular tumors (82,83).

Acute and chronic radiation nephritis are both characterized by proteinuria, azotemia, hypertension, and anemia (82,86,87). The anemia is often disproportionately severe relative to the severity of the azotemia. Acute radiation nephritis generally develops 6 to 12 months following the initiation of radiotherapy. Chronic radiation nephritis may follow acute nephritis or may first develop several years after completion of radiotherapy.

HISTOPATHOLOGY

Histologic changes in radiation nephritis, like the clinical manifestations, are variable and depend on the dose and method of irradiation as well as on the time elapsed from completion of radiation to histologic evaluation (88). Glomerular changes with mild endothelial cell swelling, basement membrane splitting, and subendothelial accumulation of electron-lucent material may be early changes. Later, more classic changes include the presence of glomeruli with hyaline obliteration of the capillary loops, marked interstitial fibrosis with tubular atrophy, and fibrinoid necrosis of arterioles or intralobular arteries (82). Endothelial cell damage by radiation with eventual vascular compromise appears to be the primary mechanism of radiation-induced renal toxicity (88).

MANAGEMENT

Treatment of radiation nephritis involves control of the associated hypertension, anemia, and renal insufficiency. Hypertension unresponsive to medical management in the setting of unilateral radiation nephritis may require nephrectomy. Although erythropoietin should be effective in the anemia of radiation nephritis, the possible exacerbation of hypertension may mitigate this benefit.

Chemoradiation Nephritis

Little information is available concerning the nephrotoxic effects of combining chemotherapy and radiation to the kidney. The combined use of chemotherapy and renal irradiation finds its most common application in the treatment of Wilms' tumor. Arneil and colleagues reported two children who developed radiation nephritis after sequential treatment with actinomycin D, radiation, and vincristine (89). The first patient was a 2-½-year-old boy who underwent a left nephrectomy for a localized Wilms' tumor. He was given actinomycin D (18μ g per kg) IV qd × 4. One week postoperatively, he began radiotherapy and received 1500 cGy to the entire abdomen followed by an additional 1500 cGy with the right kidney shielded. The radiotherapy was given in 20 fractions over 32 days. Vincristine (1.5 mg/m^2 IV every week for 5 weeks) was begun two weeks after radiotherapy was completed. Three months after completion of radiotherapy, the patient presented with severe anemia (4 g/dL), hypertension (150/100), proteinuria, and azotemia (BUN 98 mg/dL). Supportive therapy was given, and 2 years after treatment he had no evidence of tumor recurrence and only slightly impaired renal function (creatinine clearance 56 ml per minute per 1.73 meter^2). The second child, a 5-¼-year-old girl, underwent a right nephrectomy followed by similar chemotherapy and 2000 cGy to the whole abdomen in 14 fractions over 18 days. Four months after the start of radiation therapy, she developed anemia, severe hypertension, and azotemia. Sagerman reported a similar case (90). All these patients developed clinical radiation nephritis, which began less than 6 months from the start of chemoradiation.

Tefft and colleagues reported the toxicities associated with the National Wilms' Tumor Studies (NWTS) (91,92). In NWTS-1, 263 patients were evaluable and received actinomycin D, vincristine, or both, along with some form of abdominal radiation. Whole-abdominal radiation was given to 28 patients. Renal toxicity was noted in 4 patients: radiation nephritis—1, vascular thrombosis felt secondary to surgical manipulation of the renal vessels—1, and renal failure in the setting of liver failure—2. In NWTS-2, 303 patients received combined treatment with chemotherapy and radiation. Whole-abdominal radiotherapy was given to 47 patients. Three patients developed transient elevations of BUN and blood pressure after 12, 14, and 36 weeks on study.

Churchill and colleagues reported on a 29-year-old man who developed hypertension, edema, and proteinuria 5 weeks after the completion of combined chemotherapy (bleomycin-vinblastine) and abdominal radiation for testicular carcinoma (93). Abdominal radiation consisted of an initial 1450 cGy at a rate of 145 cGy per treatment over 12 days intended to cover the medial ⅔ of the kidneys and 2325 cGy over 21 days to cover the medial ⅓ of the kidneys.

Several investigators have examined the renal toxicity of combined chemotherapy and radiation in animal models (94–97). The combination of cisplatinum and radiation has been evaluated most extensively. In the mouse, cisplatinum causes dose-dependent acute renal damage which is reversible after low drug doses (95). Irradiation alone causes a dose-dependent progressive deterioration of renal function which begins 20 weeks after irradiation. Cisplatinum given 3 or 4 weeks before irradiation did not significantly increase toxicity. However, cisplatinum given 1 day before or 1 week after irradiation caused a progressive deterioration in renal function beginning at approximately 7 weeks. In the rat model low-dose cisplatinum given immediately before, or as long as 9 months after, irradiation causes a decrease in the latent period for radiation nephritis and an increase in its severity (96). Whether chemotherapy and radiation produce more than additive toxicity to the kidney has not been established with certainty. In the clinic, shielding of at least one kidney is advisable in patients receiving chemotherapy plus abdominal radiation to preserve as much renal function as possible.

BLADDER TOXICITY

Chemotherapy-Induced Cystitis

Cyclophosphamide

Cyclophosphamide is associated with hemorrhagic cystitis in approximately 0.5 to 15% of patients (98–100). Stillwell and Bernson retrospectively examined 100 patients with cyclophosphamide-induced hemorrhagic cystitis that developed after an average total cyclophosphamide dose of 57 g given over an average of 27 months (101). Hemorrhagic cystitis often appears to be more severe after high dose cyclophosphamide, and several studies have shown a positive correlation with dose (100,102,103). Other reports, however, have found hemorrhagic cystitis to be unrelated to dosage or duration of therapy (99,104,105). Stillwell and Benson reported that hemorrhagic cystitis developed within 24 hours of a single intravenous dose in 3 of their 100 patients (101). Patients commonly present with gross hematuria alone or with dysuria. Symptoms may develop months to years following therapy, and a late recurrence months to years after the initial episode of hemorrhagic cystitis is common.

Johnson and Meadows examined at autopsy the bladders of 40 children who had received cyclophosphamide for a childhood malignancy (103). Fibrosis was found in 10 of the 40 bladders, occurring when the total dose exceeded 6 g/m^2. Hemorrhagic cystitis had developed in five of the 10 children with fibrotic bladders prior to death.

Worth reported the first case of transitional cell carcinoma of the bladder following cyclophosphamide in 1971 (106). In 1985, Samra and colleagues reviewed 34 cases that had been reported (107). These bladder tumors included 23 transitional cell carcinomas, six squamous cell carcinomas, one papillary carcinoma, one adenocarcinoma, one undifferentiated carcinoma, and two fibrosarcomas. The total dose of cyclophosphamide administered was over 100 g in nearly all of these patients. Twenty (58%) of the 34 patients had experienced an episode of hemorrhagic cystitis months to years prior to diagnosis of their bladder tumor.

In Stillwell and Benson's review of 100 patients with hemorrhagic cystitis, 29 underwent bladder biopsy (101). In this group of 29 patients, focal epithelial atypia was present in six and transitional cell carcinoma was found in five.

In patients with hemorrhagic cystitis, cystoscopic findings include diffuse mucosal edema, erythema, sloughing, ulceration, and multiple punctate small-vessel hemorrhages. Cystoscopy may, on occasion, reveal a contracted fibrotic bladder or a secondary bladder tumor. Cystoscopic abnormalities frequently persist for months to years. Microscopic examination of bladder biopsies characteristically shows a hyperplastic or ulcerated mucosa, submucosal edema, inflammation, hemorrhagic dilated vascular spaces, and fibrosis (101). Epithelial atypia or transitional cell carcinoma may be present.

MECHANISMS

The urotoxic effects of cyclophosphamide appear to result from exposure of the uroepithelium to acrolein or other drug metabolites (45,108). Viral infection has been proposed as a cause of persistent hemorrhagic cystitis after cyclophosphamide. Viral isolates have included BK virus, JC virus, adenovirus, and CMV (109–111). Despite these findings, the significance of viral infection in hemorrhagic cystitis after cyclophosphamide remains controversial.

MANAGEMENT

Treatment of hemorrhagic cystitis involves discontinuing the cyclophosphamide and increasing hydration in an attempt to decrease the concentration of toxic metabolites in contact with the uroepithelium. Urethral catheters with continuous bladder irrigation may help decrease clot formation, but occlusion of the catheter by blood clots is a frequent problem. Cystoscopy with cauterization of areas of active bleeding may be helpful, but the source of hemorrhage is often diffuse. In persistent or severe hemorrhage the instillation of 1% formalin is often effective (112,113) although severe bladder fibrosis can result. Further information regarding the treatment of hemorrhagic cystitis may be found in two recent reviews (114,115). The treatment of established hemorrhagic cystitis is often a prolonged frustrating ordeal for both patient and physician, with cystectomy sometimes being the only solution.

Prevention of hemorrhagic cystitis includes hydration, diuresis, and frequent voiding in order to decrease the concentration and duration of contact of cyclophosphamide metabolites with the uroepithelium. Droller and colleagues used this approach and noted a decrease in "massive clot-producing hemorrhage" from eight of 97 patients to one of 198 patients (116). These patients had all received high-dose cyclophosphamide (50 mg/kg for each of 4 consecutive days). The possible hyponatremia effect of cyclophosphamide must be considered during aggressive hydration.

MESNA (2-mercaptoethane sulfonate) is a sulfhydryl-containing compound with a short plasma half-life ($t^{1/2} = 1.5$ h), little tissue penetration, and minimal clinical toxicity. It is rapidly oxidized to the chemically stable unreactive disulfide in blood with subsequent reduction to the active parent sulfhydryl in the urine (117,118). MESNA binds extracellular acrolein within the urine, thus reducing toxicity. MESNA does not appear to alter the cytotoxic effects of cyclophosphamide or radiation (119).

Early clinical trials were conducted in Europe. MESNA was statistically superior to forced diuresis in preventing macroscopic hematuria ($p < 0.05$) in a group of 34 patients undergoing allogeneic bone marrow transplantation (120). Gross hematuria developed in two of 18 patients treated with Mesna, and in seven of 16 patients treated with forced diuresis.

Although MESNA appears to reduce the risk of hemorrhagic cystitis following cyclophosphamide treatment, it clearly has not eliminated the problem. Brugières and colleagues did not find any correlation between the use or dose of MESNA and the incidence of hemorrhagic cystitis in their pediatric patients treated with high-dose chemotherapy and bone marrow transplantation (100).

Ifosfamide

Ifosfamide differs from cyclophosphamide in that one of ifosfamide's chlorethyl groups is shifted to the endocyclic nitrogen. Larger amounts of 4-hydroxy-ifosfamide and acrolein are formed after administration of ifosfamide compared with cyclophosphamide. The urotoxicity of ifosfamide, like that of cyclophosphamide, is felt to be related to production of acrolein. Hemorrhagic cystitis was quickly recognized in phase I trials of ifosfamide (121). Hematuria was dose-dependent and occurred with increasing frequency about 2.2 g/m^2 given as a single intravenous bolus (122). Administration of ifosfamide in divided doses (1000 to 1200 $mg/m^2 \times 5$ days) has allowed increasing doses to be delivered, but hematuria remains dose-limiting (123).

The routine use of MESNA along with ifosfamide has allowed an approximate doubling of ifosfamide dose. When MESNA is given in amounts equal to 60 to 100% of ifosfamide dose, the latter can be administered in doses up to 8 to 10 gm/m^2 per course. In a study of patients with non-oat-cell lung cancer, ifosfamide 1.8 g/m^2 was administered with MESNA on 5 consecutive days (124). Gross hematuria was observed in 2% of the cases, and myelosuppression was deemed the limiting toxicity by the investigators. Methods of prevention, diagnosis, and treatment of ifosfamide-induced hemorrhagic cystitis are identical to those used with cyclophosphamide.

Other Drugs

Busulfan has been associated with hemorrhagic cystitis after prolonged therapy and large cumulative doses (125,126). Thiotepa given intravesically has infrequently been associated with bladder hemorrhage (127). Intravesical mitomycin C has been reported to cause bladder fibrosis (128).

Radiation Cystitis

The urinary bladder is frequently exposed to radiation during treatment of cancer of the rectum, prostate, cervix, or bladder. Radiation-induced changes appear to be dose-dependent with complications occurring in 50% of patients given over 7500 cGy (129,130). The complication rate appears to increase rapidly above 7000 cGy, and complications tend to be more frequent after intracavity radiation. Radiation-induced changes may be divided into early changes, which occur days to weeks after irradiation, and late changes, which occur months to years after irradiation.

Initially, radiation injury of the bladder may produce symptoms of increased bladder irritability such as spasm or dysuria, although many patients are asymptomatic (131). Cystoscopically, the bladder first shows a blanching of the irradiated mucosa, and there may be a slight reduction in bladder capacity. This may be followed later by an erythematous reaction with microscopic findings of acute inflammation.

Late changes occur in approximately 5% of patients who receive 6000 cGy and 50% of patients who receive over 7000 cGy (130,131). Hematuria may present months to years following irradiation, and varies greatly in severity (132). Cystoscopy and microscopic examination of bladder biopsies demonstrate vascular telangiectasia, submucosal hemorrhage and interstitial fibrosis. Heavily irradiated areas often appear pale and atrophic. Ulcers may develop and persist for many years. These late changes may be a result of an obliterative endarteritis and subsequent epithelial ischemia (133).

Radiation cystitis is generally treated in the same manner as cyclophosphamide-induced hemorrhagic cystitis. Orgotein, a metalloprotein anti-inflammatory agent, and sodium pentosulfanpolysulfate, a semisynthetic polyionic compound, have been used with some success in Europe (134,135). Recently, several encouraging reports using hyperbaric oxygen have appeared (136–139).

Chemoradiation Cystitis

As in renal toxicity, relatively little information is available concerning the combined effects of chemotherapy and radiation of the bladder and the anecdotal reports in the literature do not allow clear conclusions to be drawn as to whether these treatment modalities are additive or synergistic in producing toxicity. Complications reported with combined chemotherapy and radiation are primarily hematuria and bladder fibrosis. These have occurred with many different chemotherapeutic agents administered with radiation.

Zende and colleagues reported the development of chronic hematuria following combined cyclophosphamide and radiation (140). The patient was a 13-year-old boy with Ewing sarcoma of the right pubic and ischial bones. He received 5400 cGy in 27 fractions over 7 weeks to the right side of the pelvis, along with weekly intravenous cyclophosphamide at 500 mg/m^2. Three months after completion of radiotherapy, while continuing weekly cyclophosphamide, he developed gross hematuria. Cyclophosphamide was continued for two additional doses, after which chemotherapy was changed to BCNU and Adriamycin. Cystoscopy 2 weeks after the onset of hematuria showed severe necrotic, hemorrhagic, and edematous changes on the right side of the bladder. Six months later, there were patchy areas of submucosal hemorrhage and necrosis with active hemorrhage and severe edema on the right side of the bladder. Four years after the onset of hematuria, there were numerous patchy telangiectatic lesions on the right lateral bladder wall. Microscopic hematuria with episodic gross hematuria had persisted for 5 years at the time of the report. A combined toxicity of cyclophosphamide and radiation seems likely in this case.

Many investigators have combined cisplatinum and bladder radiation. Jakse and colleagues treated eight patients with advanced transitional cell carcinoma of the bladder with intravenous cisplatinum 1.6 mg/kg over 15 minutes every 3 weeks for four cycles (141). Radiation was begun 8 to 10 hours after cisplatinum and consisted of 4000 cGy over the first 4 weeks and 2000 cGy over 2 weeks immediately following the last of the four cisplatinum doses. Teniposide was administered following this combined therapy. Toxicity consisted of an increased serum creatinine in two patients. Both of these patients had evidence of urinary tract obstruction, which may have contributed to the increased creatinine. All eight patients developed voiding discomfort which resolved in six patients. Two patients suffered contracted bladders. Jakse later expanded this therapy to 22 patients, and reports a contracted bladder in only 3 patients at a mean follow-up of 14 months (142).

Raghavan and colleagues treated 38 patients with cisplatinum 100 mg/m^2 intravenously in two doses separated by a 3-week interval followed by radiotherapy which consisted of 4500 to 5000 cGy to the whole pelvis with a 1000-cGy boost to the bladder (143). Radiotherapy was given via a three- or four-field technique in 200 cGy fractions, 5 days per week starting within 3 weeks of the second dose of cisplatinum. They report no unanticipated side effects from radiotherapy; however, severe chronic proctitis developed in 6 patients.

Shipley and colleagues treated 70 patients with muscle-invading bladder carcinoma (clinical stages T2 to T4) (144). The patients received cisplatinum 70 mg/m^2 intravenously every 3 weeks for eight courses. Radiation therapy was given by a four-field box technique to encompass the bladder, along with the perivesical, obturator, and distal external iliac nodes, to a dosage of 4500 cGy over 5 weeks, with treatments of 180 cGy five times per week. The field was then coned down to include only the bladder tumor and the dose increased to 6480 cGy (6120 to 6660 cGy). Radiation was completed in 62 patients, all of whom received 2 or more courses of cisplatinum. Acute toxicities included diarrhea, which required medication in 40% and an interruption in radiation therapy in 16%, and dysuria or frequency which required medication in 25% or an interruption in radiation therapy in 13% of patients. Hematuria requiring cystectomy developed in one patient. Bladder function and capacity were not found to be decreased significantly in these patients.

Sauer and colleagues treated 41 patients with invasive bladder cancers with transurethral resection, cisplatinum, and radiotherapy (145). Cisplatinum 25 mg/m^2/d was given intravenously over 30 to 60 minutes prior to irradiation on 5 consecutive days in the first and fifth treatment weeks. Radiation consisted of daily fractions of 180 cGy with the pelvis treated with a "box technique" up to 4180 cGy and the bladder boosted to 5040 cGy. Dysuria and diarrhea were frequently observed, but chronic sequelae of radiation were notably absent. Median follow-up, although not given, appeared short. These studies suggest that cisplatinum does not substantially enhance the toxicity of pelvic radiotherapy to the normal bladder.

Rotman and colleagues treated 19 patients who had invasive bladder carcinoma with radiotherapy and continuous infusion 5-FU (146). Radiation consisted of 4000 to 4500 cGy in 4.5 to 5 weeks to the whole pelvis by a four-field box technique followed by a boost dose to the bladder of 2000 to 2500 cGy in 2.5 to 3 weeks by the arc rotation technique. Chemotherapy was given concomitantly with radiotherapy and consisted of a continuous 120-hour infusion of 5-FU at 25 mg/kg/d on weeks 1, 4, and 7 or weeks 2, 5, and 8. Mitomycin C was given to five patients as an intravenous bolus (10 mg/m^2) on day 1 of radiation therapy. Acute complications included diarrhea (six patients), anorexia (two patients), and mucositis (three patients). Late complications included hemorrhagic cystitis (five patients), contracted bladder (two patients), diarrhea (three patients), and rectal bleeding requiring transfusion (one patient). Most of the patients had 3 to 5 years of follow-up.

Russell and colleagues also evaluated concurrent 5-FU and radiation (147). Fourteen patients with transitional cell carcinoma of the urinary bladder were given 2000 cGy to the pelvis over 2 weeks (200 cGy/d × 10). Chemotherapy consisted of 5-FU 1000 mg/m^2/d continuous infusion over 96 hours on days 1 through 4. Following this therapy, the patients were given 1 week of rest and the cycle was then repeated. Three weeks after the completion of therapy, patients underwent cystoscopy, and those with residual tumor then underwent cystectomy. Those without evidence of residual tumor received an additional 96-hour infusion of 5-FU, 400 cGy to the pelvis, and a 1600-cGy boost to the entire bladder and tumor. Seven of the 14 patients ultimately retained their bladders. Acute complications included dysuria, mucositis, diarrhea, and palmar desquamation. No longterm complications are noted; however, follow-up is limited (3 to 21 months) with a median of 7 months.

Marks and colleagues have investigated combined multiagent chemotherapy followed by cisplatinum and radiation in 19 patients (148). Following transurethral debulking of bladder tumors, chemotherapy consisting of methotrexate 30 mg/m^2 on days 0, 14, and 21, cisplatinum 70 mg/m^2 on day 1, and vinblastine 3 mg/m^2 on days 1, 14, 21 of 28-day cycle was administered. Two cycles were given. Patients then received cisplatinum 70 mg/m^2 on day 0 and day 21 combined with 4000 cGy to the entire bladder and pelvic lymphatics through four-field box technique with high energy photons (180 cGy per fraction, five fractions per week). Radiotherapy was not given on the days of cisplatinum treatment. Cytoscopic complete responders were given additional radiotherapy to a smaller boost field to bring the total dose to 6480 cGy. Additional cisplatinum was given on day 42 of radiation. All 19 patients received the cisplatinum × 2 and 4000 cGy. Nine patients received the boost to 6480 cGy. Acute toxicities consisted of dysuria (13 patients) and diarrhea. One patient developed a bladder perforation during cystoscopy after initial chemotherapy (MCV). He then developed a small bowel obstruction 3 months after completing 4000 cGy. Other late toxicities were not reported, but follow-up was limited. The longest available follow-up was 19 months.

Overall, acute toxicity appears to be acceptable in the combined chemotherapy and radiation studies published to date. The differences in reported toxicities are most probably a function of follow-up time. Longer periods of follow-up will be necessary to more completely define the true incidence of late toxicities associated with combined therapy.

GONADAL TOXICITY

Gonadal dysfunction has been recognized increasingly as an important toxic effect of cancer therapy. This is due primarily to the increasing number of patients with long disease-free survival following treatment for leukemia, lymphoma, testicular cancer, and other solid tumors. Important factors related to the occurrence of gonadal dysfunction following cancer therapy are the age and the pubertal and menstrual status of the patient at the time of therapy, along with the dose and type of chemotherapy or radiation administered (149). The effects of chemotherapy, radiation, and combination therapy on testicular and ovarian function will be briefly reviewed.

Testicular Dysfunction After Chemotherapy

The primary testicular lesion caused by antitumor agents is depletion of the germinal epithelium lining the seminiferous tubules. Testicular biopsy in most patients reveals complete germinal aplasia with only Sertoli cells left lining the tubular lumen. Occasionally, scattered spermatogonia, spermatocytes, or spermatids may be seen, or there may be evidence of maturation arrest at the spermatocyte stage.

Because the seminiferous tubules comprise a large proportion of the testicular mass, damage to the germinal epithelium often results in testicular atrophy that is readily detectable on physical examination. Impaired spermatogenesis is also manifest as a decrease in the number and/or motility of sperm present in the ejaculate and as an increase in serum follicle stimulating hormone (FSH) level. Leydig cell dysfunction may also occur and is detected by an increase in serum luteinizing hormone (LH) level or a fall in serum testosterone level.

Spitz, in 1948, was the first to describe changes in testicular histology following cytotoxic chemotherapy (150). Absent spermatogenesis was found at autopsy in 27 of 30 men who had received mechlorethamine. Other alkylating agents, most notably cyclophosphamide and chlorambucil, have been frequently associated with gonadal dysfunction (149). Both cyclophosphamide and chlorambucil deplete the germinal epithelium in a dose-related fashion.

Cyclophosphamide

Watson and colleagues reviewed the long-term effects of cyclophosphamide on testicular function in 30 men who had received cyclophosphamide during childhood for nephrotic syndrome (151). The drug was administered at a dose of 2 to 3 mg/kg/day for a mean of 280 days (range 42 to 556 days). The mean age at the time of treatment was 9.4 years (range 2.9 to 17.3) and the mean age at the time of evaluation was 22 years (range 17 to 29.5). Mean time from the end of cyclophosphamide treatment to the time of the study was 12.8 years (range 6.7 to 15.8). Semen analysis demonstrated that four patients were azoospermic, nine oligospermic (sperm count $< 20 \times 10^6$/mL) and 17 normospermic. Sperm density showed a significant inverse correlation with cumulative cyclophosphamide dosage. None of the patients who received less than 10 g of cyclophosphamide or were treated less than 112 days were oligospermic. All 30 patients had developed normal secondary sex characteristics and had normal basal testosterone levels. The basal LH concentrations in the azoospermic and oligospermic patients, however, were elevated, suggesting compensated Leydig cell failure.

In adults, decreased sperm counts have been noted in men treated with as little as 50 to 100 mg of cyclophosphamide per day for 2 months, but azoospermia and germinal aplasia are unusual until the cumulative dosage is at least 6 to 11 g. In mice, cyclophosphamide appears to affect primarily the later spermatogonia and spermatocytes (152). The effects of cyclophosphamide on testicular function may improve with time. In the study reported by Watson, 13 patients had undergone semen analysis on at least two occasions separated by 5.5 to 9 years (151). Nine patients remained stable over this period (four normospermic, three azoospermic, and two oligospermic), and four oligospermic patients had a return of normal sperm counts. Clearly, the germinal epithelium can regenerate and spermatogenesis can resume following single-agent chemotherapy. The rapidity with which spermatogenesis resumes appears to be related to the total dose of chemotherapy administered.

Chlorambucil

Richter and colleagues first reported testicular dysfunction associated with chlorambucil (153). Progressive but reversible oligospermia was noted in men with lymphoma treated with up to 400 mg of chlorambucil. Azoospermia was uniformly present at doses above 400 mg. Guesry and colleagues reported similar findings in 21 adolescents and young men (154). Azoospermia occurred in all patients who received more than 25 mg/kg of chlorambucil, but fertility remained intact with total doses < 7 mg/kg. As with cyclophosphamide, recovery of spermatogenesis has been reported years after completion of therapy (155).

Procarbazine

Procarbazine has been shown to be particularly toxic to the germinal epithelium in adult male monkeys (156). Combination chemotherapy including procarbazine frequently results in testicular dysfunction. In a comparison of mechlorethamine, Oncovin, procarbazine, and prednisone (MOPP) and Adriamycin, bleomycin, vinblastine, and dacarbazine (ABVD) for treatment of Hodgkin's disease, azoospermia occurred in 100% of patients after MOPP compared with 35% following ABVD (157). Antioxidants (N-acetyl cysteine and sodium ascorbate) have been used in animal models to decrease the spermatotoxic effects of procarbazine (158). Testosterone has also been protective of spermatogenesis during procarbazine treatment in a rat model (159). No studies in man are yet available to allow analysis of the clinical relevance of these observations.

Other Drugs

Though methotrexate at high dose (250 mg/kg) may produce transient oligospermia (160), most antimetabolites do not appear to be particularly toxic to the germinal epithelium. Adriamycin produces severe germinal epithelial injury, which is often reversible in younger patients (161–164). The contribution of cisplatinum to the gonadal toxicity produced by cisplatinum-based chemotherapy for testicular cancer is difficult to assess. Evaluation of gonadal function often reveals abnormalities in patients with testicular cancer even prior to chemotherapy, thus confounding the issue of chemotherapy effects. LH and FSH are frequently elevated after therapy with cisplatinum-containing regimens. Leitner and colleagues found that patients under 25 at treatment tended to have lower levels of FSH and LH and often showed a decline in levels over time suggestive of gonadal recovery (162). Other drugs with reported gonadal toxicity include actinomycin-D, bleomycin, busulfan, nitrosoureas, cytosine arabinoside, mitomycin-C, and m-AMSA (152,165–168).

Ovarian Dysfunction After Chemotherapy

The evaluation of ovarian function after chemotherapy is more difficult than evaluation of testicular function. The ovaries are neither anatomically nor functionally as accessible as the testes. Unlike semen analysis, no direct measurement of the female germ cell population is readily available. Thus, menstrual and reproductive history and determination of serum hormone levels are generally used to assess the functional status of the ovary. As with the testes, ovarian dysfunction appears most frequently after therapy with alkylating agents. Antimetabolites have not been implicated as a significant cause of ovarian dysfunction (160). For most drugs, the onset and duration of ovarian dysfunction appear to be both dose- and age-related. Generally, younger patients are able to tolerate larger cumulative drug doses before amenorrhea occurs and have a greater likelihood of resumption of menses when therapy is discontinued.

The primary manifestation of ovarian dysfunction after chemotherapy is amenorrhea. Menopausal symptoms, including hot flashes, may occur. Serum FSH and LH rise and estradiol falls, as in post-menopausal women. Estrogen deficiency may result in vaginal epithelial atrophy and endometrial hypoplasia.

Cyclophosphamide

Early menopausal symptoms and amenorrhea were first noted after cyclophosphamide in patients undergoing treatment for rheumatoid arthritis (169). Amenorrhea, decreased urinary estrogens, and increased urinary gonadotropins occurred in at least 50% of premenopausal women who received 40 to 120 mg of cyclophosphamide per day for an average of 18 months (170,171). In women who received cyclophosphamide as adjuvant chemotherapy for breast cancer, permanent cessation of menses occurred in all patients 40 years and older following a mean total dose of 5.2 g. In women under 40 years, amenorrhea developed in four of five patients after a mean cyclophosphamide dose of 9.3 g (172). Menses returned in two of these four patients within 6 months of completing therapy. It appears that alkylating agent chemotherapy accelerates the onset of menopause, particularly in older patients.

Other Drugs

Busulfan in doses ranging from 0.5 to 14 mg/day for at least 3 months produced permanent amenorrhea in many patients (173,174). Amenorrhea or oligomenorrhea occurred in 41% of 22 patients who received a mean cumulative etoposide dose of 5 g for gestational trophoblastic tumors (175). The risk of amenorrhea was age-related, as was the risk of amenorrhea in women receiving melphalan alone or in combination with 5-FU (176).

MOPP chemotherapy for Hodgkin's disease produces amenorrhea in approximately half of the women treated. In one study, 46% of MOPP-treated women had persistent amenorrhea when evaluated a median of 9 years after completion of therapy (177). Amenorrhea and the time to onset of amenorrhea following chemotherapy were both age-related. Attempts to protect against chemotherapy-induced ovarian dysfunction by use of oral contraceptives have produced conflicting results (178–180). The more recent studies do not confirm a protective effect.

Testicular Dysfunction After Radiation

The adult testis is exquisitely sensitive to the effects of radiation. The spermatogonia are the most radiosensitive of all cell types. In the rat, the LD_{50} of type B spermatogonia is estimated to be 21 cGy to 100 cGy and the LD_{50} of type A spermatogonia about 600 cGy (181). In man, a single dose of less than 10 cGy produces little change in spermatogenesis, whereas increasing the dose to just 15 cGy results in a marked reduction of spermatogenesis (182,183). Azoospermia occurs uniformly after 100 to 600 cGy of fractionated radiation directed at the testis.

Recovery of spermatogenesis following direct testicular radiation is inversely related to the dose. Following 200 to 300 cGy, sperm counts returned to baseline after approximately 30 months following 400 to 600 cGy. Recovery may not occur for 5 or more years (182,183).

Direct testicular radiation is not frequently used in clinical oncology. Testicular radiation, however, may be a consequence of beam scatter during therapy for Hodgkin's disease, sarcomas, or pelvic tumors. Shapiro and colleagues examined the presence and effects of scatter radiation to the testis in patients irradiated for soft tissue sarcomas (184). The scatter dose to a given point varies with the field size, distance from the edge of the radiation field, photon beam energy, and depth of the tissue of interest.

Scatter doses ranged from 1 to 14 cGy during treatment of soft tissue sarcomas of the head, thorax, or distal extremities. However, scatter doses as high as 27 to 2,500 cGy were noted following treatment of sarcomas of the retroperitoneum, buttock, and medial thigh. A dose-dependent increase in serum FSH and LH values occurred following irradiation with a maximum increase noted approximately 6 months after completion of therapy. Scatter doses < 50 cGy were associated with an early recovery of normal FSH levels. Scatter doses > 200 cGy were associated with statistically significant LH changes suggestive of Leydig cell dysfunction. Speiser reported similar effects in patients with Hodgkin's disease who received scatter radiation doses to the testes ranging from 140 to 300 cGy (185). No patients in this series had a normal serum FSH 40 months following therapy.

Methods to decrease testicular toxicity from radiation include appropriate shielding techniques. In animals, Schally and colleagues demonstrated radioprotection by administration of an LH-RH antagonist (186). Although the results are encouraging, clinical trials are necessary to determine the value of this approach in patients.

Ovarian Dysfunction After Radiation

As with chemotherapy, the incidence of ovarian dysfunction after radiation is dependent on radiation dosage and patient age. Peck and colleagues observed that 500 to 1000 cGy was required to induce amenorrhea in women under 40 years of age, whereas a dose over 375 cGy produced amenorrhea in nearly 100% of women over 40 years of age (187,188). Horning and colleagues examined ovarian function after total nodal radiation for Hodgkin's disease. They found that 70% of women 20 years of age or less at treatment retained regular cyclic menses following total nodal radiation, whereas after age 30 only 20% retained normal ovarian function after radiation (189). The radiation dose required to induce premature menopause appears to progressively decrease with increasing age at the time therapy is begun.

Stillman and colleagues examined 182 prepubertal girls who had received abdominal irradiation at least 6 years earlier for a childhood malignancy (187,190). They found that amenorrhea and elevated gonadotropins were present in 68% (12 of 25) when both ovaries were included in the radiation field (estimated ovarian doses of 1200 to 5000 cGy); in 14% (5 of 35) when at least one ovary was at the edge of the radiation field (estimated ovarian doses of 90 to 1000 cGy) and in none of the patients when at least one ovary was outside the treatment field (0 of 34 at doses of 5 to 150 cGy) or no abdominal radiation was given (0 of 88).

Ray and colleagues developed an operative procedure, oophoropexy, by which the ovaries are repositioned in the midline behind the uterus, providing some shielding (191). This procedure provides protection from radiation-induced ovarian dysfunction in approximately 50% of patients (192).

Gonadal Dysfunction After Chemoradiation

Limited data exist concerning gonadal function following combined chemotherapy and radiation. The use of combined or sequential testicular radiation and chemotherapy most frequently occurs as treatment of testicular relapse of childhood acute leukemia. Blatt and colleagues measured gonadotropin and testosterone levels in seven boys with ALL who had been treated with radiation for testicular relapse (193). All of the patients had previously received combination chemotherapy including vincristine, prednisone, 6-mercaptopurine, and oral and intrathecal methotrexate. Five of the patients had received L-asparaginase during induction, and six had received prophylactic CNS radiation. Testicular relapse was confirmed histologically, and patients then received testicular irradiation of 2400 cGy along with reinduction with all of the agents listed above. Two patients received daunorubicin during reinduction. In four of the seven boys, testicular relapse was bilateral. Three demonstrated delayed sexual maturation, elevated FSH and LH, and low testosterone levels. The evaluation was performed 2 to 7 years after testicular relapse, and suggests that Leydig cell damage occurred as well as impaired spermatogenesis.

Shalet and colleagues also proposed that Leydig cell damage may occur following treatment of testicular relapse of ALL (194). It is difficult to dissect the relative contributions of chemotherapy, radiation, and leukemia to the gonadal dysfunction in this clinical setting. Delic and colleagues used a rat model to demonstrate enhancement of radiation-induced testicular dysfunction by BCNU, cyclophosphamide, and procarbazine (195).

Himelstein-Braw and colleagues reported the histologic findings in the ovaries of five prepubertal girls who died following chemotherapy (vincristine and cyclophosphamide), and abdominal radiation. The radiation consisted of 2000 to 3000 cGy over 3 to 4 weeks. The ovarian morphology was described as quiescent in all five patients with a reduced number of small follicles in four of five patients (196). Hamre and colleagues reported on the Children's Cancer Study Group experience with ovarian function in longterm survivors of childhood ALL (197). Induction chemotherapy consisted of vincristine, prednisone, and L-asparaginase. Patients then received intensification consisting of one of the following: 2400 cGy craniospinal radiation plus 1200 cGy extended abdominal field including the gonads; 2400 cGy craniospinal radiation; 2400 cGy cranial radiation plus IT-MTX; 1800 cGy craniospinal radiation; or 1800 cGy cranial radiation plus IT-MTX. Median age at diagnosis was 4.8 years (range 1.6 to 15.3) and median age at evaluation was 14.0 years (range 10.2 to 26.1). Craniospinal plus abdominal radiation was significantly associated with lack of pubertal development and delayed onset of menses. Fifteen patients had received craniospinal plus abdominal radiation; 13 of 15 had elevated LH and 14 of 15 had elevated FSH.

At present, it is unclear if the ovarian dysfunction observed following treatment with chemotherapy and radiation is a temporary or permanent phenomenon. Jarrell and colleagues examined the changes in ovarian histology in rats following cyclophosphamide alone or in combination with irradiation (198). Given alone, cyclophosphamide produced antral follicular atresia in a dose-dependent manner. Concurrent administration of 0, 200, 300, 400, 500, and 600 cGy of radiation with cyclophosphamide (50 mg/kg) produced widespread loss of primordial, preantral, and antral follicles, increased FSH and LH, and decreased serum progesterone and estradiol. Additional studies of this type are necessary to determine if the combined effects of chemotherapy and radiation represent additive or synergistic toxicity to the ovary.

There are few data concerning the mutagenic properties of radiotherapy and/or chemotherapy in women who successfully conceive following cancer treatment. Although cytotoxic chemotherapy administered during pregnancy, particularly during the first trimester, is known to be teratogenic, the mutagenic properties of these drugs are poorly defined. Ancedotal reports suggest that there is no increased incidence of spontaneous abortion or fetal abnormalities in those treated with chemotherapy in comparison with the general population (199–201). One recent study, however, suggests that women previously treated with both chemotherapy and radiation have a greater chance of pregnancy ending in abortion or with delivery of an abnormal child than do sibling controls (202). At present, it is impossible to define the risk of fetal wastage or abnormality in patients previously treated with cytotoxic drugs and radiation. Moreover, although the physical and intellectual development of offspring appear to be normal, larger numbers of patients and longer-term follow-up will be necessary to make an accurate assessment of risk.

SUMMARY

Cancer chemotherapy and radiation produce a variety of acute and chronic toxicities to genitourinary organs. Acute toxicities are most often manifest as acute renal failure, electrolyte abnormalities, and hemorrhagic cystitis. Common chronic toxicities include chronic renal failure, hypertension, bladder fibrosis, and infertility. For both chemotherapy and radiation, toxic effects are related primarily to the cumulative dose administered although patient age, sex, and diagnosis may be important in determining the severity of the effects in any individual. Recognizing potential toxic effects and implementing strategies to ameliorate them are important goals of cancer treatment, particularly when the potential for cure and longterm survival exists.

REFERENCES

1. Lundberg WB, Cadman ED, Finch SC, Capizzi RL. Renal failure secondary to leukemic infiltration of the kidneys. Am J Med 62:636, 1977.
2. Cohen LF, Balow JE, McGrath IT, et al. Acute tumor lysis syndrome. Am J Med 68:486, 1980.
3. Boles J, Dutel JL, Briére J, et al. Acute renal failure caused by extreme hyperphosphatemia after chemotherapy of an acute lymphoblastic leukemia. Cancer 53:2425, 1984.
4. Band PR, Silverberg DS, Henderson JF, et al. Xanthine nephropathy in a patient with lymphosarcoma treated with allopurinol. N Engl J Med 283:354, 1970.
5. Rota S, Mougenot B, Baudouin B, et al. Multiple myeloma and severe renal failure: A clinicopathologic study of outcome and prognosis in 34 patients. Medicine 66:126, 1987.
6. Wiernik PH, Serpick AA. Clinical significance of serum and urinary muramidase activity in leukemia and other hematologic malignancies. Am J Med 46:330, 1969.
7. Schaeppi U, Heyman IA, Fleischmann RW, et al. Cis-dichlorodiammine-platinum II (NSC 119875): Pre-clinical toxicologic evaluation of intravenous injection in dogs, monkeys, and mice. Toxicol Appl Pharmacol 25:230, 1973.
8. Highby DJ, Wallace HJ, Holland JF. Cis-diamminedichloroplatinum (NSC 119875): A phase I study. Cancer Chemother Rep 57:459, 1973.
9. Litterst CL, LeRoy AF, Guarino AM. Disposition and distribution of platinum following parenteral administration of cis-dichlorodiammineplatinum (II) to animals. Cancer Treat Rep 63:1485, 1979.
10. Dentino M, Luft FC, Yum MN, et al. Long-term effect of cis-diammine dichloride platinum (CDDP) on renal function and structure in man. Cancer 41:1274, 1978.
11. Gonzalez-Vitale JC, Hayes DM, Cvitkovic E, Sternberg SS. The renal pathology in clinical trials of cisplatinum (II) diamminedichloride. Cancer 39:1362, 1977.
12. Rossof AH, Slayton RE, Perlia CP. Preliminary clinical experience with cis-diamminedichloroplatinum (II) (NSC-119875). Cancer 30:1451, 1972.
13. Jones BR, Bhalla RB, Mladek J, et al. Comparison of methods of evaluating nephrotoxicity of cisplatinum. Clin Pharmacol Ther 27:577, 1980.
14. Kuhn JA, Argy WP, Rakowski TA, et al. Nephrotoxicity of cis-diammine dichloroplatinum II as measured by urinary beta glucuronidase. Cancer Treat Rep 64:1083, 1980.
15. Cohen AI, Rose DP, Citrin DL. Abnormal β_2-macroglobulin excretion following CDDP (cisplatinum) therapy (Abstract 545). Proc Am Assoc Cancer Res 21:137, 1980.
16. Schilsky RL, Anderson T. Hypomagnesemia and renal magnesium wasting in patients receiving cisplatinum. Ann Intern Med 90:929, 1979.
17. Vogelzang NJ, Torkelson JL, Kennedy J. Hypomagnesemia, renal dysfunction, and Raynaud's phenomena in patients treated with cisplatin, vinblastine, and bleomycin. Cancer 56:2765, 1985.
18. Schilsky RL, Barlock A, Ozols RF. Persistent hypomagnesemia following cisplatinum chemotherapy for testicular cancer. Cancer Treat Rep 66:1767, 1982.
19. Cvitkovic E, Spaulding J, Bethene V, et al. Improvement of cis-dichlorodiammineplatinum (NSC 119875) therapeutic index in an animal model. Cancer 39:1357, 1977.
20. DeSimone PA, Yancey RS, Coupal JJ, et al. Effect of a forced diuresis on the distribution and excretion (via urine and bile) of ^{195}platinum when given as ^{195}platinum cis-dichloro diammineplatinum II. Cancer Treat Rep 63:951, 1979.
21. Frick GA, Ballentine R, Driever CW, Kramer WG. Renal excretion kinetics of high-dose cis-dichlorodiammineplatinum (II) administered with hydration and mannitol diuresis. Cancer Treat Rep 63:13, 1979.
22. Hayes DM, Cvitkovic E, Golbey RB, et al. High-dose cisplatinum-diamminedichloride, amelioration of renal toxicity by mannitol diuresis. Cancer 39:1372, 1977.
23. Litterst CL. Alterations in the toxicity of cis-dichlorodiammineplatinum II and in tissue localization of platinum as function of NaCl concentration of the vehicle of administration. Toxicol Appl Pharmacol 61:99, 1981.
24. Ozols RF, Corden BJ, Jacob J, et al. High dose cisplatinum in hypertonic saline. Ann Intern Med 100:19, 1984.
25. Lehane D, Winston A, Gray R, et al. The effect of diuretic pretreatment on clinical morphology, and ultrastructural cisplatinum induced nephrotoxicity. Int J Radiat Oncol Biol Phys 5:1393, 1979.
26. Pera M, Zook BC, Harder HC. Effects of mannitol or furosemide diuresis on the nephrotoxicity and physiological disposition of cis-dichlorodiammineplatinum II in rats. Cancer Res 39:1269, 1979.

27. Ward JM, Grabin ME, Berlin E, Young DM. Prevention of renal failure in rats receiving cis-diamminedichloroplatinum (II) by administration of furosemide. Cancer Res 37:1238, 1977.
28. Ostrow S, Egorin MD, Hahn D, et al. High-dose cisplatinum therapy using mannitol versus furosemide diuresis: Comparative pharmacokinetics and toxicity. Cancer Treat Rep 65:73, 1981.
29. Howell SB, Pfeifle CL, Wang WE, et al. Intraperitoneal cisplatinum with systemic thiosulfate protection. Ann Intern Med 97:845, 1982.
30. Borch RF, Katz JC, Liedr PH, et al. Effect of diethyldithiocarbamate rescue on tumor response to cisplatinum in a rat model. Proc Natl Acad Sci USA 77:5441, 1980.
31. Yuhas JM, Culo F. Selective inhibition of nephrotoxicity of cis-dichlorodiammineplatinum (II) by WR 2721 without altering in its antitumor properties. Cancer Treat Rep 64:57, 1980.
32. Ross DA, Gale GR. Reduction of renal toxicity of cis-dichlorodiammineplatinum (II) by probenecid. Cancer Treat Rep 63:781, 1979.
33. Offerman JJG, Meijer S, Sleijfer DT, et al. The influence of verapamil on renal function in patients treated with cisplatinum. Clin Nephrol 24:249, 1985.
34. Calvert AH, Harland SJ, Newell DR, et al. Early clinical studies with cis-diammine cyclobutane dicarboxylate platinum II. Cancer Chemother Pharmacol 9:140, 1982.
35. Rozencweig M, Nicaise C, Beer M, et al. Phase I study of carboplatin given on a five-day intravenous schedule. J Clin Oncol 1:621, 1983.
36. Leyvraz S, Ohnuma T, Lassus M, Holland JF. Phase I study of carboplatinum in patients with advanced cancer, intermittent intravenous bolus, and 24-hour infusion. J Clin Oncol 3:1385, 1985.
37. Ueda T, Yasumasu T, Uozumi J. Experimental studies on the pharmacokinetics and nephotoxicity of carboplatin (cis-diammine-1, 1-cyclobutane dicarboxylate platinum II) in rats. J Toxicol Sci 16:101, 1991.
38. Hande KR, Donehower RC, Chabner BA. Pharmacology and pharmacokinetics of high-dose methotrexate in man. *In:* Clinical Pharmacology of Antineoplastic Drugs. Pinedo HM (Ed): New York, Elsevier/North Holland, 1978, p. 97.
39. Pitman SW, Parker LM, Tattersall MHN, et al. Clinical trial of high dose methotrexate (NSC 740) with citrovorum factor (NSC 3590)-toxicologic and therapeutic observations. Cancer Chemother Rep 6:43, 1975.
40. Jacobs SA, Stoller RG, Chabner BA, et al. Dose-dependent metabolism of methotrexate in man and rhesus monkeys. Cancer Treat Rep 61:651, 1977.
41. Jacobs SA, Stoller RG, Chabner BA, et al. 7-hydroxy methotrexate as a urinary metabolite in human subjects and rhesus monkeys receiving high dose methotrexate. J Clin Invest 57:534, 1976.
42. Fox RM. Methotrexate nephrotoxicity. Clin Exp Pharmacol Physiol 5(Suppl):43, 1979.
43. Condit PT, Chanes RE, Joel W. Renal toxicity of methotrexate. Cancer 23:126, 1969.
44. Pitman SW and Frei E. Weekly methotrexate-calcium leucovorin rescue: Effects of alkalinization on nephrotoxicity; pharmacokinetics in the CNS; and use in CNS lymphoma. Cancer Treat Rep 61:695, 1977.
45. Brock N, Pohl J, Stekar J. Studies on the urotoxicity of oxazaphosphorine cytostatics and prevention. Eur J Cancer 17:596, 1981.
46. DeFronzo RA, Calvin OM, Braine H, et al. Cyclophosphamide and the kidney. Cancer 33:483, 1974.
47. DeFronzo RA, Braine H, Calvin OM, et al. Water intoxication in man after cyclophosphamide therapy. Ann Intern Med 78:861, 1973.
48. Harlow PJ, Declerck YA, Shore NA, et al. Fatal case of inappropriate ADH secretion induced by cyclophosphamide therapy. Cancer 44:896, 1979.
49. Green TP, Mirken BL. Prevention of cyclophosphamide-induced antidiuresis by furosemide infusion. Clin Pharmacol Ther 29:634, 1981.
50. Hilgard P, Burkert H. Sodium-2-mercaptoethane-sulfonate (MESNA) and ifosfamide nephrotoxicity. Eur J Cancer Clin Oncol 20:1451, 1984.
51. van Dyk JJ, Falkson HC, van der Merwe AM, Falkson G. Unexpected toxicity in patients treated with iphosphamide. Cancer Res 32:921, 1972.
52. Cohen MD, Creavan PJ, Tejeda F, et al. Phase I clinical trial of isophosphamide (NSC-109724). Cancer Chemother Rep 59:751, 1975.
53. Sangster G, Kaye SB, Calman KC, Dalton JF. Failure of 2-mercaptoethane sulphonate sodium (MESNA) to protect against ifosfamide nephrotoxicity. Eur J Cancer Clin Oncol 20:435, 1984.
54. Klein HO, Wickrammanayake PD, Loffler T, Hirshmann WD. High dose therapy with cytostatic drugs. Cancer Campaign 4:291, 1980.
55. Schaeppi U, Fleischman RW, Phelan RW, et al. Preclinical toxicologic evaluation of a sin-

gle intravenous infusion in dogs and monkeys. Cancer Chemother Rep 5:53, 1974.
56. Schacht RG, Feiner HD, Gallo GR, et al. Nephrotoxicity of nitrosoureas. Cancer 48:1328, 1981.
57. Harmon WE, Cohen HJ, Schneeberger EE, Grupe WE. Chronic renal failure in children treated with methyl CCNU. N Engl J Med 300:1200, 1979.
58. Broder LE, Carter SK. Pancreatic islet cell carcinoma II: Results of therapy with streptozotocin in 52 patients. Ann Intern Med 79:108, 1973.
59. Sadoff L. Nephrotoxicity of streptozotocin (NSC 85998). Cancer Chemother Rep 54:457, 1970.
60. Meyerowitz RL, Sartiano GP, Cavallo T. Nephrotoxic and cytoproliferative effects of streptozotocin. Cancer 38:1550, 1976.
61. Valavaara R, Nordman E. Renal complications of mitomycin C therapy with special reference to the total dose. Cancer 55:47, 1985.
62. Kressel BR, Ryan KP, Duong AT, et al. Microangiopathic hemolytic anemia, thrombocytopenia, and renal failure in patients treated for adenocarcinoma. Cancer 48:1738, 1981.
63. Liu K, Mittelman A, Sproul EE, et al. Renal toxicity in man treated with mitomycin C. Cancer 28:1314, 1971.
64. Price TM, Murgo AJ, Keveney JJ, et al. Renal failure and hemolytic anemia associated with mitomycin C. Cancer 55:51, 1985.
65. Ratanatharathorn V, Baker LH, Cadnapaphornchai P, et al. Clinical and pathologic study of mitomycin C nephrotoxicity. *In:* Mitomycin C: Current Status and New Developments. Carter SK, Crooke ST (Eds). New York, Academic Press, 1979, p. 219.
66. Cattell V. Mitomycin-induced hemolytic uremic kidney. An experimental model in the rat. Am J Pathol 121:88, 1985.
67. Kennedy BJ. Metabolic and toxic effects of mithramycin during tumor therapy. Am J Med 49:494, 1970.
68. Bocci V, Pacini A, Muscettola M, et al. The kidney is the main site of interferon catabolism. J Interferon Res 2:309, 1982.
69. Sumpio BE, Ernstoff MS, Kirkwood JM. Urinary excretion of interferon, albumin, and β_2-microglobulin during interferon treatment. Cancer Res 44:3599, 1984.
70. Kruschel E, Metz-Kruschel U, Hoffmann W, Niederle N. Analysis of urinary enzyme excretion as a parameter of the nephrotoxicity of human interferon alpha-2b in patients with chronic myelogenous leukemia. Klin Wochenschr 65:667, 1987.
71. Averbuch SD, Austin III HA, Sherwin SA, et al. Acute interstitial nephritis with the nephrotic syndrome following recombinant leukocyte A interferon therapy for mycosis fungoides. N Engl J Med 310:32, 1984.
72. Sriskandan K, Tee DEH, Pettingale KW. Nephrotic syndrome during treatment with interferon. Br Med J 290:1590, 1985.
73. Kramer P, Ten Kate FWJ, Bijnen AB, et al. Recombinant leucocyte interferon A induces steroid-resistant acute vascular rejection episodes in renal transplant recipients. Lancet 1:989, 1984.
74. Belldegrun A, Webb DE, Austin HA, et al. Effects of interleukin-2 on renal function in patients receiving immunotherapy for advanced cancer. Ann Intern Med 106:817, 1987.
75. Christiansen NP, Skubitz KM, Nath K, et al. Nephrotoxicity of continuous intravenous infusion of recombinant interleukin-2. Am J Med 84:1072, 1988.
76. Cutting HO. Inappropriate secretion of antidiuretic hormone secondary to vincristine therapy. Am J Med 51:269, 1971.
77. Suskind RM, Brusilow SW, Zehr J. Syndrome of inappropriate secretion of antidiuretic hormone produced by vincristine toxicity (with bioassay of ADH level). J Pediatr 81:90, 1972.
78. Kanofsky JR, Baron JM, Roth DG, et al. Treatment of lymphoid malignancies with 2′-deoxycoformycin. A pilot study. Am J Clin Oncol 5:179, 1982.
79. Peterson BA, Collins AJ, Vogelzang NJ, et al. 5-azacytidine and renal tubular dysfunction. Blood 57:182, 1981.
80. Baermann G, Linser P. Uber die lokale and allgemeine wirkung der rontgenstrahlen. Munch Med Wochenschr 7:996, 1904.
81. Domagk G. Rontgenstrahlenschadigungen der nierebeim menschen. Med Klin 23:345, 1927.
82. Luxton RW. Radiation nephritis. Q J Med 86:215, 1953.
83. Kunkler PB, Farr RF, Luxton RW. The limit of renal tolerance to x-rays. Brit J Radiol 25:190, 1952.
84. Avioli LV, Lazor MMZ, Cotlove E, et al. Early effects of radiation on renal function in man. Am J Med 34:329, 1963.
85. Willett CG, Tepper JE, Orlow EL, Shipley WU. Renal complications secondary to radiation treatment of upper abdominal malignancies. Int J Radiat Oncol Biol Phys 12:1601, 1986.
86. Schreiner BF, Greendyke RM. Radiation nephritis. Am J Med 26:146, 1959.
87. van Slyck EJ, Bermudez GA. Radiation nephritis. Yale J Biol Med 41:243, 1986.

88. Keane WF, Crosson JT, Staley NA, et al. Radiation-induced renal disease. Am J Med 60:127, 1976.
89. Arneil GC, Emmanuel GI, Flatman GE, et al. Nephritis in two children after irradiation and chemotherapy for nephroblastoma. Lancet 1:960, 1974.
90. Sagerman RH. Radiation nephritis. J Urol 91:332, 1964.
91. Tefft M. Radiation related toxicities in national Wilms' tumor study number 1. Int J Radiat Oncol Biol Phys 2:455, 1977.
92. Thomas PRM, Tefft M, D'Angio GJ, Norkool P. Acute toxicities associated with radiation in the second National Wilms' tumor study. J Clin Oncol 6:1964, 1988.
93. Churchill DN, Hong K, Gault MH. Radiation nephritis following combined abdominal radiation and chemotherapy (bleomycin-vinblastine). Cancer 41:2162, 1978.
94. Moulder JE, Holcenberg JS, Kamen BA, et al. Renal irradiation and the pharmacology and toxicity of methotrexate and cisplatinum. Int J Radiat Oncol Biol Phys 12:1415, 1986.
95. Stewart F, Bohlken S, Begg A, Bartelink H. Renal damage in mice after treatment with cisplatinum alone or in combination with x-irradiation. Int J Radiat Oncol Biol Phys 12:927, 1986.
96. Moulder JE, Fish BL. Effect of sequencing on combined toxicity of renal irradiation and cisplatin. NCI Monogr 6:35, 1988.
97. van Rongen E, van der Kogel AJ, Durham SK. The influence of cisplatin and unilateral nephrectomy on the response of the rat kidney to irradiation. Int J Radiat Oncol Biol Phys 55:661, 1989.
98. Shaw PJ, Hugh-Jones K, Hobbs JR, et al. Busulfan and cyclophosphamide cause little early toxicity during displacement bone marrow transplantation in fifty children. Bone Marrow Transplant 1:193, 1986.
99. Stillwell TJ, Benson RC Jr, Burgert EO Jr. Cyclophosphamide-induced hemorrhagic cystitis in Ewing's sarcoma. J Clin Oncol 6:76, 1988.
100. Brugières L, Hartmann O, Travagli JP, et al. Hemorrhagic cystitis following high-dose chemotherapy and bone marrow transplantation in children with malignancies: Incidence, clinical course, and outcome. J Clin Oncol 7:194, 1989.
101. Stillwell TJ, Benson RC Jr. Cyclophosphamide-induced hemorrhagic cystitis. A review of 100 patients. Cancer 61:451, 1988.
102. Slavin RE, Millan J, Mullins GM. Pathology of high dose intermittent cyclophosphamide therapy. Hum Pathol 6:693, 1975.
103. Johnson WW, Meadows DC. Urinary-bladder fibrosis and telangiectasia associated with long-term cyclophosphamide therapy. N Engl J Med 284:290, 1971.
104. Lawrence HJ, Simone J, Aur RJA. Cyclophosphamide-induced hemorrhagic cystitis in children with leukemia. Cancer 36:1572, 1975.
105. Aptekar RG, Atkinson JP, Decker JL, et al. Bladder toxicity with chronic oral cyclophosphamide therapy in non-malignant disease. Arthritis Rheum 16:461, 1973.
106. Worth PHL. Cyclophosphamide and the bladder. Br Med J 3:172, 1971.
107. Samara Y, Hartz M, Lindner A. Urinary bladder tumors following cyclophosphamide therapy: A report of two cases with a review of the literature. Med Pediatr Oncol 13:86, 1985.
108. Cox PJ. Cyclophosphamide cystitis. Identification of acrolein as the causative agent. Biochem Pharmacol 28:2045, 1979.
109. Arthur RR, Shah KV, Baust SJ, et al. Association of BK viruria with hemorrhagic cystitis in recipients of bone marrow transplants. N Engl J Med 315:230, 1986.
110. Ambinder RF, Burns W, Forman M, et al. Hemorrhagic cystitis associated with adenovirus infection in bone marrow transplantation. Arch Intern Med 146:1400, 1986.
111. Goldman RL, Warner NE. Hemorrhagic cystitis and cytomegalic inclusions in the bladder associated with cyclophosphamide therapy. Cancer 25:7, 1970.
112. Fair WR. Formalin in the treatment of massive bladder hemorrhage. Techniques, results, and complications. Urology 3:573, 1974.
113. Fair WR. Urologic emergencies. *In:* Cancer: Principles and Practice of Oncology. 3rd ed. Devita VT Jr, Hellman S, Rosenberg SA (Eds). Philadelphia, JB Lippincott, 1989, p. 2016.
114. Levine LA, Richie JP. Urologic complications of cyclophosphamide. J Urol 141:1063, 1989.
115. de Vries CR, Freiha FS. Hemorrhagic cystitis. A review. J Urol 143:1, 1990.
116. Droller MJ, Saral R, Santos G. Prevention of cyclophosphamide-induced hemorrhagic cystitis. Urology 20:256, 1982.
117. Brock N, Stekar J, Pohl J. An antidote to the urotoxic effects of the oxazaphosphorine derivatives, cyclophosphamide, ifosphamide and trofosfamide. Naturwissenschaften 66:60, 1979.
118. Brock N, Stecker J, Pohl J, et al. Acrolein, the causative factor of urotoxic side-effects of cyclophosphamide, ifosphamide, trofosfamide, and sufosfamide. Arzneimittelforschung 29:659, 1979.

119. Millar BC, Millar JL, Clutterbuck R, Jinks S. Studies on the toxicity of cyclophosphamide in combination with mesna in vitro and in vivo. Cancer Treat Rev 10(Suppl. A):63, 1983.
120. Hows J, Mehta A, Gordon-Smith EC. Mesna versus forced diuresis to prevent cyclophosphamide induced hemorrhagic cystitis in marrow transplant patients (preliminary data). Cancer Treat Rev 10(Suppl. A):53056, 1983.
121. van Dyk JJ, Flakson HC, van der Merwe AM, Flakson G. Unexpected toxicity in patients treated with iphosphamide. Cancer Res 32:921, 1972.
122. Cohen MH, Creaven PJ, Tejada F, et al. Phase I clinical trial of isophosphamide (NSC-109724) (Part 1). Cancer Chemother Rep 59:751, 1975.
123. Nelson RL, Creaven PJ, Cohen MH, Fossick BE Jr. Phase I clinical trial of a 3 day divided dose schedule of ifosfamide (NSC 109724). Eur J Cancer 12:195, 1976.
124. Virini M, et al. Ifosfamide with the uroprotective agent mesna in treatment of squamous cell carcinoma of the lung. *In:* Current Chemotherapy Proceedings of the 12th International Congress of Chemotherapy, 1982, p. 1391.
125. Pode D, Perlberg S, Steiner D. Busulfan-induced hemorrhagic cystitis. J Urol 130:347, 1983.
126. Millard RJ. Busulfan-induced hemorrhagic cystitis. Urology 18:143, 1981.
127. Treible DP, Skinner D, Kaisimain D, et al. Intractable bladder hemorrhage requiring cystectomy after use of intravesicular thiotepa. Urology 30:568, 1987.
128. Wajsman Z, McGill W, Englander L, et al. Severely contracted bladder following intravesicular mitomycin C therapy. J Urol 130:340, 1983.
129. Pourquier H, Delard R, Achille E, et al. A qualified approach to the analysis and prevention or urinary complications in radiotherapeutic treatment of cancer of the cervix. Int J Radiat Oncol Biol Phys 13:1025, 1987.
130. Rubin P. Radiation Biology and Pathology Syllabus. Chicago, American College of Radiology, 1975.
131. Pearse HD. The urinary bladder. *In:* Radiation Oncology. 6th ed. Moss WT, Cox JD (Eds). St. Louis, CV Mosby Co, 1989.
132. McGuire EJ, Weiss RM, Schiff M, Lytton B. Hemorrhagic radiation cystitis: Treatment. Urology 3:204, 1974.
133. Antonkopoulos GN, Hicks RM, Berry RJ. The subcellular basis of damage to the human bladder induced by irradiation. J Pathol 143:103, 1984.
134. Parsons CL. Successful management of radiation cystitis with sodium pentosanpolysulfate. J Urol 136:13, 1986.
135. Marberger H, Bartsch G, Huber W, et al. Orgotein. A new drug for the treatment of radiation cystitis. Curr Ther Res 18:466, 1975.
136. Rijkmans BG, Bakker DJ, Dabhoiwala NF, Kurth KH. Successful treatment of radiation cystitis with hyperbaric oxygen. Eur Urol 16:354, 1989.
137. Weiss JP, Neville EC. Hyperbaric oxygen: Primary treatment of radiation-induced hemorrhagic cystitis. J Urol 142:43, 1989.
138. Schoenrock GH, Cianci P. Treatment of radiation cystitis with hyperbaric oxygen. Urology 27:271, 1986.
139. Weiss JP, Boland FP, Mori H, et al. Treatment of radiation-induced cystitis with hyperbaric oxygen. J Urol 134:352, 1985.
140. Zende G, Wajsman Z, Thomas PRM, Freeman AL. Chronic hematuria and localized bladder damage following combined cyclophosphamide and local radiotherapy. J Surg Oncol 12:169, 1979.
141. Jakse G, Frommhold H, Marberger H. Combined cisplatinum and radiation therapy in patients with stages T3 and T4 bladder cancer. A pilot study. J Urol 129:502, 1983.
142. Jakse G, Frommhold H, Nedden DZ. Combined radiation and chemotherapy for locally advanced transitional cell carcinoma of the urinary bladder. Cancer 55:1659, 1985.
143. Raghavan D, Pearson B, Duval P, et al. Initial intravenous cisplatinum therapy. Improved management for invasive high risk bladder cancer? J Urol 133:399, 1985.
144. Shipley WU, Prout GR, Einstein A, et al. Treatment of invasive bladder cancer by cisplatinum and radiation in patients unsuited for surgery. JAMA 258:931, 1987.
145. Sauer R, Schrott KM, Dunst J, et al. Preliminary results of treatment of invasive bladder carcinoma with radiotherapy and cisplatinum. Int J Radiat Oncol Biol Phys 15:871, 1988.
146. Rotman M, Macchia R, Silverstein M, et al. Treatment of advanced bladder carcinoma with irradiation and concomitant 5-fluorouracil infusion. Cancer 59:710, 1987.
147. Russell KJ, Boileau MA, Ireton RC, et al. Transitional cell carcinoma of the urinary bladder. Histologic clearance with combined 5-FU chemotherapy and radiation therapy. Radiology 167:845, 1988.
148. Marks LB, Kaufman SD, Prout GR, et al. Invasive bladder carcinoma. Preliminary report of selective bladder conservation by transurethral surgery, upfront MCV (methotrexate, cisplatinum, and vinblastine) chemotherapy and pelvic irradiation plus cis-

platinum. Int J Radiat Oncol Biol Phys 15:877, 1988.
149. Gradishar WJ, Schilsky RL. Effects of cancer treatment on the reproductive system. Crit Rev Oncol Hematol 8:153, 1988.
150. Spitz S. The histologic effects of nitrogen mustard on human tumors and tissues. Cancer 1:383, 1948.
151. Watson AR, Rance CP, Bain J. Long term effects of cyclophosphamide on testicular function. Br J Med 291:1457, 1985.
152. Lu CC, Meistrich ML. Cytotoxic effects of chemotherapeutic drugs on mouse testis cells. Cancer Res 39:3575, 1979.
153. Richter P, Calamera JC, Morgenfeld MC, et al. Effect of chlorambucil on spermatogenesis in the human with malignant lymphoma. Cancer 25:1026, 1970.
154. Guesry P, Lenoir G, Broyer M. Gonadal effects of chlorambucil given to prepubertal and pubertal boys for nephrotic syndrome. J Pediatr 92:299, 1978.
155. Cheviakoff J, Calamera JC, Morgenfeld M, Manuini RE. Recovery of spermatogenesis in patients with lymphoma after treatment with chlorambucil. J Reprod Fertil 33:155, 1973.
156. Sieber SM, Correa P, Daigard DW, Adamson RH. Carcinogenic and other adverse effects of procarbazine in non-human primates. Cancer Res. 38:2125, 1978.
157. Bonnadonna G, Santoro A. ABVD chemotherapy in the treatment of Hodgkin's disease. Cancer Treat Rev 9:21, 1982.
158. Horstman MG, Meadows GG, Yost GS. Separate mechanisms for procarbazine spermatotoxicity and anticancer activity. Cancer Res 47:1547, 1987.
159. Delic JI, Bush C, Peckham MJ. Protection from procarbazine-induced damage of spermatogenesis in the rat by androgen. Cancer Res 46:1909, 1986.
160. Shamberger RC, Rosenberg SA, Scipp CA, Sherins RJ. Effects of high dose methotrexate and vincristine on ovarian and testicular functions in patients undergoing post operative adjuvant treatment of osteosarcoma. Cancer Treat Rep 65:739, 1981.
161. Meistrich ML, da Cunha MF, Chawla SP, et al. Sperm production following chemotherapy for sarcomas. Proc Am Assoc Can Res 26:170, 1985.
162. Leitner SP, Bosl GH, Bajorunas D. Gonadal dysfunction in patients treated for metastatic germ-cell tumors. J Clin Oncol 4:1500, 1986.
163. Tseng A, Kessler R, Freiha F, et al. Male fertility before and after treatment of testicular cancer. Proc Am Soc Clin Oncol 3:161, 1984.
164. Drasga RE, Einhorn LH, Williams SD, et al. Fertility after chemotherapy for testicular cancer. J Clin Oncol 1:179, 1983.
165. Meistrich ML, Finch M, da Cunha MF, et al. Damaging effects of fourteen chemotherapeutic drugs on mouse testis cells. Cancer Res 42:122, 1982.
166. Jackson H. The effects of alkylating agents on fertility. Br Med Bull 20:107, 1964.
167. Jackson H, Fox BW, Craig AW. Antifertility substances and their assessment in the male rodent. J Reprod Fertil 2:447, 1961.
168. da Cunha MF, Meistrich ML, Haq MM, et al. Temporary effects of AMSA chemotherapy on spermatogenesis. Cancer 49:2459, 1982.
169. Fosdick WM, Parsons JL, Hill DF. Long term cyclophosphamide therapy in rheumatoid arthritis. Arthritis Rheum 11:151, 1968.
170. Warne GL, Fairley KF, Hobbs JB, et al. Cyclophosphamide-induced ovarian failure. N Engl J Med 289:1159, 1973.
171. Uldall PR, Kerr DNS, Tacchi D. Sterility and cyclophosphamide. Lancet i:693, 1972.
172. Koyama H, Wada T, Nishizawa Y, et al. Cyclophosphamide-induced ovarian failure and its therapeutic significance in patients with breast cancer. Cancer 39:1403, 1977.
173. Louis J, Limarzi LR, Best WR. Treatment of chronic granulocytic leukemia with Myleran. Arch Intern Med 97:299, 1956.
174. Galton DAG, Till M, Wiltshaw E. Busulfan. Summary of clinical results. Ann NY Acad Sci 68:967, 1958.
175. Choo YC, Chan SY, Wong LC, Ma HK. Ovarian dysfunction in patients with gestational trophoblastic neoplasia treated with short intensive courses of etoposide. Cancer 55:2348, 1985.
176. Fisher B, Sherman B, Rockette H, et al. L-phenylalanine mustard in the management of pre-menopausal patients with primary breast cancer. Cancer 44:847, 1979.
177. Schilsky RL, Sherins RJ, Hubbard SM, et al. Long term follow-up of ovarian function in women treated with MOPP chemotherapy for Hodgkin's disease. Am J Med 71:552, 1981.
178. Chapman RM, Sutcliffe SB. Protection of ovarian function by oral contraceptives in women receiving chemotherapy for Hodgkin's disease. Blood 58:849, 1981.
179. Whitehead E, Shalet SM, Blackledge G, et al. The effect of combination chemotherapy on ovarian function in women treated for Hodgkin's disease. Cancer 52:988, 1983.
180. Specht L, Hansen MM, Geisler C. Ovarian function in young women in long term remission after treatment for Hodgkin's disease stage I and II. Scand J Hematol 32:265, 1984.

181. Lushbaugh CC, Ricks RC. Some cytokinetic and histopathological considerations of irradiated male and female gonadal tissues. Front Radiat Ther Oncol 6:224, 1972.
182. Rowley MJ, Leuch DR, Warner GA. Effect of graded doses of ionizing radiation on the human testis. Radiat Res 59:665, 1974.
183. Clifton DK, Bremner WJ. The effect of testicular irradiation on spermatogenesis in man. A comparison with the mouse. J Androl 4:387, 1981.
184. Shapiro E, Kinsella TJ, Makuch RW. Effects of fractionated irradiation on endocrine aspects of testicular function. J Clin Oncol 3:1232, 1985.
185. Speiser B, Rubin P, Casarett G. Aspermia following lower truncal irradiation in Hodgkin's disease. Cancer 32:692, 1973.
186. Schally AV, Paz-Bouza JI, Scholsser JV, et al. Protective effects of analogs of luteinizing hormone-releasing hormone against x-radiation-induced testicular damage in rats. Proc Natl Acad Sci USA 84:851, 1987.
187. Dembo AJ. Response of the normal ovary to irradiation. *In:* Radiation Oncology. 6th ed. Moss WT, Cox JD (Eds). St. Louis, CV Mosby Co, 1989.
188. Peck WS, McGreer JT, Kretzschmar NR, Brown WE. Castration of the female by irradiation. Radiology 34:176, 1940.
189. Horning SJ, Hoppe RT, Kaplan HS, Rosenberg SA. Female reproductive potential after treatment for Hodgkin's disease. N Engl J Med 304:1377, 1981.
190. Stillman RJ, Schinfeld JS, Schiff I, et al. Ovarian failure in long-term survivors of childhood malignancy. Am J Obstet Gynecol 139:62, 1981.
191. Ray GB, Trueblood HW, Enright LP, et al. Oophoropexy. A means of preserving ovarian function following pelvic megavoltage radiotherapy for Hodgkin's disease. Radiology 96:175, 1970.
192. Thomas PRH, Winstantly P, Peckham MJ, et al. Reproduction and endocrine function in patients with Hodgkin's disease. Effects of oophoropexy and irradiation. Br J Cancer 33:226, 1976.
193. Blatt J, Sherins RJ, Niebrugge D, et al. Leydig cell function in boys following treatment for testicular relapse of acute lymphoblastic leukemia. J Clin Oncol 4:1227, 1985.
194. Shalet SM, et al. Leydig cell damage after testicular irradiation for lymphoblastic leukemia. Med Pediatr Oncol 13:65, 1985.
195. Delic JL, Bush C, Steel GG. Influence of timing of cytotoxic drug treatment on the response of murine clonogenic spermatogenia to x-irradiation. Radiother Oncol 7:341, 1986.
196. Himelstein-Braw R, Peters H, Faber M. Influence of irradiation and chemotherapy on the ovaries of children with abdominal tumors. Br J Cancer 36:269, 1977.
197. Hamre MR, Robison LL, Nesbit ME, et al. Effects of radiation on ovarian function in long-term survivors of childhood acute lymphoblastic leukemia. A report from the Children's Cancer Study Group. J Clin Oncol 5:1759, 1987.
198. Jarrel J, Lai EV, Barr R, et al. Ovarian toxicity alone and in combination with ovarian irradiation in the rat. Cancer Res 47:2340, 1987.
199. Johnson SA, Goldman JM, Hawkins DF. Pregnancy after chemotherapy for Hodgkin's disease. Lancet ii:93, 1979.
200. Li FP, Fine W, Jaffee N, et al. Offspring of patients treated for cancer in childhood. J Natl Cancer Inst 62:1193, 1979.
201. van Thiel DW, Ross GT, Lipsett MB. Pregnancies after chemotherapy of trophoblastic neoplasms. Science 169:1326, 1970.
202. Holmes GE, Holmes FF. Pregnancy outcome of patients treated for Hodgkin's disease. Cancer 41:1317, 1978.

Chapter 40

NERVOUS SYSTEM TOXICITY

A. ROBERT KAGAN

RADIONECROSIS AND CHEMONECROSIS

Brain injury secondary to radiations can occur without major neurologic manifestation, but brain necrosis, fortunately rare, is usually clinically evident. A rough guess is that the risk of brain necrosis with doses below 5000 cGy in 25 fractions is less than 1%; at 6000 cGy, it is 10% (1), and it rises to 50% at 7000 cGy. The daily dose may be as important as the total dose (2). Sheline reported 89 patients with brain necrosis, of whom 22 received doses under 5000 cGy, but most with daily doses higher than 200 cGy (3). Small volumes of normal brain may not be as susceptible to severe injury relative to large volumes because in the irradiation of cancer of the nasopharynx, wherein small portions of the temporal lobes receive 6500 to 7000 cGy in 6-½ to 8 weeks, late sequelae to the brain are uncommon compared to other sites (4) (Table 40–1).

Most of the time, the changes from radiation are localized to the region of the cerebral tumor and do not involve normal irradiated brain. The commonest clinical findings are those of a mass, the differential diagnosis being recurrent glioma versus necrosis (Figs. 40–1 through 40–4), whereas diffuse demyelination is the common finding with combined chemoradiation encephalopathy, and may occur with only the chemotherapeutic agent (5) (Table 40–2). This chapter will stress these differences, that is, focal changes with radiations and diffuse changes with the addition of chemotherapy, which may be proven in the future to be more apparent than real.

Burger and colleagues described the parenchymal necrosis secondary to radiations which surround treated astrocytomas, and underscored the preferential localization of delayed radiation necrosis to the white matter (6,7) (Table 40–3). After irradiation of extracranial malignancy, Rottenberg (8) and Kagan (9) emphasized the vascular occlusive changes of the small and medium size blood vessels "causing" the necrosis of white matter in the normal brain. In radiation necrosis, the destruction is in the region of the damaged vessel. Yet this same constellation of vascular occlusive changes and white matter demyelination may be seen with high doses of chemotherapy *alone,* especially with intracarotid administration of chemotherapy (10,11) or chemotherapeutic regimens that condition patients prior to bone marrow transplantation (Fig. 40–5) (12,13). This contradicts any thesis declaring microscopic changes unique to radiation injury (Table 40–4). In truth, the histopathologic changes of radionecrosis and chemonecrosis are so similar that microscopic differentiation is not possible but is suggested by the distribu-

Table 40–1. Fatal Complications in 218 Patients with Cancer of the Nasopharynx Probably Receiving More than 6500 cGy to a Portion of the Temporal Lobes at a Rate Above 1000 cGy/Week.

Complications	Number of Patients
Stricture of pharynx	1
Spinal cord myelopathy	5
Necrosis of nasopharynx with hemorrhage	3
Cranial nerve paralysis	2
Brain necrosis	1
Radiation induced cancer	1

Modified with permission from Ballantyne AJ. Am J Surg 130:433, 1978.

A

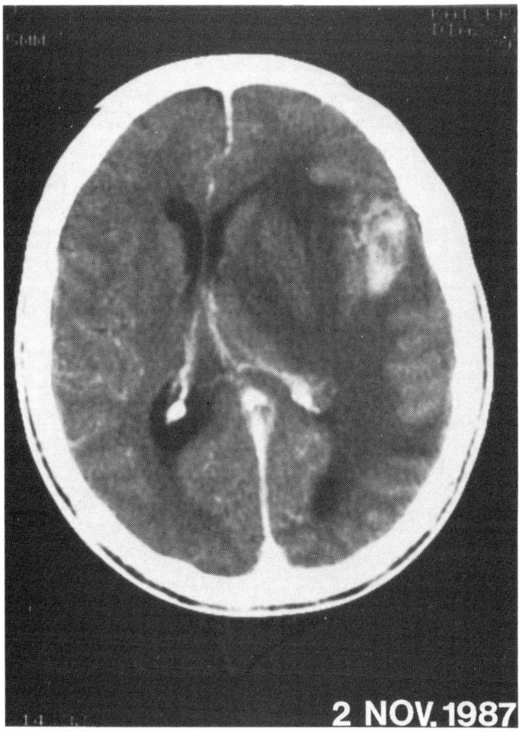

B

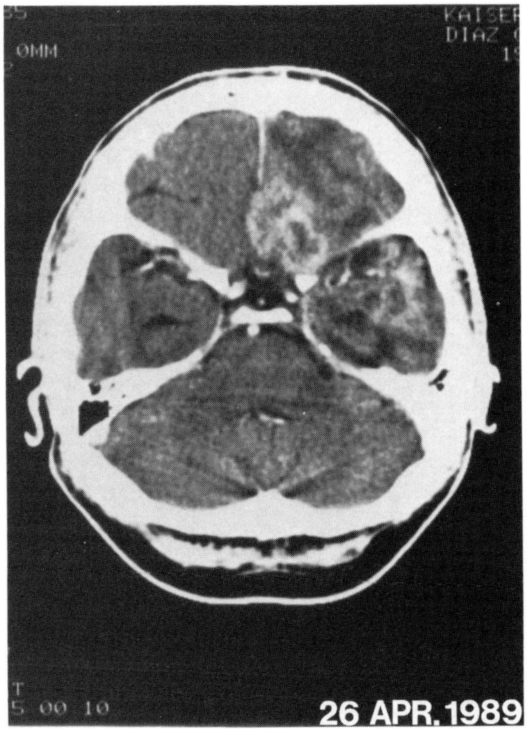

C

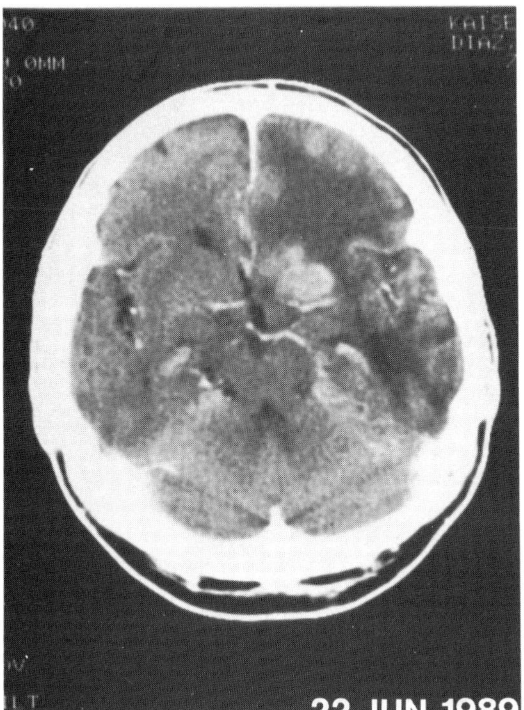

Fig. 40–1. A, B & C—CT scans at different levels with contrast enhancement over 20 months showing brain necrosis simulating a mass lesion. Patient had a history of irradiation for a large cancer of ethmoidomaxillary sinus.

tion of injury: focal in radionecrosis and symmetrical in chemonecrosis.

TYPES OF CEREBRAL INJURY

The commoner nervous system injuries secondary to chemoradiation treatment malignancies in children and adults are presented in Table 40–5 (14).

Children

The changes seen with intrathecal methotrexate (MTX) and brain irradiation in children do not mimic those seen in brain necrosis (14). Symmetrical areas of demyelinization (white matter necrosis) occur with relative sparing of grey matter, so-called **leukoencephalopathy.** Leukoencephalopathy is not commonly seen in adults after MTX and brain irradiation, and neither is **mineralizing microangiopathy,** which affects grey matter (commonly in the basal ganglia) and is characterized by a mineralizing destructive lesion of small vessels accompanied by dystrophic calcifications of adjacent cerebral grey tissue. The incidence of both mineralizing microangiopathy and leukoencephalopathy increases with increasing doses of intrathecal methotrexate, intravenous methotrexate, and radiation (14,15). The administration of intraventricular or intrathecal chemotherapy in the face of cerebrospinal fluid obstruction significantly increases the probability of injury with the use of MTX and ara-C ± radiation (16,17) (Table 40–6). Necrotizing leukomyelopathy and cortical atrophy can be found outside the field of radiation, implicating the chemical agent, and may not be symptomatic (18). Children with adverse neuropsychologic sequelae do not necessarily show hypodensities in the white matter, ventricular dilation, and widening of the subarachnoid space on imaging studies. Retrospective studies on small subsets of treated acute leukemic children for general intelligence, attention (reaction time), memory (verbal and nonverbal), and frontal lobe

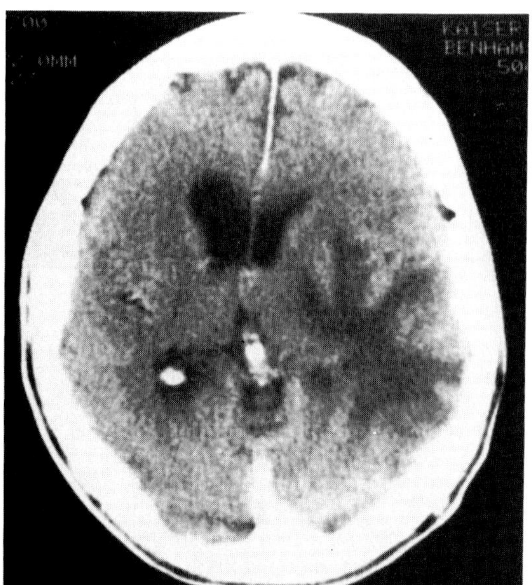

Fig. 40–2. CT scan showing "chicken foot" necrosis. Patient had a history of two courses of irradiation for cancer of external ear and mastoid.

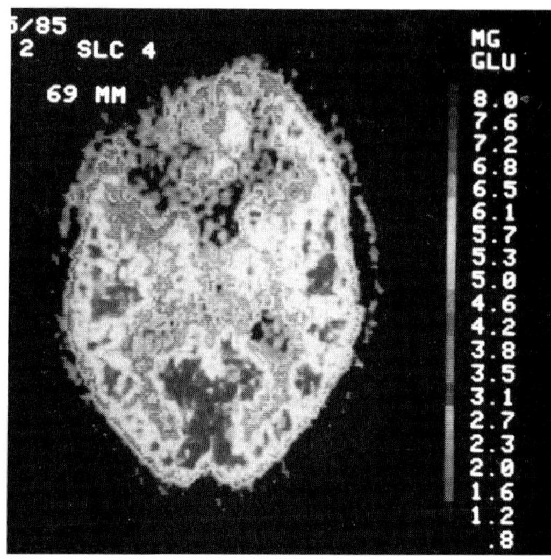

Fig. 40–3. Cerebral positron emission tomography (PET) with ^{18}F-deoxyglucose (FDG) in a 43-year-old man harboring a butterfly, bifrontal glioblastoma multiforme. Tumor had been treated with external beam radiotherapy (6300 cGy). CT shows a large bilateral frontal mass, which enhances with contrast. PET-FDG reveals marked hypometabolism in both prefrontal areas, larger on the left. Note selective sparing of interhemispheric gray matter, which is displaced toward the right. Color scale indicates range of metabolic values expressed in mg/glucose/100 g/min. (On PET scans, right side of patient is on right side of images.) Conclusion: Radiation necrosis. (Courtesy of Dr. Giovanni DiChiro, National Cancer Institute, Bethesda, Maryland.) (Figure 40–3 also appears in color in the color section.)

tasks have shown deficits; but these differences, on the whole, do not deviate from the normal to the extent that these patients would be selected out as mentally disadvantaged on first appraisal (19,20). Under age 3, the use of MTX, the presence of CNS leukemia, and cranial irradiation predispose to a clinical incidence of intellectual physiologic impairment associated with an abnormal EEG, but not necessarily an abnormal imaging study.

The growing brain is more sensitive to irradiation damage but is also more sensitive to chemotherapy. In a series of 14 patients, the majority of whom were given neoadjuvant cyclophosphamide, vincristine, VP-16 and prednisone, linear growth, adaptive behavior and mental abilities were decreased after a median of 8 months of preirradiation chemotherapy (21). With less aggressive CNS therapy, abnormal CT scans may revert to normal (22).

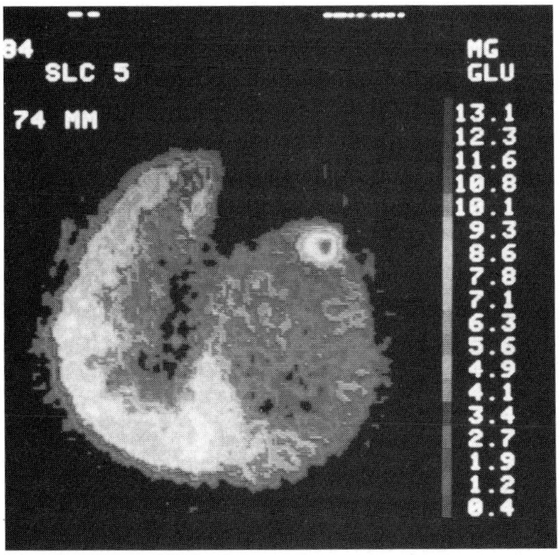

Fig. 40–4. PET-FDG scan in young female patient with a brain tumor treated with radiation plus chemotherapy. Note discrete area of intense hypermetabolism in right frontal region, behind wedge-like defect caused by previous surgery. The hypermetabolic focus indicates recurrent tumor. Vast, hypometabolic (blue) areas, most likely related to chemoradiation injury, are seen in ipsilateral as well as contralateral hemispheres. Conclusion: Radiation necrosis and recurrent tumor, which was not suspected on CT or MRI images. (Courtesy of Dr. Giovanni DiChiro, National Cancer Institute, Bethesda, Maryland.) (Figure 40–4 also appears in color in the color section.)

Neuroendocrine sequelae consist mostly of a biochemical growth hormone deficiency, but exceptions occur (23). The majority of growth problems with doses of 2400 cGy are associated with craniospinal irradiations wherein the gonads have been irradiated (24,25). Children with brain tumors receive doses above 3000 cGy and may not grow normally, especially when the hypothalamus or pituitary is in the field of irradiation (26). Although all the above cerebral-psychological-endocrine conditions have been described with single agents, the overall incidence of disabling CNS complications is below 5% and is often associated with IV MTX plus IT MTX plus cranial radiations above 1800 cGy. The incidence of leukoencephalopathy in bone marrow transplant patients for acute leukemia is 7% in a subset who received IT MTX ± radiations to the CNS prior to acceptance for bone marrow transplantation.

Recommendations for those who wish to document treatment-related cerebral injury

Table 40–2. Antineoplastic Drugs (by Category) Associated with Cerebral Encephalopathy

I. *Antimetabolites*
  - High-dose methotrexate
  - 5-Fluorouracil (with allopurinol)
  - Cytarabine (Ara-C)
  - Fludarabine
  - PALA L-aspartic acid N-(phos phono acetyl) disodium

II. *Alkylating agents*
  - Cisplatinum
  - Ifosfamide
  - BCNU (carmustine)
  - Spiromustine

III. *Plant Alkaloids*
  - Vincristine [associated with inappropriate ADH (antidiuretic hormone) secretion]

IV. *Drugs used in high doses during bone marrow transplant*
  - Nitrogen mustard
  - VP-16 (etoposide)
  - Procarbazine

V. *Miscellaneous*
  - Mitotane
  - Misonidazole
  - L-asparaginase
  - Hexamethylmelamine
  - Interleukin-2

Modified with permission from MacDonald DR. *In:* The Chemotherapy Source Book. Perry MC (Ed). Baltimore, Williams & Wilkins, 1992, p. 666.

Table 40–3. Histopathologic Findings Suggesting Radionecrosis

• Often lateralized to side of neoplasm	• Prominent foci of demyelination
• Coagulation necrosis and calcium deposition in the glioma	• Telangiectasis
• Vessels with fibrinoid necrosis	• Multilobed bizarre cells
• Discrete globoid cells with granular eosinophilic cytoplam (may be misinterpreted as gemistocytic astrocytes)	• Exudation of an amorphous, eosinophilic, structureless substance identified histochemically or immunohistochemically as fibrin

Modified with permission from Burger PC, et al. Cancer 44:1256, 1979; and Burger PC, Boyko OB. *In:* Radiation Injury to the Nervous System. Gutin P, Leibel SA, Sheline GE (Eds). New York, Raven Press, 1991, p. 191.

in children (see p. 585) are as follows: intellectual assessment tests yearly for 5 years, growth hormone if growth less than 4 cm per year and TSH, T_3, T_4 twice a year for 3 years.

Adults

Small-cell carcinoma of the lung occurs as a large unresectable mass in the mediastinum in which the natural course of events is metastasis. It metastasizes as often to the bone, liver, and lung (including pleura) as it does to the brain. Nevertheless, the brain has been singled out by many investigators as a site that merits concomitant treatment with the lung. The wide use of nitrosoureas (27), because they are lipid-soluble, in the initial therapy and large fractions (300 to 400 cGy) of cranial irradiation (28), to prevent the clinical symptoms of brain metastasis are cited as the culprit for the **dementia** demonstrated in longterm survivors. However, other studies reporting similar neurologic findings, also in longterm survivors, have used regimens excluding nitrosoureas and daily dose fractions under 300 cGy (29,30). The brain is no different from any other normal structure: the more drugs used, the higher the tissue drug concentration, the more intense the radiations, and the higher the probability of chemoradiation injury.

However, one must retain some doubt, especially in such a complex scenario as the treatment of small-cell carcinoma of the lung by multiagent chemotherapy and elective cranial irradiation. For example, out of 1200 patients with small-cell carcinoma of the lung, only 400 (⅓) patients have limited disease. Of these 400, 200 (50%) at best have a complete response, thereby being eligible for randomization to elective cranial irradiation: 100 to receive prophylactic irradiation to the brain and 100 to receive no prophylactic cranial irradiation. Of the 200 patients in complete remission, 20% are longterm

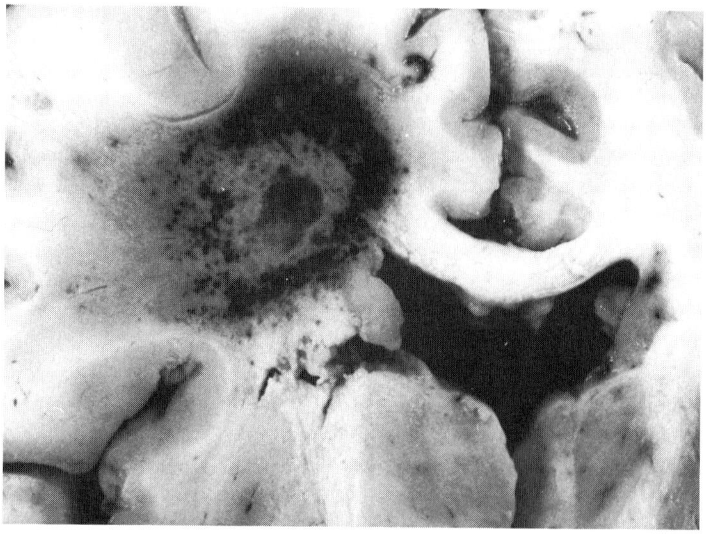

Fig. 40–5. Large area of necrotizing and hemorrhagic leukoencephalopathy in a patient who underwent bone marrow transplantation for acute lymphoblastic leukemia and received cranial irradiation and intraventricular Ara-C. The left centrum semiovale shows a necrotic hemorrhagic mass with surrounding edema. (Courtesy of Dr. Harry V. Vinters, Division of Neuropathology, UCLA Medical Center.)

Table 40–4. Histopathologic Indicators suggesting Chemonecrosis

• Vessels with fibrinoid necrosis • Symmetry of involvement • "Chemonecrosis" seen in the spinal cord	• Prominent foci of demyelination • Predilection of grey matter vasculopathy (i.e., following the distribution of an artery)

Modified with permission from Burger PC, et al. Cancer 44:1256, 1979; and Burger PC, Boyko OB. *In:* Radiation Injury to the Nervous System. Gutin P, Leibel SA, Sheline GE (Eds). New York, Raven Press, 1991, p. 191.

survivors; that is, 40 patients of whom ½ have received prophylactic irradiation (prophylactic cranial irradiation does not affect survival). Now, of the 40 patients who are longterm survivors, 20 (50%) have received prophylactic cranial irradiation of whom 10 patients (50%), at most, have treatment-induced dementia. Incidently, some of those NOT receiving cranial irradiation also sustain dementia, but the percentage is even less certain. The mean age of this group of 1200 is 60; of this group, 10 patients sustain dementia. Or, of the 400 patients with limited disease or the 200 patients who do go into complete remission, 10 patients sustain dementia. It ends up that 10 of 1200 to 10 of 200 patients have dementia, depending on what denominator is chosen. But the percentage most commonly quoted in the literature is to take 20 patients (the longterm survivors who received prophylactic cranial irradiation) as the denominator that makes the percentage of demented patients 10 of 20 or 50%.

Beginning in 1972, we treated patients with glioblastoma multiforme with whole-brain radiations and multiagent chemotherapy (31). The resultant median survival was no better or worse than our experience with radiations alone (range of median survival 10 to 12 months); hence, we stopped chemotherapy. The radiation regimens in combination with BCNU, procarbazine, and vincristine were 4000 cGy and 4800 cGy in split course, with interruptions at 2000 and 2400 cGy, respectively. For the past 10 years, our regimen has consisted of 3500 cGy in 10 fractions. Some of these patients have received postirradiation chemotherapy, most often oral CCNU. Survival in our experience seems to depend primarily on the depth of the lesion and the neurologic status and secondarily on the age of the patient and the amount of resection rather than the intensity of treatment. Of major interest to us is that fewer than 5% of patients return to work, the major neurologic disability being focal (not global as in dementia) in nature.

The results of nearly 500 patients treated by chemoradiation protocols of the Brain Tumor Cooperative Group demonstrated a

Table 40–5. The More Frequent Conditions of Cerebral Injury Secondary to Chemoradiation Treatment of a Malignancy

Condition	Imaging	Sequelae	Comment
Leukoencephalopathy	Hypodensity of white matter in both cranial hemispheres Diffuse increase in signal intensity on T_2	Death	Concurrent IV MTX, IT MTX and cranial radiations at or above 2400 cGy Intracarotid nitrosoureas
Mineralizing microangiopathy	Basal ganglia calcification (grey matter)	Serious if associated with leukoencephalopathy	High-dose IV MTX plus cranial irradiation
Dementia	Periventricular white matter hypodensity that is T_2 positive	Death	Concurrent high dose chemotherapy and daily dose radiations of 300 cGy or higher
Paraneoplastic syndromes	Not helpful		Death from co-existing cancer

IV MTX = intravenous methotrexate
IT = intrathecal
cGy = centrigray, unit of radiation dose
T_2 = tissue parameter used in magnetic resonance imaging (MRI)
Modified with permission from DeAngelis LM, Shapiro WR. *In:* Radiation Injury to the Nervous System. Gutin PH, Leibel SA, Sheline GE (Eds). New York, Raven Press, 1991, p. 361.

Table 40–6. Safe Doses (in mg) of Intrathecal Methotrexate (MTX) and Intrathecal Cytarabine (Ara-C) Given in Conjunction with 1800 cGy Brain Irradiation

	Age (Years)			Maximum Concentrations (MG/ML)
	1	1–3	3	
MTX	6	8–10	12	2.5
Ara-C	20	30–50	70	20
Comment:	In high-risk patients—under age 3, presence of altered CSF flow dynamics, intraventricular catheters—waiting 24 hours after IT MTX before irradiating decreases the probability of harmful drug-radiation interactions. IV MTX given with irradiation should not greatly exceed 20 mg/m^2.			

Modified with permission from Steinherz PG. Oncology 3:47, 1989.

Table 40–7. Grading of Treatment-Related Encephalopathy

Grade	Status
1	Transient lethargy
2	Somnolence less than 50% of the time Disorientation—moderate
3	Somnolence more than 50% of the time Disorientation—severe, characterized by babbling
4	Coma

Reprinted with permission from Ebner E, et al. AJNR 153:1283, 1989.

median survival of approximately 1 year, with nearly 20% survival at 2 years (32). Of these 100 longterm survivors, who received a total of 6000 cGy many are demented (33). Seventy-two percent of all patients in the Brain Tumor Cooperative Group Protocols received whole-brain irradiation of 4300 cGy in 25 fractions, with an additional 1720 in 10 fractions to the tumor. Whether these latter patients whose whole brain received less than 5000 cGy at conventional fractionation (with chemotherapy) will avoid dementia is to be seen.

It follows that a certain percentage of patients with treatment-related encephalopathy (grading system described in Table 40–7) recover, become obviously disabled, or die. Magnetic resonance imaging (MRI) and histologic changes in methotrexate cerebral injury have recently been demonstrated (34). The exact percentages are not available in the literature, but some guidelines may be appreciated from a study of ifosfamide encephalopathy (35). In this study, 18 patients with encephalopathy occurring after ifosfamide/MESNA chemotherapy were prospectively studied. Two of these 18 patients died. In nine of these 18 patients, the denominator was known: four of 52 patients with lung cancer and five of 30 patients with ovarian cancer for an overall incidence of nine of 82 patients. Presently, incidence data regarding chemoradiation encephalopathy are known only in small subsets of patients wherein the clinical course regarding full recovery, partial recovery, and/or fatality is often incomplete.

Further complicating the clinical differential diagnosis of chemoradiation dementia is the fact that the incidence of dementia in the elderly patient is high, Alzheimer's disease and multi-infarct dementia being the two most common causes. In addition, the radiologic diagnosis of chemoradiation dementia is disguised by the fact that periventricular lesions, seen on MRI and/or CT, are commonly found in the elderly at autopsy (36). The histopathology of these periventricular demyelinating lesions may be similar to that of those described with the leukoencephalopathy associated with chemotherapy ± irradiation as described above. Rare causes of dementia in the cancer patient are normal pressure hydrocephalus and nonbacterial thrombotic endocarditis. Progressive multifocal leukoencephalopathy has been reported in patients with AIDS (37). **Paraneoplastic syndromes** affecting the limbic system (cognitive and memory disturbances), the brain stem (eye signs), or cerebellum (ataxia) may confound recognition of syndromes of chemoradiation cerebral injury.

Treatment-induced carcinogenesis may occur but does not seem to be of clinical significance, as it is in Hodgkin's disease management by combined therapy accompanying splenectomy. In 634 children treated from 1942 to 1969 who were alive at 5 years, 32 developed a second cancer; 3 of the 32 cancers were brain tumors (38).

SUMMARY

In summary, with normal doses of chemotherapy and radiations, irradiation necrosis of the brain occurs rarely (under 5%) in adults. Therefore, in my opinion, it does not constitute a problem for the clinician or the patient over and above the increased risks of combined therapy. When high doses of many drugs are given together with concurrent high doses of radiation, the risk increases. In infants and children, systemic and intrathecal therapy combined with radiation and altered cerebrospinal fluid dynamics such as those that occur with CNS leukemia, intraventricular catheters, or partial CSF obstruction, increases the risk of CNS damage. Intracarotid drug administration also increases the risk of CNS damage.

The morphologic changes and clinical manifestations of central nervous system damage by radiotherapy and chemotherapy overlap often (6,7,39,40). Radionecrosis of the brain is rare below total doses of 6000 cGy. Many drugs can cause cerebral chemonecrosis but, like radionecrosis, it is rare unless large doses are administered. Importantly, chemoradionecrosis from concomitant or closely sequential therapies may result from seemingly low doses of each. In patients who present with signs of encephalopathy (leukoencephalopathy or dementia), the MRI shows diffuse abnormalities in the white matter, characterized by an increased signal from a T_2 weighted MRI. Mineralizing microangiopathy is characterized by multifocal intracerebral calcifications in the grey matter or at the junction of the grey and white matter. Symptoms of severe mental impairment and/or seizures are thought to be due to the presence of leukoencephalopathy. Focal areas of chemoradionecrosis may also present with cognitive, memory, and global neurological dysfunction. PET scan is the most successful imaging study for distinguishing cerebral necrosis from recurrence in patients who have been treated for brain tumors. The surgical removal of focal areas of chemoradionecrosis should be considered but subsequent significant improvement of the patient's neurologic status does not frequently occur. Major neurologic signs and symptoms may occur in paraneoplastic syndromes. The discerning feature of paraneoplastic syndromes from leukoencephalopathy, dementia or mineral microangiography is a normal MRI in the former. In some patients, the categories tend to overlap, rather than being separate, resulting in a confused clinician.

REFERENCES

1. Glanzmann C, Seelentag W. Radiotherapy for tumours of the pineal region and suprasellar germinomas. Radiother Oncol 16:31, 1989.
2. Kagan AR, Steckel RJ, Cancilla R, et al. The pathogenesis of brain necrosis: Time and dose parameters. Int J Radiat Oncol Biol Phys 1:729, 1976.
3. Sheline G. Irradiation injury of the human brain: A review of clinical experience. *In:* Radiation Damage to the Nervous System. Kagan AR, Gilberts HA (Eds). New York, Raven Press, 1980, p. 39.
4. Ballantyne AJ. Late sequelae of radiation therapy in cancer of the head and neck with particular reference to the nasophayrnx. Am J Surg 130:433, 1978.
5. MacDonald DR. Neurotoxicity of chemotherapeutic agents. *In:* The Chemotherapy Source Book. Perry MC (Ed). Baltimore, Williams & Wilkins, 1992, p. 666.
6. Burger PC, Mahaley MS Jr, Dudka L, Vogel FS. The morphologic effects of radiation administered therapeutically for intracranial gliomas. Cancer 44:1256, 1979.
7. Burger PC, Boyko OB. The pathology of central nervous system radiation injury. *In:* Radiation Injury to the Nervous System. Gutin PH, Leibel SA, Sheline GE (Eds). New York, Raven Press, 1991, p. 191.
8. Rottenberg DA, Chernik NL, Deck MDF, et al. Cerebral necrosis following radiotherapy of extracranial neoplasms. Ann Neurol 1:339, 1977.
9. Kagan AR, Bruce DW, DiChiro G. Fatal foam cell arteritis of the brain after irradiation for Hodgkin's disease: Angiography and pathology. Stroke 2:232, 1971.
10. Lee YY, Nauert C, Glass JP. Treatment-related white matter changes in cancer patients. Cancer 57:1473, 1986.
11. Kleinschmidt-DeMasters BK. Intracarotid BCNU leukoencephalopathy. Cancer 57:1276, 1986.
12. Thompson CB, Sanders JE, Flournoy N, et al. The risks of central nervous system relapse and leukoencephalopathy in patients receiving marrow transplants for acute leukemia. Blood 67:195, 1986.

13. Burger PC, Kamenar E, Schold SC, et al. Encephalomyelopathy following high-dose BCNU therapy. Cancer 48:1318, 1981.
14. DeAngelis LM, Shapiro WR. Drug/radiation interactions and central nervous system injury. *In:* Radiation Injury to the Nervous System. Gutin PH, Leibel SA, Sheline GE (Eds). New York, Raven Press, 1991, p. 361.
15. Steinherz PG. Radiotherapy vs. intrathecal chemotherapy for CNS prophylaxis in childhood ALL. Oncology 3:47, 1989.
16. Strother DR, Glyn-Barnhart A, Kovnar E, et al. Variability in the disposition of intraventricular methotrexate: a proposal for rational dosing. J Clin Oncol 7:1741, 1989.
17. Cohen ME, Duffner PK, Terplan KL. Myelopathy with severe structural derangement associated with combined modality therapy. Cancer 52:1590, 1983.
18. Bates SE, Raphaelson MI, Price RA, et al. Ascending myelopathy after chemotherapy for central nervous system acute lymphoblastic leukemia: Correlation with cerebrospinal fluid myelin basic protein. Med Pediatr Oncol 13:4, 1985.
19. Poplack DF, Brouwers P. Adverse sequelae of central nervous therapy. *In:* Clinics in Oncology. Late Effects in Successfully Treated Children with Cancer. Nesbit ME Jr (Ed). Philadelphia, WB Saunders, 1985, p. 263.
20. Copeland DR, Dowell RE Jr, Fletcher JM, et al. Neuropsychological effects on childhood cancer treatment. J Child Neurol 3:53, 1988.
21. Mulhern RK, Horowitz ME, Kovnar EH, et al. Neurodevelopmental status of infants and young children treated for brain tumors with pre-irradiation chemotherapy. J Clin Oncol 7:1660, 1989.
22. Ochs JJ, Parvey LS, Whitaker JN, et al. Serial cranial computed-tomography scans in children with leukemia given two different forms of central nervous system therapy. J Clin Oncol 7:1660, 1989.
23. Constine LS, Rubin P, Woolf PD, et al. Hyperprolactinemia and hypothyroidism following cytotoxic therapy for central nervous system malignancies. J Clin Oncol 5:1841, 1987.
24. Livesey EA, Brook CGD. Thyroid dysfunction after radiotherapy and chemotherapy of brain tumours. Arch Dis Child 64:593, 1989.
25. Livesey EA, Brook CGD. Gonadal dysfunction after treatment of intracranial tumours. Arch Dis Child 63:495, 1988.
26. Pasqualini T, Diez B, Domene H, et al. Long-term endocrine sequelae after surgery, radiotherapy and chemotherapy in children with medulloblastoma. Cancer 59:801, 1987.
27. Johnson BE, Becker B, Goff WB II, et al. Neurologic, neuropsychologic, and computed cranial tomography scan abnormalities in 2- to 10-year survivors of small-cell lung cancer. J Clin Oncol 3:1659, 1985.
28. Frytak S, Shaw JN, Lee RE, et al. Treatment toxicities in long-term survivors of limited small cell lung cancer. Cancer Invest 6:669, 1988.
29. Fleck JF, Einhorn LH, Lauer RC, et al. Is prophylactic cranial irradiation indicated in small cell lung cancer? J Clin Oncol 8:209, 1990.
30. Crino L, Meacci ML, Corgna E, et al. Long term survivors of small cell lung cancer (SCLC): Ten years experience. *In:* Proceedings of the Twenty-fifth Annual Meeting of the American Society of Clinical Oncology. Leventhal B (Ed). 1989, p. 240.
31. Gilbert HA, Sadoff L, Eder D, et al. Combination chemotherapy and delayed split course radiation therapy in malignant gliomas: A preliminary report. *In:* Proceedings of the International Conference on Adjuvant Therapy of Cancer. Salmon SE, Jones SE (Eds). Amsterdam, North-Holland Publishers, 1977, p. 487.
32. Shapiro WR, Green SB, Burger PC, et al. Randomized trial of three chemotherapy regimens and two radiotherapy regimens in post-operative treatment of malignant glioma. Brain Tumor Cooperative Group Trial 8001. J Neurosurg 71:1, 1989.
33. Shapiro WR. Personal communication. November, 1992.
34. Ebner E, Ranner G, Slavc I, et al. MR findings in methotrexate-induced CNS abnormalities. AJNR 153:1283, 1989.
35. Watkin SW, Husband DJ, Green JA, Warenius HM. Ifosfamide encephalopathy: A reappraisal. Eur J Cancer Clin Oncol 25:1303, 1989.
36. Chimowitz MI, Awad IA, Furlan AJ. Periventricular lesions on MRI. Facts and theories. Stroke 7:963, 1989.
37. Mark AS, Atlas SW. Progressive multifocal leukoencephalopathy in patients with AIDS: Appearance on MR images. Radiology 173:517, 1989.
38. deVathaire F, Francois P, Hill C, et al. Role of radiotherapy and chemotherapy in the risk of second malignancy neoplasms after cancer in childhood. Br J Cancer 59:792, 1989.
39. Lefaix JL. The pathologic characteristics of cerebral radionecrosis. Bull Cancer 79:251, 1992.
40. Kramer ED, Cohen BH, Pacher RJ. Central nervous system morbidity secondary to chemotherapy. *In:* Complications of Cancer Management. Plowman PN, McElwain T, Meadows A (Eds). Stoneham, Butterworth-Heinenann, 1991, p. 329.

Chapter 41

OCULAR TOXICITY

DAVID BARDENSTEIN AND DEVRON H. CHAR

Radiation eye damage has been a known entity for many years. In 1897, Chalupecky first described ocular radiation morbidity (1). Radiation retinopathy with visual loss was first reported in 1933 (2). However, even now, the dosage and fractionation parameters that result in many ocular complications are poorly delineated. Similarly, some ocular effects of chemotherapeutic agents have been reported, but the frequency of these complications and required dosage remains uncertain for many of these drugs. Chemoradiation has improved prognosis in many malignancies, but in most instances, even less is known about their cumulative ocular toxicities.

Fu and Phillips noted many years ago that the ocular toxicities of combination therapies were unclear for a number of reasons (3). Most pertinent reports concern patients who have been treated for nonocular tumors and who have not been monitored with systematic ophthalmologic evaluations. Often a single eye complication, most commonly a cataract, has either been evaluated by a nonophthalmologist or reported without ophthalmologic input. Much of the radiation data on ocular complications after sinus cancer irradiation are difficult to interpret because treatment planning often did not avail itself of computerized tomography (CT) simulation. We have observed many such cases with classic radiation retinopathy in which the radiation oncologist believed that no radiation had been delivered to the eye. Even recently, many reports that have discussed ocular toxicity have not included radiation dosage delivered to the eye. The latter problem is difficult to address; even with computer programs developed to delineate the radiation doses delivered to various eye structures, apparent incongruities still occur.

Comprehensive reviews of the ocular effects of either chemotherapy or radiation therapy have been published (4–10). Table 41–1 presents a compilation of the ocular side effects of chemotherapy; we have limited our list of complications to those that are known to be associated with a single agent (11–49). In many reports, it is difficult to ascribe a complication to a given agent because multidrug or multimodality treatment was used. Similarly, Table 41–2 lists ocular side effects of radiation therapy with an emphasis on those that have occurred inspite of treatment with less than 250 cGy daily fractionated megavoltage photon therapy (9,10,50–52).

Most ocular complication data on combined chemotherapy and radiation have been isolated case reports or retrospective comparative studies of chemoradiation versus single modality treatment. There is a paucity of prospective, randomized data with adequate ophthalmologic monitoring. Available data on ocular side effects from chemoradiation are primarily derived from treatment of nonocular malignancies such as acute leukemia, sinus carcinoma and central nervous system (CNS) tumors. Reports on the treatment of orbital rhabdomyosarcomas, retinoblastomas, and choroidal metastases provide supplementary data.

LEUKEMIA

Ocular toxicity occurs rarely when combined chemotherapy and prophylactic whole brain irradiation are used to treat acute lymphocytic leukemia (ALL). There

Table 41–1. Ocular Side Effects of Antineoplastic Agents

Agent	Toxicity	Reference(s)
Cytosine arabinoside	Keratitis, conjunctivitis	11–13
Adriamycin (doxorubicin)	Conjunctivitis	14
	Iritis	15
	Lacrimation	16
Nitrosoureas (BCNU/CCNU)	Neuroretinitis	17–22
	Blindness	20,21,23
	Eye pain	21,22
	Hyperemia, blurring	22
	Orbital A-V shunt	24
Cyclophosphamide	Blurred vision	25
5-Fluorouracil (5-FU)	Blepharitis	26
	Conjunctivitis	26
	Excess lacrimation	26–28
	Lacrimal stenosis	28–31
	Ectropion	30
	Optic neuropathy	32
	Epithelial defects	33
Methotrexate	Blepharitis, edema, pain, and conjunctivitis	25,34,35
	Internuclear ophthalmoplegia	36
Prednisone	Cataracts	37,38
	Elevated intraocular pressure	38,39
	Opportunistic infection	40
	Exophthalmos	41–43
	Pseudotumor cerebri	44,45
	Scleral thinning	46
Vincristine	Diplopia, ptosis	47
	Optic neuropathy	48,49

Note: Effects are those seen when the agent is used without radiation therapy, except for the nitrosoureas.

are a few cases of **optic atrophy** and visual loss after combination chemotherapy and 2400 cGy of whole brain irradiation with anterior eye shielding. In two cases there was no evidence of tumor, and histologic examinations of the optic nerves were compatible with radiation **optic neuropathy** (53,54). These cases appear to be rare examples of ocular toxicity from chemoradiation; radiation optic neuropathy has not been reported at this dose level (52). Although many of the agents used to treat leukemia, including methotrexate, cytosine arabinoside and vincristine, can produce neural damage, it is

Table 41–2. Radiation Effects on the Eye and Orbital Tissues

Tissue	Effect	Dose (cGy)	Reference(s)
Conjunctiva	Conjunctivitis	5500–7500	9
	Telangiectasis	3000	9,10
Cornea	Keratitis, edema, mild ulcer	3000–5000	10
	Ulcer, scarring, perforation	> 6000	9,10
Lens	Cataract	200 (threshold)	50
		1600	9
Retina	Retinopathy	> 4650	51
Optic nerve	Optic neuropathy	> 5500	9,52
Lacrimal system	Atrophy	5000–6000	9
	Stenosis	6500–7500	9,10
Eyelid	Lash loss	4000–6000	9,10
	Erythema	3000–4000	9,10
	Telangiectasia	> 5000	9,10
Orbit	Implant extrusion	Not specified	52

Note: These are effects seen with conventionally fractionated (< 250 cGy/day) megavoltage photon therapy.

doubtful that these agents were the sole cause of these complications. Vincristine optic neuropathy has a different histologic pattern (48) and both cytosine arabinoside and methotrexate have demonstrated CNS white matter toxicity only when used in combination with radiation (55–57).

Weaver studied 34 acute leukemia patients who were disease-free 5 years after treatment (58). Patients received either radiation plus chemotherapy (16 patients) or chemotherapy alone (18 patients). The irradiated patients received 2400 cGy of whole-brain photon therapy with shielding of the anterior portion of the globe. Two of these patients developed minimal cataracts and two patients developed varying degrees of optic atrophy (one unilateral and another minimal and bilateral). No ocular complications were noted in patients who did not receive radiation. The authors believed that the two optic neuropathies may have been due to leukemic infiltrates, although one child neither had clinical evidence of optic nerve infiltration nor developed an eventual CNS relapse. It is conceivable that at least one of these children had a chemoradiation ocular complication.

Inati and co-workers followed 215 ALL patients who received prophylactic whole brain radiation with chemotherapy and did not describe any cases of optic nerve atrophy (59). In one-half of the 69 long-term followup patients, minimal posterior **subscapular cataracts** were noted. However, they were uncertain whether these were due entirely to corticosteroids or an adjunctive radiation effect. This series points out the rarity of that problem with this treatment protocol.

The mechanisms responsible for the optic neuropathy observed in ALL chemoradiation cases are uncertain. Synergistic toxicity is possible because the threshold for damage appears to have been lowered. Possibly, radiation alters both the blood-brain and blood-retina barriers, and allows greater penetration of chemotherapeutic agents into CNS tissue. This most probably potentiated radiation damage or alternatively resulted in chemotherapeutic toxicity previously not observed when barriers are intact (55,56).

Intravenous methotrexate is an important factor in the etiology of the optic neuropathy associated with ALL therapy because optic nerve damage did not occur without it. Inati hypothesized that the low number of ocular side effects observed in her series resulted from delayed administration of intravenous methotrexate until one year after irradiation (59). Unlike the CNS, in which this drug toxicity appears to have a threshold (60), in the eye cases, doses were far lower and still were associated with damage. However, too few cases with ocular toxicity have been reported to draw significant conclusions.

In patients with leukemia and aplastic anemia treated with total body irradiation, chemotherapy, and bone marrow transplantation, anterior segment ocular complications have been described (61). Most of these are probably due to chemotherapy and compromised host immune status. Forty of 90 patients developed a **dry eye syndrome**, most likely secondary to both cyclophosphamide and a graft versus host reaction. Viral keratitis occurred in nine cases and others developed other corneal problems.

PARANASAL SINUS MALIGNANCIES

It is difficult to differentiate the ocular complications of chemotherapy from high-dose radiation effects after treatment of paranasal sinus malignancies. Most series report radiation dosages that alone were sufficient to cause major ocular complications; often one or both eyes have had to be included in the high dose field. Furthermore, ocular damage as a result of direct tumor effects can also occur. As discussed above, some of these reports were written before CT treatment planning was used, and the choice of chemoradiation versus radiation alone was not made in a randomized manner. In two of 26 patients reported by Goepfert and colleagues, contralateral optic neuritis with total loss of vision occurred after 6000 to 7000 cGy of radiation and intracarotid chemotherapy (62). Chan and Shukovsky studied 47 sinus carcinoma patients treated with 6000 cGy of photon irradiation, in 200 cGy daily fractions, along with different surgical or chemotherapeutic regimens (63). Survival was best in patients who received only radiation as compared with those who also received chemotherapy (38% versus 28% at 4 years). All of the chemoradiation group developed some eye complication compared with 30% of the irradiated group. Two of 22

(9%) patients who were treated with radiation alone versus 4 of 18 (22%) who received chemoradiation became blind. Ten percent of the radiation group and 50% of the combined group developed cataracts while 15% of the former and 100% of the latter group developed corneal problems. It is uncertain how many of the complications were due to differences in disease severity or field size and how much of the morbidity was due to at least additive adverse effects of these two modalities of treatment. The poorer survival in the combined treatment group would be consistent with disease severity being an etiologic parameter in ocular complications.

Choi et al have described chemoradiation with cisplatinum infusion being administered to 14 patients with paranasal sinus and nasopharyngeal tumors (64). Cisplatinum doses were 5 to 7 mg/m^2/day, and radiation was delivered in 120 cGy fractions twice daily to a total dose of 6000 to 6960 cGy. Four patients received less than 5500 cGy. Nine patients had either the eye or optic nerve in the radiation field. The only documented eye complication was ipsilateral corneal clouding. No information was provided about the nature of the ophthalmic evaluation.

CNS TUMORS

Various primary and secondary CNS tumors have been treated with radiation and the nitrosoureas, BCNU and CCNU. One report documented three patients who developed bilateral blindness after oral CCNU and 3000 to 4700 cGy cranial irradiation (65). The histologic examination of the optic nerves in one case showed demyelination and axonal loss of hyalinized vessels characteristic of radiation optic neuropathy. In treatment of primary or metastatic ocular tumors with radiation alone, over 5000 cGy in conventional fractions is usually needed to observe radiation vasculopathy of the retina or optic nerve (52). The fact that the neuropathy occurred at doses below the normal threshold suggests synergistic toxicity.

Glioblastoma multiforme treated with intracarotid BCNU resulted in ipsilateral visual loss in 50% of irradiated patients, but only 12.5% of patients whose radiation was given in the distant past (20). The BCNU doses varied, but there was no significant difference between any dose groups. Retinal toxicity decreased from 38 to 7% with decrease in the volume of ethanol solvent and drug administered.

Other studies have demonstrated that catheter position for intracarotid nitrosourea chemotherapy is a significant factor in ophthalmic toxicity. If the catheter was caudal to the ophthalmic artery, ocular toxicity was high. When the catheter is placed above this vessel, ocular toxicity decreased but the incidence of leukoencephalopathy increased (21). In contrast to intra-arterial chemotherapy, ocular complications after intravenous BCNU chemotherapy were significantly less; blindness occurred in 16% of the former group and 0% of the latter patients (23).

The effects of chemoradiation with bromodeoxyuridine (BUdR) and external beam therapy in 23 patients with malignant gliomas were reported (66). Patients received 400 to 500 mg/m^2 BUdR daily for 8.5 weeks by ipsilateral carotid artery injection. Focal external beam radiotherapy was delivered in 180 cGy daily fractions over 6.5 weeks to total doses of 5940 cGy. The ipsilateral face and forehead were excluded from the portals. Pretreatment and sequential ophthalmic examinations were performed. All patients developed ipsilateral eyelid erythema, forehead scaling, and dry eyes. Conjunctival hyperemia was present in 15 patients, chemosis in 9, and a mucopurulent discharge in 11. Six patients developed mechanical **ectropion** and four developed exposure keratitis. All problems had resolved by 6 months postradiation except one case of ectropion that required surgery, one case of corneal perforation, one case of trichiasis and one patient with persistent culture negative conjunctival drainage. Histopathologic examination of both eyes from one patient who died 6 weeks after treatment showed no abnormalities. Tissue from two other patients demonstrated unilateral epithelial thinning in one and changes compatible with a corneal perforation in the second. The authors calculated the enhanced radiation dose to the region, factoring in scatter and BUdR enhancement and derived a maximum of 1260 cGy. They felt that the changes were most likely due to sensitization by fluorescent or ultraviolet. Side effect severity appeared to be dose-related.

RHABDOMYOSARCOMA

The use of chemoradiation has had a profound effect on the prognosis of orbital rhabdomyosarcoma. Historically, this tumor was treated with orbital exenteration with a 50% mortality (67). Radiotherapy alone resulted in 70% survival rate (68). Chemoradiation has resulted in over 90% survival in these cases. Unfortunately, there is a paucity of data on patients treated with radiation alone. In the Intergroup Rhabdomyosarcoma Study, 50 orbital cases were followed after treatment with 5000 to 6000 cGy of unshielded photon irradiation to the orbit and Adriamycin, cyclophosphamide, vincristine and actinomycin D (69). Visually significant cataract developed in 33 of 37 patients who had visual data available for analysis. Other complications included corneal or conjunctival changes in 22, and minor lens changes in over 90% of cases. **Orbital bone dysplasia** was noted in 55% of patients and 18% had **lacrimal duct stenosis**. There are early data that timing of chemotherapy and radiation, especially with actinomycin D could influence the complication rate, but there is insufficient data on ocular morbidity of radiation alone to compare with combined therapies.

CHOROIDAL METASTASES

There is only anecdotal data on chemoradiation treatment of choroidal metastases. We have treated many patients with external radiation alone (generally 3500 to 4000 cGy over 5 weeks) without significant ocular complications. In a few patients, who either had diabetes or were on concurrent chemotherapy for breast carcinoma, we have observed that radiation **retinopathy** develops. Probably the chemotherapy, and certainly the diabetes, exacerbated the radiation vasculopathy effect.

RETINOBLASTOMA

Insights in the molecular biology of retinoblastoma have profoundly affected our understanding of the pathogenesis, inheritance and cancer diathesis associated with this disease. There are no prospective randomized data comparing radiation alone with chemoradiation in the management of retinoblastoma. Generally, only patients with poor prognosis ocular disease (large, symmetric intraocular tumors) or those with extraocular extension have received both chemotherapy and radiation. There is no meaningful data on the intraocular complications of combined chemoradiation. Some eyes have been salvaged with this technique; however, it is impossible to determine the relative contribution of the retinal tumors, chemotherapy, and radiation on the ocular morbidity observed.

The cancer diathesis associated with hereditary retinoblastoma has been known for several years (70). There is almost a 400-fold increased risk of osteosarcoma in germinal retinoblastoma survivors (71), and second tumors are more common than metastases as a cause of death in bilateral retinoblastoma patients in the United States. The importance of chemotherapy and radiation in the induction of these **second malignancies** was unclear. Recent data have demonstrated that the gene whose deletion is responsible for retinoblastoma development is on the proximal portion of the 13th chromosome (72). This gene codes a nuclear protein responsible for control of cellular proliferation. Absence of this gene on both alleles of the 13th chromosome allows tumor development. This abnormality has also been noted in osteosarcoma (68,72) small-cell carcinoma of the lung (73), breast carcinoma (74), and bladder cancer (75). In patients treated with only bilateral enucleation, three of 22 developed second tumors (76). In some series using life table analysis, up to 90% of patients followed as long as 30 years after treatment have developed second malignancies. Eighty-nine of 688 (12.9%) of these germinal mutation patients developed new nonocular neoplasms (77).

Draper, Sanders, and Kingston calculated the risk for all second tumors at 18 years after diagnosis to be 4.8% in the hereditary form of retinoblastoma (78). In this group, the 18-year risk for osteosarcomas was 2.2% outside of the orbit and rose to 3.7% in the irradiated field. Cyclophosphamide appeared to increase the second tumor risk both within and outside the radiation field. Inside the field, the tumor risk was 2.9% without chemotherapy and 4.2% with it. Outside the field, the risks were 1.0% and 4.6%, respectively.

A retrospective study of the Netherlands National Retinoblastoma Registry from 1945 to 1972 revealed conflicting data (79). Second neoplasms arose in 2 of 33 (6%) patients within the radiation field with chemotherapy and in 6 of 56 (11%) in those who did not receive drugs. This report is difficult to interpret because many clinical and treatment parameters and number of years of follow-up were not specified.

Tucker et al performed a quantitative case control study of bone sarcomas related to chemotherapy and radiotherapy in retinoblastoma patients (80). They estimated the actual radiation dose and assigned a score to reflect the quantity of alkylating agents received. Retinoblastoma patients had a 2.7 times relative risk of developing a second tumor. The risk increased with increasing radiation doses up to 6000 cGy before decreasing at doses greater than 8000 cGy. Alkylating agents increased the relative risk 4.7 fold, and this effect increased with increased dosage.

These data show that both chemotherapy and radiation additively increase the incidence of second tumors in germinal mutation retinoblastoma patients. There is an apparent difference in second tumor incidence in the Dutch and English experience when compared with the American experience, reflecting differences in the statistical manner in which the data was presented and differences in treatment technique, radiation dose and length of cohort follow-up.

CONCLUSIONS

There are no data that adequately address the mechanisms of action for either the additive tumor induction effects of chemoradiation in hereditary retinoblastoma or the ocular toxicity in patients treated with chemoradiation for nonocular malignancies. The former issue will probably be easier to resolve because the molecular basis of oncogenesis in retinoblastoma is now known.

There are insufficient randomized data with prospective ophthalmologic monitoring to determine if any ocular toxicity from chemoradiation is additive, synergistic or idiosyncratic. In many studies, selection bias cannot be factored out, and it is not entirely certain whether the combined modality therapy really produced greater ocular morbidity or whether patient selection may have been of equal or greater importance in the causation of eye damage.

REFERENCES

1. Chalupecky H. Uber die Wirkung der Rontgenstrahlen auf das Auge und die Haut. Zbl Augenheilk 21:234,267,368, 1897.
2. Stallard HB. Radiation energy as (a) a pathogenic (b) a therapeutic agent in ocular disorders. Br J Ophthalmol 7(Suppl):70, 1933.
3. Phillips TL, Fu KK. Quantification of combined radiation therapy and chemotherapy effects on critical normal tissues. Cancer 37:1186, 1976.
4. Imperia PS, Lazarus HM, Lass JH. Ocular complications of systemic cancer chemotherapy. Surv Ophthalmol 34:209, 1989.
5. Griffen JD, Garnick MB. Eye toxicity of cancer chemotherapy: A review of the literature. Cancer 48:1539, 1981.
6. Fraunfelder FT, Meyer SM. Ocular toxicity of antineoplastic agents. Ophthalmology 90:1, 1983.
7. de Schryver A, Wachtmeister L, Baryd I. Ophthalmologic observations on long-term survivors after radiotherapy for nasopharyngeal tumours. Acta Radiol Ther Phys Biol 10:193, 1971.
8. Perrers-Taylor M, Brinkley D, Reynolds T. Acta Radiol Ther Phys Biol 3:431, 1965.
9. Merriam GR Jr, Szechter A, Focht EF. The effect of ionizing radiations on the eye. Front Radiat Ther Oncol 6:346, 1972.
10. Nakissa N, Rubin P, Strohl R, et al. Ocular and orbital complications following radiation therapy of paranasal sinus malignancies and review of literature. Cancer 51:980, 1983.
11. Lass JH, Lazarus HM, Reed MD, et al. Topical corticosteroid therapy for corneal toxicity from systemically administered cytarabine. Am J Ophthalmol 94:617, 1982.
12. Ritch PS, Hansen RM, Heuer DK. Ocular toxicity from high dose cytosine arabinoside. Cancer 51:430, 1983.
13. Hopen G, Mondino BJ, Johnson BL, et al. Corneal toxicity with systemic cytarabine. Am J Ophthalmol 91:500, 1981.
14. Bonadonna G, Beretta G, Tancini G, et al. Adriamycin as a single agent in various forms of advanced neoplasia of adults and children. Tumori 60:373, 1974.
15. Curran CF, Luce JK. Ocular adverse reactions associated with adriamycin (Doxorubicin). Am J Opthalmol 108:709, 1989.
16. Blum R. An overview of studies with adriamycin in the United States. Cancer Chemother Rep 6:247, 1975.

17. Lokich J, Skarin A, Frei E. Methyl CCNU and adriamycin combination therapy. Cancer 34:1593, 1974.
18. Louie AC, Turrisi AT, Muggia FM, et al. Visual abnormalities following nitrosourea treatment. Med Pediatr Oncol 5:245, 1978.
19. McLennan R, Taylor HR. Optic neuroretinitis in association with BCNU and procarbazine therapy. Med Pediatr Oncol 4:43, 1978.
20. Greenberg HS, Ensminger WD, Chandler WF, et al. Intra-arterial BCNU chemotherapy for treatment of malignant gliomas of the central nervous system. J Neurosurg 61:423, 1984.
21. Hochberg FH, Pruitt AA, Beck DO, et al. The rationale and methodology for intra-arterial chemotherapy with BCNU as treatment for glioblastoma. J Neurosurg 63:876, 1985.
22. Shingleton BJ, Bienfand DC, Albert DM, et al. Ocular toxicity associated with high dose carmustine. Arch Ophthalmol 100:1766, 1982.
23. Shapiro WR, Green SB. Reevaluating the efficacy of intra-arterial BCNU. J Neurosurg 66:313, 1987.
24. Gebarski SS, Greenburg HS, Gabrielsen TO, et al. Orbital angiographic changes after intracarotid BCNU chemotherapy. Am J Neuroradiol 5:55, 1984.
25. Kende G, Sirkin SR, Thomas PRM, et al. Blurring of vision. A previously undescribed complication of cyclophosphamide therapy. Cancer 44:69, 1979.
26. Bonadonna G, Brusaolino E, Penuccia V, et al. Combination chemotherapy as an adjuvant treatment in operable breast cancer. N Engl J Med 294:405, 1976.
27. Haidak DJ, Hurwitz BS, Yeung KY. Tear-duct fibrosis (dacryostenosis) due to 5-fluorouracil. Ann Intern Med 88:657, 1978.
28. Christophidis N, Vajda FJE, Lucas I, et al. Ocular side effects with 5-fluorouracil. Aust NZ J Med 9:143, 1979.
29. Seiff SR, Shorr N, Adams T. Surgical treatment of punctal-canalicular fibrosis from 5-fluorouracil therapy. Cancer 56:2148, 1985.
30. Straus DJ, Mausolf FA, Ellerby RA, et al. Cicatricial ectropion secondary to 5-fluorouracil therapy. Med Pediatr Oncol 3:15, 1977.
31. Caravella LP, Burns JA, Zangmeister M. Punctual-canalicular stenosis related to systemic fluorouracil therapy. Arch Ophthalmol 99:284, 1981.
32. Adams JW, Bofenkamp TM, Kobrin J, et al. Recurrent acute toxic optic neuropathy secondary to 5-FU (letter). Cancer Treat Rep 68:565, 1984.
33. Knapp A, Heuer DK, Stern GA, et al. Serious corneal complications of glaucoma filtering surgery with postoperative 5-fluorouracil. Am J Ophthalmol 103:183, 1987.
34. Doroshow JH, Locker GY, Gasterland DE, et al. Ocular irritation from high-dose methotrexate therapy: Pharmokinetics of drug in the tear film. Cancer 48:2158, 1981.
35. Johnson DR, Burns RP. Blepharoconjunctivitis associated with cancer chemotherapy. Trans Pac Coast Otoophthalmol Soc (Ann Meeting) 46:43, 1965.
36. Lepore PE, Nissenblatt MJ. Bilateral internuclear ophthalmoplegia after intrathecal chemotherapy and cranial irradiation. Am J Ophthalmol 92:851, 1981.
37. Spaeth GL, von Sallmann L. Corticosteroids and cataracts. Int Ophthalmol Clin 6:915, 1966.
38. Burde RM, Becker B. Corticosteroid-induced glaucoma and cataracts in contact lens wearers. JAMA 213:2075, 1970.
39. Becker B. Cataracts and topical corticosteroids. Am J Ophthalmol 58:872, 1964.
40. Edward JE Jr, Foos RY, Montgomerie JZ, et al. Ocular manifestations of *Candida* septicemia. Review of seventy-six cases of hematogenous *Candida* endophthalmitis. Medicine 53:47, 1974.
41. Slansky HH, Kolbert G, Gartner S. Exophthalmos induced by steroids. Arch Ophthalmol 77:579, 1967.
42. Katz B, Carmody R. Exophthalmos induced by exogenous steroids. J Clin Neuro-Ophthalmol 6:250, 1986.
43. Cohen BA, Som PM, Haffner PH, et al. Steroid exophthalmos. J Comput Assist Tomogr 5:907, 1981.
44. Cohn GA. Pseudotumor cerebri in children secondary to administration of adrenal steroids. J Neurosurg 20:784, 1963.
45. Walker AE, Adamkiewicz JJ. Pseudotumor cerebri associated with prolonged corticosteroid therapy. JAMA 188:779, 1964.
46. Henderson RP, Lander R. Scleral discoloration associated with long-term prednisone administration. Cutis 34:76, 1984.
47. Albert DM, Wong VG, Henderson ES. Ocular complications of vincristine therapy. Arch Ophthalmol 78:709, 1967.
48. Norton SW, Stockman JA 3d. Unilateral optic neuropathy following vincristine chemotherapy. J Pediatr Ophthalmol Strabismus 16:190, 1979.
49. Sanderson PA, Kuwabara T, Cogan DG. Optic neuropathy presumably caused by vincristine therapy. Am J Ophthalmol 81:146, 1976.
50. Merriam GR Jr, Focht EF. A clinical study of radiation cataracts and the relationship to dose. Am J Roentgenol 77:759, 1957.
51. Wara WM, Irvine AR, Neger RE, et al. Radiation retinopathy. Int J Radiat Oncol Biol Phys 5:81, 1979.

52. Parsons JT, Fitzgerald CR, Hood CI, et al. The effects of irradiation on the eye and optic nerve. Int J Radiat Oncol Biol Phys 9:609, 1983.
53. Fishman ML, Bean SC, Cogan DG. Optic atrophy following prophylactic chemotherapy and cranial radiation for acute lymphocytic leukemia. Am J Ophthalmol 82:571, 1976.
54. Margileth DA, Poplack DG, Pizzo PA, et al. Blindness during remission in two patients with acute lymphoblastic leukemia. Cancer 39:58, 1977.
55. Rubinstein LJ, Herman MM, Long TF, et al. Disseminated necrotizing leukoencephalopathy. Complication of treated central nervous system leukemia and lymphoma. Cancer 35:291, 1975.
56. Price RA, Jamieson PA. The central nervous system in childhood leukemia. II. Subacute leukoencephalopathy. Cancer 35:306, 1975.
57. Band PR, Holland JF, Bernard J, et al. Treatment of central nervous system leukemia with intrathecal cytosine arabinoside. Cancer 32:744, 1973.
58. Weaver RG Jr, Chauvenet AR, Smith TJ, et al. Ophthalmic evaluation of long-term survivors of childhood acute lymphoblastic leukemia. Cancer 58:963, 1986.
59. Inati A, Sallan SE, Cassady JR, et al. Efficacy and morbidity of central nervous system "prophylaxis" in childhood acute lymphoblastic leukemia: Eight years' experience with cranial irradiation and intrathecal methotrexate. Blood 61:297, 1983.
60. Aur RJA, Simone JV, Verzosa MS, et al. Childhood acute lymphocytic leukemia. Study VIII. Cancer 42:2123, 1978.
61. Jack MK, Hicks JD. Ocular complications in high-dose chemoradiotherapy and marrow transplantation. Ann Ophthalmol 13:709, 1981.
62. Goepfert H, Jesse RH, Lindberg RD. Arterial infusion and radiation therapy in the treatment of advanced cancer of the nasal cavity and paranasal sinuses. Am J Surg 126:464, 1973.
63. Chan RC, Shukovsky LJ. Effects of irradiation on the eye. Radiology 120:673, 1976.
64. Choi KN, Rotman M, Aziz H, et al. Locally advanced paranasal sinus and nasopharynx tumors treated with hyperfractionated radiation and concomitant infusion cisplatin. Cancer 67:2748, 1991.
65. Wilson WB, Perez GM, Kleinschmidt-Demasters BK. Sudden onset of blindness in patients treated with oral CCNU and low-dose cranial irradiation. Cancer 59:901, 1987.
66. Vander JF, Kincaid MC, Hegarty TJ, et al. The ocular effects of intracarotid bromodeoxyuridine and radiation therapy in the treatment of malignant glioma, Ophthalmology 97:352, 1990.
67. Jones IS, Reese AB, Krant J. Orbital rhabdomyosarcoma. An analysis of 62 cases. Am J Ophthalmol 61:721, 1966.
68. Sagerman RH, Tretter P, Ellsworth RM. Orbital rhabdomyosarcoma in children. Trans Am Acad Ophthalmol Otolaryngol 78:OP602, 1974.
69. Heyn R, Ragab A, Raney B Jr, et al. Late effects of therapy in orbital rhabdomyosarcoma in children. Cancer 57:1738, 1986.
70. Friend SH, Bernards R, Rogelj S, et al. A human DNA segment with properties of the gene that predisposes to retinoblastoma and osteosarcoma. Nature 323:643, 1986.
71. Sagerman RH, Cassady JR, Tretter P, et al. Radiation induced neoplasia following external beam therapy for children with retinoblastoma. Am J Roentgenol Radium Ther Nucl Med 105:529, 1969.
72. Dryja TP, Rapaport JM, Epstein J, et al. Chromosome 13 homozygosity in osteosarcoma without retinoblastoma. Am J Hum Genet 38:59, 1986.
73. Harbour JW, Lai SL, Whang-Peng J, et al. Abnormalities in structure and expression of the human retinoblastoma gene in SCLC. Science 241:353, 1988.
74. Lee EY-HP, To H, Shew JY, et al. Inactivation of the retinoblastoma susceptibility gene in human breast cancers. Science 241:218, 1988.
75. Horowitz JM, Yandell DW, Park SH, et al. Point mutational inactivation of the retinoblastoma antioncogene. Science 243:937, 1989.
76. Abramson DH, Ronner JH, Ellsworth RM. Second tumors in non-irradiated bilateral retinoblastoma. Am J Ophthalmol 87:624, 1979.
77. Abramson DH, Ellsworth RM, Kitchin FD, et al. Second nonocular tumors in retinoblastoma survivors. Ophthalmology 91:1351, 1984.
78. Draper GJ, Sanders BM, Kinston JE. Second primary neoplasms in patients with retinoblastoma. Br J Cancer 53:661, 1986.
79. Derkinderen DJ, Koten JW, Wolterbeek R, et al. Non-ocular cancer in hereditary retinoblastoma survivors and relatives. Ophthalmic Pediat Genetics 8:23, 1987.
80. Tucker MA, D'Angio GJ, Boice JD Jr, et al for the Late Effects Study Group. Bone sarcomas linked to radiotherapy and chemotherapy in children. N Engl J Med 317:588, 1987.

Section B

TOXICITY GRADING CRITERIA

Chapter 42

GRADING OF CHEMORADIATION TOXICITY

MADHU J. JOHN

The earliest attempt at grading the results of cancer treatment was in 1948 by Karnofsky (1). The Karnofsky Performance Scale, frequently in use even today, is a gradient (measured in increments of 10 from 0 to 100) of the overall physical status of the cancer patient. This scale has been simplified in recent years by the American Joint Commission for Cancer (AJCC) and the Eastern Cooperative Oncology Group (ECOG) (2). The AJCC Host (H) performance scale grades patients from H_0 (normal activity) to H_4 (bedridden, may need hospitalization). The ECOG scale similarly grades the patients' physical status from 0 to 4.

In 1977, two guidelines for assessment of response to treatment for breast cancer were suggested by the UICC (Union Internationale Contre le Cancer) and the Breast Cancer Task Force Treatment Committee of the National Cancer Institute (NCI), USA (3,4). These guidelines provided the structural framework for two meetings sponsored by the World Health Organization (WHO) in Turin (1977) and Brussels (1979), on the "Standardization of Reporting Results of Cancer Treatment." These meetings had the input of several international, North American, and European health and cancer research organizations. They culminated in a summary report in 1981 with guidelines for reporting baseline data, treatment, toxicity, and response in the cancer patient (5). For the first time, a grading system attempted to accommodate the multiplicity of acute and subacute toxicities of various cancer treatment modalities (surgery, radiotherapy, chemotherapy, immunotherapy and hormonal therapy). End organs reportable by this toxicity grading system included the bone marrow, the gastrointestinal and genitourinary tracts, and the cardiac and nervous systems. It recognized the concept of "combined modality therapy" but suggested that each modality be described individually. It also suggested a means for reporting late or chronic toxicity though no grading system was offered.

Several cancer research organizations adopted these recommendations with some modifications suited to their particular needs or interest in the ensuing years. The radiotherapy community, in particular, recognized the inadequacies of the WHO grading system in relation to the wide range of radiotherapy-related toxicities. After several meetings of a task force consisting of key members of the RTOG (Radiation Therapy Oncology Group) and the EORTC (European Organization for Research on Treatment of Cancer), separate grading systems for acute and chronic/late radiation morbidity were compiled and introduced in 1987 (Tables 42–1 and 42–2) (6).

In 1988, the National Cancer Institute (USA), made available the common toxicity criteria for use by various research organizations in cancer clinical trials (Table 42–3). This was in fact, an elaboration of the WHO system (5) with recognition of a greater range in body and systemic functional toxicities. Once again, research organizations such as South West Oncology Group (SWOG), Cancer and Leukemia Group B (CALGB), and NSABP (National Surgical Adjuvant Breast and Bowel Project) adapted these common toxicity criteria to form their own set of criteria conforming to the modalities used in their own protocols.

By and large, the common toxicity criteria introduced by the NCI and adopted by some research organizations are related to chemotherapy toxicity. For example, the gradient

Table 42–1. Acute Radiation Morbidity Scoring Criteria

Toxicity Site	Grade [0]	[1]	[2]	[3]	[4]
Skin	No change over baseline	Follicular, faint or dull erythema/epilation/dry desquamation/decreased sweating	Tender or bright erythema, patchy moist desquamation/moderate edema	Confluent, moist desquamation other than skin folds, pitting edema	Ulceration, hemorrhage, necrosis
Mucous Membrane	No change over baseline	Injection/may experience mild pain not requiring analgesic	Patchy mucositis which may produce an inflammatory serosanguinous discharge/ may experience moderate pain requiring analgesic	Confluent fibrinous mucositis/may include severe pain requiring narcotic	Ulceration, hemorrhage or necrosis
Eye	No change	Mild conjunctivitis with or without scleral injection/ increased tearing	Moderate conjunctivitis with or without keratitis requiring steroids &/or antibiotics/dry eye requiring artificial tears/ iritis with photophobia	Severe keratitis with corneal ulceration/objective decrease in visual acuity or in visual fields/acute glaucoma/panophthalmitis	Loss of vision (unilateral or bilateral)
Ear	No change over baseline	Mild external otitis with erythema, pruritis, secondary to dry desquamation not requiring medication. Audiogram unchanged from baseline	Moderate external otitis requiring topical medication/serous otitis medius/hypoacusis on testing only	Severe external otitis with discharge or moist desquamation/symptomatic hypoacusis/tinnitus, not drug related	Deafness
Salivary Gland	No change over baseline	Mild mouth dryness/slightly thickened saliva/may have slightly altered taste such as metallic taste/ these changes not reflected in alteration in baseline feeding behavior, such as increased use of liquids with meals	Moderate to complete dryness/thick, sticky saliva/markedly altered taste	—	Acute salivary gland necrosis
Pharynx and Esophagus	No change over baseline	Mild dysphagia or odynophagia/may require topical anesthetic or non-narcotic analgesics/may require soft diet	Moderate dysphagia or odynophagia/may require narcotic analgesics/may require puree or liquid diet	Severe dysphagia or odynophagia with dehydration or weight loss (>15% from pretreatment baseline) requiring N-G feeding tube, I.V. fluids, or hyperalimentation	Complete obstruction, ulceration, perforation, fistula
Larynx	No change over baseline	Mild or intermittent hoarseness/cough not requiring antitussive/erythema of mucosa	Persistent hoarseness but able to vocalize/referred ear pain, sore throat, patchy fibrinous exudate or mild arytenoid edema not requiring narcotic/ cough requiring antitussive	Whispered speech, throat pain or referred ear pain requiring narcotic/confluent fibrinous exudate, marked arytenoid edema	Marked dyspnea, stridor or hemoptysis with tracheostomy or intubation necessary
Upper G.I.	No change	Anorexia with <=5% weight loss from pretreatment baseline/ nausea not requiring antiemetics/abdominal discomfort not requiring parasympathetic drugs or analgesics	Anorexia with <=15% weight loss from pretreatment baseline/ nausea &/or vomiting requiring antiemetics/abdominal pain requiring analgesics	Anorexia with >15% wt. loss from pretreatment baseline or requiring N-G tube or parenteral support. Nausea &/or vomiting requiring N-G tube or parenteral support/abdominal pain, severe despite medication/hematemesis or melena/abdominal distention (flat plate radiograph demonstrated distended bowel loops)	Ileus, subacute or acute obstruction, perforation, GI bleeding requiring transfusion/abdominal pain requiring tube decompression or bowel diversion
Lower GI including pelvis	No change	Increased frequency or change in quality of bowel habits not requiring medication/rectal discomfort not requiring analgesics	Diarrhea requiring parasympatholytic drugs (e.g. Lomotil)/mucous discharge not necessitating sanitary pads/rectal or abodminal pain requiring analgesics	Diarrhea requiring parenteral support/severe mucous or blood discharge necessitating sanitary pads/abdominal distention (flat plate radiograph demonstrates distended bowel loops)	Acute or subacute obstruction, fistula or perforation GI bleeding requiring transfusion abdominal pain or tenesmus requiring tube decompression or bowel diversion

Table 42–1. (cont.)

Toxicity Site	Grade [0]	[1]	[2]	[3]	[4]
Lung	No change	Mild symptoms of dry cough or dyspnea on exertion	Persistent cough requiring narcotic, antitussive agents/dyspnea with minimal effort but not at rest	Severe cough unresponsive to narcotic antitussive agent or dyspnea at rest/ clinical or radiologic evidence of acute pneumonitis/intermittent 0_2 or steroids may be required	Severe respiratory insufficiency/continuous oxygen or assisted ventilation
Genitourinary	No change	Frequency of urination or nocturia twice pretreatment habit/dysuria, urgency not requiring medication	Frequency of urination or nocturia which is less frequent than every hour. Dysuria, urgency, bladder spasm requiring local anesthetic (e.g. Pyridium)	Frequency with urgency and nocturia hourly or more frequently/dysuria, pelvis pain or bladder spasm requiring regular, frequent narcotic/Gross hematuria with/without clot passage	Hematuria requiring transfusion/acute bladder obstruction not secondary to clot passage, ulceration or necrosis
Heart	No change over baseline	Asymptomatic but objective evidence of ECG changes or pericardial abnormalities without evidence of other heart disease	Symptomatic with ECG changes and radiologic findings of congestive heart failure or pericardial disease/no specific treatment required	Congestive heart failure, angina pectoris, pericardial disease responding to therapy	Congestive heart failure, angina pectoris, pericardial disease, arrhythmias not responsive to nonsurgical measures
CNS	No change	Fully functional status (i.e., able to work) with minor neurologic findings, no medication needed	Neurologic findings present sufficient to require home care/nursing assistance may be required/meds. including steroids/anti-seizure agents may be required.	Neurologic findings requiring hospitalization for initial management	Serious neurologic impairment which includes paralysis, coma or seizures > 3 per week despite medication/ hospitalization required
Hematologic					
WBC (× 1000)	≥4.0	3.0–<4.0	2.0–<3.0	1.0–<2.0	<1.0
Platelets (× 1000)	>100	75–<100	50–<75	25–<50	<25 or spontaneous bleeding
Neutrophils (× 1000)	≥1.9	1.5–<1.9	1.0–<1.5	0.5–<1.0	<0.5 or sepsis
Hemoglobin (GM %)	>11	11–9.5	<9.5–7.5	<7.5–5.0	—
Hematocrit (%)	≥32	28–<32	28	Packed cell transfusion required	—

GUIDELINES
The acute morbidity criteria are used to score/grade toxicity from radiation therapy. The criteria are relevant from day 1, the commencement of therapy, through day 90. Thereafter, the EORTC/RTOG Criteria for Late Effects are to be utilized.
The evaluator must attempt to discriminate between disease and treatment related signs and symptoms.
An accurate baseline evaluation prior to commencement of therapy is necessary.
All toxicities Grade 3, 4 or 5* must be verified by the Principal Investigator.
*ANY TOXICITY THAT CAUSED DEATH IS GRADED 5.
Reproduced with permission from the Radiation Therapy Oncology Group (RTOG) and European Organization for Research on Treatment of Cancer (EORTC).

of bone marrow (hemoglobin) and gastrointestinal (vomiting/diarrhea) toxicity is different for radiotherapy and chemotherapy (compare Tables 42–1 and 42–3). The differences, obviously, relate to the localized (radiotherapy) and systemic (chemotherapy) effects of the two modalities. Even so, these differences do not appear to be insurmountable; most toxicities resulting from either modality appear to be akin, particularly when one considers the result in functionality of the patient. In fact, representatives of the RTOG, EORTC, and the NCI are currently in the process of defining a new set of common toxicity criteria, which would more truly reflect chemoradiation effects.

Table 42–2. RTOG/EORTC Late Radiation Morbidity Scoring Criteria

Organ/Tissue	0	Grade 1	Grade 2	Grade 3	Grade 4	Grade 5
Skin	None	Slight atrophy Pigmentation change Some hair loss	Patchy atrophy Moderate telangiectasia Total hair loss	Marked atrophy Gross telangiectasia	Ulceration	
Subcutaneous tissue	None	Slight induration (fibrosis) and loss of subcutaneous fat	Moderate fibrosis but asymptomatic/Slight field contracture/<10% linear reduction	Severe induration and loss of subcutaneous tissue Field contracture >10% linear measurement	Necrosis	
Mucous membrane	None	Slight atrophy and dryness	Moderate atrophy and telangiectasia/Little mucous	Marked atrophy with complete dryness/Severe telangiectasia	Ulceration	
Salivary glands	None	Slight dryness of mouth/ Good response on stimulation	Moderate dryness of mouth/ Poor response on stimulation	Complete dryness of mouth/ No response on stimulation	Fibrosis	DEATH DIRECTLY RELATED TO RADIATION LATE EFFECT
Spinal cord	None	Mild L'hermitte's syndrome	Severe L'hermitte's syndrome	Objective neurological findings at or below cord level treated	Mono, para quadraplegia	
Brain	None	Mild headache/Slight lethargy	Moderate headache/ Great lethargy	Severe headache/Severe CNS dysfunction (partial loss of power or dyskinesia)	Seizures or paralysis/coma	
Eye	None	Asymptomatic cataract Minor corneal ulceration or keratitis	Symptomatic cataract Moderate corneal ulceration/Minor retinopathy or glaucoma	Severe keratitis Severe retinopathy or detachment/Severe glaucoma	Panophthalmitis Blindness	
Larynx	None	Hoarseness/Slight arytenoid edema	Moderate arytenoid edema/ Chondritis	Severe edema/Severe chondritis	Necrosis	
Lung	None	Asymptomatic or mild symptoms (dry cough) Slight radiographic appearances	Moderate symptomatic fibrosis or pneumonitis (severe cough) Low grade fever/Patchy radiographic appearances	Severe symptomatic fibrosis or pneumonitis/Dense radiographic changes	Severe respiratory insufficiency/ Continuous O_2/ Assisted ventilation	
Heart	None	Asymptomatic or mild symptoms/Transient T wave inversion and ST changes/Sinus tachycardia >110 (at rest)	Moderate angina on effort/ Mild pericarditis/Normal heart size/Persistent abnormality T wave and ST changes/Low QRS	Severe angina/Pericardial effusion/Constrictive pericarditis/Moderate heart failure/Cardiac enlargement/ECG abnormalities	Tamponade/Severe heart failure Severe constrictive pericarditis	
Esophagus	None	Mild fibrosis/Slight difficulty in swallowing solids/No pain on swallowing	Unable to take solid food normally/Swallowing semi-solid food/Dilatation may be indicated	Severe fibrosis/Able to swallow only liquids/May have pain on swallowing Dilatation required	Necrosis/ perforation/ fistula	
Small/large intestine	None	Mild diarrhea/Mild cramping/Bowel movement 5 times daily Slight rectal discharge or bleeding	Moderate diarrhea and colic/Bowel movement >5 times daily/Excessive rectal mucus or intermittent bleeding	Obstruction or bleeding requiring surgery	Necrosis/ Perforation/ Fistula	
Liver	None	Mild lassitude/Nausea dyspepsia/Slightly abnormal liver function	Moderate symptoms/Some abnormal liver function tests/Serum albumin normal	Disabling hepatitic insufficiency/Liver function tests grossly abnormal/Low albumin/ Edema or ascites	Necrosis/Hepatic coma or encephalopathy	
Kidney	None	Transient albuminuria No hypertension/Mild impairment renal function/urea 25–35 mg% Creatinine 1.5–2.0 mg% Creat. clearance >75%	Persistent moderate albuminuria (2+)/Mild hypertension/No related anemia/Moderate impairment renal function/Urea >36–60 mg% Creatinine clearance (50–74%)	Severe albuminuria/Severe hypertension/Persistent anemia (<10G%) Severe renal failure/Urea >60 mg% Creatining >4.0 mg% Creatinine clearance <50%	Malignant hypertension/ Uremic coma Urea >100%	
Bladder	None	Slight epithelial atrophy/ Minor telangiectasia (microscopic hematuria)	Moderate frequency/ Generalized telangiectasia Intermittent macroscopic hematuria	Severe frequency & dysuria Severe generalized telangiectasia (often with petechiae) Frequent hematuria. Reduction in bladder capacity (<150 cc)	Necrosis/Contracted bladder capacity (<100 cc) Severe hemorrhagic cystitis	
Bone	None	Asymptomatic/No growth retardation Reduced bone density	Moderate pain or tenderness/Growth retardation Irregular bone sclerosis	Severe pain or tenderness Complete arrest of bone growth Dense bone sclerosis	Necrosis/Spontaneous fracture	
Joint	None	Mild joint stiffness Slight limitation of movement	Moderate stiffness/ Intermittent or moderate joint pain/Moderate limitation of movement	Severe joint stiffness/Pain with severe limitation of movement	Necrosis/Complete fixation	

Reproduced with permission from the Radiation Therapy Oncology Group (RTOG) and European Organization for Research on Treatment of Cancer (EORTC).

Table 42–3. Common Toxicity Criteria (NCI)

		Grade				
	Toxicity	0	1	2	3	4
Blood/Bone Marrow	WBC (× 1000)	≥4.0	3.0–3.9	2.0–2.9	1.0–1.9	<1.0
	PLT (× 1000)	WNL	75.0–normal	50.0–74.9	25.0–49.9	<25.0
	Hgb (Gm %)	WNL	10.0–normal	8.0–10.0	6.5–7.9	<6.5
	Granulocytes/Bands (× 1000)	≥2.0	1.5–1.9	1.0–1.4	0.5–0.9	<0.5
	Lymphocytes (× 1000)	≥2.0	1.5–1.9	1.0–1.4	0.5–0.9	<0.5
	Hemorrhage (clinical)	None	Mild, no transfusion	Gross, 1–2 units transfusion per episode	Gross, 3–4 units transfusion per episode	Massive, >4 units transfusion per episode
	Infection	None	Mild	Moderate	Severe	Life-threatening
Gastrointestinal	Nausea	None	Able to eat, reasonable intake	Intake significantly decreased but can eat	No significant intake	—
	Vomiting	None	1 episode in 24 hrs	2–5 episodes in 24 hrs	6–10 episodes in 24 hrs	>10 episodes in 24 hrs or requiring parenteral support
	Diarrhea	None	Increase of 2–3 stools/day over pre-Rx	Increase of 4–6 stools/day, or nocturnal stools, or moderate cramping	Increase of 7–9 stools/day, or incontinence, or severe cramping	Increase of ≥10 stools/day or grossly bloody diarrhea or need for parenteral support
	Stomatitis	None	Painless ulcers, erythema, or mild soreness	Painful erythema, edema, or ulcers, but can eat	Painful erythema, edema, or ulcers, and cannot eat	Required parenteral or enteral support
Liver	Bilirubin	WNL	—	<1.5 × N	1.5–3.0 × N	>3.0 × N
	Transaminase (SGOT, SGPT)	WNL	≤2.5 × N	2.6–5.0 × N	5.1–20.0 × N	>20.0 × N
	Alk Phos or 5′ nucleotidase	WNL	≤2.5 × N	2.6–5.0 × N	5.1–20.0 × N	>20.0 × N
	Liver—clinical	No change from baseline	—	—	Precoma	Hepatic coma
Bladder/Kidney	Creatinine	WNL	<1.5 × N	1.5–3.0 × N	3.1–6.0 × N	>6.0 × N
	Proteinuria	No change	1+ or <0.3 g% or <3 g/l	2–3+ or 0.3–1.0 g% or 3–10 g/l	4+ or >1.0 g% or >10 g/l	Nephrotic syndrome
	Hematuria	Neg	Micro only	Gross, no clots	Gross + clots	Requires transfusion
	Alopecia	No loss	Mild hair loss	Pronounced or total hair loss	—	—
	Pulmonary	None or no change	Asymptomatic with abnormality in PFT's	Dyspnea on significant exertion	Dyspnea at normal level of activity	Dyspnea at rest
Heart	Cardiac dysrhythmias	None	Asymptomatic, transient requiring no therapy	Recurrent or persistent, no therapy required	Requires treatment	Requires monitoring; or hypotension, or ventricular tachycardia, or fibrillation
	Cardiac	None	Asymptomatic, decline of resting ejection fraction by less than 20% of baseline value	Asymptomatic, decline of resting ejection fraction by more than 20% of baseline value	Mild CHF, responsive to therapy	Severe or refractory CHF
	Cardiac—ischemia	None	Non-specific T-wave flattening	Asymptomatic, ST and T wave changes suggesting ischemia	Angina without evidence for infarction	Acute myocardial infarction
	Cardiac—pericardial	None	Asymptomatic effusion, no intervention required	Pericarditis (rub, chest pain, ECG changes)	Symptomatic effusion; drainage required	Tamponade; drainage urgently required
Blood Pressure	Hypertension	None or no change	Asymptomatic, transient increase by greater than 20 mm Hg (D) or to >150/100 if previously WNL. No treatment required	Recurrent or persistent increase by greater than 20 mm Hg (D) or to >150/100 if previously WNL. No treatment required	Requires therapy	Hypertensive crisis
	Hypotension	None or no change	Changes requiring no therapy (including transient orthostatic hypotension)	Requires fluid replacement or other therapy but not hospitalization	Requires therapy and hospitalization; resolves within 48 hrs of stopping the agent	Requires therapy and hospitalization for>48 hrs after stopping the agent
Neurologic	Neuro—sensory	None or no change	Mild paresthesias, loss of deep tendon reflexes	Mild or moderate objective sensory loss; moderate paresthesias	Severe objective sensory loss or paresthesias that interfere with function	—
	Neuro—motor	None or no change	Subjective weakness; no objective findings	Mild objective weakness without significant impairment of function	Objective weakness with impairment of function	Paralysis
	Neuro—cortical	None	Mild somnolence or agitation	Moderate somnolence or agitation	Severe somnolence, agitation, confusion, disorientation, or hallucinations	Coma, seizures, toxic psychosis

Table 42–3. (cont.)

		Grade				
	Toxicity	0	1	2	3	4
Neurologic	Neuro—cerebellar	None	Slight incoordination, dysdiadokinesis	Intention tremor, dysmetria, slurred speech, nystagmus	Locomotor ataxia	Cerebellar necrosis
	Neuro—mood	No change	Mild anxiety or depression	Moderate anxiety or depression	Severe anxiety or depression	Suicidal ideation
	Neuro—headache	None	Mild	Moderate or severe but transient	Unrelenting and severe	—
	Neuro—constipation	None or no change	Mild	Moderate	Severe	Ileus > 96 hrs
	Neuro—hearing	None or no change	Asymptomatic, hearing loss on audiometry only	Tinnitus	Hearing loss interfering with function but correctable with hearing aid	Deafness not correctable
	Neuro—vision	None or no change			Symptomatic subtotal loss of vision	Blindness
	Skin	None or no change	Scattered macular or papular eruption or erythema that is asymptomatic	Scattered macular or papular eruption or erythema with pruritus or other associated symptoms	Generalized symptomatic macular, papular, or vesicular eruption	Exfoliative dermatitis or ulcerating dermatitis
	Allergy	None	Transient rash, drug fever <38c, 100.4F	Urticaria, drug fever = 38c, 100.4F mild bronchospasm	Serum sickness, bronchospasm, req parenteral meds	Anaphylaxis
	Fever in absence of infection	None	37.1–38.0c 98.7–100.4F	38.1–40.0c 100.5–104.0F	>40.0c >104.0F for less than 24 hours	>40.0c (104.0F) for more than 24 hrs or fever accompanied by hypotension
	Local	None	Pain	Pain and swelling, with inflammation or phlebitis	Ulceration	Plastic surgery indicated
Metabolic	Weight gain/loss	<5.0%	5.0–9.9%	10.0–19.9%	≥ 20.0%	—
	Hyperglycemia	<116	116–160	161–250	251–500	>500 or ketoacidosis
	Hypoglycemia	>64	55–64	40–54	30–39	<30
	Amylase	WNL	<1.5 × N	1.5–2.0 × N	2.1–5.0 × N	>5.1 × N
	Hypercalcemia	<10.6	10.6–11.5	11.6–12.5	12.6–13.5	≥13.5
	Hypocalcemia	>8.4	8.4–7.8	7.7–7.0	6.9–6.1	≤6.0
	Hypomagnesemia	>1.4	1.4–1.2	1.1–0.9	0.8–0.6	≤0.5
Coagulation	Fibrinogen	WNL	0.99–0.75 × N	0.74–0.50 × N	0.49–0.25 × N	≤0.24 × N
	Prothrombin time	WNL	1.01–1.25 × N	1.26–1.50 × N	1.51–2.00 × N	>2.00 × N
	Partial thromboplastin time	WNL	1.01–1.66 × N	1.67–2.33 × N	2.34–3.00 × N	>3.00 × N

Reproduced with permission from the National Cancer Institute (NCI) USA.

REFERENCES

1. Karnofsky DA, Abelman WH, Craver LF, et al. The use of nitrogen mustards in the palliative treatment of carcinoma. Cancer 1:634, 1948.
2. UICC. TNM Classification of Malignant Tumors. 3rd ed. Geneva, International Union Against Cancer, 1978.
3. Hayward JL, Carbone PP, Heuson JC, et al. Assessment of response to therapy in advanced breast cancer. Cancer 39:1289, 1977.
4. Breast Cancer Task Force Treatment Committee, National Cancer Institute. Report from the combination chemotherapy trials working group. U.S. Department of Health Education and Welfare. DHEW, Publication No. (NIH) 77-1192, 1977.
5. Miller AB, Hoogstraten B, Staquet M, Winkler A. Reporting results of cancer treatment. Cancer 47:207, 1981.
6. Stetz J, Director, Data Management, Radiation Therapy Oncology Group. Personal communication. May 1992.

Section C

POTENTIAL METHODS OF DECREASING CHEMORADIATION TOXICITY

Chapter 43

MULTIPLE RADIOTHERAPY FRACTIONATION SCHEDULES

RITSUKO KOMAKI AND JAMES D. COX

The aim of chemotherapy and radiation therapy combinations is to improve the therapeutic ratio. Normal tissue effects are of paramount concern, whether the intent of combined modality treatment is a greater effect on the local-regional tumor or its semi-independent actions (spatial cooperation).

Combinations of chemotherapy and radiation therapy have become well-established in neoplastic diseases of childhood such as acute leukemia, Ewing's sarcoma, Wilms' tumor, and embryonal rhabdomyosarcoma, and such malignant tumors in adults as Hodgkin's disease, malignant lymphoma, and small-cell carcinoma of the lung. In each of these conditions, therapeutic success has been accompanied by well-characterized acute and late morbidity. Such morbidity has led to studies to determine whether radiation therapy can be eliminated, at least in favorable subsets of patients. Few efforts have been directed toward altering fractionation to diminish toxicity, but such efforts deserve consideration when radiation therapy continues to be an indispensable part of a treatment program.

A BRIEF HISTORY OF FRACTIONATION

Fractionation is a general term that encompasses the near-limitless variations of total dose of radiations, numbers of individual treatments or fractions, and the time in which they are administered. For the first two decades after the discovery of x-rays and radium, there was no consistent application of ionizing radiations for treatment. The most common method was a single, prolonged treatment, made popular in Germany, which resulted in necrosis and a prolonged period of healing. Regaud (1) and his younger colleague Coutard (2), espoused a method of short, repeated applications of radiations, based on observations of the dissociation of radiation effects on spermatogonia and scrotal skin which resulted from differences in inherent sensitivities of the two types of epithelium, and in their proliferative capacities. They applied this method to carcinomas of the larynx and tonsillar fossa and, for the first time, observed permanent control of these tumors by ionizing radiations, with complete healing of the surrounding tissues.

In the third, fourth, and fifth decades of this century, a wide variety of fractionation regimens was tried, including more than one treatment per day. Formulations that reduced total dose and numbers of fractions to an expression, graphic or numerical, purported to define the same endpoint and, thus, to be isoeffective (for tumor control, moist desquamation, necrosis, etc.) were put forward. They were eventually found to be simplistic and inaccurate (3).

THE BIOLOGIC BASIS FOR FRACTIONATION

The following summary of some basic considerations in fractionation necessarily oversimplifies the results of a host of laboratory findings. The interested reader is encouraged to consult standard texts (4) for a comprehensive review and discussion, as well as a listing of primary sources.

Cells that survive doses of ionizing radiations in the therapeutic range can be shown to recover in a matter of hours. There are at least two components of this recovery: **sublethal damage repair (SLDR)**, which occurs in 3 to 6 hours; and **potentially lethal damage repair (PLDR)**, in which alterations in the environment of cells following exposure can be shown to affect the proportion of cells surviving irradiation. SLDR and especially PLDR may have immediate relevance to the presence of an intrinsically cytotoxic agent such as that which would be present when radiation therapy and chemotherapy are combined.

Reassortment of cells occurs after radiation therapy due to different sensitivities of cells by virtue of their positions in the cell cycle: cells in mitosis are demonstrably more sensitive than those, for example, in the late phase of DNA synthesis. Drugs which might be effective in less radiosensitive phases of the cycle, or which could synchronize cells in a radiation sensitive phase could enhance cell killing.

Repopulation occurs from division of surviving cells both in tumors and in normal tissues. This is favorable insofar as it is an essential element in repair of normal tissues, but is obviously unfavorable in tumors. An argument against prolonged interruptions (splits) during a course of radiation therapy is repopulation in tumors. It might also suggest a disadvantage to 72+-hour interruptions of radiation therapy on weekends and even a full 24 hours between fractions.

Current constructs of tumor cell kinetics include the phenomenon of **accelerated repopulation** (5). Proliferation of tumor cells is thought to be slower when tumors are smaller. Therefore, an insult which leads to a decrease in tumor cells is thought to stimulate a surviving subset. If insufficient cell killing is achieved in a short period, the proliferating compartment (perhaps consisting of a selection of resistant clonogens) could determine the failure of the treatment. Insults that might lead to accelerated proliferation are a first dose of radiation or drugs, or even subtotal resection of a tumor.

Each of the three phenomena noted above—repair, reassortment, and repopulation—is thought to occur both in tumors and normal tissues. **Reoxygenation** is usually considered to occur only in tumors as they shrink or metabolic demands decrease. Most tumors are thought to contain a substantial proportion of hypoxic cells, and hypoxia protects cells from radiation. The addition of radiation therapy to drugs which are equally effective in well oxygenated and hypoxic cells, or drugs that are selectively toxic to hypoxic cells or that sensitize them to radiations, may thus be beneficial.

ACUTE AND LATE EFFECTS OF RADIATION

Differences in repair and perhaps reassortment of cells lead to different dose-response relationships in acute-responding and late-responding tissues. Acute-responding tissues include the bone marrow, testis, gut, squamous mucous membranes, and skin. Late-responding tissues include thyroid, breast, bone, pancreas, and uterus. Tumors are thought to behave more like acute-responding tissues.

The size of radiation fractions is considered far more important for late-responding than for acute-responding tissues, i.e., large size fractions cause more profound late effects than acute effects. This is explained by a linear-quadratic relationship between radiation dose and effect, reflecting the greater degree of cell-killing in late-responding tissues with large-size fractions. Thus, the acute-responding tissues have alpha/beta ratios near 2, whereas late-responding tissues have ratios greater than 5.

DEFINITIONS FOR FRACTIONATION

Standard or common fractionation consists of a single treatment per day, 5 days per week, for a period of several (usually 2 to 8) weeks. A few institutions treat for 4 or 6 days per week, but the standard work week in the United States is a compelling justification for 5 fractions per week at roughly 24 hour intervals. Fractions of 150 cGy to 200 cGy are most commonly used.

Hypofractionation usually means larger fractions (from 300 cGy to 1000 cGy) administered less often than 5 times weekly. In the era when isoeffect formulae were popular (6), fractions of 300 cGy given 3 times per week and fractions of about 400 cGy twice weekly, given over a 6-week period, were considered comparable (isoeffective) to 200 cGy, 5 times per week, for 30 fractions in 6 weeks. A wide variety of hypofractionation treatment schedules were tried, the published reports of which, taken in toto, showed a lessening of tumor control, presumably due to repopulation between fractions, and an increase in late effects in normal tissues, seemingly the consequence of the larger-size fractions (7). In fact, the simultaneous decreasing of tumor control and increasing of normal tissue effects, taken together as a lessening of therapeutic ratio, suggested the possibility of benefit from a larger number of smaller-size fractions (Table 43–1).

Hyperfractionation refers to an increased number of small-size fractions delivered over a period comparable to that which would be used with standard or common fractionation. For example, if a standard regimen for squamous carcinoma of the upper aerodigestive tract were 7000 cGy in 35 fractions of 200 cGy in 7 weeks, a hyperfractionation regimen with the aim of decreasing late effects in normal tissues could consist of 70 fractions of 100 cGy given twice daily, 5 days per week, also in 7 weeks. Alternatively, one might be satisfied with an already acceptably low level of normal tissue effects and, therefore, try to increase tumor control while maintaining the low risk of normal tissue damage: one might elect to give 110 cGy or 120 cGy per fraction twice daily, and increase the total dose to 7700 cGy or 8400 cGy, respectively, in 70 fractions in 7 weeks. If more than one fraction is given per day, there needs to be an interval of 3 to 6 hours between fractions to permit repair of sublethal damage. With the uncertainties attending the rate of repair in normal tissues in man, a 6-hour interval is probably safer. As might be expected from considerations of alpha/beta ratios for acute-responding tissues, hyperfractionated radiation therapy

Table 43–1. Summary of Studies of Reduced Numbers of Large Fractions

Regimen	Tumor Control	Late Effects*
3 times/week	NC or ↓	NC
2 times/week	↓	↑
1 time/week	NC or ↓	↑ ↑
Rapid	NC or ↓	NC
Rapid-split	NC or ↓	NC or ↑

*Relative to common fractionation
NC: No change
Reprinted with permission from Cox JD. Cancer 55(S):2105, 1985.

with fractions of 110 cGy or 120 cGy, twice daily, results in increased acute reactions in normal tissues (3), and, hopefully, increased effects on tumors.

Accelerated fractionation refers to the use of fractions nearly the same size as those administered with common fractionation, but given more often than 5 times per week. The result is a total dose near that with common fractionation, but with a considerable shortening of the actual treatment time. In actuality, the acute reactions from accelerated fractionation are usually so marked that, depending upon the normal tissues included with the field of irradiation, an interruption or split is necessary to permit reactions to subside and patients to tolerate the treatment. Such is the case in treatment of squamous carcinoma of the upper aerodigestive tract if fractions of 150 cGy or 160 cGy are administered twice daily, 5 days per week: an interruption is required beginning in the third week of treatment (8). It is possible to avoid the interruption with a lesser degree of acceleration such as, for example, that employed with the "concomitant boost": a large field is treated daily, five times per week, and a smaller field (including all known tumor and within the larger field) is treated 1, 2, or 3 times per week by treating more than once a day with a 3- to 6-hour interval.

It may be argued that the repopulation of normal tissues after acute effects is a rapid, effective response, with a homeostatic aim of restoring anatomic and functional integrity, and that tumors cannot mount such a proliferative response because they have escaped normal control mechanisms. However, there are ample laboratory and clinical data to document accelerated proliferation in tumors. To assume that tumors cannot repopulate as efficiently and completely as normal tissues during an interruption of treatment is, at least, risky and may be disastrous for a patient. For example, the introduction of an interruption of 2 weeks in a course of radiation therapy for squamous carcinoma of the upper aerodigestive tract led to a decrease in tumor control (9). Compensation for the split may be possible by increasing fraction size (10) or accelerating fractionation (8).

INTEGRATED CHEMORADIATION

Integration of chemotherapy and radiation therapy is used only to distinguish a planned combination of the modalities with a well-thought-out sequence and careful timing, as opposed to an arbitrary use of both treatments. Several studies have shown that the simultaneous administration of chemotherapy and radiation therapy may result in alarming, if not actually harmful effects (11,12). The simultaneous use of chemotherapy and either hyperfractionated or accelerated radiation therapy increases acute reactions even further (13). Unless the site to be irradiated has a few or no acute-responding normal tissues or patient and physicians are prepared to cope with extraordinarily intense acute effects, usually requiring hospitalization, these forms of altered fractionation should not be combined with cytotoxic drugs. There is every reason to expect acceptable effects of altered fractionation integrated with chemotherapy if an interval is permitted between the administration of either modality. This has been well documented in the systematic use of alternating chemotherapy and radiation therapy for small-cell carcinoma of the lung (14).

It is conceivable that hyperfractionation could reduce or eliminate the adverse late effects of treatment with integrated chemoradiation, but no clinical data are available to provide documentation. For example, it is now widely accepted that radiation therapy alone, or interacting with intravenous and intrathecal methotrexate, has longterm effects on neuropsychologic function in children treated for acute lymphocytic leukemia (ALL) (15). Hyperfractionation has been better tolerated by the central nervous system (CNS), notably in the brain stem, than would have been considered possible with standard fractionation. It is likely that hyperfractionated prophylactic cranial irradiation (PCI) for ALL would reduce late effects on neuropsychologic function. Similarly, PCI for small-cell carcinoma of the lung using, for example, 150 cGy twice daily to a total dose of 3000 cGy would afford greater protection than the usual 300 cGy per fraction widely reported in the literature.

CLINICAL APPLICATIONS OF HYPERFRACTIONATED RADIOTHERAPY ± CHEMOTHERAPY

Although there is a risk, at least with regard to acute reactions, in simultaneous chemotherapy and radiation therapy, there are also concerns in separating their use. Interruptions in a course of radiation therapy, as noted, permit the possibility of repopulation of tumors as well as normal tissues. Indeed, accelerated proliferation may defeat radiation therapy and tumor control may decrease. Previous efforts to compensate for the split by increase in fraction size carried risks of increased late effects (10). Multiple fractions per day as a means of compensating for the split carry the highest probability of maintaining tumor control at levels equal or superior to those with common fractionation without increasing the probability of late effects. Thus, alternating cycles of radiation therapy and chemotherapy, studied extensively in the laboratory by Looney and Hopkins (16), would be expected to produce the best results in human malignant tumors by using accelerated radiation therapy.

In malignant tumors of children, in whom radiation volumes necessarily includes growing bones and the tumors are thought to have especially short cell doubling times, a real gain in therapeutic ratio could be anticipated from hyperfractionation. Improvements in tumor control have, in fact, been described in B-cell lymphoma (Burkitt's) of African children (17), but late effects have not been reported.

A small but important experience with accelerated fractionation and systemic chemotherapy, has been reported in small-cell carcinoma of the lung by Turrisi et al (13). Fractions of 150 cGy were given twice daily to a total dose of 4500 cGy in 3 weeks, combined with cisplatinum and etoposide. There were 23 patients treated by this protocol. The actuarial 2-year survival for all patients was 57% with a median follow-up of 22 months. No patients failed within the radiation field. The earliest death was at day 93 in a apparently disease-free patient dying of an infectious complication. Six of eight patients remain free of disease at or beyond 24 months. Tumor control was achieved in all patients at considerable cost in acute reactions; late effects have not accompanied the increased acute effects. It is not surprising to find a disassociation between acute and late effects; this phenomenon may be exploited further in the interests of increased tumor control without increased late effects.

A phase I_{late}/II trial of hyperfractionation (HFX) radiation therapy for nonsmall-cell carcinoma of the lung (NSCLC) was conducted by the Radiation Therapy Oncology Group (RTOG) between 1983 and 1987. Twice-daily fractions (120 cGy/fraction) were delivered with a 4-hour or longer interval between fractions. Patients were randomized to receive minimal total doses of 6000, 6480, and 6960 cGy. After acceptable risks of acute and late effects were found, two additional arms using 7440 and 7920 cGy were added, and the two lowest total dose arms were closed.

No significant differences in the risks of acute or late effects in normal tissues were found among the 848 patients analyzed in the five arms; risks of severe or life-threatening pneumonitis were 2.6% for 6000 to 6480 cGy, 5.7% for 6960 to 7440 cGy, and 8.1% for 7920 cGy. Among 350 patients who had the same criteria as in the Cancer and Leukemia Group B (CALGB) protocol 84-33 (namely, American Joint Committee on Cancer Staging, 1984, stage III; Karnofsky Performance Status 70–100; < 6% weight loss), there was a dose response for survival: survival with 6960 cGy (median, 13.0 months; 29% at 2 years), was significantly better ($p = 0.02$) than with the lower total doses. There were no differences in survival among the three highest total-dose arms. Comparisons with results in similar patients treated with 6000 cGy in 30 fractions of 200 cGy, 5 days per week, for 6 weeks suggest benefit from HFX radiation therapy with 6960 cGy. Improvement in survival with HFX radiation therapy at 6960 cGy total dose without increase in normal tissue effects, justifies phase III comparison with standard fractionation alone and combined with systemic chemotherapy in this common presentation of NSCLC (18).

RTOG protocol 88-08 (Table 43–2) was a study for the improvement of survival by using HFX RT, compared to standard RT or neoadjuvant chemotherapy followed by standard RT. There have been 500 patients entered into this study; however, results of the study are not yet available.

RTOG protocol 90-15 (Table 43–3) was designed to test toxicity and efficacy of HFX with concomitant chemotherapy consisting of vinblastine and cisplatinum. Forty-five patients have been entered. Results of the study are not yet available.

Table 43–2. Schema of Radiation Therapy Oncology Group Protocol 88-08: Intergroup Phase II Study of Twice-daily Fractionation vs. Conventional Radiation Therapy Alone or in Combination with Chemotherapy for Patients with Locally Advanced Non-small Cell Lung Cancer

S	*Cell Type*	R	(1) Standard RT alone, 200
T	Squamous	A	cGy/day, 5 days a week,
R	vs. other	N	total dose 6000 cGy in 6
A		D	weeks
T	*Performance*	O	(2) Vinblastine weekly for 5
I	*Status*	M	weeks, Cisplatinum days
F	70–80 vs.	I	1 and 29. RT as in Arm 1
Y	90–100	Z	begins day 50
	AJCC Stage	E	(3) 120 cGy twice daily, total
	II vs. IIIA vs.		6960 cGy/58 fx/29 Rx
	IIIB		days/6 weeks
			(Hyperfractionated RT)

RTOG protocol 91-06 was developed to test more effective chemotherapy, oral VP-16 and IV cisplatinum combined with concomitant HFX RT. This study is ongoing and the major toxicity appears to be esophagitis; however, tumor reduction seems to be rapid among the 22 patients entered to date.

Table 43–3. Schema of Radiation Therapy Oncology Group Protocol 90-15: Phase I/II Study of Concurrent Radiation Therapy and Chemotherapy for Patients with Non-small Cell Lung Cancer

T	Vinblastine weekly for 5 weeks
R	plus Cisplatinum on days
E	1, 29, and 50
A	RT begins day 1 of chemotherapy
T	
M	RT and chemotherapy will be given
E	on the same days
N	
T	

Radiation Therapy

RT dose to primary and mediastinum: 5040 in 4 weeks at 120 cGy twice daily (at least 6 hours apart) × 42 fx

Booster dose: 1920 cGy in 16 fractions in 8 treatment days at 120 cGy twice daily (at least 6 hours apart)

Total Dose: 6960 cGy in 58 fractions in 29 treatment days in 6 weeks

Chemotherapy

Vinblastine 5 mg/m^2 IV bolus weekly × 5 weeks

Cisplatinum 75 mg/m^2 over 30 to 60 minutes IV on days 1, 29, and 50

Dose calculations are based on actual body weight

CONCLUSIONS

The biologic rationale for improved therapeutic ratios using multiple fractions of radiation therapy per day is well described in the literature. Preliminary results in the clinic are just emerging. Laboratory studies of integrated chemotherapy and radiation therapy have been followed by parallel results in several malignant tumors of children, less so in adults. There is ample justification to pursue clinical trials integrating hyperfractionated radiation therapy with chemotherapy, especially in children, to try to achieve high levels of tumor control with low risks of late effects. In adults, accelerated fractionation perhaps holds more promise, with the emphasis more on tumor control, accepting increased acute reactions, but not late effects. Alternating chemotherapy and radiation therapy is best accomplished with accelerated fractionation whereby the interruption or split is compensated by the increased dose per day, without the potential burden of increased late effects from fraction sizes as has been widely used in the past.

REFERENCES

1. del Regato JA. Claudius Regaud. Int J Radiat Oncol Biol Phys 1:933, 1976.
2. del Regato JA. Henri Coutard. Int J Radiat Oncol Biol Phys 13:433, 1987.
3. Cox JD. Presidential address. Fractionation: A paradigm for clinical research in radiation oncology. Int J Radiat Oncol Biol Phys 13:1271, 1987.
4. Hall EJ. Radiobiology for the radiologist. 3rd ed. Philadelphia, JB Lippincott, 1988, p. 240.
5. Withers HR, Taylor JMG, Maciejewski B. The hazard of accelerated tumor clonogen repopulation during radiotherapy. Acta Oncologia 27:131, 1988.
6. Ellis F. The relationship of biological effect to dose-time-fractionation factors in radiotherapy. *In:* Current Topics in Radiation Research. Ebert M, Howard A (Eds). Amsterdam, Holland Publishing Co., 1968, p. 359.
7. Cox JD. Large dose fractionation (hypofractionation). *In:* Proceedings of National Conference on Radiation Oncology. Cancer 55S:2105, 1985.
8. Wang CC, Blitzer PH, Suit HD. Twice-a-day radiation therapy for cancer of the head and neck. Cancer 55:2100, 1985.
9. Parsons JT, Bova F, Million RR. Re-evaluation of split-course technique for squamous cell carcinoma of the head and neck. Int J Radiat Oncol Biol Phys 6:1645, 1980.
10. Marcial VA. Split-course radiation therapy of carcinoma of the base of the tongue. Results of a prospective national collaborative clinical trial of the Radiation Therapy Oncology Group. Int J Radiat Oncol Biol Phys 9:437, 1983.
11. Perry MC, Eaton WL, Propert KJ, et al. Chemotherapy with or without radiation therapy in limited small-cell carcinoma of the lung. N Engl J Med 316:912, 1987.
12. Johnson RE, Brereton HD, Kent CH. Small-cell carcinoma of the lung: Attempt to remedy causes of past therapeutic failure. Lancet ii:289, 1976.
13. Turrisi AT, Glover DJ, Mason BA. A preliminary report: Concurrent twice-daily radiotherapy plus platinum-etoposide chemotherapy for limited small cell lung cancer. Int J Radiat Oncol Biol Phys 15:183, 1988.
14. Arriagada R, Pellae-Cosset B, Ladron de Guevara C, et al. Alternating radiotherapy and chemotherapy with doxorubicin, etoposide, cyclophosphamide, and cisplatin in limited small cell lung cancer. Cancer Treat Symp 2:115, 1985.
15. Bleyer WA, Poplack DC. Prophylaxis and treatment of leukemia in the central nervous system and other sanctuaries. Semin Oncol 12:131, 1985.
16. Looney WB, Hopkins HA. Alternation of chemotherapy and radiotherapy in cancer management. III. Results in experimental solid tumor systems and their relationship to clinical studies. Cancer Treat Rep 70:141, 1986.
17. Norin T, Onyango J. Radiotherapy in Burkitt's lymphoma. Conventional or superfractionated regime—early results. Int J Radiat Oncol Biol Phys 2:399, 1977.
18. Cox JD, Azarwia N, Byhardt RW, et al. A randomized Phase I/II trial of hyperfractionated radiation therapy with total doses of 60.0 Gy to 79.2 Gy: Possible survival benefit with greater than or equal to 69.6 Gy in favorable patients with Radiation Therapy Oncology Group Stage III non-small-cell lung carcinoma: Report of Radiation Therapy Oncology Group 83-11. J Clin Oncol 8:1543, 1990.

Chapter 44

INFUSIONAL CHEMOTHERAPY

SEWA S. LEGHA

Because both chemotherapy and radiotherapy are more toxic to the rapidly proliferating tissues of the body, the acute toxic effects of both modalities of treatment are generally additive. The side effects common to both treatments include myelotoxicity and mucosal toxicity. However, the toxic effects of radiation are generally limited to the anatomic area included in the radiation field, whereas the effects of chemotherapy are more generalized. Some of the chemotherapeutic agents are more prone to cause mucosal toxicity but do not cause significant myelosuppression. Examples of the latter class include 5-fluorouracil (5-FU) administered as a continuous infusion and bleomycin. On the other hand, there is enhancement of local toxicity of radiation therapy by the addition of chemotherapeutic drugs such as Adriamycin and Actinomycin D.

Besides the acute toxicity, there is potential for additive or enhanced chronic toxicity when chemotherapy and radiotherapy are combined simultaneously or sequentially. This problem is uncommon but can create serious complications because it frequently involves the vital organs. Examples of the latter situation include cardiotoxicity of anthracyclines and radiation therapy and pulmonary toxicity of bleomycin and radiation therapy. Fortunately, much of the acute toxicity of chemotherapy is reversible, leaving few or no permanent effects. On the other hand, radiation therapy does leave behind residual subacute or chronic toxicity in most organs exposed to it. This is especially the case with bone marrow effects of radiotherapy, which are persistent and probably permanent, whereas the bone marrow effects of a majority of chemotherapeutic agents are entirely reversible except for drugs such as mitomycin-C and nitrosoureas, which do have longterm effects similar to those of radiotherapy.

A great deal of attention has been devoted to reducing the toxicity of the commonly used chemotherapeutic agents. This has included the development and utilization of analogs with reduced toxicity, utilization of antidotes as blocking agents to prevent target organ toxicity and clinical manipulations in the methods and schedules of drug administration. The area of analog development has not been particularly fruitful except with recent development of platinum analogues, which are clearly less toxic than cisplatinum. Blocking of target organ toxicity for chemotherapy has not been successful despite its extensive evaluation in the prevention of cardiac toxicity of anthracyclines and the nephrotoxicity of cisplatinum.

The most fruitful area in reducing the toxicity of chemotherapy has been schedule manipulations of various cytotoxic agents which have influenced their acute and frequently their chronic toxicity, resulting in significant enhancement of their therapeutic index. Nearly all classes of drugs have been evaluated by different schedules of administration (1,2). By and large, there is no significant change in the toxicity pattern of alkylating agents with a change in their schedule of administration. The drugs that are most influenced by schedule alterations are antimetabolites, particularly 5-FU, and cytosine arabinoside. Anthracyclines, bleomycin, and plant alkaloids such as vinblastine and vincristine have also been tested extensively and are favorably influenced by their schedule of administration. Although splitting the total dose over a few days as opposed to bolus administration generally reduces the acute toxicity, the schedule that has had a major impact on drug toxicity is the continuous-infusion delivery which generally eliminates plasma peak-related acute toxicity and has salutary effects on the chronic toxicity of several drugs (1,3). The clinical experience with infusion delivery of cytotoxic agents as a method of reducing their toxicity will be described in this chapter.

ANTHRACYCLINES

Daunomycin and adriamycin (ADR), widely used in the treatment of cancer, are both limited by cardiac toxicity which prevents their use after a cumulative dose level of 450 to 550 mg/m^2 (4). Cardiac toxicity manifests as an impairment of left ventricular function leading to congestive heart failure. Radiotherapy used alone rarely produces left ventricular dysfunction, although vascular complications from its use can cause myocardial infarction and varying degrees of subclinical cardiac damage (5). Cardiac toxicity of ADR is clearly enhanced by prior irradiation of the mediastinum as well as the left anterior chest wall, which is frequently done for the treatment of lymphomas and breast cancer, respectively. Because of an increased risk of heart failure in such patients, the cumulative dose of ADR, which can be safely used, must be kept lower, generally in the range of 400 to 450 mg/m^2 as opposed to 550 to 600 mg/m^2 in patients without prior radiation therapy (6–8) (see Chapter 35 on cardiac toxicity of chemoradiation for more details and recommendations). Among the many analogues of ADR developed with an aim to reduce cardiotoxicity, epirubicin is the only one which has a significantly lower risk of cardiotoxicity. But its advantage over ADR is modest, and this drug is still cardiotoxic, albeit after a cumulative dose that is 25% to 30% higher than that of ADR (9).

Based on recent clinical experience and experimental evidence, it appears that the cardiac toxicity of ADR is proportional to the plasma peak produced by bolus doses of the drug (10,11). Accordingly, fractionation of the dose either by using a weekly schedule or delivery of ADR as a continuous infusion have both resulted in significant reduction in its cardiac toxicity (10,12,13). The reduction in cardiac toxicity is most pronounced when ADR is delivered as a continuous infusion over 48 to 96 hours which results in a marked reduction in the risk of heart failure, so that cumulative dose levels two times as high as the bolus dose can be used with a lower risk of cardiac toxicity than that expected from the bolus administration (14). A more protracted venous infusion over periods of 2 to 3 weeks or longer has also been used with a similar reduction in the cardiac toxicity of ADR (15). The total dose of ADR per course is similar, that is, 60 to 90 mg/m^2 over a period of three weeks, but the drug has to be delivered through a central venous catheter in order to avoid extravasation which can cause serious tissue necrosis.

In addition to a reduction in cardiac toxicity, continuous infusion use of ADR is associated with a marked reduction in nausea and vomiting. Myelosuppression and alopecia are ADR toxicities that are not altered by these schedule manipulations. One disadvantage of continuous infusion delivery of ADR is an increase in the incidence of stomatitis, which is proportional to the duration of infusion. Approximately 30 to 40% of the patients experience stomatitis when ADR is given over 96 hours as opposed to 5 to 10% of the patients receiving it by bolus administration.

Based on these data, it is possible to make full use of ADR without a major risk of cardiac toxicity in patients who have had radiation therapy to the cardiac area. Such patients should preferably receive their ADR therapy by a 48- or 96-hour infusion, which will allow the use of ADR in a cumulative dose range of 500 to 600 mg/m^2 without an unduly high risk of heart failure. However, one must be cautious in using simultaneous administration of ADR and radiotherapy because of increased skin, mucosal, and pulmonary toxicity when these two treatment modalities are used simultaneously (16,17). In such situations, bolus administration of ADR on either a single dose every 3 weeks or weekly may be preferred until radiation therapy is completed, at which time further administration of ADR could be changed over to continuous infusion delivery. Because of the enhancement of skin and mucosal toxicities when simultaneous use is contemplated, the dose of ADR should be reduced by 50% or the cumulative dose of radiation must be reduced by 25 to 30% (16,17).

BLEOMYCIN

Bleomycin (BLM) is commonly used in the treatment of germ-cell tumors, lymphomas, and squamous cell carcinomas of the head and neck and genitourinary areas. The main side effects of BLM are skin rashes, stomatitis, and pulmonary fibrosis, but the drug is free from bone marrow toxicity. The pulmonary toxicity of BLM is the most serious complication and can be fatal. The incidence of lung toxicity is related to the cumulative dose with a risk of 3 to 5% for a BLM dose of 400 units, which is a commonly used dose limit not to be exceeded (18). The risk of lung toxicity is higher in older individuals and is clearly increased by radiotherapy to the mediastinum and the lung parenchyma.

The change in the schedule of administration of BLM from bolus to continuous infusion appears to significantly decrease the incidence of lung toxicity and allows administration of a higher cumulative dose (19–21). This has been established in experimental animals by Sikic et al (19) and in the clinic by Cooper et al (20) in head and neck cancer and in germ cell tumors by Samuels et al (21). The dose of BLM used by continuous infusion per course is similar to that used for bolus administration, that is, 20 to 30 units daily for 5 days, at 3- to 4-week intervals. Besides increased risk of lung toxicity when BLM and radiotherapy are used sequentially or concurrently, there is suggestive evidence of enhancement in their skin toxicity resulting in delayed fibrosis in patients with head and neck cancer exposed to both radiotherapy and BLM (22). Consequently, patients who are at high risk of BLM toxicity are best treated with the drug used as a continuous infusion. Because there is no risk of extravasation, BLM infusion can be delivered through a peripheral vein.

ANTIMETABOLITES

Because of the short elimination half-life of antimetabolites such as 5-FU and cytosine arabinoside, continuous-infusion delivery of these drugs results in marked alterations in their toxicity and efficacy. Cytosine arabinoside, which is widely used in the treatment of acute leukemias, is the best example of enhancement of therapeutic efficacy when a drug is given as a continuous infusion as opposed to bolus administration (23). Because radiation therapy has limited use in the treatment of acute leukemias, simultaneous use of radiation therapy and cytosine arabinoside is rarely practiced. On the other hand, 5-FU is a widely used anti-cancer drug for the treatment of several solid tumors including gastrointestinal malignancies, breast cancer, nonsmall-cell carcinoma of the lung, and squamous cell cancers of the head and neck region. The major side effect of 5-fluorouracil, when used as a bolus, is myelosuppression, whereas the continuous-infusion administration is associated with minimal or no myelosuppressive toxicity. The maximum tolerated dose on the bolus schedule is 500 mg/m^2 daily for 5 days; the continuous infusion delivery of 5-FU allows doubling of the dose to 1000 mg/m^2/day for 5 days, without causing significant change in the blood counts (24). The dose-limiting toxicity of continuous infusion of 5-FU is mucositis. This remarkable effect on the myelotoxicity of 5-FU by using it as a continuous infusion allows simultaneous administration of radiotherapy and full dosage of 5-FU.

The combination of 5-FU and simultaneous radiation therapy has found widespread usage in the treatment of malignancies of the GI tract, particularly of the esophagus and anal canal (25–29). These results, of improved therapeutic index, have generated a great deal of interest in simultaneous utilization of these two agents in the treatment of head and neck cancers and nonsmall-cell carcinoma of the lung (30,31). The lack of myelosuppression from continuous infusion of 5-FU allows it to be used in its full dose, which is 1,000 mg/m^2/day for 4 to 5 days repeated at 2- to 3-week intervals. It has also been used on a protracted continuous infusion schedule where the optimum dose of 300 mg/m^2/day, which can be used daily for 4- to 6-week periods without encountering any major toxicity (27,30). The dose-limiting toxicity of protracted-infusion 5-FU is on the skin, resulting in erythematous and sometimes painful changes on the palms and soles of feet. This toxicity, however, is rapidly reversible on temporary withholding of drug administration for 7 to 10 days.

CISPLATINUM

The major toxicity of cisplatinum is acute nausea and vomiting immediately following its bolus administration. The subacute toxicities include modest myelosuppression and nephrotoxicity, and chronic toxicity in the form of peripheral neuropathy occurs after prolonged usage. Cisplatinum has been used on a number of dose schedules, but most commonly it is used as a single dose of 100 mg/m^2 to 120 mg/m^2 over 30 to 120 minutes, which is associated with very severe nausea and vomiting. This has led to usage of fractionated doses of either bolus administration over 5 days or weekly administration, both of which reduce the severity of nausea and vomiting significantly. Cisplatinum has also been used as a 5-day continuous infusion using the same dose per course (32,33). This has led to a marked reduction in nausea and vomiting but no significant change in its myelosuppressive and other side effects. More recently, a protracted daily infusion of cisplatinum has also been investigated when a daily dose of 5 to 7 mg/m^2 can be used for periods of 3 to 4 weeks at a time (34). Once again, nausea and vomiting constitute a dose-limiting toxicity and tends to be quite significant despite the relatively low daily dose used. Accordingly, the best way to ameliorate the acute nausea and vomiting of cisplatinum is daily administration over 5 days given as a continuous infusion. The antitumor activity of cisplatinum is not altered by schedule alterations and appears to be maintained whether the drug is given as a single dose or in daily or weekly fractionated boluses or as a continuous infusion.

Simultaneous use of cisplatinum and radiotherapy is becoming popular due to the radiation-enhancing properties of cisplatinum and lack of any overlapping toxicity of these two therapies. The optimum schedule of cisplatinum when combined with radiotherapy remains to be defined.

VINCA ALKALOIDS

Vinblastine and vincristine are widely used in the treatment of solid tumors and hematologic malignancies. They are singularly free of acute toxicity of nausea and vomiting; furthermore, no myelosuppression is experienced with the use of vincristine although vinblastine is highly myelotoxic. The major toxicity of vincristine is neurotoxicity. Based on experimental evidence of enhanced antitumor activity when vinca alkaloids were used as a prolonged exposure to cell lines in vitro, several clinical trials have been conducted with continuous infusion schedules of vincristine, vindesine as well as vinblastine (35–39). Although the overall results of antitumor activity have been variable, there does appear to be some increase in the response rates, particularly in breast cancer when vinblastine is used as a continuous infusion as opposed to its bolus usage (37,40). Whether fractionation of a dose over 5 days will do as well as a 5-day continuous infusion of vinblastine, is still unclear. Similarly, there is a suggestion of enhanced efficacy when vincristine is used as a continuous infusion, particularly in the treatment of hematologic malignancies such as lymphomas and multiple myeloma (41). Because the vinca alkaloids have no mucosal or skin toxicity, there is no enhancement of local toxicity with the simultaneous use of radiation therapy and vinca alkaloids. However, the myelosuppression from vinblastine certainly will add to myelosuppression induced by simultaneous radiation therapy.

EPIPODOPHYLLOTOXINS

The two members of this class, VP-16 (etoposide) and VM26 (teniposide) are drugs with significant activity in the treatment of solid tumors and lymphomas. VP-16 has been widely used in the treatment of lung cancer, both small-cell and nonsmall-cell varieties. VM26 also has significant activity in small-cell lung cancer but is largely used in the treatment of acute lymphoblastic leukemia in children. Both drugs are limited by myelosuppressive toxicity but cause little nausea or other GI side effects. A change in schedule of epipodophyllotoxins from bolus administration to continuous infusion has not been associated with any significant changes in their toxicity pattern (42). However, these drugs are best used in 5-day courses as opposed to a single dose administration which appears to be less efficacious. The experience with continuous infusion of VP-16 however, shows no particular advantage to this schedule of drug administration (43). VM26 has not been explored in the continuous-infusion schedule.

Table 44–1. Clinical Experience with Infusion Therapy

Drugs	Efficacy	Acute Toxicity	Chronic Toxicity	Improvement in Therapeutic Index*
Adriamycin	Same or improved	Reduced	Reduced	+++
Bleomycin	Improved	Reduced	Reduced	++
Cytosine arabinoside	Improved	Reduced	None	++
5-Fluorouracil	Same or improved	Altered	None	+
Vinblastine	Same or improved	Unchanged	None	+
Cisplatinum	Same	Reduced	Reduced (±)	+

*Key:
± = Uncertain
\+ = Some Improvement
++ = Considerable Improvement
+++ = Marked Improvement

SUMMARY

The overall impact of infusion schedules of chemotherapy on the efficacy and toxicity of various drugs is summarized in Table 44–1 . There is clearly a significant reduction in acute toxicity of drugs such as Adriamycin, cisplatinum and 5-fluorouracil. Reduction in longterm toxicity is the major advantage for using infusion schedules of administering Adriamycin and bleomycin. Although simultaneous usage of radiotherapy and chemotherapy is largely useful only with 5-FU and cisplatinum, the reduced cardiac and pulmonary effects of infusion Adriamycin and bleomycin respectively should be capitalized whenever possible in anticipation of any future application of radiotherapy to the thoracic region. These considerations will allow optimum usage of these drugs and radiotherapy.

REFERENCES

1. Carlson RW, Sikic BI. Continuous infusion or bolus injection in cancer chemotherapy. Ann Intern Med 99:823, 1983.
2. Vogelzang NJ. Continuous infusion chemotherapy: A critical review. J Clin Oncol 2:1289, 1984.
3. Kramer AM, Legha SS. Continuous venous infusion chemotherapy: An overview. Cancer Bull 38:179, 1986.
4. von Hoff DD, Layard MW, Basa P, et al. Risk factors for doxorubicin-induced congestive heart failure. Ann Intern Med 91:710, 1979.
5. Stewart RJ, Fajardo LF. Radiation-induced heart disease. Radiol Clin North Am IX:511, 1971.
6. Kinsella TJ, Ahmann DL, Giuliani ER, Lie JT. Adriamycin cardiotoxicity in stage IV breast cancer: Possible enhancement with prior left chest radiation therapy. Int J Radiat Oncol Biol Phys 5:1997, 1979.
7. Gilladoga AC, Manuel C, Tan CC, et al. Cardiotoxicity of adriamycin (NSC-123127) in children. Cancer Chemother Rep 6:209, 1975.
8. Minnow RA, Benjamin RS, Lee ET, Gottlieb JA. Adriamycin cardiomyopathy-risk factors. Cancer 39:1397, 1977.
9. Torti FM, Bristow MM, Lum BL, et al. Cardiotoxicity of epirubicin and doxorubicin. Assessment by endomyocardial biopsy. Cancer Res 46:3722, 1986.
10. Legha SS, Benjamin RS, Mackay B, et al. Reduction of doxorubicin cardiotoxicity by prolonged continuous intravenous infusion. Ann Intern Med 96:133, 1982.
11. Pacciarini MA, Barbieri B, Colombo T, et al. Distribution and antitumor activity of adriamycin given in a high-dose and a repeated low-dose schedule to mice. Cancer Treat Rep 62:791, 1978.
12. Weiss AJ. Studies on cardiotoxicity and antitumor effect of doxorubicin administered weekly. Cancer Treat Symp 3:91, 1984.
13. Legha SS, Benjamin RS, Mackay B, et al. Adriamycin therapy by continuous intravenous infusion in patients with metastatic breast cancer. Cancer 49:1762, 1982.
14. Benjamin RS, Chawla SP, Ewer MS, et al. Adriamycin cardiac toxicity—An assessment of approaches to cardiac monitoring and cardioprotection. *In:* Organ Directed Toxicities of Anticancer Drugs. Hacker MP, Lazo JS, Tritton TR (Eds). Boston, Martin Nijhoff Publishing, 1988.
15. Samuels BL, Vogelzang NJ, Ruane M, Simon MA. Continuous venous infusion of doxorubicin in advanced sarcomas. Cancer Treat Rep 71:971, 1987.
16. Mayer EG, Poulter CA, Artistizabal SA. Complications of irradiation related to apparent

drug potentiation by adriamycin. Int J Radiat Oncol Biol Phys 1:1179, 1976.

17. Cassady JR, Richter MP, Piro AJ, Jaffe N. Radiation-adriamycin interactions: Preliminary clinical observations. Cancer 36:946, 1975.
18. Blum RH, Carter SK, Agre K. A clinical review of bleomycin—A new antineoplastic agent. Cancer 31:903, 1973.
19. Sikic BI, Collins JM, Mimnaugh EG, Gram TE. Improved therapeutic index of bleomycin when administered by continuous infusion in mice. Cancer Treat Rep 62:2011, 978.
20. Cooper KR, Hong WK. Prospective study of the pulmonary toxicity of continuously infusion bleomycin. Cancer Treat Rep 65:419, 1981.
21. Samuels ML, Johnson DE, Holoye PY, Lonzotti VJ. Large-dose bleomycin therapy and pulmonary toxicity. JAMA 235:1117, 1976.
22. Peters LJ, Harrison ML, Dimery IW, et al. Acute and late toxicity associated with sequential bleomycin-containing chemotherapy regimens and radiation therapy in the treatment of carcinoma of the nasopharynx. Int J Radiat Oncol Biol Phys 14:623, 1988.
23. Rai KR, Holland JF, Glidewell OJ, et al. Treatment of acute myelocytic leukemia. A study by Cancer and Leukemia Group B. Blood 58:1203, 1981.
24. Seifert P, Baker LH, Reed ML, Vaitkevicius VK. Comparison of continuously infused 5-fluorouracil with bolus injection in treatment of patients with colorectal adenocarcinoma. Cancer 36:123, 1975.
25. Franklin R, Steiger Z, Vaishampayan G, et al. Combined modality therapy for esophageal squamous cell carcinoma. Cancer 51:1062, 1983.
26. John MJ, Flam MS, Mowry PA, et al. Radiotherapy alone and chemoradiation for nonmetastatic esophageal carcinoma. Cancer 63:2397, 1989.
27. Rich TA, Lokich JJ, Chaffey JT. A pilot study of protracted venous infusion of 5-Fluorouracil and concomitant radiation therapy. J Clin Oncol 3:402, 1985.
28. Nigro ND, Seydel HG, Considine B, et al. Combined preoperative radiation and chemotherapy for squamous cell carcinoma of the anal canal. Cancer 51:1826, 1983.
29. Sischy B, Doggett RLS, Krall JM, et al. Definitive irradiation and chemotherapy for radiosensitization in management of anal carcinoma. Interim report on Radiation Therapy Oncology Group Study No. 8314. J Natl Cancer Inst 81:850, 1989.
30. Lokich J, Chaffey J, Neptune W. Concomitant 5-fluorouracil infusion and high-dose radiation for stage III non-small cell lung cancer. Cancer 64:1021, 1989.
31. Taylor SG, Murthy AK, Bonomi P, et al. Concomitant therapy with infusion of cisplatin and 5-fluorouracil plus radiation in stage III non-small cell lung cancer. NCI Monogr 6:327, 1988.
32. Yap HY, Salem P, Hortobagyi GN, et al. Phase II study of cis-dichlorodiammine-platinum (II) in advanced breast cancer. Cancer Treat Rep 62:405, 1978.
33. Lokich JJ. Phase I study of cis-diammine-dichloroplatinum (II) administered as a constant 5-day infusion. Cancer Treat Rep 64:905, 1980.
34. Lokich JJ, Zipoli TE. Phase I study of protracted infusion of cisplatin. Cancer Drug Delivery 1:247, 1984.
35. Jackson DV Jr, Sethi VS, Spurr CL, et al. Intravenous vincristine infusion: Phase I trial. Cancer 48:2559, 1981.
36. Yap HY, Blumenschein GR, Bodey GP, et al. Vindesine in the treatment of refractory breast cancer: Improvement in therapeutic index with continuous 5-day infusion. Cancer Treat Rep 65:775, 1981.
37. Fraschini G, Yap HY, Hortobagyi GN, et al. Five-day continuous-infusion vinblastine in the treatment of breast cancer. Cancer 56:225, 1985.
38. Lokich JJ, Zipoli TE, Perri J, Bothe A. Protracted vinblastine infusion—phase I-II study in malignant melanoma and other tumors. Am J Clin Oncol 7:551, 1984.
39. Zeffren J, Yagoda A, Kelsen D, Winn R. Phase I-II trial of a 5-day continuous infusion of vinblastine sulfate. Anticancer Research 4:411, 1984.
40. Tannir, N, Yap HY, Hortobagyi GH, et al. Sequential continuous infusion with doxorubicin and vinblastine: An effective chemotherapy combination for patients with advanced breast cancer previously treated with cyclophosphamide, methotrexate, 5-FU, vincristine and prednisone. Cancer Treat Rep 68:1039, 1984.
41. Barlogie B, Smith L, Alexanian R. Effective treatment of advanced multiple myeloma refractory to alkylating agents. N Engl J Med 310:1353, 1984.
42. Bennet CL, Sinkule JA, Schilsky RL, et al. Phase I clinical and pharmacological study of 72-hour continuous infusion of etoposide in patients with advanced cancer. Cancer Res 47:1952, 1987.
43. Schell FC, Yap HY, Hortobagyi GN, et al. Phase II study of VP16-213 (etoposide) in refractory metastatic breast carcinoma. Cancer Chemother Pharmacol 7:223, 1982.

Chapter 45

CHEMORADIATION PROTECTORS

SEWA S. LEGHA AND THEODORE L. PHILLIPS

The spectra of toxicity from chemotherapy and radiotherapy are similar and often overlapping. Both modalities of treatment have potential to cause significant toxicity to the rapidly dividing tissues of the body including bone marrow, mucosa of the gastrointestinal tract, gonads, and skin. Additionally, the various organ systems can suffer varying degrees of delayed injury from radiation therapy and sometimes from chemotherapy as well. These organ toxicities may include cardiac, pulmonary, hepatic, renal, and bladder toxicities and damage to the central nervous system and the peripheral nerves. Because of the overlapping toxicities of chemotherapy and radiotherapy, their effects tend to be addictive when both modalities are used simultaneously, thus sometimes requiring a temporal separation between these therapies. Besides the temporal separation of the two modalities of treatment and other maneuvers such as drug selection, schedule manipulations for chemotherapy, and fractionation of radiation therapy, several protective agents have been developed to reduce the undesirable side effects of chemotherapy and radiotherapy. In this chapter, the results of experience with the various protective agents aimed at different organ system toxicities will be described.

PROTECTION FROM HEMATOLOGIC TOXICITY

The most common and frequently dose-limiting toxicity of chemotherapy is myelosuppression. The myelotoxicity of radiotherapy is usually less significant because of the limited extent of bone marrow within the field of conventional radiation therapy. However, hemi-body or total body radiation therapy, depending on the extent and the dosage used, can result in varying degrees of bone marrow ablation. The myeloid toxicity of chemoradiation results in varying degrees of leukopenia, anemia, and thrombocytopenia. Recent developments in understanding of the physiology of hematopoiesis have led to the discovery of hematopoietic growth factors which are now available in sufficient quantities to be used as antidotes to the bone marrow toxicity from chemotherapy and possibly from radiotherapy (1). The hematopoietic factors, also called colony stimulating factors (CSFs), are quite specific in their proliferative effects and generally affect a single lineage of blood cells (2). For the red cell series, erythropoietin provides the major proliferative stimulus and has been found to be useful in the treatment of anemia from various causes. The white cell series can be stimulated by a number of interleukins which operate at different levels of cellular differentiation from the totipotent stem cells to the more differentiated myeloid precursors and the most differentiated neutrophils (3). The growth factors for the megakaryocytic precursors are still in the experimental stages of development and no single thrombopoietic factor has yet been shown to be clinically useful. The subject of hematopoiesis is covered in greater detail in Chapter 31 on bone marrow toxicity.

Erythropoietin

Produced in the kidneys, erythropoietin regulates the production of red cells in the human bone marrow. Recombinant human erythropoietin has been available since 1985 and is now in common usage for the treatment of anemia in patients with chronic renal failure (4). It is commonly used in a dosage of 50 to 100 U/kg IV or subcutaneously 3 times a week and results in a rapid increase in hemoglobin starting within 2 to 3 weeks of initiation of therapy and maintains its effectiveness over prolonged periods of time (5). In cancer patients with anemia from either their primary disease or their treatment with chemotherapy or radiotherapy, the experience with the use of erythropoietin is still limited, but its effectiveness has been shown in preliminary trials (6,7). The dosage of erythropoietin used in patients receiving chemotherapy has generally been higher than in patients with renal failure, ranging from 150 to 300 U/kg daily or 3 times a week started along with a course of chemotherapy (6,7). Approximately 50 to 60% of the patients respond to erythropoietin by showing an increase in their hemoglobin so that they do not require repeated blood transfusions (7). Erythropoietin therapy is not associated with any significant side effects and promises to become an important component of overall management of patients receiving chemotherapy regimens that are associated with significant anemia requiring RBC transfusions.

Myeloid Growth Factors

The proliferation and differentiation of white blood cells is regulated by a number of myeloid growth factors which act at different stages of differentiation. Several of these growth factors have been recently cloned using recombinant DNA technology and made available in large quantities for clinical trials (1–3). A summary of their cellular sources of origin and the targets of their action is provided in Table 45–1. The granulocyte colony stimulating factor (G-CSF) controls the terminal differentiation of neutrophils whereas the granulocyte macrophage colony stimulating factor (GM-CSF) causes proliferation of granulocytes, macrophages, and eosinophils. Based on the favorable results of extensive clinical experience during the past 3 years, both of these growth factors were marketed recently. Although their ultimate role in the management of patients with cancer is still being defined, it is clear that both G-CSF and GM-CSF are effective in causing leukocytosis and have been found to be useful in amelioration of neutropenia induced by chemotherapy (8). Although they do not completely abrogate neutropenia, which fol-

Table 45–1. Characteristics of Human Hematopoietic Growth Factors

Growth Factor	Acronym	Cellular Source	Progenitor–Cell Target	Cells Stimulated
Erythropoietin	EPO	Peritubular cells in the kidneys	Erythroblasts	Red blood cells
Granulocyte–macrophage colony stimulating factor	GM-CSF	T-lymphocytes, monocytes, fibroblasts, endothelial cells	Myeloblasts Erythroblasts Megakaryocytes	Granulocytes Eosinophils Monocytes
Granulocyte colony stimulating factor	G-CSF	Monocytes, fibroblasts, endothelial cells	Myeloblasts and other myeloid precursors	Granulocytes
Multipotential colony stimulating factor (Interleukin-3)	Multi-CSF (IL-3)	T-lymphocytes	Myeloid, erythroid, and megakaryocytic progenitors	Granulocytes Eosinophils Monocytes Platelets
Stem cell factor* (mast cell growth factor)	SCF (MGF)	Most tissues	Pluripotent stem cells and progenitors for myeloid and lymphoid cells and megakaryocytes	Red blood cells, all types of white cells including lymphocytes and platelets

*Data derived from primates, no human data yet.

lows each course of chemotherapy, there is significant reduction in the severity and duration of neutropenia and an associated reduction in the frequency of infections in patients treated with either of these growth factors (9,10). In order to achieve this protective effect, patients require daily treatment with G-CSF or GM-CSF, starting approximately 24 hours after each course of chemotherapy and continuing for periods of 10 to 15 days or until the recovery of neutrophil count to > 5000/mm^3. Because of the shortened duration of neutropenia, patients can usually be treated with a shorter interval between courses of chemotherapy and at somewhat higher doses, thus allowing an increase in the dose intensity of chemotherapy.

Although their utility following radiation therapy has not been formally tested, the myeloprotective effects of myeloid CSFs should be equally applicable to patients treated with radiotherapy as they are to patients receiving chemotherapy. Because the nadir of neutropenia is not completely abrogated by the CSFs, patients are not completely protected from infections, but there is about 50% reduction in the incidence of infections in the clinical trials reported to date (9,10). The dose levels of G-CSF and GM-CSF utilized and found to be biologically optimum are similar. A dose range of 5 to 10 μg/kg (200 to 400 μg/m^2) daily is commonly used, and can be administered subcutaneously or intravenously. Because the half-life of these growth factors is quite short, the subcutaneous route is preferred over IV administration in order to maximize their biologic effects.

G-CSF and GM-CSF are selective in their effects, primarily causing neutrophilic leukocytosis which, in patients with normal bone marrow, begins within 24 to 48 hours following drug administration and is associated with a clear dose response effect. However, a daily maintenance dose is required to sustain the leukocytic stimulation, which frequently abates within 48 to 96 hours after stopping therapy with the growth factor. Furthermore, their effects are limited predominantly to neutrophilic leukocytosis and neither G-CSF nor GM-CSF stimulate production of red cells or platelets. Consequently, other growth factors would have to be used for stimulation of platelet production before more intensive chemotherapy can be used routinely. Two potential candidates for this purpose include interleukin-3 and interleukin-1. In experimental animal studies, both of these growth factors provide proliferative stimulus for the pluripotent stem cells in the bone marrow leading to a multilineage response in the form of leukocytosis, thrombocytosis, and erythrocytosis (11,12). In early clinical trials, there appears to be a modest increase in platelet production with the use of both IL-3 and with IL-1 (13,14). Furthermore, IL-3 is also synergistic with G-CSF and GM-CSF (15). Sequential combinations of interleukin-3 followed by GM-CSF or G-CSF are currently in clinical trials and offer the potential for multilineage stimulation of the bone marrow. In the future, we can envision using combinations of growth factors for red cells, white cells and megakaryocytic series that may allow delivery of more intensive chemotherapy but with less morbidity from hematopoietic toxicity of chemoradiation.

GASTROINTESTINAL TOXICITY

The manifestations of gastrointestinal toxicity from chemoradiation include nausea and vomiting, mucosal toxicity in the form of stomatitis or ulceration of the anal/genital region, and diarrhea. These are described in greater detail in Chapter 32 on gastrointestinal toxicity. The nausea and vomiting tend to be more frequent and severe with chemotherapy compared to those experienced from radiation therapy. In fact, nausea and vomiting are rarely encountered from radiation therapy except when the abdominal viscera are in the radiation field. On the other hand, mucosal toxicity is invariably present when the mucosal surfaces of the body are in the radiation field, whereas stomatitis is relatively uncommon in patients receiving chemotherapy except with the use of antimetabolites such as 5-fluorouracil or methotrexate. Diarrhea is relatively uncommon from chemotherapy but is not uncommon in patients receiving radiation therapy to the abdomen or the pelvic regions.

Antiemetics

Nausea and vomiting engender the most fear in the patient's mind when the topic of chemotherapy is discussed. Consequently, there has been an ongoing search for antiemetics ever since the beginnings of cancer chemotherapy. The first class of drugs to be used to control nausea and vomiting were the phenothiazines, including prochlorperazine and chlorpromazine. Their antiemetic effects were modest, and the drugs produced considerable neurologic side effects including sedation, extrapyramidal reactions, and hypotension, especially with the use of chlorpromazine. During the last decade, several new antiemetics have been developed and have been found to be more effective than the phenothiazine (16). The most effective of these drugs is metoclopramide (Reglan), which is highly effective, particularly against the nausea and vomiting produced by the severely emetogenic drugs such as cisplatinum (17). Two other drugs that have found common usage recently include dexamethasone, which has an antiemetic potency equivalent to that of metoclopramide (18) and lorazepam (Ativan), which, besides having a modest degree of antiemetic activity, produces a significant tranquilizing effect, a desirable feature, especially in patients who are prone to anxiety under stressful situations (19). The most recent and currently a popular antiemetic is ondansetron (Zofran) which belongs to a class of serotonin antagonists which block the 5-hydroxytryptamine-3 receptors involved in triggering the emetic response from chemotherapy (20). The relative efficacy of the antiemetic agents along with their commonly used dose schedules are summarized in Table 45–2.

The choice of a particular antiemetic agent has to be tailored to the emetogenic potential of chemotherapy used for an individual patient. Accordingly, the chemotherapeutic agents that produce mild or no nausea may not need any antiemetics or at most a mild antiemetic agent such as Ativan or low-dose Reglan. The cytotoxic agents in this category include the vinca alkaloids, 5-fluorouracil, methotrexate and bleomycin. For drugs with moderately severe emetic potential, a more potent antiemetic regimen including Ativan and a second agent such as Reglan or dexamethasone can provide sufficient antiemetic coverage (21). For drugs with severe emetic potential such as cisplatinum, dacarbazine and cyclophosphamide, potent antiemetic agents such as Zofran alone or in combination with another antiemetic agent such as dexamethasone are recommended (22).

Antiemetic agents must be used judiciously and as a preventive measure rather than reserved for use only if the patient experiences nausea and vomiting. The prevention of nausea and vomiting right from the start of chemotherapy prevents the develop-

Table 45–2. Antiemetic Agents

Antiemetic Agent	Dose, Route, and Schedule	Relative Efficacy and Toxicity
Phenothiazines:		
Prochlorperazine	10–25 mg I.V. q 4–6 hrs	Mild to moderately active; well tolerated
Chlorpromazine	25–50 mg q 6 hr (oral/rectal)	Causes hypotension and sedation
Butyrophenones:		
Haloperidol	1–2 mg oral or I.V. q 2–6 hr	Moderately active, causes sedation
Droperidol	0.5–2 mg I.V. q 4 hr	Moderately active, causes sedation
Benzodiazepines:		
Lorazepam	1–2 mg I.V. q 8 hr	Mild activity; anxiolytic and causes amnesia
Cannabinoid:		
THC (Dronabinol)	5–10 mg/m^2 q 4–6 hr	Moderate activity, neurologic toxicity
Corticosteroids:		
Dexamethasone	4–20 mg PO or I.V. q 24 hr	Moderately active, causes insomnia
Substituted Benzamide:		
Metoclopramide	1–3 mg/kg I.V. q 2–3 hr	Highly active, controls nausea and vomiting in 40–50% of patients, can cause neurologic complications
Serotonin antagonists:		
Ondansetron	10–20 mg I.V. q 8 hr	Most active antiemetic, controls nausea and vomiting in 60–75% of patients, has minimal toxicity

ment of a conditioned response of anticipatory nausea and vomiting, which can become very difficult to control once they have set in. The proper choice of an antiemetic agent can completely abrogate the unpleasantness of nausea and vomiting and have a major impact on the quality of life in patients receiving cancer chemotherapy (23). The lack of CNS side effects from the newly discovered antiemetic agents allows patients to function at their normal potential and not interfere with their daily activities. This was not possible in the past, when most antiemetic agents produced significant sedation such that patients had to literally sleep through the period of chemotherapy administration, usually covering a period of several days out of a month.

Because the emetic response to radiation therapy is generally mild or nonexistent, antiemetic agents are generally not required. A few of the patients receiving radiation therapy to the gastrointestinal tract regions may require some mild antiemetic agents. However, in some instances, nausea and vomiting can be marked with radiotherapy, for example, in patients with seminoma receiving para-aortic irradiation. In these cases, control is generally achieved with the drugs described above for chemotherapy with phenothiazines effective for mild nausea and metoclopramide for more severe nausea. Recently, experience with ondansetron suggests that it is an effective agent in radiation-induced nausea and vomiting and that it can be used in the rare severe case and most certainly in cases in which radiation is combined with chemotherapy. However, patients receiving combined chemoradiation require appropriate antiemetic therapy in order to allow continued therapy without interruptions.

Mucositis

Mucosal ulceration is not an infrequent complication of treatment with radiation therapy as well as some of the chemotherapeutic agents. The worst manifestation of mucosal toxicity is stomatitis, which can cause severe oral pain and lead to marked impairment of oral intake and consequently compromise the nutritional status of patients experiencing this toxicity. It is a frequent side effect of cytotoxic agents such as 5-fluorouracil and methotrexate. The likelihood of developing mucositis is clearly dose-related and frequently the dose-limiting factor in the use of these drugs. Stomatitis from 5-fluorouracil is related to the schedule of administration. It is uncommon when the drug is used by the bolus schedule compared to the continuous infusion schedule, which is often limited by stomatitis. Other anticancer drugs which have a lesser incidence of stomatitis include bleomycin, actinomycin-D and Adriamycin when used at high dose levels.

Radiotherapy, especially to the head and neck regions, is frequently associated with varying degrees of stomatitis and pharyngitis. Mucositis is a frequent dose rate (i.e., dose per day) limiting factor in the delivery of radiation therapy to organs where the mucous membranes are in the field. Reduction of the daily dose or a short break in treatment is sometimes required. Utilization of chemotherapy and radiotherapy together often produces more severe mucosal toxicity, and the ulceration of the mucous membrane becomes a major limiting factor in their use.

The available treatments for established mucositis are not satisfactory (24). Symptomatic relief is possible with local anesthetic solutions or gels applied orally for moderately severe degrees of stomatitis. For more severe cases, parenteral analgesics have to be used around the clock for a few days until mucosal healing takes place. Local application of anesthetic preparations such as 2% xylocaine viscous is frequently used but provides only modest and short-lived relief from pain. More recently, sucralfate (Carafate) has been claimed to be useful and is a popular choice. It has to be used as a suspension, which provides a protective coating to the mucosa and has a modest degree of soothing effect (25,26).

Although there are no ideal protective agents against stomatitis, the dose and schedule of drug administration, particularly of the antimetabolites, are amenable to adjustment and are frequently useful in minimizing the severity of stomatitis. The most effective pharmacologic agent in prevention of stomatitis is folinic acid (calcium leucovorin) for patients treated with antifolates such as methotrexate and related drugs. The availability of folinic acid (leucovorin rescue) provides the best example of pharmacologically blocking the toxicity of methotrexate and permits administration of very high doses of methotrexate, frequently more than 100-fold higher than the dose tolerable without folinic acid (27). This has therapeutic implications in diseases such as osteogenic sarcoma and high-grade lymphomas, in which methotrexate is frequently used in a high-dose schedule without significant toxicity and permits use of full dosage of other cytotoxic agents. Folinic acid (10 mg/m^2 q 6 hr) is also useful in conjunction with standard-dose methotrexate when it is combined with other drugs such as 5-fluorouracil and Adriamycin and allows their use in full dosage on account of complete blockage of toxicity from methotrexate (28).

More recently, hematopoietic growth factors have also been claimed to provide some protection from the stomatitis induced by chemotherapeutic agents (8). The degree of protection and the mechanism of protective effect are still not clearly defined and require further study. It appears that the hematopoietic growth factors such as G-CSF and GM-CSF might also provide a proliferative stimulus for the stem cells in the mucosal layer of the oral cavity and the gastrointestinal tract. These agents are currently under investigation for use in radiation-induced stomatitis.

PROTECTIVE AGENTS AGAINST ORGAN DIRECTED TOXICITIES

Besides the toxicities described in the previous section, several chemotherapeutic agents can potentially cause toxicities to the vital organs. Examples include the cardiotoxicity of anthracyclines, pulmonary toxicity of bleomycin, nephrotoxicity of cisplatinum, and bladder toxicity from cyclophosphamide and ifosfamide. The various protective agents currently available and their efficacy are discussed in this section.

Cardioprotective Agents

The clinical utility of both daunomycin and Adriamycin (ADR) are limited by the development of cardiotoxicity at cumulative doses .exceeding 550 mg/m^2. Some patients are more susceptible and have developed cardiotoxicity at lower cumulative doses; others can tolerate somewhat higher doses without experiencing significant cardiac damage. Cardiac toxicity of anthracyclines is exacerbated by radiation therapy as described in greater detail in Chapter 35. The cardiac toxicity of anthracyclines has been thought to involve formation of free radicals that, in the presence of iron, act as oxidizing agents in the heart.

Several potentially cardioprotective agents have been tested in animals and in clinical trials (29). The earliest drug tested was alpha-tocopherol, which produced significant protective effects in mice but failed to provide meaningful cardioprotection in humans (30,31). Other free radical scavengers such as N-acetylcysteine and coenzyme Q-10 have similarly been tested in clinical trials and produced no major protection from cardiac toxicity of ADR (29,32). The most interesting recent compound that has shown substantial cardioprotective activity in experimental animals is ICRF-187 (33,34). It is a piperazine derivative of ethylenediamine tetracetic acid (EDTA) and is a potent chelating agent of both free iron and iron that has formed a complex with the anthracycline. The cardioprotective effect in animals is reproducible in several species and does not interfere with the antitumor effect. This compound has also shown significant cardiac protection in recent clinical trials reported by Speyer and associates from New York (34–36). Patients with breast cancer received ICRF-187 (ADR-529) as a 1 g/m^2 bolus half an hour prior to each dose of ADR, which was used in combination with 5-FU and cyclophosphamide (FAC). In this randomized prospective trial, ICRF-187 provided substantial cardioprotection. Among 76 women receiving FAC with ICRF-187, only 5 (6%) developed cardiac toxicity compared to 35 (47%) of 74 given FAC alone. Furthermore, ICRF-187 allowed 22 patients to receive cumulative ADR dose beyond 600 mg/m^2 and 10 patients to receive doses beyond 1000 mg/m^2 (36). Other investigations are currently under way to independently confirm the magnitude of cardiac protection provided by the ICRF-187.

Uroprotective Agents

The urinary tract, including kidneys and bladder, is not an infrequent target of toxicity from chemoradiation. Alkylating agents such as cyclophosphamide and ifosfamide and cisplatinum are the major drugs causing toxic damage to bladder and kidneys, respectively. Several drugs have been tested as protective agents against these toxicities. These include WR-2721, sodium thiosulfate, sodium diethyldithiocarbamate (DDTC), sodium-2-mercaptoethanesulfonate (MESNA), and N-acetylcysteine (NAC). Although these compounds have all shown significant protection in the experimental animal studies, their effectiveness in man has been established only for WR-2721, sodium thiosulfate, and MESNA. The guidelines for their use and the degree of protection provided are briefly described in this section.

WR-2721 (Amifostine, Ethiofos, Ethylol)

WR-2721, S-2-(3-aminopropylamino) ethyl phosphorothioic acid is an organic thiophosphate compound that selectively protects normal tissues against the toxicity of radiation and alkylating agents (37–42). Besides the protection against the myelosuppressive toxicity of alkylating agents such as cyclophosphamide (43), WR-2721 improves the renal tolerance to cisplatinum by factors of 1.3 to 1.7 (44). The mechanism of selective protection has not been exactly defined but appears in part to be related to the preferential absorption of WR-2721 into normal tissues relative to the malignant tissues. In Phase I clinical trials, WR-2721 in conjunction with radiotherapy has been well tolerated in the dose range of 450 to 950 mg/m^2 when given IV over 15 minutes (45). The side effects associated with its use consist of mild nausea and vomiting, hypocalcemia and hypotension at the highest dose levels (1100 mg/m^2 to 1330 mg/m^2). WR-2721 has had Phase I-II trials in combination with cyclophosphamide and with cisplatinum and the preliminary results indicate modest degree of protection from myelosuppression and from nephrotoxicity of cisplatinum and possibly some reduction in the neurotoxicity of cisplatinum (43,44,46,47). Phase III studies to determine the degree of myeloprotection provided by WR-2721 are currently ongoing in several institutions and cooperative groups. The maximum tolerated single dose of WR-2721 is 910 mg/m^2 (45). A lower dose level of 750 mg/m^2 is suggested for patients who are at high risk for hypotension. A daily dose of 340 mg/m^2 is tolerable for 5 weeks and is recommended for patients receiving radiotherapy (48). The ultimate clinical applications of ethiofos await results of ongoing Phase III clinical trials (49).

Sodium Thiosulfate

Sodium thiosulfate is an excellent neutralizing agent that reacts covalently with cisplatinum, forming a complex that neither is toxic nor has antitumor activity (50). This has allowed a selective rescue of cisplatinum toxicity for patients given intracavitary therapy with high-dose cisplatinum (51–53). This treatment approach has been largely applicable to patients with intra-abdominal malignancies such as ovarian carcinoma and mesothelioma. Cisplatinum in a dose of 225 to 270 mg/m^2 intraperitoneally has been used with minimal nephrotoxicity provided patients concurrently received intravenous thiosulfate in a dose range of 9 g/m^2 to 12 g/m^2 over 4 to 6 hours. This approach to protection from cisplatinum toxicity, of course, has limitations in that it is not useful for a majority of the patients requiring intravenous cisplatinum for metastatic solid tumors. Furthermore, a sufficient amount of cisplatinum is absorbed from the peritoneal surface to result in moderate degrees of myelotoxicity and nephrotoxicity to preclude therapy beyond 4 to 5 courses (52,53).

Sodium 2-Mercaptoethanesulfonate (MESNA)

High-dose cyclophosphamide therapy and utilization of its analog, ifosfamide, are limited by bladder toxicity in the form of hemorrhagic cystitis leading to hematuria. The causative agent of bladder toxicity is acrolein, a major oxazaphosphorine metabolite (54,55). Because thiol compounds are good scavengers of free radical damage, several sulfhydryl compounds have been tested as uroprotective agents (56,57). Among these, MESNA has been found to be the most effective and is largely free from toxicity (58). Although hemorrhagic cystitis is a rare complication of standard dose therapy with cyclophosphamide, doses in excess of 5 g/m^2, which are commonly used in bone marrow transplantation programs, have a significant risk of hemorrhagic cystitis (54). Ifosfamide is associated with a much higher incidence of hemorrhagic cystitis in the commonly used dose schedules of 1 g/m^2 to 1.5 g/m^2 daily for 5 days. In fact, ifosfamide was almost discarded as an anticancer drug due to its bladder toxicity but was rescued from oblivion when MESNA became available. Utilization of MESNA allowed a two-fold dose escalation of ifosfamide which clearly enhanced its therapeutic index in a major way and made it a very useful anticancer drug in the treatment of several malignancies (59,60).

Because MESNA has a short half-life, it has to be given at 4-hour intervals, generally as a short IV infusion in a dose of 400 mg/m^2 to 500 mg/m^2, which is approximately 20% of the corresponding dose of ifosfamide (61). With the use of MESNA, the incidence of hemorrhagic cystitis is reduced to <5% compared to an expected risk of 40 to 50% in patients receiving ifosfamide without the use of this uroprotective agent. As a short bolus injection, MESNA is generally used immediately preceding ifosfamide and for two additional doses at 4-hour intervals following each dose of ifosfamide. Alternatively, it can be mixed in the same bag of ifosfamide in an equimolar concentration and given as a continuous infusion over 24 hours. Because both cyclophosphamide and ifosfamide are physically inert formulations and have to be activated in the body, MESNA can be mixed with them in the same IV bag without concern for incompatibility (62,63). Besides MESNA, other thiol compounds such as cysteine and N-acetylcysteine have been tested as uroprotective agents, but their efficacy is marginal and clearly inferior to that of MESNA (64,65). The risk of hemorrhagic cystitis from ifosfamide or cyclophosphamide is greatly enhanced by exposure of the bladder to radiation therapy before or during their use (66). Hence such patients require extra precaution in using ifosfamide and even standard dose cyclophosphamide, and should be given MESNA on a prophylactic basis.

RADIOPROTECTIVE AGENTS

Chapter 31 discusses the possible use of ethiofos, or WR-2721, in conjunction with chemotherapy. This drug has considerable potential for not only reducing radiation injury but perhaps allowing greater tumor response through the delivery of higher doses. It was initially discovered that sulfhydryl compounds would protect against whole-body lethality in frogs and rodents by Patt in the 1940s (67). This subsequently lead to a large effort on the part of the U.S. Army to develop radioprotective compounds. A large synthesis and testing program identified many classes of compounds. The first group were cysteamine and related analogs, which gave significant protection. Subsequently, thiophosphates were discovered. They were somewhat less toxic and could be given in higher doses and gave even greater degrees of protection. Several of these compounds are shown with their chemical structures in Table 45–3 (68). As these compounds became available, they were found by Yuhas and Storer to protect differentially the normal tissues vis-a-vis tumor (37). Shortly after this discovery, Harris and Phillips tested two thiophosphates in both aerated and hypoxic cells derived from mouse bone marrow colony-forming units and found that there was far greater protection of aerated than of hypoxic cells (69) (Fig. 45–1). They also found that the difference in protection between tumor and normal tissue was not due to different enzymatic breakdown of the thiophosphates. A wide range of tissues was tested (70) (Fig. 45–2). Subsequent pharmacologic studies indicated that, because of its partition coefficient, ethiofos is excluded from brain and from most tumors, at least during the first 30 minutes after injection. Thus, the differential radioprotection originally described by Yuhas and Storer appears to be due to two factors, i.e., pharmacologic distribution favoring normal tissue and decreased effectiveness in the protection of hypoxic cells.

What remains to be done is to take advantage of the potential shown by ethiofos, i.e., the ability to protect normal tissue and allow either a reduction of morbidity or an escalation of dose with equal morbidity to achieve greater tumor response than that achieved now with conventional radiotherapy. The latter would seem to be the approach of choice because current radiotherapy is delivered at doses that cause acceptable morbidity. In order to establish the agent, however, it will be necessary first to prove that doses tolerated by humans, summarized above as single or multiple administrations, do indeed provide measurable protection of the various organs that limit radiotherapy. Animal experiments have proven that, with fractionated irradiation, one still achieves

Table 45–3. Thiophosphate Radioprotective Agents and Their Chemical Structures

Designation	Chemical Name	Structure
MEA	β-mercaptoethylamine (cysteamine)	$H_2NCH_2CH_2SH$
WR-2529	3-(2-mercaptoethylamino) propionamide p-toluenesulfonate	$HSCH_2CH_2NH\ \ CH_2CH_2\overset{\overset{O}{\Vert}}{C}NH_2 \mid CH_3C_6H_4SO_3H$
WR-2721	S-2-(3-aminopropylamino) ethyl phosphorothioic acid hydrate	$H_2NCH_2CH_2CH_2\ \ NHCH_2CH_2S\ \ PO_3H_2 \mid XH_2O$
WR-2823	S-2-(5-aminopentylamino) ethyl phosphorothioic acid monohydrate	$H_2N(CH_2)_5\ \ NHCH_2CH_2S\ \ PO_3H_2 \mid H_2O$
WR-638	Sodium hydrogen S-(2-aminoethyl) phosphorothioate	$H_2NCH_2CH_2S\ \ \overset{\overset{O}{\Vert}}{P}\text{-}(OH)\ \ (ONa)$

Reproduced with permission from Phillips TL. Radiation sensitizers and protectors. *In:* Cancer: Principles and Practice of Oncology. DeVita VT, et al (Eds). Philadelphia, JB Lippincott, 1982, p. 1822.

protection. If the maximum tolerated doses described above of 750 mg/m^2 single dose or 340 mg/m^2 4 days a week for 5 weeks (45) are compared to mouse doses on an mg/m^2 basis, they should be highly protective. On the other hand, if the distribution of protection follows a more uniform distribution throughout the total body pharmacologic space, one would see little protection. Pharmacologic studies have indicated a rapid disappearance of ethiofos from the blood as it is taken up by tissues and converted to other thiols which are, in many cases, also radioprotective.

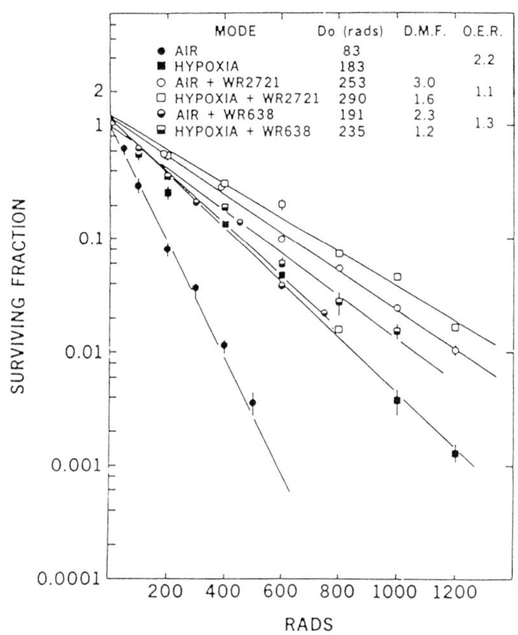

Fig. 45–1. Survival of mouse CFU bone marrow cells as a function of radiation dose and chemical radioprotector administration. Treatment was delivered in the donor mouse, breathing air or made hypoxic through the breathing of 5.5% nitrogen. Note the very low OER for CFUs irradiated in the presence of WR-2721 and the markedly low-dose modifying factor for both protectors shown in hypoxic cells. (From Harris JW, Phillips TL. Radiat Res 46:362, 1971.)

The initial clinical trials have established the maximum tolerated dose for single and fractionated experiments. One study in dogs by Halberg et al has indicated that intraluminal ethiofos significantly protects the duodenum in the situation of intraoperative irradiation without significant system dosage (71). Constine et al have shown that there is apparent protection of human bone marrow during hemi-body irradiation by using 750 to 900 mg/m^2 and radiation doses up to 700 cGy (42).

The efficacy of ethiofos with fractionated radiotherapy is yet to be evaluated. Suitable sites appear to be the head and neck and pelvic regions, where reactions of several tissues could be carefully observed and calibrated in ethiofos-treated and control patients. These include reactions of skin, mucosa, subcutaneous tissue, and bone during treatment of head and neck cancers. During treatment of pelvic neoplasms, one could evaluate rectal and bladder mucosa, skin,

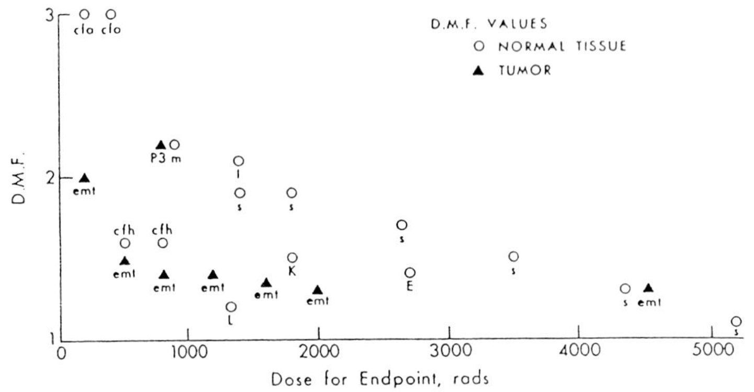

Fig. 45–2. Dose-modifying factor values for normal tissue and tumor as a function of the dose size required for a given end-point in control animals. (cfa = aerated CFUs; cfh = hypoxic CFUs; emt = EMT6/S.F. carcinoma; P3 = P388 leukemia; I = intestinal crypts; L = lung $LD_{50/160}$; K = kidney $LD_{50/365}$; s = skin reaction grade, days 16–40; E = esophageal $LD_{50/28}$; m = $LD_{50/30}$ in DBA/2 mice). (From Phillips TL, et al. Cancer 32:528, 1973.)

small intestinal, vaginal, and cervical reactions. Accelerated hyperfractionation schedules such as 370 cGy b.i.d. for 2 days with 2-week breaks, repeated 3 times, have been applied both in the pelvis and head and neck regions. These regimens are tolerated overall but do cause significant acute reactions. Phase II testing of ethiofos in this setting followed by randomized trials should lead to the answer as to whether it provides protection of human tissues. Following this, it would be necessary to escalate the radiation dose to the point where the same degree of reaction occurred as was seen in radiation patients in the control group. This work is yet to be done, and one would hope that it is organized in the near future. The moderate to significant toxicity of multidose ethiofos is a limiting factor, and therefore short course, accelerated fractionation regimens may be optimal.

REFERENCES

1. Metcalf D. The colony stimulating factors. Discovery development and clinical applications. Cancer 65:2185, 1990.
2. Morstyn G, Burgess AW. Hemopoietic growth factors. A review. Cancer Res 48:5624, 1988.
3. Groopman JE, Molina JM, Scadden DT. Hematopoietic growth factors. Biology and clinical applications. N Engl J Med 321:1449, 1989.
4. Eschbach JW, Egrie JC, Downing MR, et al. Correction of the anemia of end-stage renal disease with recombinant human erythropoietin. N Engl J Med 316:73, 1987.
5. Erslev AJ. Erythropoietin. N Engl J Med 324:1339, 1991.
6. Platanias LC, Miller CB, Mick R, et al. Treatment of chemotherapy-induced anemia with recombinant human erythropoietin in cancer. J Clin Oncol 9:2021, 1991.
7. Doweiko JP, Goldberg MA. Erythropoietin therapy in cancer patients. Oncology 5:31, 1991.
8. Gabrilove JL. Effects of granulocyte colony-stimulating factor on neutropenia and associated morbidity due to chemotherapy for transitional-cell carcinoma of the urothelium. N Engl J Med 318:1414, 1988.
9. Crawford J, Ozer H, Stoller R, et al. Reduction by granulocyte colony-stimulating factor of fever and neutropenia induced by chemotherapy in patients with small-cell lung cancer. N Engl J Med 325:164, 1991.
10. Nemunaitis J, Rabinowe SN, Singer JW, et al. Recombinant granulocyte-macrophage colony-stimulating factor after autologous bone marrow transplantation for lymphoid cancer. N Engl J Med 324:1773, 1991.
11. Clark-Lewis I, Aebersold R, Ziltener H, et al. Automated chemical synthesis of a protein growth factor for hemopoietic cells, Interleukin-3. Science 231:134, 1986.
12. Platanias LC and Vogelzang NJ. Interleukin-1. Biology, pathophysiology, and clinical prospects. Am J Med 89:621, 1990.
13. Tewari A, Buhles Jr WC, Starnes Jr HF. Preliminary report. Effects of interleukin-1 on platelet counts. Lancet 336:712, 1990.
14. Ganser A, Lindemann A, Seipelt G, et al. Effects of recombinant human interleukin-3 in

patients with normal hematopoiesis and in patients with bone marrow failure. Blood 76:666, 1990.
15. Donahue RE, Seehra J, Metzger M, et al. Human IL-3 and GM-CSF act synergistically in stimulating hematopoiesis in primates. Science 241:1820, 1988.
16. Gralla RJ, Tyson LB, Kriss MG, Clark RA. The management of chemotherapy-induced nausea and vomiting. Med Clin North Am 71:289, 1987.
17. Kris MG, Gralla RJ, Tyson LB, et al. Improved control of cisplatin-induced emesis with high-dose metoclopramide and with combinations of metoclopramide, dexamethasone, and diphenhydramine. Results of consecutive trials in 255 patients. Cancer 55:527, 1985.
18. Gagen M, Gochnour D, Yound D, et al. A randomized trial of metoclopramide and a combination of dexamethasone and lorazepam for prevention of chemotherapy-induced vomiting. J Clin Oncol 2:696, 1984.
19. Laszlo J, Clark RA, Hanson DC, et al. Lorazepam in cancer patients treated with cisplatin. A drug having antiemetic, amnesic, and anxiolytic effects. J Clin Oncol 3:864, 1985.
20. Hainsworth J, Harvey W, Pendergrass K, et al. A single-blind comparison of intravenous ondansetron, a selective serotonin antagonist, with intravenous metoclopramide in the prevention of nausea and vomiting associated with high-dose cisplatin chemotherapy. J Clin Oncol 9:713, 1991.
21. Kris MG, Gralla RJ, Clark RA, et al. Antiemetic control and prevention of side effects of anticancer therapy with lorazepam or diphenhydramine when used in combination with metoclopramide plus dexamethasone. A double-blind, randomized trial. Cancer 60:2816, 1987.
22. Roila F, Tonato M, Cognetti F, et al. Prevention of cisplatin-induced emesis: A double-blind multicenter randomized crossover study comparing ondansetron and ondansetron plus dexamethasone. J Clin Oncol 9:675, 1991.
23. Gralla RJ. An outline of anti-emetic treatment. Eur J Cancer Clin Oncol 25(Suppl 1):11, 1989.
24. Loprinzi CL. A controlled evaluation of an allopurinol mouthwash as prophylaxis against 5-FU-induced stomatitis. Cancer 65:1879, 1990.
25. Pfeiffer P, Madsen EL, Hansen O, May O. Effect of prophylactic sucralfate suspension on stomatitis induced by cancer chemotherapy. A randomized, double-blind cross-over study. Acta Oncologica 29:171, 1989.
26. Solomon MA. Oral sucralfate suspension for mucositis. N Engl J Med 315:459, 1986.
27. Frei III E. High dose methotrexate with leucovorin rescue. Rationale and spectrum of antitumor activity. Am J Med 68:370, 1980.
28. Jolivet J. The pharmacology and clinical use of methotrexate. N Engl J Med 309:1094, 1983.
29. Green MD, Speyer JL, Muggia FM. Cardiotoxicity of anthracyclines. Eur J Cancer Clin Oncol 20:293, 1984.
30. Myers CE, McGuire W, Young R. Adriamycin: amelioration of toxicity by α-Tocopherol. Cancer Treat Rep 60:961, 1976.
31. Legha SS, Wang YM, Mackay B, et al. Clinical and pharmacologic investigation of the effects of α-tocopherol on adriamycin cardiotoxicity. Ann NY Acad Sci 393:411, 1982.
32. Dresdale AR, Barr LH, Bonow RO, et al. Prospective randomized study of the role of N-acetylcysteine in reversing doxorubicin-induced cardiomyopathy. Am J Clin Oncol 5:657, 1982.
33. Herman EH, Ferrans VJ, Meyers CE, van Vleet JF. Comparison of the effectiveness of (±)-1, 2-Bis (3,5-dioxopiperazinyl-1-yl) propane (ICRF-187) and N-Acetylcysteine in preventing chronic doxorubicin cardiotoxicity in beagles. Cancer Res 45:276, 1985.
34. Green MD, Alderton P, Gross J, et al. Evidence of the selective alteration of anthracycline activity due to modulation by ICRF-187 (ADR-529). Pharmacol Ther 48:61, 1990.
35. Speyer JL, Green MD, Kramer E, et al. Protective effect of the bispiperazinedione ICRF-187 against doxorubicin-induced cardiac toxicity in women with advanced breast cancer. N Engl J Med 319:745, 1988.
36. Speyer JL, Green MD, Sanger J, et al. A prospective randomized trial of ICRF-187 for prevention of cumulative doxorubicin-induced cardiac toxicity in women with breast cancer. Cancer Treat Rev 17:161, 1990.
37. Yuhas JM and Storer JB. Differential chemoprotection of normal and malignant tissues. J Natl Cancer Inst 42:331, 1969.
38. Ito H, Meistrich ML, Barkley HT, et al. Protection of acute and late radiation damage of the gastrointestinal tract by WR-2721. Int J Radiat Oncol Biol Phys 12:211, 1985.
39. Shaw LM, Glover D, Turrisi A, et al. Pharmacokinetics of WR-2721. Pharmacol Ther 39:195, 1988.
40. Coia LR, Brown DQ, Hardiman J. WR-2721 as cytotoxic and radioprotective agent in treatment of murine lymphoma with total body irradiation. NCI Monogr 6:235, 1988.
41. Takahashi I, Nagai T, Miyashi K, et al. Clinical study of the radioprotective effects of amifost-

ine (YM-08310, WR-2721) on chronic radiation injury. Int J Radiat Oncol Biol Phys 12:935, 1986.
42. Constine LS, Zagars G, Rubin P, Kligerman M. Protection by WR-2721 of human bone marrow function following irradiation. Int J Radiat Oncol Biol Phys 12:1505, 1986.
43. Glover D, Glick JS, Weiler C, et al. WR-2721 protects against the hematologic toxicity of cyclophosphamide: A controlled phase II trial. J Clin Oncol 4:584, 1986.
44. Glover D, Fox KR, Weiler C, et al. Clinical trials of WR-2721 prior to alkylating agent chemotherapy and radiotherapy. Pharmacol Ther 39:3, 1988.
45. Turrisi AT, Glover DJ, Glick JH, et al. Final report of the phase I trial of single-dose WR-2721 (S-2-(3-Aminopropylamino) ethylphosphorothioic acid). Cancer Treat Rep 70:1389, 1986.
46. Kemp GM, Glover DJ, Schein PS. The role of WR-2721 in the reduction of combined cisplatin and cyclophosphamide toxicity. Proc Am Soc Clin Oncol 9:67, 1990.
47. Mollman JE, Glover DJ, Hogan WM, Furman RE. Cisplatin neuropathy. Risk factors, prognosis, and protection by WR-2721. Cancer 61:2192, 1988.
48. Kligerman MM, Turrisi AT, Urtasun RC, et al. Final report on phase I trial of WR-2721 before protracted fractionated radiation therapy. Int J Radiat Oncol Biol Phys 14:1119, 1988.
49. Schein PS. WR-2721: A chemotherapy and radiation protective agent. Clin Investig 8:265, 1990.
50. Shea M, Koziol JA, Howell SB. Kinetics of sodium thiosulfate, a cisplatin neutralizer. Clin Pharmacol Ther 35:419, 1984.
51. Howell SB, Pfeifle CE, Wung WE, Olshen RA. Intraperitoneal cis-Diamminedichloroplatinum with systemic thiosulfate protection. Cancer Res 43:1426, 1983.
52. Howell SB, Pfeifle CL, Wung WE, et al. Intraperitoneal cisplatin with systemic thiosulfate protection. Ann Intern Med 97:845, 1982.
53. Pfeifle CE, Howell SB, Felthouse RD. High-dose cisplatin with sodium thiosulfate protection. J Clin Oncol 3(2):237, 1985.
54. Hows JM, Mehta A, Ward L, et al. Comparison of mesna with forced diuresis to prevent cyclophosphamide induced haemorrhagic cystitis in marrow transplantation: A prospective randomized study. Br J Cancer 50:753, 1984.
55. Hilgard P, Herdrich K, Brade W. Ifosfamide—current aspects and perspectives. Cancer Treat Rev 10:183, 1983.
56. Scheef W, Klein HO, Brock N, et al. Controlled clinical studies with an antidote against the urotoxicity of oxazaphosphorines: Preliminary results. Cancer Treat Rep 63:501, 1979.
57. Brock N, Pohl J, Stekar J, Scheef W. Studies on the urotoxicity of oxazaphosphorine cytostatics and its prevention-III. Profile of action of sodium 2-mercaptoethane sulfonate (Mesna). Eur J Cancer Clin Oncol 18:377, 1982.
58. Shaw IC, Graham MI. Mesna—a short review. Cancer Treat Rev 14:67, 1987.
59. Elias AD, Eder JP, Shea T, et al. High-dose ifosfamide with mesna uroprotection. A phase I study. J Clin Oncol 8:170, 1990.
60. Zalupski M, Baker LH. Ifosfamide. J Natl Cancer Inst 80:566, 1988.
61. Burkert H. Clinical overview of mesna. Cancer Treat Rev 10:175, 1983.
62. Colvin M. The comparative pharmacology of cyclophosphamide and ifosfamide. Semin Oncol 9:2, 1982.
63. Klein HO, Wickramahayake PD, Coerper C, et al. High-dose ifosfamide and mesna as continuous infusion over five days—a phase I/II trial. Cancer Treat Rev 10:167, 1983.
64. Brock B, Pohl J, Stekar J. Comparative study on the uroprotective efficacy of thiols and other sulfur compounds. Eur J Cancer Clin Oncol 17:1155, 1981.
65. Morgan LR, Donley PJ, Harrison EF, Hunter HL. The control of ifsosfamide-induced hematuria with N-acetylcysteine in patients with advanced carcinoma of the lung. Semin Oncol 9:71, 1982.
66. Jayalakshmamma B, Pinkel D. Urinary-bladder toxicity following pelvic irradiation and simultaneous cyclophosphamide therapy. Cancer 38:701, 1976.
67. Patt HM, Tyree EB, Straube RL, et al. Cysteine protection against x-irradiation. Science 110:213, 1949.
68. Phillips TL. Radiation sensitizers and protectors. *In:* Cancer: Principles and Practice of Oncology. (1st ed). DeVita VT, Hellman S, Rosenberg SA (Eds). Philadelphia, JB Lippincott, 1982, p. 1822.
69. Harris JW, Phillips TL. Radiobiological and biochemical studies of thiophosphate radioprotective compounds related to cysteamine. Radiat Res 46:362, 1971.
70. Phillips TL, Kane L, Utley JF. Radioprotection of tumor and normal tissues by thiophosphate compounds. Cancer 32:528, 1973.
71. Halberg FE, La Rue SM, Rayner AA, et al. Intraoperative radiotherapy with localized radioprotection: Diminished duodenal toxicity with intraluminal WR2721. Int J Radiat Oncol Biol Phys 21:1241, 1991.

Part V

FUTURE TRENDS

Chapter 46

COMPENDIUM OF SELECT CURRENT CLINICAL TRIALS

This compendium lists a number of current (or recently completed) investigative protocols being conducted through the auspices of various national and international research groups listed below. These, we believe, are examples of the variegated clinical research in chemoradiation today. Treatment schemas are given in abbreviated form; eligibility criteria, dose-modification factors, follow-up, and other specifications have been omitted. The glossary of chemotherapeutic agents at the end of this book explains the abbreviations used in this compendium.

You are encouraged to contact the respective research groups (addresses and telephone numbers provided) for further details and updates of protocols that interest you. Moreover, you are strongly urged *not* to conduct these studies on your own without official approval from these research groups; you would do so at considerable risk to your patient.

The Editors

RESEARCH GROUPS

Brain Tumor Cooperative Group (BTCG)
Information Management Services (IMS)
1400 Spring Street, Suite 500
Silver Spring, MD 20910
(301) 495-0444

Cancer and Leukemia Group B (CALGB)
Data Management and Data Processing
Frontier Science and Technical Research Foundation, Inc.
O. Ross McIntyre, M.D.
Chairperson
303 Boyiston Street, First Floor
Brookline, MA 02146

Children's Cancer Study Group (CCG)
G. Denman Hammond, M.D.
Chairperson
440 E. Huntington Drive, Suite 300
P.O. Box 60012
Arcadia, CA 91066-6012
(818) 447-1674

Community Oncology Program (COP)
Roger Winn, M.D.
Chairperson
University of Texas, M.D. Anderson
1515 Holcombe Boulevard
Houston, TX 77030
(713) 792-8515

Eastern Cooperative Oncology Group (ECOG)
Douglas Tormey, M.D., Ph.D.
Chairperson
Operations Office
Medical Science Center, Room 4765
420 N. Charter Street
Madison, WI 53706
(608) 263-6650

European Organization for Research and Treatment of Cancer (EORTC)
P. Auerbacher
Executive Director
Avenue E. Mounier, 83
1200 Brussels, Belgium
(2) 535 34 80

Gynecologic Oncology Group (GOG)
Operations Office
Robert C. Park, M.D.
Chairperson
1234 Market Street, Suite 1945
Philadelphia, PA 19107
(800) 225-3053

Intergroup Testicular Cancer Study
Operations Office
c/o Marsha Denekas
11325 Seven Locks Road, Suite 214
Potomac, MD 20854
(301) 299-8655

The Clinical Trials Group
National Cancer Institute of Canada
82-84 Barrie Street
Queens University
Kingston, Ontario, Canada K7L3N6
(613) 545-6430

National Surgical Adjuvant Breast Project (NSABP)
Dr. Bernard Fisher
Chairman
Room 914 Scaife Hall
3550 Terrace Street
Pittsburgh, PA 15261
(412) 648-9720

North Central Cancer Treatment Group (NCCTG)
Charles Moertel, M.D.
Professor
Department of Medical Oncology
Mayo Clinic
200 First Street SW
Rochester, MN 55905
(507) 284-2511

Northern California Cancer Program (NCCP/NCOG/NCCC)
1301 Shoreway Road, Suite 425
Belmont, CA 94002
(415) 591-4484

Pediatric Oncology Group (POG)
Jeffrey Krischer, Ph.D.
Department of Pediatrics
University of Florida
4110 S.W. 34th Street, Suite 22
Gainesville, FL 32608-2516
(904) 392-5198

Radiation Therapy Oncology Group (RTOG)
J. Cox, M.D.
Chairman
American College of Radiology
1101 Market Street, 14th Floor
Philadelphia, PA 19107
(215) 574-3150

Sarcoma Intergroup
Wayne State University School of Medicine
Division of Medical Oncology
P.O. Box 02188
Detroit, MI 48201
(313) 745-4862

Southwest Oncology Group (SWOG)
Charles A. Coltman, Jr., M.D.
Chairperson
5430 Fredrickson, Suite 618
San Antonio, TX 78229-6197
(512) 366-9300

United Kingdom Medical Research Council (MRC)
D. Rees, M.D.
Chief Executive
20 Park Crescent
London W1N 4AL
United Kingdom
071 636 5422

HEAD AND NECK

1. **E-1392/EST-1389/INT-0126/SWOG-9059**
   Phase III Randomized Study of Standard Radiotherapy Alone vs. Standard Radiotherapy plus CDDP vs. Split-Course Radiotherapy plus CDDP/5-FU in Patients with Unresectable Squamous Cell Carcinoma of the Head and Neck.

   Lead Organization: Eastern Cooperative Oncology Group

   SCHEDULE:

   Arm I: 7000 cGy delivered as a continuous 7-week course in daily fractions of 200 cGy, 5 days/week.

   Arm II: Radiotherapy as in Arm I; CDDP —100 mg/sqm in NS IV over 15–20 minutes on days 1, 22, and 43 of radiotherapy, with vigorous forced hydration.

   Arm III: Radiotherapy—7,000 cGy to the fields described in Arm I, delivered as a split-course in daily fractions of 200 cGy, 5 days/week, as follows: 3000 cGy over 3 weeks in 15 daily fractions; a second course, consisting of 4000 cGy, including the entire operative field and incisions, begins on day 56 or 2–6 weeks postoperatively in patients undergoing resection. CDDP—75 mg/sqm IV over 15 minutes with hydration, diuresis, and antiemetic therapy as on Arm II on days

1 (day 1 of the first course of radiotherapy), 29, and 56.

After completion of all planned therapy on any arm, patients with residual disease considered curatively resectable may undergo salvage resection.

2. EORTC-24891
Phase III Randomized Comparison of Induction Chemotherapy with CDDP/5-FU Followed by Definitive Radiotherapy vs. Surgery and Postoperative Radiotherapy in Patients with Squamous Cell Carcinoma of the Hypopharynx.

Lead Organization: European Organization for Research and Treatment of Cancer

SCHEDULE:

Arm I: Total laryngectomy and partial pharyngectomy (without a distant flap for closure) with permanent tracheostomy plus neck dissection; followed by Radiotherapy—5000 cGy in 25 fractions of 200 cGy, 5 days/week, delivered to the remaining pharynx, the neck bilaterally, and the tracheostomy followed by a boost of 1400 cGy to high-risk sites.

Arm II: CDDP—100 mg/sqm IV on day 1; 5-FU—1,000 mg/sqm/day by continuous infusion over 5 days on day 1. Courses repeat q 21 days for a maximum of three courses. Following course 1, patients with progressive disease proceed to surgery and postoperative radiotherapy (vide infra), while those with SD, PR, and CR receive a second course of chemotherapy. Following course 2, patients with progressive disease and SD proceed to surgery and postoperative radiotherapy, while those with PR receive a third course of chemotherapy and those in CR proceed to definitive radiotherapy (vide infra). Following course 3, patients in CR proceed to definitive radiotherapy, while all others undergo surgery and postoperative radiotherapy.

Surgery following chemotherapy is carried out after hematologic recovery but no sooner than 3 weeks following the last dose of cytotoxic agents.

Definitive radiotherapy for patients achieving CR on chemotherapy consists of 5000 cGy in 25 fractions of 200 cGy, 5 days/week delivered to the entire hypopharynx and the neck bilaterally followed by a boost of 2000 cGy in 10 fractions delivered over 2 weeks to the tumor site and (if present originally) areas of palpable adenopathy.

3. EST-2388/INT-0099/RTOG-8817/SWOG-8892
Phase III Study of Radiotherapy With vs. Without Concurrent CDDP Followed by CDDP/5-FU in Previously Untreated Patients with Stage III/IV Carcinoma of the Nasopharynx.

Lead Organization: Southwest Oncology Group

<u>**Schema:**</u> (Protocol No. 3)

<u>**Arm I:**</u>

<u>**Arm II:**</u>

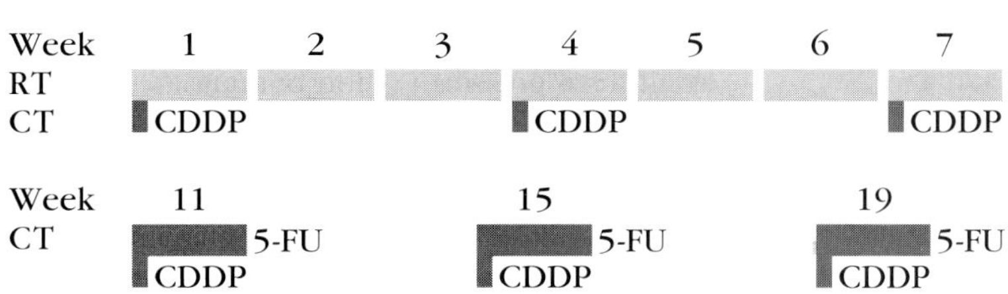

SCHEDULE:

Arm I: Total tumor dose of 7000 cGy over 7–8 weeks delivered as follows: 5000 cGy in daily fractions of 180–200 cGy, 5 days/week, delivered to the primary and neck. A boost volume consisting of the primary tumor and any enlarged neck nodes is treated further to 6600 cGy, after which the field is again reduced to include the primary and any nodes larger than 2 cm and treated to a total of 7000 cGy.

Arm II: Radiotherapy as in Arm I. Concurrent chemotherapy: CDDP—100 mg/sqm IV over 15–20 minutes on days 1, 22, and 43 of radiotherapy with hydration/diuresis. Subsequent chemotherapy: CDDP—80 mg/sqm IV over 15–20 minutes on days 70, 98, and 126, with hydration and diuresis; 5-FU 1 $g/m^2/24$ hours by continuous IV infusion on days 70 through 73, 98 through 101, and 126 through 129.

4. **EORTC-24844**
Phase III Randomized Comparison of Induction Chemotherapy with CDDP/5-FU Followed by Surgery and Postoperative Radiotherapy vs. Surgery and Radiotherapy Alone in the Treatment of Patients with Advanced Squamous Cell Carcinoma of the Lateral Oropharynx and Lateral Posterior Oral Cavity.

Lead Organization: European Organization for Research and Treatment of Cancer

SCHEDULE:

Arm I: CDDP—100 mg/sqm IV on day 1 with pre- and posthydration. 5-FU—1,000 mg/sqm/day for 120 hours (5 days). Beginning on day 22, a second course is administered to responding patients and those with stable disease, while patients with progressive disease proceed to surgery after hematologic recovery. Beginning on day 22 after the second course, a third course is administered to patients in PR and CR, while those with stable or progressive disease proceed to surgery. Surgery—en bloc resection of primary and nodal disease with radical or modified neck dissection and segmental mandibulectomy but no sooner than 3 weeks after the last course of chemotherapy. Radiotherapy—5000 cGy in 25 daily fractions of 200 cGy, delivered in 5 fractions/week to the resected area of the primary tumor and the neck beginning when wound healing is complete, but in no case more than 10 weeks postoperatively. A boost dose of 1400 cGy in 7 fractions is delivered to the primary tumor areas and to the site of neck node metastases under certain conditions.

Arm II: Surgery and radiotherapy as in Arm I.

CENTRAL NERVOUS SYSTEM

5. **RTOG-8905**
Phase III Randomized Comparison of Conventional-Fractionation Radiotherapy With vs. Without Radiosensitization with 5-Bromodeoxyuridine in Patients with Solid Tumors Metastatic to the Brain.

Lead Organization: Radiation Therapy Oncology Group

Schema: (Protocol No. 5)

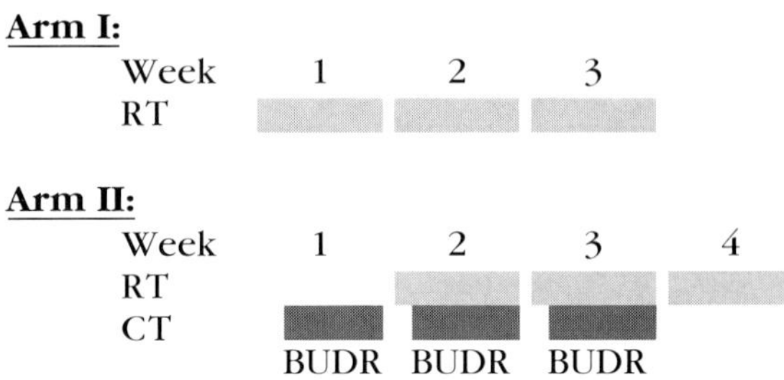

SCHEDULE:

Arm I: 3750 cGy over 3 weeks delivered to the whole brain in 15 fractions of 250 cGy, 5 days/week. Treatment must begin on a Monday.

Arm II: Whole-brain irradiation as on Arm I; BUDR—800 mg/sqm/day by continuous IV infusion over 96 hours (total dose 3,200 mg) beginning on the Thursday or Friday prior to initiation of radiotherapy and repeated (beginning on Thursday or Friday) during the first and second week of radiotherapy. Once radiotherapy has begun, it should be continued on schedule regardless of drug schedule. If radiotherapy is terminated for any reason, BUDR must also be terminated, but if BUDR is terminated or delayed, radiotherapy must proceed on schedule.

6. **NCI-T91-00560/NCOG-6G903**
Phase III Randomized Study of Radiotherapy Alone vs. Radiotherapy/BUDR vs. Radiotherapy/IUDR Followed by PCV (PCB/CCNU/VCR) in Patients with Anaplastic Astrocytomas.

Lead Organization: Northern California Cancer Program

SCHEDULE:

Radiotherapy should begin within 4 weeks of the first craniotomy.

Arm I: Radiotherapy—6,000 cGy to the contrast-enhanced CT- or MRI-defined tumor plus a 3-cm margin delivered in daily fractions of 180-200 cGy, 5 days/week for 6-7 weeks. Chemotherapy begins within 2 weeks of completion of radiotherapy, as follows: PCV: CCNU—110 mg/sqm po on day 1; PCB—60 mg/sqm po daily on days 8 through 21; VCR—1.4 mg/sqm IV push on days 8 and 29. Courses repeat q 6–8 weeks.

Arm II: Radiotherapy—as in Arm I; BUDR—0.8 g/sqm/day by continuous IV infusion over 96 hours, beginning 3 or 4 days prior to radiotherapy (i.e., on the Thursday or Friday prior to the first Monday of radiotherapy) and repeated weekly through week 5; PCV—as in Arm I.

Arm III: Radiotherapy—as in Arm I; IUDR—0.8 g/sqm/day by continuous IV infusion over 96 hours, beginning 3 or 4 days prior to radiotherapy (i.e., on the Thursday or Friday prior to the first Monday of radiotherapy) and repeated weekly through week 5; PCV—as in Arm I.

7. **BTCG-8901**
Phase III Comparison of Surgery and External Radiotherapy Combined With Intravenous BCNU vs. Intravenous BCNU/Intra-arterial CDDP vs. Intravenous Piroxantrone (PXT) in Patients With Malignant Glioma.

Lead Organization: Brain Tumor Cooperative Group

SCHEDULE:

Regimen A: Maximum tumor resection with internal cerebral decompression is performed initially. A second procedure is carried out if the CT or MRI scan 48 hours postoperatively suggests that this would be beneficial.

Regimen B: Newly diagnosed patients should begin therapy within 6 weeks of initial surgery. Radiotherapy—6,020 cGy over 7–8 weeks in 35 daily fractions of 172 cGy, 5 days/week, delivered to a target volume.

In newly diagnosed patients, chemotherapy begins concomitantly with the first radiotherapy treatment.

Arm I: BCNU—200 mg/sqm IV over 30–60 minutes on day 1 or 2 q 8 weeks for 8 courses. The first course should be administered approximately 16 hours prior to the initiation of radiotherapy if possible.

Arm II: BCNU—as in Arm I; CDDP—60 mg/sqm, 3–4 ml/minute, via the carotid artery prior to BCNU on day 1 and on day 22 of the first 3 BCNU courses (i.e., total of 6 doses of CDDP).

Arm III: PXT—150 mg/sqm in 250 ml D5W IV over 1 hour q 3 weeks. Treatment continues until development of progressive disease or unacceptable toxicity.

8. **NCI-T91-00470/NCOG-6G901**
Phase III Trial of Accelerated Hyperfractionation With or Without DFMO vs. Single Fraction Radiotherapy With or With-

out DFMO in Patients with Newly Diagnosed Glioblastoma Multiforme.

Lead Organization: Northern California Cancer Program

SCHEDULE:

Radiotherapy should begin within 4 weeks following surgery and may be initiated as early as 2 weeks post surgery.

Arm I: 7040 cGy administered in 44 fractions of 160 cGy twice daily (a minimum of 6 and a maximum of 8 hours apart), 5 days/week, to the contrast-enhanced CT- or MRI-defined tumor plus 3-cm margins.

Arm II: Radiotherapy—as in Arm I; DFMO—1.8 g/sqm po q 8 hours, beginning 1 week prior to initiation of radiotherapy and continuing throughout radiotherapy.

Arm III: 5940 cGy administered in 33 daily fractions of 180 cGy to the contrast-enhanced CT- or MRI-defined tumor plus 3-cm margins.

Arm IV: Radiotherapy—as in Arm III; DFMO—as in Arm II. No adjuvant chemotherapy is permitted on this study; however, patients should be treated, at the investigator's discretion, at the time of tumor progression.

9. MAYO-887252/NCCTG-887252
Phase III Randomized Comparison of Radiotherapy Plus BCNU vs. Radiotherapy plus BCNU/IFN-A in the Treatment of Adults With Newly Diagnosed High-Grade Gliomas.

Lead Organization: North Central Cancer Treatment Group

SCHEDULE:

Regimen A: Radiotherapy—5,040 cGy in single daily fractions of 180 cGy, 5 days/week, followed by 1,440 cGy to a reduced target volume, for a total tumor dose of 6,480 cGy; BCNU—200 mg/sqm IV over 90 minutes within 48 hours of initiation of radiotherapy. All patients treated on regimen A; randomized to Arm I or II.

Arm I: BCNU—200 mg/sqm administered as in Regimen A q 7 weeks for up to 1 year (maximum 6 doses after randomization) or until disease progression.

Arm II: Interferon A (IFN-A)—12 × 10 to the sixth U/sqm sc on days 1, 2, and 3 of weeks 1, 3, and 5 of each 7-week course for 1 year; BCNU—150 mg/sqm administered as in Regimen A immediately after the day-3 IFN-A q 7 weeks for up to 1 year (maximum 6 doses after randomization) or until disease progression.

10. POG-8633/POG-8633/34/POG-8634
Phase II Postoperative Chemotherapy With VCR/CTX Alternating With CACP/VP-16 Prior to Radiotherapy in Children Less Than 3 Years of Age With Malignant Brain Tumors.

Lead Organization: Pediatric Oncology Group

SCHEDULE:

Surgery: Maximum surgical removal of tumor is recommended where possible; tumor resection in the brain stem, thalamus, and dominant hemispheres may be limited because of anatomic factors.

Chemotherapy (regimen closed as of April 1990): VCR—0.065 mg/kg (maximum dose 1.5 mg) IV push over 5 minutes on days 1 and 8; CTX—65 mg/kg IV over 30 minutes on day 1 with adequate post-hydration. Course repeats in 28 days. After 2 courses of VCR/CTX have been given, one course of CDDP/VP-16 is given as follows: CDDP—4 mg/kg in 1,000 ml/sqm IV over 6 hours on day 1 with adequate pre- and post-hydration; VP-16—6.5 mg/kg IV over 1 hour on days 3 and 4. Entire cycle repeats in 28 days (2 courses VCR/CTX followed by one course of CDDP/VP-16 at 28-day intervals); children continue therapy for 24 months or 12 months, depending on age. Patients completing the prescribed chemotherapy treatment are treated with Radiotherapy beginning 3–4 weeks after the last course of Chemotherapy.

Radiotherapy: Patients with medulloblastoma, IVth ventricular anaplastic ependymoma, or malignant astrocytoma/glioblastoma of the cerebellum receive 3520 cGy in 22 160-cGy fractions to the cranium and spine. Such patients receive a boost to the posterior fossa of 1800 cGy in 10 180-cGy fractions (total posterior fossa dose of 5320 cGy). Patients with IVth ventricular ependymoma receive 5400 cGy in thirty 180 cGy fractions to the posterior fossa only. Patients with supratentorial primitive neuroectodermal tumors, germ cell tumors (except germinoma), or pineoblastoma receive 3520 cGy in 22 160-cGy fractions to the cranium and the spine, plus a boost to the primary of 1800 cGy in 180-cGy fractions to a total local dose of 5320 cGy. Patients with brainstem glioma or supratentorial malignant astrocytoma/glioblastoma receive 4,140 cGy in 23 180-cGy fractions to the primary field with a boost of 1260 cGy in 7 180-cGy fractions to the primary tumor for a total local dose of 5400 cGy. Primary and primary boost fields should include the preoperative/prechemotherapy tumor volume with 2-cm margins in all directions beyond initially identifiable tumor.

SOFT-TISSUE SARCOMAS

11. NCI-0264N/NCI-83-C-212

Phase III Study of Adjuvant Chemotherapy With ADR/CTX With or Without Radiotherapy Following Surgery for Grade II/III Soft Tissue Sarcomas of the Extremities.

Lead Organization: Community Oncology Program

SCHEDULE:

Regimen A: Wide local excision of the primary tumor with an attempt to remove all gross tumor and approximately 3–5 cm of normal tissue in every direction from the lesion. Patients are then treated on Arm I or II at the time of wound healing; those who require amputation receive no further therapy.

Arm I: ADR—70 mg/sqm IV push over 3–5 min on day 1; CTX—700 mg/sqm IV over 15–20 min on day 1, with adequate pre- and post-hydration. Courses repeat q 28 days for a total of 5 courses.

Arm II: ADR and CTX as in Arm I; Radiotherapy—4500 cGy in fractions of 180 cGy/day over 5 weeks beginning 48–72 hours after initiation of chemotherapy. An additional 1500–2500 cGy is delivered to the tumor bed using a shrinking field technique over weeks 6 and 7.

12. NCI-T86-0281N/NCI-86-C-191

Phase III Randomized Trial of Surgery and Radiotherapy With vs. Without Adjuvant Chemotherapy With CTX/ADR in Patients with Soft-Tissue Sarcomas of the Head, Neck, Breast, or Trunk.

Lead Organization: Community Oncology Program

SCHEDULE:

Arm I: Surgery—removal of as much malignant tissue as is possible consistent with reasonable morbidity (extensive morbid resections of soft tissue will not be undertaken to obtain negative margins). Patients referred to the NIH who have undergone local excision of their

<u>**Schema:**</u> (Protocol No. 11)

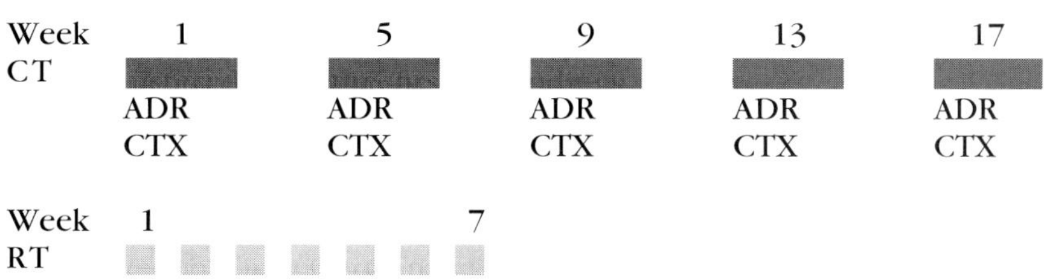

sarcoma elsewhere will, in general, undergo a reresection of the involved areas at the NIH unless pathologic reexamination of submitted slides reveals that a maximum of tumor has been removed. As soon as the wound has healed, patients undergo radiotherapy—5000 cGy over 6–7 weeks to a wide field of the involved area; when possible, a total of 6000–7000 cGy should be delivered to the tumor bed. It will not be possible to deliver these doses in many patients because of the location of the lesion on the trunk or head and neck, and such patients will receive the maximum tolerated dose. Treatment technique will be varied to maximize exposure to the tumor bed and suspected points of invasion and to minimize normal tissue toxicity; details of radiotherapy are at the discretion of the radiotherapist. Chemotherapy is initiated concomitantly with radiotherapy—CTX—750 mg/sqm IV over 15–20 minutes with adequate pre- and post-hydration on day 1; ADR—70 mg/sqm slow IV push on day 1. Course repeats q 28 days until a total dose of 350 mg/sqm ADR has been given or 5 courses have been administered.

Arm II: Surgery—as in Arm I; Radiotherapy—as in Arm I.

LYMPHOMAS

13. SWOG-8736

Phase III Randomized Comparison of Eight Courses of CHOP (CTX/ADR/VCR/PRED) vs. Three Courses of CHOP Plus Involved-Field Radiotherapy in Patients with Stages I/IE/II/IIE Intermediate- or High-Grade Non-Hodgkin's Lymphoma.

Lead Organization: Southwest Oncology Group

SCHEDULE:

Arm I: CHOP: CTX—750 mg/sqm IV over 60–90 minutes on day 1; ADR—50 mg/sqm IV bolus on day 1 VCR—1.4 mg/sqm IV bolus on day 1; PRED (omitted in patients with active peptic ulcer disease)—100 mg po on days 1 through 5. Courses repeat q 21 days for a total of 8 courses.

Arm II: CHOP—as in Arm I for 3 courses; Radiotherapy— 4000–4600 cGy with an optional small boost volume to 5000–5500 cGy delivered to involved fields (defined prior to any therapy, including surgical resection) in daily fractions of 180–200 cGy, 5 days/week, beginning at approximately week 10.

14. EST-1484

Phase III Randomized Comparison of Chemotherapy With CHOP (CTX/ADR/VCR/PRED) Alone vs. CHOP plus Radiotherapy Consolidation for Unfavorable Early Stage Non-Hodgkin's Lymphoma.

Lead Organization: Eastern Cooperative Oncology Group

SCHEDULE:

Arm I: CHOP—CTX—750 mg/sqm IV on day 1 with adequate pre- and post-hydration; ADR—50 mg/sqm IV on day 1; VCR—1.4 mg/sqm (maximum dose 2.0 mg) IV on day 1; PRED—100 mg/sqm/day po on days 1 through 5. Courses repeat q 21 days for 8 courses. Patients are restaged following 8 courses; those in CR are observed with no further treatment.

Arm II: CHOP—as in Arm I. Following eight courses and restaging, patients in CR receive radiotherapy—3000 cGy to areas of pretreatment involvement, delivered in fractions of 150–200 cGy, 5 fractions/week. On both arms, patients in stable PR after eight courses of chemotherapy are restaged 4 weeks after the last course; if PR is documented and no new areas of disease have appeared, patients are treated on Regimen A. Patients with progressive disease after two courses of chemotherapy or no change after four courses go off study and may be treated at the discretion of the investigator. Regimen A: radiotherapy—4000 cGy to areas of pretreatment involvement and contiguous uninvolved regions with at least a 3-cm margin, delivered in fractions of 150–200 cGy, 5 fractions/week. Patients who achieve a CR will be observed; those who remain in PR go off study.

15. EORTC-20871

Phase III Randomized Comparison of Modified CHVmP-BV vs. Abdominal Radiotherapy in Stage pI Adult Intermediate- and High-Grade NHL of the GI Tract and of Adjuvant Radiotherapy vs. No Adjuvant Therapy in Patients with Stage pII Gastrointestinal NHL in Remission Following 6 Courses of Modified CHVmP-BV.

Lead Organization: European Organization for Research and Treatment of Cancer

SCHEDULE:

Regimen A: Total resection of tumor and lymphatic drainage areas is performed using an en bloc technique. Splenectomy is highly recommended with antipneumococcal immunization. Radical surgery such as total gastrectomy is not performed. Treatment on Arms I and II is initiated 4–6 weeks after surgical staging.

Arm I: CHVmP-BV: ADR—50 mg/sqm IV on day 1; VM-26—60 mg/sqm IV on day 1; CTX—600 mg/sqm IV on day 1; PRED—40 mg/sqm po on days 1 through 5 (and optionally on day 15 as prophylaxis for BLEO-induced chills and fever); VCR—1.4 mg/sqm (maximum dose 2 mg) IV on day 15; BLEO—10 mg total dose on day 15. Courses repeat q 21 days for 3 courses.

Arm II: Radiotherapy—2000 cGy in daily fractions of 150 cGy, 5 days/week, to the whole abdomen. Followed by a boost dose of 2000 cGy in daily fractions of 200 cGy, 5 days/week, delivered to the primary site and regional nodes with as a margin of 3 cm.

Regimen B: CHVmP-BV—drugs and doses as for Arm I. Courses repeat q 3 weeks for a total of 6 courses, after which patients in CR are randomized for treatment on Arms III and IV and those not in CR go off study.

Arm III: Radiotherapy—3000 cGy delivered in daily fractions of 200 cGy, 5 days/week, to the primary site and regional lymph nodes as defined by laparotomy, x-rays, and/or CT scan plus a margin of 3 cm.

Arm IV: Observation.

16. POG-8725

Phase III Randomized Study of Combination Chemotherapy With MOPP/ABV(D) (NM/VCR/PRED/PCB Alternating With ADR/BLEO/VBL/DTIC or ADR/BLEO/VBL) With or Without Low-Dose Total Nodal Irradiation in Children With Stages IIB, IIIA, IIIB, and IV Hodgkin's Disease.

Lead Organization: Pediatric Oncology Group

SCHEDULE:

Regimen A: MOPP/ABV(D): MOPP—NM—6 mg/sqm IV push on days 1 and 8; VCR—1.5 mg/sqm IV push on days 1 and 8; PCB—100 mg/sqm po on days 1 through 14; PRED—40 mg/sqm po in 3 divided doses on days 1 through 14; alternating q 28 days with ABVD or ABV: ADR—25 mg/sqm IV push on days 1 and 15; BLEO—10 mg/sqm IV push on days 1 and 15; VBL—6 mg/sqm IV push on days 1 and 15; with or without DTIC—375 mg/sqm IV push on days 1 and 15. Courses of MOPP and ABVD or ABV alternate q 28 days until 8 courses of chemotherapy (4 of each combination) have been administered.

Clinical restaging is carried out at 3, 6, and 9 months after initiation of treatment, and those patients in CR at 9 months who were randomized to receive radiotherapy begin radiotherapy on Arm I.

Arm I: Radiotherapy—2100 cGy in daily fractions of 150 cGy, 5 days/week, over 2.8 weeks (14 treatment sessions) to each of 3 fields (mantle, para-aortic nodes and spleen, and pelvic field) sequentially with a 2-week rest separating treatment of each field. The dose to extranodal sites that were involved pretreatment is 1050 cGy (2100 cGy to bone lesions).

Arm II: Observation only.

17. Phase III Comparison of CHOP (CTX/DOX/VCR/PRD_2) vs. No Chemotherapy following Radiotherapy in Patients with Primary Cerebral Lymphoma.

Lead Organization: United Kingdom Medical Research Council

BREAST

18. POR-BCCG-006

Phase III Study of FNM (5-FU/DHAD/MTX) Alone vs. FNM Plus Radiotherapy in Patients With Locally Advanced Breast Cancer.

Lead Organization: Portugal Breast Cancer Cooperative Group

SCHEDULE:

Arm I: FNM: 5-FU—750 mg/sqm (maximum dose 1200 mg) in 100 ml NS IV over 60 minutes on day 1; DHAD—10 mg/sqm in 100 ml NS over 30 minutes on day 1; MTX—35 mg/sqm IV bolus on day 1. Courses repeat q 21 days, toxicity permitting, for a total of 3 courses. Beginning 3 weeks after the first day of the last chemotherapy course, patients receive radiotherapy to the breast and regional lymph node areas as follows: 6000 cGy over 6 weeks to the mammary area and 5000 cGy (or biologically equivalent doses) over 5 weeks to the lymph node chain. Patients who achieve a CR or PR enter Regimen A; those with stable or progressive disease go off study.

Arm II: FNM—5-FU, DHAD, and MTX as in Arm I. Patients who achieve a CR or PR enter Regimen A. Patients with no response receive two additional courses of therapy and are then reevaluated; those who achieve a CR or PR enter Regimen A, and those with stable or progressive disease go off study.

Regimen A: Surgery—modified radical mastectomy (Madden or Pattey technique); FNM—5-FU, DHAD, and MTX as in Arm I for a total of 6 courses.

19. CLB-8944/EST-6189/INT-0112

Phase II Combined Modality Treatment of Patients With Stage III Adenocarcinoma of the Breast: Intensive ADR Chemotherapy Followed By Definitive Surgery, CMF (CTX/MTX/5-FU), and Radiotherapy.

Lead Organization: Cancer and Leukemia Group B

SCHEDULE:

Regimen A: ADR—30 mg/sqm IV bolus at the same time on days 1, 2, and 3. Courses repeat q 28 days for a total of 4 courses, with escalation of the daily dose by 5 mg/sqm on successive courses to a maximum of 40 mg/sqm/day in the absence of limiting toxicity.

Regimen B: Modified radical mastectomy or (if tumor broadly involves the pectoralis major but is otherwise resectable) radical mastectomy is carried out after four courses of ADR if technically feasible.

Regimen C: Treatment begins 14–21 days postoperatively. CMF: CTX—2 mg/kg/day po in divided doses for 16 weeks; MTX—0.7 mg/kg IV weekly for 8 doses, then biweekly until week 16; 5-FU—12 mg/kg IV weekly for 8 doses, then biweekly until week 16.

Regimen D: Treatment begins in the fourth week following the last dose of CTX on Regimen C. All radiotherapy is delivered in a single fraction/day, 5 fractions/week; without interruption, the maximum 36 fractions would be delivered in 7 weeks and 1 day. Treatment volumes include the chest wall and supraclavicular fossa in all patients and the axilla and internal mammary nodes (IMN) in selected patients, with supplemental fields to the chest wall, part of the mastectomy scar, and IMN in a few patients. Total doses are as follows: chest wall, supraclavicular nodes, and internal mammary nodes—5040 cGy in 28 fractions of 180 cGy; axillary nodes—5040 cGy in 28 fractions of 180 cGy, with the contribution from the supraclavicular field calculated at mid-separation over the axilla and the number of fractions via the posterior supplemental axillary field adjusted so that the mid-axilla receives no more than 200 cGy/fraction; chest-wall boost—1504 cGy in 8 fractions of 188 cGy (total dose to the boosted area 6544 cGy in 36 fractions); mastectomy scar—5040 cGy in 28 fractions of 180 cGy; IMN boost—1504 cGy in 8 fractions of 188 cGy.

Regimen E: Treatment begins after completion of radiotherapy. TMX—10 mg po BID for 5 years.

20. EST-2190/INT-0121/SWOG-9061

NCI HIGH PRIORITY CLINICAL TRIAL—Phase III Study of Adjuvant CAF

(CTX/ADR/5-FU) vs. Adjuvant CAF Followed by Intensification With High-Dose CTX/TSPA Plus Autologous Bone Marrow Rescue in Patients With Stage II/III Breast Cancer at High Risk of Recurrence.

Lead Organization: Eastern Cooperative Oncology Group

SCHEDULE:

Arm I: CAF—CTX—100 mg/sqm po on days 1 through 14; ADR—30 mg/sqm IV on days 1 and 8; 5-FU—500 mg/sqm IV on days 1 through 8. Courses repeat q 4 weeks for a total of 6 courses, with escalation of all three agents by 20% if possible. Bone marrow harvest is instituted no sooner than 4 weeks and no later than 8 weeks following the last dose of CAF.

Arm II: CAF—CTX, ADR, and 5-FU as in Arm I. High-dose chemotherapy and ABM infusion is initiated following bone marrow harvest. CTX—6,000 mg/sqm by continuous iv infusion over 96 hours, beginning on day 6 (1,500 mg/sqm/day in 250–500 ml D5W); TSPA—800 mg/sqm by continuous IV infusion over 96 hours via a separate line, beginning on day 6 (200 mg/sqm/day in 500 ml D5W), with continuous bladder irrigation (500 ml NS/hour) beginning with CTX and continuing until 24 hours after CTX; ABM—nucleated cells thawed and infused as rapidly as possible 48–72 hours after completion of chemotherapy; GM-CSF—250 mcg/sqm beginning 2–4 hours after ABM infusion and continuing for 28 days.

Arm III: CAF—CTX, ADR, and 5-FU as in Arm I. High-dose chemotherapy and ABM infusion is initiated following bone marrow harvest. CTX, TSPA, and ABM as in Arm II; GM-CSF as in Arm II but administered as a 6-hour infusion.

Arm IV: CAF—CTX, ADR, and 5-FU as in Arm I. High-dose chemotherapy and ABM infusion is initiated following bone marrow harvest. CTX, TSPA, and ABM as in Arm II; GM-CSF as in Arm II but administered as a 24-hour infusion.

Patients on Arm I begin radiotherapy within 4 weeks of completing chemotherapy or when WBC and platelets have recovered. Patients on Arms II, III, and IV begin radiotherapy within 8 weeks following ABM or when WBC and platelets have recovered.

Regimen A: 5000 cGy in 25 daily fractions of 200 cGy, 5 days/week, over 5 weeks. In lumpectomy patients, the field includes the entire remaining breast and underlying chest wall. In mastectomy patients, the field includes the entire chest wall.

Regimen B: Treatment begins 28 days after the start of the last CAF course for patients on Arm I and following ABM when the WBC exceeds 4,000 or the ANC exceeds 2,000 for patients on Arms II, III, and IV. TMX—20 mg/day (or 10 mg BID) po for 5 years.

GASTROINTESTINAL TRACT

21. RTOG-9207

Phase I/II Study of External-Beam Radiotherapy, Esophageal Brachytherapy, and CDDP/5-FU in Patients with Localized Cancer of the Esophagus.

Lead Organization: Radiation Therapy Oncology Group

Schema: (Protocol No. 21)

Regimen A:

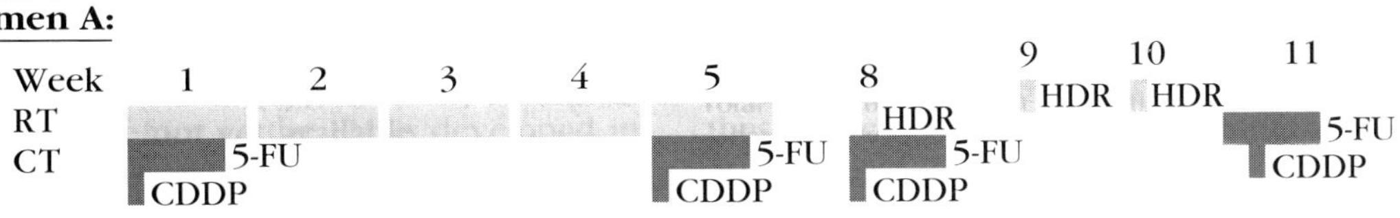

Regimen B:

Same as above except for HDR given in 1 dose on week 8.

SCHEDULE:

Regimen A: CDDP—75 mg/sqm IV on day 1 of weeks 1, 5, 8, and 11, with adequate hydration and diuresis. 5-FU—1,000 mg/sqm/day by continuous IV infusion on days 1 through 4 of weeks 1, 5, 8, and 11. External-beam radiotherapy—3000 cGy in daily fractions of 200 cGy, 5 days/week starting on day 1, delivered to the tumor volume with margins. A boost of 2000 cGy to a similar target volume (excluding supraclavicular nodes) is delivered.

Following external-beam radiotherapy, patients receive brachytherapy—1500 cGy delivered to the pretreatment tumor with a 1-cm margin in 3 fractions (6–8 days apart) of 500 cGy at a dose rate of 20–500 cGy/min during weeks 8, 9, and 10, beginning 24–48 hours after initiation of the 5-FU infusion on week 8.

Regimen B: CDDP/5-FU—as in Regimen A; external-beam radiotherapy—as in Regimen A; brachytherapy — 2000 cGy to the treatment volume as in Regimen A delivered in a single fraction at a rate of 50–100 cGy/hour, 24–48 hours after initiation of the 5-FU infusion on week 8.

22. **EORTC-40881**
Phase III Comparison of Neoadjuvant Chemoradiotherapy Using CDDP Plus Split-Course Radiotherapy vs. No Neoadjuvant Therapy Prior to Surgical Resection of Stage I/II Squamous Cell Carcinoma of the Thoracic Esophagus.

Leading Organization: EORTC, Gastrointestinal Tract Cooperative Group

SCHEDULE:

Arm I: Radiotherapy—3700 cGy in 10 daily fractions of 370 cGy on days 1 through 5 and 22 through 26 delivered with a three- or four-field technique to a target tumor volume. CDDP—80 mg/sqm in 250 ml NS IV over 30 minutes within 3 days prior to each course of radiotherapy, with pre- and posthydration.

Surgery — Surgical resection with a 5-cm tumor-free superior margin is carried out 2–4 weeks after completion of the second course of radiotherapy.

Arm II: Surgical resection as in Arm I.

23. **EST-7290**
Phase II Study of Combination Chemotherapy With 5-FU/MITO in Conjunction With Radiotherapy Followed by Esophagogastrectomy in Patients With Adenocarcinoma of the Esophagus and Gastroesophageal Junction.

Lead Organization: Eastern Cooperative Oncology Group

SCHEDULE:

Radiotherapy: 6000 cGy in fractions of 200 cGy/day over 6 weeks. An initial 4000 cGy is delivered to the tumor plus 2–5 cm margins plus the periesophageal and celiac nodes followed by a cone-down of 2000 cGy to the tumor with 2-cm margins and including at least the distal 2/3 of the stomach.

Chemotherapy: Beginning within 24 hours after initiation of radiotherapy, patients receive 5-FU—1000 mg/sqm/day in D5W by continuous IV infusion on days 2 through 5 and 28 through 31; MITO—10 mg/sqm IV bolus on day 2.

Surgery: Patients who complete chemoradiation and achieve a CR, PR, or stable disease undergo esophagogastrectomy. Either a right thoracotomy and laparotomy or a transhiatal esophagectomy may be performed.

24. **CLB-9195/EST-6290/INT-0116/NCCTG-904151/RTOG-9018/SWOG-9008**
NCI HIGH PRIORITY CLINICAL TRIAL—Phase III Randomized Study of Adjuvant Chemoradiotherapy with 5-FU/CF in Patients with Resected Gastric Cancer.

Lead Organization: Southwest Oncology Group

SCHEDULE:

Treatment must begin no later than 48 days postgastrectomy and within 7 working days of registration.

Arm I: Observation only.

Arm II: 5-FU—425 mg/sqm IV bolus on days 1 through 5; CF—20 mg/sqm IV bolus immediately prior to each dose of 5-FU. Beginning 4 weeks after initiation of 5-FU/CF. Patients begin radiotherapy—4500 cGy in daily fractions of 180 cGy, 5 days/week for 5 weeks, to the entire preoperative location of the stomach plus perigastric tumor extension and draining lymph nodes. Concomitantly, chemotherapy is administered as follows: 5-FU—400 mg/sqm IV bolus on days 1 through 4 of the first radiotherapy week and on days 1 through 3 of the fifth radiotherapy week; CF—20 mg/sqm IV bolus immediately before each dose of 5-FU. Beginning 28–35 days after completion of radiotherapy, patients receive two additional courses of 5-FU/CF, 4 weeks apart, on the same dose and schedule as the preradiotherapy course.

25. EORTC-40891

Phase III Randomized Comparison of Adjuvant Radiotherapy With 5-FU Sensitization vs. No Adjuvant Therapy Following Potentially Curative Resection of Pancreatic or Periampullary Cancer.

Lead Organization: European Organization for Research and Treatment of Cancer

Schema: (Protocol No. 25)

Arm I:

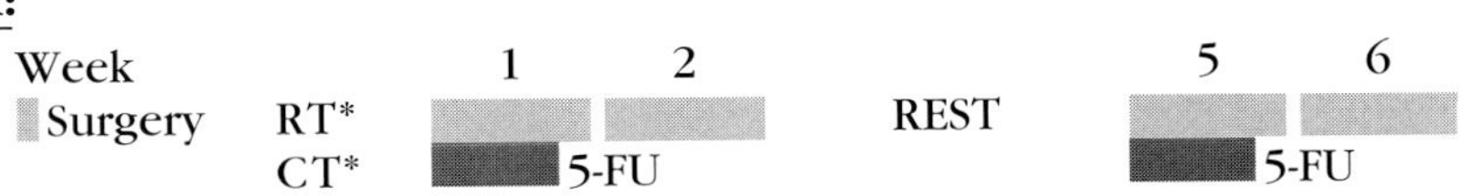

*RT and CT 2-8 weeks postoperatively

SCHEDULE:

Arm I: Treatment should begin on a Monday within 2–8 weeks postoperatively. Radiotherapy—4000 cGy total dose over 6 weeks in daily fractions of 200 cGy, 5 days/week, with a 2-week rest period after the first 2000 cGy, delivered to a volume determined by the findings at surgery, 5-FU—25 mg/kg/day by continuous IV infusion on days 1–4 of the first course of radiotherapy and 0, 3, or 5 days of the second course.

Arm II: Observation.

26. EORTC-40873

Phase II Study of Combination Chemotherapy With EP (EPI/CDDP) Followed by Split-Course Radiotherapy Plus 5-FU in Patients With Locally Advanced, Nonresectable Pancreatic Cancer.

Lead Organization: European Organization for Research and Treatment of Cancer

SCHEDULE:

Chemotherapy: EPI—60 mg/sqm slow IV push during hydration over 4 hours with 1 liter NS on day 1 (hours 10:00 to 14:00); CDDP—100 mg/sqm in 1 liter NS IV over 4 hours on day 1 (hours 14:00 to 18:00) followed by hydration and diuresis. Cycle repeats q 3 weeks for a total of 3 cycles.

Radiotherapy: Four weeks after completion of the third EP cycle patients undergo radiotherapy—a total of 4000 cGy to the whole pancreas (including the tumor) with a 2-cm margin. The total radiotherapy dose is delivered in two 2-week courses of 2000 cGy each in daily fractions of 200 cGy, 5 days/week; a 2-week rest period is observed between the two radiotherapy courses. Patients concurrently receive 5-FU—500 mg/sqm/day IV bolus administered 30–60 minutes before the radiotherapy fraction on days 1 through 3 of each course of radiotherapy. Three more cycles of EP are given q 3 weeks starting 6 weeks after completion of radiotherapy.

27. **NCOG-NSABP-R-02/NSABP-R-02**
NCI HIGH PRIORITY CLINICAL TRIAL—Phase III Randomized Comparison of Adjuvant Chemotherapy with MOF (MeCCNU/VCR/5-FU) with and without Radiotherapy vs 5-FU plus High-Dose CF with and without Radiotherapy Following Curative Resection of Dukes' B and C Adenocarcinoma of the Rectum.

Lead Organization: National Surgical Adjuvant Breast and Bowel Project

SCHEDULE:

Arm I: MOF: 5-FU—325 mg/sqm IV bolus on days 1 through 5 and 375 mg/sqm IV bolus on days 36 through 40; MeCCNU — 130 mg/sqm po on day 1; VCR—1 mg/sqm (maximum single dose 2.0 mg) IV on days 1 and 36 prior to other agents. Course repeats q 10 weeks for a total of 5 courses.

Arm II: MOF as in Arm I except that the second course consists of 5-FU only—400 mg/sqm IV on each of the first and last 3 days of Radiotherapy. Radiotherapy—4,500 cGy in 25 fractions to the pelvis, including the entire tumor bed with a margin plus the nodal groups, followed by an additional 540 cGy in 3 fractions to a cone-down field that excludes the small bowel for a total of 5040 cGy to the smaller volume. Radiotherapy is delivered 5 days/week. Radiotherapy begins following the first course of MOF when peripheral counts recover (usually 3–5 weeks following day 40 of the first course). The third course of MOF begins after hematologic recovery following completion of Radiotherapy.

Arm III: CF—500 mg/sqm in 250 ml NS IV over 2 hours on days 1, 8, 15, 22, 29, and 36; 5-FU—500 mg/sqm IV bolus 1 hour after the beginning of the CF infusion (i.e., midway through the CF infusion) on days 1, 8, 15, 22, 29, and 36. Course repeats q 8 weeks for a total of six courses.

Arm IV: CF and 5-FU as in Arm III, except that the second course consists of 5-FU only—400 mg/sqm IV on each of the first and last 3 days of Radiotherapy. Radiotherapy—as in Arm II.

Regardless of dosage modifications or delays, neither MOF nor CF/5-FU may continue beyond 1 year from the time of randomization.

28. **RTOG-8902**
Phase I/II Study of Sphincter-Sparing Local Excision Combined With Postoperative Adjuvant Radiotherapy and Concurrent 5-Fluorouracil in Patients With Limited Adenocarcinoma of the Rectum.

Lead Organization: Radiation Therapy Oncology Group

SCHEDULE:

Regimen A: Surgery—en bloc full-thickness excision of the rectal wall. Patients with incomplete excisions are removed from study; those whose excised tumor has pathologically negative margins and other specific criteria remain on observation. All other patients receive concomitant radiotherapy and radiosensitization.

Regimen B: Radiotherapy—4500–5040 cGy in daily fractions of 180–225 cGy, 4 or 5 days/week (total weekly dose of 900–1000 cGy) over 5 weeks to a target volume with a cone-down boost to a total dose of 5000–5600 cGy to the area of excision with a 3.0 cm margin. A further cone-down to a total dose of 5940–6500 cGy is given if there is microscopic tumor within 3.0 mm of the excision margin; 5-FU—1,000 mg/sqm/day by continuous IV infusion over 96 hours on weeks 1 and 5 of radiotherapy, to be administered only on days when radiotherapy is also delivered.

29. **RTOG 92-08**
A Phase II Pilot Study Employing 5-Fluorouracil, Mitomycin-C and 5940 cGy Radiotherapy in Carcinoma of the Anal Canal.

Lead Organization: Radiation Therapy Oncology Group

Schema: (Protocol No. 29)

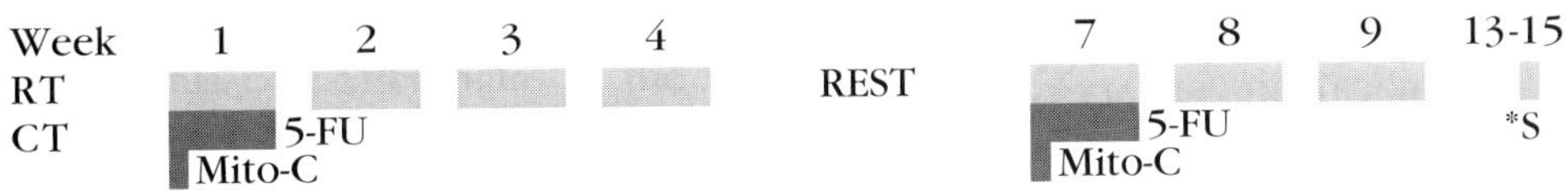

*Full-thickness biopsy 4–6 weeks after last RT fraction.

SCHEDULE:

Chemotherapy: 5-FU 1000 mg/m^2/24 hrs, continuous IV for 96 hours, during weeks 1 and 7 during radiation therapy (2000 mg maximum daily dose. Mitomycin-C 10 mg/m^2 IV bolus on day 1 of each 5-FU course (20 mg maximum per cycle).

Radiation: 180 cGy daily 5 times per week to 5940 cGy in 33 fractions over 9 weeks. Rest during weeks 5 and 6 (after 3600 cGy). Two field reductions specified.

Surgery: Biopsy of palpable inguinal lymph nodes prior to treatment. Full-thickness biopsy to be performed 4–6 weeks after completion of radiation and chemotherapy when there is any palpable residual abnormality.

30. EORTC-22861
Phase II Randomized Trial of Radiotherapy Plus Concomitant Chemotherapy with 5-FU/MITO vs. Radiotherapy Alone in Patients with Anal Carcinoma.

Lead Organization: European Organization for Research and Treatment of Cancer

SCHEDULE:

Arm I: Radiotherapy—4500 cGy in 180 cGy fractions delivered 5 days/week over 5 weeks to the anus and pelvic lymph nodes; a boost of 1500 cGy (if there is macroscopic CR) or 2000 cGy (if there is PR) is delivered to the initial tumor plus a 1-cm margin 6 weeks following completion of the initial 4500 cGy; the boost may be given by Iridium 192 implant or in 180 cGy external beam (electrons or Co60) fractions. Lymph nodes are included in the boost volume if they were enlarged prior to treatment or are suspected of containing a tumor.

Arm II: Radiotherapy—as in Arm I; 5-FU—750 mg/sqm by continuous IV infusion on days 1 through 5, beginning on the same day as radiotherapy; MITO—15 mg/sqm IV bolus on day 1. Treatment with 5-FU alone is repeated once during the last full week of radiotherapy. Patients who experience progressive disease or no change after the initial 4500 cGy of radiotherapy should undergo surgery and are considered treatment failures.

LUNG

31. MAYO-902452/NCCTG-902452
Phase II Pilot Study of IFN-G and Accel-

Schema: (Protocol No. 30)
Arm II:

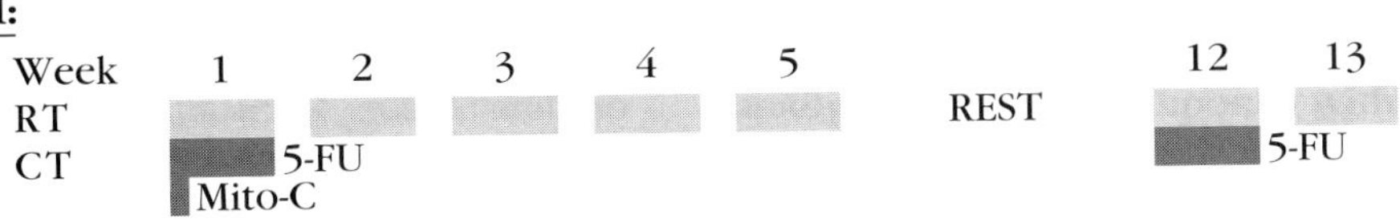

erated, Hyperfractionated Thoracic Irradiation in Patients with Inoperable Stage III M_0 Non-Small Cell Carcinoma of the Lung.

Lead Organization: North Central Cancer Treatment Group

Arm I: Surgery—thoracotomy with resection of primary tumor and complete mediastinal node dissection. Patients in CR and in PR proceed to consolidation chemotherapy 4–6 weeks postoperatively.

Schema: (Protocol No. 31)

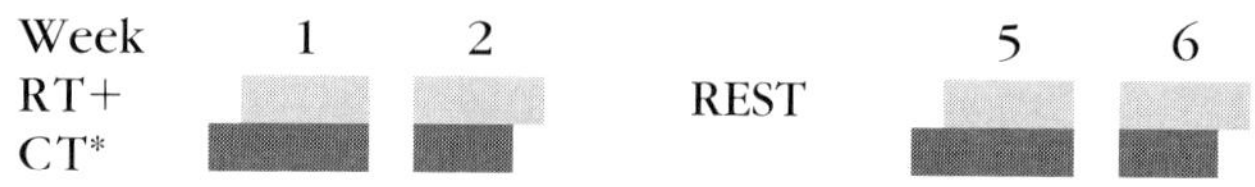

RT+ – RT given b.i.d.
*Immunotherapy = Interferon starts 1-3 days before each RT course, and given before each morning RT fraction.

SCHEDULE:

Treatment begins no more than 7 days after registration. Interferon (IFN-G)—0.2 mg sc daily at 8 am beginning 1–3 days prior to the initiation of each radiotherapy treatment period and continuing until the last day of each radiotherapy treatment period. Radiotherapy—6000 cGy to the thorax delivered in 40, twice-daily fractions of 150 cGy each (at 3–4 hours and 8–9 hours following IFN-G administration) and administered in two, 2-week treatment periods (3000 cGy each) with a 2-week break between periods. RT fields reduced at 4500 cGy total dose.

32. EST-2591/RTOG-8901

Phase III Comparison of Surgical Resection vs. Radiotherapy Following Initial Chemotherapy With CDDP/VBL in Patients with Non-Small Cell Lung Cancer with Ipsilateral Mediastinal Node Involvement.

Lead Organization: Radiation Therapy Oncology Group

SCHEDULE:

Induction: CDDP—120 mg/sqm or 3 mg/kg (whichever is less) IV over 20–30 minutes on day 1 with pre- and posthydration. VBL—4.5 mg/sqm IV on days 1 and 15. A second course is initiated on day 29. Patients proceed to surgery (Arm I) 4–6 weeks or radiotherapy (Arm II) 2–4 weeks after the second course of induction chemotherapy.

Arm II: Radiotherapy—5000 cGy in 25 daily fractions of 200 cGy, 5 fractions/week, to the primary tumor and all regional nodes followed by 1400 cGy (total tumor dose 64 cGy) to a field defined by all gross disease seen on chest CT prior to initiation of chemotherapy.

Consolidation: Day 1 of consolidation is treatment day 99 for Arm I patients and treatment day 141 for Arm II patients. CDDP—100 mg/sqm IV over 20–30 minutes on day 1, with hydration and mannitol-induced diuresis as in Induction; VBL—4.5 mg/sqm IV on days 1 and 15. A second course is initiated on day 29.

33. EST-4588/RTOG-8808/SWOG-8992

NCI High Priority Clinical Trial—Phase III Comparison of Standard-Fractionation Radiotherapy Alone vs. VBL/CDDP Followed by Radiotherapy vs. Hyperfractionated Radiotherapy Alone in Patients with Nonresectable Stages II/IIIA/IIIB Non-Small Cell Lung Cancer.

Lead Organization: Radiation Therapy Oncology Group

SCHEDULE:

Arm I: Radiotherapy: 5000 cGy in daily fractions of 200 cGy, 5 days/week, delivered over 5 weeks to the primary tumor and nodal target areas. An additional 1000 cGy (total dose 6000 cGy) is delivered as a boost to the initial tumor volume.

Arm II: VBL—5 mg/sqm IV bolus on days 1, 8, 15, 22, and 29; CDDP—100 mg/sqm IV over 30–60 minutes on days 1 and 29 with hydration. Radiotherapy as in Arm I begins on day 50.

Arm III: Radiotherapy—5040 cGy delivered to the large target volume defined on Arm I in 2 daily fractions of 120 cGy separated by 4–6 hours, 42 fractions in 21 treatment days over 4 weeks, followed by a boost to the primary of 1920 cGy on the same fractionation schedule over 14 days (total tumor dose 6960 cGy in 58 fractions on 29 treatment days over 6 weeks).

34. MDA-DM-87044/NCI-T87-0266D
Phase III Randomized Comparison of Adjuvant Combination Chemotherapy With CEP (CTX/VP-16/CDDP) Followed by Chest Irradiation vs. No Adjuvant Therapy in Patients With Totally Resected Stage II/III Limited Non-Small Cell Lung Cancer.

Lead Organization: University of Texas, M.D. Anderson Cancer Center

SCHEDULE:

Arm I: Treatment should be initiated within 6 weeks postoperatively. CEP: CTX—500 mg/sqm IV over 30 minutes on day 1; VP-16—100 mg/sqm IV over 3 hours on day 1 and 200 mg/sqm po on days 2 and 3 following an overnight fast. CDDP—80 mg/sqm IV over 4 hours on day 1 with hydration during the 24 hours prior to and after CDDP. Courses repeat q 4 weeks for a total of 6 courses. Patients are restaged at the conclusion of chemotherapy. Radiotherapy begins at week 25 or, if there were treatment delays during chemotherapy, within 1 week of restaging. Chest irradiation—5000 cGy in 25 fractions of 200 cGy over 32–37 days.

Arm II: Observation.

35. EST-3588/INT-0096/RTOG-8815/SWOG-8991
NCI High Priority Clinical Trial—Phase III Study of CDDP/VP-16 Combined With Standard Fractionation Thoracic Radiotherapy vs CDDP/VP-16 Combined With Hyperfractionated Thoracic Radiotherapy for Limited Stage Small Cell Lung Cancer.

Lead Organization: Eastern Cooperative Oncology Group

SCHEDULE:

Arm I: CDDP—60 mg/sqm in 1 liter NS IV over 1–2 hours on day 1 with additional hydration VP-16—120 mg/sqm/day IV on days 1, 2, and 3. Courses repeat q 3 weeks for a total of 4 courses, toxicity permitting. Thoracic irradiation—4500 cGy in 25 daily fractions of 180 cGy, 5 days/week, over 5 weeks, beginning on day 1 of course 1 of chemotherapy or within 24 hours. Radiotherapy should begin on Monday, Tuesday, or Wednesday to permit the required minimum of 3 days of concurrent therapy.

Arm II: Chemotherapy as in Arm I. Thoracic irradiation to the volume specified in Arm I—4500 cGy in 30 twice-daily fractions of 150 cGy administered between 4 and 8 hours apart, 5 days/week over 3 weeks, beginning on day 1 of course 1 of chemotherapy or within 24 hours. Radiotherapy should begin on Monday, Tuesday, or Wednesday to permit the required minimum of 3 days of concurrent therapy.

Regimen A: Prophylactic cranial irradiation—2500 cGy in 10 fractions over 2 weeks to the entire cranial contents.

36. EORTC-08877
Phase III Randomized Trial of Radiotherapy and Chemotherapy With CDE (CTX/DOX/VP-16) Given on Sequential vs. Alternating Schedules in Patients with Limited Small Cell Lung Cancer.

Lead Organization: European Organization for Research and Treatment of Cancer

SCHEDULE:

Arm I: CDE: CTX—1,000 mg/sqm IV into the tube of a running infusion of NS on day 1; DOX—45 mg/sqm IV into the tube of a running infusion of NS on day 1; VP-16—100 mg/sqm in 250 ml NS IV over at least 30 minutes on days 1, 3, and 5; Mesna—60% of CTX dose IV concurrently with CTX and 4 and 8 hours thereafter. Courses repeat q 4 weeks for a total of 5 courses in the absence of disease progression. Radiotherapy—1250 cGy in 5 fractions of 250 cGy, beginning on day 15 of courses 2 through 5 (total dose 5000 cGy).

Arm II: CDE—as in Arm I but q 3 weeks for a total of 5 courses in the absence of disease progression; radiotherapy—5000 cGy in 20 fractions of 250 cGy over 5 weeks, beginning exactly 2 weeks after the first day of the last course of chemotherapy.

Regimen A: Patients who develop cerebral metastases during chemotherapy are treated with steroids and radiotherapy (3000 cGy in 12 daily fractions); chemotherapy should be continued if symptoms and signs of CNS disease respond to treatment. Patients without evidence of metastases after 5 courses of CDE may receive prophylactic cranial irradiation (3000 cGy in 12 fractions of 250 cGy).

37. BGSM-62286/NCI-T86-0119D
Phase III Randomized Study of Split-Course vs. Continuous Radiotherapy Plus Chemotherapy With VP-16/CDDP and CTX/ADR/VCR in Patients With Limited Small Cell Lung Cancer.

Lead Organization: Comprehensive Cancer Center of Wake Forest University Bowman Gray School of Medicine

<u>**Schema:**</u> (Protocol No. 37)

<u>**Arm I:**</u>

Week	1	4	7	10	13	16
CT	CDDP	CDDP	CTX	CTX	CDDP	CTX
	VP-16	VP-16	ADR	ADR	VP-16	ADR
			VCR	VCR		VCR

Week	1	2	3	4	5	20
RT						PCI

<u>**Arm II:**</u>

Week	1	4	7	10	13	16
CT	CDDP	CDDP	CTX	CTX	CDDP	CTX
	VP-16	VP-16	ADR	ADR	VP-16	ADR
			VCR	VCR		VCR

Week	2,3	5,6	8	20
RT				PCI

PCI = Prophylactic cranial irradiation

SCHEDULE:

Arm I: Six courses of chemotherapy are delivered at 3-week intervals, with courses 1, 2, and 5 consisting of CDDP/VP-16 and courses 3, 4, and 6 consisting of CTX/ADR/VCR. CDDP/VP-16: CDDP—60 mg/sqm IV on day 1 after adequate hydration; VP-16—120 mg/sqm IV on days 1, 2, and 3. CTX/ADR/VCR: CTX—750 mg/sqm IV on day 1; ADR—60 mg/sqm IV on day 1; VCR—2.0 mg IV on day 1. Radiotherapy is initiated on the first treatment day: 5000 cGy in 25 equal fractions delivered 5 days/week through parallel opposed anterior and posterior fields. Three weeks after the last course of chemotherapy, patients in CR receive prophylactic cranial irradiation—2400 cGy in 12 equal fractions through opposed lateral portals.

Arm II: Six courses of chemotherapy are delivered as in Arm I. Three courses of radiotherapy are delivered as follows: 2000 cGy in eight fractions of 250 cGy beginning on day 8 of the first and second chemotherapy courses; 1000 cGy in 4 fractions of 250 cGy beginning on day 8 of the third chemotherapy course. Radiotherapy guidelines as in Arm I are followed, and patients in CR following chemotherapy may receive prophylactic cranial irradiation as in Arm I.

Therapy is continued until all planned therapy has been delivered (approximately week 20).

GYNECOLOGY

38. GOG-109/INT-0107/RTOG-9112/SWOG-8797
Phase III Randomized Comparison of Radiotherapy With vs. Without Continuous Infusion 5-FU/Bolus CDDP Following Radical Hysterectomy and Node Dissection in High-Risk Patients With Stages IA2, IB, and IIA Carcinoma of the Cervix.

Leading Organization: Southwest Oncology Group

SCHEDULE:

Arm I: Radiotherapy—4930 cGy over 6 weeks delivered to the whole pelvis and iliac nodes in 29 daily fractions of 170 cGy, 5 days/week. 5-FU—1000 mg/sqm/day by continuous IV infusion over days 1 through 4 beginning on day 1 of radiotherapy; CDDP—70 mg/sqm IV on day 1; with hydration and diuresis. 5-FU/CDDP courses repeat q 3 weeks for a total of 4 courses.

Arm II: Radiotherapy—as in Arm I.

39. RTOG-9001
Phase III Comparison of Pelvic Irradiation With Concurrent CDDP/5-FU vs. Pelvic and Para-Aortic Irradiation Without Chemotherapy in Patients With High-Risk Carcinoma of the Cervix.

Lead Organization: Radiation Therapy Oncology Group

SCHEDULE:

Arm I: Radiotherapy—external beam irradiation—4500 cGy over 5 weeks to the whole pelvis delivered in daily fractions of 180 cGy, 5 days/week. Involved lateral parametrium and/or involved pelvic nodes should be boosted to achieve a total dose (including that from intracavitary application) of 6000 cGy. Intracavitary applications—two applications using standard intracavitary systems are employed to deliver a total dose (external and intracavitary) of 8500 cGy to point A.

Schema: (Protocol No. 38)
Arm I:

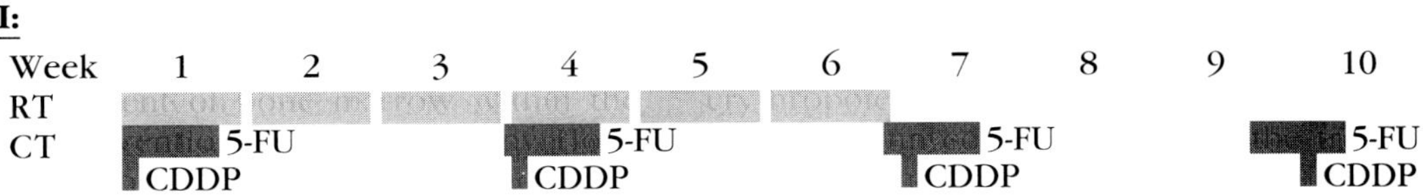

Chemotherapy: CDDP—75 mg/sqm (maximum dose 150 mg) IV over 4 hours on days 1 (within 16 hours of the first radiation fraction) and 22 of radiotherapy with hydration. 5-FU—1,000 mg/sqm/day (maximum daily dose 2,000 mg) by continuous 96-hour infusion on days 2 through 5 and 23 through 26 (beginning 1–36 hours after completion of the CDDP infusion) of radiotherapy. A third course of CDDP/5-FU identical to the first two is administered in conjunction with the second course of brachytherapy.

Arm II: Radiotherapy—as in Arm I, with the external beam field extended to include the para-aortic area.

40. GOG-9001
Phase I Limited-Access Study of Weekly Cisplatin and Whole-Abdominal Irradiation in Patients with Stage III/IV Endometrial Carcinoma.

Lead Organization: Gynecologic Oncology Group

SCHEDULE:

Patients who have not previously undergone surgery as specified on protocol undergo *total abdominal hysterectomy* and extrafascial bilateral salpingo-oophorectomy, with pelvic and para-aortic lymph node sampling and removal of all resectable gross tumor. Patients proceed to radiotherapy/chemotherapy if tumor is debulked to 2 cm or less and eligibility criteria for extent of disease are met.

Radiotherapy and concomitant chemotherapy are initiated within 8 weeks following surgery, whether surgery is performed on protocol or off. Radiotherapy—3000 cGy in 20 fractions of 150 cGy to the whole abdomen, 5 days/week over 4–5 weeks, followed by a boost to the pelvis of 1980 cGy in 11 fractions of 180 cGy for a total of 4980 cGy over 6–7 weeks. Patients with positive para-aortic nodes receive a boost of 1500 cGy for a total dose of 4500 cGy to the para-aortic field. CDDP—15 mg/sqm IV at a rate of 1 mg/min q 7 days during radiotherapy, with hydration.

41. GOG-8812
Phase II Study of Sequential CDDP/CTX and Hyperfractionated Radiotherapy in Patients With Optimally Debulked Epithelial Ovarian Cancer.

Lead Organization: Gynecologic Oncology Group

SCHEDULE:

Chemotherapy must begin within 6 weeks of the last surgical procedure. CDDP—75 mg/sqm IV; CTX—750 mg/sqm IV. Patients are treated q 21 days, toxicity permitting, for 3 courses. Within 4–6 weeks after the third course of chemotherapy, second-look surgery is performed with maximum debulking of gross disease if positive, and the amount of residual disease is documented. Radiotherapy must begin within 8 weeks of second-look surgery.

Whole-abdominal irradiation—3040 cGy in 38 twice-daily fractions of 80 cGy, administered 4–8 hours apart 5 days a week, delivered to an abdominal field. Small field (4 × 4 cm) boosts to extrapelvic sites of gross residual disease (1 cm or less) are encouraged. Boost fields receive 1440 cGy in 18 fractions of 80 cGy twice a day, with an interval of 4–8 hours between doses.

42. GOG-101
Phase II Evaluation of Preoperative Radiotherapy Plus CDDP/5-FU in Patients With Advanced Vulvar Cancer.

Lead Organization: Gynecologic Oncology Group

SCHEDULE:

Nonrandomized study. Patients with T_4 or unresectable T_3 primaries and N_0 or resectable N_2 groin nodes are treated on regimen A, while those with unresectable $N_{2\text{-}3}$ groin nodes are treated on regimen B.

Regimen A: Split-course external beam radiotherapy — 2380 cGy to the midplane of the vulva in twice-daily fractions (separated by a minimum of 6 hours) of 170 cGy on days 1–4 and once daily fractions of 170 cGy on days 5 and 8–12. The course is repeated after 1.5–2.5 weeks of rest for a total dose of 4,760 cGy. CDDP—50 mg/sqm IV on day 1, 5-FU—1,000 mg/sqm/day in 1 liter NS by continuous IV infusion over 24 hours on days 1–4. Course repeats once to coincide with the second course of twice-daily radiotherapy. Four to eight weeks following the completion of chemoradiation, patients considered to have resectable disease without need for an exenterative procedure undergo resection. Patients with unresectable primaries receive additional radiotherapy—2000 cGy through reduced AP/PA and/or a direct perineal portal with photons in daily fractions of 170–200 cGy or with electrons such that the dose at the deepest point within the tumor is at least 80% of the surface dose or by interstitial or intracavitary methods.

Regimen B: Split-course external beam radiotherapy — doses as in Regimen A to the vulva, inguinal-femoral lymph nodes, and low pelvic lymph nodes (electron beams may be used for the inguinal fields at the discretion of the radiation oncologist); CDDP—as in Regimen A; 5-FU—as in Regimen A; Surgery—as in Regimen A. Patients with unresectable lymph nodes receive additional radiotherapy as in Regimen A.

Patients treated on Regimen A who are found to have three or more positive nodes in the resected specimen, or extracapsular invasion, receive postoperative radiotherapy—4400–4500 cGy in single daily fractions of 170–200 cGy to the inguinal and low pelvic nodes, with blocking of the previously irradiated area. Patients in whom further resection is not feasible receive additional radiotherapy—1000–1500 cGy through reduced AP/PA and/or a direct peritoneal portal by photon or electron beam or by interstitial or intracavitary methods.

At the conclusion of chemo- and radiotherapy, if there has been a complete clinical response, patients undergo a groin node dissection with at least a biopsy or excision of the primary tumor site.

GENITOURINARY SYSTEM

43. RTOG 92-02

A Phase III Trial of the Use of Long Term Total Androgen Suppression Following Neoadjuvant Hormonal Cytoreduction and Radiotherapy in Locally Advanced Carcinoma of the Prostate.

Lead Organization: Radiation Therapy Oncology Group

SCHEDULE:

Radiation: 4400–4600 cGy (180–200 cGy/day four to five times a week) to regional lymphatics followed by 2000–2900 cGy (180–200 cGy/day) for a total of 6500–7000 cGy to the prostate for Stage T_{2b} and 6750–7000 cGy for Stages T_3 and T_4.

Total Androgen Suppression (TAS): Patients will receive Flutamide (250 mg t.i.d., p.o.) and Zoladex, (3.6 mg s.c. monthly), beginning 2 months before RT and continuing until RT is completed. Randomization will assign half the patients to additional Zoladex to begin after the completion of RT and continuing monthly at least for 2 years.

Arm I: TAS 2 months before and during RT.

Arm II: TAS 2 months before and during RT. Then Zoladex alone at least for 2 years after RT ends.

44. CAN-NCIC-BL5/EORTC-30894/MRC-BA06

Phase III Randomized Comparison of Neoadjuvant Chemotherapy With CMV (CDDP/MTX/VBL) vs. No Neoadjuvant Chemotherapy Prior to Definitive Surgery or Radiotherapy in Patients With Resectable Transitional Cell Carcinoma of the Bladder.

Lead Organization: European Organization for Research and Treatment of Cancer

SCHEDULE:

Arm I: MTX—30 mg/sqm IV bolus on days 1 and 8; VBL—4 mg/sqm IV bolus on days 1 and 8; CF—15 mg po or IV q 6 hours for 4 doses beginning 24 hours after MTX administration; CDDP—100 mg/sqm IV over 4 hours on day 2 after hydration. Courses repeat q 3 weeks for a total of 3 courses. Definitive therapy follows 3–4 weeks after the last dose of chemotherapy and consists of either total (simple) or radical cystectomy with urinary diversion according to institutional practice or radiotherapy—6000–6400 cGy delivered to the whole bladder in daily fractions of 200 cGy, 5 days/week. Either of two schemes of preoperative irradiation will be accepted: 2000 cGy in 5 consecutive daily fractions of 4000 cGy or 4000 cGy over 28 days in daily fractions of 2000 cGy.

Arm II: Cystectomy or whole-bladder irradiation as in Arm I as soon as possible (no longer than 4 weeks) after randomization.

45. RTOG-8903

Phase III Randomized Study of Neoadjuvant Chemotherapy With MCV (MTX/CDDP/VBL) vs. No Neoadjuvant Chemotherapy Followed by Radiotherapy plus CDDP for Selective Bladder Preservation Following TURB in Patients With Muscle-Invading Bladder Cancer.

Lead Organization: Radiation Therapy Oncology Group

SCHEDULE:

Arm I: Chemotherapy begins 2–4 weeks following entry TURB. MCV: MTX—30 mg/sqm IV bolus on days 0, 14, and 21; VBL—3 mg/sqm IV bolus on days 1, 14, and 21; CDDP—70 mg/sqm in 250 ml NS IV on day 1 with hydration. A second course of MCV is initiated on day 28. Radiotherapy begins 2–3 weeks after completion of the second course of chemotherapy, 3960 cGy over 450–5 weeks in 22 daily fractions of 180 cGy, 5 days/week, delivered to the small pelvic field. CDDP—100 mg/sqm IV with hydration as above on days 1 and 21 of radiotherapy.

Arm II: Radiotherapy and CDDP as in Arm I, beginning 2–4 weeks following staging cystoscopy.

After completion of initial treatment on Arm I or II, patients with incomplete response who are suited for surgery undergo radical cystectomy. Complete responders and those incomplete responders unsuited for surgery enter consolidation therapy.

Consolidation: Treatment begins 1–2 weeks after documentation of complete regression following initial radiotherapy/CDDP. CDDP—100 mg/sqm IV with hydration as in Arm I; Radiotherapy—540 cGy to the small pelvic field to a total dose of 4500 cGy followed by 1980 cGy over 2.5–3 weeks in 11 daily fractions of 1800 cGy, 5 days/week, to a cone-down volume (total tumor dose of 6480 cGy).

MISCELLANEOUS

46. RTOG-9017

Phase II Pilot Study of CAPPr (CTX/ADR/CDDP/PRED) Followed by Surgery and Radiotherapy in Patients With Locally Advanced Thymoma.

Lead Organization: Radiation Therapy Oncology Group

SCHEDULE:

Patients undergo surgical exploration via median sternotomy for assessment of tumor resectability. If possible, resection will be attempted; patients with greater than 50% of the tumor remaining following exploration and attempted resection are considered to have unresectable disease and proceed to induction chemotherapy on Regimen A within 6 weeks following surgery.

Regimen A: CAPPr—CTX—500 mg/sqm IV over 30 minutes on day 1; ADR—20 mg/sqm/day by continuous IV infusion on days 1 through 3; CDDP—30 mg/sqm IV over 2 hours on days 1 through 3, with prehydration; PRED—100 mg po on days 1 through 5. Courses repeat q 3 weeks, toxicity permitting, for a total of 3 courses.

Following completion of Regimen A, patients are restaged; those with a response proceed to Regimen B and then to Regimens C and D, while those with no response proceed to Regimen C only.

Regimen B: Surgery—patients undergo surgical reexploration via median sternotomy 2 weeks after completion of chemotherapy and, if possible, resection is attempted.

Regimen C: Patients with no response to induction chemotherapy begin radiotherapy within 3–4 weeks following completion of Regimen A. Patients with a response to induction chemotherapy who underwent complete or partial tumor resection on Regimen B begin radiotherapy within 4 weeks following surgery; those who on Regimen B were biopsied only (with no further attempt at resection) begin radiotherapy within a few days following surgery. Radiotherapy—5000 cGy in 25 daily fractions of 200 cGy in patients with complete resections and pathologic CR (6000 cGy in 30 daily fractions of 200 cGy in all other patients) delivered to the surgical bed with 2-cm margins and mediastinal lymph nodes and bilateral hilar lymph nodes with margins of 1 cm or less. Patients who had no response to the chemotherapy may have tumor resection attempted after delivery of 5000 cGy, if feasible.

Regimen D: (only in patients with a response to initial induction chemotherapy): CAPPr—as in Regimen A, beginning 2–4 weeks following completion of radiotherapy on Regimen C. Courses begin 2–4 weeks following radiotherapy and repeat q 3 weeks, toxicity permitting, for a total of 3 courses.

47. EST-1380/INT-0014/RTOG-8107/SEG-INT-81304/SWOG-8094
Phase III Radiotherapy With and Without Chemotherapy With ADR for Pleural Mesothelioma Localized to One Hemithorax.

Lead Organization: Eastern Cooperative Oncology Group

SCHEDULE:

Arm I: Radiotherapy—4680 cGy to the hemithorax in 26 fractions over a 5-week period. Patients are treated 5 times a week at a daily dose of 180 cGy. Treatment with a combination of photon and electron beams or photon beam only is acceptable. Two weeks after hemithorax irradiation, an additional boost of 1440 cGy will be given to areas of known residual disease in the pleura (not pericardium or mediastinum) in 8 fractions at a daily dose of 180 cGy. Chemotherapy (ADR—60 mg/sqm IV on day 1 q 3 weeks) is initiated no sooner than 21 days and no later than 6 weeks following the completion of radiotherapy; the total dose administered must not exceed 420 mg/sqm.

Arm II: Radiotherapy as in Arm I.

48. NCI-T89-0208D/UPCC-3489
Phase II Pilot Study of High-Dose Cytoxan/Radiotherapy, Peripheral Blood Stem Cell Rescue, and GM-CSF in Patients with Relapsing or Plateau-Phase Multiple Myeloma.

Lead Organization: University of Pennsylvania Cancer Center

SCHEDULE:

Peripheral Stem Cell Harvest: Beginning 3 days prior to and continuing throughout the harvest period, patients receive GM-CSF (10 mcg/kg/day sc). Peripheral blood mononuclear cells are harvested 3 times weekly by 4-hour continuous flow leukophoresis until at least 10 to the ninth nucleated cells/kg are obtained. The cells are diluted with autologous plasma to a concentration of approximately 8 × 10 to the seventh cells/ml and cryopreserved in 100-ml aliquots.

Local Radiotherapy: 2,000 cGy to all areas of active bone disease (greater than 2 cm) or sites of prior massive involvement (masses greater than 5 cm) in fractions of 180–200 cGy each, 5 days/week, over 12–14 days (6–8 areas are treated simultaneously to limit overall elapsed time of radiotherapy to less than 1 month).

High-Dose Chemo/Radiotherapy: Treatment begins within 1 week following completion of local radiotherapy. CTX—60 mg/kg in 250 ml D5W IV over 2 hours on days 5 and 4 with IV hydration/diuresis. TBI—1200 cGy in 6 fractions of 200 cGy, 2 fractions/day, on days 3, 2, and 1.

Peripheral Stem Cell Rescue and Hematologic Toxicity Attenuation: Prehydration with 0.5 NS and sufficient $NaHCO_3$ to ensure an alkaline urine is initiated 12 hours prior to stem cell infusion at a rate sufficient to ensure a urinary output of at least 3 ml/kg/hour. Patients are pretreated with mannitol (12.5 g IV), Benadryl (50 mg IV), and Solu-Cortef (250 mg IV) 15 minutes prior to stem cell infusion. Stem cells are infused via a central venous catheter on day 0 at a rate of 50 ml/3–5 minutes, with a rest of 30–60 minutes after 300–400 ml. GM-CSF—10 mcg/kg/day sc beginning on day + 1 and continuing until the granulocyte count exceeds 1,000.

Chapter 47

PERSPECTIVE AND THOUGHTS FOR THE FUTURE

STEPHEN K. CARTER

Combining chemotherapy with surgery and/or irradiation has been a major therapeutic strategy for nearly two decades and part of the clinical research scene from the earliest days of cytotoxic chemotherapy in the 1950s. In the last two decades, it has received tremendous attention because micrometastases have become an important conceptual focus. In this view, surgery and x-ray are local and regional modalities and fail to eradicate many tumors because of the existence of micrometastases outside their therapeutic range. In this construct, chemotherapy, which is a systemic modality, can be used to eradicate the micrometastatic foci and therefore achieve a cure where relapse would otherwise occur with surgery and/or x-ray alone. This has been an attractive approach because it is strongly supported by data from rodent, particularly murine, transplantable tumor systems. In addition, the logic of the cell-kill hypothesis, as expounded by Skipper and Schabel, stated that micrometastases should be kinetically more sensitive to cytotoxic drugs and eradicated more easily.

In the 1970s, surgical adjuvant chemotherapy data from trials in breast cancer and osteogenic sarcoma led to an era of tremendous optimism about the strategy. With longer follow-up, the data on overall survival did not fulfill all of the promise of the early relapse-free survival data. It became clear that adjuvant chemotherapy was not a panacea but a strategy that achieved some success but still required a great deal more before it would dramatically affect overall cancer mortality.

BASIC STRATEGIES

Combining chemotherapy and irradiation has been much more complicated than either modality alone. The reason for this is that drugs and x-ray can biologically interact at the tumor cell and normal cell level, in ways that are not relevant when surgery and drugs are combined. Because of this interaction, the concepts of sensitization and potentiation enter into the equation and must be integrated into the planning and analytic strategies along with the concept of adjuvant cell kill (Table 47–1).

The experimental data base for combining drugs and x-ray is vaster and also more

Table 47–1. Conceptual Strategies of How X-ray and Chemotherapy can Interact

1. Sensitization	The drug interacts biologically with the DNA of the tumor cell and makes it more vulnerable to cell killing by x-ray Manifested by enhanced local control
2. Additive killing	The drug kills tumor cells that would otherwise not be killed by the x-ray Manifested by enhanced local control
3. Neoadjuvant cell kill	The drug kills tumor cells outside the radiation field Manifested by enhanced relapse-free survival (RFS) The drug can also sensitize or give additive killing manifested by enhanced local control
4. Adjuvant	The drug eradicates micrometastatic disease not within the area of local-regional control Manifested by enhanced RFS. The drug mops up residual viable tumor cells within the field Manifested by enhanced local control

Table 47–2. Simple Sequences of Chemotherapy and X-ray

Sequence	Theoretical Strategy	Biologic End Point for Efficacy
C→X	1. Sensitize tumor cells to x-ray 2. Additive tumor cell killing within the field 3. Neoadjuvant cell kill	1. Local control 2. Local control 3. RFS
C + X	1. Sensitization 2. Additive tumor cell kill 3. Minor adjuvant kill	1. Local control 2. Local control 3. RFS
X→C	1. Adjuvant cell kill 2. Killing of residual tumor cells in the field	1. RFS 2. Local control

C = chemotherapy; X = x-rays/radiotherapy; RFS = relapse-free survival.

complex than for surgery and drugs. The data base involves a heavy emphasis on in vitro systems along with varied in vivo models. In addition, the experiments involve biologic interactions from both an efficacy (tumor cell) and a toxicity (normal cell) perspective. When in vitro systems are used, the two limbs of the therapeutic index equation are examined in isolation. Even when in vivo systems are studied, there is a tendency to look at efficacy and side effects separately, although the concept of therapeutic index is intrinsic in any survival model.

When radiation and drugs are combined, there are basic sequences that can be utilized and each of these sequences can be related to a conceptual strategy (Table 47–2). The first sequence is drugs first followed by x-ray. In modern thought processes, this could be viewed as neoadjuvant or induction chemotherapy, in line with the Goldie-Coldman hypothesis, which emphasizes the importance of treating before tumor cells mutate to become drug-resistant. In more traditional thinking, it could be viewed as accomplishing one or more of the following objectives.

1. Killing tumor cells outside of the treatment field to be used.
2. Killing tumor cells inside the area to be irradiated.
3. Sensitizing the tumor cells to be irradiated to enhance the killing action of x-ray.

In reality, when a clinical trial is analyzed, it is difficult, if not impossible, to clearly dissect out the three mechanisms.

The second basic sequence involves drugs and x-ray administered concomitantly. This could be viewed as the classic sequence for sensitization. Despite this, it is highly problematic, when an active cytotoxic drug is used, to state that what is happening is sensitization and not killing of the tumor cells intrinsically refractive to x-ray eradication. In addition, the drugs could still be potentially killing cells in an adjuvant fashion outside of the field to be treated.

The third basic sequence involves irradiation followed by drugs. This is the classic adjuvant sequence and is conceptually viewed as designed to kill cells outside of the treated area. Drugs used in this sequence could also eradicate remaining viable tumor cells within the treated field and thus enhance local control. What is hard, if not impossible, to conceptualize with this sequence is a sensitization strategy, at least within the realm of the view of the drug sensitizing the cell for x-ray kill.

These three basic sequences lend themselves to mixtures that can lead to four ad-

Table 47–3. Complex sequences of chemotherapy and x-ray

1. C → X + C	Combines sensitization and neoadjuvant strategies
2. C → X → C	Combines sensitization, neoadjuvant and adjuvant strategies
3. C → X + C → C	Combines all strategies
4. X + C → C	Combines sensitization and adjuvant strategies

C = chemotherapy; X = x-rays/radiotherapy.

ditional complex sequences (Table 47–3). These complex sequences would obviously be even more difficult to dissect out as they involve almost all the conceptual strategies that can be applied. When the additional variables of drug schedule, fractionation scheme, and relative dose intensity are added into the analytical pot, two things become blatantly obvious: clinical trials are designed with more empiricism than most investigators care to admit, and a closer interaction between the experimentalist and the clinician is valuable.

EVALUATION OF CLINICAL TRIALS

In the analysis of clinical trials combining irradiation and chemotherapy, as in any trial, there are two perspectives to be taken. The first is the research orientation and the second is the patient care therapeutic index orientation. The research perspective emphasizes the testing of biologic principles and the patient care perspective is focused on what the practicing oncologist should do to optimally care for patients outside a clinical research milieu. Although it is of the utmost importance to strive for the ideal of every patient participating in clinical research, one cannot escape the reality that most patients are treated pragmatically in a nonclinical research milieu. A criticism that can be made of the clinical oncology literature is that, in the reporting the clinical trial data, there is little patient-care-oriented therapeutic index perspective, particularly in the discussion section and in the summary.

From a research perspective, there are two critical end-points in a combined drug and x-ray trial. In a broad sense, one can be viewed as relating predominantly to enhanced action of irradiation. This end-point is **local control** or complete response. Ideally, a combined-modality regimen should achieve a higher percentage of complete remissions than would be obvious with x-ray alone. As discussed previously, this could be due to sensitization of additional cell kill by drugs within the field. Regardless of which mechanism is dominating, enhanced local control would imply the biologic principle that the chemotherapy is improving the activity of the radiation.

The second end-point is **relapse-free survival.** This could be viewed as the end-point related to adjuvant drug effect if the relapses are diminished outside of the radiation treatment field. In this situation, the distant or metastatic relapse-free survival should be greater in the combined modality arm. If this were observed, the biologic principles of adjuvant cell kill could be presumed to be in effect. If the relapses are diminished within the treatment area, the analysis, as related to biologic principle, becomes more complex. In this situation, the drug effect has to be viewed as being related to improving the biologic activity of the irradiation. Because the proof of biologic principle should be a paramount research aspect of combined-modality trials, it would be helpful if trial analysis and reporting would clearly delineate the relapse rates between local and distant and relate them to the investigator's view of the biologic principles involved.

From the patient care therapeutic index perspective, **overall survival** and **quality of life** become the critical parameters of efficacy. Because combined-modality treatment involves more therapy, which will have psychosocial and socioeconomic impacts, in addition to any additional side effects, there must be some benefit to the patient as a trade-off. As important as local control is, as a biologic end-point, and as a prerequisite for meaningful patient benefit, it does not help the patient per se. The patient is only helped by local control if he or she feels better and/or lives longer. The assumption of response and patient-care benefit is so ingrained in oncologists who have been trained to rigorously measure objectively, that there is a tendency to downplay the reality that the benefit may be slight and the cost to the patient great enough to cancel it out, from a practice-oriented point of view.

The toxicity aspect of a combined trial of chemotherapy and radiation therapy must be viewed in comparative terms to radiation therapy and/or drug alone and viewed from a biologic (research) and patient-care perspective. From a biologic point of view, toxicity can be dichotomized into two essential components. The first component involves the normal tissue tolerance within the radiated field. Here, the question is whether the chemotherapy is either sensitizing the normal tissue to x-ray damage or causing additive damage. Regardless of the biologic mechanism, which clinically is difficult to dissect out, the bottom line is whether local toxicity is worse within the radiated area or the systemic side effects of radiation are increased. The second component involves side effects of the chemotherapy that are in addition to, and unrelated to, the toxicities caused by x-ray. Examples could be the neurologic side effects of vincristine and platinol, the cardiac toxicity of Adriamycin, and the pulmonary toxicity of bleomycin in situations in which radiation could not be possibly implicated as playing a role. From the research viewpoint, this kind of dissection of side effects is important and is usually absent from clinical research reports. From the patient care therapeutic index orientation, what counts are the acute and chronic impacts on the quality of life caused by side effects and an equation that balances this against the prolongation of survival resulting from the therapy.

At this time, a massive data base exists on the combination of x-ray and chemotherapy. This volume is a testament to that data base and its importance. The critical questions are (1) Is the strategy working? and (2) Where do we go from here? The answer to the first question depends on your expectations and perspective. There is no question that selective trials exist in a range of tumors, such as small-cell lung cancer, head and neck cancer, and ovarian and rectal cancer, which demonstrate results with combined therapy being superior to x-ray or drug alone. None of these is dramatic in the sense of doubling or tripling the cure rates. There also exists a large number of negative trials. Every negative trial can be criticized from the perspective of its design, execution, and analysis to vitiate its impact on the critical biologic questions that require answering. Even in recognition of that reality, the current clinical trial data base indicates that the strategy of combining drugs and x-ray has been only a limited success. It has not achieved the gains hoped for by its enthusiastic pioneers and predicted by the experimental data base. In many situations in which both the drugs and x-ray are effective when used alone, e.g., small-cell lung cancer, the effect of combining the two is less than additive ($2 + 2 = 3$). Although this is still of clinical importance, it is clearly less than was originally expected by both the radiation and medical oncologists who designed the trials.

Another area of relative disappointment is malignant lymphomas. These tumors are highly sensitive to irradiation, and chemotherapy induces a high response rate, with many complete responses. The combined strategy in the lymphomas has been mainly adjuvant, with the goal being to diminish systemic relapses. What the majority of trials show in both Hodgkin's disease and the non-Hodgkin's lymphomas is an improvement in relapse-free survival, which does not translate into improved overall survival. The optimistic view can be that biologic effects are being demonstrated. The pessimistic view can be that, for most patients, combined therapy does not demonstrate overall therapeutic superiority to sequential use of the modalities, which in many cases would spare the patient the exposure and risk of one of the modalities in question.

The lymphoma trials exemplify an important aspect of analyzing combined modality trials when curative, or salvage, second-line therapeutic options exist. In a tumor situation such as Stage I–II Hodgkin's disease, it is not enough to compare irradiation and combined chemotherapy to irradiation alone. The comparison is the cleanest test of the biologic question focusing on relapse-free survival. The critical practical comparison is irradiation and chemotherapy versus irradiation, followed by chemotherapy in those who relapse. The comparison is then relative efficacy (RFS and OS) versus acute and chronic toxicities for both therapeutic strategies. If the efficacy is comparable for the sequence (x-ray followed by drug in those who relapse), the sequence must be superior from a side-effects perspective, particularly when combined with socioeconomic considerations.

FUTURE PROSPECTS

The best hope for the future resides in the ability to improve the capabilities of radiation alone and chemotherapy alone, so that their combined effects, even if only additive or less than additive, will result in a significant increase in the total eradication of the existing tumor cell burden. Empirical clinical trials combining existing drug regimens will and should continue until newer and more interesting options come to the fore. In a sense, every drug and drug combination has the potential to be combined with various fields of radiation designed for specific tumor types. In truth, only a tiny fraction of all the possible combinations can be clinically evaluated, and the choices will be, at least in the near future, made by clinicians in the style of rational empiricism, which integrates clinical intuition with an individualistic understanding and interpretation of the existing experimental and clinical data base.

In terms of improving the effectiveness of chemotherapy, there exists a range of approaches and hopes. The search for new chemotypes continues. There had been a plateau of more than 10 years in which no new major cytotoxic drug has been discovered. With the discovery of Taxol, a new and exciting chemotype has been found. This has not diminished the search, although it has altered the strategy, which is now focusing on using panels of human tumor-derived cell lines. These panels have been developed with two broad goals in mind. The first is to bring more solid tumor specificity and diversity into the screening mix. The second is to attack the problem of resistance, which is the generic stumbling block to chemotherapy's improved success. The importance of an in vivo counterpart to in vitro screening has led to a greater utilization of heterotransplantation rodent models. Gone are the days of screening using one or two murine transplantable leukemias such as P-388 and L-1210, although it should not be forgotten that nearly all the major drugs that are effective in solid tumors have activity in one or both of these old model systems.

A second approach involves the search for improved analogs of the existing active agents. The greatest successes have occurred historically in the area of the anthracyclines and alkylating agents. Adriamycin was a significant improvement over daunomycin in that it greatly broadened the spectrum of antitumor activity. Newer anthracyclines have been disappointing in terms of improved efficacy and broader spectrum but have diminished selected side effects to some degree. Cyclophosphamide was a significant improvement over nitrogen mustard and thiotepa in terms of both broader spectrum of activity and greater clinical versatility. More recently, ifosfamide, combined with uroprotection, has led to even greater activity in some tumor types. The most recent success of analog development involves carboplatin (CBCDA, paraplatin) as a cisplatinum second-generation drug. Carboplatin, with its minimal renal and neurologic toxicity, combined with its lessened emetogenic activity, offers a significant improvement in the patient care-oriented therapeutic index from the toxicity end of the equation. Here again, the screening approach is moving away from dependence on a small number of murine transplatable systems and is shifting toward panels of cell lines and heterotransplantation models.

A third approach involves greater specificity of drug delivery to the tumor site. Two broad strategies are involved. The first attempts to link cytotoxic drugs to monoclonal antibodies and utilize the antibodies as warheads to deliver the drugs to the tumor site. This strategy must overcome both immunogenic and antigenic heterogeneity, in addition to significant chemical challenges, but is now being vigorously pursued by many groups. The second strategy includes encapsulating the drugs in liposomes designed so that a greater amount of drug is sent to the tumor cells and kept away from critical normal tissues. If either of these approaches were to be successful, the more specific delivery of higher drug concentrations ought to augur positively for an improved effect when combined with radiotherapy.

A fourth approach involves supportive care allowing higher doses of drugs to be administered and therefore higher concentrations of the active moiety of the drug reaching the tumor tissue. Again, there are two broad strategies. The first involves autologous bone marrow transplantation, which protects against what would otherwise be marrow-lethal drug doses. This can be successfully achieved, and a range of drugs and regimens have been given at lethal marrow doses with protection. The new dose-limiting toxicity becomes organ damage in the lung, liver, kidney, central nervous system, etc., depending on the drugs used. The current results indicate that higher response rates can result from this strategy. What has been disappointing is that the complete remission rate has not been dramatically raised and that, when achieved, the remission tends to be of short duration. The second strategy involves the use of colony-stimulating factors (CSFs) to stimulate bone marrow recovery. The results so far are encouraging with bone granulocyte CSF (G-CSF) and granulocyte-macrophase CSF (GM-CSF), in that bone marrow toxicity can be diminished. It is too early to say whether this protection will lead to higher doses, giving superior efficacy. The evidence from autologous marrow transplantation studies is not too encouraging because organ damage, outside of the marrow, also limits drug doses given in conjunction with CSFs. The ease of CSF administration, however, in comparison to autologous marrow, should allow broader testing of high-dose strategies. Other supportive care approaches that might allow more effective or higher dosing include toxicity protectants such as MESNA for ifosfamide, WR 2721, and newer antiemetics of the 5HT3 mechanism of action type. Again, if these are successful, the implication for combined-modality trials is obvious.

In conclusion, the combination of radiation therapy and chemotherapy is both intuitively logical and supported by an extensive experimental data base. The clinical trials of the last decades have attempted to exploit the pragmatic value of combining two distinct modalities of therapy utilizing the experimental logic to the extent deemed possible. Although true synergism or potentiation (2 + 2 = 5) has not been observed, there is a range of clinical situations in which the combination of modalities has achieved results superior to the best of either one used alone. From the research perspective, a continuation of empirically designed trials, combining x-ray with drug regimens active in the particular tumor under study, is reasonable as long as expectations are not too great and a superior research strategy does not exist. The hope for the future lies in strategies that will improve the efficacy of each modality alone and then bring them together, hopefully in a more specifically rational manner derived from more clinically relevant experimental systems.

GLOSSARY OF CHEMOTHERAPEUTIC AGENTS AND OTHER PERTINENT DRUGS

Generic Name	Trade Names (Abbreviations)
Aminoglutethimide	Cytadren (AG)
Asparaginase	Elspar, L-Asparaginase
Azathioprine	Imuran (AZ)
Bacillus Calmette-Guérin	TheraCys (TICE, BCG-MER)
Bleomycin Sulfate	Blenoxane (BLEO)
Busulfan	Myleran (BUS)
Buthionine Sulfoximine	(BSO)
Carboplatin	Paraplatin (PP)
Carmustine	1,3bis-(2-chloroethyl)-1-nitrosourea (Bicnu, BCNU)
Chlorambucil	Leukeran (CLB)
Chromic Phosphate P^{32}	Phosphocol P32
Cisplatin	Platinol, Cisplatinum (CDDP, P, DDP)
Citrovorum Factor	(CF)
Cyclophosphamide	Cytoxan, Neosar (CTX, CP)
Cytarabine Hydrochloride (cytosine arabinoside)	Cytosar-U (ara-C)
Dacarbazine	Dtic-Dome (DTIC)
Dactinomycin	Actinomycin D, Cosmegen (Act-D)
Daunorubicin	Cerubidine, Daunomycin (DNR)
Dexamethasone	Decadron (DEX)
Diethylstilbestrol Diphosphate	Diethylstilbestrol, Stilphostrol (DES)
Doxorubicin Hydrochloride	Adriamycin, Rubex (ADR)
Epirubicin Hydrochloride	Pharmorubicin (EPI)
Epoetin Alfa	Epogen, Procrit
Estramustine Phosphate Sodium	Emcyt (EP)
Estrogens	Conjugated, Esterified
Estrone	
Ethinyl Estradiol	Estinyl
Etidronate Disodium	Didronel
Eteposide	VePesid (VP-16, E, VP-16-213)
Filgrastim	Neupogen
Floxuridine	(FUDR)
Fludarabine Phosphate	Fludara (FLU)
5-Fluorouracil	Fluorouracil, Adrucil (5-FU, FUra)
Flutamide	Eulexin (FLU)
Ftorafur	Tegafur
Gallium Nitrate	Ganite
Goserelin	Zoladex (ZOL)
Halotestin	Fluoxymesterone (HALO)
Hexalen	Altretamine (HMM)

Generic Name	Trade Names (Abbreviations)
Hydroxyprogesterone Caproate	Prodox
Hydroxyurea	Hydrea (HU)
Idarubicin Hydrochloride	Idamycin (IDA)
Ifosfamide	Ifex (IFEX)
Immune Globulin	Gammagard, Gamimune N
Interferon Alfa-2A	Roferon-A
Interferon Alfa-2B	Intron-A
Interferon Alfa-N3	Alferon N
Ketoconazole	Nizoral
Leucovorin Calcium	Wellcovorin, folinic acid
Leuprolide Acetate	Lupron, Lupron Depot (LU)
Levamisole Hydrochloride	Ergamisol (LEV)
Lomustine	(CeeNU, CCNU)
Mechlorethamine Hydrochloride	Mustargen, nitrogen mustard, (HN_2)
Medroxyprogesterone Acetate	Provera, Depo-Provera
Megestrol Acetate	Megace (MEG)
Melphalan (L-phenylalanine mustard)	Alkeran (L-PAM)
6-Mercaptopurine	Purinethol (6-MP)
Mesna	Mesnex, MESNA
Methotrexate	Folex, Mexate (MTX)
Methyl CCNU	Semustine (MeCCNU)
Methyltestosterone	
Mitomycin C	Mutamycin, Mitomycin (MITO, Mito C)
Mitotane	Lysodren (LYS)
Mitoxantrone Hydrochloride	Novantrone (NOV, DHAD)
Nandrolone	
Ondansetron Hydrochloride	Zofran
Piroxantrone Hydrochloride	(PXT)
Plicamycin	Mithracin, Mithromycin, Mithramycin (MITH)
Prednisone	Deltasone (PRED)
Procarbazine Hydrochloride	Matulane (PCZ)
Sargramostim	Leukine, Prokine
Sodium Iodide ^{131}I	Idotope
Sodium Phosphate P32	P32
Streptozocin	Zanosar (STN)
Tamoxifen Citrate	Nolvadex, Tamofen (TMX)
Taxol	(TAX)
Teniposide	(VM-26)
6-Thioguanine	Tabloid-6, Thioguanine (6-TG)
Thiotepa	(TT)
Vinblastine Sulfate	Velban, Velsar (VLB, VBL)
Vincristine Sulfate	Oncovin, Vincasar (VCR)
Vindesine Sulfate	Eldisine (VDS)

INDEX

Page numbers in *italics* indicate illustrations; pages followed by "t" indicate tables.